P9-AGM-063

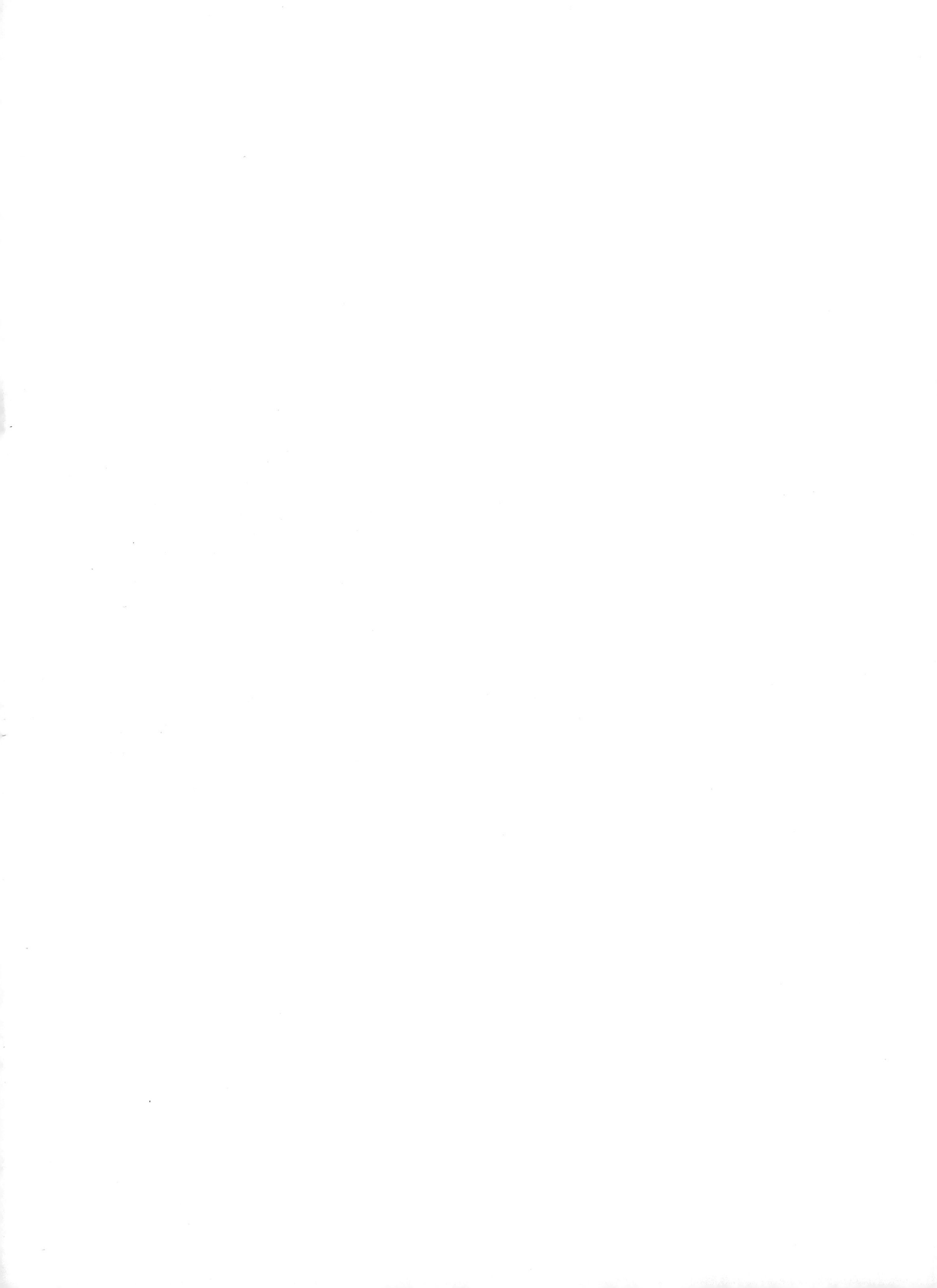

The 5-Minute Sports Medicine Consult

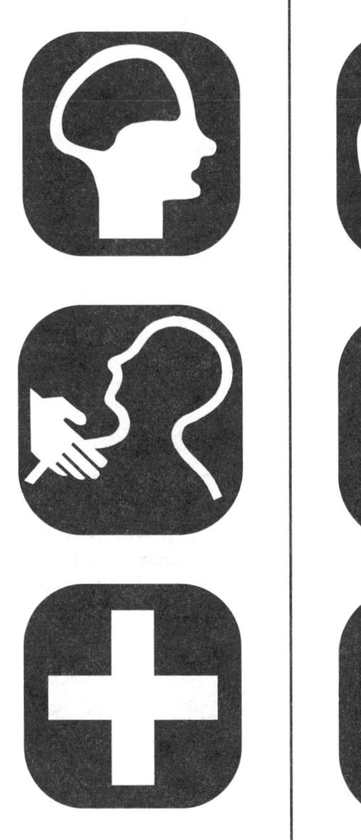

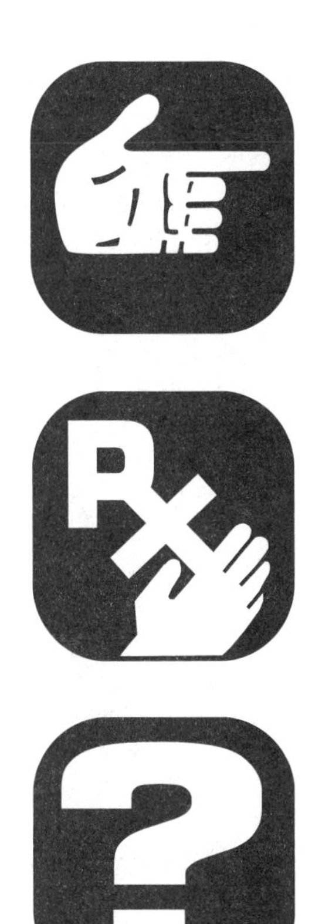

The 5-Minute Sports Medicine Consult

EDITOR

MARK D. BRACKER, M.D.

DIRECTOR

PRIMARY CARE SPORTS MEDICINE FELLOWSHIP

UNIVERSITY OF CALIFORNIA, SAN DIEGO

SAN DIEGO, CALIFORNIA

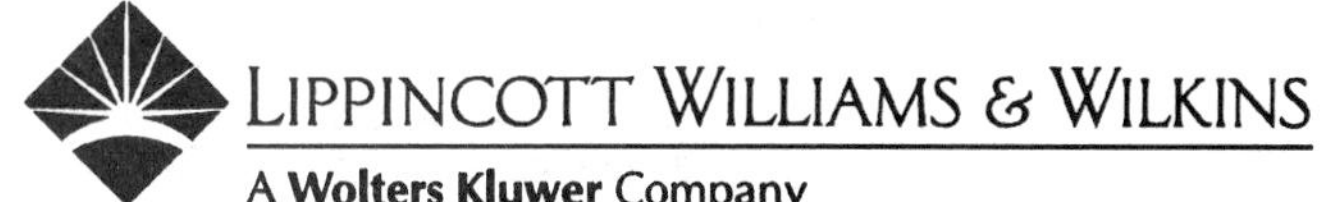

Philadelphia • Baltimore • New York • London
Buenos Aires • Hong Kong • Sydney • Tokyo

Acquisitions Editor: Timothy Y. Hiscock
Developmental Editor: Selina M. Bush
Supervising Editor: Mary Ann McLaughlin
Manufacturing Manager: Tim Reynolds
Production Service: Colophon
Compositor: TechBooks
Printer: R.R. Donnelley/Willard

530 Walnut Street
Philadelphia, PA 19106-3780
lww.com

Printed in the USA

Library of Congress Cataloging-in-Publication Data

The 5 minute sports medicine consult / editor, Mark D. Bracker.—1st ed.
p. ; cm.
Includes bibliographical references and index.
ISBN 0-7817-3045-7 (alk. paper)
1. Sports medicine—Handbooks, manuals, etc. I. Title: Five minute sports medicine consult. II. Bracker, Mark D.
[DNLM: 1. Sports Medicine—Handbooks. QT 29 Z999 2001]

RC1211 .A145 2001
617.1'027—dc21 2001029912

---

10 9 8 7 6 5 4 3 2 1

This book is dedicated to the entire team of health care professionals who work with athletes in all phases of training in an atmosphere where time becomes essential, and rapid diagnosis and intervention are expected. *The 5-Minute Sports Medicine Consult* is ideal for this setting. It is our hope that the information contained in this book will help guide you and your patient along the path to recovery and peak performance.

Preface

The basic idea for *The 5-Minute Sports Medicine Consult* comes, in part, from an educational technique that has been used since 1991 for sports medicine fellows in training at the University of California, San Diego (UCSD) called the "How I Manage Series." As part of our regular weekly didactic program for the fellowship, faculty and fellows are asked to present a lecture on a single topic related to their sports medicine clinical practice, covering the essential elements in the diagnosis and management of problems as seen through the eyes of a primary care physician. In the audience would be experienced clinicians, including orthopedic surgeons, radiologists, physical therapists, and athletic trainers who would give input as part of the "Sports Medicine Team."

Over the years, the "How I Manage Series" has grown into a formidable collection of common and unusual problems that has become a very useful learning resource for our fellows in training. The idea for publishing a sports medicine text using this format has been a desire of mine for several years. As a clinician myself, I needed a book that would answer my questions quickly, and also serve as an educational guide for my patients to better understand their problem and my treatment approach.

In the early development stage of this book, three important things happened to make an idea become a reality. First was the decision to have Lippincott Williams & Wilkins as the publisher and to use *The 5-Minute Consult* series format. Fortunately, a group of emergency medicine physicians at UCSD had just gone to press with *The 5-Minute Emergency Medicine Consult,* which paved the way for this book from the university to the publisher's desk. Second was our ability to join forces with other sports medicine training programs across the country to assemble a team of chapter authors from this group of talented clinician-educators. The organization for this was made possible through the American Medical Society for Sports Medicine (AMSSM), which has developed the leadership format for fellowship training programs in North America. The final key ingredient was the ability to produce this book "on-line" using the latest Internet website technology, which was not previously available.

With these pieces of the puzzle in place, our website was born, and we were "off to the races." The road has had its bumps and detours along the way, but our team was able to complete the 275 chapters of the first edition on schedule. What we have generated is what I believe to be an up-to-date reference guide to the management of sports medicine problems. Included are special sections of physical therapy, and algorithms linked to specific chapters to help guide the workup of presenting complaints.

Thanks to the hard work of 200 contributing authors, 30 chapter editors, and 6 section editors, what we have developed is an essential reference that will find its way to the bedside in our care of patients.

Mark D. Bracker, M.D.

Acknowledgments

I know now that bringing a textbook to press requires a lot of hard work and a serving of good luck thrown in. Linking up with the publisher was the result of Drs. Steve Hayden and Mary Anne Fuchs, who had worked on *The 5-Minute Emergency Medicine Consult* here at UCSD for two years. Having their initial guidance was essential to getting started on the right foot. The decision to use the website to write and edit the manuscript was a leap of faith that could not have happened without the technical expertise, foresight, and dedication of Dr. Patrick Yassini (who at the beginning of the project was a second-year resident in Family Medicine at UCSD!). Without his tireless work on this project from beginning to end, this book would have never been completed on time. Finally, I owe a special debt of gratitude to Tim Hiscock and Selina Bush at LWW for their guidance every step of the way, and their encouragement to not give up on my dreams.

Contributing Authors

ABDULRAZAK ABYAD, M.D., M.P.H., A.G.S.F.
Director
Adyad Medical Center
Coordinator
Ain WaZein Comprehensive Geriatric Program
Abyad Medical Center, Ain WaZein Hospital
Tripoli, Lebanon

SURAJ ACHAR, M.D.
Sports Medicine Fellow
Clinical Instructor
School of Medicine
University of California at San Diego
San Diego, California

SURITI KUNDU ACHAR
Clinical Instructor
Department of Family Medicine
University of California, San Diego
San Diego, California

MICHAEL T. ANDARY, M.D.
Associate Professor
Department of Physical Medicine and Rehabilitation
Michigan State University
Lansing, Michigan

VENU AKUTHOTA, M.D.
Attending Physician
Center of Spine, Sports, and Occupational Rehabilitation
Clinical Instructor in Rehabilitation Medicine
Northwestern Memorial Hospital
Chicago, Illinois

JOSEPH ARMEN, D.O.
Family Practice Resident
Carolinas Medical Center
Mooresville, North Carolina

THOMAS D. ARMSEY, M.D.
Program Director
Kentucky Clinic
University of Kentucky
Lexington, Kentucky

PAUL ARNOLD, M.D.
Department of Emergency Medicine
The Toronto Hospital
Toronto, Ontario
Canada

ELIZABETH AUSTIN, M.D.
Epidemiology Unit
Medical Center
University of California at San Diego
San Diego, California

ROBERT BAKER, M.D., PH.D., A.T.C.
Director of Sports Medicine
Department of Family Practice
Kalamazoo Family Practice
Kalamazoo Center for Medical Studies
University of Michigan
Kalamazoo, Michigan

THOMAS A. BALCOM, M.D.
Director
Sports Medicine Clinic
Branch Medical Clinic
Marine Corps Recruit Depot
San Diego, California

LISA BARKLEY, M.D.
Director
Christiana Care Health Services
Wilmington Hospital
Wilmington, Delaware

JAMES BARRETT, M.D.
Director
Department of Family and Preventive Medicine
University of Oklahoma at Oklahoma City
Oklahoma City, Oklahoma

B. BAYDOCK, M.D., C.C.F.D., DIP. SPORT MED
Hargrave Sports Medicine Clinic
Winnipeg, Manitoba
Canada

DAVID BAZZO, M.D.
Assistant Clinical Professor of Family Medicine
Department of Family and Preventive Medicine
University of California at San Diego
La Jolla, California

DAVID T. BERNHARDT, M.D.
Director
Department of Pediatrics
Childrens Hospital and Clinic
University of Wisconsin Hospital
Madison, Wisconsin

ANTHONY BEST

KENNETH BIELAK, M.D.
Director
Assistant Professor
University of Tennessee at Knoxville
Primary Care Sports Medicine Fellowship
Department of Family Medicine
Knoxville, Tennessee

JAMES BLOUNT, M.D.
Resident
Carolinas Medical Center/Family Practice
Charlotte, North Carolina

KRISTEN L. BODINE

DELMAS J. BOLIN, M.D., PH.D.
Associate Faculty
Primary Care Sports Medicine Fellowship
UMPC-St. Margaret Hospital
Family Practice Residency
Pittsburgh, Pennsylvania

MARK D. BRACKER, M.D.
Director of Sports Medicine
Clinical Professor
University of California at San Diego
Division of Family Medicine
La Jolla, California

KENNETH BRAMWELL, M.D.
Department of Emergency Medicine
San Diego Medical Center
University of California at San Diego
San Diego, California

JAMES BRAY, M.D.
Moses Cone Family Practice Resident
Moses Cone Family Practice
Greensboro, North Carolina

FRED H. BRENNAN JR.

WILLIAM W. BRINER JR., M.D.
Director
Department of Family Practice
Lutheran General Hospital
Park Ridge, Illinois

MELISSA BROKAW
Department of Emergency Medicine
Strong Memorial Hospital
University of Rochester
Rochester, New York

PER BROLINSON, D.O.
Director
Department of Sports Medicine
The Toledo Hospital
Toledo, Ohio

STEVE BROOK

BRIAN I. BROWN

DAVID BROWN, M.D.
Department of Emergency Medicine
Massachusetts General Hospital
Boston, Massachusetts

DOUGLAS BROWNING, M.D., A.T.C.
Director of Sports Medicine
Department of Family and Community Medicine
School of Medicine
Wake Forest University
Winston-Salem, North Carolina

JASON BRYANT, M.D.
Intern
Department of Surgery
Harbor–UCLA Medical Center
Torrance, California

SEAN BRYANT, M.D.
Chief Resident
Emergency Medicine Resident
Department of Emergency Medicine
Wright State University School of Medicine
Dayton, Ohio

J.C. BULLER, M.D.
Fellow
Primary Care Sports Medicine
San Diego Sports Medicine Center
Stanford University/Grossmont Hospital
San Diego, California

KEVIN BURROUGHS, M.D.
Sports Medicine Fellow
Moses Cone Sports Medicine Fellowship
Team Physician
Elon College
Greensboro, North Carolina

WALTER L. CALMBACH, M.D.
Director
Department of Family Practice
University of Texas Health Science Center
San Antonio, Texas

TERESA CARLIN, M.D.
Department of Emergency Medicine
Johns Hopkins Hospital
Baltimore, Maryland

NICK CARTER, M.D. M.R.C.P.
Fellow
Specialist in Rheumatology
Allan McGavin Sports Medicine Centre
University of British Columbia
Vancouver, British Columbia
Canada

WALLACE CARTER, M.D.
Department of Emergency Medicine
Bellevue Hospital Center
New York University
New York, New York

THEODORE C. CHAN, M.D.
Department of Emergency Medicine
San Diego Medical Center
University of California at San Diego
San Diego, California

ROBERT CHANG, M.D.
Department of Emergency Medicine
Bellevue Hospital Center
New York University
New York, New York

GORDON CHEW, M.D.
Department of Emergency Medicine
San Diego Medical Center University of California at San Diego
San Diego, California

LARRY CHOU, M.D.
Assistant Professor
Department of Rehabilitation Medicine
Penn Medicine at Radnor
University of Pennsylvania Health System
Radnor, Pennsylvania

ANDREA CLARKE, M.D.
Family Practice Physician
San Diego, California

DANIEL CLINKENBEARD, M.D.
Sports Medicine Fellow
Department of Family Medicine
Primary Care Sports Medicine Fellowship
Family Medicine Center
University of Oklahoma
Oklahoma City, Oklahoma

PHILIP H. COHEN, M.D.
Primary Care Sports Medicine Fellow
Department of Family Medicine
University of California at Los Angeles
Beverly Hills, California

ANGELO J. COLOSIMO, M.D.
Co-Director
Assistant Professor of Orthopaedic Surgery
The Christ Hospital Bone and Joint Institute
University of Cincinnati
Cincinnati, Ohio

ANDREW CONCOFF, M.D.
Associate Professor
Rheumatology and Orthopedics
University of Texas–Houston Medical School
Houston, Texas

FRANCIS COUNSELMAN, M.D.
Department of Emergency Medicine
Eastern Virginia Medical School
Norfolk, Virginia

DAVID CRANE, M.D.
Director
Primary Sports Medicine
Washington University
St. Louis, Missouri

NEIL CRATON, M.D.
Director
University of Manitoba
Musculoskeletal Fellowship
Winnipeg, Manitoba
Canada

ALAN J. CROPP, M.D., F.C.C.P.
Associate Professor of Internal Medicine
Northeastern Ohio Universities College of Medicine
Youngstown, Ohio

GREG CROVETTI, M.D.
Fellow
Sports Medicine
University of Kentucky
Lexington, Kentucky

ANDREW R. CURRAN, D.O.
Orthopedic Sports Medicine Fellow
New England Baptist Hospital
Newton, Massachusetts

ANDREW DAHLGREN, M.D.
Clinical Fellow, Sports Medicine
Department of Family Medicine
University of Michigan
Ypsilanti, Michigan

MARK R. DAMBRO, M.D., F.A.A.F.P., F.A.B.H.P.M.
Private Practice
Fort Worth, Texas

CARA DECKELMAN

RANIA L. DEMPSEY, M.D.
Clinical Instructor
Sports Medicine Fellow
Medical College of Wisconsin
Pewaukee, Wisconsin

MATT DESJARDINS, M.D.
House Officer
Wake Forest University
Department of Family Medicine
Baptist Medical Center
Winston-Salem, North Carolina

WILLIAM W. DEXTER, M.D.
Director
Maine Medical Center
Sports Medicine Fellowship Program
Department of Family Practice
Portland, Maine

JOHN P. DIFIORI, M.D.
Associate Professor
Division of Sports Medicine
Department of Family Medicine
Team Physician
Department of Intercollegiate Athletics
University of California, Los Angeles
Los Angeles, California

JOHN P. DORMANS

JONATHAN DREZNER, M.D.
Assistant Professor
Department of Family Practice and Community Medicine
University of Pennsylvania
Philadelphia, Pennsylvania

AYSE DURAL, M.D.

JONATHAN EDLOW, M.D.
Division of Emergency Medicine
Beth Israel Hospital
Boston, Massachusetts

JAMIE EDWARDS, M.D.
Family Practice Resident
Street Luke's Medical Center
University of Wisconsin
Milwaukee, Wisconsin

JEFFREY ELLIS, M.D.
Department of Emergency Medicine
University Medical Center
Las Vegas, Nevada

T. JEFF EMEL, M.D.
Director
College of Medicine at Tulsa
University of Oklahoma
Tulsa, Oklahoma

JAMES FAMBRO, M.D.
Department of Sports Medicine
Marshall University
Huntington, West Virginia

PAUL FAVORITO, M.D.
Wellington Orthopedic and Sports Medicine
Department of Orthopedics
University of Cincinnati
Cincinnati, Ohio

KARL B. FIELDS, M.D.
Director of Family Medicine
Sports Medicine Fellowship
Associate Chair
Department of Family Medicine
Moses H. Cone Memorial Hospital
School of Medicine
University of North Carolina at Chapel Hill
Greensboro, North Carolina

SCOTT FLINN, M.D.
Director
Sports Medicine Clinic
Senior Medical Officer
BMC Parris Island
Beaufort Naval Hospital
Parris Island, South Carolina

KELLY ANNE FOLEY, M.D.
Department of Emergency Medicine
Eastern Virginia Medical School
Norfolk, Virginia

AARICK FOREST

ROBERT GALLI, M.D.
Department of Emergency Medicine
University of Mississippi
Jackson, Mississippi

COLEY GATLIN, M.D.
Sports Medicine Fellow
Moses Cone Hospital
Family Practice Residency
Greensboro AHEC
Greensboro, North Carolina

KEVIN B. GEBKE, M.D.
Assistant Professor of Family Medicine
Department of Family Medicine
School of Medicine
Indiana University
Indy, Indiana

DELARAM GHADISHAH, M.D.
Department of Emergency Medicine
Irvine Medical Center
University of California at Irving
Orange, California

SUSAN GLOCKNER
Volunteer Faculty
Former Sports Medicine Fellow
Encinitas, California

MARSHALL GODWIN, M.D.
Hotel Dieu Family Medicine Center
Queen's University
Kingston, Ontario
Canada

WILLIAM GOLDBERG, M.D.
Department of Emergency Medicine
Bellevue Hospital Center
New York University
New York, New York

JEFFREY GORDON
Department of Emergency Medicine
Resurrection Hospital
Chicago, Illinois

GARY GREEN, M.D.
Associate Professor
Division of Sports Medicine
Department of Family Medicine
University of California, Los Angeles
Los Angeles, California

MARK HALSTEAD, M.D.
Pediatric Resident
University of Wisconsin Hospital and Clinics
Madison, Wisconsin

NICHOLAS K. HAN
Department of Emergency Medicine
Beth Israel Medical Center
New York, New York

MATTHEW R. HARMODY

KIMBERLY HARMON, M.D.
Clinical Assistant Professor
Department of Family Medicine
Clinic Instructor
Department of Orthopedics
University of Washington
Seattle, Washington

BENJAMIN HASAN, M.D.
Family Practice and Sports Medicine
Associate Director
Resurrection Family Practice Residency
Chicago, Illinois

SUZANNE HECHT

ROBERT S. HEIDT JR., M.D.
Co-Director
Sports Medicine Fellowship
Team Physician
Cincinnati Bengals
The Christ Hospital Bone and Joint Institute
Wellington Orthopaedic and Sports Medicine
Cincinnati, Ohio

MICHAEL J. HENEHAN, D.O.
Director
Sports Medicine Fellowship Program
San Jose Medical Center
Clinical Assistant Professor in Family Medicine
Stanford University School of Medicine
San Jose, California

JOHN HILL, D.O.
Director
University of Colorado
Primary Sports Medicine Fellowship
Denver, Colorado

CHRIS HO, M.D.
Department of Emergency Medicine
San Diego Medical Center
University of California at San Diego
San Diego, California

JEFFREY HORTON, M.D.
Department of Emergency Medicine
Beth Israel Medical Center
New York, New York

ROBERT G. HOSEY, M.D.
Assistant Professor of Family Medicine
Associate Director Primary Care Sports Medicine
Kentucky Clinic
University of Kentucky
Lexington, Kentucky

BRIAN A. JACOBS, M.D., F.A.C.S.M.
Head Team Physician
Clinical Assistant Professor
Department of Family Medicine
University of Indiana
South Bend, Illinois

CARRIE JAWORSKI, M.D.
Sports Medicine Fellow
Family Physician
Kaiser Permanente
Fontana, California

ERIC JENKINSON, M.D.
Orthopedics Northeast
Fort Wayne, Indiana

GARY JOHNSON, M.D.
Department of Emergency Medicine
University of Maryland
Baltimore, Maryland

JASON D. JOHNSON, M.D.
Resident 3, Family Practice
Incoming Sports Medicine Fellow
Lutheran General Hospital
Park Ridge, Illinois

PAUL JOHNSON, M.D.
South Bend Primary Care Sports Medicine Fellowship
South Bend, Indiana

ANNETTE Q. JONES, M.S., P.T., A.T., C.
Staff Physical Therapist
Mountain View Physical Therapy
Upland, California

KIRK D. JONES, M.S., A.T., C.
Head Athletic Trainer
Pomona College
Claremont, California

ROBERT L. JONES, M.D.
Director
Miller Orthopaedic Clinic
Sports Medicine Fellowship
Department of Family Medicine
Carolinas Medical Center
Charlotte, North Carolina

PASCAL S. C. JUANG, M.D.
Department of Emergency Medicine
Brigham and Women's Hospital
Boston, Massachusetts

A. ANTOINE KAZZI, M.D.
Department of Emergency Medicine
Irvine Medical Center
University of California at Irving
Orange, California

GREGORY F. KEENAN, M.D.

SHAWN KERGER

JULIE KERR, M.D.
Director, Medical Education
Akron Children's Hospital Sports Medicine Center
Akron, Ohio

AHMED KHALIFA, M.D., MPH
Director
Houston Health Science Center
Department of Physical Medicine and Rehabilitation
University of Texas
Houston, Texas

THOMAS KIM, M.D.
Fellow, Sports Medicine
Boston Children's Hospital/Harvard University
Brookline, Massachusetts

TAMAKI KIMBRO, M.D.
Department of Emergency Medicine
San Diego Medical Center
University of California at San Diego
San Diego, California

BRADLEY KOCIAN, M.D.
Sports Medicine Fellow
University of Tennessee
Knoxville, Tennessee

GEORGE KONDYLIS
Department of Emergency Medicine
State University of New York Health Science Center
Syracuse, New York

CHRIS KOUTURES, M.D.
Gladstien and Koutures
Irvine, California

PETER KOZISEK, M.D.
Family Practice Residency of Idaho
Boise, Idaho

BERENT KRUMM, M.D.
Family Practice Residency
St. Joseph Regional Medical Center
South Bend, Illinois

GEOFFREY KUHLMAN, M.D.
Associate Director
Director of Sports Medicine
Hinsdale Family Practice Residency
Hinsdale, Illinois

NANCY KWON, M.D.
Department of Emergency Medicine
Bellevue Hospital Center
New York University
New York, New York

ALEX LAI, M.D.
Fellow
University of California Los Angeles
Los Angeles, California

PHILLIP W. LANDES, M.D.
Sports Medicine Fellow
Kessler Institute
West Orange, New Jersey
Department of Physical Medicine and Rehabilitation
UMDNJ–New Jersey Medical School
Newark, New Jersey

JOHN LANGLAND, M.D.
Orthopedic Surgeon
The Christ Hospital
Sports Medicine Fellowship
Steindler Orthopedic Clinic, P.L.C.
Iowa City, Iowa
The Christ Hospital Bone and Joint Institute
Cincinnati, Ohio

MARK LAVALLEE, M.D.
Co-Director
Director
South Bend Primary Care Sports Medicine Fellowship
Sports Medicine, Memorial Family Practice Residency
South Bend, Indiana

HARVEY LEO, M.D.
Pediatric Resident
Department of Pediatrics
Children's Hospital and Clinics
University of Wisconsin
Madison, Wisconsin

DAVID LEVINE, M.D.
Department of Emergency Medicine
Cook County Hospital
Chicago, Illinois

SAM LIN, M.D.
University of Kentucky
Primary Care Sports Medicine
Kentucky Clinic, Family Medicine
Lexington, Kentucky

TIMOTHY J. LINKER, M.D.
Family Practice Resident
Miami Valley Hospital
Associate Clinical Instructor
Wright State School of Medicine
Berry Family Health Center
Dayton, Ohio

EVAN LIU
Department of Emergency Medicine
Hahnemann Division
Allegheny University Hospital
Philadelphia, Pennsylvania

JOHN LOMBARDO, M.D.
Director
OSU Sports Medicine Center
Ohio State University
Columbus, Ohio

MICHELLE LOOK
Sports Medicine Fellowship Faculty
Scripps Clinic
San Diego, California

JOSEPH P. LUFTMAN, M.D.
Fellow
Division of Sports Medicine
Department of Family Medicine
UCLA School of Medicine
Los Angeles, California

JOHN MACKNIGHT, M.D.
Assistant Team Physician
Primary Care Sports Medicine
UVA Health Sciences Center
University of Virginia
Charlottesville, North Carolina

CHRISTOPHER MADDEN, M.D.
Medical Center Shadyside
University of Pittsburgh
Pittsburgh, Pennsylvania

MARK L. MADENWALD, M.D.
Department of Emergency Medicine
Naval Medical Center
Portsmouth, Virginia

TIMOTHY J. MADER, M.D.
Department of Emergency Medicine
Baystate Medical Center
Springfield, Massachusetts

DANIELLE MAHAFFEY, M.D.
Sports Medicine Fellow
Moses Cone Family Practice Residency
Greensboro, North Carolina

GERALD MALANGA, M.D.
Director
Sports, Spine and Orthopedic Rehabilitation
Kessler Institute
West Orange, New Jersey
Associate Professor
Department of Physical Medicine and Rehabilitation
UMDNJ–New Jersey Medical School
Newark, New Jersey

LINDA MANSFIELD, M.D.
Sports Medicine Fellow
South Bend Primary Care Sports Medicine Fellowship
South Bend, Indiana

ALLEN MARINO, M.D.
Department of Emergency Medicine
San Diego Medical Center
University of California at San Diego
San Diego, California

TODD MAY, D.O.
Sports Medicine Fellow
Staff FP Naval Hospital
Camp Pendleton
San Diego, California

ANDREW T. McAFEE, M.D.
Department of Emergency Medicine
Brigham and Women's Hospital
Boston, Massachusetts

DOUGLAS McKEAG, M.D., M.S.
Director
Indiana University School of Medicine
Family Sports Medicine
Long Hospital
Indianapolis, Indiana

DOMINIC McKINLEY, M.D.
Sports Medicine Fellow
Moses Cone Hospital
Family Practice Residency
Greensboro AHEC
Greensboro, North Carolina

MATTHEW P. MELANDER

WILEM MEEUWISSE, M.D.
Sport Medicine Center
University of Calgary
Calgary, Alberta
Canada

ROBIN MERKET, M.D.
Sports Medicine Fellow
University of Tennessee at Knoxville
Knoxville, Tennessee

LYLE J. MICHELI, M.D.
Director
Division of Sports Medicine
Boston Children's Hospital
Associate Clinical Professor
Harvard Medical School
Boston Children's Hospital
Harvard Medical School
Boston, Massachusetts

MICHAEL MIKUS, M.D.
Clinical Instructor
School of Medicine
University of California at San Diego
San Diego, California

LARRY MILIKAN, M.D.
Chairman
Department of Dermatology
Tulane University School of Medicine
New Orleans, Louisiana

JEFFREY F. MINTEER, M.D.
Associate Director
Family Practice Residency Program
The Washington Hospital
Washington, Pennsylvania

SCOTT MITCHELL

GUY MONTELEONE, M.D.
Director
Department of Family and Community Medicine
School of Medicine
Wake Forest University
Winston-Salem, North Carolina

DAVID W. MUNTER, M.D., M.B.A., F.A.C.E.P.
Department of Emergency Medicine
Naval Medical Center
Portsmouth, Virginia

ANTHONY J. MUSIELEWICZ, M.D.
Department of Emergency Medicine
United States Naval Hospital
Guam

GREG NAKAMOTO, M.D.
Clinical Instructor
School of Medicine
University of California at San Diego
La Jolla, California

ISAM NASR, M.D.
Department of Emergency Medicine
Cook County Hospital
Chicago, Illinois

AURELIA NATTIV, M.D.
Associate Professor
Department of Family Medicine, Division of Sports Medicine, and Department of Orthopaedic Surgery
Team Physician
Department of Intercollegiate Athletics
University of California, Los Angeles
Los Angeles, California

SEAN-XAVIER NEATH, M.D.
Department of Emergency Medicine
San Diego Medical Center
University of California at San Diego
San Diego, California

ROSCOE NELSON, M.D.
San Diego Medical Center
Department of Emergency Medicine
University of California at San Diego
San Diego, California

ED NEWTON, M.D.
Department of Emergency Medicine
Los Angeles County/University of Southern California Medical Center
Los Angeles, California

MARK W. NIEDFELDT, M.D.
Assistant Professor
The Medical School of Wisconsin
Milwaukee, Wisconsin

RICHARD NORENBERG, M.D.
Sports Medicine Fellow
Fellow, American College of Surgeons
Bayfront Medical Center
St. Petersburg, Florida

STACY NUNBERG, M.D.
Department of Emergency Medicine
Long Island Jewish Medical Center
New Hyde Park, New York

RYAN O'CONNOR, D.O.
Assistant Professor
Department of Physical Medicine and Rehabilitation
Team Physician
Michigan State University Spartans
Michigan State University College of Osteopathic Medicine
College of Osteopathic Medicine
East Lansing, Michigan

DAN OSTLIE, M.D.
Central Indiana Sports Medicine
Muncie, Indiana

DAVID PACHOLKE, M.D.
Senior Medical Student
Indiana University
Bloomington, Indiana

ROSS M. PATTON, M.D.
Director
Marshall University School of Medicine
Department of Family and Community Health
Huntington, West Virginia

W. MARK PELUSO, M.D.
Medical Director/Team Physician
Middlebury College
Middlebury, Vermont

SOURAV PODDAR, M.D.
University of Colorado
Primary Sports Medicine Fellowship
Denver, Colorado

THOMAS L. POMMERING, D.O.
Family Practice Residency
Grant Medical Center
Columbus, Ohio

MICHAEL B. POTTER

JOEL M. PRESS, M.D.
Director
Center for Spine Sports and Occupational Rehabilitation
Rehabilitation Institute of Chicago
Chicago, Illinois

JAMES C. PUFFER, M.D.
Director
Department of Family Medicine
University of California at Los Angeles
Los Angeles, California

MARTHA PYRON, M.D.
Kalamazoo Center for Medical Studies
Michigan State University
Kalamazoo, Michigan

DOUGLAS REEVES JR., M.D.
Sports Medicine Fellow
Eastern Oklahoma Orthopedic Center
Tulsa, Oklahoma

KEVIN REILLY, M.D.
Department of Emergency Medicine
Albany Medical Center
Albany, New York

ANDREW REISMAN, M.D.
Christiana Care Health System
Primary Care Sports Medicine Fellowship
Wilmington Hospital
Wilmington, Delaware

ALLEN RICHBURG, M.D., M.S.
Family Practice/Sports Medicine
San Diego Sports Medicine and Family Health Center
San Diego, California

CARLTON A. RICHIE III, M.D.
Clinical Faculty Member
Family Medicine/Sports Medicine
Midwestern University
Tempe, Arizona

LELAND S. RICKMAN, M.D.
Associate Clinical Professor of Medicine
Division of Infectious Diseases
University of California, San Diego
San Diego, California

JAMES B. RIVAS
Department of Emergency Medicine
Palomar Hospital
Escondido, California

GREGORY N. ROCCO, M.D.
Fellow
Department of Family Practice
Lutheran General Hospital
Parkridge, Illinois

MICHAEL ROLNICK, M.D.
Division of Emergency Medicine
University of Maryland
Baltimore, Maryland

CARLO ROSEN, M.D.
Department of Emergency Medicine
Massachusetts General Hospital
Boston, Massachusetts

DARYL A. ROSENBAUM, M.D.
Team Physician
Western Carolina University
Cullowhee, North Carolina

GLEN ROSS, M.D.
Orthopedic Surgeon
Department of Sports Medicine
New England Baptist Hospital
Team Physician
Northeastern University
Assistant Team Physician
Boston Celtics
ProSports Orthopaedics
Boston, Massachusetts

AARON L. RUBIN, M.D.
Director
Kaiser Permanente
SPORT Medicine Fellowship Program
Fontana, California

DARIN RUTHERFORD, M.D.
Mercy Sports Medicine
Janesville, Wisconsin

WILLIAM SABINA, M.D.
Department of Emergency Medicine
Rhode Island Hospital
Providence, Rhode Island

ANNIE JEWEL SADOSTY, M.D.
Division of Emergency Medicine
University of Maryland
Baltimore, Maryland

MARC R. SAFRAN, M.D.
Co-Director, Sports Medicine
Associate Professor
Department of Orthopaedic Surgery
University of California, San Francisco
San Francisco, California

DEBORAH SANDERS, M.D.
Department of Emergency Medicine
University of Mississippi Medical Center
Jackson, Mississippi

MARCELO SANDOVAL, M.D.
Department of Emergency Medicine
Beth Israel Medical Center
New York, New York

DANIEL L. SAVITT, M.D.
Department of Emergency Medicine
Rhode Island Hospital
Providence, Rhode Island

AENOR SAWYER, M.D.
Fellow
Department of Sports Medicine
Children's Hospital
Boston, Massachusetts

ASSAAD J. SAYAH, M.D.
Department of Emergency Medicine
Brigham and Women's Hospital
Boston, Massachusetts

SHARI SCHABOWSKI
Department of Emergency Medicine
Cook County Hospital
Chicago, Illinois

ARNOLD D. SCHELLER JR., M.D.
Director
New England Baptist Hospital
Sports Medicine Fellowship
Chestnut Hill, Massachusetts

NILESH SHAH, M.D.
Chief Resident
Grant Medical Center
Columbus, Ohio

MARC J. SHAPIRO, M.D.
Department of Emergency Medicine
Rhode Island Hospital
Providence, Rhode Island

JOHN SHELTON, M.D.
Director
Halifax Medical Center
Sports Medicine Fellowship
Daytona Beach, Florida

IAN SHRIER, M.D., PH.D.
Assistant Professor
McGill University
Centre for Clinical Epidemiology and Community Studies
SMBD-Jewish General Hospital
Montreal, Quebec
Canada

STEPHEN SIMONS, M.D.
Co-Director
South Bend Primary Care Sports Medicine Fellowship
South Bend, Indiana

GREGORY SKAGGS, M.D.
Bend Memorial Clinic
Bend, Oregon

EDWARD SNELL, M.D.
Director
The Human Motion Center at Allegheny University Hospital
Sports Medicine Graduate Fellowship
Pittsburgh, Pennsylvania

MARK SNOWISE, M.D.
The Family Doctors
Swampscott, Massachusetts

DAN SOMOGYI, M.D.
Program Director
University of Pennsylvania Medical Center at Shadyside
Primary Care Sports Medicine Fellowship
Pittsburgh, Pennsylvania

JOYCE SOPRANO, M.D.
Fellow
Primary Care Sports Medicine
Attending Physician
Pediatric Emergency Medicine
Children's Hospital
Harvard Medical School
Boston, Massachusetts

KURT SPINDLER, M.D.
Vanderbilt Sports Medicine Center
Vanderbilt University
Nashville, Tennessee

THOMAS OSBORNE STAIR, M.D.
Division of Emergency Medicine
University of Maryland
Baltimore, Maryland

JEFFREY A. STEARNS, M.D.
Associate Chair and Campus Director
Milwaukee Clinical Campus
University of Wisconsin Medical School
Milwaukee, Wisconsin

BRADFORD STILES, M.D.
Education Director
UCSD Primary Care Sports Medicine Fellowship
Kaiser Permanente
Clinical Instructor
Department of Family and Preventive Medicine
University of California, San Diego
San Diego, California

DAVID A. STONE, M.D.
Program Director
University of Pennsylvania Medical Center–St. Margarets
Primary Care Sports Medicine Fellowship
Pittsburgh, Pennsylvania

MARK STOVAK, M.D.
Medical Director
Department of Sports Medicine
Associate Director
Family Practice Residency Program
Associate Director
Family Practice Residency
Via Christi Regional Medical Center
Wichita, Kansas

PAUL STRICKER, M.D.
Director
Associate Professor and Team Physician
Vanderbilt Sports Medicine Center
Vanderbilt University
Nashville, Tennessee

KEITH STUESSI, M.D.
LCDR
Primary Care Sports Medicine Fellow
U.S. Navy
Del Mar, California

JAMES E. STURMI, M.D.
Director
Grant Hospital
Sports Medicine Fellowship at Grant
Columbus, Ohio

TOD SWEENEY, M.D.
Resident Physician
Family Practice Department
Maine Medical Center
Portland, Maine

JEFF TAYLOR

KEN TAYLOR, M.D.
University of California, San Diego
Scripps Clinic Medical Group
Solana Beach, California

R. THOLE, M.D.
Sports Medicine Fellow
Kaiser Permanente
Riverside, California

JOHN TIERNEY, D.O.
Orthopaedic Surgeon
ProSports Orthopedics
New England Baptist Hospital
Brookline, Massachusetts

THOMAS TROJIAN, M.D.
Assistant Professor
Team Physician
Saint Francis MC&H Family Practice Residency
University of Connecticut Health Center
University of Connecticut
Hartford, Connecticut

ANDREW TUCKER, M.D.
Program Director
Primary Care Sports Medicine
University of Maryland
Baltimore, Maryland

SHANNON M. URTON

RAJIV R. VARMA, M.D.
Associate Professor
Division of Gastroenterology and Hepatology
Medical College of Wisconsin
Froedt Hospital
Milwaukee, Wisconsin

RAYMOND A. VIDUCICH, M.D.
University of Pittsburgh School of Medicine
Pittsburgh, Pennsylvania

ROBERT J. VISSERS, M.D.
Department of Emergency Medicine
University of North Carolina Hospitals
University of North Carolina
Chapel Hill, North Carolina

DAVID WALLIS, M.D.
Residency Program
University of California at Santa Monica
Orange, California

DONALD H. WALLIS, D.D.S.
Private Practice
Santa Clare, California

QUINCY WANG, M.D.
Sports Medicine Fellow
Family and Sports Medicine
Kaiser Permanente
Long Beach, California

JOSEPH WATHEN, M.D.
Department of Emergency Medicine
Children's Hospital
Denver, Colorado

KATHLEEN WEBER, M.D., M.S.
Clinical Instructor
School of Medicine
Sports Medicine Fellow
University of California at San Diego
San Diego, California

ROBERT L. WESTON, M.D.
Associate Clinical Professor
Division of International Health and Cross Cultural Medicine
School of Medicine
University of California at San Diego
President
International Healthcare Division
International SOS Assistance, Inc.
Trevose, Pennsylvania

RUSSELL D. WHITE, M.D.
Director
Associate Director
Sports Medicine Fellowship
Family Practice Residency
Bayfront Medical Center - FHC
St. Petersburg, Florida

GREGORY A. WHITLEY,
Sports Medicine Fellow
San Jose Medical Center
Emergency Physician
Santa Clara Valley Medical Center
San Jose, California

RICHARD WOLFE, M.D.
Residency Director
Department of Emergency Medicine
Harvard Medical School
Brigham and Women's Hospital
Boston, Massachusetts

CRAIG C. YOUNG, M.D.
Medical and Fellowship Director
Associate Professor
Department of Orthopaedic Surgery
Medical College of Wisconsin
Milwaukee, Wisconsin

RICHARD D. ZANE

Contents

SECTION II: POPULATION-SPECIFIC MUSCULOSKELETAL INJURIES / 327

SECTION III: GENERAL MEDICINE / 361

SECTION I

General Musculoskeletal Topics

Abdominal Muscle Strains

Basics

DEFINITION

- Acute or chronic muscle-tendon injury involving the abdominal wall musculature

INCIDENCE/PREVALENCE

- Relatively uncommon muscle-tendon injury
- Usually seen with running and cutting sports, e.g., soccer, football, or lacrosse
- May occur with training and conditioning, e.g., weight training or abdominal exercises

SIGNS AND SYMPTOMS

- Acute or subacute abdominal wall pain worsened with contraction of the abdominal wall muscles
- Swelling more likely seen with blunt trauma mechanism
- Disability dependent on the extent of the muscle injury

RISK FACTORS

- Poorly conditioned abdominal musculature
- Previous abdominal wall muscle strain/tear
- Poor weight training or conditioning techniques

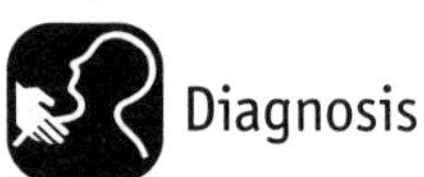

Diagnosis

DIFFERENTIAL DIAGNOSIS

- Abdominal wall contusion
- Abdominal wall hematoma
- Abdominal wall hernia (umbilical, Spigelian)
- Intra-abdominal injury (contusion, laceration, perforation)
- Intra-abdominal process (e.g., infection, mass, etc.)
- Iliac apophysitis

HISTORY

- Acute abdominal wall pain associated with stretching or twisting mechanism
- Pain usually focal; may be diffuse and associated with spasm
- Variable disability may exceed objective findings
- Pain with active contraction of affected muscle; often pain with cough, sneeze, or Valsalva

PHYSICAL EXAMINATION

- With severe injury, may splint toward affected side
- Usually no to minimal swelling; hematoma formation possible
- Point tenderness over affected muscle
- Muscle defect possible with severe injury
- Variable pain and weakness with active contraction of affected muscle group(s)
- Possible spasm, but negative peritoneal signs

IMAGING

- Plain films, computed tomographic scan indicated if intra-abdominal process being considered
- Magnetic resonance imaging of abdominal wall difficult due to motion

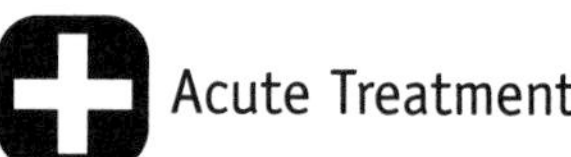

Acute Treatment

ANALGESIA

- Ice
- Compression
- Nonsteroidal antiinflammatory drugs: Some prefer to avoid their use in the first 24–48 hours to avoid potential bleeding.
- Narcotics usually not necessary in acute setting

IMMOBILIZATION

- Compressive wrap for support of injured area may be helpful in the acute setting.

SPECIAL CONSIDERATIONS

- Corticosteroid injection at the site of muscle tear/strain may be performed for subacute or chronic pain.

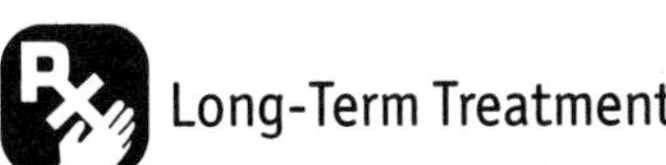

Long-Term Treatment

REHABILITATION

- Local modalities for moderate-to-severe injuries
- Gradual stretching
- Progressive strengthening with advancement to functional sport-specific rehabilitation

SURGERY

- May be applicable in cases of hernia or intra-abdominal process

REFERRAL/DISPOSITION

- For cases of suspected hernia or intra-abdominal process

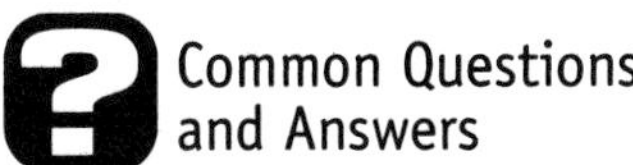

Common Questions and Answers

Physician responses to common patient questions:
Q: Return to play?
A: Minimal-to-no tenderness, normal muscle strength and stamina, performance of sport-specific tasks

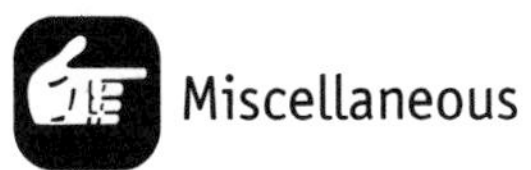

Miscellaneous

SYNONYMS

- abdominal wall injury
- abdominal muscle cramp or "stitch"

ICD-9 CODE

848.8

BIBLIOGRAPHY

Mellion MB, ed. *Sports medicine secrets*. Philadelphia: Hanley and Belfus, 1999.

Safran MB, McKeag BB, Van Camp SP. *Manual of sports medicine*. Philadelphia: Lippincott-Raven Publishers, 1998

Author: Andrew Tucker

Achilles' Tendinitis

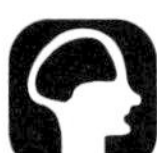

Basics

DEFINITION

Achilles' tendinitis is an overuse injury of the leg muscles that causes pain in the posterior calf and heel.

INCIDENCE/PREVALENCE

- Occurs in sports that require running and jumping
- Accounts for 6.5% to 11% of lower extremity injuries in runners

SIGNS AND SYMPTOMS

- Pain 2–6 cm above Achilles' tendon insertion
- Pain with running, especially sprinting

RISK FACTORS

- Training errors: recent increase in distance, intensity, or length of activity
- Worn, old shoes
- Inflexibility, especially tight heel cords
- Malalignment of the leg, ankle, and foot
- Fluoroquinolones: Recent use of these antibiotics has been associated with increased risk for Achilles' tendinitis.

ASSOCIATED INJURIES AND COMPLICATIONS

- Retrocalcaneal bursitis
- Superficial Achilles' bursitis ("pump bump")
- Achilles' tendon rupture: Chronic changes in tendon may predispose to rupture.

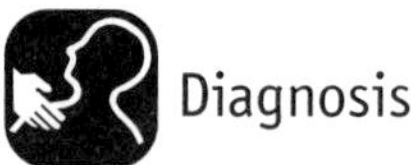

Diagnosis

DIFFERENTIAL DIAGNOSIS

- Retrocalcaneal bursitis
- Superficial Achilles' bursitis
- Haglund deformity: prominent superior tuberosity of calcaneus
- Achilles' tendon rupture
- Gastroc-soleus tear
- Overuse myositis
- Exertional compartment syndrome
- Os trigonum irritation or posterior ankle impingement syndrome

HISTORY

- Pain that initially subsides with use, but returns with continued use or after use, suggests an overuse injury.
- Pain usually is 2–6 cm above insertion.
- Morning stiffness is a hallmark of Achilles' tendinitis.
- Training errors are a factor in a large percentage of cases.
- Shoes need to be changed every 250–500 miles because of shoe padding breakdown.
- Patients may report weakness and intermittent swelling.

PHYSICAL EXAMINATION

- Tenderness over the distal Achilles' tendon (2–6 cm above the insertion)
- Thickening of the distal Achilles' tendon (chronic injury)
- Tenderness with resisted plantar flexion
- Crepitus with ankle motion
- Negative Thompson's test: Compression of the calf will cause normal passive plantar flexion of the foot.
- Decreased ankle dorsiflexion (from tight heel cord)

IMAGING

- Not usually needed for initial treatment. X-rays should be obtained if other potential injuries are suspected (e.g., fracture or tumor) or if injury is not responding to appropriate treatment.
- Standard ankle series (anteroposterior, lateral, and mortise) may show calcification of tendon; however, presence of calcification does not affect initial treatment.

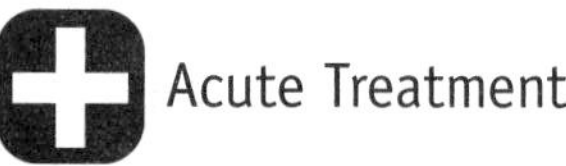

Acute Treatment

ACTIVITY MODIFICATION

- Relative rest: especially eliminate sprinting, speedwork, and running hills or stairs. Overall decrease in running intensity, duration, and/or frequency.
- New shoes: Avoid shoes with structures that place pressure over irritated area.
- Use of heel lifts or high heels often can acutely decrease symptoms.

ANTI-INFLAMMATORY TREATMENT

- Ice after activity
- Anti-inflammatory medications: Consider nonsteroidal anti-inflammatory agents
- Modalities: Consider the use of ultrasound or phonophoresis. Although some studies have shown that these modalities are useful in returning an athlete to activity sooner, they also show no long-term benefit.

OTHER TREATMENTS

- Hamstring and calf stretching and strengthening program
- Orthotics or arch supports may be useful in patients with low foot arches and those who overpronate.
- Night splints or walking boots may be useful in patients with recalcitrant symptoms.
- Short-term immobilization (7–10 days) for severe acute symptoms or recalcitrant symptoms

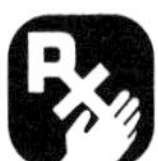

Long-Term Treatment

REHABILITATION

- Stretching: Ensure athlete is on appropriate conditioning program, preactivity warmup, and postactivity cooldown programs.
- Strengthening, including a gastrocnemius and soleus strengthening program with emphasis on eccentric exercises

SURGICAL TREATMENT/REFERRAL

Consider referral for surgical debridement for individuals whose symptoms have not responded to 3–6 or more months of conservative treatment.

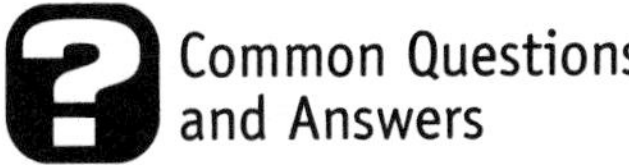

Common Questions and Answers

Physician responses to common patient questions:
Q: Can you just give me a cortisone injection?
A: Because of the high stresses placed upon the Achilles' tendon with weight-bearing activities and the risk of rupture, corticosteroid injection into the Achilles' tendon should be avoided.

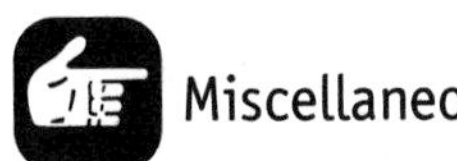

Miscellaneous

SYNONYMS

- Achilles' tendinosis

ICD-9 CODE

726.71

BIBLIOGRAPHY

Marks RM. Achilles tendinopathy: peritendinitis. *Foot Ankle Clin* 1999;4(4):789–809.

Myerson MS, McGarvey W. Disorders of the Achilles tendon insertion. *Instructional Course Lectures* 1999;48:211–218.

Saltzman CL, Tearse DS. Achilles tendon injuries. *J Am Acad Orthop Surg* 1998;6(5):316–325.

Authors: Craig C. Young and Mark W. Niedfeldt

Achilles' Tendon (Gastrocnemius Rupture)

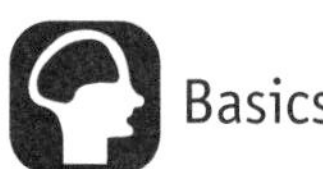

Basics

DEFINITION

- Achilles' tendon rupture is a complete disruption of the Achilles' tendon, usually occurring 2–6 cm proximal to its calcaneal insertion, where blood supply is the poorest.
- It can be associated with preexisting tendon degeneration and microtrauma.
- It most commonly occurs in 30- to 40-year-old men.

ANATOMY

- Is the largest tendon in the human body. It is designed to endure stresses up to ten times the body's weight.
- Is formed by the confluence of the tendons of the gastrocnemius and soleus muscles. The gastrocnemius medial and lateral heads originate from the medial and lateral femoral condyles, respectively. The soleus originates from a large attachment on the posterior tibia and fibula. Together, these tendons insert onto the calcaneus to form the Achilles' tendon.
- Receives its blood supply intrinsically from both the musculotendinous junction and the osteotendinous insertion site.
- Additional vascular supply comes from an external source known as the paratenon. The paratenon is a thin layer of areolar tissue that encases the Achilles' tendon. The further the tendon is from its musculotendinous origin and calcaneal insertion, the more it relies on the paratenon for vascular support.
- The area with the poorest vascular supply is approximately 2–6 cm proximal to the calcaneal insertion site.
- Prior to inserting into the calcaneus, the Achilles' tendon internally rotates, which imparts a structural torque stress in the tendon. This is thought to contribute to decreased vascularity in the tendon and ensuing tendon failure.

INCIDENCE/PREVALENCE

- More than 75% of Achilles' tendon ruptures occur in patients 30 to 40 years old while they partake in sports activities.
- Males >> females: Ratio ranges from 1.7:1 to 19:1.
- Left Achilles' >> right Achilles': thought to be due to higher prevalence of right-side dominant individuals using left lower limb to push off during activity

RISK FACTORS

- Disease processes: connective tissue disorders, seronegative spondylopathies, rheumatoid arthritis, collagen vascular disease, diabetes mellitus, gout, hyperparathyroidism, renal insufficiency
- Medications: Anabolic steroids or prolonged oral corticosteroid usage leads to degradation of collagen fibrils and decreased Achilles' tendon strength. Corticosteroid injections weaken tendon structure. Fluoroquinolone antimicrobials lead to ischemia of tendon.
- Disuse atrophy and sedentary lifestyle
- Prolonged immobilization
- Advanced age
- History of Achilles' tendonitis regardless of history of injection therapy
- Mechanical imbalances (i.e., decreased flexibility of gastrocnemius-soleus complex)
- Body weight/obesity
- Possibility of genetic predisposition (possibility of association with HLA-B27, blood group O)

MECHANISM

- Achilles' tendon ruptures are caused laceration or by indirect forces applied to the tendon.
- Three types of indirect forces have been described:
  —Pushing off with the weight-bearing forefoot while extending the knee, such as with sprint starts and the pushoff in basketball
  —Sudden, unexpected dorsiflexion of the ankle, as when the foot slips in a hole
  —Violent dorsiflexion of a plantar flexed foot, as with a fall from a height

SIGNS AND SYMPTOMS

- Acute complete rupture of the Achilles' tendon involves a sudden, sharp pain behind the ankle, usually associated with a painful, palpable defect in the tendon.
- Swelling and/or ecchymosis

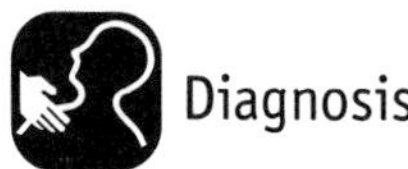

Diagnosis

DIFFERENTIAL DIAGNOSIS

- Achilles' tendinitis
- Ankle sprain
- Peritendonitis
- Retrocalcaneal bursitis
- Superficial Achilles' bursitis
- Periostitis
- Plantar tendon rupture
- Calcaneal avulsion

HISTORY

- Patients commonly report feeling as if they have been kicked or struck in the back of the heel, only to find no one is nearby.
- May feel, or hear, a "pop" or snap
- Pain with weight-bearing
- Weakness or stiffness of posterior ankle
- May give history of chronic Achilles' tendinitis with or without history of injection therapy

PHYSICAL EXAMINATION

- "Hatchet strike" defect: palpable, tender defect, usually 2–6 cm from the tendon insertion site
- Swelling and/or ecchymosis
- Positive Thompson test is diagnostic. Have patient lie prone, or kneel, with ankles clear of the table. Squeeze bulk of calf muscle and observe for plantar flexion. Perform on uninvolved side first for comparison. Absence of plantar flexion is consistent with complete tendon rupture.
- Note that only 25% of the fibers is needed for Achilles' to function normally; therefore, partial tears may be missed on examination.
- Plantar flexion strength and ability to toe rise may be decreased compared to unaffected side.*
- Passive dorsiflexion may be increased compared to unaffected side.*

* These signs may be absent because of recruitment of other intact muscles, such as tibialis posterior, peroneus longus and brevis, and flexor digitorum and hallucis longus.

IMAGING

- Routine plain films should be obtained to avoid missing a calcaneal avulsion rupture, which would require surgical treatment. This finding usually can be appreciated on the lateral ankle radiograph.
- Ultrasound and magnetic resonance imaging should be reserved for when the diagnosis of a complete rupture is questionable or if one is considering a partial tear.

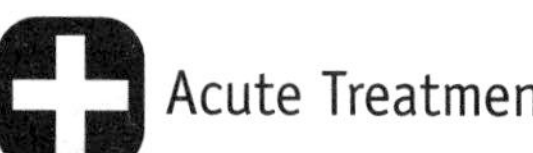

Acute Treatment

ANALGESIA

- Analgesia should be based on the patient's degree of pain.
- Rest, ice, compression, and elevation (RICE) should be used in the initial treatment of complete and partial tears.

ACTIVITY

- The foot should be kept in slight plantar flexion and crutches should be used.
- No activity until definitive treatment is under way and cleared by physician

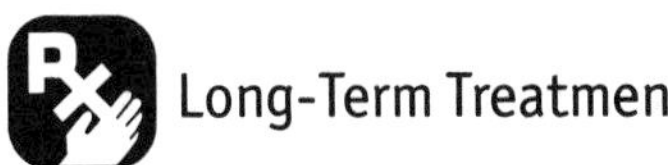

Long-Term Treatment

TREATMENT OPTIONS

- Controversy in the literature exists as to the best treatment approach for Achilles' tendon rupture.
- Careful patient selection is based on the patient's activity level and goals.
- The two treatment options are surgical repair and casting.

NONSURGICAL APPROACH

- Offers quicker return to work
- Fewer complications than surgery
- Risk of rerupture greater than with surgical repair: 13% for nonsurgical versus 5% for surgical repair
- Risk of deep venous thrombosis (DVT) with prolonged casting; warfarin prophylaxis for high-risk patients
- Usually recommended for less active or elderly patients, those with medical contraindications to surgery, or those with a history of multiple, chronic tears
- Partial tears, or a tear in continuity diagnosed by magnetic resonance imaging, also treated conservatively

CONSERVATIVE MANAGEMENT TIMELINE

- 0–4 weeks: long-leg cast with knee at 45 degrees and foot in gravity equinus. Can use short-leg cast nonweight-bearing (SLC NWB) if patient avoids any leg extension. This prevents pull on the Achilles' from the gastrocnemius attachment at the femoral condyles.
- 4–8 weeks: short-leg walking cast (SLWC) in slightly less equinus/neutral position
- 8–10 weeks: continuous active motion (CAM) walker with gradual increases in dorsiflexion as tolerated. Approximately 10 degrees every 2–3 days. Discontinue CAM walker when full dorsiflexion is achieved.
- 10 weeks: 2- to 2.5-cm heel lift gradually decreased over next several weeks/months and aggressive rehabilitation for range of motion then strengthening
- ~6 months: return to full activity

SURGICAL APPROACH

- Open repair or closed, percutaneous technique
- Associated with a lower incidence of rerupture
- Increased restoration of calf strength/less loss of pushoff power
- More likely to return to preinjury level: 57% surgical versus 29% nonsurgical
- Surgical complications can include infection, DVT, pulmonary embolism, and death.
- Other postoperative risks include delayed healing, scar adhesions, infection, persistent equinus, overlengthening, and fistulas.
- Usually recommended for high-level athletes, those returning to high-risk activities (basketball, tennis, soccer, and sprinting), and for treatment of rerupture

SURGICAL MANAGEMENT TIMELINE

- 0 weeks: surgical repair
- 0–2 weeks: SLC NWB in gravity equinus
- 2–4 weeks: SLC NWB foot 50% to neutral
- 4–6 weeks: SLWC in neutral position
- 6–8 weeks: CAM walker with free plantar flexion and 0 degree dorsiflexion
- 8 weeks: heel lift and nonresisted ROM
- 12 weeks: resisted calf strengthening
- 6 months: return to sports

REHABILITATION

- Both treatment approaches should be followed by a well-outlined rehabilitation program.
- Advances in therapy should be supervised by the treating physician.
- Cardiovascular fitness during treatment can be sustained through arm ergometer use, then recumbent cycling once weight-bearing is initiated.
- Once the cast is removed, passive, then active, dorsiflexion and plantar flexion stretches for range of motion should be initiated.
- Strengthening is achieved through resisted range of motion exercises and heel rises.

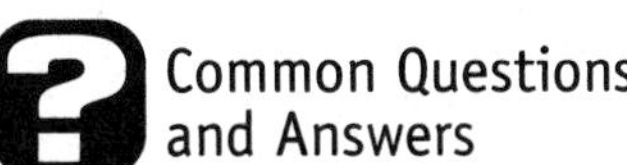

Common Questions and Answers

Physician responses to common patient questions:

Q: Do I need surgery?

A: This is an ongoing debate. The literature varies in its reported success and failure rates for both the surgical and nonsurgical approaches. Physicians need to be aware of both treatment options and their risks/benefits in order to help their patients make an informed decision (see "Long-Term Treatment").

Q: How long will I need to be in a cast?

A: If casting is the treatment choice, typically 4 weeks of nonweight-bearing, then 4 weeks in an SLWC. After a patient has surgery, this is also generally the routine. Recently, however, earlier mobilization with special braces that allow passive plantarflexion have been used. It is best to discuss surgical treatment approaches with your local orthopaedic group to determine their philosophy (see "Long-Term Treatment").

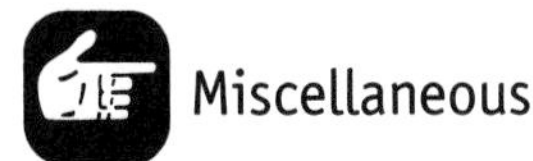

Miscellaneous

SYNONYMS

- Heel-cord rupture, Achilles' tear

ICD-9 CODE

845.09 Achilles' tendon injury, rupture

BIBLIOGRAPHY

Benedetti R, Sallis RE. Achilles tendon: to cut or not to cut. Kaiser Permanente Sports Medicine Symposium-Southern California Permanente Medical Group. Symposium, March 25, 2000.

Cetti R, Christensen S, Ejsted R, et al. Operative versus nonoperative treatment of Achilles tendon rupture: A prospective randomized study and review of the literature. *Am J Sports Med* 1993;21(6): 791–799.

Myerson MS. Achilles tendon ruptures. *AAOS Instructional Course Lectures* 1999;48: 219–230.

Authors: Carrie Jaworski and Aaron L. Rubin

Acromioclavicular Dislocations (Types 1–6)

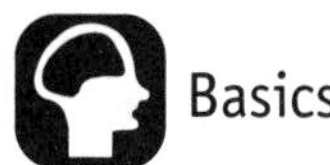

Basics

DEFINITION

- Separation of the clavicle and acromion due to injury of the acromioclavicular (AC) and coracoclavicular (CC) ligaments
- Classified based on the degree of separation and the anatomical structures that are involved (types I–VI)

INCIDENCE/PREVALENCE

- Males are five times more likely to suffer injuries than females.
- Type I and II injuries are two times as likely as types III, IV, V, and VI.

SIGNS AND SYMPTOMS

- Pain in the AC joint
- Pain during forward flexion and/or adduction of shoulder
- Deformity of AC joint with type III injuries and higher

MECHANISMS

- Direct trauma to an unprotected shoulder, such as when tackling or blocking an opponent
- Falling onto the shoulder with the arm adducted

TYPES

- Type I: mild sprain of the AC ligament
- Type II: tear of the AC ligament with a mild CC ligament sprain (clavicle to coracoid distance unchanged compared to unaffected side)
- Types III–VI: all involving complete tears of both ligaments with varying positions of clavicular displacement
- Type III: mild superior clavicle displacement
- Type IV: posterior displacement of the clavicle, occasionally displacing through the trapezius
- Type V: severe superior clavicular displacement, disrupting the deltoid and trapezius attachments to the clavicle
- Type VI: severe inferior clavicle displacement with potential damage to the underlying brachial plexus and subclavian vessels

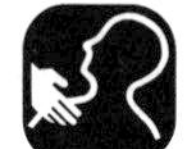

Diagnosis

DIFFERENTIAL DIAGNOSIS

- Fractures of the coracoid, acromion, or clavicle
- Rotator cuff injuries
- Glenohumeral dislocation
- Burner/stinger
- Cervical spine injuries

HISTORY

- Exact mechanism of injury (to assess how severe the injury is and whether there is a possibility of associated injuries)
- Neurologic symptoms or vascular symptoms (indicates a more severe injury that might require immediate surgery)

PHYSICAL EXAMINATION

- Inspection (asymmetry of the shoulders)
- Palpation (point tenderness of the affected AC joint)
- Range of motion (pain with shoulder adduction)
- Crossover or scarf test: Flexion of shoulder to 90 degrees and forced adduction across chest reproduce pain at the AC joint.
- Neurovascular examination

RADIOGRAPHY

- Anteroposterior (AP) of both shoulders: evaluate separation of AC joint and CC ligament disruption, and identify fractures of the clavicle, acromion, coracoid
- Lateral Y view if suspect glenohumeral instability
- Stress views (weighted views) can be used to differentiate types I–III, but are not recommended, as the results do not affect treatment, and disruption of the CC ligament (larger space between coracoid and clavicle on the affected side) can be seen on the standard AP.

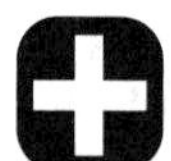

Acute Treatment

TYPES I AND II

- Shoulder sling for several days for pain reduction and comfort
- Ice and analgesics for pain and swelling
- Range of motion exercises early in course
- Shoulder and trunk strengthening exercises as pain resolves

TYPE III

- Controversial: nonsurgical versus surgical repair. Studies indicate good outcome with nonsurgical management, as detailed under types I and II.
- Consider surgical referral, particularly in heavy manual laborers, high-level athletes, patients unwilling to tolerate cosmetic deformity, and those who fail conservative management.

TYPES IV–VI

- Surgical referral

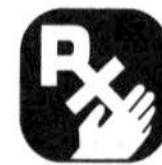

Long-Term Treatment

REHABILITATION

- Types I and II: Shoulder range of motion and strengthening exercise are introduced as pain subsides. Full return to contact when full painless range of motion and normal strength.
- Type III: Shoulder strengthening exercises are introduced when range of motion and pain are improved. Return to contact sports usually is anticipated in 2–6 months, depending on resumption of full painless range of motion and normal strength.

SURGERY

- Types IV–VI usually require operative treatment.

REFERRAL TO ORTHOPAEDICS

- Type IV–VI
- Type III in high-level athletes, patients unwilling to have conservative therapy, heavy manual laborers, patients unwilling to tolerate the deformity, and patients who have failed conservative treatment after 3–6 months

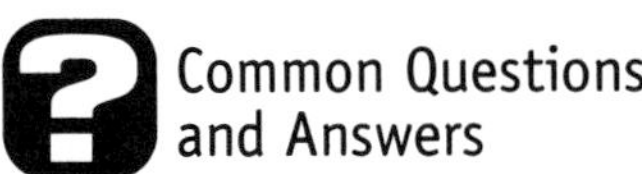

Common Questions and Answers

Physician responses to common patient questions:
Q: When can I return to play contact sports?
A: Full return to contact when painless range of motion and normal strength are achieved is a general guide. However, type I sprains are stable, so the athlete may return immediately if strength is normal and pain is not too severe.
Q: What complications are likely?
A: Cosmetic deformity and AC joint arthritis are common complications.

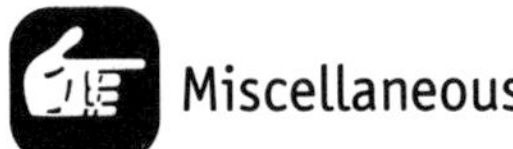

Miscellaneous

SYNONYMS

- Shoulder separation
- Shoulder sprain
- AC sprain
- AC dislocation
- Shoulder dislocation (misname, usually refers to glenohumeral dislocation)

ICD-9 CODE

831.04 Acromioclavicular dislocation

BIBLIOGRAPHY

Lemos MJ. The evaluation and treatment of the injured acromioclavicular joint in athletes. *Am J Sports Med* 1998;26(1): 137–144.

Press J, Zuckerman JD, Gallagher M, et al. Treatment of Grade III acromioclavicular separation. *Bull Hosp Joint Dis* 1997;56(2): 77–83.

Snider R, ed. *Essentials of musculoskeletal care.* Rosemont, IL: American Academy of Orthopaedic Surgeons, 1997.

Turnbull JR. Acromioclavicular joint disorders. *Med Sci Sports Exerc* 1998;30[4 Suppl]: S26–S32.

Yap JJ, Curl LA, Kvitne RS, et al. The value of weighted views of the acromioclavicul. *Am J Sports Med* 1992;27(6):806–809.

Author: James Barrett

Adductor Thigh Strain

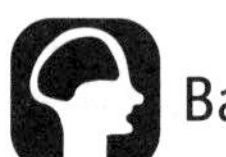

Basics

DEFINITION

- Medial thigh/adductor pain and weakness resulting from injury to muscle
- Usually adductor longus muscle, but also may include gracilis, iliopsoas, rectus femoris, or sartorius

INCIDENCE/PREVALENCE

- Most common cause of groin pain in athletes, but symptoms overlap with a wide differential

SIGNS AND SYMPTOMS

- Classic triad of tenderness to palpation in the muscle and its insertion, pain with passive stretching, and pain with resisted contraction
- Usually acute episode is noted, but symptoms may become chronic after initial injury if undertreated and repeatedly strained.

RISK FACTORS

- Eccentric loading of muscle (muscle is passively being stretched while it is contracting) is usual mechanism of injury.
- Inactive or fatigued muscles have less ability to absorb energy and are more likely to undergo acute strain.

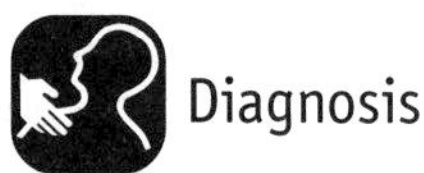

Diagnosis

DIFFERENTIAL DIAGNOSIS

- Osteitis pubis
- Stress fracture of femoral neck or pubic ramus
- Iliopsoas bursitis
- Avascular necrosis of femoral head
- Groin disruption (a.k.a., sports hernia, Gilmore's groin)
- Myositis ossificans
- Adductor tendinitis
- Avulsion fracture (especially in an adolescent)
- Slipped capital femoral epiphysis (usually seen in early teens)
- Inguinal hernia
- Lymphadenopathy
- Nerve entrapment
- Referred pain from spine or genitourinary tract

HISTORY

- Acutely, often a stretch injury with an abrupt cutting motion, or straddling injury as in gymnastics, cheerleading, or horseback riding
- Also can result from overuse, as in skating or rollerblading
- May have only minor discomfort with walking, but pain and weakness develop with cutting or running
- If symptoms do not respond to initial therapy, need to consider other diagnoses.

PHYSICAL EXAMINATION

- Tenderness along proximal third of medial thigh and tendinous origin in pubic region
- Pain with passive abduction
- Pain with resisted adduction
- Swelling and ecchymosis increase suspicion for tear
- With complete rupture, palpable depression and knot of torn muscle may be present.

IMAGING

- Generally not necessary in straightforward cases, but may be part of workup if appropriate
- Hip and pelvis films recommended to rule out other conditions
- Bone scan if stress fracture suspected

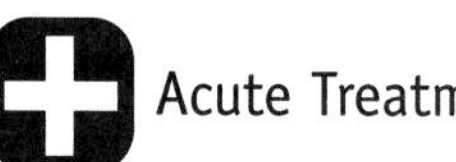

Acute Treatment

ANALGESIA

- Over-the-counter analgesics usually are sufficient.
- Some sources recommend avoiding nonsteroidal anti-inflammatory drugs with antiplatelet properties to help prevent bleeding into tissue
- Topical anesthetics
- Muscle relaxants may provide some benefit.

IMMOBILIZATION

- Strict immobilization generally is not recommended, and rehabilitation should be initiated early in the first few days.
- Subpain activity for 1–2 weeks; longer for more protracted cases
- For severe, incomplete tears, crutches for walking while symptomatic with ambulation
- Gentle compression with compression shorts, Neoprene sleeve, or elastic wrap

SPECIAL CONSIDERATIONS

- Ice for approximately 20 minutes every 2–3 hours for the first 2–3 days
- Heat may be added after 2–3 days.
- Gentle stretching exercises may be instituted after the first few days.

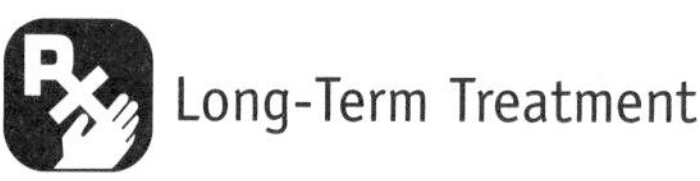

Long-Term Treatment

REHABILITATION

- Gentle stretching and low-intensity isotonic strengthening can be instituted as symptoms subside.
- Physical therapy modalities, such as ultrasound or electrical stimulation, may benefit in more chronic cases.
- Correction of predisposing factors, such as muscle tightness, weakness, or imbalance, should be addressed.
- Adequate stretching and warmup may help prevent reinjury.

SURGERY

- Surgical repair may be required for complete avulsion from the femur.
- Early repair is generally recommended.

REFERRAL/DISPOSITION

- Except for significant tears, referral to a specialist generally is not necessary unless another diagnosis is being considered and requires evaluation.

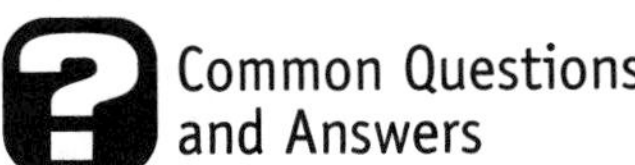

Common Questions and Answers

Physician responses to common patient questions:
Q: When can I return to play?
A: Decision on return to play depends on extent of injury and underlying predisposing factors. Pain is usually a fair measure, so unrestricted play is generally permitted if pain-free, which may take weeks.
Q: Can't I just "play through the pain"?
A: Although initial symptoms may not be debilitating enough to impair performance, pain is a marker for injury, which left untreated can become chronic and ultimately take longer to rehabilitate.

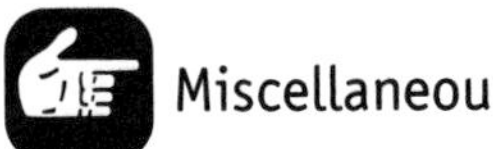

Miscellaneous

SYNONYMS

- Groin strain
- Pulled groin

ICD-9 CODE

843.8 Adductor thigh sprain

BIBLIOGRAPHY

Garrett WE. Muscle strain injuries. *Am J Sports Med* 1996;24[6 Suppl]:S2–S8.

Gilmore J. Groin pain in the soccer athlete. *Clin Sports Med* 1998;17(4):787–793.

Lacroix VJ. A complete approach to groin pain. *Physician Sports Med* 2000;28(1):online.

Ruane JJ, Rossi TA. When groin pain is more than "just a strain." *Physician Sports Med* 1998;26(4):online.

Sim FH, Nicholas JA, Hershman EB. *The lower extremity and spine in sports medicine.* St. Louis: Mosby, 1995.

Author: Michael Mikus

Adhesive Capsulitis

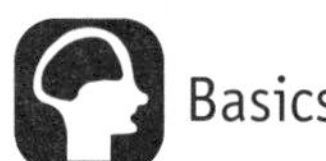

Basics

DEFINITION

- The presence of glenohumeral capsular restrictions accompanied by pain and decreased active and passive range of motion. It can occur with no obvious cause or be associated with any condition causing relative immobility of the shoulder. Most cases are idiopathic in nature.

INCIDENCE/PREVALENCE

- The highest incidence occurs in the fifth and sixth decades of life. Women are at increased risk. Involvement of the nondominant arm is higher than that of the dominant arm. About 12% of patients will develop bilateral symptoms.
- The reported incidence in the general population is approximately 3%.

SIGNS AND SYMPTOMS

- The hallmark of adhesive capsulitis is a decreased glenohumeral range of motion associated with pain. The loss of motion occurs earliest in external rotation, but later in the disease course all ranges of motion are affected.
- Adhesive capsulitis follows a progression comprised of an early painful loss of motion (freezing), an intermediate stiff stage (frozen), and a recovery stage (thawing). The mean duration of this condition was found to be 30 months, but a significant number of patients (up to 60%) will have ongoing loss of shoulder range past symptom resolution.

RISK FACTORS

- Include voluntary immobilization, rotator cuff tendonopathy, cervical radiculitis, hemiplegia, coronary artery disease, cervical herpes zoster infection, mastectomy, thoracic surgery, pulmonary infection, and medical conditions such as diabetes mellitus and hyperthyroidism.
- Female gender and age are also risk factors for adhesive capsulitis.

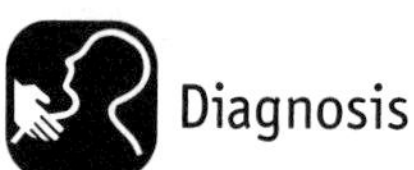

Diagnosis

DIFFERENTIAL DIAGNOSIS

- Rotator cuff tendonopathy
- Degenerative arthrosis of the glenohumeral joint
- Fracture of the humerus or glenoid
- Referred pain from the cervical spine, thorax, or abdomen
- Polymyalgia rheumatica
- Unrecognized posterior shoulder dislocation

HISTORY

- Patients will tend to have symptoms of pain and stiffness for weeks to months prior to presentation to a physician.
- Early symptoms may mimic rotator cuff tendonopathy. Little loss of range of motion will be present.
- Pain usually is present in the region of the deltoid, but also may radiate into the upper arm and neck regions. Pain is worsened by movement and relieved by limiting use of the extremity. Pain is worse at night and may interfere with sleep.
- Common functional impairments include difficulty dressing, combing one's hair, reaching into one's back pocket for a wallet, or fastening a brassiere.
- A careful medical history to exclude associated conditions should be conducted.

PHYSICAL EXAMINATION

- Observation usually reveals limited use of the limb and lack of arm swing in walking.
- The scapula usually is elevated, laterally placed, and protracted. Wasting of the shoulder girdle muscles may be present due to disuse atrophy.
- The range of motion will be limited and, in early stages, painful. The greatest limitation is usually seen in external rotation and abduction. In later stages, all ranges of motion usually are limited.
- A capsular pattern of restriction characterized by a "leathery," hard end feel has been described. Anecdotally, a hard end point and a greater limitation in external rotation than any other range of motion can be strongly suggestive of adhesive capsulitis.

IMAGING

- Results of laboratory investigations usually are normal unless there is an associated illness.
- Radiographs are useful to assess the presence of alternate diagnoses. No specific findings on radiographs correlating with a diagnosis of adhesive capsulitis have been reported.
- Arthrography has been described as sensitive in making the diagnosis where the joint capsule volume is decreased. However, a loss of volume of the shoulder capsule is not always present, and the test carries risks that have led some authors to recommend avoiding its use in diagnosis.
- Technetium scans reportedly have been useful for diagnosing the condition in early presentations but presently lack sufficient confirmation.
- Magnetic resonance imaging recently has been shown to have appropriate specificity and sensitivity to diagnose this condition.

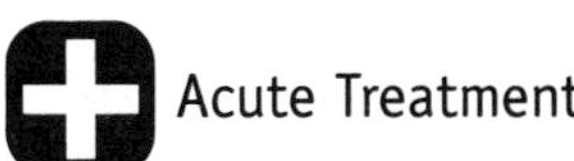

Acute Treatment

TREATMENT

- A high rate of spontaneous recovery for this condition should be kept in mind when choosing treatment options. Treatment should be focused on relief of symptoms and optimization of ranges of motion.
- A program of therapeutic exercise comprised of gentle range of motion exercises, stretching, and graded resistance training has been associated with increased range of motion and decreased pain. The program should be guided by the patient, and vigorous programs that increase symptoms should be avoided.
- Joint mobilization may be helpful in improving scapular mechanics, increasing range of motion, and decreasing pain.
- Manipulation under anesthesia has been described and has been both condemned and praised by some authors. It should not be used early in the treatment and should be reserved for refractory cases, as manipulation is associated with a high risk of complications.
- Intra-articular and subacromial corticosteroid injections have been shown to decrease pain but have not been shown to affect recovery. Suprascapular nerve blocks may decrease pain but presently are considered investigational procedures.
- Therapeutic modalities have not been shown to significantly affect the outcome of this condition. Their use would be considered elective.
- Other options such as distention arthrography and surgery have been proposed, but their merits have been questioned in a condition that is considered relatively self-limited.
- Recently, active release techniques (ART) have been proposed as a conservative treatment option. Further investigation into this modality is needed.

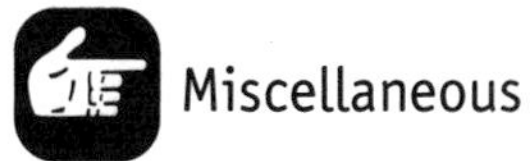

Miscellaneous

ICD-9 CODE

726.0

BIBLIOGRAPHY

Emig EW, Schweitzer ME, Karasick D, et al. Adhesive capsulitis of the shoulder: MR diagnosis. *Am J Roentgenol* 1995;164(6): 1457–1459.

Grubbs N. Frozen shoulder syndrome: a review of literature. *JOSP* 1993;18(3):479–487.

Rogers LF, Hendrix RW. The painful shoulder. *Radiol Clin North Am* 1988;26(6): 1359–1371.

Shaffer B, Tibone JE, Kerlan RK. Frozen shoulder. *J Bone Joint Surg* 1992;74A(5): 738–746.

Authors: Neil Craton and B. Baydock

Ankle Sprains, Lateral

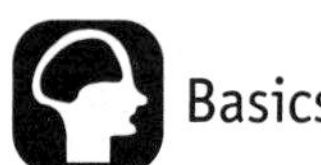

Basics

DEFINITION

- Occurs when the ankle is forced into excessive inversion, stretching or tearing one or more of the lateral ankle ligaments

INCIDENCE/PREVALENCE

- Lateral ankle sprains are the most common sprains.
- Lateral ankle sprains occur more than four times as frequently as medial ankle sprains.
- Lateral ankle sprains are the most common injury in sports, especially basketball (almost half of injuries), soccer, cross-country running, and dance.

SIGNS AND SYMPTOMS

- Pain over the lateral ankle, inferior to the lateral malleolus
- Localized swelling over the area of pain
- Pain usually exacerbated with weight-bearing or movement

RISK FACTORS

- Ligamentous laxity may be from natural hypermobility or from previous lateral ankle sprains.

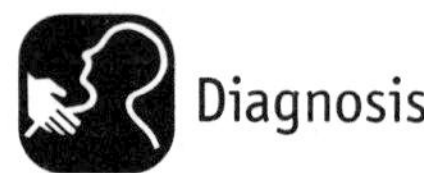

Diagnosis

DIFFERENTIAL DIAGNOSIS

- Fracture of the distal fibula
- Fracture of the talus
- Fracture of the calcaneus
- Fracture of the proximal fifth metatarsal
- Strain or subluxation of the peroneal tendon
- Stretch neurapraxia of the sensory nerves of the foot

HISTORY

- Acute inversion of the ankle
- Varying amounts of early swelling over the lateral ankle
- May hear a "pop" at the time of injury

PHYSICAL EXAMINATION

- Observation of gait abnormalities
- Amount and location of localized swelling
- Check distal neurovascular status
- Active range of motion
- Passive range of motion
- Palpate to localize the tenderness to specific anatomical structure(s): anterior talofibular, calcaneofibular, posterior talofibular, and tibiofibular ligaments
- Tibiofibular squeeze test to assess for syndesmosis involvement
- Anterior drawer test of the ankle to assess degree of ligamentous laxity
- Talar tilt test (inversion of the ankle) to assess degree of ligamentous laxity

IMAGING

- The "Ottawa Ankle Rules" recommend x-raying the ankle if the patient complains of pain on either side of the ankle and either the posterior aspect of the distal 6 cm of the fibula is tender, the posterior aspect of the distal 6 cm of the tibia is tender, or the patient is unable to bear weight on the injured ankle.
- Typical x-ray series of the ankle includes anteroposterior (AP), lateral, and ankle mortise views
- Consider x-ray of any ankle injury that does not resolve within approximately 10 days

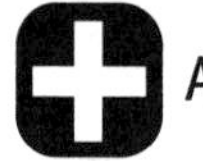

Acute Treatment

ANALGESIA

- Ice for 20 minutes at a time, repeating up to every hour for the first 24–48 hours, will reduce pain and swelling.
- Acetaminophen or mild narcotic analgesics may be required in the first 24–48 hours following injury.
- Nonsteroidal anti-inflammatories (especially COX-1 inhibitors) may increase bleeding and swelling immediately following an injury, but may be considered after acute bruising and swelling has stabilized.

SPECIAL CONSIDERATIONS

- Always evaluate neurovascular status immediately following an ankle sprain to rule out any associated neurovascular damage.
- Prolonged immobilization increases the risk of deep vein thrombosis.

PROTECT

- Immediate immobilization or splinting to protect from further injury

REST

- Relative rest: reduce level of activity to prevent aggravation of injury
- Avoid activities that have a high risk of lateral ankle injury (i.e., activities with running, jumping, etc.)
- Encourage quick (within 1–2 days) resumption of low-level of activity, such as walking as tolerated, as early weight-bearing can be beneficial in strengthening the ankle, reducing swelling, and thus speeding recovery.

ICE

- Apply ice to the lateral ankle (ice in plastic bag, commercial cold pack, ankle immersed in a bucket of ice water).
- Ice for 15–20 minutes usually is enough to promote vasoconstriction and reduce swelling, without significant risk of frost bite.
- Repeat icing at least 3–4 times a day until all swelling is gone.

COMPRESSION

- Elastic ankle wrap (Ace bandage) or pneumatic compression splint over the ankle to reduce swelling
- Increases the interstitial hydrostatic pressure, pushing edema in the tissue back into the lymphatic and venous system, where it can drain away from the injury

ELEVATION

- Elevation of the ankle will help to reduce swelling.
- Elevate the injured ankle above the level of the heart as possible
- Elevation above the level of the heart increases the interstitial hydrostatic pressure to a level that is greater than the pressure within the lymphatic and venous systems, thus encouraging drainage of swelling away from the injured ankle.

SUPPORT

- Support with tape or brace as level of activity increases
- Functional support reduces the risk of reinjury as patient is able to return to activities.

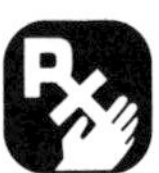

Long-Term Treatment

REHABILITATION

- Functional support (tape, brace)
- Range of motion, active and passive, concentrating on plantar flexion and dorsiflexion in the early phases of rehabilitation
- Strengthen evertors and dorsiflexors with low-resistance, high-repetition progressive resistance exercises
- Proprioception training (e.g., balance board) improves neuromotor control and strengthens the lateral ankle with eccentric contractions.
- Agility drills
- Endurance training
- Return to normal activity/sport
- Consider continuing functional support during competitive training or activity with taping or bracing for a period of 3–6 months

SURGERY

- May consider surgical repair of the lateral ligaments if there is gross instability in the high-level athlete, or if there is a concomitant unstable fracture of the ankle or a subluxation/tear of the peroneal tendon
- Open reduction and internal fixation with a syndesmosis screw usually are indicated for injuries that involve widening of the ankle mortise on x-ray with a tibiofibular diastasis.

REFERRAL/DISPOSITION

- Early aggressive physical therapy for range of motion, edema reduction, and progressive strengthening of the ankle may help reduce acute symptoms and hasten return to normal activity/sport.
- Consider surgical referral with gross instability or concomitant significant injuries.

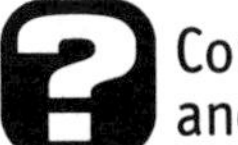

Common Questions and Answers

Physician responses to common patient questions:

Q: How long before I can play again?
A: Most athletes with mild ankle sprains improve with proper treatment and rehabilitation within 1–2 weeks, and can return to participation at that time with appropriate taping or bracing to reduce the risk of further injury.
Q: Will my ligaments tighten back up after an ankle sprain?
A: Sprained ligaments will tighten up some as they scar down and heal, but some laxity will probably remain.
Q: How can I prevent reinjuring my ankle?
A: Nothing can totally prevent ankle injury and reinjury, but in the short-term, taping or bracing may reduce the risk of reinjury. In the long-term, the best method of reducing the risk of reinjury to the ankle is a progressive ankle strengthening program with proprioception training.

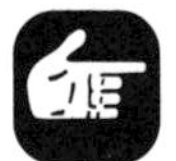

Miscellaneous

SYNONYMS

- Ankle sprain
- Inversion ankle sprain
- Common ankle sprain

ICD-9 CODE

845.02 Sprain of the ankle, calcaneofibular (lateral) ligament
845.00 Sprain of the ankle, unspecified site

BIBLIOGRAPHY

Liu SH, Jason WJ. Lateral ankle sprains and instability problems. *Clin Sports Med* 1994;13(4):793–809.

Safran MR, Benedetti RS, Bartolozzi AR III, et al. Lateral ankle sprains: a comprehensive review. Part I: etiology, pathoanatomy, histopathogenesis, and diagnosis. *Med Sci Sports Exerc* 1999;31[7 Suppl]:S429–S437.

Safran MR, Zachazewski JE, Benedetti RS, et al. Lateral ankle sprains: a comprehensive review. Part 2. *Med Sci Sports Exerc* 1999;31[7 Suppl]:S429–S437.

Stiell IG, Wells G, Laupicus A, et al. A multicentre trial to introduce clinical decision rules for the use of radiography in acute ankle injury. *Br Med J* 1995;311: 594–597.

Authors: Douglas Browning and Michael B. Potter

Ankle Sprains, Medial

Basics

DEFINITION

- Injury to the deltoid ligament of the ankle that occurs from a pronation/external rotation injury of the foot. Deltoid ligament injury usually is a more serious injury than lateral ankle sprain. Most often, deltoid ligament injuries are associated with concomitant injury to the lateral ligaments or fibula.
- Grade I sprain involves stretching of deltoid ligament.
- Grade II sprain involves a tear of some portion of the deltoid ligament with associated pain and swelling.
- Grade III sprain is complete disruption of the superficial and deep deltoid ligament.

INCIDENCE/PREVALENCE

Isolated deltoid ligament injuries constitute less than 10% of all ankle sprains.

SIGNS AND SYMPTOMS

- Medial ankle pain
- Swelling on the medial aspect of ankle
- Ecchymosis around the medial malleolus

RISK FACTORS

- Previous ankle injuries
- High-risk sports, including football, basketball, and long-jumping

ASSOCIATED INJURIES AND COMPLICATIONS

- Talar dome lesions
- Syndesmosis sprain
- Fractures of the fibula and tibia
- Chronic deltoid insufficiency, functional instability, and recurrent sprains

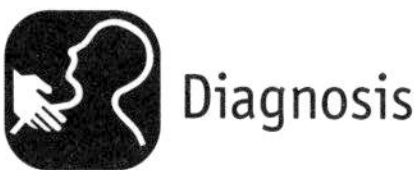

Diagnosis

DIFFERENTIAL DIAGNOSIS

- Syndesmosis sprain
- Posterior tibial tendon injuries
- Flexor hallucis longus tendon injuries
- Distal tibia fracture
- Proximal fibular fracture (Maisonneuve fracture)
- Osteochondral fracture

HISTORY

Athlete reports an eversion injury with the foot abducted from landing or stepping on another opponent's foot.

PHYSICAL EXAMINATION

- Careful palpation to identify tender structures
- Tenderness over the deltoid ligament
- Check for tenderness over the anterior syndesmosis ligament, lateral ankle, and fibula (distal and proximal)
- Check posterior tibial tendon function-resisted eversion
- Check flexor hallucis longus tendon function-resisted flexion of great toe
- Squeeze test and external rotation test to rule out syndesmotic injury
- Reverse talar tilt test to test the stability of the deltoid ligament, done with passive eversion of the ankle

IMAGING

- Anteroposterior, lateral, and mortise views of injured ankle are essential to rule out fracture (60% of patients with a deltoid rupture have an associated avulsion fracture of the medial malleolus, diastasis, or fibular fracture).
- Mortise view: Greater than 4 mm of medial clear space between lateral border of the medial malleolus to the medial border of the talus at the level of talar dome is abnormal and indicates the possibility of an unstable joint.
- Weight-bearing views are recommended to rule out instability with physiologic stress.
- Consider reverse talar tilt stress radiograph to assess for significant instability and possible surgical treatment: More than 10 degrees of abduction tilt of the talus is abnormal (only do if there is no associated fractures).
- Consider magnetic resonance imaging if the extent of deltoid ligament rupture is unclear (partial vs. complete) and surgical treatment is considered.

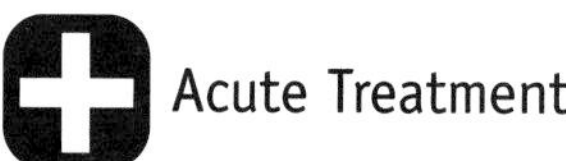

Acute Treatment

GENERAL PRINCIPLES

- Prevention/reduction of swelling: elevation, compression, and ice for 20 minutes 3–4 times a day until swelling is gone
- Protection: Ace wrap, stirrup brace, tibial walker, or short-leg cast (may need crutches if unable to bear weight)
- Restoration of motion: active range of motion as soon as tolerated

ANALGESIA

- Nonsteroidal anti-inflammatory drugs and ice

GRADE I SPRAIN

- Functional management in a stirrup brace, with the recognition that return to sports is generally more delayed (3–6 weeks) than a lateral sprain (1–3 weeks)

GRADE II SPRAIN

- Same as grade I, but may need a short period of immobilization in posterior splint or short-leg cast

GRADE III SPRAIN

Treatment is controversial. Requires immobilization (6–8 weeks) or may need operative repair (see "Referral/Disposition").

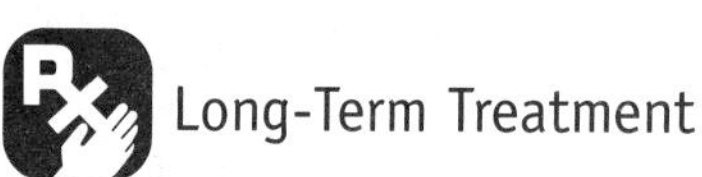

Long-Term Treatment

REHABILITATION

- Recommend teaching the athlete a home rehabilitation program
- Range of motions exercises until patient achieves full range of motion
- Progressive resistance exercises for 4–6 months
- Proprioception exercises for 4–6 months
- Protection with sporting activities for 6–9 months

REFERRAL/DISPOSITION

- Greater than 4 mm of medial clear space on the mortise view
- Significant instability on reverse talar tilt stress radiograph or weight-bearing views
- Grade III injury may need operative repair to prevent long-term complications.
- Medial malleolus fracture
- Displaced lateral malleolus fracture

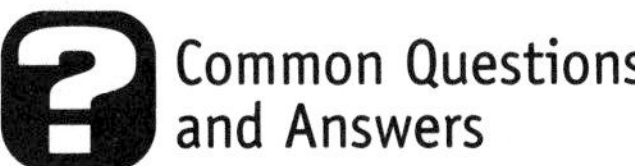

Common Questions and Answers

Physician responses to common patient questions:
Q: When can I return to activity?
A: An athlete may return to full activity once the swelling is gone and he or she is able to do a progressive running program without pain and instability. Return to sports may be prolonged more than 3 months depending on the degree of injury.
Q: How can I prevent future injuries?
A: Wear an ankle brace for sporting activities and complete rehabilitation.

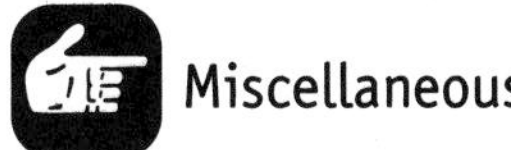

Miscellaneous

SYNONYMS

- Medial ankle sprain
- Deltoid ligament sprain

ICD-9 CODE

845.01 Deltoid ligament sprain

BIBLIOGRAPHY

Birrer RB, Dellacorte MP. *Common foot problems in primary care,* 2nd ed. Philadelphia: Hanley & Belfus, 1998.

Birrer RB, Fani-Salek MH, Totten UY. Managing ankle injuries in the emergency department. *J Emerg Med* 1999;17;651–660.

Clanton TO, Porter DA. Primary care of foot and ankle injuries in the athlete. *Clin Sports Med* 1997;16:435–466.

DeLee JC, Drez D. *Orthopaedic sports medicine: principles and practice.* Philadelphia: WB Saunders, 1994.

Stiehl JB. Complex ankle fracture dislocations with syndesmotic diastasis. *Orthop Rev* 1990;14:499–507.

Authors: Daniel Clinkenbeard and James Barrett

Ankylosing Spondylitis

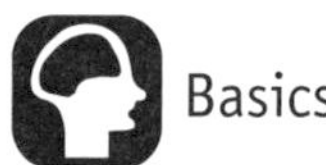

Basics

DEFINITION

Ankylosing spondylitis is an inflammatory arthritis that tends to be asymmetric peripherally and to involve the insertion of tendons, ligaments, as well as the sacroiliac joints and spine.

CAUSES

- Idiopathic

PATHOLOGY

- Inflammatory synovitis of joints and calcification of the anterior and posterior longitudinal ligaments of the spine

EPIDEMIOLOGY

- Typically affects adolescent males
- About 1 per 1000 white boys
- Much less common in blacks

GENETICS

- HLA-B27 associated

COMPLICATIONS

- Acute anterior uveitis
- Aortic insufficiency

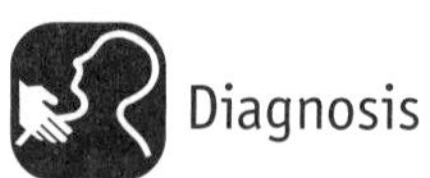

Diagnosis

INFECTION

- Reiter syndrome caused by *Enterobacteriaceae* or *Chlamydia*
- Whipple disease
- Intestinal-bypass—associated arthritis
- Diskitis
- Pott disease

TUMORS

- Osteoid osteoma

TRAUMA

- Traumatic injury causing low back pain/spasm
- Herniated disk

METABOLIC

- Ochronosis

CONGENITAL

- Kyphosis

IMMUNOLOGICAL

- Inflammatory bowel disease—associated arthropathy
- Pauciarticular juvenile rheumatoid arthritis

PSYCHOLOGICAL

- Feigning low back pain/stiffness

MISCELLANEOUS

- Psoriasis-associated arthritis
- SEA (seronegative enthesopathy and arthropathy) syndrome

DATA GATHERING

History

Question: Ankylosing spondylitis
Significance: Signified by back pain of insidious onset that has been present for at least 3 months. There is usually a familial history of a male relative with disease and inactivity stiffness resulting in gelling of peripheral joints and back.

PHYSICAL EXAMINATION

Finding: Sacroiliac tenderness
Significance: Indicates site of inflammation
Finding: Pain on direct palpation at insertion of Achilles tendon and plantar fascia at calcaneal insertion
Significance: Indicates site of inflammation
Finding: Schober test of lumbar spine flexibility
Significance: Mark 15-cm span at mid-low back at level of iliac crest while patient is standing. Have patient flex back as far as possible. Remeasure span. Abnormal if less than 5 cm increase in span.

LABORATORY AIDS

Test: CBC, ESR, HLA-B27, rheumatoid factor (RF), and antinuclear antibody (ANA) tests should be done.
Significance: Note that ESR is occasionally not elevated. RF and ANA are typically negative.
Test: Imaging
Significance: Sacroiliac views should be obtained to demonstrate evidence of pseudowidening and/or sclerosis.
Test: False Positives
Significance: HLA-B27 occurs in 8% of whites and 6% of blacks.

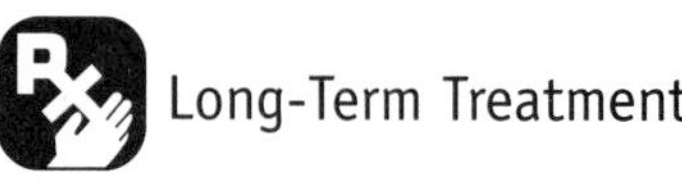

Long-Term Treatment

DRUGS

- NSAIDs: naproxen, indomethacin, meclofenemate
- Disease-modifying drugs: sulfasalazine, methotrexate

PHYSICAL THERAPY

- Physical therapy is an essential component of treatment
- Must encourage range-of-motion exercises and avoid prolonged neck flexion.

DURATION OF THERAPY

- May be lifelong

DIET

- Food intake should be good with NSAIDs
- Ensure folate intake with methotrexate

WHEN TO EXPECT IMPROVEMENT

Over weeks to several months one should see some improvement in stiffness, synovitis, and range of motion.

SIGNS TO WATCH FOR TO INDICATE PROBLEMS

- Worsening stiffness
- Acute or chronic eye pain
- Chest pain or shortness of breath

PROGNOSIS

- Poor if disease remains active for 10 years or more

PITFALLS

Overdiagnosis in HLA-B27-positive individuals in whom other causes for joint swelling should be considered.

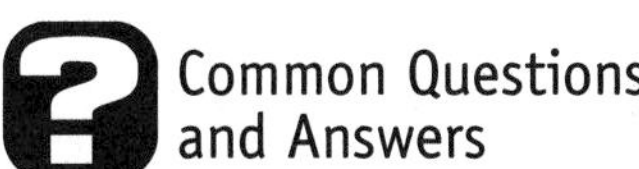

Common Questions and Answers

Q: Should HLA-B27 be checked routinely in boys with back pain?
A: Detection of HLA-B27 alone should not precipitate an extensive work-up because it is so common in the normal healthy population. However, the risk for developing a spondyloarthropathy is 16 times greater than in the HLA-B27-negative individual.

Q: Can affected individuals play contact sports?
A: This is probably not a good idea because as the spine fuses, the risk for fracture of the spine (especially the C-spine) increases.

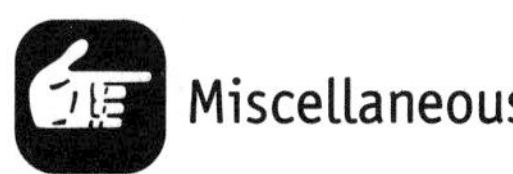

Miscellaneous

ICD-9 CODE

720.0

BIBLIOGRAPHY

Cabral DA, Malleson PN, Petty RE. Spondyloarthropathies of childhood. *Pediatr Clin North Am* 1995;42(5):1051–1070.

Case records of the Massachusetts General Hospital. Weekly clinicopathological exercises. Case 17-1990. A 16-year-old boy with painful swelling of the left knee joint and calf. *N Engl J Med* 1990;322:1214–1223.

Flato B, Aasland A, Vinje O, Forre O. Outcome and predictive factors in juvenile rheumatoid arthritis and juvenile spondyloarthropathy. *J Rheumatol* 1998;25(2):366–375.

Spondyloarthropathies and psoriatic arthritis in children. *Curr Opin Rheumatol* 1993;5:634–643.

Author: Gregory F. Keenan

Anterior Interosseous Syndrome

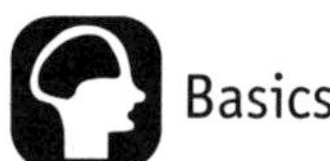

Basics

DEFINITION

- The anterior interosseous nerve is a pure motor branch of the median nerve as it divides 4 to 6 cm below the elbow.
- The anterior interosseous nerve usually innervates the flexor pollicis longus, the flexor digitorum profundus of the index finger, and the pronator quadratus.
- Anterior interosseous syndrome is a rare compression neuropathy of the corresponding nerve.

SIGNS AND SYMPTOMS

- Pain in the forearm
- No objective sensory findings
- Inability to make the "OK" sign because of loss of thumb-index finger pinch strength

RISK FACTORS

- Tendinous bands
- Accessory muscles
- Vascular abnormalities
- Trauma including fractures or penetrating injuries
- Throwers, weight lifters, and racquet sports

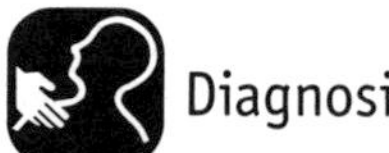

Diagnosis

DIFFERENTIAL DIAGNOSIS

- Brachial plexus neuritis (Neuritis of Parsonage and Turner)
- Mannerfelt syndrome (attrition rupture of the flexor pollicis longus in patients with rheumatoid arthritis)
- Congenital absence of the flexor digitorum longus and flexor pollicis longus
- Partial lesion of the median nerve

HISTORY

- Pain in the forearm that is aggravated by upper extremity exercise and relieved with rest
- Difficulty picking up small objects with first two digits

PHYSICAL EXAMINATION

- Sensation intact
- Weakness in flexion of the distal interphalangeal joint of the second and third digits due to weakness of the flexor digitorum profundus
- Pronator quadratus weakness, detected by flexing the forearm and asking the patient to resist supination
- Inability to make "OK" sign

DIAGNOSTIC TESTING

- EMG testing confirms the diagnosis in 80% to 90% of cases.
- EMG testing is carried out by stimulating at the elbow and recording from the pronator quadratus muscle
- The latency and amplitude of compound muscle action potential are compared with the unaffected side.
- Needle examination reveals abnormalities in the flexor pollicis longus, radial part of the flexor digitorum profundus, and pronator quadratus.
- Sensory nerve action potentials are normal.

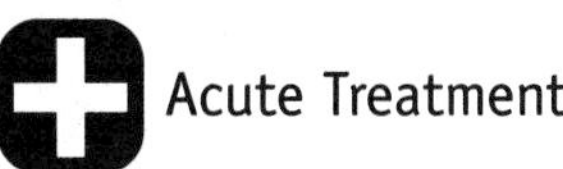

Acute Treatment

SPECIAL CONSIDERATIONS

- Treatment consists of 8 to 12 weeks of rest and splinting
- Anterior interosseous nerve exploration may be considered when conservative treatment fails to result in improvement.

ICD-9 CODE

354.1 Other lesion of median nerve
355.9 General

BIBLIOGRAPHY

Bracker MD, Ralph LP. The numb arm and hand. *American Family Physician* 51(1): 103–116.

Authors: Suraj Achar, Ahmed Khalifa, and Ayse Dural

Anterior Metatarsalgia (Submetatarsal Head Pain)

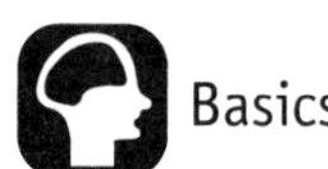

Basics

DEFINITION

- Refers to pain in the plantar aspects of the metatarsal heads. Metatarsalgia is not an anatomical diagnosis. It can be divided into primary and secondary metatarsalgia.
- Primary metatarsalgia develops from intrinsic factors, such as a long first ray, hallux valgus, and other congenital deformities.
- Secondary metatarsalgia may result from trauma, sesamoiditis, or neurogenic disorders.

INCIDENCE/PREVALENCE

- Common

SIGNS AND SYMPTOMS

- Pain is predominantly located in the plantar forefoot, especially in the distal half of the metatarsal shaft. Such pain may be described as "walking with a pebble in the shoe."
- May be associated with swelling, tenderness, and occasionally erythema.
- Frequently, plantar keratoses (calluses under the metatarsal heads) will be found and will be variable in location, size, and shape.

RISK FACTORS

- Pronation
- Pes planus (flat foot)
- Old or poorly fitted shoes
- Tight Achilles' tendon
- High heels
- Morton's foot with a short first metatarsal and a relatively long second metatarsal
- Hallux valgus or rigidus
- Abnormal gait or stance due to intrinsic or extrinsic factors
- Hammertoe
- Obesity
- Fat pad atrophy or displacement

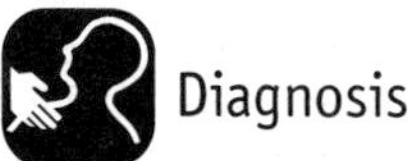

Diagnosis

DIFFERENTIAL DIAGNOSIS

- Neuroma (plantar or Morton's)
- Idiopathic metatarsophalangeal joint synovitis
- Freiberg disease: ischemic epiphyseal necrosis of the second metatarsal
- Inflammatory arthritis of metatarsophalangeal joints (rheumatoid arthritis, seronegative spondyloarthropathy, crystalline-induced arthritis)
- Stress fracture
- Traumatic arthritis
- Foreign body
- Cellulitis or infection
- Tumor (rare)

HISTORY

- Variable
- May be acute or progressive in onset
- Patient may have history of repetitive stress with unaccustomed walking and running.

PHYSICAL EXAMINATION

- Palpation of painful area will help determine whether this represents a soft tissue injury or one primarily involving the bony metatarsal head.
- Examination for the presence of callus, edema, erythema, swelling, gross deformity, breaks in the skin, and/or abnormal foot mechanics should be performed.
- Range of motion of the phalanges, metatarsophalangeal joint, and ankle, especially to dorsiflexion, should be examined.
- Gait analysis should be performed.
- Diagnostic injection (metatarsophalangeal joint) with local anesthetic sometimes can help differentiate intra-articular pathology (synovitis, capsulitis) from extra-articular pathology (neuroma).

IMAGING

- Routine anteroposterior and lateral foot x-rays should be normal.
- Bone scan is indicated if there is a high index of suspicion for stress fracture. Triple-phase bone scan will help delineate soft tissue from bony pathology.
- Magnetic resonance imaging is indicated if a mass lesion is suspected.

LABORATORY

- White blood cell count may be elevated in infection, but is normal in metatarsalgia.
- Sedimentation rate will be normal, barring infection or arthritis.
- Consider testing for gout or systemic disease if history and physical examination support these diagnoses.

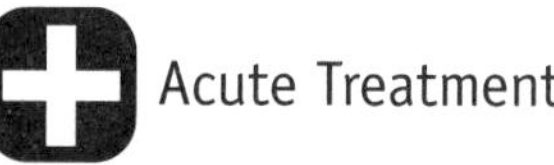

Acute Treatment

- Calluses should be pared down, preferably after soaking the foot in warm water and using a stone or emery board.
- A metatarsal pad may be placed just proximal to the metatarsal heads to relieve pressure. A common error is to place the pad directly beneath the metatarsal heads, which will exacerbate the symptoms.
- Nonsteroidal anti-inflammatory drugs may be of benefit.
- Good, supportive, well-cushioned athletic shoes should be worn.
- Stretching a tight Achilles' tendon may help reduce metatarsal loading acutely.

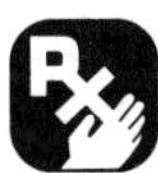

Long-Term Treatment

- Arch support and a well-fitted, low heel shoe for daily wear
- Energy-absorbing sole on shoe
- Enhance gastroc-soleus mechanism flexibility
- Correction of postural or gait imbalance
- Rarely, a cam walker boot, cane, or crutch may be necessary.
- Progressive return to sports activities as tolerated
- Orthotics/over-the-counter arch support and/or metatarsal pad for recalcitrant symptoms
- Replace daily and sports shoes frequently.
- Physical therapy may be helpful.
- Avoid hard surfaces and prolonged standing.

Miscellaneous

ICD-9 CODE

726.70 Metatarsalgia, not otherwise specified

SPECIAL CONSIDERATIONS

Corticosteroid injection should be avoided because it may cause fat pad atrophy.

BIBLIOGRAPHY

Baker CL. Reactive synovitis of the foot—metatarsalgia. In *The Hughston Clinic sports medicine field manual.* Baltimore: Williams & Wilkins, 1996:270.

Cailliet R. *Foot and ankle pain,* 2nd ed. Philadelphia: FA Davis Company, 1983.

Cohen RT. *Griffith's 5-minute clinical consult—1998.* Baltimore: Williams & Wilkins, 1998.

Hockenbury RT. Forefoot problems in athletes. *Med Sci Sports Exerc* 1999; July 31(7 suppl): S448–458.

Authors: Per Brolinson and Shawn Kerger

Atlantoaxial Instability

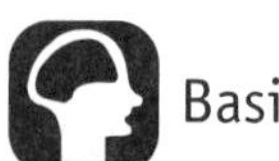

Basics

DEFINITION

- The atlantoaxial joint (C1-2) is not inherently stable and depends on the integrity of the surrounding ligaments and joint capsule.
- Congenital, inflammatory, traumatic, or infectious conditions may weaken the supporting structures to the C1-2 joint leading to atlantoaxial instability (AAI).
- Instability may be acute or chronic.

INCIDENCE/PREVALENCE

- From 10% to 25% of Down syndrome patients have AAI.
- Incidence of AAI increases with age and may occur during growth spurts.

SIGNS AND SYMPTOMS

- Patients with AAI most often are asymptomatic.
- Symptomatic patients initially may present with fatigue, headache, or paresthesias in the arms or legs with neck flexion.
- Symptoms may progress to cord compression, with neck pain, bowel and bladder incontinence, ataxia, hyperreflexia, weakness, spasticity, and varying degrees of quadriplegia.
- In patients with cord compression, symptoms may be unilateral.

RISK FACTORS

- Down syndrome
- Rheumatoid arthritis
- Dwarfism
- Marfan syndrome

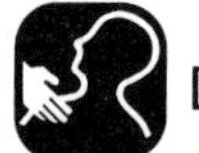

Diagnosis

DIFFERENTIAL DIAGNOSIS

- Neck sprain
- Torticollis
- Vertebral fracture
- Ligamentous laxity
- Spinal contusion
- Epidural hemorrhage

HISTORY

- Patients may present with chronic neurologic symptoms for months or even years.
- Acute AAI may result from indirect trauma due to hyperflexion, hyperextension, or vertical compression of the neck.

PHYSICAL EXAMINATION

- Cervical neck examination may be normal.
- Evaluate for paresthesias with neck flexion.
- Reflexes, muscle strength, and gait should be documented.

IMAGING

- Instability is evaluated by lateral neck radiographs in flexion and extension.
- AAI is defined as >4.0-mm distance between the odontoid process of the axis and the anterior arch of the atlas.
- Computed tomography/magnetic resonance imaging may be indicated to rule out additional injuries.

SCREENING EVALUATION

- Screening x-rays for AAI in patients with Down syndrome is controversial.
- Lateral flexion/extension views may be indicated as part of a preparticipation physical examination or as part of a preoperative evaluation. Currently, the Special Olympics requires all athletes with Down syndrome to receive radiographs of the cervical spine.
- Some authors suggest screening lateral x-rays in patients with Down syndrome during periods of rapid growth at ages 5, 12, and 18 years.

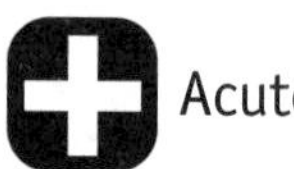

Acute Treatment

ACUTE MANAGEMENT

- With acute neck trauma in a patient with known AAI or risk factors, a potentially unstable injury is present until proven otherwise.
- The cervical spine must be stabilized in the field.
- Protect the airway if respiratory difficulties arise.
- High-dose intravenous steroids often are given for suspected spinal cord injury.

SPECIAL CONSIDERATIONS

- Blind endotracheal intubation of a patient with AAI should be avoided.
- Tracheal intubation with a flexible bronchoscope under topical anesthesia avoids neck flexion and maintains cervical spine stability.
- Regional anesthesia with minimal sedation is another option.

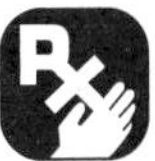

Long-Term Treatment

LONG-TERM MANAGEMENT

- Treat the underlying condition.
- An abnormal atlas-dens interval on lateral flexion/extension views constitutes an absolute contraindication to collision activity.

SURGERY

- Cervical spine fusion should be considered for patients with marked instability and for those with significant myelopathy.
- Nonoperative management is recommended for most patients without neurologic symptoms, because surgical complications are common, myelopathic findings often do not improve, and data on long-term surgical outcomes are lacking.

REFERRAL/DISPOSITION

- Immediate referral is indicated for acute spinal cord injury.
- Asymptomatic patients with demonstrated instability should be referred for confirmation of diagnosis.

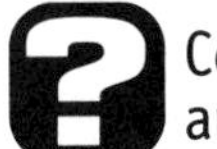

Common Questions and Answers

Physician responses to common patient questions:

Q: If I have AAI, can I play noncontact sports?

A: From the available scientific evidence, asymptomatic patients with AAI may participate in noncontact sports and exercise activities. Further studies are needed for risk stratification.

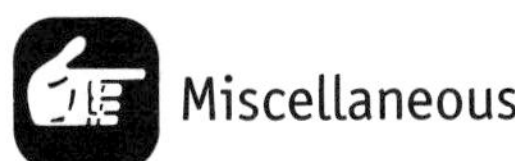

Miscellaneous

SYNONYMS

- Atlantoaxial subluxation

ICD-9 CODE

847.00 Sprain/strain
952.00 Cervical spine injury

BIBLIOGRAPHY

American Academy of Pediatrics Committee on Sports Medicine and Fitness. Atlantoaxial instability in Down syndrome: subject review. *Pediatrics* 1995;96[1 Pt 1]:151–154.

Cremers MJ, Bol E, Roos FS, et al. Risk of sports activities in children with Down's syndrome and atlantoaxial instability. *Lancet* 1993;342:511–514.

Epps HR, Salter RB. Orthopedic conditions of the cervical spine and shoulder. *Pediatr Clin North Am* 1996;43:919–927.

Torg JS, Ramsey-Emrhein JA. Suggested management guidelines for participation in collision activities with congenital, developmental, or postinjury lesions involving the cervical spine. *Med Sci Sports Exerc* 1997;29:S256–S272.

Authors: Suraj Achar and Suriti Kundu Achar

Biceps Tendinitis

Basics

DEFINITION

- Inflammation of the long head of the biceps tendon as it courses through the biceps groove
- Rarely occurs as a primary tendinitis

INCIDENCE/PREVALENCE

- Typically seen in adults over the age of 40 years
- Most commonly seen in combination with rotator cuff impingement

SIGNS AND SYMPTOMS

- Patients complain of pain over the anterior shoulder.
- Can radiate into the biceps muscle
- Usually described as a dull ache

RISK FACTORS

Because the biceps assists in deceleration of the humerus, any throwing, overhead hitting, or racquet sports can contribute to its development.

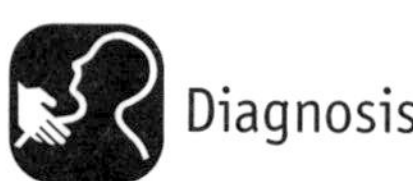

Diagnosis

DIFFERENTIAL DIAGNOSIS

- Rotator cuff tendinitis or impingement
- Thoracic outlet syndrome
- Cervical disc disease
- Rheumatoid arthritis
- Pancoast tumor

HISTORY

- Patient will complain of pain with overhead movements
- Patient may experience pain with supination of the forearm and contraction of the biceps.
- Determine which movements elicit the pain, especially throwing and racquet sports.

PHYSICAL EXAMINATION

- Palpation of the long head of the biceps in the bicipital groove will elicit pain. External rotation will expose the bicipital groove. Caution is needed, as the area is tender in most people.
- Speed test: The straight arm is forward flexed to 60 degrees at the shoulder with the hand supinated. Then have the patient resist downward pressure. Pain at biceps tendon insertion site suggests tendinitis.
- Yergason test: Resisted supination of the forearm with the elbow at 90 degrees and the elbow placed comfortably at the side. This is the most specific test for tendinitis.
- Yergason test also has been described by Hoppenfeld. It is used to test the long head of the biceps to see if it is stable in the bicipital groove. This is done by having the patient fully flex the elbow, with the elbow at the patient's side. Then grasp the wrist with one hand and stabilize the elbow with the other, attempt to extend the elbow, and externally rotate the arm while the patient resists. If positive, this action elicits pain.
- General shoulder range of motion, impingement signs, and strength of internal and external rotators should be included in the examination.

IMAGING

- Initial trauma radiographs include anteroposterior, axillary, and scapular Y views. Internal and external rotation views can be used to evaluate the shoulder.
- Occasionally a calcified tendon will be seen.
- If pain persists, then magnetic resonance imaging or magnetic resonance arthrogram should be considered.

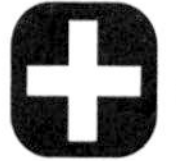

Acute Treatment

ANALGESIA

- Nonsteroidal anti-inflammatory drugs can be given.
- Ice is helpful.

IMMOBILIZATION

- Immobilization can be considered. Caution must be exercised, as patients who are immobilized too long will lose range of motion.
- May lead to adhesive capsulitis
- 1–2 weeks for comfort only
- The patient should use the arm in a pain-free range of motion. If the elbow is in a sling, the elbow should come out several times a day, and range-of-motion exercises should be done.

SPECIAL CONSIDERATIONS

- If pain still persists despite therapy, consider a corticosteroid injection. However, not all authorities recommend this. Care must be exercised not to inject into the tendon. Strenuous activity should be avoided for about 72 hours.
- If tendinitis is due to long-standing impingement, rupture of the tendon can occur. This is seen as a second bulge in the muscle belly.
- Functional impairment is rare, as the short head remains intact. Patients may have a few weeks of mild-to-moderate pain, which resolves with rest.

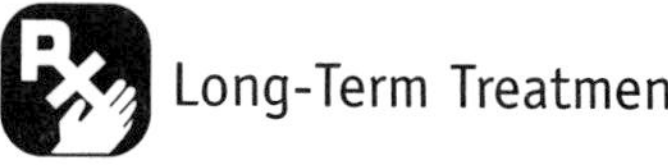

Long-Term Treatment

REHABILITATION

- Therapy should be started early. In the early phase, range of motion needs to be preserved and slowly increased before any strengthening is undertaken.
- Examples of range-of-motion exercises: Have the patient lean on a chair and hang the arm down. Then perform clockwise and counterclockwise concentrically larger circles. Also, use the arm as a pendulum and use body momentum to move the arm. The patient can perform wall walking, i.e., walking the fingers up a wall toward the ceiling.

STRETCHING

Can be done in several ways:

- Options are: Have the patient place a towel on a wall. Then slide the towel up the wall to achieve a stretch. Hold for 5–10 seconds and slide back down. Then repeat. The patient also can slide and hold for longer periods of time. This should be done several times per day.
- Another option: Have the patient lay supine on the floor or table. Hold a broom stick, golf club, or similar object, then use the good arm as the force to move the affected arm through flexion, abduction, and external and internal rotation.
- Final option: Fasten a pulley to a door with two rope ends. The good arm functions as the force to take the affected arm through a range of motion, achieving a gentle stretch.

MODALITIES

- After the acute phase, several modalities can be used. First would be regular ultrasound, which uses a sound wave to heat up the affected tissues.
- Phonophoresis: Using an ultrasound wave to push hydrocortisone cream into the affected area sometimes can be helpful.
- Iontophoresis: Uses an electric current to drive hydrocortisone cream into the affected tissues.

THERAPEUTIC EXERCISES

- Because this disorder coexists with rotator cuff disease, it is best to follow a generalized strengthening program.

- Dumbbell weights or Thera-Bands can be used for resistance. Lighter weights with higher repetitions are best.
- Internal and external rotators should be worked. Start with one set of 15 repetitions and work up to three sets of 15 repetitions.
- Scapular stabilizers need to be worked. These can be done with cable rows, shoulder shrugs, and reverse flies.
- The strengthening program should be supervised by a physical therapist. Often this can be done with one or two visits and then having the patient follow a home program.

SURGERY

If conservative treatment fails, surgery to transfer the tendon may be helpful.

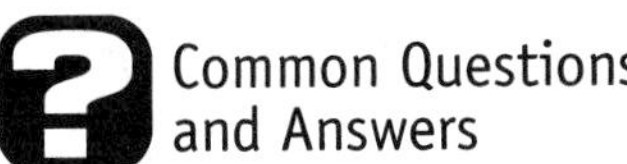

Common Questions and Answers

Physician responses to common patient questions:

Q: What are the long-term problems?
A: If left alone, it can progress to adhesive capsulitis.

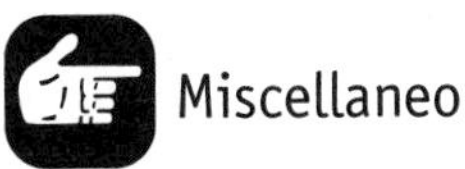

Miscellaneous

ICD-9 CODE

726.12 Biceps tendinitis

BIBLIOGRAPHY

Barry NN, McGuire JL. Overuse syndromes in adult athletes. *Rheum Dis Clin North Am* 1996;22:515–530.

Daigneault J, Cooney LM Jr. Progress in geriatrics: shoulder pain in older people. *J Am Geriatr Soc* 1998;46:1144–1157.

Hoppenfeld S, ed. *Physical examination of the spine and extremities.* East Norwalk, CT: Appleton-Century-Crofts, 1976.

Mercier LR, Pettid FJ, Tamisiea DF, et al. *Practical orthopedics.* St. Louis: Mosby, 1995.

Woodward TW, Best TM. The painful shoulder. *Am Fam Physician* 2000;61:3291–3300.

Author: Todd May

Biceps Tendon Rupture

Basics

DEFINITION

- Complete or partial disruption of either the proximal long head or distal biceps tendon. The proximal long head of the biceps tendon usually ruptures in the region of the bicipital groove of the humerus. The distal biceps tendon ruptures at the elbow.

INCIDENCE/PREVALENCE

- From 90% to 97% of biceps ruptures are proximal.
- From 3% to 10% occur at the elbow.
- Biceps muscle ruptures are rare and usually are associated with direct injury or trauma to the contracted muscle belly.

SIGNS AND SYMPTOMS

Proximal Rupture

- Acute pain, ecchymosis, and swelling around the anterior shoulder
- Visible "lump" in the mid-upper arm anteriorly, giving a "Popeye" appearance; secondary to muscle belly retracting distally

Distal Rupture

- Acute sharp pain, ecchymosis, and swelling in the antecubital fossa
- Patient may have heard a "pop" at the time of the injury.
- Sometimes a visible defect or asymmetry in the distal biceps is seen when compared to the opposite arm.
- Ruptures can be relatively pain-free after the acute injury, especially if they are associated with preexisting degenerative tendon changes.

RISK FACTORS

- Male
- Age over 30 years
- Prior tendinopathy or degenerative change
- Prior steroid injections
- Anabolic steroids

ASSOCIATED INJURIES AND COMPLICATIONS

- Rotator cuff impingement: Subacromial impingement in combination with repetitive overhead motion, such as with throwing, can lead to proximal biceps tendon degeneration.
- Superior labrum anterior to posterior (SLAP) lesions: Lesions of the superior glenoid labrum from the 10-o'clock to the 2-o'clock position. SLAP lesions may involve the biceps anchor.
- Subscapularis rupture/partial rupture: Following subscapularis tears, the biceps tendon can sublux medially out of the bicipital groove, causing a painful clicking sensation.
- Rotator interval lesions: The biceps tendon can sublux medially over the lesser tuberosity after tears to the rotator interval, but there usually is an associated subscapularis injury.

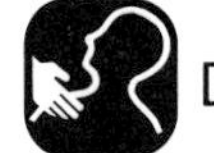

Diagnosis

DIFFERENTIAL DIAGNOSIS

Proximal Rupture

- SLAP lesion
- Subscapularis injury
- Rotator cuff/rotator interval injury
- Biceps tendon subluxation (rupture of transverse ligament)
- Long head of biceps tendinitis or tendinosis; onset usually insidious
- Greater or lesser tuberosity fractures may occur following shoulder dislocation.

Distal Rupture

- Distal biceps tendinitis or tendinosis; onset usually insidious
- Partial distal biceps tendon rupture
- Anterior capsule strain. Occurs with hyperextension injuries, and tenderness is more diffuse anteriorly.
- Coronoid process fractures, directly tender over coronoid process; no palpable biceps defect
- Lateral antebrachial cutaneous nerve entrapment syndrome
- None of these problems demonstrate absence of a palpable biceps tendon in the antecubital fossa. Partial ruptures can be difficult to diagnose, and magnetic resonance imaging (MRI) often is required.

HISTORY

Q: Where is the pain?
A: Proximal versus distal
Q: How did the injury occur?
A: Ruptures occur commonly after a forceful eccentric biceps contraction with the elbow flexed.
Q: When did the injury occur?
A: Best surgical outcomes in acute setting
Q: Any prior symptoms?
A: Indicative of prior tendinitis or tendinosis
Q: Any treatment?
A: Prior steroid injections for tendinopathy; physical therapy for current problem
Q: Is the injury affecting functional activities?
A: May be less likely to repair minimally painful rupture in an elderly patient with enough strength to function adequately.

PHYSICAL EXAMINATION

- Inspect for ecchymosis, swelling, and tenderness at the site of the injury
- Range of motion: With distal ruptures, a visible deformity may be noted distally with active elbow flexion. A proximal defect associated with a mid-upper arm "bulge" occurs after proximal tendon ruptures.
- Strength: Proximal ruptures exhibit mild weakness of elbow flexion and supination. Distal ruptures frequently have more marked weakness. The brachialis and supinator muscles preserve some elbow flexion and supination strength, respectively. However, flexion and supination endurance may be greatly reduced.
- Palpate the biceps tendons: With distal ruptures, the distal biceps tendon often is not palpable as it traverses the antecubital fossa. Proximal ruptures exhibit tenderness in the bicipital groove, but the long head of the biceps tendon is more difficult to palpate.
- Speed, Yergason, O'Brien, and lift-off tests can result in pain with biceps tendon ruptures, but more commonly are used to assess other lesions, such as tendinitis, labral tears, and subscapularis tears.

IMAGING

- Standard elbow x-ray series for distal injuries. Check for avulsion fragment of radial tuberosity. Degenerative changes or lipping at the radial tuberosity can be associated with biceps tendinopathy.
- Shoulder x-rays often are normal with proximal injuries.
- MRI to confirm diagnosis, especially if partial ruptures or other soft tissue restraints prevent muscle retraction and obvious deformity. MRI with shoulder contrast is best for suspected SLAP lesions.

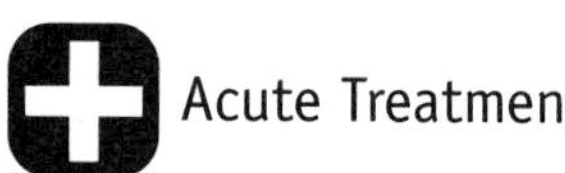

Acute Treatment

ANALGESIA

Nonsteroidal anti-inflammatory drugs can be used to reduce pain and swelling, but likely will not change overall outcomes.

REDUCTION TECHNIQUES

- Proximal biceps tendon ruptures can occur with anterior shoulder dislocation.
- Biceps tendon subluxation can occur after subscapularis or rotator interval tears. The tendon sometimes "pops" as it slides over the lesser tuberosity with shoulder internal and external rotation, and with the elbow flexed 90 degrees. Reduction (e.g., tenodesis) is performed surgically.

IMMOBILIZATION

Proximal Rupture

- Place in a sling with the elbow flexed to 90 degrees for comfort. Some advocate more aggressive immobilization with the forearm in supination using a posterior elbow splint.
- Older patients, especially over 50–60 years, should be immobilized for a brief period (e.g., 2–6 weeks) until they can tolerate rehabilitation with minimal or no discomfort.
- Younger athletic individuals can be placed in a sling initially for pain control, but often require surgical fixation to return to their previous level of functioning.

Distal Rupture

- Place in a posterior elbow splint with the elbow flexed 90 degrees and the forearm in supination. A sling can be used if there will be immediate surgical repair.
- Most patients require surgical repair. However, elderly patients who do not require full flexion or supination strength to function may be managed conservatively with continued immobilization for 6–8 weeks, followed by rehabilitation.

SPECIAL CONSIDERATIONS

The main complaint after conservative management of biceps tendon ruptures, especially distal ruptures, is loss of elbow flexion and forearm supination strength, especially endurance. Most young people and athletes require surgical repair of complete biceps tendon injuries. Many advocate surgical repair of partial ruptures in this population, especially if the ruptures are distal.

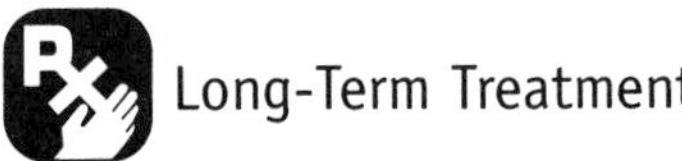

Long-Term Treatment

REHABILITATION

Conservative Management

- The initial goal is to regain elbow extension and forearm pronation. A generalized elbow and forearm strengthening program should be started as soon as symptoms will allow.
- For distal biceps tendon injuries, active elbow flexion or forearm supination against loads should be avoided for at least 6–8 weeks
- Therapy progresses until strength and endurance return to normal or to a functional level. Regular applications of ice, preferably three times daily and after activity, can reduce swelling.

Postoperative Management

The specific therapy program should be tailored to the surgical technique and the preference of the surgeon, but most rehabilitation programs start 2–6 weeks after the repair. Range of motion can be started as early as 2–3 weeks, but some advocate immobilization for as long as 6–8 weeks. Active strengthening exercises are almost never started prior to 6 weeks.

SURGERY

Proximal Rupture

The type of repair or surgery often will depend on associated problems, such as subacromial impingement, rotator cuff tears, SLAP lesions, or subscapularis/rotator interval lesions. Isolated long head biceps tendon ruptures can be treated surgically with a tenodesis.

Distal Rupture

- Conventional and modified Boyd-Anderson repairs result in the most successful clinical outcomes for distal ruptures.
- The one-incision technique recently gained popularity secondary to a possible increased incidence of radioulnar synostosis and heterotopic ossification following two-incision techniques. The technique used will depend on the preference and experience of the managing physician.

REFERRAL/DISPOSITION

- Consider orthopaedic referral for all complete biceps tendon ruptures. All complete distal ruptures in young people should be referred immediately.
- The one exception may be elderly patients who agree to conservative management, especially those with proximal tendon ruptures. Associated injuries should be screened, although many still respond to conservative measures.

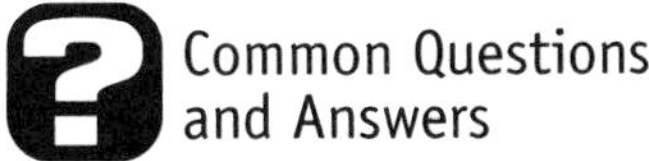

Common Questions and Answers

Physician responses to common patient questions:

Q: When can athletes return to sports after biceps tendon ruptures?
A: Forceful biceps activity should be avoided for 3–6 months after surgical repair. Patients often feel "normal" sooner than this, but should still be restricted. Proximal fixations may heal more quickly.

Q: What are the most common complaints after conservative management?
A: Patients may note decreased elbow flexion and supination strength, especially manifested as fatigue with these movements. These findings are more pronounced after distal ruptures. Surgical management often results in normal to near-normal strength and endurance.

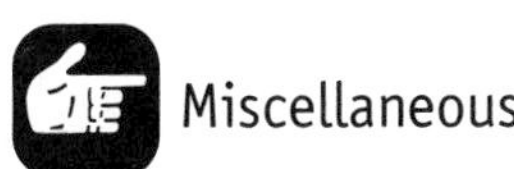

Miscellaneous

ICD-9 CODE

840.9

See also: Glenoid Labral Tears (SLAP Lesions); Impingement, Subacromial Bursitis, and Rotator Cuff Tendonitis

BIBLIOGRAPHY

Arendt EA, ed. *Orthopaedic knowledge update sports medicine 2.* Rosemont, IL: American Academy of Orthopaedic Surgeons, 1999.

D'Arco P, Sitler M, Kelly J, et al. Clinical, functional, and radiographic assessments. *Am J Sports Med* 1998;26:254–261.

DeLee JC, Drex D Jr, eds. *Orthopaedic sports medicine: principles and practice.* Philadelphia: WB Saunders, 1994.

Mellion MB, Walsh WM, Shelton GL, eds. *The team physician's handbook,* 2nd ed. Philadelphia: Hanley & Belfus, 1997.

Morrey BD, Askew LJ, An KN, et al. Rupture of the distal tendon of the biceps brachii. *J Bone Joint Surg Am* 1985;67:418–421.

Authors: Christopher Madden and Dan Somogyi

Brachial Plexus Injuries ("Burners" and "Stingers")

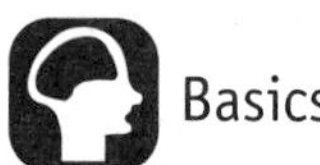

Basics

DEFINITION

- Acute trauma to the neck and shoulder area injuring the brachial plexus
- Typically causes burning or stinging pain radiating down the entire upper extremity, hence the names "burner" and "stinger"
- Most commonly involves the upper trunk of the plexus or cervical nerve roots C5 and C6

MECHANISMS

- Traction to the plexus when the shoulder is depressed and the head is forced away from the injured side
- Compression of cervical roots when the head is forced toward the side of injury
- Direct blow to the supraclavicular fossa

INCIDENCE/PREVALENCE

- Exact incidence unknown due to underreporting by athletes
- Common in contact sports (football, wrestling, hockey); football career incidence reported between 49% and 65%
- Frequent recurrence, reported as high as 87%

SIGNS AND SYMPTOMS

- Burning or stinging pain radiating down one arm circumferentially (i.e., nondermatomal pattern)
- Sometimes numbness, paresthesias, and weakness in the extremity
- Acutely holds the arm close to the body
- Symptoms often last a few minutes but can persist for weeks, particularly in recurrent episodes.

RISK FACTORS

- Previous burner
- Limited range of motion of the neck or shoulder

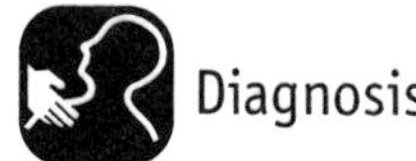

Diagnosis

DIFFERENTIAL DIAGNOSIS

- Cervical injury (fracture, dislocation, spinal cord injury, disc herniation)
- Glenohumeral dislocation
- Acromioclavicular separation
- Clavicle fracture
- Thoracic outlet syndrome (when chronic, recurrent)

HISTORY

- Mechanism of injury (falling on an outstretched arm suggests alternative injury)
- Details of symptom type, location, and quality (bilateral or lower extremity symptoms indicate cervical fracture or cord injury until proven otherwise; symptoms not typical of burners mandate search for an alternative diagnosis)
- Initial versus recurrent injury (recurrence typically requires more aggressive rehabilitation)

PHYSICAL EXAMINATION

- Inspection (asymmetry or postural abnormality to address in therapy)
- Palpation (tenderness suggests alternative diagnosis; spasm is consistent with burners or other)
- Neurologic examination (localize injury, rule out cord injury)
- Weakness most common in deltoid, biceps, and rotator cuff
- Tinel sign at the supraclavicular fossa (positive result indicates plexus injury)
- Spurling test, after serious cervical injury is ruled out (disc herniation, burner from cervical foraminal stenosis)

DIAGNOSTIC TESTS

- Not routine
- X-ray cervical spine if fracture, dislocation, or cervical instability suspected (anteroposterior, lateral, oblique, flexion, extension)
- Magnetic resonance imaging or computed tomography typically not needed; many false-positive results
- Electromyogram (EMG) if symptoms last 3 weeks for confirmation, localization, and prognosis (EMG normalization lags far behind clinical and neurologic recovery, so follow-up EMG generally not indicated)

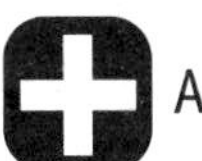

Acute Treatment

MANAGEMENT

- Stretch tight muscles at neck and shoulder
- Strengthen neck, shoulder, and muscles weakened by injury

SPECIAL CONSIDERATIONS

- No competition until asymptomatic and normal neurologic examination

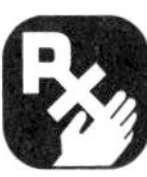

Long-Term Treatment

GENERAL

- Chest-out posture
- Ensure correct playing technique
- Maintain strength and flexibility of neck and shoulder

PROTECTIVE EQUIPMENT

- Neck roll, shoulder pad lifter, or cowboy collar in football

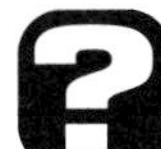

Common Questions and Answers

Physician responses to common patient questions:

Q: Is the nerve damage permanent?

A: Generally not, but a few patients have symptoms lasting months to years.

Q: When can I practice?

A: Conditioning and rehabilitation should begin immediately. You can return to contact activity when the symptoms are gone and your strength and sensation are back to normal.

Q: How long do I need to stretch and strengthen?

A: Continue at least the rest of the season. If you can continue the exercises throughout your career, you will lower the chance of having another burner.

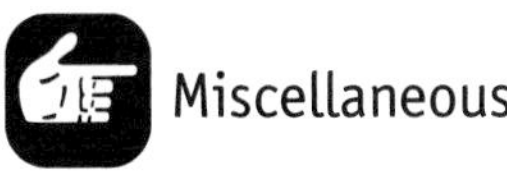

Miscellaneous

ICD-9 CODE

953.4

BIBLIOGRAPHY

Clancy WG, Brand RL, Bergfeld JA. Upper trunk brachial plexus injuries in contact sports. *Am J Sports Med* 1997;5:209–216.

Hershman EB. Brachial plexus injuries. *Clin Sports Med* 1990;9:311–329.

Kuhlman GS, McKeag DB. The "burner": a common nerve injury in contact sports. *Am Fam Physician* 1999;60:2035–2040.

Sallis RE, Jones K, Knopp W. Burners: an offensive strategy for an underreported injury. *Physician Sports Med* 1992;20:47–55.

Authors: Geoffrey Kuhlman and James Barrett

Bursitis

Basics

SIGNS AND SYMPTOMS

- Localized pain that worsens with movement of structures adjacent to affected bursae
- Usually presents with acute onset, but may be chronic (especially in hip)
- May have low-grade temperature
- Localized swelling may be present with superficial bursal involvement
- Overlying erythema or skin trauma may be present with infectious bursitis
- Traumatic bursitis often follows specific traumatic event or recent overuse of related joints

MECHANISM/DESCRIPTION

- Bursae are sacs lined with synovial membrane. There are approximately 150 in the body located at sites of friction between bones, ligaments, tendons, muscles, and skin. They provide lubrication for movement
- Bursitis-inflammation of the bursae caused by trauma (acute or chronic), infection, crystal deposition, or systemic disease

ETIOLOGY

- Trauma (both acute and chronic)—most common cause
- Infection—may be obvious or microscopic
  —Higher risk in diabetes, chronic alcohol abuse, uremia, and gout
  —Staphylococci cause 90%
- Crystal deposition—calcium phosphate, urate
- Systemic disease—rheumatoid, gout, ankylosing spondylitis, psoriatic arthritis, lupus, rheumatic fever

AFFECTED JOINTS

- Potentially any bursa may be affected
- Commonly affected joints
  —Shoulder
  —Elbow—usually secondary to trauma; high incidence of infection
  —Wrist and hand
  —Hip—more common in older women
  —Knee—often secondary to chronic trauma or arthritis
  —Foot—calcaneal bursitis is almost always from improper shoes/high heels

CAUTIONS

- May be difficult to distinguish from fractures. Suspicious joints should be immobilized, particularly in the setting of trauma

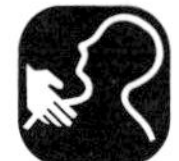

Diagnosis

ESSENTIAL WORKUP

- Full assessment of regional musculoskeletal function
- Any suspicion of infection warrants aspiration of bursae (especially olecranon and prepatellar bursae)
- Aspiration of hip and other deep bursae should be deferred to orthopedics or rheumatology, or may be guided in ED by ultrasound

LABORATORY TESTS

- For infection: CBC with differential
- Evaluation of related disease (e.g., uric acid level for gout)
- If joint aspiration is done, serum glucose should be sent
- Fluid analysis
  —Analysis of bursa fluid: cell count with differential, glucose and total protein, crystal determination, Gram stain, culture
  —Normal fluid is clear yellow and has 0–200 WBC; 0 RBC; low protein and glucose is same as serum
  —Traumatic bursitis: fluid is bloody/xanthochromic and has <1200 WBC; many RBCs; low protein and normal glucose
  —Infective bursitis: fluid is yellow, cloudy, and has 50,000–200,000 WBC; few RBCs; slightly increased protein and decreased glucose; bacteria on Gram stain
  —Rheumatoid and microcrystalline inflammation: Fluid is yellow to cloudy and has 1000–40,000 WBC; few RBCs; slightly increased protein and variable glucose
  —Because infection and inflammation may be difficult to differentiate, cultures must always be sent

IMAGING/SPECIAL TESTS

- X-rays may demonstrate chronic arthritic changes or calcium deposits
- Recommended when trauma is involved to rule out fracture

DIFFERENTIAL DIAGNOSIS

- Arthritis, gout
- Tendinitis
- Fracture, tendon/ligament tear, contusion, sprain
- Also in hips: neuritis, lumbar spine disease, sacroiliitis

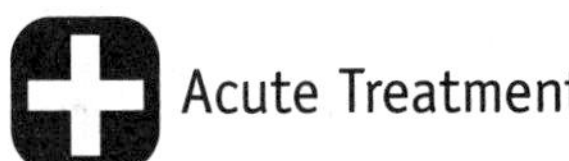

Acute Treatment

INITIAL STABILIZATION

- Immobilize joint if pain is severe

ED TREATMENT

- Shoulders should not be immobilized for more than 2–3 days due to the risk of adhesive capsulitis
- Ice affected areas for 10 minutes, 4 times a day until improved
- NSAIDs for at least 7 days; best if continued for 5 days after improvement to help prevent recurrence
- If no improvement within 5–7 days and infection has been ruled out (by culture) injection of lidocaine or steroids may be considered
  —Mix 2 ml of 2% lidocaine with 20–40 mg of depoglucocorticoid and inject 1–3 ml of this mixture into the bursae using sterile technique
  —Steroid injections should not be repeated until at least 2 weeks have passed and no more than two injections into one joint should be performed without rheumatologic or orthopedic consultation
- Treat associated diseases as needed (e.g., gout)
- Septic bursitis should be treated with antibiotics and drainage of bursae
  —Antibiotics treatment for septic bursitis should be based on the Gram stain
  —Penicillinase-resistant antistaphylococcal drug may be used if Gram stain is negative or shows Gram-positive cocci
  —If Gram-negative organisms are found, blood cultures should be done and another primary source for the infection should be sought
  —Antibiotics should be continued for 5–7 days beyond the sterilization of bursal fluid

MEDICATIONS

- Nonsteroidal anti-inflammatory agents (there are many choices, a few are listed below)
  —Diclofenac: 50 mg po bid tid
  —Ibuprofen: adult: 600 mg po q 6 hrs; pediatric: 5–10 mg/kg po q 6 hrs
  —Ketorolac: 30 mg IV/IM q 6 hrs or 10 mg po q 4–6 hrs
  —Piroxicam: 20 mg po qd
- Most patients may be treated as an outpatient

HOSPITAL ADMISSION CRITERIA FOR SEPTIC BURSITIS

- Patients with high fevers and chills/rigors, large surrounding cellulitis, unable to take oral antibiotics, failed outpatient therapy, or immunosuppressed
- Unusual organisms, extrabursal primary site or deep bursal involvement

FOLLOW-UP

- Most patients respond to therapy in 3–4 days and may follow-up with primary care provider within a week.
- Septic bursitis requires repeated bursal aspiration every 3–5 days
- Rheumatology or orthopedic referral is recommended for patients who do not respond to intrabursal steroids or recurrent bursitis

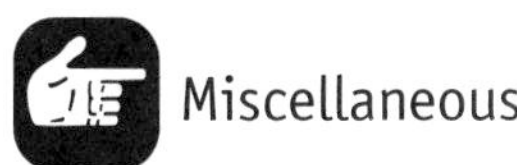

Miscellaneous

ICD-9 CODE

727.3

CORE CONTENT CODE

10.4.2

BIBLIOGRAPHY

Butcher JD, et al. Lower extremity bursitis. *Am Fam Physician* 1996;53(7):2317–2324

Kopicky-Burd J. Nonarticular rheumatic disorders. In: Barker LR, ed. *Principles of ambulatory medicine*. 3rd ed. Baltimore: Williams & Wilkins, 1991:827–835

Talbot-Stern JK. Arthritis, tendonitis, and bursitis. In: Rosen P, ed. *Emergency medicine*. 3rd ed. St. Louis: Mosby-Yearbook 1992:822–826

Author: Melissa Brokaw

Bursitis, Trochanteric and Iliopsoas

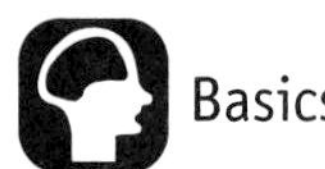

Basics

DEFINITION

- Bursitis is inflammation and secondary pain in a bursal structure.
- It is a common cause of lower extremity pain in people of all ages and activity levels.
- Two types of bursae have been described, constant and adventitial. Constant bursae are formed in embryogenesis and are endothelial-lined, sac-like structures (e.g., iliopsoas and trochanteric). Adventitial bursae form later in life through myxomatous degeneration of fibrous tissues at sites of friction (e.g., bunion).
- The iliopsoas bursa is the largest synovial bursa in the body and is present in over 95% of all adults. It averages 6 cm x 3 cm in size. There often is communication with the hip joint capsule.
- Four bursae usually are present around the greater trochanter; three are constant (two major, one minor). The subgluteus maximus and medius bursae are considered the major bursae, the subgluteus minimus the minor.

INCIDENCE/PREVALENCE

Bursitis is reported to account for 0.4% of all visits to primary care, but in runners the incidence may be as high as 10%.

Iliopsoas Bursitis

- Reported in patients of all ages
- Stronger prevalence in those with osteoarthritis or rheumatoid arthritis

Trochanteric Bursitis

- Most commonly reported in middle-aged, overweight women
- Reportedly the second most common cause of lateral hip pain, after osteoarthritis

SIGNS AND SYMPTOMS

Iliopsoas Bursitis

- If pain is the predominant feature, it is in the anterior thigh secondary to inflammatory irritation of the femoral nerve.
- If there is remarkable bursal swelling, a pelvic or inguinal mass may be palpated.
- Stride may be abbreviated during gait to avoid extension.

Trochanteric Bursitis

- Chronic, intermittent aching pain over the lateral aspect of the hip
- Occasionally, onset of pain is acute or subacute, with sharp lancinating or burning pain, especially if the patient lies on the affected side.
- Causes symptoms along the L-2 dermatomal pattern

RISK FACTORS

Iliopsoas Bursitis

- Osteoarthritis, rheumatoid arthritis, pigmented villonodular synovitis, synovial chondromatosis, infection, trauma, status post total hip arthroplasty, avascular necrosis of the femoral head

Trochanteric Bursitis

- Ipsilateral or contralateral hip arthritis, degenerative arthritis of the lower lumbar spine, degenerative joint disease of the knees, chronic mechanical low back pain, leg length discrepancy, obesity, fibromyalgia, iliotibial band syndrome, status post total hip arthroplasty, pes planus
- Acute trauma, overuse, or mechanical factors (tightened hip adductors or external rotators, varus leg alignment)

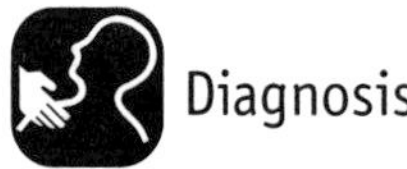

Diagnosis

DIFFERENTIAL DIAGNOSIS

Iliopsoas Bursitis

- Inguinal mass present: lymphadenopathy, malignant tumor, hernia, vascular malformation, hematoma
- Pain or paresthesia present: L-1 dermatomal disease, meralgia paresthetica, hip arthritis, stress fracture of the hip, acetabulum labral tear, proximal rectus femoris avulsion fracture at the anterior inferior iliac spine in an adolescent

Trochanteric Bursitis

- Lumbar facet arthropathy, lumbar disc disease (particularly L-2, L-3 distribution), sacroiliac dysfunction or inflammation, osteoarthritis or rheumatoid arthritis of the hip, stress fracture of the hip, meralgia paresthetica

HISTORY

Q: What are the characteristics of the pain and possible radiations?
A: The characteristics can help differentiation from lumbar disease.
Q: What movements of the hip cause pain?
A: Repetitive motions with pain on the lateral side of the hip may be indicative of trochanteric bursitis, as would pain with external rotation of the hip. Pain in the inguinal region or front of leg with hip flexion or extension may indicate iliopsoas bursitis.

PHYSICAL EXAMINATION

Iliopsoas Bursitis

- Local tenderness to pressure beneath the midpoint of the inguinal ligament
- The hip may be passively held in flexion, and the gait may be shortened to avoid hip extension.
- Pain is present in the inguinal region with resisted external rotation in a seated position. Pain in same location with passive hip extension or internal rotation, but there should not be a fixed limitation of motion.

Trochanteric Bursitis

- With patient in contralateral recumbent position (painful side uppermost), palpate for area of maximal tenderness. It should be over the greater trochanter at the most proximal aspect of femur.
- Patient may be tender to palpation just posterior or superior to the trochanter.
- Patient may have lateral hip pain with resisted abduction from an adducted position.

IMAGING

Iliopsoas Bursitis

- X-rays: Anteroposterior view of the pelvis may show osteoarthritis of the hip (associated cause) or other bony pathology.
- Ultrasound: Perform if there is a palpable inguinal mass.
- Contrast bursography: Not often used. It will not show communication with hip joint if present.
- Arthrography: Clearly shows communication of bursa with hip joint.
- Computed tomography: More commonly reported in the literature than magnetic resonance imaging to detect presence, delineate size, and establish if there is communication with the hip joint.

Trochanteric Bursitis

- X-rays: Anteroposterior view (internal or external rotation), usually normal; may show roughening of the trochanter. An area of calcification is present if long-standing (up to 40% of cases).
- Radioisotope bone scan: May show increased uptake in the region of the greater trochanter, which usually is linear. This can help differentiate bursitis from hip stress fracture.
- Magnetic resonance imaging/magnetic resonance angiography: Magnetic resonance imaging is a more specific means of identifying lesions other than bursa as the source of hip pain. Magnetic resonance angiography may be required to rule out acetabular labral tear.

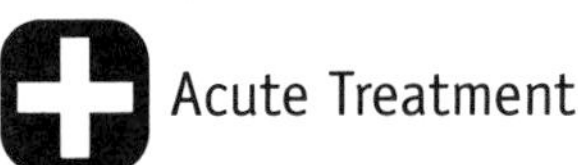

Acute Treatment

BASICS

- Two basic premises: reduce pain and inflammation and rehabilitation and prevention of reinjury.
- Treatment depends on the severity and nature of the underlying cause.

RECOMMENDATIONS

Iliopsoas Bursitis

- In mild cases, relative rest, nonsteroidal anti-inflammatory drugs, and heat or other physical therapy modalities.
- If there is a palpable mass or remarkable enlargement of the bursa by imaging, computed tomography or ultrasound-guided aspiration and instillation of a steroid preparation may be indicated.

Trochanteric Bursitis

- In mild cases, relative rest, nonsteroidal anti-inflammatory drugs, and heat or other physical therapy modalities (including phonophoresis or iontophoresis).
- Stretching is especially directed at the iliotibial band, gluteal musculature, and strengthening at the hip adductors.
- Corticosteroid injection can be used initially if symptoms warrant, or if conservative therapy fails.

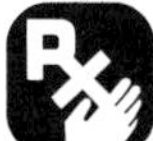

Long-Term Treatment

REHABILITATION

Stretching and strengthening, along with modification of any underlying mechanical abnormality (i.e., correcting leg length discrepancy), is the cornerstone of injury prevention.

SURGERY

- Typically only as a last resort, and after several attempts at conservative measures

REFERRAL/DISPOSITION

Iliopsoas Bursitis

- Referral to interventional radiologist if bursal enlargement results in substantial mass that must be drained and injected
- Referral to orthopedic surgeon if above fails

Trochanteric Bursitis

- Referral to orthopaedic surgeon if conservative therapy fails

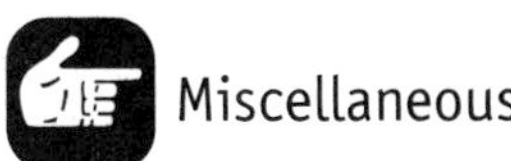

Miscellaneous

SYNONYMS

"Snapping hip syndrome" has been described as being caused by either condition.

ICD-9 CODE

726.5 Enthesopathy of the hip region
Includes bursitis (hip, ischiogluteal, and trochanteric area); tendinitis (gluteal, psoas, trochanteric)

BIBLIOGRAPHY

Binek R, Levinsohn EM. Enlarged iliopsoas bursa: an unusual cause of thigh mass and hip pain. *Clin Orthop* 1987;224:158–163.

Butcher JD, Salzman KL, Lillegard WA. Lower extremity bursitis. *Am Fam Physician* 1996;53:2317–2324.

Flanagan FL, Sant S, Coughlin RJ, et al. Symptomatic enlarged iliopsoas bursae in the presence of a normal plain hip radiograph. *Br J Rheumatol* 1995;34:365–369.

Jones DL, Erhard RE. Diagnosis of trochanteric bursitis versus femoral neck stress fracture. *Phys Ther* 1997;77:58–67.

Little H. Trochanteric bursitis: a common cause of pelvic girdle pain. *CMA* 1979;120:456–458.

McBeath AA. Some common causes of hip pain. *Postgrad Med* 1985;77:189–192, 194–195, 198.

Penkaya RR. Iliopsoas bursitis demonstrated by computed tomography. *AJR Am J Roentgenol* 19 80;135:175–1766.

Schon L, Zuckerman JD. Hip pain in the elderly: evaluation and diagnosis. *Geriatrics* 1988;43:48–52, 54, 56, 58, 60–62.

Shapira D, Nahir M, Scharf Y. Trochanteric bursitis: a common clinical problem. *Arch Phys Med Rehabil* 1986;67:815–817.

Shbeeb MI, Matteson EL. Trochanteric bursitis (greater trochanteric pain syndrome). *Mayo Clin Proc* 1996;71:565–569.

Toohey AK, LaSalle TL, Martinez S, et al. Iliopsoas bursitis: clinical features, radiographic findings and disease associations. *Semin Arthritis Rheum* 1990;20:41–47.

Author: Kevin Burroughs

Calcium Pyrophosphate Deposition Disease

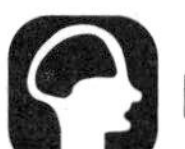

Basics

DEFINITION

Calcium pyrophosphate deposition disease (CPPD) is a crystal arthropathy characterized by deposition of calcium pyrophosphate dihydrate crystals in joints.

INCIDENCE/PREVALENCE

- Prevalence of chondrocalcinosis is 5% to 8% in the general population, but 15% by the ninth decade
- Female-to-male ratio: 2–7:1
- Peak age: 65–75 years

SIGNS AND SYMPTOMS

- Pseudogout: acute self-limiting monoarthritis lasting one day to a few weeks. May be severe and associated with malaise and fever. Patients often are symptom-free between attacks. Knee involved in 50%, then wrist, shoulder, ankle, and elbow.
- Chronic CPPD: symmetrical polyarthritis affecting knees, metacarpophalangeal joints, wrists, ankles, and shoulders. May involve the spine. Affected joints show signs of osteoarthritis with varying degrees of synovitis. Predominantly affects women.
- Pseudorheumatoid arthritis: severe synovitis in rheumatoid pattern
- Uncommon presentations include tendinopathy, tenosynovitis, and bursitis.

RISK FACTORS

- Gout (20% may be hyperuricemic)
- Hemochromatosis
- Hypothyroidism
- Trauma
- Osteoarthritis
- Hyperparathyroidism
- Hemosiderosis
- Hypophosphatasia
- Hypomagnesemia
- Ageing
- Amyloidosis

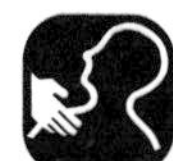

Diagnosis

DIFFERENTIAL DIAGNOSIS

- Gout (can coexist)
- Septic arthritis (can coexist)
- Rheumatoid arthritis
- Osteoarthritis
- Trauma (hemarthrosis)
- Human leukocyte antigen (HLA) B27-related peripheral arthritis (psoriatic arthritis, ankylosing spondylitis, reactive arthritis)
- Hypertrophic osteoarthropathy

HISTORY

- Acute joint swelling in one or more joints with previous episodes involving the same joint (characteristic of crystal arthropathies)
- Period of previous episodes (typically several days to weeks)
- Past medical history of gout, thyroid disease, diabetes, or hemochromatosis (risk factors)
- Fever, trauma, other arthropathies, extra-articular features of HLA B27 arthropathies (eye, bowel, skin, nail involvement) (differential diagnosis)

PHYSICAL EXAMINATION

- Involved joint: hot, swollen, tender, limited range of motion
- Locomotor examination: other joint involvement (differential diagnosis)
- Skin, nails: rheumatoid nodules, psoriasis, gouty tophi (differential diagnosis)
- Temperature: high fever with septic arthritis, mildly raised in acute gout

INVESTIGATIONS

- Synovial fluid microscopy (compensated polarized light microscopy: weakly positive birefringent rhomboidal shaped crystals), gram stain and culture (septic arthritis)
- Erythrocyte sedimentation rate, C-reactive protein, rheumatoid factor, uric acid, white cell count (leukocytosis), blood cultures (differential diagnosis)
- X-ray: calcification of articular fibrocartilage (chondrocalcinosis) in menisci of the knee, triangular fibrocartilage complex in the wrist. Other sites include glenoid and acetabular labra and symphysis pubis.
- X-ray changes of osteoarthritis often are pronounced.
- X-ray hands (second/third metacarpophalangeal "hook" osteophytes in hemochromatosis)

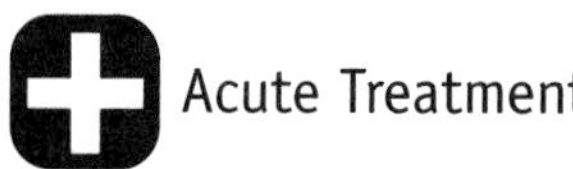

Acute Treatment

ANALGESIA

- Joint aspiration (often significantly reduces pain)
- Joint rest and splinting
- Nonsteroidal anti-inflammatory drugs and oral analgesia
- Colchicine and systemic corticosteroids can be used if other treatments are contraindicated.

SPECIAL CONSIDERATIONS

- Antibiotics if septic arthritis is suspected until joint and blood cultures return negative
- Intra-articular local anesthetic and corticosteroid injection, plus splinting until joint settles
- Repeat joint aspiration may be required.

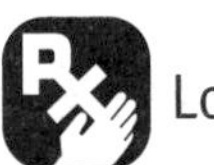

Long-Term Treatment

REHABILITATION

- Once acute attacks have settled, the aims of treatment are to relieve symptoms and regain function.
- No specific treatment exists for chronic CPPD, and no treatments are available that reverse joint damage.
- Although acute pseudogout usually responds well to therapy, chronic CPPD often is progressive and may cause considerable disability.

SURGERY

Joint arthroplasty may be required for severely damaged joints.

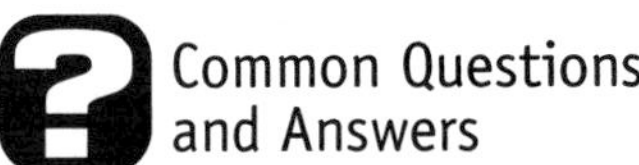

Common Questions and Answers

Physician responses to common patient questions:
Q: Are there drugs available (as in gout) that can prevent recurrent attacks of acute pseudogout?
A: The cause of CPPD is unknown (unlike gout, in which hyperuricemia leads to precipitation of uric acid crystals into joints). Therefore, there is no preventative treatment for recurrent attacks, although colchicine may be useful as prophylaxis in those with frequent recurrences

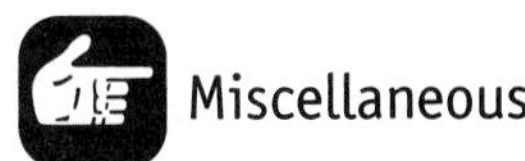

Miscellaneous

SYNONYMS

- Pseudogout
- Chondrocalcinosis
- Pyrophosphate arthropathy

ICD-9 CODE

712.2 Pseudogout CPPD
712.3 Chondrocalcinosis

BIBLIOGRAPHY

Doherty M. Crystal arthropathies: calcium pyrophosphate dihydrate. In: Klippel JH, Dieppe PA, eds. *Rheumatology*. London: Mosby-Year Book Europe Limited, 1994:7.13.1–7.13.12.

Ryan LM, McCarty DJ. Calcium pyrophosphate crystal deposition disease, pseudogout and articular chondrocalcinosis. In: Koopman WJ, ed. *Arthritis and allied conditions: a textbook of rheumatology,* 13th ed. Baltimore: Williams & Wilkins, 1997:2103–2125

Author: Nick Carter

Carpal Tunnel Syndrome

Basics

DEFINITION

- Clinical condition that may include characteristic symptoms of numbness on the palmar surface of the first 3½ digits, dysesthesias, and wrist pain caused by entrapment of the median nerve at the wrist

INCIDENCE/PREVALENCE

- The lifetime incidence of carpal tunnel syndrome (CTS) in the general population is approximately 10%. It is the most frequently encountered entrapment neuropathy in medical practice. When present, it is more likely to occur in the dominant extremity and is bilateral up to 50% of the time.
- The female-to-male ratio of CTS has been reported in ranges from 3:1 to as high as 10:1.
- Few studies have been performed relating the prevalence of CTS among athletes in particular sports. However, the prevalence of CTS in paraplegic wheelchair basketball players has been observed to be as high as 52% in one study. CTS also has been reported to be high among competitive race car drivers as well as bodybuilders who have trained for >6 years.

SIGNS AND SYMPTOMS

- There is considerable variability in the presenting symptoms for CTS. Numbness and paresthesias on the palmar aspect of the thumb, index, and middle fingers, as well as the radial half of the ring finger, can characterize compromise to the median nerve-innervated structures of the hand. Symptoms may worsen during the nighttime hours.
- Pain may be present across the region of the carpal tunnel on the palmar surface of the wrist and distal forearm. It is exacerbated by activities that involve flexion and extension of the wrist.
- Flick sign, in which a patient may demonstrate vigorous shaking of the hand and wrist in order to relieve symptoms, may be present.
- In cases of severe CTS, atrophy may be seen over the muscles of the thenar eminence, with weakness demonstrated in the abductor pollicis brevis muscle. Patients may complain of "dropping things."

RISK FACTORS

- Diabetes, thyroid disease, and rheumatoid arthritis have all been associated with the development of CTS.
- Activities involving repetitive wrist motion, vibration, and excessive forces through the wrist
- Narrow bony measurements of the wrist, elevated body mass index, increased age, female gender, and pregnancy

PATHOPHYSIOLOGY

The carpal tunnel is a longitudinally positioned canal in the palmar wrist that is bordered by the scaphoid and trapezium bones on its radial aspect, and the pisiform and hook of the hamate bones on its ulnar aspect. The roof of the carpal tunnel is formed by the transverse carpal ligament. The structures that pass through the carpal tunnel include the median nerve, the four tendons of the flexor digitorum superficialis, the four tendons of the flexor digitorum profundus, and the flexor pollicis longus tendon. The synovial membranes of these tendons can thicken, and the transverse carpal ligament can compress the median nerve as it passes through the carpal tunnel. Compartmental pressure can be increased within the carpal tunnel by sustained wrist flexion or extension, thus causing additional strain to the median nerve in an anatomically compromised canal space. The damage that occurs to the median nerve within the carpal tunnel is primarily a demyelinating lesion, but severe compression can cause an axonotmetic lesion (loss of median nerve axons.) The nerve fiber type affected can include both sensory and motor fibers, with sensory symptoms presenting in milder lesions.

ASSOCIATED INJURIES AND COMPLICATIONS

- Traumatic carpal bone dislocation or wrist fracture can disrupt the median nerve through the carpal tunnel.
- Lipomas, ganglion cysts, or other anatomical anomalies can grow and directly compress the median nerve.
- Proximal upper extremity nerve entrapment or nerve root compression, the double crush syndrome

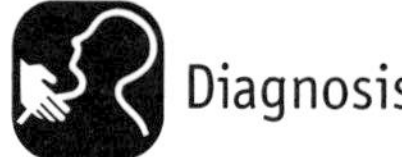

Diagnosis

DIFFERENTIAL DIAGNOSIS

- de Quervain tenosynovitis
- Cervical radiculopathy
- Proximal median nerve entrapment, pronator teres syndrome, or anterior interosseous syndrome
- Ulnar neuropathy at the elbow or wrist
- Generalized peripheral polyneuropathy
- Upper motor neuron pathology
- Wrist arthritis or other lesions in the wrist

HISTORY

Q: What activities exacerbate symptoms?
A: Determine specific wrist motion in sport, occupational task, sleeping, driving, etc.
Q: Associated with neck/shoulder pain or "shooting pain"?
A: Suggests cervical root pathology or radiculopathy
Q: Are symptoms present in the feet?
A: Possible generalized peripheral polyneuropathy
Q: Do symptoms become apparent at night, and are they improved with "shaking of the hands"?
A: Consistent with CTS.

PHYSICAL EXAMINATION

- Carpal compression test: Press with thumbs over the carpal tunnel for 30 seconds to elicit symptoms. Test has reported 87% sensitivity and 90% specificity for CTS.
- Phalen test: Position wrists against each other in complete flexion for up to 60 seconds to elicit symptoms. Test has reported 70% sensitivity and 84% specificity for CTS.
- Tinel sign: Percussion over the region of the carpal tunnel at the wrist to elicit symptoms. Test has reported 56% sensitivity and 80% specificity for CTS.
- Observe and palpate region of thenar muscle mass for evident atrophy.
- Strength testing of the abductor pollicis brevis muscle
- Sensory testing, especially in median nerve distribution

IMAGING

- Plain films generally are normal. Occasionally they can be helpful to rule out anatomical variants, fractures in trauma, and calcification in carpal tunnel.
- Magnetic resonance imaging has been used to visualize median nerve compression and synovial thickening of tendon sheaths. It may show the presence of space-occupying masses within the carpal tunnel. Its sensitivity and specificity for this purpose have not been assessed.
- Cost may limit its diagnostic practicality. It cannot assess the physiologic integrity of the median nerve across the carpal tunnel segment.

ELECTRODIAGNOSTIC STUDIES

- Sensory nerve conduction studies with or without motor nerve conduction studies provide a highly sensitive and specific means for assessing the physiologic integrity of the median nerve across the carpal tunnel segment.
- It can be used to classify severity of CTS and to monitor progression of median nerve entrapment.
- Needle electromyography is useful for documenting the presence of axonal loss to intrinsic hand muscles innervated by the median nerve distal to the carpal tunnel segment and identifying other or coexisting neuromuscular pathology (e.g., cervical radiculopathy).

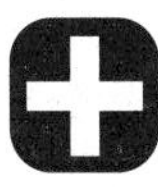

Acute Treatment

SPLINTING

Wrist splinting during the day, night, or both, with the wrist positioned in neutral, may provide relief of symptoms in mild cases of CTS.

MEDICATION

Nonsteroidal anti-inflammatory drugs can provide analgesia and may reduce inflammation within the carpal tunnel.

INJECTION

Injection of a corticosteroid preparation with or without lidocaine has been reported to be effective for short-term symptomatic relief of CTS; however, symptoms often recur over a variable period of time.

EXERCISE

- Stretching of the carpal tunnel segment via the opponens roll technique has been used to mobilize the transverse carpal ligament and relieve median nerve compression.
- Restriction of precipitating activities may relieve symptoms.

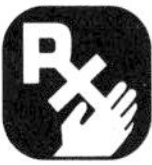

Long-Term Treatment

SURGERY

- Surgical decompression of the carpal tunnel segment by sectioning of the transverse carpal ligament has been reported to result in good symptomatic improvement in 85% to 90% of cases and may prevent further median nerve axon loss.
- Both open and endoscopic carpal tunnel surgical procedures currently are used. Although controversy exists over the optimum technique for successful outcomes, the open technique remains the most widely practiced.
- Distal latencies of the median nerve as measured by nerve conduction studies may improve after carpal tunnel surgery, but may not necessarily return to normal.

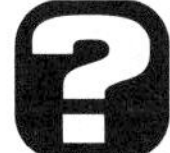

Common Questions and Answers

Physician responses to common patient questions:
Q: How can I minimize symptom exacerbation of CTS during athletic activities?
A: Use of wrist wraps and taping may minimize forces through the carpal tunnel by limiting excessive motion through the wrist in upper extremity weight-bearing sports such as gymnastics and weight lifting.
Q: When may I begin to experience improvements in my symptoms after CTS surgery?
A: Improvements in wrist pain and paresthesias may be noted within a few weeks after CTS surgery, but maximal improvements in thenar strength and numbness may take as long as 9 months.

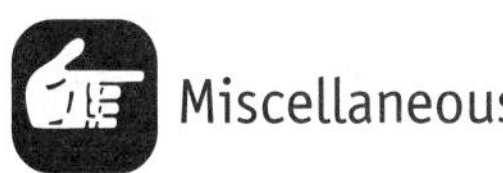

Miscellaneous

ICD-9 CODE

354.0 Carpal tunnel syndrome

BIBLIOGRAPHY

Burnham RS, Steadward RD. Upper extremity nerve entrapments among wheelchair athletes: prevalence, location and risk factors. *Arch Phys Med Rehabil* 1994;75:519–524.

Gellman H, Gelberman RH, Tan AM, et al. Carpal tunnel syndrome: an evaluation of the provocative diagnostic tests. *J Bone Joint Surg* 1986;68:735–737.

Kerwin G, Williams CS, Seiler JG. The pathophysiology of carpal tunnel syndrome. *Hand Clin* 1996;12:243–251.

Mesgarzadeh M, Triolo J. Carpal tunnel syndrome: MR imaging diagnosis. *Magn Reson Imaging Clin North Am* 1995;3:249–264.

Palmer D. Carpal tunnel syndrome in athletes. *Op Tech Sports Med* 1996;4:33–39.

Sucher BM. Palpatory diagnosis and manipulative management of carpal tunnel syndrome. *J Am Osteopath Assoc* 1994;8:647–663.

Authors: Ryan O'Connor and Michael T. Andary

Central Slip Avulsion and Pseudoboutonniere Deformities

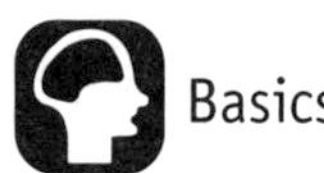

Basics

DEFINITION

- Boutonniere or "buttonhole" deformity is a delayed chronic complication of the acute injuries that cause central slip avulsion.
- Several mechanisms produce central slip avulsion. Most common is forced flexion of the proximal interphalangeal (PIP) joint during active extension causing avulsion. Avulsion also occurs after dislocation of the PIP joint and blunt trauma to the dorsal PIP joint.
- Avulsion of the central slip compromises the "roof" of the PIP capsule, allowing gradual dorsal buttonholing of the joint between the lateral bands that gradually migrate volarly.
- Pseudoboutonniere deformity is a complication of PIP volar plate injuries, including dislocations, if not treated correctly in the acute stages. Gradual flexion contracture occurs at the PIP joint during scarring of the volar plate. In these cases, the central slip is intact.

INCIDENCE/PREVALENCE

Rupture of the central slip is the second most common closed tendon injury in athletes. In sports, dorsal dislocations are reported more frequently than volar dislocations.

SIGNS AND SYMPTOMS

- The PIP joint is always acutely injured preceding these late developing deformities. After acute injury, tenderness and swelling occur over the entire PIP joint, including the dorsal base of the middle phalanx at site of avulsion of central slip, along collateral ligaments, lateral bands, and volar plate.
- With acute central slip avulsion, the dorsal PIP joint is tender. Active extension of the PIP joint is lost, but passive extension is intact. Active DIP joint extension and flexion usually are limited by pain.
- On the field, the finger may show good alignment, but collateral ligament injury or fracture must be considered. Integrity of PIP joint collateral ligaments is assessed with the joint in full extension and 30 degrees flexion.
- In central slip avulsion, PIP joint extension remains weak as time passes after the injury.
- Weeks later, insidious development of classic "boutonniere" deformity occurs. The lateral bands migrate volarly, converting into flexors of the PIP. The PIP joint flexes, "buttonholing" between these bands. The DIP joint is pulled into extension by the process.
- Presentation of pseudoboutonniere deformity after acute injury is the same as a true boutonniere, except active PIP joint extension may be possible early and late, as the central slip is intact. Later, the joint will remain painful with progressive flexion contracture from the scarring volar plate if not managed appropriately.

RISK FACTORS

- Sports involving use of a ball, and contact sports. The PIP joint is forced into flexion during active extension. Axial forces of a ball to a finger that is in full extension when struck can produce dislocations leading to either deformity.

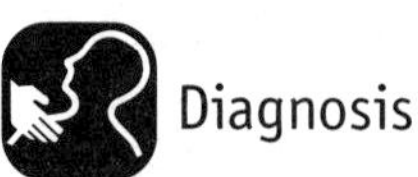

Diagnosis

DIFFERENTIAL DIAGNOSIS

- Fracture, dislocation, collateral ligament tears, volar plate disruption

HISTORY

- Finger injury with forced flexion while athlete is actively extending the finger. May be a "jammed" finger with possible dislocation, reduced on the field. Athlete may not have been evaluated by a physician until difficulty with PIP joint range of motion or slow recovery was noted.

PHYSICAL EXAMINATION

- Acute presentation: swollen, slightly flexed, and tender PIP joint with point tenderness over dorsum of base of middle phalanx. Difficulty with active extension of PIP joint. Assess neurovascular status before and after attempting reduction
- Late presentation: Classic boutonniere; may be relatively painless but has a flexion contracture of PIP joint with hyperextension of DIP joint.

IMAGING

- Plain films may reveal a dorsal fleck avulsed proximally with the central slip, fractures, and dislocations. Volar avulsion fragments suggest volar displacement injury.
- Appropriate alignment

POSTREDUCTION VIEWS

- Same as "Imaging" above
- Generally good alignment, depending on associated fractures

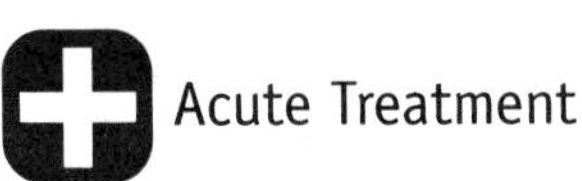

Acute Treatment

ANALGESIA

- Narcotics, nonsteroidal anti-inflammatory drugs, or digital block may help with reduction.
- Splinting is the most effective analgesia and is the necessary treatment.
- Rest, ice, compression, and elevation

IMMOBILIZATION

- Splint PIP joint in full extension, allowing flexion of DIP joint, for 4 to 8 weeks

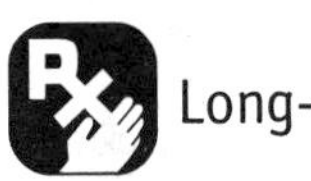

Long-Term Treatment

REHABILITATION

- Maintain range of motion, especially extension, with passive then active therapy when out of splint to avoid contracture of volar plate.
- Active extension with a small rubber band around fingers in grasp position is easy to perform all day.
- Graded grip putty is available for flexion rehabilitation.

SURGERY

- Avulsion fractures involving more than one third of the joint surface may require surgery.
- Maintain range of motion, especially extension, with passive and active therapy when out of splint to avoid contracture of volar plate.

REFERRAL/DISPOSITION

- Consultation with a hand surgeon confirms appropriate management.
- Orthopaedic surgery consultation is warranted with associated phalangeal fracture.
- Advise on return to play that another injury with a similar mechanism will reproduce the injury.

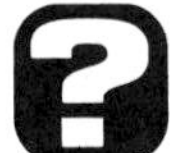

Common Questions and Answers

Physician responses to common patient questions:
Q: How long before I can return to play?
A: Depending on function and stability, may begin some position specific rehabilitation in 4–8 weeks. Avoidance of repeat trauma (forced flexion) is essential to allow healing of the central slip. Full pain-free function may take 12 weeks or more.
Q: Are x-rays needed?
A: Yes, to assure no fractures occurred.

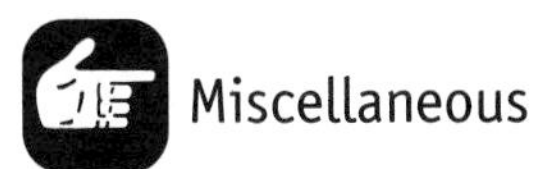

Miscellaneous

ICD-9 CODE

736.21 Boutonniere deformity
No code for pseudoboutonniere, same deformity

BIBLIOGRAPHY

Aronwitz A, Leddy JP. Closed tendon injuries of the hand and wrist in athletes. *Clin Sports Med* 1998;17:449–467.

Bach AW. Finger joint injuries in active patients: pointers for acute and late phase management. *Phys Sports Med* 1999;3:89–104.

Eaton RG. *Joint injuries of the hand.* Springfield, IL: Charles C Thomas Publisher, 1971.

Sallis R, ed. *ACSM essentials of sports medicine.* Fontana, CA: Mosby, 1996.

Author: John Shelton

Cervical Stenosis

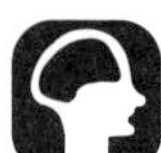

Basics

DEFINITION

- A congenital or acquired narrowing of the cervical spine canal. However, this problem has several definitions. This definition is based on magnetic resonance evidence from the National Center for Catastrophic Sports Injury Research (NCCSIR).
- Functional spinal stenosis is the loss of cerebral spinal fluid cushion around the spinal cord or a clear deformation of the cord demonstrated by computed tomography (CT), magnetic resonance imaging (MRI), or myelography.

INCIDENCE/PREVALENCE

The incidence of cervical stenosis is unknown. However, Torg reported that, in a single football season, 6 of 10,000 exposures resulted in transient paresthesia in all four extremities and 1.3 of 10,000 exposures resulted in transient quadriplegia. This describes cervical cord neurapraxia (CCN), which is thought to be a sequela of stenosis.

SIGNS AND SYMPTOMS

- Unfortunately, cervical stenosis is asymptomatic until forced hyperflexion or hyperextension occurs with an axial load. This causes CCN.
- The athlete develops acute transient sensory paresthesia and/or motor paresis.
- Finding are always bilateral.
- Paresthesia is described as burning pain, numbness, tingling, or loss of sensation.
- Motor changes can range from weakness to complete paralysis.
- Neurapraxia commonly lasts 10 to 15 minutes, but can take up to 36 hours to resolve.

RISK FACTORS

- Congenital defects; or acquired defects, which include bulging disc, hypertrophied or unstable ligaments, and degenerative changes
- Involvement in sports that engage in potential axial loading, i.e., football, ice hockey, diving, head-first sliding in baseball, wrestling, soccer, gymnastics, rugby

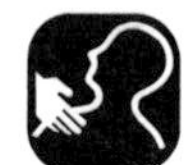

Diagnosis

DIFFERENTIAL DIAGNOSIS

- Stable spinal fracture
- Any cause of permanent spinal cord injury
- Spear tacklers spine
- Unstable fracture
- Spinal fracture with dislocation
- Ligamentous injury
- Herniated cervical disk

HISTORY

- During preparticipation physical examination, determination of any prior history of neurologic events, such as burners/stingers, or transient neurologic events is critical.
- If the athlete gives a positive response, all data from previous evaluations must be reviewed. If no workup has been done, then seriously consider starting one before allowing an athlete to begin contact/collision sports.
- If the athlete has a condition such as Down syndrome, odontoid abnormality, atlantooccipital fusion, or Klippel-Feil anomaly, these will give clues to having developmental cervical stenosis. The athlete should be evaluated for the existence of stenosis.

PHYSICAL EXAMINATION

- During the preparticipation physical examination, the Spurling test can be done. If symptoms are elicited, further workup can be started. The yield is very low unless the patient already has stenosis. It should be done on any athlete who gives a history of neurologic events.
- If the initial event occurs on the field, start with assessment of the athlete's level of consciousness. If unconscious, immobilize and transport. If conscious, proceed to asses neck pain.
- If neck pain is present or absent and athlete has neurologic symptoms, immobilize and transport for further workup.

IMAGING

- The initial radiographic examination should start with cervical spinal x-rays, which can be used to evaluate for gross fracture or dislocation. In addition, some measurements of the spinal canal can be done. The normal canal measures >15 mm; <13 mm is considered spinal stenosis.
- On the lateral x-ray, the Torg ratio can be calculated. Measure (in millimeters) the distance from the posterior aspect of the vertebral body to the spinolaminar line (a) and the width of the vertebral body (b), then calculate the ratio a/b. A value <0.8 is abnormal and needs further evaluation.
- A large vertebral body can result in a false-positive result; the false-positive rate has been reported as 88%. If the patient has spinal stenosis, the ratio almost always is abnormal.
- The next step is to use MRI, CT, or myelography.

- Resnick reports that CT with myelography is the most sensitive measure for spinal stenosis. Ladd and Scranton argue metrizamide-enhanced myelography is needed in the injured athlete because CT alone fails to reveal neural compression adequately; however, this is an invasive procedure.
- MRI can evaluate spinal stenosis caused by most abnormalities. It is not as effective as CT in evaluating bony lesions. According to Cantu, MRI is sufficient in most cases.
- MRI is done in neutral position. With hyperextension, spinal canal diameter decreases by 30% due to infolding of the interlaminar ligaments.

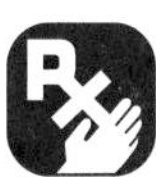

Long-Term Treatment

REHABILITATION

- After the first episode of CCN, if the initial workup is negative for stenosis, a generalized neck strengthening program should be started.
- Athletes involved in collision sports should be able to support their body weight with the cervical spine in neutral in all directions when positioned at a 45-degree angle.

SURGERY

If an acquired cause for spinal stenosis is detected, consultation with a neurosurgeon or orthopaedic spine surgeon for consideration of surgery can be undertaken. However, after surgery, the athlete probably cannot participate in contact/collision sports.

REFERRAL/DISPOSITION

- Cantu argues that team physicians should be concerned with functional spinal stenosis. If present, and the athlete incurs spinal cord symptoms, the athlete should not continue in contact/collision sports, as such activities predispose athletes to a worse neurologic outcome in the context of cervical spine injuries.
- Data collected by the NCCSI from 1987 to 1996 showed no athlete with functional spinal stenosis and cervical spinal fracture recovered from quadriplegia.
- This finding needs to be compared with nearly 20% of athletes with cervical spinal fracture and normal canal sizes who had initial quadriplegia and recovered fully.
- During the same period, in all cases of quadriplegia without cervical spinal fracture dislocation, severe spinal stenosis was present.
- If the athlete redevelops CCN, the workup should proceed again, from plain radiographs to MRI or CT with myelography.

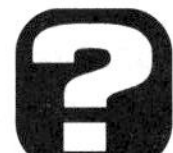

Common Questions and Answers

Physician responses to common patient questions:

Q: When can I return to play?

A: Cantu (1997) gives the following guidelines.

- Canal/vertebral body ratio of 0.8 or less in asymptomatic individuals: no contra-indication
- Ratio of 0.8 or less with one episode of CCN: relative contraindication
- Documented episodes of CCN associated with intervertebral disc disease and/or degenerative changes: relative contraindication
- Documented episode of CCN associated with MRI evidence of cord defect or cord edema: relative/absolute contraindication
- Documented episode of CCN associated with ligamentous instability, symptoms, or neurologic findings lasting >36 hours, and/or multiple episodes: absolute contraindication
- Any episode in which, during the evaluation, functional stenosis is detected: absolute contraindication

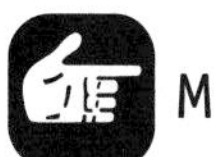

Miscellaneous

SYNONYMS

- Cervical cord neurapraxia, any transient neurologic deficits

ICD-9 CODE

723.0

BIBLIOGRAPHY

Cantu RC. Cervical spinal injuries in the athlete. *Semin Neurol* 2000;20:173–178.

Cantu RC. The cervical spinal stenosis controversy. *Clin Sport Med* 1998;17:121–126.

Cantu RC. Stingers, transient quadriplegia, and cervical stenosis: return to play criteria. *Med Sci Sports Exerc* 1997;29 [7 Suppl]:233–235.

Cantu RC, Bailes JE, Wilberger JE Jr. Guidelines for return to contact or collision sport after a cervical spine injury. *Clin Sport Med* 1998;17:137–146.

Maroon JC, Bailes JE. Athletes with cervical spine injury. *Spine* 1996;21:2294–2299.

Torg JS. Cervical spinal stenosis with cord neuropraxia and transient quadriplegia. *Clin Sport Med* 1990;9:279–296.

Wilberger JE Jr. Athletic spinal cord and spine injuries. *Clin Sport Med* 1998;17:111–120.

Zachazewsia JE, Magee DJ, Quillen WS. *Athletic injury and rehabilitation.* Philadelphia: WB Saunders, 1996.

Author: Todd May

Cervical Strains

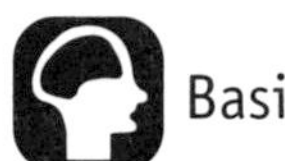

Basics

DEFINITION

Cervical strain refers to musculotendinous injury of the cervical region. It commonly occurs in conjunction with ligamentous injury.

INCIDENCE/PREVALENCE

- Most frequently caused by whiplash injury, i.e., hyperextension of the cervical spine from a rear-end motor vehicle collision. More than one million cases per year are reported in the United States. More common in urban areas with high concentrations of motor vehicles. Higher incidence seen in females and in persons ages 30–50 years.
- Incidence associated with sports is unknown.

SIGNS AND SYMPTOMS

- Cardinal symptoms: neck pain and headache
- Neck fatigue, stiffness, pain at rest and/or with movement
- Pain may be referred to shoulder, upper limb, and head.
- Other symptoms may include unusual skin sensations at head/face, dizziness, light-headedness, concentration and memory deficits, tinnitus, blurred vision, hearing difficulties, and other cranial nerve deficit complaints.
- Limitation in range of motion at neck and tenderness at cervical paraspinal muscles, often with hypertonicity or "spasm"
- Generally normal neurologic examination, although subjective sensory deficits may be present.

RISK FACTORS

- Speculated: age, level of conditioning, prior history of neck injury, cervical spondylosis, cervical degenerative disc disease, head position at time of impact, mechanism of injury, personality traits, and psychosocial factors

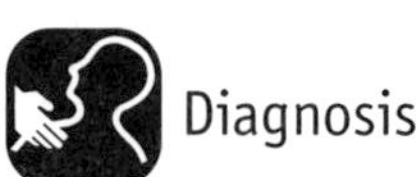

Diagnosis

DIFFERENTIAL DIAGNOSIS

- Other musculoskeletal disorders involving neck or shoulder: disc annulus fibrosis injury, facet joint injury, rotator cuff injury, myofascial pain
- Neurologic injury: cervical radiculopathy, myelopathy, brachial plexus injury, thoracic outlet syndrome, peripheral nerve entrapment (e.g., suprascapular nerve)
- Cervical fracture and cervical instability

HISTORY

- Main complaint and location of symptoms. Anatomical pain drawings may be helpful in providing an overview of the pain pattern.
- Neurologic symptoms and course, including changes in gait, bowel or bladder dysfunction, upper or lower extremity sensory changes or weakness
- Activities and head positions that aggravate or alleviate symptoms
- Onset, mechanism, and time course of injury or symptoms
- Prior episodes of similar symptoms and of neck injury or surgery
- Previous treatment, including modalities, medications, physical therapy, traction, manipulation, injection, and surgical treatments
- Social history, including level of physical activity, occupation, job satisfaction, ongoing litigation, and use of nicotine and/or alcohol

PHYSICAL EXAMINATION

- Observation of head and neck posture, movement during normal conversation, presence of head list and stiff movement
- Active range of motion, usually reduced, particularly in directions stretching the injured muscles
- Palpation: Tenderness, usually noted along the cervical paraspinal muscles, may be present along muscles where symptoms are referred, associated hypertonicity, or "spasm."
- Careful manual muscle testing for evidence of deficits in myotomal distribution
- Sensory examination for dermatomal deficits in sensation, hyperesthesia, inconsistent or "nonanatomical" pattern
- Deep tendon reflexes/muscle stretch reflexes and Hoffman or Babinski signs, helpful in identifying myelopathy, radiculopathy, and brachial plexopathy
- Special provocative tests: Spurling sign, Lhermitte sign, and Adson test. All provocative tests are negative. Spurling test is performed by extending the neck and rotating the head, and then applying downward pressure on the head. Considered positive if pain radiates into the limb ipsilateral to the side the head is rotated. Specific but not sensitive in diagnosing acute radiculopathy. Lhermitte sign is performed by passively flexing the neck. Considered positive if "electric-like" sensation radiates down the spine. Positive with cervical stenosis, myelopathy, spinal cord injury due to tumor, multiple sclerosis, and other conditions. Manual distraction often greatly reduces neck and limb symptoms in patients with radiculopathy.

IMAGING

- Plain radiographs: anteroposterior, lateral, and oblique cervical spine views for evidence of acute fracture or subluxation with trauma. Open mouth view for evidence of atlantoaxial instability. Flexion and extension views for evidence of spinal instability. The latter views are performed in the acute setting.
- Computed tomography: offers superior sensitivity and specificity for acute fractures and for radiculopathy and stenosis, when combined with myelography. Performed as indicated.
- Magnetic resonance imaging: study of choice to detect soft tissue pathology, including disc and ligament disruption and nerve root or spinal cord compression/injury. Performed as indicated, not in acute setting.

ELECTRODIAGNOSTIC STUDIES

- Used to diagnose nerve root dysfunction when the diagnosis is uncertain or to distinguish a cervical radiculopathy from other lesions that are unclear on physical examination.
- Ideally performed 3 or more weeks after injury, as diagnostic abnormalities will first be seen 18–21 days after the onset of radiculopathy.

OTHER STUDIES

Diagnostic fluoroscopic-guided medial branch anesthetic block may be performed to assess for facet-mediated pain in patients resistant to treatment.

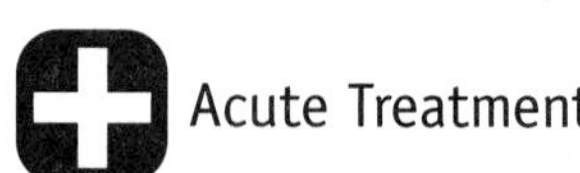

Acute Treatment

ACUTE PHASE

- Directed at reducing pain and inflammation. Therapies include local icing, nonsteroidal anti-inflammatory drugs, relative rest, avoiding positions that increase symptoms, and manual or mechanical traction.
- Modalities such as electrical stimulation may be helpful in reducing the associated muscle pain and spasm. Should be limited to the initial pain control phase of treatment.

- Consider myofascial trigger pain injections for severe pain not controlled by initial therapies in the acute phase.
- Gentle stretching; first passive mobilization and then active to begin to reestablish nonpainful range of motion
- Gentle strengthening: isometric cervical strengthening in a single plane (flexion, extension, lateral flexion, rotation), scapular stabilization, and cervicothoracic stabilization programs. All exercises should be performed without pain.
- Low-level aerobic cross-training (e.g., stationary bike, stair stepper, treadmill, aquatic running, etc.) begun as soon as tolerated to avoid deconditioning.

RECOVERY PHASE

- Directed toward normalizing active range of motion, neuromuscular control, strength, and posture
- Progressive passive and active stretching, mobilization, and manipulation as appropriate
- Progressive strengthening (isometric to isotonic) with independent single-plane and complex multiple-plane coordinated motions to include cervicothoracic, scapulothoracic, and scapulohumeral stabilization activities
- Continued aerobic cross-training

MAINTENANCE PHASE

- Directed toward sport/activity-specific training
- Protected padding often helpful: neck rolls/collars, interval pads, and customized orthoses
- Flexibility and strength balance postural training
- Power and endurance training, including strenuous upper extremity strengthening and plyometric activities
- Patterned motion training
- Continued aerobic training
- Stretching and strengthening should be continued indefinitely to minimize injury recurrence.
- Guidelines for returning to competition: no pain at rest, full pain-free range of motion, normal posture, normal strength, and normal physical examination

Common Questions and Answers

Physician responses to common patient questions:

Q: What is the prognosis?

A: At 1–10 years after whiplash injury associated with motor vehicle trauma: 60% to 80% of patients are asymptomatic, and only 5% to 15% are severely symptomatic. Prognosis associated with sports activities is believed to be excellent, although no data are available.

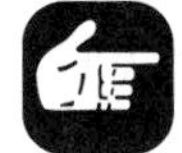

Miscellaneous

SYNONYMS

- Cervical sprain, whiplash

ICD-9 CODE

847.0

BIBLIOGRAPHY

Bogduk N, Teasell R. Whiplash: the evidence for an organic etiology. *Arch Neurol* 2000;57:590–591.

Cole AJ, et al. Cervical spine athletic injuries. *Phys Med Rehabil Clin North Am* 1994;5:37–68.

Gore DR, Murray MP, Sepic SB, Gardner G. Neck pain: a long term follow up of 250 patients. *Spine* 1987;12:1–5.

Johnson G. Hyperextension soft tissue injuries of the cervical spine—a review. *J Accid Emerg Med* 1996;13:3–8.

Jonnson H, Cesarini K, Sahlstedt B, Rauschning T. Findings and outcome in whiplash type neck distortions. *Spine* 1994;19:2733–2743.

Lagattuta FP, Falco FJE. Assessment and treatment of cervical spine disorders. In: Braddom RL, ed. *Physical medicine rehabilitation,* 1st ed. Philadelphia: WB Saunders, 1996:747–748.

Malanga GA. The diagnosis and treatment of cervical radiculopathy. *Med Sci Sports Exerc* 1997;29[7 Suppl]:S236–S245.

Panjabi M, et al. Cervical spine biomechanics. *Semin Spine Surg* 1994;5:10–16.

Pettersson K, Hildingson C, Toolanen G, et al. Disc pathology after whiplash injury: a prospective magnetic resonance imaging and clinical investigation. *Spine* 1997;22: 283–288.

Phull PS. Management of cervical pain. In: De Lisa JA, ed. *Rehabilitation medicine: principles and practice,* 1st ed. Philadelphia: JB Lippincott, 1988:757–758.

Ronnen HR, de Korte PJ, Brink PR, et al. Acute whiplash injury: is there a role for MRI imaging? A prospective study of 100 patients. *Radiology* 1996;201:93–96.

Squires B, Gargan MF, Bannister GC. Soft-tissue injuries of the cervical spine: 15-year follow-up. *J Bone Joint Surg Br* 1996;78:955–957.

Sturzenegger M, Di Stefano G, Radanov BP, Schnidrig A. Presenting symptoms and signs after whiplash injury: the influence of accident mechanisms. *Neurology* 1994;44:688–693.

Torg JS, Glasgow SG. Criteria for return to contact activities following cervical spine injury. *Clin J Sports Med* 1991;1:12–26.

Authors: Gerald Malanga and Phillip W. Landes

Compartment Syndrome, Anterior

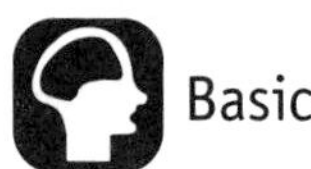

Basics

DEFINITION

- Compartment syndrome is a condition in which increased tissue pressure within a limited space compromises the circulation and function of the contents of that space. Exertional compartment syndrome occurs during exercise when muscles swell and may cause pain and/or neurologic symptoms.
- The diagnosis is based primarily on the history and physical examination, with the assistance of intracompartmental monitoring. The potential for irreversible ischemic damage is infrequent but depends on prompt recognition and institution of treatment.

INCIDENCE/PREVALENCE

- More frequent in distance runners and endurance athletes (i.e., soccer players)

SIGNS AND SYMPTOMS

Leg pain after prolonged exercise, often associated with a recent change in training (increase in distance or intensity). Onset of pain occurs predictably within the same time period from the onset of exercise. The pain is relieved with rest but may take several hours to completely resolve. There may be numbness or tingling in the foot.

RISK FACTORS

- Endurance athletes or long distance runners

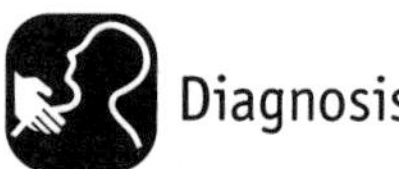

Diagnosis

DIFFERENTIAL DIAGNOSIS

- Stress fractures, periostitis, nerve entrapment syndromes, or claudication

HISTORY

Q: When does pain begin and end?
A: Frequently, pain occurs during exercise, predictably at the same time from the onset of the activity, and is relieved only by cessation of activity.
Q: Is there numbness or tingling in the foot at rest and during exercise?
A: Tingling that begins during exercise is consistent with exertional compartment syndrome. Tingling at rest is related to nerve entrapment syndromes.
Q: Where do you feel symptoms (in the leg and/or foot)?
A: Most frequently, the anterior and lateral compartments are involved and the leg pain will be anterolateral. The superficial (lateral compartment) or deep peroneal (anterior compartment) nerves, which provide sensation to the first web space and dorsum of the foot, respectively, may be involved.
Q: Do you have symptoms in both legs?
A: From 75% to 90% may have bilateral symptoms.

PHYSICAL EXAMINATION

Examination immediately after exercise is more valuable than examination with the patient at rest. Occasionally, there may be fascial defects or the compartments may feel tense. Neurovascular examination of the leg and foot may suggest irritation of the nerves that traverse the affected compartment.

ANCILLARY STUDIES

- Intracompartmental pressure monitoring before, during, and after exercise is the most beneficial test. A positive test has a resting pressure $\geq$15 mm Hg or 1- and 5-minute postexercise measurements $\geq$30 and 20 mm Hg, respectively.
- Radiographs are helpful in excluding stress fractures or neoplastic processes.

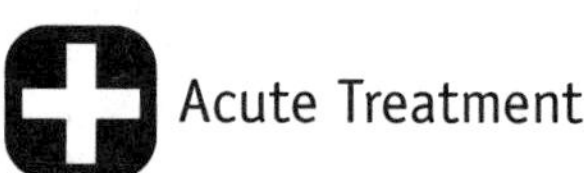

Acute Treatment

ANALGESIA

- Rest and activity modification
- Nonsurgical treatment usually is not effective for competitive athletes.

SPECIAL CONSIDERATIONS

Acute compartment syndrome is a surgical emergency and must be treated with emergent fasciotomy to avoid muscle necrosis.

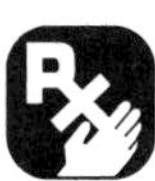

Long-Term Treatment

SURGERY

- If there is no improvement in symptoms and intracompartmental measuring is positive, fasciotomies of involved compartments are indicated. The goal is to release the investing muscular fascia and allow the muscle to increase in size during exercise.
- Fasciotomies are effective treatment in 80% to 90% of cases.

REHABILITATION

After a compartment syndrome has been recognized and fasciotomies performed, returning to the previous level of activity becomes a priority.

Common Questions and Answers

Physician responses to common patient questions:

Q: After fasciotomies are performed, when can I resume activities?

A: Most athletes will return to light jogging in 4–6 weeks. Training may begin around 8 weeks.

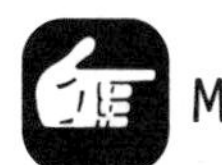

Miscellaneous

ICD-9 CODE

729.8
958.8

BIBLIOGRAPHY

Eisele SA, Sammarco GJ. Chronic exertional compartment syndrome. In: *Instructional course lectures.* Rosemont, IL: American Academy of Orthopedic Surgeons, 1993:213–217.

Pedowitz RA, Hargens AR, Mubarak SJ, et al. Modified criteria for the objective diagnosis of chronic compartment syndrome of the leg. *Am J Sports Med* 1990;18:35–40.

Schepsis AA, Martini D, Corbett M. Surgical management of exertional compartment syndrome of the lower leg. Long-term followup. *Am J Sports Med* 1993;21: 811–817.

Authors: Paul Favorito, Angelo J. Colosimo, and Robert S. Heidt Jr.

Concussion

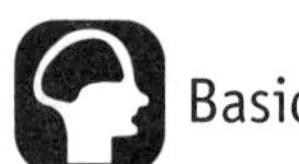

Basics

DEFINITION

- Transient impairment of mental status as a result of a blow to the head

INCIDENCE/PREVALENCE

- National Football Head and Neck Injury Registry estimates that ~250,000 concussions occur in football each year, or ~20% of football players will sustain a concussion each year.
- National Football Head and Neck Injury Registry reported an average of eight deaths per year in football due to head injury between 1971 and 1984.
- An athlete with a previous concussion is four times more likely to have a repeat concussion than an athlete without a history of a concussion.
- Much more common in contact and collision sports, although concussion may occur in any sport

SIGNS AND SYMPTOMS

- An athlete with a concussion can display a wide range of symptoms consistent with alteration in mental status.
- In many instances, the athlete will not know that the symptoms represent a concussion.
- Possible symptoms include headache, confusion, difficulties with concentration, disorientation, amnesia, slowness of thought, dizziness, irritability, fatigue, or changes in personality.
- The range and potential vague nature of symptoms can make the diagnosis difficult.
- The athlete may or may not have a loss of consciousness.

RISK FACTORS

- Previous concussion
- Improperly maintained head gear (loose fitting, pneumatic compartments not filled, damaged)
- Failure to wear mouth guard
- Improper technique (e.g., tackling with head down or "spearing")

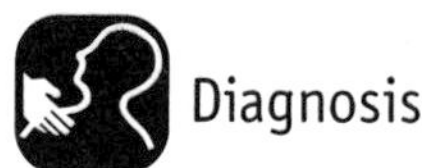

Diagnosis

DIFFERENTIAL DIAGNOSIS

- Subdural hematoma, which may be acute or subacute
- Epidural hematoma, which results from tear of middle meningeal artery causing rapid deterioration (may or may not occur after a "lucid interval")
- Diffuse axonal injury, which leads to prolonged loss of consciousness that often causes residual deficits

HISTORY

- Direct blow to the head
- Presume any unconscious athlete has suffered trauma to the head and neck
- Athlete with amnesia following a concussion may not remember a blow to the head. This should be presumed in anyone demonstrating signs of a concussion.
- Athlete with prior concussion is four times more likely to suffer a repeat concussion.

PHYSICAL EXAMINATION

- Presume any athlete with a head injury may have a cervical spine injury as well, until proven otherwise
- Assess ABCs (airway, breathing, circulation)
- Determine level of consciousness (alert, responds to verbal stimuli, responds to painful stimuli, or unconscious)
- Assess pupils for symmetry and reactivity to light. "Blown" pupil (asymmetrically dilated and nonreactive to light) in an unconscious athlete may indicate a transtentorial herniation. Hyperventilate patient and transport emergently.
- Evaluate athlete for other injuries, including skull fracture, scalp laceration, or signs of basilar skull fracture, including postauricular hematoma (Battle sign), rhinorrhea, otorrhea, periorbital ecchymosis (raccoon eyes), or hemotympanum
- If athlete is conscious and cervical spine injury has been reasonably ruled out, take athlete to sideline for observation and reevaluation.
- Evaluate for changes in mental status (loss of orientation, amnesia, or confusion)

CLASSIFICATION

- Classification systems for grading severity are based on duration of unconsciousness and duration of mental status changes.
- Multiple classification systems currently exist (American College of Sports Medicine ("Modified Cantu"), Colorado Medical Society, American Academy of Neurology). None are yet universally accepted.
- Mild (grade I): transient confusion, no amnesia, no loss of consciousness. Symptoms and mental status abnormalities usually resolve within 15–20 minutes.

- Moderate (grade II): transient confusion, amnesia, no loss of consciousness. Symptoms and mental status abnormalities last >20–30 minutes.
- Severe (grade III): loss of consciousness. Disagreement exists whether this includes concussions with brief (few seconds) loss of consciousness in which symptoms totally resolve within a few minutes. Some clinicians chose to treat these as "mild," but some argue that any loss of consciousness constitutes a "severe" concussion.

IMAGING

- Cranial computed tomography (CT): useful in acute imaging to rule out intracranial bleed. Consider if symptoms are worsening or fail to resolve in a timely manner.
- Magnetic resonance imaging (MRI): useful in acute trauma if available to rule out intracranial bleed. More commonly used to evaluate continuing symptoms in the subacute phase ("postconcussion syndrome").

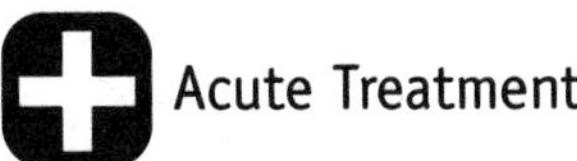

Acute Treatment

ON-FIELD MANAGEMENT

- Presume every unconscious athlete has a cervical spine injury and stabilize spine until x-rays are obtained
- Presume any athlete who complains of neck pain, numbness, weakness, or paralysis has a cervical spine injury until proven otherwise
- Assess ABCs (airway, breathing, circulation)
- Perform baseline neurologic evaluation
- Evaluate athlete for associated and other injuries
- If athlete is conscious and cervical spine injury has been reasonably ruled out, take athlete to sideline for observation and reevaluation.

SIDELINE MANAGEMENT

- Determine orientation to time, person, and place
- Determine if confusion and/or amnesia are present
- Observe gait
- Asymptomatic athlete should not have any headache, confusion, dizziness, impaired orientation, impaired concentration, or memory dysfunction.
- Asymptomatic athletes should be tested with exertion to see if any symptoms occur.
- Athlete with persistence of symptoms should not return to play.
- Athlete with any loss of consciousness (even if only for a few seconds) probably should not be allowed to return to play that day.
- Observe and reexamine the asymptomatic athlete for symptom recurrence at least every 5 minutes for ~20 minutes before considering return to play

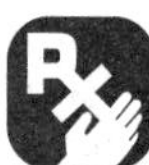

Long-Term Treatment

POSTCONCUSSION SYNDROME

- Diagnose when symptoms (e.g., headache, dizziness, irritability, fatigue, impaired memory, impaired concentration, or slow decision-making) persist for weeks to months
- Symptoms may be aggravated by exercise.
- Perform CT or MRI to exclude intracranial lesions.
- No specific treatment other than rest
- May use neuropsychiatric tests to monitor recovery
- Athlete should not return to competition until all symptoms resolve, both at rest and with exertion.

SECOND-IMPACT SYNDROME

- Rapid swelling of the brain from second mild head injury while still symptomatic from first head injury
- Often is fatal
- May occur from even a very mild (often unnoticed or not felt to be significant) direct or indirect trauma to a previously concussed brain
- One of the primary reasons to use extreme caution in returning athletes to play

RETURN TO PLAY

- Management guidelines for return to participation after concussion are generally based on presence or absence of confusion, amnesia, or loss of consciousness.
- Multiple recommendations exist regarding return to participation in sports after concussion. There are no current universally accepted guidelines. Current guidelines in use include those from the American College of Sports Medicine ("Modified Cantu Guidelines"), Colorado Medical Society, and American Academy of Neurology. New guidelines are under evaluation by the American Medical Society for Sports Medicine and the National Collegiate Athletic Association.
- After an initial mild concussion in which symptoms completely resolve within minutes, the athlete may return to play after being totally asymptomatic for ~15–20 minutes.
- Following an initial moderate concussion or a repeat mild concussion, remove the athlete from participation until the athlete has been completely asymptomatic for ~1 week.
- Following an initial severe concussion or a repeat moderate concussion, remove the athlete from participation for ~2–4 weeks. The athlete may return to participation if the athlete has been completely asymptomatic for ~1–2 weeks (may allow conditioning after ~1 asymptomatic week).
- Following repeat severe concussion or >2 mild or moderate concussions, terminate season.
- Terminate season if any abnormality is present on CT or MRI that is consistent with brain contusion or other intracranial lesion.
- Discuss possible termination of involvement in contact/collision sports, and potential risks of further and permanent injury, with any athlete who has experienced multiple recurring concussions.
- No guidelines or recommendations are universally accepted at this point. Any decision regarding return to play ultimately rests with the supervising physician, who should take into consideration these guidelines (and be comfortable in defending any deviation from them), the individual circumstances regarding the athlete and the injury, and the physician's own level of expertise and comfort with the individual situation.
- Concussions are injuries to the brain and can have lasting, deleterious effects. They have the potential to be fatal. Always err on the side of conservative management if any uncertainty exists.

PREVENTION

- Athletes in collision sports (e.g., football, boxing, lacrosse, ice hockey) should wear properly maintained protective head gear.
- Pneumatic pocket helmets appear to provide superior protection than strap-type suspension helmets.

- Helmets should be fully intact and properly fitted. Defective or damaged helmets should be replaced.
- Well-fitted mouth guards and padded chin straps may help minimize concussions.
- Rule changes to enforce safe and proper technique and prevent dangerous techniques (e.g., spearing was outlawed in football) can help decrease head and neck injuries.
- Strengthening neck muscles may reduce the number and severity of head and neck injuries.

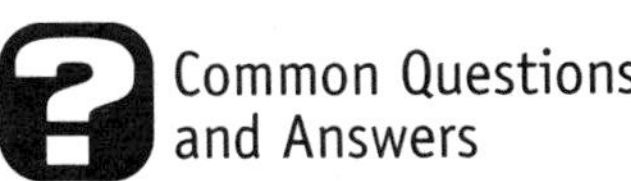

Common Questions and Answers

Physician responses to common patient questions:

Q: When can I return to play after a concussion?
A: Receiving a second blow to the head (even a minor one) while still suffering from the effects of the original concussion can lead to a condition called second-impact syndrome, which results in severe brain swelling and usually death. No one should return to play while still having the signs or symptoms of a concussion. The more severe the original concussion, the longer your doctor may require you to be symptom-free before returning.

Q: How many concussions can I have before I can no longer play sports?
A: As of yet, there is no specific cutoff number of concussions used to permanently disqualify an athlete. However, mounting evidence exists that the more concussions a person suffers, the worse he or she tends to do on various tests of brain function. Athletes should consider this risk of cumulative brain injury from multiple concussions when deciding whether or not to return to play.

Q: How can I prevent concussions?
A: Using proper equipment is the most obvious step. When indicated, wear protective head gear that meets the safety specifications for that sport. Head gear should be held in place by a snugly fitting, padded chin strap. Mouth pieces also help by absorbing force from a blow to the head. Learning safe fundamentals of a given sport, such as proper head-up tackling position in football and heading technique in soccer, can help to reduce the occurrence and severity of concussions.

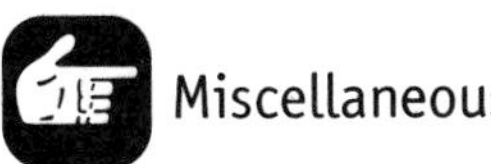

Miscellaneous

SYNONYMS

- "Bell ringer"
- Mild traumatic brain injury (TBI)
- Commotio cerebri
- Cerebral contusion
- "Brain bruise"
- "Head injury"

ICD-9 CODE

850.0 Concussion, with no loss of consciousness
850.1 Concussion, with brief loss of consciousness (<1 hour)
850.9 Concussion, unspecified

BIBLIOGRAPHY

Practice parameter: the management of concussion in sports (summary statement). Report of the Quality Standards Subcommittee. *Neurology* 1997;48:581–585.

Cantu RC, Micheli LJ, eds. *American College of Sports Medicine's guidelines for the team physician.* Philadelphia: Lea & Febiger, 1991.

Kelly JP, Nichols JS, Filley CM, et al. Concussion in sports. Guidelines for the prevention of catastrophic outcome. *JAMA* 1991;266:2867–2869.

McCrea M, Kelly JP, Kluge J, et al. Standardized assessment of concussion in football players. *Neurology* 1997;48:586–588.

Torg JS. *Athletic injuries to the head, neck, and face.* St. Louis: Mosby, 1991.

Wojtys EM, Hovda D, Landry G, et al. Concussion in sports. *Am J Sports Med* 1999;27:676–687.

Authors: Douglas Browning and Daryl A. Rosenbaum

Cuboid Subluxation and Fracture

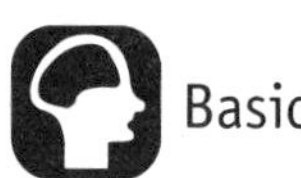

Basics

DEFINITION

Subluxation and Dislocation

- Midfoot injury that disrupts the ligamentous structures around the cuboid allowing subluxation and, rarely, complete dislocation of the cuboid. Both subluxation and dislocation usually occur in the plantar direction, but one case of dorsal subluxation has been reported. Mechanism of injury is often an inversion ankle sprain.

Fracture

- Fracture of the tarsal cuboid bone is thought to be due to indirect compression usually after significant traumatic force causing abduction of the forefoot. Has been reported in the literature to occur after falls or motor vehicle accidents. Other types of cuboid fractures include avulsion fractures and stress fractures.

INCIDENCE/PREVALENCE

Subluxation and Dislocation

- Both subluxation and complete dislocation are rare, but some propose that these injuries are underdiagnosed. One study of 3,600 athletes found 4% of foot problems stemmed from instability of the cuboid.

Fracture

- Rare

SIGNS AND SYMPTOMS

- Pain in lateral midfoot or over fourth and/or fifth metatarsal, exacerbated with activity
- Patient with subluxation or dislocation may have difficulty with ambulation. Most patients with fractures are unable to bear weight.
- Initial midfoot swelling often is present.

RISK FACTORS

- Pronated feet
- Tight peroneal longus tendon

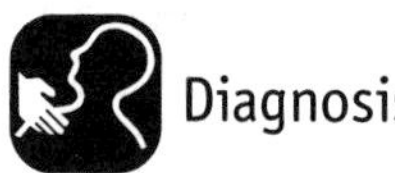

Diagnosis

DIFFERENTIAL DIAGNOSIS

- Peroneus longus tenosynovitis
- Base of fourth and fifth metatarsal stress fracture
- Calcaneonavicular coalition
- Peroneal longus tendon subluxation
- Os peroneum fracture

HISTORY

Subluxation and Dislocation

- May follow inversion ankle injury
- Determine new or increased activity
- Subluxation may be precipitated by increased routine activity, increased activity on uneven terrain, or initiation of new activity, especially for patient with excess pronation.

Fracture

- Substantial traumatic force needed due to stable ligamentous attachments

PHYSICAL EXAMINATION

- Midfoot swelling
- Tenderness to palpation over cuboid (dorsal and/or plantar surface)
- With complete dislocation, abnormal indentation in lateral midfoot occasionally noted

IMAGING

- Recommend anteroposterior, lateral, and oblique views
- Subluxation often not seen
- Oblique view usually demonstrates a cuboid fracture.
- Computed tomographic scan often beneficial if fracture present

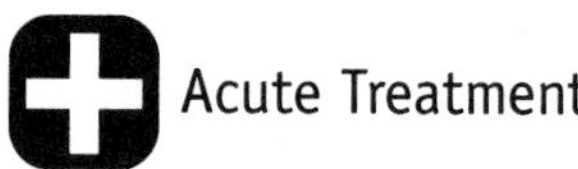

Acute Treatment

SUBLUXATION

- Literature suggests repeated manipulation, "the cuboid whip" or "cuboid squeeze" that attempts to reestablish proper alignment of the calcaneocuboid joint
- Patient stands with support, affected leg with knee bent to 90 degrees. Examiner grasps forefoot with fingers and places thumbs (one over the other) on plantar aspect of cuboid. Cuboid is manipulated with a quick downward thrust of the thumbs in a dorsal and lateral direction.
- Orthotics, use of cuboid pad, or taping recommended
- Strength and proprioception rehabilitation.

DISLOCATION

- Controversial
- Open fixation followed by short leg casting and nonweight-bearing for 6 weeks
- Closed reduction with local anesthesia

FRACTURE

- Controversial
- Open reduction with internal fixation, possibly requiring a bone graft, is the most commonly accepted treatment.
- Other options include conservative treatment with immobilization and surgical arthrodesis

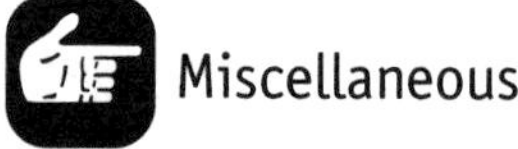

Miscellaneous

SYNONYMS

Subluxation and Dislocation

- Cuboid syndrome
- Locked cuboid
- Calcaneal cuboid fault syndrome
- Lateral plantar neuritis

Fracture

- Nutcracker fracture

ICD-9 CODE

755.69 Subluxation
838.01 Dislocation
825.23 Fracture

BIBLIOGRAPHY

Hunter JC, Sangeorzan BJ. A nutcracker fracture. *Am J Roentgenol* 1996;4:888.

Littlejohn SG, Line LL, Yerger LV Jr. Complete cuboid dislocation. *Orthopedics* 1995;19:175–176.

Main BJ, Jowett RL. Injuries of the midtarsal joint. *J Bone Joint Surg* 1975;57-B:89–97.

Mooney M, Maffey-Ward L. Cuboid plantar and dorsal subluxations: assessment. *J Orthopaed Sports Phys Ther* 1994;20(4): 220–226.

Newell SG, Woodle A. Cuboid syndrome. *Phys Sports Med* 1981;9:71–76.

Omey ML, Micheli LJ. Foot and ankle problems in the young athlete. *Med Sci Sports Exerc* 1999;31[7 Suppl]:S470–S486.

Sangeorzan BJ, Swintkowski MF. Displaced fractures of the cuboid. *J Bone Joint Surg* 1990;72-B:376–378.

Authors: Danielle Mahaffey and Karl B. Fields

Dental Trauma

Basics

SIGNS AND SYMPTOMS

- History of facial trauma
- Facial pain
  - —Tooth
  - —Jaw
  - —Ear
  - —Throat
- Exacerbating factors
  - —Chewing
  - —Drinking
  - —Extremes of temperature
- Pain on palpation
- Facial swelling
- Loose or avulsed tooth
- Oral or facial laceration

MECHANISM/DESCRIPTION

- Ellis classification
  - —Class I fracture
    - —Only involves the enamel
    - —Fracture line appears chalky white
    - —Painless to percussion
  - —Class II fracture
    - —Involves the enamel and dentin
    - —Ivory/yellow appearance
    - —Sensitive to cold
  - —Class III fracture
    - —Involves enamel, dentin, and pulp
    - —Exquisitely painful or desensitized
    - —Pinkish blush of blood after wiping the tooth
- Alveolar bone fractures
- Associated with dental fractures, avulsions, or subluxations
- Anterior overbite makes this part of dentition more susceptible to fractures in children
- With avulsed teeth, a 1% chance for successful reimplantation is lost every minute

ETIOLOGY

- Isolated injuries
- Fall
- Athletic event
- Assault
- Laryngoscopy
- Childhood activities
- Child abuse
- Multiple trauma

PRE-HOSPITAL

- Maintain a patent airway
- Account for all teeth
- Immediate reimplantation of tooth if possible
- Otherwise place in a transport solution
  - —Hanks solution (TPS—"tooth preserving system")
  - —Milk
  - —Saline
  - —Saliva (patient or parent's mouth)

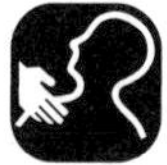

Diagnosis

ESSENTIAL WORKUP

- Time of injury
- Mechanism
- Changes in occlusion
- Account for all missing teeth
- Careful inspection of the oral cavity
  - —Soft tissue injuries
  - —Embedded fragments
  - —Associated injuries
  - —Salivary glands
  - —Ducts
  - —Nerves
  - —Blood vessels

IMAGING/SPECIAL TESTS

- Plain dental radiograph
  - —Ellis class III fractures
  - —Assess for associated root or alveolar fracture
- Panorex
  - —Indicated if there is a suspicion of associated injuries
    - —Foreign bodies
    - —Displacement of teeth
    - —Alveolar or jaw fractures
- Chest radiograph
  - —Indicated if a tooth or tooth fragment is missing
  - —Bronchoscopic removal is indicated for dental aspiration

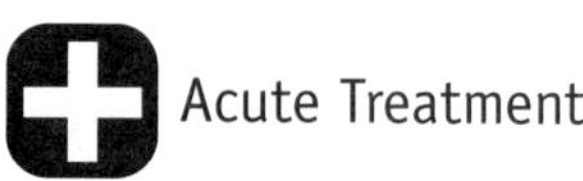

Acute Treatment

INITIAL STABILIZATION

- Ensure patent airway as needed
- Control bleeding by having the patient bite on gauze
- Account for all teeth and fragments
- Immediate reimplantation of avulsed tooth

ED TREATMENT

- Ellis class I
  - —Smooth sharp edges with an emory board
  - —Dental referral for cosmetic repair
- Ellis class II
  - —Dressing of calcium hydroxide paste
  - —Cover with dry foil, a metal band, or an enamel-bonded plastic
  - —Dental referral within 24 hours

- Ellis class III
    - —Immediate dental referral when available
        - —Pulpotomy by dentist
    - —If dental consultation is unavailable
        - —Place a piece of moist cotton over the exposed pulp
        - —Cover with dry foil
- Subluxed tooth
    - —Soft diet if minimally mobile
    - —Stabilization for more mobile teeth
- Tooth avulsion
    - —Rinse (do not scrub) in saline
    - —Administer local anesthesia
    - —Reinsert holding the tooth by the crown
    - —Temporary stabilization with a periodontal pack such as a "Coe-Pak"
        - —Mix resin and catalyst in even amounts to a firm consistency
        - —Apply to anterior and posterior surface of the avulsed tooth and adjacent two teeth
    - —Prophylactic antibiotic coverage
    - —Definitive stabilization by a dentist
- Alveolar fracture
    - —Oral surgery consult for stabilization
    - —Prophylactic antibiotic coverage

MEDICATIONS

- Clindamycin: adult: 300 mg po q 8 hrs; peds: 25–30 mg/kg/24 hrs po q 8 hrs
- Erythromycin: adult: 500 mg po q 6 hrs; peds: 30–50 mg/kg/24 hrs (max 2 g) po q 6 hrs
- Penicillin V: adult: 500 mg po q 6 hrs; peds: 25–50 mg/kg/24 hrs (max 3 g) po q 6 hrs
- Tylenol #3: adult: 2 tablets po q 4–6 hrs PRN; peds: codeine: 2.5–5.0 mg/kg/24 hrs (max 30 mg) po q 4–6 hrs for children 2–6 years old
- Tylenol and oxycodone: adult: 2 tablets po q 8 hrs PRN; peds: oxycodone: 0.05–0.15 mg/kg/dose (max 10 mg/dose)

HOSPITAL ADMISSION CRITERIA

- Admission for other associated injuries
- Suspected child abuse and no safe environment available

HOSPITAL DISCHARGE CRITERIA

- Isolated dental fractures
- Follow-up with a dentist
- Within 24 hours for avulsions, Ellis class II and Ellis class III fractures

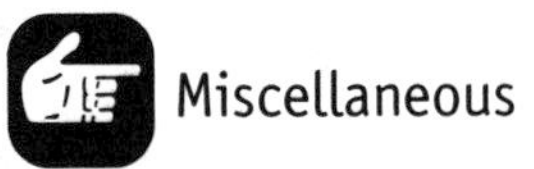

Miscellaneous

ICD-9 CODE

525.0

CORE CONTENT CODE

18.4.4.6

BIBLIOGRAPHY

Amsterdam JT. Dental disorders. In: Rosen P, et al., eds. *Emergency medicine: Concepts and clinical practice*. 4th ed. St. Louis: CV Mosby, 1998:2680–2697.

Medford HM. Acute care of avulsed teeth. *Ann Emerg Med* 1982;11:559.

Medford HM, Curtis JW. Acute care of severe tooth fractures. *Ann Emerg Med* 1983;12:364–365.

Powers MP. Diagnosis and management of dentoalveolar injuries. In: Fonseca RJ, Walker RV, eds. *Oral and maxillofacial trauma*. Philadelphia: WB Saunders, 1991:323–358.

Author: Marc J. Shapiro

de Quervain Tenosynovitis

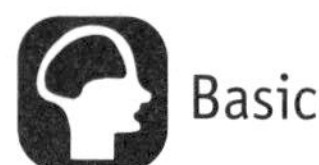

Basics

DEFINITION

- de Quervain tenosynovitis is an inflammation of the tendons and tendon sheaths of the first dorsal compartment of the wrist.
- It is the most frequently encountered tendonitis on the dorsal side of the wrist.
- The abductor pollicis longus (APL) and extensor pollicis brevis (EPB) tendons are involved.
- de Quervain tenosynovitis is typically an overuse injury, but may result from direct trauma.

INCIDENCE/PREVALENCE

- Usually seen in adults aged 30–50 years
- Ten times more common in females

SIGNS AND SYMPTOMS

- Pain near the radial styloid of the wrist
- Pain may radiate up the radial side of the forearm.

RISK FACTORS

- Activities requiring forceful grasp with excessive ulnar wrist deviation or repetitive use of the thumb, e.g., golfing, bowling, wrestling, fly fishing, racquet sports (squash, badminton, tennis), javelin or discus throwing

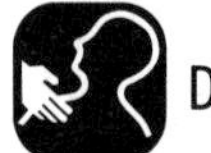

Diagnosis

DIFFERENTIAL DIAGNOSIS

- Trigger thumb
- Thumb carpometacarpal joint arthritis
- Intersection syndrome
- Flexor carpi radialis tendonitis
- Radial styloid fracture
- Scaphoid fracture
- Avascular necrosis of the scaphoid

HISTORY

- Pain for several weeks to months, felt near the radial styloid and aggravated by moving the wrist or thumb
- Pain may radiate up the dorsoradial aspect of the arm.

PHYSICAL EXAMINATION

- Tenderness to palpation of the APL and EPB tendons near the radial styloid process
- Positive Finkelstein test confirms diagnosis.
- Finkelstein test is performed by tucking the thumb into the palm and having the patient make a fist. Passive ulnar deviation will stretch the inflamed tendons and cause pain.

IMAGING

- Usually none needed
- If patient has history of trauma, obtain wrist x-rays to rule out fracture.

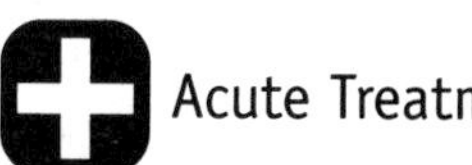

Acute Treatment

ANALGESIA

- Rest from offending activity for 2–3 weeks
- Ice most beneficial when used early
- Nonsteroidal anti-inflammatory drugs
- Immobilization
- Splinting (thumb spica) relieves pain, but may actually increase recovery time.

SPECIAL CONSIDERATIONS

- Corticosteroid injection is the most effective treatment.
- A 2-mL mixture of one third each lidocaine, bupivacaine, and dexamethasone phosphate can be injected into the first dorsal compartment at the point of maximum tenderness through a 25-gauge needle at a 45-degree angle, infiltrating the sheath from distal to proximal and causing a fusiform swelling if properly placed.
- Pain relief is immediate.
- Patient must be cautioned against overuse after an injection. Consider immobilization to minimize chance of tendon rupture.
- If no improvement is seen in 2 weeks, assume patient has an anatomical variant with two tendon sheaths in the first dorsal compartment. Can inject again in the same manner, but redirect needle to enter both tendon sheaths.
- Refer if second injection fails
- Anatomical variants seen in up to 40% of patients

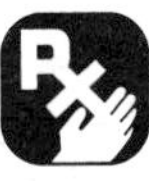

Long-Term Treatment

SURGERY

If conservative therapy is ineffective, surgical release of the fibrous first dorsal compartment may be considered.

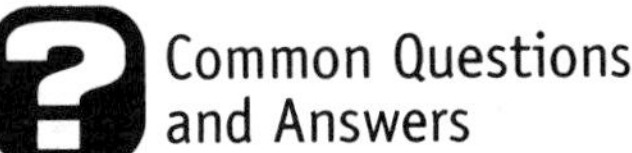

Common Questions and Answers

Physician responses to common patient questions:

Q: What is tenosynovitis?
A: Inflammation involving the tendon and its sheath. Occurs from either direct trauma or from repetitive overuse.
Q: How can I prevent recurrence of de Quervain syndrome?
A: Change your technique when doing repetitive wrist activities.
Q: Why did the injection fail?
A: Two separate sheaths for the APL and EPB may be present. Anatomical variants are seen in up to 40% of patients. Sometimes takes >1 injection, even in cases without anatomical variant.

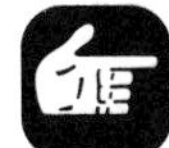

Miscellaneous

SYNONYMS

- Extensor tendonitis
- Stenosing tenosynovitis

ICD-9 CODE

727.04

BIBLIOGRAPHY

Aluisio FV, Christensen CP, Urbaniak JR. De Quervain's stenosing tenosynovitis. *Orthopedics,* 2nd ed. Baltimore: Williams & Wilkins, 1998:200–201.

Andersen B, Manthey R, Brouns M. Treatment of De Quervain's tenosynovitis with corticosteroids. *Arthritis Rheum* 1991;34:793–798.

Dvorkin ML. De Quervain's syndrome. *Office Orthoped* 1993;124–126.

Harvey FJ, Harvey PM, Horsley MW. De Quervain's disease: surgical or nonsurgical treatment. *J Hand Surg* 1990;15A:83–87.

Mercier LR. Stenosing tenosynovitis. *Pract Orthoped* 1994;106–107.

Paget S, Pellicci P, Beary JF III, eds. *Manual of rheumatology and outpatient orthopedic disorders.* New York: Little Brown and Company, 1993.

Urbaniak JR, Roth JH. Tendinitis and tenosynovitis. *Orthoped Clin North Am* 1982;13(3):483–485.

Weiss AP, Akelman E, Tabatabai M. Treatment of De Quervain's disease. *J Hand Surg* 1994;19A:595–598.

Witt W, Pess G, Gelberman RH. Treatment of de Quervain tenosynovitis. *J Bone Joint Surg* 1991;73A:219–222.

Zingas C, Failla JM, Van Holsbeeck M. Injection accuracy and clinical relief of de Quervain's tendinitis. *J Hand Surg* 1998;23A:89–96.

Authors: Gregory N. Rocco, Carlton A. Richie III, William W. Briner Jr., and Thomas A. Balcom

DIP Dislocation

Basics

DEFINITION

- Dislocations of distal interphalangeal (DIP) or first interphalangeal (IP) joints
- Mechanism is typically a hyperextension injury of the DIP joint.

INCIDENCE/PREVALENCE

- Pure DIP dislocations are uncommon. Dislocations usually are accompanied by a bony avulsion fracture.
- Most are acute dorsal dislocations.
- Simultaneous DIP and PIP dislocations are rare, occurring most commonly in ring and small fingers.

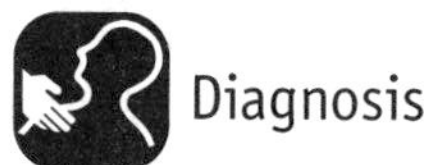

Diagnosis

DIFFERENTIAL DIAGNOSIS

- Fracture of distal or middle phalanx
- Flexor digitorum profundus (FDP) rupture (i.e., jersey finger)
- Extensor mechanism rupture (i.e., Mallet finger)
- Bony Mallet finger (bony avulsion of the insertion of extensor mechanism at the dorsal base of the distal phalanx)
- Fracture-dislocation
- Collateral ligament disruption
- Chronic dislocation

HISTORY

- Mechanism of injury (i.e., hyperextension)
- Presence of an obvious deformity (e.g., distal phalanx positioned above or below the plane of the middle phalanx)
- Often self-reduced by the patient

PHYSICAL EXAMINATION

- Obvious deformity if not already reduced: distal phalanx sitting above (dorsal dislocation) or below (volar dislocation) the plane of the middle phalanx
- Careful neurologic examination: Check flexor and extensor function (with the PIP joint held in extension) of the DIP joint and sensation at the tip of the finger.
- Check collateral ligament: Place radial and ulnar stress across DIP joint with joint in full extension and 30 degrees flexion looking for increased laxity.
- Check volar plate: Increased hyperextension of joint is indicative of a volar plate injury.

IMAGING

- Radiographs: at least two views, anteroposterior and lateral; oblique view is useful if fracture is suspected but not seen on other two views
- Look carefully for any bony avulsion.

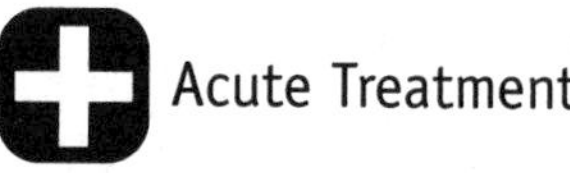

Acute Treatment

REDUCTION TECHNIQUES

- On-field reduction should be attempted to reduce pain and usually is easily performed when done acutely.
- Apply forceful longitudinal traction
- May require a digital block if dislocation is prolonged or associated with significant pain

POSTREDUCTION EVALUATION

- Careful examination as above, especially checking neurovascular status
- Postreduction radiographs from at least two views

IMMOBILIZATION

- Splint only the DIP joint in slight extension for 2–3 weeks
- Can use a dorsal or volar splint

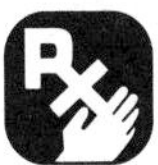

Long-Term Treatment

REHABILITATION

- Range of motion (ROM) exercises after splint removal
- Both active and passive ROM initially
- Start resisted ROM as soon as active and passive motions are pain-free

REFERRAL/DISPOSITION

- Inability to reduce dislocation closed
- Open fracture-dislocation
- Chronic dislocations
- FDP rupture
- Unstable collateral ligaments

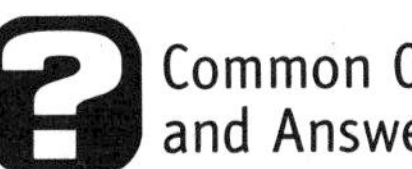

Common Questions and Answers

Physician responses to common patient questions:
Q: When can I return to play?
A: Immediately, if dislocation is uncomplicated and reduced and the athlete is allowed to play with a splint
Q: How do I treat thumb IP dislocations?
A: Treat exactly the same as for DIP dislocations

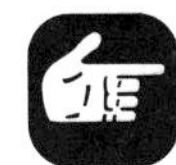

Miscellaneous

SYNONYMS

- Jammed finger

ICD-9 CODE

843.02

BIBLIOGRAPHY

Eiff MP, Hatch RL, Calmbach WL. *Fracture management for primary care: finger fractures.* Philadelphia: WB Saunders, 1998.

Green DP, Butler TE. *Rockwood and Green's fractures in adults, vol. 1,* 4th ed. Philadelphia: Lippincott-Raven Publishers, 1996.

Green DP, Strickland JW. *Orthopaedic sports medicine: principles and practice, the hand.* Philadelphia: WB Saunders, 1994.

Palmer RE. Joint injuries of the hand in athletes. *Clin Sports Med* 1998;17:513–531.

Author: William W. Dexter

Dislocation, Hip, Posterior

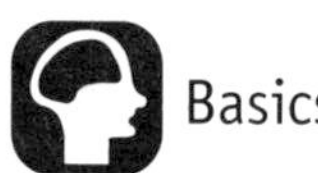

Basics

DEFINITION

- Posterior hip dislocation is an orthopaedic emergency in which the femoral head is displaced posteriorly relative to the acetabulum.
- Of primary concern when evaluating the patient with a posterior hip dislocation is the search for additional injuries (often life or limb threatening due to the excessive forces necessary to create this injury) and the attainment of early reduction (within 12 hours) to prevent long-term sequelae.
- In the case of posterior dislocation without fracture, the experienced physician may perform one attempt at closed reduction. If reduction is not accomplished with ease or if there is an associated fracture of the hip, then urgent orthopaedic consultation is warranted.

INCIDENCE/PREVALENCE

- Because of the forces required for this injury, it is relatively uncommon in contact sports. Seen more often in high-energy trauma such as with motor sports, equestrian events, and high-speed mountain sports.
- Accounts for about 90% of all hip dislocations

SIGNS AND SYMPTOMS

- Immediate severe pain and disability
- Limb shortening with hip flexion, internal rotation, and adduction
- Classic position may be absent if there is an associated femoral shaft fracture

RISK FACTORS

- High-energy trauma
- Most common mechanism is knee striking the dashboard in a head-on motor vehicle accident (depending on the position of the hip, this can result in either anterior or posterior dislocation)

ASSOCIATED INJURIES AND COMPLICATIONS

- Life-threatening internal organ damage, bleeding, and shock
- Ipsilateral sciatic nerve injured in 10% to 14% of cases; changes a posterior hip dislocation from an orthopaedic urgency to a true surgical emergency
- Irreducible dislocations occur in up to 16% of simple posterior dislocations
- Fractures of the pelvis, acetabulum, femoral head/neck, and femoral shaft
- Ligamentous injury to the ipsilateral knee not uncommon when the mechanism of injury involves a blow to the anterior knee
- Delayed reduction increases risk of avascular necrosis
- Other chronic complications include recurrent posterior dislocation, posttraumatic arthritis, and myositis ossificans of the thigh or buttocks

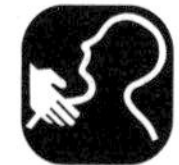

Diagnosis

DIFFERENTIAL DIAGNOSIS

- Anterior dislocation of the hip
- Combined fracture-dislocation
- Fracture of the pelvis, acetabulum, or femur
- Gastrointestinal or genitoureteral visceral injury

HISTORY

Q: Mechanism?
A: Can help guide the search for associated visceral and orthopaedic injuries
Q: Position at time of injury?
A: Simple posterior dislocation most commonly occurs with force on a flexed knee with the hip in varying degrees of flexion and adduction. Addition of hip abduction increases the risk of associated acetabular fracture or anterior dislocation.

PHYSICAL EXAMINATION

- Vital signs and complete trauma evaluation essential because of the high association with life-threatening injuries
- Look for classic presenting position as described above. Femoral head may be palpable in the buttocks.
- Pelvic rocking and pubic compression tests to examine for associated pelvic rim fractures
- Distal neurovascular examination to assess for sciatic nerve or vascular injures, which merit more urgent reduction

IMAGING

- Initial x-rays: anteroposterior (AP) and lateral views of the pelvis. AP often reveals the dislocation, but a true lateral may be needed to confirm the direction.
- Search for associated pelvic rim, acetabular, femoral head/neck, and femoral shaft fractures generally merits additional x-rays, including three-quarter internal and external obliques of the pelvis as well as femur films.

POSTREDUCTION VIEWS

- X-rays to ascertain adequacy of reduction
- Computed tomographic (CT) scan to evaluate for presence of osteochondral fragments and acetabular fractures; should be part of the standard postreduction evaluation

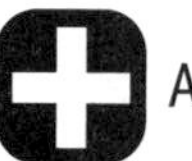

Acute Treatment

ANALGESIA

- Will often require intravenous analgesics and muscle relaxants to overcome severe pain and muscular spasm before closed reduction can be attempted
- May require spinal or general anesthesia to achieve closed reduction

REDUCTION TECHNIQUES

- Simple posterior dislocation without fracture should be reduced by closed reduction as early as possible.
- Allis method: An assistant stabilizes the pelvis of the supine patient with downward pressure on the anterior superior iliac spines. The operator applies axial traction in line with the deformity by pulling with his or her hands from behind the flexed knee. While maintaining this traction, the hip is gently flexed to 90 degrees and then gently internally and externally rotated until reduction occurs.
- Posterior fracture-dislocations, or simple dislocations that are not easily reducible with one attempt, should be referred for orthopaedic consultation.

POSTREDUCTION EVALUATION

- Repeat AP and lateral x-rays immediately, as well as CT scan within hours as described above
- Repeat neurovascular examination of the injured limb

IMMOBILIZATION

After successful closed reduction, start light skin traction of 5 to 8 lb to prevent hip flexion, internal rotation, and adduction (protects the hip from recurrent dislocation while the capsule heals). Early pain-free range of motion is encouraged. Traction is maintained for a few days to 2 weeks, until the hip is pain free through full range of motion.

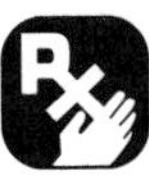

Long-Term Treatment

REHABILITATION

- Physical therapy should start with range of motion exercises while the patient is still in traction and continue to include muscle rehabilitation and strengthening once out of traction.
- Weight-bearing can start as soon as the patient is comfortable. Exceptions to early weight-bearing are those patients at increased risk for AVN, including those in whom reduction was not achieved in the first 12 hours (in these patients, weight-bearing may be delayed up to 6–12 weeks depending of risk of AVN).

SURGERY

Urgent referral should be made for any patient in whom closed reduction does not result in easy reduction or in any case of fracture-dislocation. Reduction in <12 hours is the goal to reduce the risk of AVN. More urgent reduction is needed if there is associated neurovascular compromise.

REFERRAL/DISPOSITION

- Admission, often to trauma service, for continued evaluation and treatment of associated injuries
- In the case of isolated posterior dislocation managed with closed reduction, patient can be discharged when outpatient traction devices, physical therapy, and caregiver support have been arranged.

Common Questions and Answers

Physician responses to common patient questions:
Q: When can I start walking again?
A: In an isolated posterior dislocation without fracture treated with closed reduction within 12 hours of injury, the patient may start weight-bearing as soon as comfort allows. This may be as early as 2 weeks after injury.
Q: Will I have chronic problems because of this injury?
A: Whereas a significant delay between dislocation and reduction may increase the risk of AVN, the overall long-term prognosis is most dependent on the severity of the initial trauma.

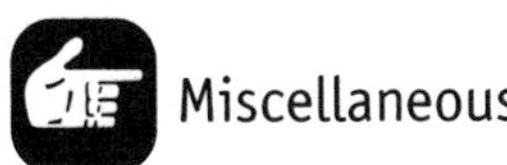

Miscellaneous

ICD-9 CODE

835.01 Dislocation of hip, closed, posterior
835.11 Dislocation of hip, open, posterior

BIBLIOGRAPHY

Kum C, Tan S. Traumatic posterior dislocation of the hip. *Singapore Med J* 1990;31:22–25.

Rockwood C, Green D, Bucholz R, et al., eds. *Rockwood and Green's fractures in adults,* 4th ed. Philadelphia: Lippincott-Raven Publishers, 1996.

Schlickewei W, Elseasser B, Mullaji A, et al. Hip dislocation without fracture. *Injury* 1993;24:27–31.

Author: Greg Nakamoto

Distal Clavicular Osteolysis

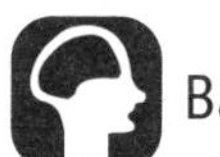

Basics

DEFINITION

- A loss of subchondral bone detail with osteoporosis, cystic changes, osteolysis, and osteophyte formation of the distal clavicle while sparing the acromion
- Although the specific pathophysiologic cause has not been determined, it is thought to start as a stress fracture of the distal clavicle from repetitive microtrauma.

INCIDENCE/PREVALENCE

- Not common
- Usually seen in power weight-lifters. Can be seen as a result of trauma. First described in an air-hammer operator.
- In one study of 25 Danish weight-lifters and 25 age-matched controls, 28% had classic radiographic changes and 16% had symptoms with x-ray changes.
- In another study of 46 men with radiologic evidence, 45 engaged in weight-training.

SIGNS AND SYMPTOMS

- Patient complains of a dull ache over the acromioclavicular (AC) joint.
- Mild swelling of the joint may be present.
- Pain usually is worse at the beginning of the exercise period.
- Any movement of the arm requiring 90 degrees or more of abduction causes pain.
- Pain can radiate to the adjacent superior trapezius border and deltoid muscles.

RISK FACTORS

- Any activity putting excessive repetitive force on the AC joint
- Occasionally will result from blunt trauma to the shoulder. Can be seen in hockey, football, rugby, wrestling, skiing, skating, and bicycling.
- Traumatic injuries include AC joint dislocation and separation, as well as clavicle fractures.

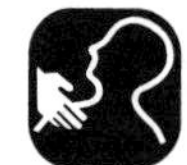

Diagnosis

DIFFERENTIAL DIAGNOSIS

- Includes hyperparathyroidism, connective tissue disorders, and infection
- Other shoulder pathology should be considered, i.e., instability, impingement, rotator cuff tears, tendinitis, and labral disease.

HISTORY

- Slow onset of ache to AC joint
- Can have history of remote trauma
- Will engage in activities placing repetitive stress to the joint
- In weight-lifters, bench press, military press, shoulder shrugs, and clean-and-jerk cause pain.

PHYSICAL EXAMINATION

- Tenderness over the AC joint
- Positive cross-arm test: Forward flexion to 90 degrees and adduction of the arm causes pain. This compresses the AC joint.
- Sometimes a trapezius spasm will be palpated.

IMAGING

- Clavicular view: 35 degrees of cephalic tilt. Distal clavicular end will appeared frayed. Will see bony osteolysis, cystic changes, and translucency of the bone.
- Technetium bone scan can be helpful as an additional test.

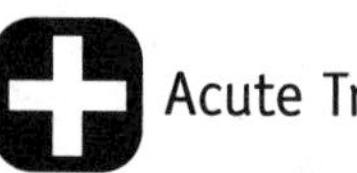

Acute Treatment

ANALGESIA

- Nonsteroidal anti-inflammatory drugs or other pain medications can be given, but currently no studies evaluating efficacy have been reported.
- Cessation of activity is the best medicine.
- Ice in the acute phase almost always is helpful.

SPECIAL CONSIDERATIONS

If rest and activity modification do not produce relief, then AC joint injection including steroids can be attempted.

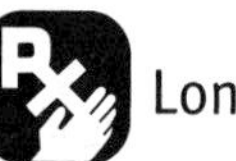

Long-Term Treatment

- Rehabilitation
- Behavior modification is the cornerstone. This is the main reason for nonsurgical failure.
- Activity modification by weight-lifters should include decreased weight with increased repetitions or substitution of exercises.

- Other aspects should include range of motion therapy and strengthening exercises for the rotator cuff and scapulothoracic stabilizer muscles.
- Once the offending activity is discontinued, it takes 4-6 months for the degenerative stage to decrease and reparative change to occur.

SURGERY

- Currently surgery produces the best results.
- Can be done arthroscopically. This allows for smaller section of bone to be resected. Patients who do best with this procedure are those without other shoulder pathology.
- The most common technique is the Mumford. This requires an open incision and removal of 1–2 cm of the distal clavicle. This is especially useful if transfer of the coracoacromial ligaments is needed to stabilize the clavicle.

REFERRAL/DISPOSITION

- Referral to orthopedic surgeon for nonsurgical failure

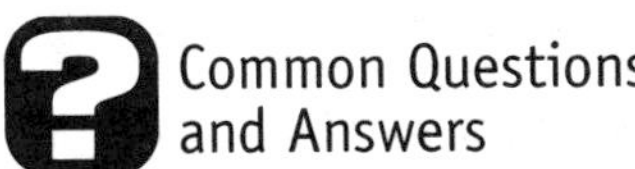

Common Questions and Answers

Physician responses to common patient questions:
Q: Will this go away without surgery?
A: Yes, but only a minority of cases produce satisfactory results, mostly because the athlete did not want to stop training long enough for the AC joint to heal.

Q: Will I ever be able to compete at the same level?
A: Yes, studies have shown athletes can return to their former level of competition after surgical resection.

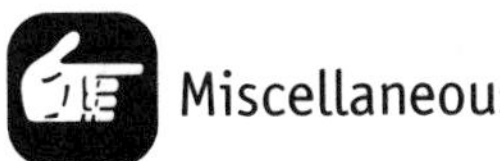

Miscellaneous

ICD-9 CODE

No specific ICD-9 code

- 810.03 Fracture clavicle AC end
- 716.91 Shoulder arthritis
- 840.9 Shoulder sprain

BIBLIOGRAPHY

Auge WK II, Fischer RA. Arthroscopic distal clavicle resection for isolated atraumatic osteolysis in weight lifters. *Am J Sports Med* 1998;26:189–192.

Cahill BR. Osteolysis of the distal part of the clavicle in male athletes. *J Bone Joint Surg* 1982;64A:1053–1058.

Hawkins BJ, Covey DC, Thiel BG. Distal clavicle osteolysis unrelated to trauma, overuse, or metabolic disease. *Clin Orthop* 2000;370:208–211.

Scavenius M, Iversen BF. Nontraumatic clavicular osteolysis in weight lifters. *Am J Sports Med* 1992;20:463–467.

Scuderi GR, McMann PD, Bruno PJ. *Sports medicine principles of primary care.* St. Louis: Mosby, 1997.

Woodward TW, Best TM. The painful shoulder. *Am Fam Physician* 2000;61:3291–3300.

Author: Todd May

Dupuytren's Contracture

Basics

DESCRIPTION

Contracture of the palmar fascia due to fibrous proliferation resulting in flexion deformities and loss of function. Similar change may rarely occur in plantar fascia. It usually appears simultaneously.

System(s) affected: Musculoskeletal

Genetics:

- Autosomal dominant with variable penetrance
- 10% of patients have a positive family history

Incidence/Prevalence in USA:

- Unknown
- Norway—9% males and 3% females

Predominant age: 50 for males; 60 for females

Predominant sex: Male Female (ranges from 2:1 to 10:1)

SIGNS AND SYMPTOMS

- Typical
  - —Caucasian male 50–60
  - —Bilateral with one hand more involved
  - —Family history
  - —Unilateral or bilateral (50%)
  - —Right hand more frequent
  - —Ring finger more frequent
  - —Ulnar digits more affected than radial
  - —Mild pain early
  - —Later painless plaques or nodules in palmar fascia
  - —Extends into a cord-like band in the palmar fascia
  - —Skin adheres to fascia and becomes puckered
  - —Nodules can be palpated under the skin
  - —Digital fascia becomes involved as disease progresses
  - —Web space contractures
  - —Dupuytren's diathesis can involve plantar (Ledderhose's—10%) and penile (Peyronie's—2%) fascia
  - —Knuckle pads
- Atypical
  - —No age, gender differences
  - —No family history
  - —May have systemic disease (see Risk Factors)
  - —May have a history of trauma
  - —More common unilateral
  - —No ectopic manifestations (Ledderhose's or Peyronies)
  - —Nonprogressive

CAUSES

- Unknown
- Ischemia to the fascia with oxygen free radical formation
- Possibly related to release of angiogenic basic fibroblast growth factor
- Related to microhemorrhage and release of growth factors

RISK FACTORS

- Smoking (mean 16 pack-years, odds ratio 2.8)
- Alcohol intake
- Increasing age
- Male/Caucasian
- Diabetes mellitus (one-third affected, increases with time, usually mild; middle and ring finger involved)
- Epilepsy
- Chronic illness (e.g., pulmonary tuberculosis, liver disease)
- Hypercholesterolemia
- Liver disease
- HIV infection

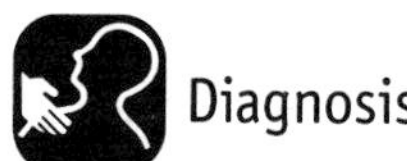

Diagnosis

DIFFERENTIAL DIAGNOSIS

- Early for callosity
- Tendon abnormalities
- Camplodactyly—early teens tight facial bands ulnar side of small finger

LABORATORY

N/A

Drugs that may alter lab results: N/A
Disorders that may alter lab results: N/A

PATHOLOGICAL FINDINGS

- Myofibroblasts
- First stage (proliferative)—increased myofibroblasts
- Second stage (residual)—dense fibroblast network
- Third stage (involutional)—myofibroblasts disappear

SPECIAL TESTS

N/A

IMAGING

MR can assess cellularity of lesions which correlate with higher recurrence after surgery

DIAGNOSTIC PROCEDURES

N/A

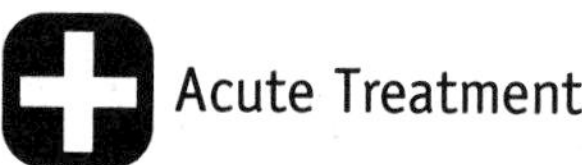

Acute Treatment

APPROPRIATE HEALTH CARE

- Outpatient monitoring and physical therapy
- Inpatient if surgery indicated

GENERAL MEASURES

- Steroid injection for acute tender nodule
- Physiotherapy is ineffective alone
- Isolated involvement of palmar fascia can be followed
- Metacarpophalangeal (MP) joint involvement can be followed if flexion contracture is 30 degrees

SURGICAL MEASURES

- Surgery—selective fascial ray release
  - —Indications: Any involvement of the proximal interphalangeal (PIP) joints. Hueston's table-top test, if positive, consider surgery (when the palm is placed on a flat surface, the digits can not be simultaneously placed fully on the same surface as the palm because of flexion contractures).
  - —May require skin grafts for wound closure with severe cutaneous shrinkage
  - —80% have full range of movement if operated on early
  - —Continuous elongation technique is useful to prepare a severely contracted PIP joint for surgery. The digit can frequently be completely extended, however, will relapse if surgery not performed.
  - —Amputation of little finger, if severe and deforming

ACTIVITY

- No restrictions
- Physical therapy after surgery—started 3–5 days after surgery (passive and active exercises, posterior dynamic extension splints)

DIET

No special diet

PATIENT EDUCATION

- Avoid risk factors especially with a strong family history
- Regular follow-up by physician every 6 months–1 year

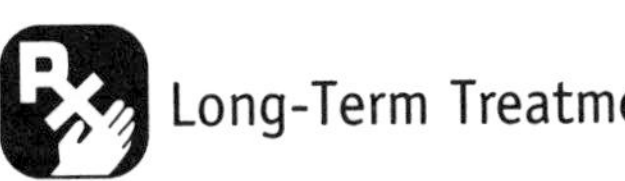

Long-Term Treatment

DRUG(S) OF CHOICE

Steroid injection for an acute tender nodule, painful knuckle pad

ALTERNATIVE DRUGS

Topical high-potency steroids—case report of improvement with clobetasol 0.1% bid and hs for 2–4 weeks

PATIENT MONITORING

Follow patient in early stages of disease.

PREVENTION/AVOIDANCE

None known. Avoid risk factors when possible.

POSSIBLE COMPLICATIONS

- Postsurgery development of reflex sympathetic dystrophy
- Postoperative recurrence or extension 46–80%
- Postoperative hand edema and skin necrosis
- Digital infarction

EXPECTED COURSE/PROGNOSIS

- Typical
  —Unpredictable, but usually slowly progressive
  —Patients likely to have aggressive disease (one or more) 40 at onset, knuckle pads, positive family history, bilateral disease involving radial side of hand
  —Reports of clinical regression with continuous passive skeletal traction in extension and under a skin graft
  —Recurrence rate after surgery is 10–34%
  —Prognosis better for MP joint vs PIP joint after surgery
- Atypical
  —Nonprogressive
  —Surgery rarely needed
  —Recurrence unlikely if surgery performed

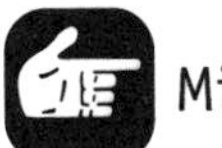

Miscellaneous

ASSOCIATED CONDITIONS

- Alcoholism
- Epilepsy
- Diabetes mellitus
- Chronic lung disease
- Occupational hand trauma (vibration white finger)
- Shoulder-hand syndrome
- Status post myocardial infarction
- Hypercholesterolemia

AGE-RELATED FACTORS

Pediatric: N/A
Geriatric: Primarily in this age group
Others: N/A

ICD-9 CODE

728.6 Contracture of palmar fascia (Dupuytren's)

ABBREVIATIONS

MP = Metacarpophalangeal
PIP = proximal interphalangeal

BIBLIOGRAPHY

Attali P, Ink O, et al. Dupuytren's contracture, alcohol consumption and chronic liver disease. *Arch Intern Med* 1987;147: 1065-67.

Hill N, Hurst L. Dupuytren's contracture. *Hand Clinics* 1989;5(3):349-57.

Hueston JT. Repression of Dupuytren's contracture. *J of Hand Surg* 1992;17(4): 453-57.

McFarlane RM. The current status of Dupuytren's disease. *J of Hand Surg* 1995;8(3):181-4.

Rayan G. Clinical presentation of Dupuytren's disease. *Hand Clinics* 1999;15(1):87-96.

Way LW. *Current surgical diagnosis & treatment*. 8th Ed. Los Altos, CA, Lange, 1989.

Internet references: http://www.5mcc.com

Author: Jeffrey F. Minteer

Elbow Dislocation

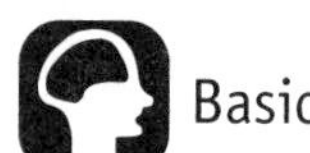

Basics

DEFINITION

- Consists of complete dissociation of the ulnohumeral joint of the elbow
- Simple dislocation implies no significant associated fracture.
- Complex dislocation has an associated fracture often requiring surgical treatment.

INCIDENCE/PREVALENCE

- The elbow is the second most frequently dislocated major joint after the shoulder.
- Comprises 10% to 25% of all elbow injuries
- More frequently seen in wrestling, gymnastics, football, falls, and motor vehicle accidents

SIGNS AND SYMPTOMS

- Diagnosis usually can be made clinically, but radiographs are important.
- Almost all dislocations are posterior (i.e., the olecranon is posterior to the humerus). The majority are posterolateral or posteromedial. Anterior dislocations are extremely rare.
- An obvious visual deformity usually is present.

RISK FACTORS

- Anatomical risk factors include a shallow olecranon fossa and a prominent olecranon tip.
- Age and sports activity

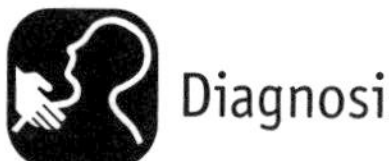

Diagnosis

DIFFERENTIAL DIAGNOSIS

- Elbow fracture
- Elbow subluxation
- Spontaneous elbow dislocation and reduction
- Be especially cautious in the pediatric age group, as supracondylar elbow fractures are common in 5- to 10-year-olds.

HISTORY

- Participation in wrestling, gymnastics, or contact sports
- Involvement in motor vehicle accidents or significant falls

PHYSICAL EXAMINATION

- First inspect the injured extremity and check for other injuries.
- Note the condition of the skin; look for wounds or an open dislocation.
- Perform a careful neurovascular examination. Injury to the brachial artery has been described.

IMAGING

- Biplanar radiographs are critical. The vast majority are posterior dislocations.
- Look for associated fractures. If suspicious, obtain radiographs of the wrist to evaluate for possible associated injury.

POSTREDUCTION VIEWS

- Postreduction radiographs should show a stable concentrically reduced elbow. The capitellum should point to the radial head on all views.
- Be alert for associated fractures.

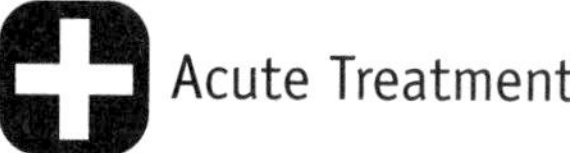

Acute Treatment

ANALGESIA

- In experienced hands, attempted reduction may be performed on the field without analgesia. Otherwise, transport patient to a medical facility where radiographs can be obtained before reduction.
- Intravenous midazolam supplemented with a narcotic medication can be useful for providing adequate analgesia during reduction. Appropriate monitoring is required and proper resuscitation equipment should be available.
- In rare instances, general anesthesia in the operating room may be required.

REDUCTION TECHNIQUES

- Reduction can be performed using several different techniques.
- Our preferred method is to place the patient in a prone position. Correct medial or lateral translation. Initiate gentle traction on the proximal forearm, with an assistant holding countertraction on the brachium. Gently supinate the arm. Apply direct pressure to the olecranon. A nice "clunk" will signify reduction.

POSTREDUCTION EVALUATION

- Check elbow stability and document range of motion
- Obtain postreduction radiographs
- Immobilize the elbow in a posterior splint at 90 degrees flexion
- Perform a postreduction neurovascular examination

IMMOBILIZATION

Duration of elbow immobilization is a controversial issue. Recommendations vary from 1 day to 2 weeks. We advocate initiating immediate active range of motion for simple elbow dislocations beginning on the first postreduction day.

SPECIAL CONSIDERATIONS

A follow-up radiograph should be obtained 1 and 2 weeks after injury. A small percentage of patients will develop recurrent instability, which can be due to insufficiency of the lateral ulnar collateral ligament. These patients may require surgical reconstruction to restore stability.

Long-Term Treatment

REHABILITATION

Rehabilitation after simple elbow dislocation requires 1–3 months to return to preinjury status. Typically, the outcome is good, with most athletes experiencing little morbidity or loss of function. The most common problem is loss of extension, which is minimized with an active, aggressive early rehabilitation program.

SURGERY

- Surgery is indicated only in select circumstances. Complex dislocations with fractures, including significant radial head, olecranon, and coronoid fractures, require surgical stabilization.
- Grossly unstable elbows may require acute ligament repair to confer early stability to allow for motion and rehabilitation.
- Chronically unstable elbows may require reconstruction of the lateral ulnar collateral ligament.

REFERRAL/DISPOSITION

Consultation with an orthopaedic surgeon should be obtained in most cases.

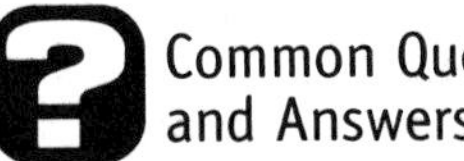

Common Questions and Answers

Physician responses to common patient questions:

Q: How long should a simple elbow dislocation be immobilized?

A: Our recent data indicate that, in most cases, the earlier active motion is initiated, the better the overall outcome.

Q: What are some of the complications of elbow dislocations?

A: Stiffness is the most common problem. Other complications are neurologic injury, heterotopic ossification, wrist ligament injuries, and recurrent instability.

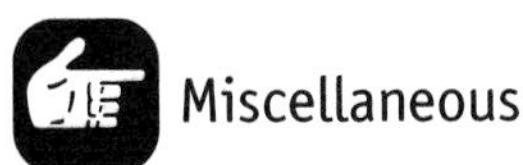

Miscellaneous

ICD-9 CODE

823.00 Closed
832.11 Open

BIBLIOGRAPHY

Cohen MS, Hastings H. Acute elbow dislocation: evaluation and management. *J Am Acad Orthopaed Surg* 1998;6:15–23.

Mehlhoff TL, Noble P, Bennet J, et al. Simple dislocation of the elbow in the adult. *J Bone Joint Surgery Am* 1988;70:244–249.

Morrey BF, ed. *The elbow and its disorders.* Philadelphia: WB Saunders, 1993.

Ross G, Chronister R, Ove P, et al. Treatment of elbow dislocation utilizing an immediate motion protocol. *Am J Sports Med* 1999;3: 308–311.

Wadstrom J, Kinast J, Pfeiffer K. Anatomical variations of the semilunar notch in elbow dislocations. *Arch Orthop Trauma Surg* 1986; 105:313–315.

Authors: Glen Ross, Andrew R. Curran, and Arnold D. Scheller Jr.

Extensor Tendon Avulsion from the Distal Phalanx/Mallet Finger

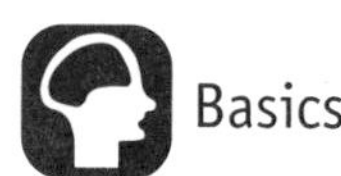

Basics

DEFINITION

The so-called "mallet finger" injury occurs when the extensor tendon is avulsed from the dorsal aspect of the base of the distal phalanx. The extensor tendon is avulsed when the distal interphalangeal (DIP) joint is forcibly flexed while being actively extended by the patient, as when catching a ball.

SIGNS AND SYMPTOMS

- Symptoms: Patient reports pain at the dorsum of the DIP joint.
- Signs: Patient is tender at the dorsum of the DIP joint and is unable to extend the DIP joint.

RISK FACTORS

- Sports (i.e., catching a ball)

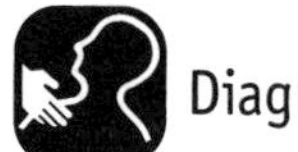

Diagnosis

DIFFERENTIAL DIAGNOSIS

- Tuft fracture deformity

HISTORY

- Patient reports forced flexion of DIP joint while it is being held in extension (e.g., when catching a ball).
- Patient reports pain at DIP joint, especially the dorsal aspect.

PHYSICAL EXAMINATION

- Tender at dorsum of DIP joint
- Lack of active extension at DIP joint. Examiner should isolate extension at the affected DIP joint by placing all fingers in the flexed position.

IMAGING

- Three views of the affected finger: anteroposterior, lateral, oblique
- Three patterns: no avulsion fracture; small avulsion fracture (<30% articular surface); large avulsion fracture (>30% articular surface)

POSTREDUCTION VIEWS

- Not necessary

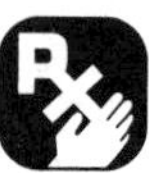

Acute Treatment

- Splint DIP joint in extension for 6–10 weeks
- Instruct patient to maintain extension when changing the splint.
- Recheck patient at 1 week.

ANALGESIA

- Usually not necessary

IMMOBILIZATION

Splint DIP joint in extension for 6–10 weeks: 6 weeks for bony avulsion; 10 weeks for tendon avulsion (without bony avulsion)

SPECIAL CONSIDERATIONS

- Strict extension of DIP joint (i.e., teach patient how to change splints without testing range of motion at DIP joint)
- No avulsion fracture
- More difficult to heal; requires prolonged immobilization (i.e., 10 weeks)

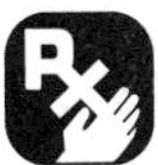

Long-Term Treatment

- Prolonged immobilization
- No avulsion fracture: splint in extension for 10 weeks
- Small avulsion fracture: splint in extension for 6 weeks
- Large avulsion fracture: consider pin fixation

REHABILITATION

DIP joint often is stiff after prolonged immobilization and requires physical therapy to regain full range of motion.

SURGERY

- Not usually indicated. Pin fixation usually causes bony overgrowth and limited range of motion at the DIP joint.
- Indicated only if large avulsion fragment causes joint instability

REFERRAL/DISPOSITION

- Large avulsion fragment
- Failed 10 weeks of splinting

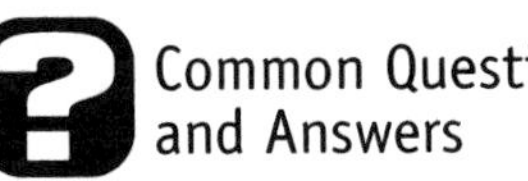

Common Questions and Answers

Q: Is the mallet deformity apparent after the injury?
A: The typical "mallet finger" appearance is sometimes not present until 6–8 weeks after injury. Early diagnosis requires a high index of suspicion and testing of active extension at the DIP joint.
Q: How long should the patient splint the DIP joint in extension?
A: For extensor tendon avulsions with bony avulsions, the DIP joint should be splinted in extension for 6 weeks; for tendon avulsions without bony avulsion, the DIP joint should be splinted in extension for 10 weeks.

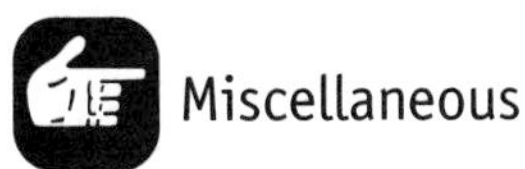

Miscellaneous

SYNONYMS

- Mallet finger

ICD-9 CODE

736.1 Mallet, finger (acquired)

BIBLIOGRAPHY

Green DP, Rowland SA. Fractures and dislocations in the hand. In: Rockwood CA Jr, Green DP, Bucholz RW, eds. *Rockwood and Green's fractures in adults*, 3rd ed. Philadelphia: JP Lippincott, 1991:441–561.

Green DP, Strickland JW. The hand. In: DeLee JC, Drez D Jr, eds. *Orthopaedic sports medicine: principles and practice.* Philadelphia: WB Saunders, 1994:945–1017.

Author: Walter L. Calmbach

Flexor Tendon Avulsion/Jersey Finger

Basics

DEFINITION

- Flexor digitorum profundus (FDP) avulsion from its distal phalanx insertion

INCIDENCE/PREVALENCE

- Relatively rare injury in general population and most sports
- Known to occur primarily in rugby players due to loose-fitting jerseys and the nature of tackling in this sport. Very common in flag football. Occurs less commonly in American tackle football.
- Most common finger affected is "ring" or fourth finger, approximately 80% to 90% of the time.

SIGNS AND SYMPTOMS

- Pain and swelling in distal phalanx
- Often discoloration out of proportion to simple tendon laceration due to bony avulsion
- Inability to flex distal interphalangeal (DIP) joint

RISK FACTORS

- Participation in any sport where tackling occurs by grabbing another player's jersey

CLASSIFICATION OF INJURY

- Type I: tendon retraction into palm
- Type II: tendon retracts to level of proximal interphalangeal (PIP) joint
- Type III: large bony avulsion causing a hang-up of the tendon at the distal pulley

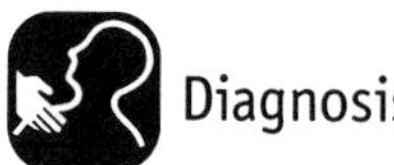

Diagnosis

DIFFERENTIAL DIAGNOSIS

- DIP joint dislocation
- Distal phalanx fracture
- Flexor digitorum superficialis avulsion

HISTORY

Q: Mechanism of injury?
A: While attempting to maintain a grasp, the flexed finger is forcibly extended.
Q: Time of injury?
A: Important because early surgical correction usually is necessary.
Q: Mobility of DIP joint?
A: Useful in narrowing the differential diagnosis
Q: Type of sport playing at the time of injury?
A: Useful in narrowing the differential diagnosis

PHYSICAL EXAMINATION

- Evaluate patient's inability to actively flex DIP joint
- Often tender to palpation at the site of avulsion
- Usually most tender at the location of the distal tip of the avulsed tendon. This is either at the level of the PIP joint or the A1 pulley in the palm.

IMAGING

Lateral and oblique radiographs of the affected digit are essential to evaluate for a bony avulsion; however, usually no deformity is seen on x-ray.

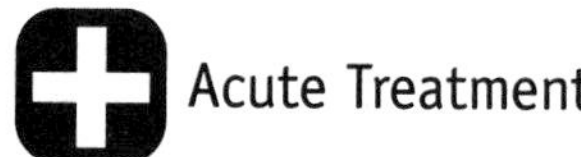

Acute Treatment

ANALGESIA

- Ice
- Nonsteroidal anti-inflammatory drugs

IMMOBILIZATION

- Buddy taping to "middle" or third phalanx

SPECIAL CONSIDERATIONS

- Immediate surgical repair is important for type I lesions; repair may be impossible after 7–10 days.
- Early surgical repair is advisable for type II lesions; repair can be successful 3 months after injury.
- Type III injuries must be surgically repaired as soon as possible; one should not wait longer than 2 weeks.

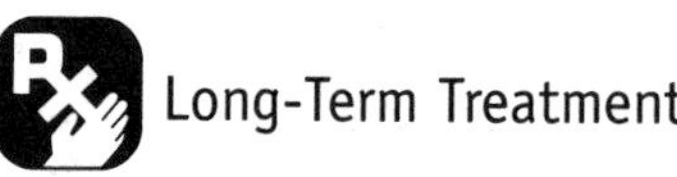

Long-Term Treatment

REHABILITATION

- Range of motion and strengthening after surgery
- If surgical correction was not done, then work should focus on trying to get full range of motion and strength of the PIP joint with exercise and splinting. Flexion contraction of this joint is common in type II injuries.

SURGERY

- Type II injuries can be repaired 3 months after injury.
- Arthrodesis of the DIP joint can be done for hyperflexion instability.
- Resection of the FDP stump at the PIP joint or palm due to chronic pain in these areas
- PIP joint volar scar release is done in refractory cases where range of motion cannot be regained with exercises and splinting.
- Only a few patients may be able to regain active motion of the DIP joint after FDP tendon grafting. This procedure often limits PIP joint motion.

REFERRAL/DISPOSITION

- Immediate referral for surgical evaluation in all patients is imperative.
- Early referral to physical therapy for patients developing PIP joint flexion contractures is important.

Common Questions and Answers

Physician responses to common patient questions:

Q: Can surgical repair wait until after the season is over?

A: Waiting in type I injuries most likely will result in permanent inability to actively flex DIP joint.

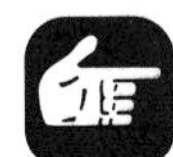

Miscellaneous

SYNONYMS

- Rugby jersey finger
- FDP avulsion

ICD-9 CODE

842.13 Finger interphalangeal ligamentous sprain

BIBLIOGRAPHY

Leddy JP. Avulsions of the flexor digitorum profundus tendon insertion in athletes. *J Hand Surg* 1977;2:66–69.

Reef TC. Avulsion of the flexor digitorum profundus: an athletic injury. *Am J Sports Med* 1977;5:281–285.

Rockwood CA Jr, ed. *Rockwood and Green's fractures in adults,* 3rd ed. Philadelphia: JB Lippincott, 1991.

Author: Suraj Achar

Flexor Tendinitis

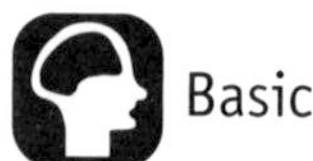

Basics

DEFINITION

- Acute, subacute, or chronic inflammation with subsequent degenerative changes in tendon or peritendinous structures, usually from repetitive stress
- Initially, tissue inflammation may be present, but chronically, tissue becomes more degenerative, so the term tendinitis is somewhat controversial (some authors prefer the term tendinopathy or tendinosis).

INCIDENCE/PREVALENCE

- Flexor carpi ulnaris (FCU) is the most commonly involved wrist flexor, but symptoms also may be found with the flexor carpi radialis (FCR).
- Less commonly, Linburg syndrome, an anomalous tendon interconnection between the thumb's flexor pollicis longus and the index finger's flexor digitorum profundus, which occurs in 25% to 30% of individuals, may lead to symptoms with activities.

SIGNS AND SYMPTOMS

- Inflammation along volar side of wrist
- Pain with wrist movement, often with proximal radiation

RISK FACTORS

- Repetitive strain with activities such as typing or using mouse, especially if no pad or support is used
- Racquet sports
- Improper technique
- Rollerblading, skateboarding, or snowboarding for acute injuries

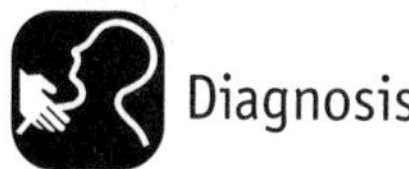

Diagnosis

DIFFERENTIAL DIAGNOSIS

- Arthritis of joints between bones in wrist
- Carpal tunnel syndrome
- Fracture of bone in wrist
- Ganglion cyst
- Scapholunate dissociation
- Tendon rupture
- Triangular fibrocartilage complex tear
- Synovitis, as in rheumatoid arthritis
- Cellulitis/lymphangitis

HISTORY

- Possible acute trauma to volar aspect of wrist
- Repetitive trauma or strain from work or recreational activities
- Pain with wrist motion, often radiating proximally

PHYSICAL EXAMINATION

- FCU: tenderness with or without swelling along tendon of ulnar volar wrist proximal to pisiform; pain with abrupt passive extension or resisted ulnar deviation/wrist flexion
- FCR: tenderness with or without swelling along tendon of radial volar wrist proximal to crease; pain with abrupt passive extension or resisted radial deviation/wrist flexion
- Crepitation in severe, chronic inflammation
- In acute calcific tendinitis, occasionally redness, warmth, and swelling along tendon extending into hand and forearm without lymphadenopathy, fever, or other signs of infection
- Linburg syndrome: Pathognomonic sign is simultaneous index finger interphalangeal flexion with active flexion of thumb across palm that becomes painful if finger flexion is inhibited.

IMAGING

- Wrist anteroposterior, lateral, and oblique views
- Calcific deposits may be evidenced in chronic cases.

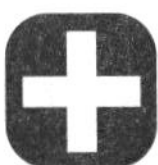

Acute Treatment

ANALGESIA

- Nonsteroidal anti-inflammatory drugs (NSAIDs)

IMMOBILIZATION

- Wrist splint in 25 degrees of flexion for 3–6 weeks with repetitive activity or while symptomatic

SPECIAL CONSIDERATIONS

- Cessation of aggravating activities is recommended.
- Corticosteroid injection may be beneficial.
- Gel keyboard/wrist pads may be helpful.
- Topical NSAIDS may provide benefit.

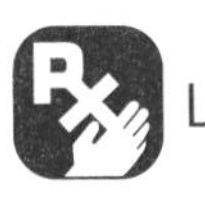

Long-Term Treatment

REHABILITATION

- Physical therapy for stretch/strength exercises
- Evaluation and alteration of ergonomics or technique may help reduce chance of recurrence.

SURGERY

- Surgical decompression with or without lengthening of tendon may be indicated in chronic, refractory cases.
- Surgical release of tendinous interconnection often is successful in treating Linburg syndrome.

REFERRAL/DISPOSITION

Referral to hand surgeon is appropriate for failure of conservative therapy.

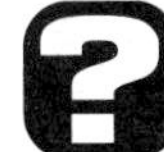

Common Questions and Answers

Physician responses to common patient questions:
Q: When can I return to play?
A: This decision depends on the severity and extent of disease, but as a general rule, participation may be resumed when activities are no longer painful. Correction of predisposing factors such as technique or ergonomics should be addressed.
Q: Can't I just "play through the pain"?
A: Although initial symptoms may not be debilitating enough to impair performance, pain is a marker for injury, which left untreated can become chronic and ultimately take longer to rehabilitate.

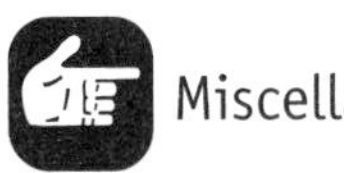

Miscellaneous

ICD-9 CODE

727.05 Wrist tenosynovitis

BIBLIOGRAPHY

Fulcher SM. Upper extremity tendinitis and overuse syndromes in the athlete. *Clin Sports Med* 1998;17:433–448.

Posner MA, Nicholas JA, Hershman EB, eds. *The upper extremity in sports medicine.* St. Louis: Mosby, 1995.

Verdon ME. Overuse syndromes of the hand and wrist. *Prim Care* 1996;23:305–319.

Author: Michael Mikus

Fracture, Avulsion

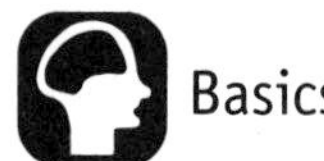

Basics

DEFINITION

Avulsion fractures occur when either the tendon–bone or ligament–bone interface is ruptured by forceful muscle contraction or undue ligament stress.

INCIDENCE/PREVALENCE

- Avulsion fractures of the anterior cruciate ligament (ACL) attachment to the tibial eminence are most prevalent in children <14 years, but are seen in adults >35 years who have low bone density.
- ACL avulsion from the femoral attachment is less common.

SIGNS AND SYMPTOMS

- Presence of a large, tense knee effusion (especially in a child <16 years) should raise concern of a potential ACL avulsion fracture.
- Examination findings of an ACL tear should raise suspicion.

RISK FACTORS

- Children <16 years
- Adults >35 years who are osteopenic

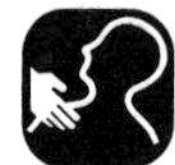

Diagnosis

DIFFERENTIAL DIAGNOSIS

- Mid-substance anterior cruciate ligament tear
- Congenital absence or deficiency of the anterior cruciate ligament
- Avulsion or mid-substance tear of the posterior cruciate ligament
- Tibial plateau fracture
- Patellar dislocation or subluxation
- Osteochondral fracture of the femoral condyle

HISTORY

- In children aged 8–11 years, often due to hyperflexion injury
- Above this age, due to either hyperextension injury or single-leg landing from a jump, both associated with a rotational or twisting stress to the knee
- Audible "pop" at the time of injury may be present.
- Immediate (within 1–2 hours) prominent swelling of the knee (acute hemarthrosis)
- Frequently unable to bear weight after injury

PHYSICAL EXAMINATION

- Large, tense effusion noted with loss of full range of motion
- ACL stress tests (Lachman, anterior drawer, and pivot shift) show more forward translation of the tibia compared to the noninjured side.
- Evaluate for other ligament and meniscal structures for concomitant pathology

IMAGING

- Plain radiographs should include anteroposterior, lateral, and tunnel views. The latter outlines the femoral notch and tibial eminence.
- Grades of tibial eminence avulsion fractures are based on displacement: type 1: minimal displacement of the anterior eminence; type 2: elevation of the anterior third to half of the eminence with hinging on posterior eminence; type 3: complete displacement of separation of fragment. Types 2 and 3 are of equal incidence and are more common than type 1.

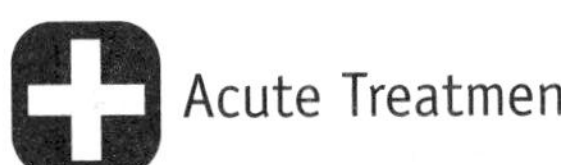

ANALGESIA

- Nonsteroidal anti-inflammatory and narcotic medications initially are used for pain control. Frequent application of ice for 20-minute periods is recommended.
- Aspiration of the joint may enhance comfort and allow further knee extension. Lack of full knee extension may imply a mechanical block (i.e., fracture fragment or meniscal tear).

IMMOBILIZATION

Initial care includes complete knee immobilization with minimal knee flexion for 2–3 days until effusion begins to resolve. Crutch ambulation is recommended in this initial stage.

SPECIAL CONSIDERATIONS

- Nondisplaced type 1 injuries eventually require long leg cast immobilization for 4–6 weeks after the effusion resolves.
- Displaced tibial eminence avulsion fractures (types 2 and 3) often require open reduction and internal fixation. Better results are obtained if surgery is done within the first week after injury; thus, prompt surgical referral is essential. The knee should be immobilized while awaiting surgical consultation.

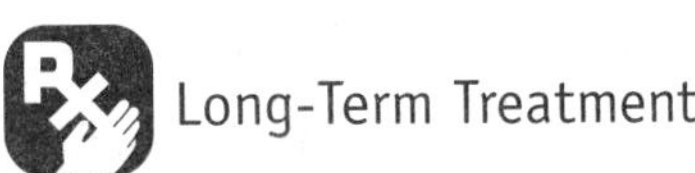

REHABILITATION

- After completion of cast immobilization, focus should be on recovering full knee range of motion followed by strengthening of knee extensors.
- Proprioception is another key part of the rehabilitation process.

REFERRAL

- All suspected ACL avulsion fractures should be referred to an orthopaedic surgeon.
- Patients with open growth plates would benefit from consultation with a pediatric orthopaedist.

SURGERY

Displaced type 2 or 3 avulsion fractures require closed or open reduction and internal fixation. Many authors prefer arthroscopic reduction due to less surgical trauma and easier postoperative rehabilitation course.

LONG-TERM PROGNOSIS

Even with true anatomical reduction, about 50% of patients may have mild measurable ACL laxity likely due to interstitial ligament damage that occurs before the avulsion but does not result in functional instability.

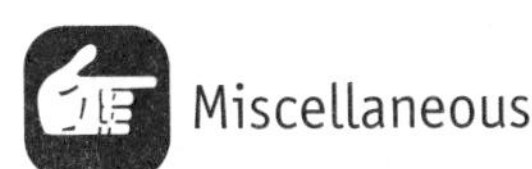

ICD-9 CODE

824.8 Closed
824.9 Open

BIBLIOGRAPHY

Lastihenos M, Nicholas SJ. Managing ACL injuries in children. *Physician Sportsmed* 1996;24:59–70.

Stanitski C, Sherman C. How I manage physeal fractures about the knee. *Physician Sportsmed* 1997;25:108–121.

Author: Chris Koutures

Fracture, Avulsion: ASIS, AIIS, Ischial Tuberosity, Iliac Crest

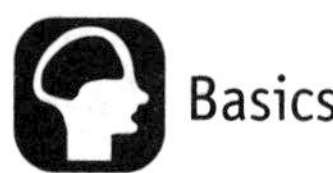

Basics

DEFINITION

- Injury occurs about the apophysis (secondary growth center); results from sudden, violent concentric, or eccentric muscular contraction without external trauma. May occur from sudden excessive passive lengthening of a muscle.
- Chronic injury may occur as a result of repetitive microtrauma or overuse.
- Anterior superior iliac spine (ASIS): forceful overpull of sartorius muscle with hip in extension and knee in flexion
- Anterior inferior iliac spine (AIIS): forceful extension of hip resulting in avulsion of straight head of rectus femoris.
- Ischial tuberosity: sudden, forceful eccentric contraction of hamstring with knee extended and hip flexed
- Iliac crest: avulsion of abdominal muscles

INCIDENCE/PREVALENCE

- Account for 13% to 40% of pediatric pelvic fractures
- More common in males
- More common among adolescents than young children
- May occur in adults ("weekend warriors")

SIGNS AND SYMPTOMS

- Pain and localized tenderness at avulsion site
- Limitation of motion about the site of avulsion injury

RISK FACTORS

- Athletes involved in strenuous sporting activities (soccer, football)
- Sprinters (ASIS, AIIS)
- Gymnasts, hurdlers, long-jumpers (ischial tuberosity)

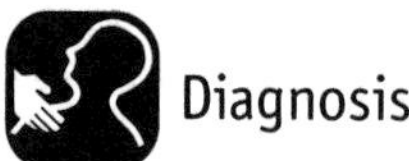

Diagnosis

DIFFERENTIAL DIAGNOSIS

- Apophysitis
- Muscle strain

HISTORY

Q: Activity at time of injury?
A: Helps define the mechanism of injury: attempting to kick a soccer ball (AIIS); clearing a hurdle (ischial tuberosity).
Q: Radiation of pain?
A: May have pain into posterior thigh with ischial tuberosity avulsion; pain into anterior thigh with AIIS avulsion.

PHYSICAL EXAMINATION

- Palpate regions of suspected avulsion. Acute localized tenderness to palpation present over involved apophysis; avulsed apophyseal fragment may be palpated.
- Assess active and passive range of motion of involved muscle(s). ASIS: pain on passive extension or active flexion of hip. AIIS: pain with passive hyperextension and active flexion of hip. Ischial tuberosity: pain with passive hip flexion and active hip extension. Iliac crest: pain with contraction of abdominal muscles, lateral bending of torso, resisted hip abduction.

IMAGING

- AP pelvis: Will demonstrate avulsion of a portion of involved apophysis. Fragments may be mildly to severely displaced. Chronic avulsions may result in prominent bone formation and nonunion. Fracture without a clear history of injury may be confused with Ewing sarcoma, osteosarcoma, or osteomyelitis.
- Oblique view of pelvis: May better demonstrate avulsions of iliac crest.
- Computed tomographic scan: May be helpful in chronic cases or those without a clear history. May aid in managing cases of impingement of sciatic nerve (ischial tuberosity avulsions).

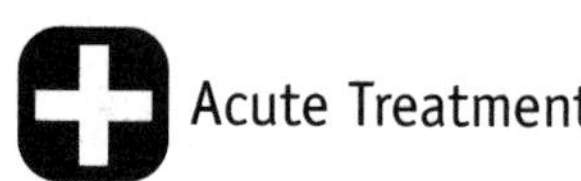

Acute Treatment

ANALGESIA

- Ice application
- Analgesics

IMMOBILIZATION

- Rest
- Positioning of the limb to relieve tension on the involved muscle group
- Crutch therapy may be required initially, with progressive weight-bearing as pain decreases and range of motion improves.

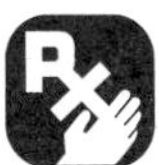

Long-Term Treatment

REHABILITATION

- Gradual increase in active and passive excursion of involved muscle group to achieve full active range of motion
- Progressive resistance exercise program, followed by integration of injured musculotendinous unit with the other muscles of the hip and pelvis
- Sport-specific training followed by return to sport when pain-free, and with normal motion and strength of involved muscle

SURGERY

- Open reduction internal fixation considered when fragment displaced >2 cm, especially for ischial tuberosity avulsion

REFERRAL/DISPOSITION

- Majority of fractures heal with conservative treatment

Common Questions and Answers

Physician responses to common patient questions:
Q: How long before I can return to play?
A: Depending on fracture location, most can return by 4–8 weeks.

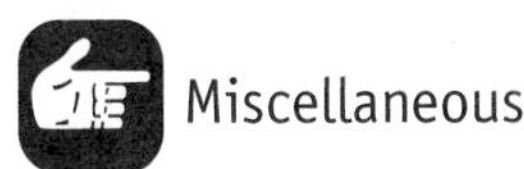

Miscellaneous

SYNONYMS

- Hip pointer

ICD-9 CODE

808.49 Pelvic rim, closed fracture

BIBLIOGRAPHY

Paletta GA, Andrish JT. Injuries about the hip and pelvis in the young athlete. *Clin Sports Med* 1995;14:591–628.

Stevens MA, El-Khoury GY, Kathol MH, et al. Imaging features of avulsion injuries. *Radiographics* 1999;19:655–672.

Winfield C, Salis RE, Massimino F, eds. *ACSM's essentials of sports medicine.* St. Louis: Mosby, 1997.

Author: Robin Merket

Fracture, Blow Out

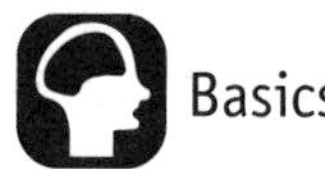

Basics

SIGNS AND SYMPTOMS

- Periorbital tenderness, swelling, ecchymosis
- Impaired ocular mobility or diplopia
  —Upward gaze due to inferior rectus entrapment
  —Ipsilateral lateral gaze with medial rectus entrapment
- Infraorbital hypoesthesia
  —Due to compression/contusion of infraorbital nerve
- Enophthalmos
  —Due to herniation of orbital fat through fracture
- Periorbital emphysema
- Normal visual acuity (unless associated ocular injury)
- Epistaxis

Associated Injuries

- Ocular injuries
  —Ruptured globe
    —Incidence 5–10% of blow out fractures
    —Ophthalmologic emergency
  —Subconjunctival hemorrhage
  —Corneal abrasion/laceration
  —Hyphema
  —Iridodialysis
  —Traumatic iridocyclitis (uveitis)
  —Traumatic mydriasis
  —Retinal detachment
  —Vitreous hemorrhage
  —Compressive orbital emphysema
  —Retrobulbar hemorrhage
  —Optic nerve injury
- Facial fractures
  —Nasal bones
  —Zygomatic arch fracture
- Neck injuries
- Intracranial injury

Late Complications

- Sinusitis
- Orbital infection
- Permanent restriction of extraocular movement
- Enophthalmos

MECHANISM/DESCRIPTION

- Defined as an orbital floor fracture without orbital rim involvement due to blunt trauma to the orbit
- Caused by blunt trauma to the orbit
- Force transmitted through the orbital structures to the weakest structural point—the orbital floor
  —Results in fracture of the orbital floor
- Orbital floor serves as roof to air filled maxillary and ethmoid.
  —Communication between the spaces results in orbital emphysema.
- Orbit contains fat which holds the globe in place.
  —Orbital floor fracture may result in herniation of the fat on the inferior orbital surface into the maxillary or ethmoid sinuses.
  —Leads to enophthalmos due to orbital volume loss
  —Sinus congestion and fluid collection occur secondary to edema.
- Infraorbital nerve runs through the bony canal 3 mm below the orbital floor.
  —Injury results in hypoesthesia of the ipsilateral cheek.
  —Distinguished from hypoesthesia due to swelling by testing for decreased sensation on the ipsilateral gingiva which is within the infraorbital nerve distribution
- Inferior rectus and the inferior oblique muscle run along the orbital floor.
  —Restriction of these extraocular muscles occurs due to entrapment within the fracture, contusion, or cranial nerve dysfunction.
  —Diplopia on upward gaze
  —Inability to elevate the affected eye normally on exam
- Medial rectus located above the ethmoid sinus
  —Less commonly entrapped
  —Diplopia on ipsilateral lateral gaze

ETIOLOGY

- Most commonly caused by handballs, baseballs, or fists.

PEDIATRIC CONSIDERATIONS

- Orbital floor fractures—extremely unlikely before 7 years of age
- Lack of pneumatization of the paranasal sinuses—orbital floor is not a weak point in the orbit
- Orbital roof fractures with associated CNS injuries more common

PRE-HOSPITAL

- Metal protective eyeshield if possible globe injury
- Place in supine position.

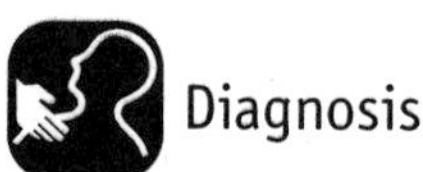

Diagnosis

ESSENTIAL WORKUP

- Thorough ophthalmologic examination
  —Visual acuity (should not be affected)
  —Test extraocular movements for disconjugate gaze or diplopia.
  —Palpate bony structures for evidence of step-off.
  —Test sensation in inferior orbital nerve distribution.
  —Examine lid and adnexa.
  —Careful attention not to place pressure on the globe until ruptured globe excluded
  —Slitlamp and funduscopic examination to identify associated injuries

LABORATORY

- Preoperative laboratory studies if indicated

IMAGING/SPECIAL TESTS

- Plain radiographs
  —Facial films
  —Orbits
  —Water's view and exaggerated Water's view
    —Classic "teardrop sign" illustrates herniated mass of orbital contents in the ipsilateral maxillary sinus.
    —Opacification of or air fluid level in the ipsilateral maxillary sinus (less specific)
    —Orbital floor bony fracture
    —Lucency in orbits consistent with orbital emphysema
- Diagnostic in up to 97%
- 10% false-positives and false-negative rate
- Tomograms helpful when available
- CT orbits
  —If diagnosis in question and for follow-up
  —Defines involved anatomy
  —Obtain 1.5-mm cuts
- Forced duction test
  —Distinguishes nerve dysfunction from entrapment
  —Topical anesthesia applied to the conjunctiva on the opposite side and the globe is pulled away from the expected point of entrapment. If the globe is not mobile, the test is positive.

DIFFERENTIAL DIAGNOSIS

- Retrobulbar hemorrhage
- Periorbital contusion/ecchymosis
- Cranial nerve palsy
- Ruptured globe
- Orbital cellulitis
- Periorbital cellulitis

PEDIATRIC CONSIDERATION

- Immature facial skeleton with lack of pneumatization of the paranasal sinuses makes plain radiographs of limited value.
- Orbital CT—study of choice

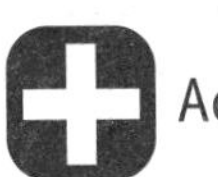

Acute Treatment

INITIAL STABILIZATION

- Initial approach and immediate concerns
  - —Rule out ruptured globe
  - —Assess for associated intracranial or cervical spine injuries
  - —Test visual acuity
    - —Decreased visual acuity suggestive of associated ocular injury

ED TREATMENT

- Apply cool compresses for the first 24–48 hours to decrease swelling in order to minimize/reverse herniation and avoid surgical intervention.
- Avoid Valsalva maneuvers and nose blowing to prevent compressive orbital emphysema.
- Prophylactic antibiotics (amoxicillin, cephalexin, erythromycin) to prevent infection
- Nasal decongestants (phenylephrine nasal spray)
- Analgesics
- Tetanus prophylaxis

MEDICATIONS

- Phenylephrine nasal spray: BID for 10–14 days
- Amoxicillin: 250–500 mg po TID 10–14 days
- Cephalexin: 250–500 mg po QID 10–14 days
- Erythromycin: 250–500 mg po QID 10–14 days

HOSPITAL ADMISSION CRITERIA

- Rarely indicated except with
  - —Severe herniation of orbital contents threatening vision
  - —Cosmetically enophthalmos typically 5 mm
  - —Associated injuries which mandate admission

HOSPITAL DISCHARGE CRITERIA

- Consultation with facial trauma service
  - —Arrange follow up evaluation within 1–2 weeks of injury and to determine need for surgery.
- Immediate ophthalmology evaluation if patient has evidence of visual loss or within 24 hours for complete retinal evaluation
- Need for surgical intervention
  - —Rarely indicated immediately
  - —85% resolve without surgical intervention
  - —Typically observe for 10–14 days until swelling resolves
  - —Surgery indications
    - —Persistent diplopia
    - —Restricted extraocular movements
    - —Cosmetically significant enophthalmos

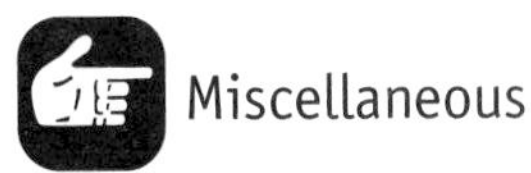

Miscellaneous

ICD-9 CODE

829.0

CORE CONTENT CODE

18.4.4.1.5

BIBLIOGRAPHY

Anderson PJ, Poole MD. Orbital floor fractures in young children (Rev). *J Craniomaxillofac Surg* 1995;23(3):151–154.

Joondeph BC. Blunt ocular trauma. *Emerg Med Clin North Am* 1988;6(1):151.

Koltai PJ, Amjad I, Meyer D. Orbital fractures in children. *Arch Otolaryngol Head Neck Surg* 1995;121(12):1375–1379.

Linden JA, Renner GS. Trauma to the globe. *Emerg Med Clin North Am* 1995;13(3): 581–605.

Author: Shari Schabowski

Fracture, Calcaneus

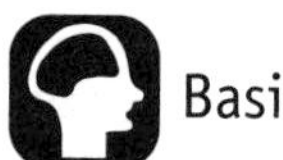

Basics

DEFINITION

Injury can occur secondary to either acute trauma or recurrent stress (calcaneal stress fracture). Of primary concern when evaluating the acute calcaneus fracture is determining whether the fracture is extra- or intra-articular. Most extra-articular fractures can be managed conservatively. Fractures that extend intra-articularly (involve the subtalar joint) should be referred for surgical management.

INCIDENCE/PREVALENCE

- Common in adults; calcaneal fractures relatively rare in children
- 25% to 30% of calcaneal fractures are extra-articular; 70% to 75% are intra-articular.
- Approximately 90% of all calcaneal fractures are either two- or three-part fractures.

SIGNS AND SYMPTOMS

- Heel pain
- Swelling
- Ecchymosis

RISK FACTORS

- Fall from a height
- Osteoporosis can predispose to calcaneal fractures despite seemingly trivial mechanism of injury.

ASSOCIATED INJURIES AND COMPLICATIONS

- Up to 70% of patients have an additional lower extremity or spinal fracture.
- Often associated with significant local soft tissue injury
- Acute compartment syndrome of the foot
- Open fracture
- Can lead to chronic pain and arthritis

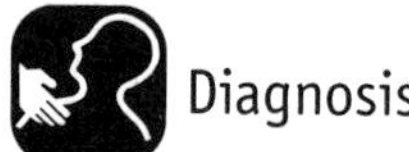

Diagnosis

DIFFERENTIAL DIAGNOSIS

- Talar fracture
- Cuboid fracture
- Malleolar fracture
- Ankle dislocation
- Ankle sprain

HISTORY

Q: Mechanism?
A: Extra-articular fractures are more commonly due to an indirect mechanism such as a twisting injury or muscular avulsion. Intra-articular fractures are due to high-energy accidents; history of a fall from a height is particularly concerning for additional lower extremity and lumbar spine injury.

PHYSICAL EXAMINATION

- Look for associated soft tissue injury. Excessive soft tissue injury and swelling will influence duration of time in a splint before placing into a cast for those being treated conservatively or may delay definitive surgical treatment if not addressed early in those being treated operatively.
- Check for evidence of lower extremity compartment syndrome. Requires emergent surgical referral even if the fracture itself is nonoperative.
- Look for associated lower extremity and lumbar bony injury because of high incidence of additional injury.

IMAGING

- Goal of imaging is to confirm diagnosis of calcaneus fracture and to determine whether the fracture is intra- or extra-articular.
- Standard initial x-rays: anteroposterior, lateral, and axial calcaneus (Harris) views
- Bohler tuber joint angle: complement of the angle between (a) the line drawn from the highest part of the anterior process and the highest part of the posterior articular surface and (b) the line drawn between the same point on the posterior articular surface and the most superior point of the tuberosity. Measures between 25 and 40 degrees, with a similar angle found in the two calcanei in any one person. Decrease of 10 degrees versus the uninjured side is considered a significant difference.
- "Crucial angle" of Gissane: on the lateral x-ray, the angle formed by the wedge in which the lateral process of the talus sits. This angle is disrupted when axial compressive forces drive the talus as a wedge into this space.
- Obliques (Broden) views can be helpful in assessing involvement of the articular surfaces.
- Additional x-rays to consider based on history and physical examination include views of the contralateral foot (because of the significant incidence of bilateral injury and to compare Bohler and Gissane angles with the injured foot); ipsilateral ankle; and lumbar spine and pelvis (because of high frequency of associated fractures).
- Computed tomographic (CT) scan: If plain films show articular involvement or if suspicion of articular involvement remains high despite equivocal plain films, then a CT scan is essential for a more specific analysis of the subtalar and calcaneocuboid joints, as displacement of either will likely require surgical management. Should include axial and coronal cuts.

POSTREDUCTION VIEWS

Repeat the standard radiographs to assess adequacy of reduction after closed manipulation. Comparison with the opposite foot often is useful.

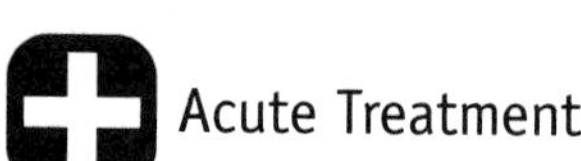

Acute Treatment

ANALGESIA

Ice and oral analgesics are useful in the prehospital setting, and oral analgesics may be required for some time after casting.

REDUCTION TECHNIQUES

Mediolateral compression of the heel with the palms of the hands can be applied to reduce displaced extra-articular body fractures.

POSTREDUCTION EVALUATION

Repeat x-rays in 1 week in any patient requiring closed manipulation.

IMMOBILIZATION

- Usually begins with splinting or Bulky Jones dressing to accommodate changes in soft tissue swelling
- In patients who require casting, the splint can be changed to a short-leg cast after the initial soft tissue injury has stabilized after approximately 3–5 days.
- In patients who require operative treatment, splinting is appropriate until the patient can see an orthopaedic surgeon.

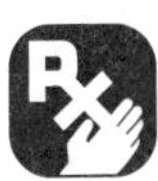

Long-Term Treatment

INJURY-SPECIFIC RECOMMENDATIONS

- Nondisplaced extra-articular fractures of the body of the calcaneus: can be treated with 2–3 days of rest, ice, compression, and elevation (RICE) and a Bulky Jones dressing followed by active range of motion and toe-touch ambulation for 4–6 weeks.
- Displaced extra-articular fractures of the body requiring closed manipulation (e.g., extra-articular calcaneal body fractures with significant widening of the heel requiring closed manipulation): generally can be treated conservatively, usually in a short-leg cast for 4–6 weeks, followed by gradual return to full activity.
- Exceptions: Extra-articular fractures with a decrease of Bohler angle by 10 degrees versus the contralateral side or displaced avulsions of the Achilles' tendon insertion from the tuberosity should be referred for reduction and fixation.
- Intra-articular fractures, or extra-articular fractures as listed above, should be referred for orthopaedic consultation.

REHABILITATION

After removal from splinting/casting, patient should be referred to physical therapy to restore normal flexibility and strength before returning to play.

SURGERY

- In cases requiring operative treatment, referral should be made promptly so that fixation can occur within 5–7 days.
- All cases of compartment syndrome require emergent referral.

REFERRAL/DISPOSITION

Conservative treatment should be reserved for cases of extra-articular fracture only. All cases of intra-articular fracture, or the specific extra-articular fractures listed above, should be referred for consideration of surgical fixation.

Common Questions and Answers

Physician responses to common patient questions:
Q: When can I return to play?
A: In nonoperative cases, athletes may be ready to return to play in as little as 8 weeks. In operative cases, the duration of immobilization and recovery is more variable and depends on the particulars of the fracture.

Q: What are the chances that I will have chronic problems because of this fracture?
A: Long-term outcome is mainly determined by the degree of joint destruction at the time of injury. About 90% of all calcaneus fractures are two- or three-part fractures. In these two groups, patients achieve a 70% rate of good or excellent results.

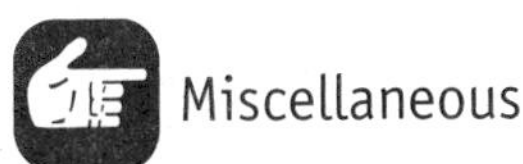

Miscellaneous

SYNONYMS

- Os calcis fracture
- Heel bone fracture

ICD-9 CODE

825.0 Fracture of calcaneus, closed
825.1 Fracture of calcaneus, open

BIBLIOGRAPHY

Lewis G. Biomechanics as a basis for management of intra-articular fractures. *J Am Podiatr Med Assoc* 1999;89:234–246.

Miric A, Patterson B. Pathoanatomy of intra-articular fractures of the calcaneus. *J Bone Joint Surg* 1998;80A:207–212.

Rockwood C, Green D, Bucholz R, et al., eds. *Rockwood and Green's fractures in adults,* 4th ed. Philadelphia: Lippincott-Raven Publishers, 1996.

Thermann H, Krettek C, Heufner T, et al. Management of calcaneal fractures in adults: conservative versus operative treatment. *Clin Orthop* 1998;353:107–124.

Author: Greg Nakamoto

Fracture, Carpal Bone (Other)

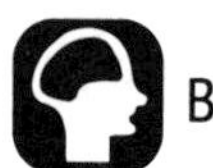

Basics

DEFINITION

- Fracture of the carpal bones of the wrist, excluding those of the hamate and scaphoid
- Includes Kienbock disease

INCIDENCE/PREVALENCE

- The carpal bones consist of the scaphoid, lunate, triquetrum, and pisiform in the proximal row and the trapezoid, trapezium, capitate, and hamate in the distal row.
- Carpal fractures make up 2% to 4% of fractures of the hand and wrist.
- Frequency of fracture seen in carpal bones is scaphoid ~80%, triquetrum ~6%, hamate ~5%, trapezium ~4%, lunate <3%, and capitate, trapezoid, and pisiform, <1% each.
- Carpal fractures are caused by trauma from either a fall on the extended wrist or a direct blow.
- Kienbock disease in 75% of the cases is preceded by severe trauma with the wrist in extreme dorsiflexion.

SIGNS AND SYMPTOMS

- Pain and tenderness over the dorsum of the wrist
- Localized swelling and limited range of motion; a prominence may be present.
- Muscle strength testing of the attachment of the tendon units inserted on or supported by the injured structure may help localize the injury.
- Neurovascular signs are unusual, except for injury of the pisiform, which may affect the ulnar nerve and artery.

RISK FACTORS

Fractures of the carpal bones other than the scaphoid and lunate bones are seen often in sports using a stick (e.g., hockey, lacrosse).

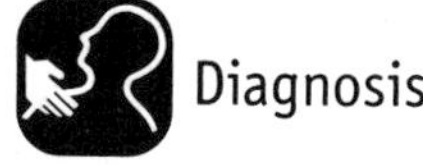

Diagnosis

DIFFERENTIAL DIAGNOSIS

- Ligamentous injury (wrist sprain)
- Contusion
- Carpal dislocation
- Metacarpal fracture
- Distal radioulnar fracture

HISTORY

- Athlete usually will present with a fall on the outstretched hand. However, direct trauma or a fall on a flexed wrist can cause a fracture. Pain and restricted motion often are presenting complaints.
- Mechanism of injury can help localize the injury to a specific carpal bone.
- Determine when the wrist began to hurt; recent versus prolonged is important.
- Determine location of pain, whether ulnar or radial, at rest or with motion.
- An occult fracture often will present as a persistent wrist sprain. Carefully examine the patient, as Kienbock disease and small chip fractures of the triquetrum can present in this manner.

PHYSICAL EXAMINATION

- Inspect for swelling, deformity, and ecchymosis (the latter usually not seen with carpal fractures).
- Evaluate movement of wrist in flexion, extension, and ulnar and radial deviation.
- Palpate individual carpal bones to determine tenderness.
- Test strength of muscles that attach to carpal bones.
- Assess neurovascular integrity (fracture of the pisiform may affect the ulnar nerve and a lunate dislocation may compress the median nerve).
- Axial loading of metacarpals above the carpal bones may help in diagnosis.

IMAGING

- Radiographs consisting of six views: anteroposterior (AP) and lateral, each taken in an exact neutral position; motion views of maximal radial deviation and maximal ulnar deviation; lateral views in maximal flexion and maximal extension.
- Additional radiographic views may be needed if a fracture is suspected for certain carpal bones: pisiform (carpal tunnel views, oblique view with forearm in 20 degrees supination), triquetrum (slightly oblique, pronated lateral view), trapezium (carpal tunnel views and true AP [Robert] view), and trapezoid (oblique views).
- Computed tomographic scanning should be considered if a fracture of the capitate, lunate, or trapezoid is suspected and negative plain films are seen.
- Postreduction views should be obtained to confirm reduction and correct anatomical alignment.

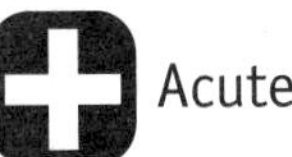

Acute Treatment

ANALGESIA

- Immobilization of the wrist should eliminate the pain of the fracture.
- Nonsteroidal anti-inflammatory drugs or narcotics can be added as needed.

REDUCTION TECHNIQUES

- Should not be necessary. All displaced or dislocated fractures should be splinted and referred for surgery.
- Lunate dislocation may need immediate reduction if median nerve or artery is involved.

Fracture, Carpal Bone (Other)

POSTREDUCTION EVALUATION

Immobilization

- All treatments are for nondisplaced fractures.
- Triquetrum: short arm cast for 4–6 weeks for transverse body fracture; short arm cast or splint for 2–4 weeks for dorsal avulsion
- Trapezium: short arm thumb spica cast for 4–6 weeks
- Pisiform: short arm cast or splint for 3–4 weeks
- Trapezoid: short arm cast for 4–6 weeks
- Capitate: short arm cast for 6–8 weeks. Some recommend long arm with finger extension. Consider referral because of possible AVN.
- Lunate: short arm cast or splint until referred; prolonged immobilization of 12–16 weeks, often in long arm cast with finger extension

SPECIAL CONSIDERATIONS

- Triquetrum
  —Dorsal chips of the triquetrum are easily missed on AP view and may be the only sign of a fracture.
  —Persistent pain after appropriate treatment should alert the treating physician that a concurrent injury (pisiform fracture, triangular fibrocartilage complex injury, and/or lunate-triquetrum ligament tear) was initially not noticed.
- Capitate
  —Most often fractured with the scaphoid or metacarpal
  —Consider all capitate fractures unstable
- Trapezium
  —Easily missed; patients will describe a localized pain at base of the thenar eminence.
  —Missed fractures cause on-going pain at base of the thumb.
  —Carpal tunnel view demonstrates fracture of the palmar ridge.
- Pisiform
  —Usually caused by direct blow to hand
  —Can compress the ulnar nerve or artery
- Trapezoid
  —Rarely fractured; patients describe pain at the base of the second metacarpal.
  —Axial compression of second metacarpal will elicit tenderness.
- Lunate
  —Lunate fractures can be occult.
  —AVN is seen in 20% of lunate fractures.
  —Kienbock disease may be secondary to lunate injury.
  —Kienbock disease has a high association with ulna-minus variant.

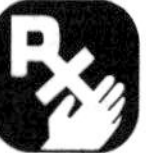

Long-Term Treatment

REHABILITATION

- Initially, while in cast, the athlete needs to continue fitness training. Constant monitoring of the cast and frequent (weekly) changes may be needed to maintain skin and cast integrity.
- Once out of the cast, range of motion (ROM) then strengthening of the wrist need to be done until restoration of a painless, functional arc of wrist motion and near-normal strength are obtained.

SURGERY

Surgery is needed for displaced fractures(s) through the metacarpocarpal joint articulation.

REFERRAL/DISPOSITION

- Any displaced fracture of the carpal bones should be referred to an orthopaedic surgeon.
- Lunate fractures may develop AVN (avascular necrosis of the hip, Kienbock disease) and should be considered for referral even if not displaced.

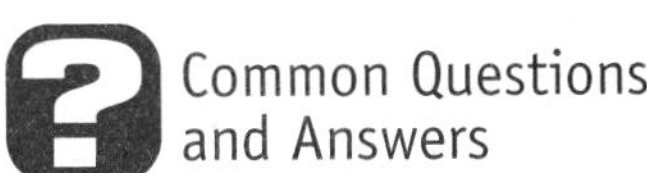

Common Questions and Answers

Physician responses to common patient questions:

Q: How long until I can play?

A: This varies with the degree of injury and casting. In lunate fractures, it is up to 6 months; in triquetrum fractures, it is 4 weeks, possibly less, in cast. General requirements for returning to play are complete healing of the fracture and any concurrent soft tissue injuries. Thorough rehabilitation with restoration of a painless, functional arc of wrist motion and near-normal strength are essential.

Q: Will I have pain when I am done?

A: Wrist stiffness is a common problem after casting, and physical therapy for ROM and strengthening is essential after cast removal. When rehabilitation is done, the wrist is most often free of pain.

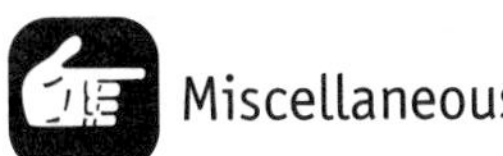

Miscellaneous

SYNONYMS

- Wrist fracture

ICD-9 CODE

814.00 Fracture, carpal bones unspecified
814.02 Fracture, carpal bones lunate
814.03 Fracture, carpal bones triquetral
814.04 Fracture, carpal bones pisiform
814.05 Fracture, carpal bones trapezium
814.06 Fracture, carpal bones trapezoid
814.07 Fracture, carpal bones capitate

BIBLIOGRAPHY

Cooney WP III, Linscheid RL, Dobyns JH. Fractures and dislocations of the wrist. In Rockwood A Jr and Green DP, eds. *Rockwood and Green's fractures in adults,* 4th ed. Philadelphia: Lippincott-Raven Publishers, 1996:822–827.

Culver JE, Anderson TE. Fractures of the hand and wrist in the athlete. *Clin Sports Med* 1992;11:101–128.

DeHaven KE, Lintner DM. Athletic injuries: comparison by age, sport, and gender. *Am J Sports Med* 1986;14:218–224.

Eisenhauer MA. Wrist and forearm. In: Rosen P, ed. *Emergency medicine: concepts and clinical practice,* 4th ed. St. Louis: Mosby-Year Book, 1998:673–677.

Rettig AC. Epidemiology of hand and wrist injuries in sports. *Clin Sports Med* 1998;17: 401–406.

Rettig ME, Dassa GL, Raskin KB, et al. Hand and wrist injuries. *Clin Sports Med* 1998;17: 469–489.

Wright PE II. Wrist. In: Canale T, ed. *Campbell's operative orthopaedics,* 9th ed. St. Louis: Mosby, 1998:3455–3476.

Author: Thomas Trojian

Fracture, Clavicle

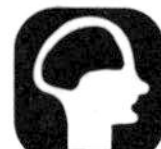 Basics

DEFINITION

Classification

- ***Group I***: fracture of the middle third
- ***Group II***: fracture of the distal third
  —Type I: minimal displacement
  —Type II: displaced secondary to a fracture medial to the coracoclavicular ligaments
  —Type III: fractures of the articular surface
  —Type IV: ligaments intact to the periosteum (children), with displacement of the proximal fragment
  —Type V: comminuted, with ligaments attached neither proximally nor distally, but to an inferior, comminuted fragment
- ***Group III***: fracture of the proximal third
  —Type I: minimal displacement
  —Type II: displaced (ligaments ruptured)
  —Type III: intra-articular
  —Type IV: epiphyseal separation (children and young adults)
  —Type V: comminuted

INCIDENCE/PREVALENCE

- Most frequently broken bone in children and adolescents
- More frequent in males
- The highest incidence of clavicle injury occurs in the sports of ice hockey, lacrosse, wrestling, spring football, gymnastics, and football, respectively.
- Some martial arts have a high incidence of clavicle injury.
- Group I (middle third) accounts for 80%; group II (distal third) accounts for 12% to 15%; group III (proximal third) accounts for 5% to 6%.

SIGNS AND SYMPTOMS

- Clinical deformity that may be out of proportion to the amount of discomfort the patient experiences
- The overlying skin may be tented from the proximal fragment, which is displaced upward and backward.
- Patient usually holds the injured shoulder and arm close to the body and supports the arm.

RISK FACTORS

- Contact sports and stick sports (football, lacrosse, hockey), during which an athlete sustains a direct blow to the clavicle

ASSOCIATED INJURIES AND COMPLICATIONS

- Acromioclavicular (AC) injury or separation
- Proximal humeral fractures

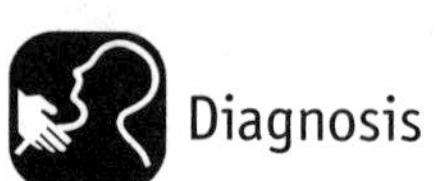

Diagnosis

DIFFERENTIAL DIAGNOSIS

- AC joint separation
- Sternoclavicular (SC) joint injury
- Humeral head fracture
- Glenohumeral dislocation

HISTORY

- May result from direct or indirect trauma
- May occur from a direct blow, a fall onto the clavicle, or a fall onto the outstretched arm or lateral aspect of the shoulder. Fractures to the middle third frequently are seen in falls onto outstretched arm. Fractures of the distal third most often are associated with loads transmitted to the lateral aspect of the shoulder.
- Pain at the fracture site
- May support the arm on the affected side

PHYSICAL EXAMINATION

- A complete neurovascular examination must be performed to identify possible brachial plexus or vascular injuries.
- Careful chest auscultation must be performed to evaluate for pulmonary injury.
- Likely able to visualize and palpate a deformity
- May see ecchymosis or tenting of the skin over the fracture
- Careful palpation along the entire clavicular complex can identify focal tenderness at the AC joint, SC joint, or fracture site.
- Pressure along the clavicle may reveal fracture motion or crepitus at a fracture site.

IMAGING

- An anteroposterior (AP) view and a 45-degree cephalic tilt AP view (apical lordotic view) are recommended. This should include the upper third of the humerus, shoulder girdle, and upper lung field.
- For fractures of the distal third, consider adding oblique views.
- Medial fractures will likely require a 45-degree cephalic tilt view, in addition to the standard views. If clinical suspicion of medial clavicular injury is high, a thin-cut computed tomographic (CT) scan usually is indicated to ensure that underlying structures are not at risk and to evaluate the proximal clavicular physis.
- Articular fractures of the distal clavicle may require CT scan.
- Arteriography is warranted if an ipsilateral asymmetrical bruit or abnormal vascular findings is appreciated.
- For AC injuries, comparison views of the opposite side are indicated.

POSTREDUCTION VIEWS

The same standard views may be used for postreduction views as were used for diagnosis.

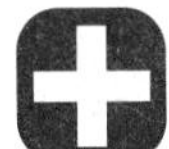

Acute Treatment

ANALGESIA

- Consider hematoma block
- Narcotic analgesics as appropriate
- Nonsteroidal anti-inflammatory drugs of choice

REDUCTION TECHNIQUES

Middle Third (Group I)

- Goal of treatment for midshaft fractures is reduction of motion at the fracture site, which rarely requires surgical intervention.
- For moderately displaced midshaft fractures with no neurovascular compromise, a well-padded, tightly fitting, figure-of-eight harness used for 3–6 weeks serves to reduce the fracture by longitudinal traction.
- Nondisplaced or minimally displaced fractures of the midclavicle can be treated symptomatically with a sling or figure-of-eight harness for 3–6 weeks in young adults and 6 weeks or longer in older adults.

Distal Third (Group II)

- Nondisplaced fractures of the distal clavicle are best treated with a sling or figure-of-eight brace and early rehabilitation.
- Consider early referral for type II distal clavicle fractures for possible internal fixation.

Proximal Third (Group III)

- Most proximal fractures are treated successfully with ice, analgesics, and sling or figure-of-eight immobilization.
- Reduction of posterior fracture dislocations of the clavicle requires great care and should be done in the presence of a thoracic surgeon in the operating room.

POSTREDUCTION EVALUATION

- Follow-up visits should be scheduled 1–2 weeks after injury to assess clinical symptoms, then every 2–3 weeks until the patient is asymptomatic.
- Radiographic union progresses more slowly than clinical union.
- A final radiograph should be performed at 6 weeks and when clinical union is definite to assess callus formation.

IMMOBILIZATION

- The value of a figure-of-eight harness over a sling increases with the degree of displacement of the fracture.
- Middle third: 3–6 weeks or until the fracture site is nontender; may need 4–8 weeks in older adults
- Distal third (types I and III): 3–6 weeks or until fracture site is nontender
- Distal third (type II): 6–8 weeks
- Proximal third: 3–6 weeks or until fracture site is nontender

SPECIAL CONSIDERATIONS

The proximal clavicular epiphysis is the last growth plate in the body to fuse (approximately age 22 years). Therefore, many injures involving the SC joint in athletes probably are physeal injuries and should be evaluated by thin-cut CT scan.

COMPLICATIONS

- Nonunion (degree of displacement most important factor)
- Malunion (rarely troublesome), resulting in angulation, shortening, and a poor cosmetic appearance
- Neurovascular injury (uncommon)
- Posttraumatic arthritis, which may be proximal or distal; may respond to nonoperative measures, but in certain circumstances, the lateral 2 cm of the clavicle can be excised

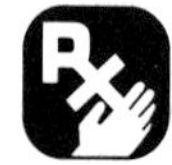

Long-Term Treatment

REHABILITATION

- When the acute pain has resolved, may begin gentle pendulum exercises of the ipsilateral shoulder, active use of the shoulder up to 40 degrees of flexion, isometric deltoid and rotator cuff strengthening, and normal use of the ipsilateral elbow and hand.
- Should not start range of motion (ROM) exercises beyond 40–45 degrees of flexion until there is clinical evidence that healing is occurring, typically 4–6 weeks.
- As union progresses, ROM may be increased and resistive exercises instituted.
- When radiographic union is present, full active use of the arm is allowed.

SURGERY

- Open reduction for any fracture site if complete displacement persists for longer than 3 weeks of figure-of-eight splinting
- Clavicle nonunions can be treated using a variety of surgical techniques, including ORIF with dynamic compression plates and intramedullary devices.
- Indications for early operative treatment include open fractures, multiple trauma when closed means are impossible, neurovascular compromise requiring immediate exploration, severe tenting of the skin that fails to respond to closed reduction, completely displaced fractures of the middle third of the clavicle in selected patients, displaced distal fractures with rupture of the coracoclavicular ligaments, and completely displaced, irreducible distal fractures in which the coracoclavicular ligaments are intact.

REFERRAL/DISPOSITION

- Conservative treatment of clavicle fractures usually leads to excellent prognosis and full return to sports.
- Consider surgical referral for those reasons noted above.

Return to Play

- Athletes should not be allowed to return to play until the fracture is clinically and radiographically healed (typically 6–8 weeks).
- Noncontact and throwing athletes should have full, painless ROM and at least 90% strength compared to the uninjured arm (usually requires approximately 6 weeks).
- Return to contact/collision sports should be managed on an individual basis.
- Donut pads may be used to protect the clavicle from reinjury.

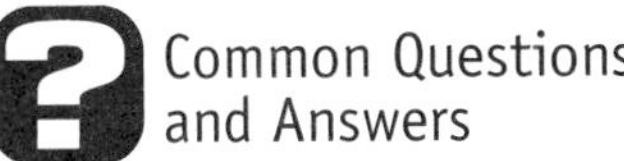

Common Questions and Answers

Physician responses to common patient questions:
Q: While my arm is immobilized, is it allowable to periodically remove my arm from the sling to stretch?
A: Yes. The patient may periodically use the extremity as symptoms allow, but strenuous activity should be avoided. Patients should be instructed to perform elbow ROM exercises to maintain normal function and prevent stiffness.

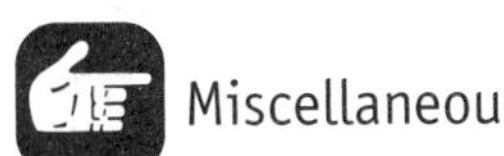

Miscellaneous

ICD-9 CODE

810.00 Clavicle fracture (interligamentous part)(closed)
810.10 Clavicle fracture (open)
810.03 Clavicle fracture, acromial end
810.13 Clavicle fracture, acromial end (open)
810.02 Clavicle fracture, shaft
810.01 Clavicle fracture, sternal end
810.11 Clavicle fracture, sternal end (open)

BIBLIOGRAPHY

Craig EV. In: Rockwood CA and Green DP, eds. *Rockwood and Green's fractures in adults.* Philadelphia: Lippincott-Raven Publishers, 1996.

Eiff MP. Management of clavicle fractures. *Am Fam Physician* 1997;55:121–128.

Hutchinson MR, Ahuja GS. Diagnosing and treating clavicle injuries. *Phys Sports Med* 1996;24:26–36.

McKoy BE, Bensen CV, Hartsock LA. Fractures about the shoulder–conservative management. *Orthop Clin North Am* 2000;31:205–216.

Young DC, Rockwood CA Jr. *Orthopedic sports medicine: principles and practice.* Philadelphia: WB Saunders, 1994.

Authors: Timothy J. Linker and James E. Sturmi

Fracture, Coccyx

Basics

SIGNS AND SYMPTOMS

- Tenderness localized to coccyx
- Low back pain, buttock pain, rectal bleeding (if associated rectal tear)
- Ecchymosis and localized tenderness along gluteal crease
- Pain when sitting or defecating

MECHANISM/DESCRIPTION

- Fall landing in sitting position is most common.
- Also can occur during childbirth
- Surgical procedures performed in area of coccyx
- Fractures of the coccyx are usually transverse.
- More common in women

CAUTIONS

- Although the mechanism may be low impact, patients should be immobilized until other spine injuries are properly evaluated.

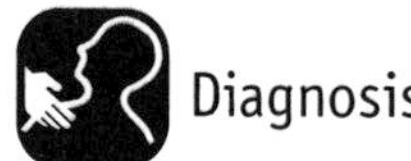

Diagnosis

ESSENTIAL WORKUP

- History and examination
- Exam reveals ecchymosis and tenderness in the gluteal fold.
- Rectal examination is diagnostic and reveals tenderness and crepitus of coccyx.
- Anoscopy should be performed if gross blood is present to evaluate for possible rectal perforation (very rare).
- Examination of entire spine is necessary to evaluate for concomitant injury.

IMAGING/SPECIAL TESTS

- Radiographs will identify other suspected spine injuries.
- Displaced coccyx fractures can be seen on the lateral view.
- Radiographs are not necessary if isolated coccyx fracture is apparent on rectal exam.
- Nondisplaced fractures are difficult to see on x-ray.

DIFFERENTIAL DIAGNOSIS

- Contusion, hematoma
- Pilonidal cyst

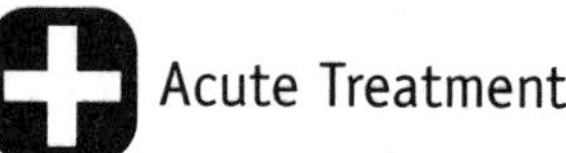

Acute Treatment

INITIAL STABILIZATION

- Spine immobilization for suspected concomitant cervical, thoracic, or lumbar injuries
- Pain control with NSAID or narcotic analgesics

ED TREATMENT

- Symptomatic treatment
- Bedrest initially until ambulation can be tolerated
- Reduction of displaced coccygeal fractures is not necessary.
- If associated rectal injury, surgical consult is required
  —Antibiotics to cover enterics; cefoxitin, cefotetan, metronidazole
- Cushions ("doughnuts")
- Sitz baths
- Stool softeners

MEDICATIONS

- Cefotetan: adult: 2 g IV; peds: 80 mg/kg/day div q 6–8 hrs
- Cefoxitin: adult: 2 g IV; peds: 80–160 mg/kg/day div q 6 hrs
- Metronidazole: adult: 500 mg–1 g IV; peds: 30 mg/kg/day div q 12 hrs

HOSPITAL ADMISSION CRITERIA

- Virtually all patients can be managed as outpatients
- Only patients with severe pain, inability to walk or to take care of themselves, or other serious injury need admission.

HOSPITAL DISCHARGE CRITERIA

- Vast majority can be managed as outpatients with appropriate follow-up.
- Healing is slow.
- Pain may be chronic.
- Orthopedic consultation and possible coccygectomy may be required in severe cases.

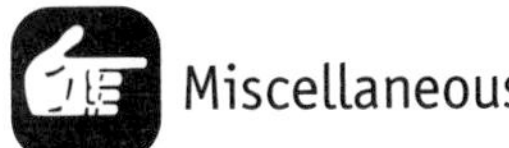

Miscellaneous

ICD-9 CODE

805.6

CORE CONTENT CODE

18.4.3.1.4

BIBLIOGRAPHY

Cwinn AA. Pelvis and hip. In Rosen P, et al., eds. *Emergency medicine: Concepts and clinical practice*. 4th ed. St. Louis: CV Mosby, 1998:739–762.

Pollack C. Pelvic trauma. In: Harwood-Nuss, A, et al., eds. *The clinical practice of emergency medicine*. 2d ed. Philadelphia: Lippincott-Raven, 1996.

Simon R, Koenigsknecht SJ. *Emergency orthopedics: The extremities*. 4th ed. E. Norwalk, CT: Appleton & Lange, 1996.

Rockwood C, Green D, eds. *Fractures in adults*. 4th ed. Philadelphia: Lippincott-Raven, 1996.

Authors: Jaime B. Rivas and Teresa Carlin

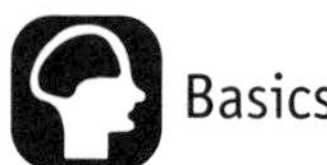

Basics

DEFINITION

- Compression fracture is defined as failure of the anterior vertebral column of the spine. Thoracolumbar spine is divided into anterior column (anterior portion of vertebral body, anterior longitudinal ligament, and anterior annulus fibrosus); middle column (posterior longitudinal ligament, posterior annulus fibrosus, and posterior wall of vertebral body); and posterior column (posterior arch and posterior ligamentous complex).
- Two subtypes: anterior caused by anterior flexion and lateral caused by lateral flexion
- Three locations: cervical, thoracolumbar, and lower lumbar vertebrae
- If anterior and middle columns are involved, the fracture is termed burst. A similar classification system was developed by the Orthopedic Trauma Association for cervical spine injuries.

INCIDENCE/PREVALENCE

- About 50% of spinal column injuries and fractures result from motor vehicle accidents. Sports-related activities account for only 6% to 7% of spine injuries.
- Spine injuries make up about 10% of all athletic injuries.
- Compression fractures made up 48% of thoracolumbar spinal fractures in Denis' series; most commonly injured was the L-1 vertebral body.
- Most common cervical compression fracture is anterior wedge fracture, usually of C-5, as a result of axial loading as might occur in football or diving
- Approximately 10% of cervical spine fractures have an associated, noncontiguous spinal column fracture.
- 15% of female population >50 years will suffer a compression fracture secondary to osteoporosis, usually nontraumatic.

SIGNS AND SYMPTOMS

- Sudden localized pain immediately following direct trauma or axial loading injury

RISK FACTORS

Cervical spine injuries are most common in diving, American football (poor tackling technique), and wrestling.

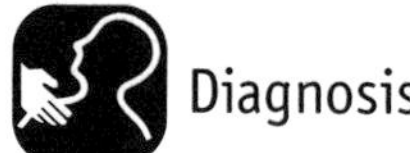

Diagnosis

DIFFERENTIAL DIAGNOSIS

- Burst fracture (anterior and middle column disrupted with or without posterior involvement)
- Fracture-dislocation (anterior, middle, and posterior columns disrupted)
- "Tear-drop" fracture (triangular fracture of anteroinferior vertebral body)
- Transverse process or spinous process fracture
- Lumbar or cervical strain or sprain
- Spondylolysis and/or spondylolisthesis
- Scheuermann disease: kyphosis >50 degrees, wedging of at least three vertebral bodies by at least 5 degrees, disk space narrowing, irregularity of end-plates
- Spear tackler spine: Radiographic evidence of
  —Developmental narrowing of the cervical spinal canal (<13-mm anteroposterior [AP] diameter of spinal canal on plain film or impedence of contrast medium on myelography)
  —Straightening or reversal of the normal cervical lordotic curve
  —Preexisting minor posttraumatic radiographic evidence of bony or ligamentous injury
  —History of repeated spear tackling. Some authors believe that these findings absolutely prohibit return to contact sports. Others believe that if normal cervical lordosis is restored by treatment and the athlete refrains from further spear tackling, then there is not a high risk of injury in returning to athletic activity.
- Burning hands syndrome: variant of central cord syndrome with characteristic complaint of burning paresthesia and dysesthesia in both arms or hands and occasionally legs. Associated with bony or ligamentous spine injury in 50% of cases.

HISTORY

Q: What was the mechanism of injury?
A: Hyperflexion and axial loading injuries such as with "spear tackling" in football or striking the forehead on the bottom of the pool typically cause cervical compression fractures. Hyperextension mechanism suggests a "tear-drop" fracture or defect of posterior spinal elements or pars interarticularis.

Q: Are there any neurologic symptoms?
A: Transient or permanent paralysis and/or sensory deficits can occur with compression fractures but are rare. Neurologic deficits imply spinal cord injury due to retropulsion of disk material or the fracture fragment, i.e., burst fracture.

PHYSICAL EXAMINATION

- Palpate the spinal column for "step-off" defect or tenderness.
- Careful neurologic examination including sensation, motor function, and reflexes. Should be completely intact, but occasionally transient neurologic symptoms occur in an isolated compression fracture.

IMAGING

- AP radiograph: buckling of lateral vertebral cortex next to end-plate with decreased interspinous distance. May show lateral wedging with lateral flexion injury.
- Lateral radiograph: height of anterior vertebral body is decreased while posterior height is unchanged, causing increased density of vertebral body from bony impaction and prevertebral swelling. No subluxation of vertebral bodies.
- Flexion-extension views: evaluate cervical ligamentous instability (>3.5 mm horizontal or 11 degree angular displacement between adjacent vertebrae).

ADDITIONAL IMAGING

- Computed tomographic (CT) scan: should confirm intact vertebral ring (posterior wall, pedicles, and lamina), but up to 25% of compression fractures identified on plain films will be reclassified as burst fractures after CT scanning
- Myelography: rules out osseous protrusion into spinal canal and better evaluates neural compression than CT.
- Magnetic resonance imaging: recommended if neurologic symptoms present or plain films are abnormal to evaluate extrinsic cord or nerve root compression and intrinsic cord abnormalities

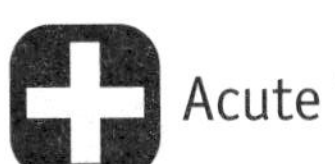

Acute Treatment

ANALGESIA

- Nonsteroidal anti-inflammatory drugs
- Consider narcotics

IMMOBILIZATION

Initial full spinal immobilization with a firm cervical orthosis and back board are necessary in all cases of suspected spine injury.

SPECIAL CONSIDERATIONS

- If spinal cord injury is suspected, then airway should be established and protected, breathing maintained, and circulation supported. If available, methylprednisolone 30 mg/kg can be given.
- If the player is wearing a helmet, it should *not* be removed unless airway is protected. Care must be taken to keep the neck in neutral position, as the helmet will tend to force the neck into flexion. Leaving the shoulder pads on will help keep the neck extended.

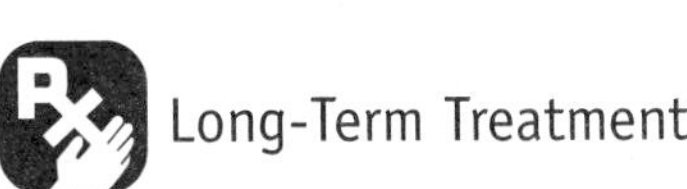

Long-Term Treatment

REHABILITATION

- Cervical compression fractures in the absence of subluxation are treated with a rigid brace for 8–12 weeks with or without halo.
- Thoracic fractures are relatively stable because of surrounding chest cage and strong costovertebral ligaments and can be treated conservatively with relative rest.
- Thoracolumbar injuries (T11-L5) are inherently more unstable and require a longer recumbency and possible immobilization in thoracolumbar spinal orthosis.

SURGERY

- Isolated fractures with <25% anterior compression are considered stable and can be treated with orthotic immobilization.
- A >50% loss of anterior vertebral height, multiple adjacent compression fractures, or angulation >20 degrees at the thoracolumbar junction are associated with segmental instability due to posterior ligamentous injury. This requires surgery to prevent formation of chronic instability and possible further kyphotic deformity. The procedure of choice is usually posterior segmental interspinous wiring and fusion.

REFERRAL/DISPOSITION

Any patient with unstable radiographic abnormalities should be seen by an orthopaedist or neurosurgeon for complete evaluation.

Common Questions and Answers

Physician responses to common patient questions:
Q: Can I play again?
A: Compression fractures without neurologic injuries are considered stable and, once healed completely, should allow the player to return to action when neck pain is gone, range of motion is complete, muscle strength is normal, and fusion is solid (if done). However, athletes with significant vertebral injury requiring a halo brace or surgical stabilization are considered not to have adequate strength to return to contact sports.

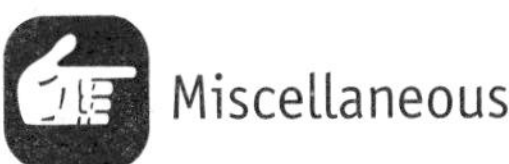

Miscellaneous

SYNONYMS

- Wedge fracture

ICD-9 CODE

805.0 Cervical fracture, closed
805.2 Thoracic fracture, closed
805.4 Lumbar fracture, closed

BIBLIOGRAPHY

Cantu R, Bailes JE, Wilberger JE Jr. Guidelines for return to contact or collision sports after a cervical spine injury. *Clin Sports Med* 1998;17:137–146.

Denis F. The three column spine and its significance in the classification of acute thoracolumbar spinal injuries. *Spine* 1983;8: 817–831.

Maroon JC, Bailes J. Athletes with cervical spine injury. *Spine* 1996;21:2294–2299.

Nicholas J, Nuber G, eds. *The lower extremity and spine in sports medicine.* St. Louis: Mosby, 1995.

Authors: David Bazzo and Jason Bryant

Fracture, Coronoid

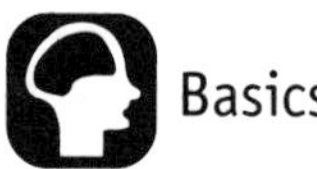

Basics

DEFINITION

- The coronoid process is part of the sigmoid notch, the portion of the proximal ulna that articulates with the humerus.
- Insertion site of the brachialis muscle is just distal to the coronoid process.
- Anterior bundle of the ulna collateral ligament and the middle of the anterior capsule attach at the coronoid process.
- Fractures are categorized according to initial radiographs.
  —Type I: avulsion fractures of the tip of the coronoid process
  —Type II: single or comminuted fragment involving <50% of the coronoid process.
  —Type III: single or comminuted fragment involving >50% of the coronoid process
- All fractures are subclassified.
  —Type A: isolated fractures
  —Type B: fractures associated with dislocation

INCIDENCE/PREVALENCE

- Uncommon, rarely occurring as an isolated injury
- In elbow dislocations, 2% to 15% of cases have coronoid process fractures.

SIGNS AND SYMPTOMS

- Diffuse swelling.
- Tenderness in the anterior elbow over the antecubital fossa
- Limited range of motion for flexion-extension and pronation-supination
- Crepitus may be present.
- Anterior-posterior instability may be present.

RISK FACTORS

- Displacement of large coronoid process fracture fragments has been associated with recurrent dislocation.
- No known significant risk factors to date.

ASSOCIATED INJURIES AND COMPLICATIONS

- Elbow instability
- Radial head fracture
- Olecranon fracture
- Loss of range of motion
- Degenerative joint disease (posttraumatic arthritis)
- Ulnar, median, radial, and anterior interosseous nerve injury
- Brachial artery injury
- Heterotopic ossification

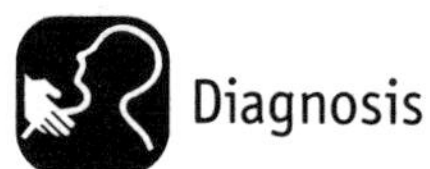

Diagnosis

DIFFERENTIAL DIAGNOSIS

- Elbow subluxation
- Ulnar collateral ligament sprain
- Radial head fractures
- Hyperextension injuries to the anterior joint capsule

HISTORY

- Mechanism of injury usually is impaction.
- Avulsion of the brachialis muscle may be a mechanism.

PHYSICAL EXAMINATION

- If elbow dislocated, perform neurologic and vascular examinations before and after reduction.
- If elbow reduced, check range of motion after reduction to determine stability.
- Palpate radial head and olecranon to look for accompanying fractures.

IMAGING

- Standard elbow x-ray series (anteroposterior, lateral, and one or both obliques) should be requested at the time of evaluation.
- If radial head tenderness, radial head view should be added to x-ray series to increase yield of radial head fractures.

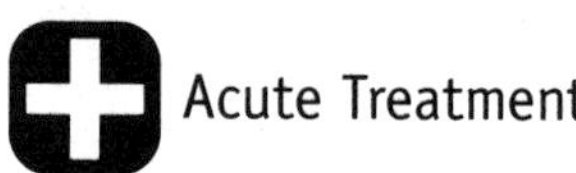

Acute Treatment

IMMOBILIZATION

- Patients should be treated with elbow splints pending definitive care. Immobilization in flexion >90 degrees has been advocated as the optimal position.
- Type I fractures usually are immobilized up to 2 weeks.
- Type II fractures with no or minor displacement are immobilized 3–4 weeks.
- Displaced type II and III fractures are controversial injuries that may predispose the patient to recurrent dislocations. These patients should have a surgical consult to discuss open reduction internal fixation.

SPECIAL CONSIDERATIONS

- Length of immobilization correlates with posttreatment range of motion.
- Presence of posttraumatic arthritis correlates with patient age.
- Pain is a common complaint in at least half of all patients after treatment.

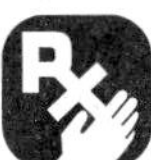

Long-Term Treatment

REHABILITATION

- Gentle active range of motion exercises should be started after immobilization and progress as tolerated.
- Passive range of motion is associated with heterotopic bone formation.
- When full range of motion is present, gentle progressive resistive and stretching exercises can be instituted.

SURGERY

Elective surgical stabilization should be considered in all type III injuries and fractures that are widely displaced.

REFERRAL/DISPOSITION

- Vascular and neurologic injuries
- Complex dislocations with loss of range of motion and stability
- Persistent pain and loss of range of motion after treatment

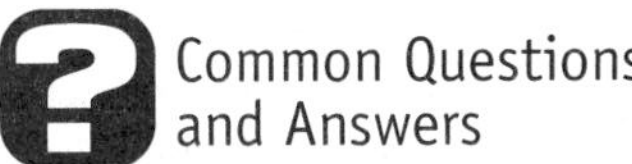

Common Questions and Answers

Physician responses to common patient questions:
Q: How long before I play again?
A: Return to play is based on fracture healing and restoration of functional range of motion, strength, and function. Usually about 6–8 weeks.

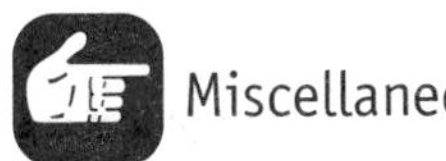

Miscellaneous

ICD-9 CODE

813.02 Fracture coronoid process of ulna

BIBLIOGRAPHY

Regan W, Morrey B. Fractures of the coronoid process of the ulna. *J Bone Joint Surg* 1989;71A:1348–1354.

Rockwood C, Green D, eds. *Rockwood and Green's fractures in adults,* 4th ed. Philadelphia: Lippincott-Raven Publishers, 1996:929–1025.

Selesnick FH, Dolitsky D, Haskell SS. Fracture of the coronoid process requiring open reduction with internal fixation. *J Bone Joint Surg* 1984;66A:1304–1305.

Authors: David A. Stone and Delmas J. Bolin

Fracture, Distal Femur

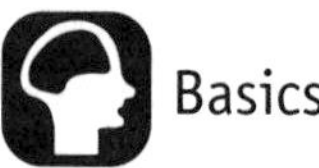

Basics

SIGNS AND SYMPTOMS

- Usually obvious with pain, deformity, swelling, and thigh shortening
- Patient unable to move hip or knee
- Commonly presents with associated injuries: chest or abdominal trauma, hip or knee injury, including dislocation
- Rarely open fracture unless injury is due to penetrating trauma
- Patient may be hypotensive due to hemorrhagic into the thigh.
- Patient may have impaired circulation in the foot due to vascular compromise.

MECHANISM/DESCRIPTION

- Fractures classified according to
  —Location
  —Proximal third (subtrochanteric region)
  —For fractures of the femoral head, neck, and intertrochanteric regions, see topic on Hip Injury
  —Middle third
  —Distal third (distal metaphyseal-diaphyseal junction)
  —Geometry of major fracture line
  —Transverse, oblique, spiral, longitudinal, or segmental
  —Degree of comminution-Winquist and Hansen classification
  —Grade I: small fragment of bone has been broken off; stable lengthwise and rotationally
  —Grade II: >50% contact between abutting cortices; stable lengthwise; may or may not have rotational stability
  —Grade III: <50% contact between abutting cortices; unstable lengthwise and rotationally
  —Grade IV: circumferential loss of cortex; unstable lengthwise and rotationally
- Usually requires major trauma
- Patients are mostly young adults with high-energy injuries (MVAs, GSWs, falls).
- Occasionally seen as a pathologic fracture
- Rarely seen as a stress fracture

PEDIATRIC CONSIDERATIONS

- 70% of femoral fractures in children 3 years old are the result of nonaccidental trauma.
- Spiral fractures of the femur strongly suggest child abuse.

PRE-HOSPITAL

- Immobilization of the extremity and application of a traction splint is important as it can tamponade further blood loss into the thigh.
- Contraindications to traction
  —Fractures close to the knee
  —Fracture or dislocation of the ipsilateral hip
  —Fractures of the pelvis
  —Fractures of the lower leg

CAUTIONS

- Do not attempt to reduce open fractures in the field; cover open wounds with sterile dressings.

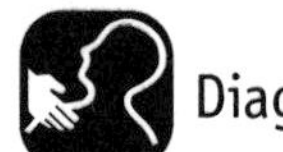

Diagnosis

ESSENTIAL WORKUP

- Radiographs (see below)
- Assess distal pulses, palpate compartments, evaluate sensation and motor function
- If pulses are not equal or palpable, bedside Doppler may be necessary.
- Search for associated injuries.
- In suspected child abuse, obtain skeletal survey or bone scan.

LABORATORY

- CBC, type, and crossmatch

IMAGING/SPECIAL TESTS

- AP pelvis; true lateral of the hip; AP and lateral views of the femur; and complete knee series
- Baseline CXR, other films as indicated trauma protocols

DIFFERENTIAL DIAGNOSIS

- Hip fracture or dislocation
- Knee fracture or dislocation
- Thigh contusion or hematoma

PEDIATRIC CONSIDERATIONS

- Cartilaginous components of the proximal and distal ends of the developing femur alter the fracture patterns seen in hip and knee injuries in children.

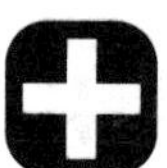

Acute Treatment

INITIAL STABILIZATION

- ABCs of trauma care
- Monitor blood pressure continuously; the thigh can contain 4–6 units of blood

ED TREATMENT

- Pain control is essential; parenteral analgesia acceptable in isolated femur injuries
  —A femoral nerve block can be performed in multiple trauma patients or pediatric patients.
- Orthopedic consultation is necessary for all femoral fractures and is emergent in cases of fracture with neurovascular compromise.
- Femur fractures with diminished or absent distal pulses, an expanding hematoma, or a palpable pulsatile mass require immediate angiography or femoral artery exploration.

- Skeletal traction should be applied if the patient will not go to the OR immediately.
- For closed fractures that require internal fixation, give cefazolin within 24 hours prior to operation.
- Open fractures must go directly to the OR for irrigation and débridement.
  —For open fractures with a laceration of >1 cm, extensive soft-tissue injury, or obvious contamination, give cefazolin and gentamicin or tobramycin in the ED, as well as tetanus booster if indicated.
  —For injuries with highly contaminated wounds add penicillin G to cover Clostridial species.
  —For gunshot wounds to the femur, culture the missile track and cover with an iodine dressing.

MEDICATIONS

- Cefazolin: adult: 2 g IM/IV; peds: 20 mg/kg IM/IV
- Gentamicin/tobramycin: 1.5 mg/kg IV
- Penicillin G: adults: 2 million IU IV; peds: 25,000 IU/kg/day IV divided q 8 hrs

PEDIATRIC CONSIDERATIONS

- Assess markers for nonaccidental trauma
  —Delay in presentation; history of mechanism inconsistent with the injury
  —Isolated trauma to the thigh, associated burns, bruises, or linear abrasions
- Assess for dislocation of the femoral capital epiphysis
- Depending on the age of the patient and the fracture type, pediatric femoral fractures may not require operative treatment.

HOSPITAL ADMISSION CRITERIA

- All femur fractures must be admitted except as noted below in discharge criteria.
- Any suspicion of nonaccidental trauma in children

HOSPITAL DISCHARGE CRITERIA

- In certain rare circumstances of pathologic fracture, or femur fractures in patients that are not ambulatory and would not undergo operative fixation, discharge can be considered in consultation with orthopedics if adequate pain control can be achieved and proper follow-up assured.

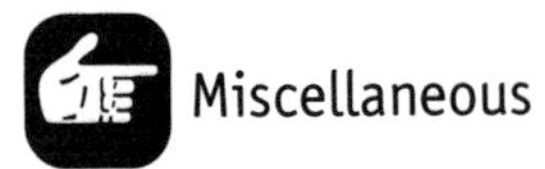

Miscellaneous

ICD-9 CODE

821.00

CORE CONTENT CODE

18.4.13.1.7

BIBLIOGRAPHY

Brien W, et al. Management of gunshot wounds to the femur. *Orthop Clin North Am* 1995;26(1):133–138.

Buckley S. Current trends in the treatment of femoral shaft fractures in children and adolescents. *Clin Orthop* 1997;338:60–73.

Rockwood C, et al. Fractures of the femoral shaft. Chap. 19. In: Rockwood CA, Green DP, eds. *Rockwood and Green's Fractures in adults and children*. Philadelphia: Lippincott-Raven, 1991.

Author: Chris Ho

Fracture, Distal Phalanx

Basics

INCIDENCE/PREVALENCE

- Seen more with contact sports where direct trauma is more likely (e.g., football) or with sports where the hand is exposed to projectiles (e.g., baseball)

SIGNS AND SYMPTOMS

- Pain, swelling, and ecchymosis
- Loss of range of motion
- Obvious deformity, especially if associated with dislocation
- Subungual hematomas
- Traumatic swelling and tenderness over the volar aspect of the distal phalanx with additional palmar pain is a rupture of the flexor digitorum profundus (FDP) until proven otherwise.

RISK FACTORS

- Crush injury to tip of finger (e.g., getting stepped on by opponent's spiked shoes) results in comminuted fracture or tuft injury.
- Acute flexion of an extended distal interphalangeal (DIP) joint (e.g., catching a ball on the tip of the finger or striking an object with the finger extended) results in mallet finger.
- Forced extension while actively flexing the DIP joint (e.g., grabbing a jersey of a ball carrier in football or catching the rim while dunking a basketball) results in jersey finger.

CLASSIFICATION

- Class A: Extra-articular is divided into
  —Type I: longitudinal
  —Type II: transverse
  —Type III: comminuted
  —Type IV: displaced; distal phalanx fractures that are transverse with angulation or displacement
- Class B: Intra-articular avulsion fracture of the dorsal surface (mallet fracture), results when the extensor digitorum is avulsed from its dorsal insertion on the distal phalanx.
- Subclassified into
  —Type IA: <25% of articular surface
  —Type IB: >25% of articular surface; often associated with some degree of subluxation making proper treatment important to prevent a hyperextension proximal interphalangeal joint deformity.
- Mallet finger injury without obvious bony avulsion (tendon stretch or tear) is essentially treated as a class B: type IA distal phalanx fracture.
- Class B: Intra-articular avulsion fractures of the volar surface occurs when the FDP avulses from its site of insertion at the base of the distal phalanx. A bony fragment need not be apparent on x-rays if the clinical signs and symptoms are present.

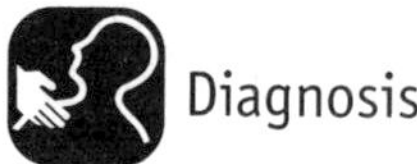

Diagnosis

DIFFERENTIAL DIAGNOSIS

- Fracture or sprain
- Tendon rupture or avulsion

PHYSICAL EXAMINATION

- Include sites of tenderness, range of motion, evidence of instability, and neurovascular examination
- Radiographs should be obtained before any manipulative examination
- Mallet finger: 40 to 45 degree loss of extension at the DIP joint with inability to extend the distal phalanx. There also is pain and swelling over the dorsal aspect of the joint.
- Jersey finger: inability to flex the distal phalanx with tenderness over the volar aspect of the joint and in the palm secondary to retraction of the tendon after rupture.

IMAGING

- Anteroposterior and true lateral views usually adequate; oblique views sometimes helpful
- Consider comparison views of the unaffected side when skeletal immaturity is involved.

POSTREDUCTION VIEWS

- View that best depicts the injury

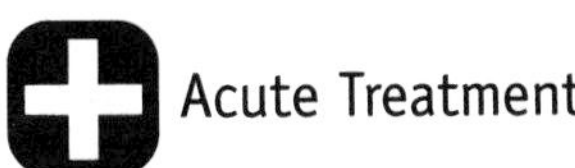

Acute Treatment

ANALGESIA

- If reduction is needed or repair of associated soft tissue injuries (e.g., nail bed laceration), a hematoma block, digital block, or wrist block can be used.
- Nonsteroidal anti-inflammatory drugs with or without narcotics.
- Conscious sedation or reduction under general anesthesia may be needed.

REDUCTION TECHNIQUES

- Class A: type I, II, and II (longitudinal, transverse, and comminuted) distal phalanx fractures: No reduction usually is required; only protective splinting for 3–4 weeks, elevation, and analgesics. Treat associated subungual hematomas.
- Class A: type IV (displaced) distal phalanx fractures with anterior-posterior displacement: Apply traction to the distal aspect and mold the fragments by squeezing the end of the finger between your thumb and index finger. Lateral displacement is corrected by compressing the lateral borders of the terminal phalanx with your thumb and index finger. Be aware that these can be difficult to reduce when soft tissues become interposed between fragments. If uncorrected, this may lead to nonunion.

POSTREDUCTION EVALUATION

- Repeat radiographs
- Neurovascular examination

IMMOBILIZATION

- Class A
  —Type I, II, and III distal phalanx fractures: treated with 3–4 weeks of protective volar or dorsal splinting
  —type IV: reduced and placed into a volar splint for 3–4 weeks.
- Class B
  —Type IA (mallet finger): If seen within 12 weeks of initial injury, splint the DIP joint in extension (not hyperextension) for a minimum of 6 weeks (if associated fracture) or at least 8 weeks (with a pure tendon injury). This usually is accomplished by using a dorsal aluminum splint or a stack splint with strict instructions that the DIP joint remain in continuous extension at all times. Any momentary loss of extension (e.g., during changing or removal of splint for hygiene) mandates restarting back at day 1 of immobilization. This initial treatment often is followed by 2–4 weeks of nighttime-only splinting. The PIP joint is always left free. Some extension lag after treatment is expected.
  —Type IB mallet fractures: Controversy exists between conservative versus surgical treatment. The goal is to prevent a hyperextension PIP deformity (swan-neck deformity). Because the surgery often is deceptively difficult to perform and is associated with several possible complications, operative management is reserved for those injuries with volar subluxation of the distal phalanx. Discussion with your consultant is advised.
  —Acute type II (FDP avulsion) injuries: Initial volar splinting and surgical referral since early operative repair (within 7–10 days) yields best results.

Fracture, Distal Phalanx

SPECIAL CONSIDERATIONS

- With fractures associated with subungual hematomas involving >30% to 50% of the nail, concomitant nailbed lacerations should be suspected and repaired if present. This is usually done using 5-0 or 6-0 dissolvable sutures and replacing the nail plate if possible. This is treated as an open fracture in the sense that it should be done under sterile conditions followed by antibiotic coverage for 7–10 days.
- Complications of distal phalanx fractures include osteomyelitis (open fractures), nonunion, delayed union, osteoarthritis, loss of normal function, and hyperextension deformities of the PIP joint.

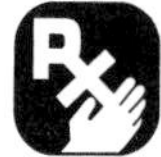

Long-Term Treatment

REHABILITATION

- Physical therapy with a qualified hand therapist is recommended in postoperative cases, after prolonged immobilization, and after splinting mallet finger if return to full range of motion is not progressing
- With mallet finger, patients should be warned against strong passive range of motion in an attempt to hasten flexion, due to the risk of additional damage to the extensor insertion. Gradual progression is usually the rule.

SURGERY

- FDP tears or jersey finger
- Mallet finger injury with volar subluxation of the distal phalanx
- Minimally comminuted distal phalanx fracture with significant displacement (Tuft fracture)
- Any distal phalanx fracture not correctable by closed methods

REFERRAL/DISPOSITION

- Referral is indicated for any injury where surgery is a possible indication.
- Injuries showing poor progression or in patients who are not good candidates for conservative treatment
- For mallet finger injuries not requiring surgery (most of them), return to play depends on the sport and position played and whether the athlete can be reliably padded and splinted once the acute pain and swelling have dissipated.
- If the athlete is in a sport and position where immobilization of the DIP joint would be prohibitive (e.g., basketball player or quarterback) and there is only 4–6 weeks left in the season, it may be reasonable to defer treatment until after the season since "late mallet finger" injuries (seen after 12 weeks) still do very well with conservative treatment, unlike late FDP injuries.

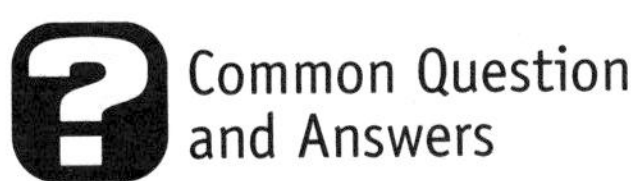

Common Questions and Answers

Physician responses to common patient questions:

Q: If I come out of my stack splint during the treatment of my mallet finger, even for a moment, do I really have to start over at day 1 of treatment?

A: Unfortunately, *yes*. Proper healing is dependent on continuous splinting of the DIP joint for 6–10 weeks. To ensure this, patients are shown how to change their splints while keeping the DIP joint extended against a hard surface before splint application. Patients are seen again after 1–2 weeks to be sure they have complied or can comply with strict protocol.

Q: Does an "old or late" mallet finger need to be splinted?

A: Late, untreated mallet fingers with no functional problems need not be treated.

Q: With mallet finger, what happens if I still have significant extensor lag after an initial trial of splinting?

A: Some experts recommend a second course (8 weeks) of full-time splinting.

Q: Can athletes compete with uncomplicated distal phalanx fractures (class A, types I, II, III)?

A: It depends on several factors. (i) What are the athlete's (and parent's, if a minor) wishes and expectations? They need to be involved in the decision and understand the risks and benefits. (ii) What are the rules governing the athlete's sport? Can you fabricate an effective splint that meets the safe play criteria? (iii) In what position/sport does the athlete compete? Can you realistically place a splint that will protect the DIP joint and allow the athlete to play at a competitive level? Depending on the athlete, their age and maturity, many times they can return to play in a protective splint once the initial swelling and pain have subsided.

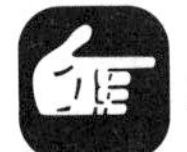

Miscellaneous

SYNONYMS

- Mallet finger: Extensor digitorum avulsion or tear
- Jersey finger: FDP rupture
- Swan-neck deformity: reverse boutonniere deformity; hyperextension of PIP joint caused by disruption of the volar plate attachment to the middle phalanx causing relaxation of the extensor mechanism and allowing the unapposed flexor digitorum to draw the distal phalanx into flexion

ICD-9 CODE

842.10 Finger sprain
816.02 Fracture phalanx, distal (closed)
816.12 Fracture phalanx, distal (open)

BIBLIOGRAPHY

Connolly JF. *Fractures and dislocations: closed management.* Philadelphia: WB Saunders, 1995.

Delee JC, Drez DD, eds. *Orthopedic sports medicine: principles and practices.* Philadelphia: WB Saunders, 1994.

Lairmore JR, Engber WD. Serious, often subtle, finger injuries: avoiding diagnosis and treatment pitfalls. *Physician Sportsmed* 1998;26:57–69.

Pappas AM, ed. *Upper extremity injuries in the athlete.* New York: Churchill Livingstone, 1995.

Reider B, ed. *Sports medicine: the school aged athlete.* Philadelphia: WB Saunders, 1996.

Sallis RE, Massimino F, eds. *ACSM's essentials of sports medicine.* St. Louis: Mosby, 1997.

Simon RR, Koenigsknecht SJ. *Emergency orthopedics: the extremities.* New York: McGraw-Hill, 1994.

Author: Thomas L. Pommering

Fracture, Distal Radius

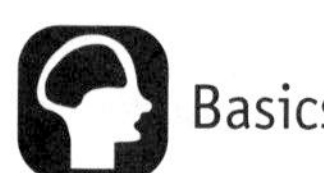

Basics

DEFINITION

- Commonly sustained by falling onto an outstretched hand with the wrist in extension
- Classically, the fractured distal portion will be dorsally displaced and angulated ("silver-fork deformity"); commonly referred to as Colles fracture.
- Other variations include Smith fracture (volar displacement and angulation), Barton fracture (dorsal fracture-dislocation involving displacement of carpus with distal fragment), reverse Barton (Barton fracture with volar displacement), Hutchinson fracture (lateral oriented fracture through radial styloid process extending into radiocarpal articulation), and Galeazzi fracture-dislocation (fracture of distal third of radius with associated dislocation of distal radioulnar joint).
- Key is to always describe fracture location, angulation, displacement, and involvement of either radiocarpal or radioulnar joints.

INCIDENCE/PREVALENCE

- Most common fracture of the upper extremity
- More frequently seen in patients >50 years old
- Female predominance

SIGNS AND SYMPTOMS

- Pain, swelling, and limitation of movement of distal upper extremity
- Paresthesias, weakness, or coolness to touch (associated neurologic or vascular injury)

RISK FACTORS

- Decreased bone mineral density
- Unsteady gait

ASSOCIATED INJURIES AND COMPLICATIONS

- Vascular injury
- Compartment syndrome
- Nonunion
- Arthrosis secondary to poor joint approximation at radioulnar or radiocarpal joint
- Joint stiffness or weakness
- Median nerve dysfunction
- Reflex sympathetic dystrophy

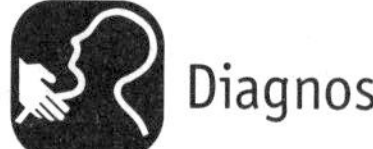

Diagnosis

DIFFERENTIAL DIAGNOSIS

- Carpal fracture
- Ulnar fracture
- Radiocarpal sprain
- Radioulnar sprain
- Soft tissue/bony contusion

HISTORY

- Elicit specific details regarding fall or trauma involved (high vs. low impact)
- Comorbid conditions such as osteoporosis or malignancy

PHYSICAL EXAMINATION

- Gross visualization of the involved extremity for bony deformity and evidence of open injury
- Neurologic evaluation including median and ulnar nerve testing
- Vascular evaluation including radial and ulnar pulses

IMAGING

- Posteroanterior (PA) view: useful for identifying Colles and Hutchinson fractures, and Galeazzi fracture-dislocation
- Lateral view: useful for identifying Colles, Smith, Barton, and reverse Barton fractures, and Galeazzi fracture-dislocation
- Ancillary imaging techniques, including arthrography, bone scan, tomography, or magnetic resonance imaging: may be necessary in subtle or complex cases for further evaluation

POSTREDUCTION VIEWS

PA and lateral views should be obtained after reduction to evaluate correction of radial length and angulation of distal articular surface.

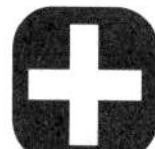

Acute Treatment

ANALGESIA

- Local anesthetic injection into hematoma at fracture site
- Conscious sedation
- General anesthesia for open reduction and internal fixation

REDUCTION TECHNIQUES

- Goal is to achieve anatomical alignment to allow proper healing of the fragments and eventual restoration of normal function.
- Reduction should always be accomplished in a timely manner before soft tissue inflammatory changes progress.
- Closed reduction of displaced distal radial fractures frequently can be accomplished using manual traction of the extremity in combination with manipulative maneuvers to restore alignment.
- Pinning and external fixation frequently are used when there is concern of loss of reduction, especially for intra-articular fracture requiring maintenance of perfect alignment.
- Open reduction and internal fixation are required when a closed reduction cannot be achieved.

POSTREDUCTION EVALUATION

- Repeat neurovascular examination
- Postreduction x-rays (PA and lateral) after application of immobilizing device to assure maintenance of reduction

IMMOBILIZATION

- Nondisplaced fractures allow for adequate immobilization with short arm splint followed by casting when swelling decreases.
- Reducible fractures that are maintained require a sugar-tong splint to reduce supination and pronation. Splint may be exchanged for short arm cast if no displacement on follow-up at 7–10 days.
- Unstable, unreducible, and complex injuries require percutaneous pinning, open reduction internal fixation, and/or external fixation.

SPECIAL CONSIDERATIONS

- Symptomatic patients with open physes should invoke a high suspicion of Salter fracture and should be immobilized with short arm cast for 3–4 weeks.
- Reevaluation and repeat films are recommended at 3, 7, and 21 days to ensure maintenance of reduction.
- If a distal radial fracture is suspected during event coverage, splinting should be applied after careful neurovascular assessment. Transport for radiographic evaluation.

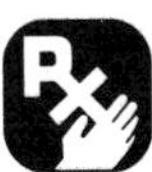

Long-Term Treatment

REHABILITATION

- Physical therapy should be initiated immediately after reduction and immobilization.
- Therapy should focus on mobilization of metacarpophalangeal, proximal interphalangeal, and distal interphalangeal joints.
- Union generally is achieved within 6–8 weeks, after which the patient should begin range of motion of the forearm and wrist.
- Return to sport or usual activities is individualized per patient and should follow appropriate recovery of range of motion and strength.

SURGERY

- Percutaneous pinning, external fixation, and open reduction and internal fixation procedures as outlined in the Immobilization section.

REFERRAL/DISPOSITION

- Orthopaedic surgery referral indicated for fractures involving displacement not easily reducible or with lack of stability (greater displacement increases urgency).
- Surgical procedures optimally performed within 7–10 days.

Common Questions and Answers

Physician responses to common patient questions:

- Physician should be proactive in educating patients on issues of potential adverse outcomes with noncompliance.
- With appropriate intervention, long-term functional deficits are minimized for uncomplicated fractures.
- Duration of casting for Salter fractures and adult fractures average 3–4 weeks and 6–8 weeks, respectively.

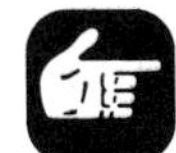

Miscellaneous

SYNONYMS

- Colles fracture
- Smith fracture
- Barton fracture
- Reverse Barton fracture
- Hutchinson fracture
- Galeazzi fracture-dislocation

ICD-9 CODE

813.21 Radius shaft fracture (closed)
813.31 Radius shaft fracture (open)

BIBLIOGRAPHY

Connolly JF, ed. *DePalma's the management of fractures and dislocations.* Philadelphia: WB Saunders, 1981.

Fu FH, Stone DA, eds. *Sports injuries: mechanisms, prevention, and treatment.* Baltimore: Williams & Wilkins, 1994.

Greenspan A. *Orthopedic radiology: a practical approach.* Philadelphia: Lippincott-Raven Publishers, 1996.

Harries M, Williams C, Stanish WE, et al., eds. *Oxford textbook of sports medicine.* Oxford: Oxford University Press, 2000.

Newport ML. Colles fracture: managing a common upper-extremity injury. *J Musculoskel Med* 2000;5:292–301.

Rikli DA, Kupfer K, Bodoky A. Long-term results of the external fixation of distal radius fractures. *J Trauma* 1998;44: 970–976.

Stoffelen D, Broos P. Minimally displaced distal radius fractures: do they need plaster treatment. *J Trauma* 1998;44:503–505.

Stoffelen DV, Broos PL. Kapandji pinning or closed reduction for extra-articular distal radius fractures. *J Trauma* 1998;45: 753–757.

Authors: Douglas McKeag and Kevin B. Gebke

Fracture, Fibula

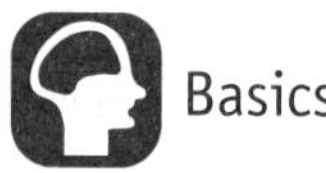

Basics

DEFINITION

An isolated fibula shaft fracture involves the diaphysis only, not ligamentous injury to the tibia or ankle.

INCIDENCE/PREVALENCE

Isolated fibula shaft fractures are rare, usually the result of acute, specific trauma.

SIGNS AND SYMPTOMS

- Acute fibula fractures: swelling, pain, and tenderness over the fracture site
- Isolated shaft fractures: should not present with associated ankle or knee pain or swelling.

RISK FACTORS

- Any sport that may result in direct trauma to the fibular shaft, e.g., direct hit from baseball or puck

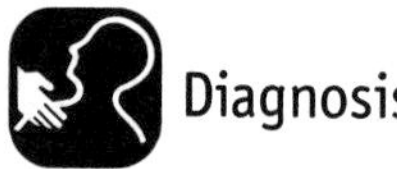

Diagnosis

DIFFERENTIAL DIAGNOSIS

- Concomitant injuries to the knee and ankle
- Rule out pathologic fractures that may occur with such conditions as Ewing sarcoma.

HISTORY

Patients presenting with an isolated fibula fracture typically will give a history of blunt trauma directly to the area of involvement.

PHYSICAL EXAMINATION

- Physical examination of a suspected fibular fracture involves a detailed neurovascular examination. Particular attention to the peroneal nerve should be given, especially with more proximal fractures.
- Direct palpation over the fracture site should reveal point tenderness. No tenderness over the tibia should be present.
- Ankle stability should be assessed to rule out any associated ligamentous injuries that can occur with indirect fibular shaft fractures.

IMAGING

- Anteroposterior and lateral views of the fibula are sufficient for isolated fractures.
- If any ankle tenderness or swelling is present, then three views of the ankle should be obtained.
- Stress view of the ankle may be necessary if ligamentous injury is suspected.

POSTREDUCTION VIEWS

Isolated fibula shaft fractures do not need to be reduced.

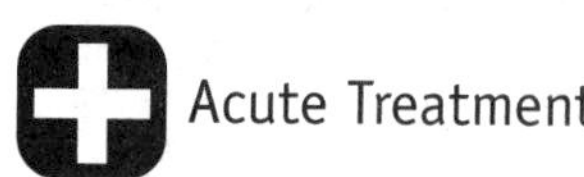

Acute Treatment

ANALGESIA

Nonsteroidal anti-inflammatory drugs or acetaminophen are the treatment of choice. Narcotics rarely are needed.

IMMOBILIZATION

A well-padded splint or cast may be used for comfort, but this is not required. If the patient is comfortable, a lightly wrapped elastic bandage support is applied over adequate padding.

SPECIAL CONSIDERATIONS

Special considerations are only given to fibula fractures associated with fractures to the tibia or ankle.

FIXATION

Isolated fibula fractures require no internal fixation.

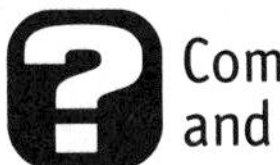

Common Questions and Answers

Physician responses to common patient questions:
Q: Do I need surgery?
A: No, these fractures will heal on their own without surgery.
Q: How long will it take to heal?
A: Most fibula fractures will completely heal in 6–8 weeks. Most patients will be relatively asymptomatic within 1–2 weeks.

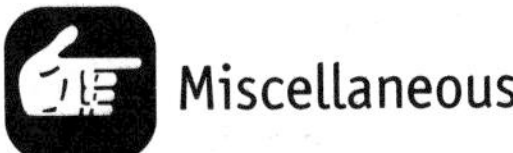

Miscellaneous

SYNONYMS

- Fibula shaft fracture
- Fibula diaphyseal fracture

ICD-9 CODE

823.91

BIBLIOGRAPHY

al-Awami SM, Sadat-Ali M, Sankaran-Kutty M. Arterial injury complicating fracture of the fibula: A case report. *Injury* 1987;18(3): 214–215.

Bostman O, Kyro A. Delayed union of fibular fractures accompanying fractures of the tibial shaft. *J Trauma* 1991;31(1):99–102.

Browner BD, Jupiter JB, Levine AM, et al. *Skeletal trauma.* Philadelphia: WB Saunders, 1998.

Mino DE, Hughes EC Jr. Bony entrapment of the superficial peroneal nerve. *Clin Orthop* 1984;185:203–206.

Morrison KM, Ebraheim NA, Southworth SR, et al. Plating of the fibula: its potential value as an adjunct to external fixation of the tibia. *Clin Orthop* 1991;266:209–213.

Rockwood CA, Green DP, Bucholz RW, et al., eds. *Rockwood and Green's fractures in adults.* Philadelphia: Lippincott-Raven Publishers, 1996.

Shen WJ, Shen YS. Fibular nonunion after fixation of the tibia in lower leg fractures. *Clin Orthop* 1993;287:231–232.

Takebe K, Nakagawa A, Minami H, et al. Role of the fibula in weight bearing. *Clin Orthop* 1984;185:289–292.

Authors: Andrew R. Curran, Arnold D. Scheller Jr., Glen Ross, and Matthew P. Melander

Fracture, Fifth Metatarsal (Avulsion, Jones Fractures)

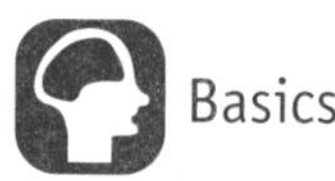

Basics

DEFINITION

- There are two subtypes of fractures involving the fifth metatarsal of the foot.
  —Avulsion fracture of the tuberosity: Near splayed insertion of the peroneus brevis tendon (within 0.5 cm from proximal tip of fifth metatarsal)
  —Jones fracture (metaphyseal/diaphyseal junction): Measuring from the proximal tip of the fifth metatarsal, >0.5 cm and <1.5 cm. Subtypes are
  —***Type 1*** (acute): acute without prior pain. X-rays show clean fracture without sclerosis
  —***Type 2*** (delayed union): involve prior symptoms or a known stress fracture. X-rays show medullary sclerosis and a widened fracture line
  —***Type 3***(nonunion): involves prior symptoms or a known stress fracture. X-rays show evidence of repeated trauma, widened fracture line, and exuberant sclerosis (suggesting fracture nonunion)

INCIDENCE/PREVALENCE

- Avulsion fractures of the fifth metatarsal are the more common of the two types of fractures.
- Fractures of the fifth metatarsal are common foot fractures.

SIGNS AND SYMPTOMS

- Patient may complain of pain over the lateral aspect of foot, especially when weight-bearing on plantar-flexed foot.
- Avulsion fractures often are associated with lateral ankle sprain.
- Jones fractures often occur as a result of a pivot in the direction opposite the planted foot.
- Patient is tender to palpation over the proximal fifth metatarsal.
- Often there may be swelling or ecchymosis of the proximal fifth metatarsal.

RISK FACTORS

- Previous fracture to the fifth metatarsal
- Concurrent, undiagnosed stress fracture of the fifth metatarsal
- Lateral ankle instability

ASSOCIATED INJURIES AND COMPLICATIONS

- Lateral ankle sprain: The anterior talofibular and calcaneofibular ligaments often are injured, and there may be swelling and ecchymosis just anterior and distal to the lateral malleolus.
- Fifth metatarsal stress fracture: Patient may have had a previously undiagnosed and slightly symptomatic stress fracture of the fifth metatarsal.

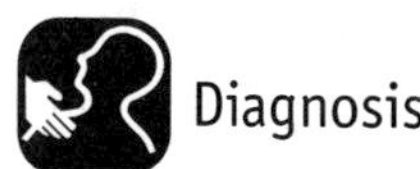

Diagnosis

DIFFERENTIAL DIAGNOSIS

- Peroneus brevis tendon injury
- Diaphyseal stress fracture of the fifth metatarsal
- Apophysis (secondary ossification center closes between ages 9–11 years in girls, 11–14 years in boys)
- Apophysitis (Iselin disease)
- Accessory ossicles
- Hematoma of lateral proximal foot
- Diaphyseal fracture of the fifth metatarsal

HISTORY

Q: How and when did it occur?
A: Mechanism of injury is important to determine
Q: Did athlete injure this foot previously?
A: Determine presence of fracture of the fifth metatarsal
Q: Was there a recent history of ankle sprain prior to this injury?
A: Loss of proprioception and reflex inhibition may have predisposed athlete to this injury.
Q: History of other medical conditions?
A: Diabetes or other causes of peripheral neuropathy

PHYSICAL EXAMINATION

- Check neurovascular status: posterior tibial, dorsalis pedis pulses and normal capillary refill
- Palpate the peroneus brevis tendon to assesses its integrity
- Resisted external rotation of foot activates the peroneus brevis muscle and checks its strength
- Full examination of the distal fibular, lateral ligaments, and foot helps identify associated ankle or foot injury
- Check sensation: if decreased around lateral aspect of foot, the lateral dorsal cutaneous nerve, a branch off the sural nerve, may be injured.

IMAGING

- Standard x-ray films: anteroposterior (AP), lateral, and oblique views of the foot. If findings are suggestive of ankle trauma meeting the Ottawa criteria, ankle films (AP, lateral, and oblique views) also should be taken.
- Avulsion fracture are often extra-articular; involvement of the cubometatarsal joint is not uncommon.

POSTREDUCTION VIEWS

Only applicable when clinician attempts to reduce a significantly displaced fracture of the fifth metatarsal. Most displaced fractures are best treated operatively. Views would be AP, lateral, and oblique.

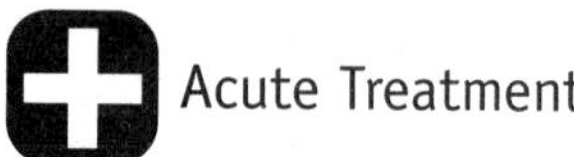

Acute Treatment

ANALGESIA

- Apply ice, rest, and elevate foot
- Oral pain relief (acetaminophen, aspirin, nonsteroidal anti-inflammatory drugs, or narcotics) often sufficient if reduction not necessary
- If reduction is needed, give oral pain relief before performing a hematoma block (2–5 mL of 1% lidocaine). Significantly displaced fracture warrants an orthopaedic referral for possible surgery.

REDUCTION TECHNIQUES

- Generally, not recommended, if surgical fixation is an option.
- Grab the fifth toe and distract in a longitudinal plane. Apply plantar or dorsal pressure to the proximal portion of the fifth metatarsal.

POSTREDUCTION EVALUATION

Check alignment via postreduction radiographs.

IMMOBILIZATION

- Avulsion fractures: Place in a hard-soled shoe for 3–4 weeks. Can place in a walking boot or walking cast if worried about patient compliance.
- Jones (metaphyseal/diaphyseal) fractures:
  —***Type 1:*** Place in a nonweight-bearing short leg cast for 6–8 weeks.
  —***Type 2:*** May place in a nonweight-bearing short leg cast for 8–12 weeks. Conservative treatment has variable outcomes. Many consider surgical fixation because of better prognosis and quicker return to activity.
  —***Type 3:*** Consider surgical fixation.

SPECIAL CONSIDERATIONS

When deciding on treatment for type 2 Jones fractures, take into account athlete's time table and previous medical history. Occasionally after conservative treatment a nonunion develops secondary to "distal-to proximal" vascular supply to the bone and requires surgery.

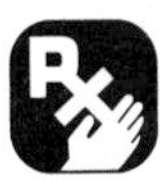

Long-Term Treatment

REHABILITATION

- Avulsion fractures: Start with range of motion and progress to strengthening of the peroneus brevis (external rotation and pronation of the foot). Patient may return to play after 3–4 weeks and when no longer symptomatic.
- Jones fractures: Once no longer immobilized, start with range of motion and progress to strengthening. Electrical stimulation may help patient initially learn to reactivate musculature.

SURGERY

- Consider surgical fixation (open reduction, internal fixation with a cannulated screw) with type 2 and 3 Jones fracture.
- If the fracture is significantly displaced or comminuted, consider surgery.

REFERRAL/DISPOSITION

- Orthopaedic referral for surgery as indicated above and for avulsion fracture that are displaced (rare), comminuted (rare), or involve >30% of the cubometatarsal articulation.
- Patients not responding to home exercise programs after immobilization is complete may benefit from referral to physical therapy.
- Type 1 Jones fractures should be referred to an orthopaedist if patient prefers surgery in order to return to play quicker or the fracture is displaced or comminuted.

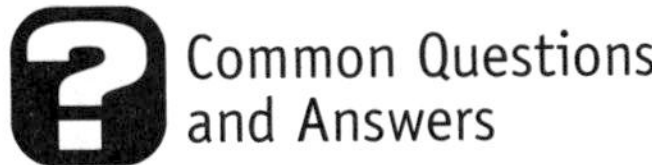

Common Questions and Answers

Physician responses to common patient questions:
Q: How long until I can play again?
A: Avulsion fractures: about 3–4 weeks. Jones fractures: up to 20 weeks with conservative therapy. Type 1: ≥8 weeks. Types 2 and 3: if casted, 3–5 months and 8 weeks for surgery

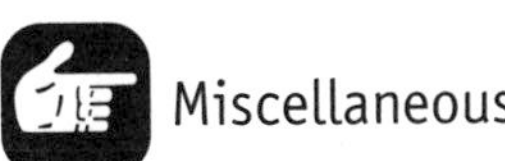

Miscellaneous

SYNONYMS

Dancers or tennis fracture: avulsion fracture of base of the fifth metatarsal

ICD-9 CODE

825.25 Metatarsal fracture, closed
825.35 Metatarsal fracture, open

BIBLIOGRAPHY

Clapper MF, O'Brien TJ, Lyons PM. Fractures of the fifth metatarsal. *Clin Orthop* 1995;315: 238–241.

Lawrence SJ, Botte MJ. Jones fractures and related fractures of the proximal fifth metatarsal. *Foot Ankle* 1993;14:358–365.

Leddy JJ. Imaging ankle injuries. *Am J Sports Med* 1998;26:158–165.

Quill GE. Fractures of the proximal fifth metatarsal. *Ortho Clin NA* 1995; 26(2):353–361.

Simons SM. Foot injuries in the recreational athlete. *Physician Sportsmed* 1999;27: 57–70.

Strayer SM, Reece SG, Petrizzi MJ. Fractures of the proximal fifth metatarsal. *Am Fam Physician* 1999;59:2516–2522.

Torg JS, Baldvini FC, Zelko RR, et al. Fractures of the base of the fifth metatarsal distal to the tuberosity. Classification and guidelines for nonsurgical and surgical management. *J Bone Joint Surg* 1984;66(2):209–214.

Author: Mark Lavallee

Fracture, Frontal Sinus

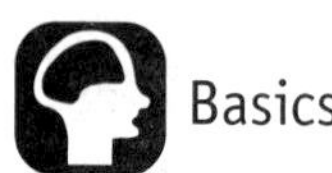

Basics

SIGNS AND SYMPTOMS

- Contusion, bruise, or laceration on the forehead overlying the frontal sinus
- Depression or swelling over the frontal sinus area
- Crepitus over the frontal sinus
- Loss of consciousness or altered mental status secondary to associated brain injury or posterior table fracture
- Associated facial trauma with supraorbital, orbital, nasal, frontonasoethmoid, or maxillary fractures
- Associated ocular trauma may be present.
- Bloody discharge from the nose, without visible nasal source
- Clear rhinorrhea indicative of cerebrospinal fluid leak
- Absent tearing which may be indicative of nasofrontal duct injury

MECHANISM/DESCRIPTION

- Typically due to high-velocity blunt trauma localized to the frontal sinus area
- Because the anterior table is thick it requires 800–2200 pounds of force to cause frontal sinus fracture (twice the force required to fracture other facial bones).
- Most frontal sinus fractures are from motor vehicle accidents, although altercations or assaults, usually with a weapon such as a cue stick or baseball bat, can also create enough localized force to cause the injury.

PEDIATRIC CONSIDERATIONS

- The frontal sinuses are not fully formed in children and this is a rare injury. The force required to create this injury is usually transmitted to the frontal bones and brain.

CAUTIONS

- Airway control takes precedence
  - —Associated facial injuries may preclude the use of oral intubation.
  - —Nasotracheal intubation is contraindicated in massive facial or nasal trauma.
  - —Cricothyrotomy is the airway of choice if intubation using RSI cannot be performed.
- Most patients with frontal sinus fractures have serious associated injuries due to amount of force needed to create the injury.
  - —If associated injuries are present, protect the cervical spine.
- 75% of patients with frontal sinus fractures lose consciousness.
- The frontal sinus fracture is not the immediate concern in a multiple trauma victim.

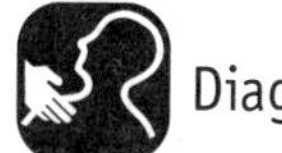

Diagnosis

ESSENTIAL WORKUP

- The physical examination is the most important aspect of the evaluation. Failure to diagnose a frontal sinus fracture can lead to abscess formation, meningitis, mucocele formation, osteomyelitis of the calvarium, or permanent cosmetic deformity.
- Look for more serious injuries first, and treat life-threats.
- Carefully palpate the frontal area for crepitus or depression.
- Lacerations over the frontal sinus area mandate digital palpation for a fracture line and a careful visual exploration for underlying fractures.
- Perform a nasal speculum examination looking for blood, septal hematoma, or CSF high in the nasal cavity.
- Perform a careful neurologic examination to look for CNS injury.
- Perform a careful ophthalmologic exam.

IMAGING/SPECIAL TESTS

- Caldwell and lateral views are good for preliminary evaluation but frontal sinus fractures can be subtle on these films.
- *CT scanning is the imaging modality of choice.* Altered mental status or history of loss of consciousness, or discovery of an anterior table fracture by exam or on plain films should be further investigated by CT to rule out associated posterior table fracture or intracranial injury.
  - —Associated intracranial injuries on CT may include subdural hemorrhage or pneumocephalus.

ASSOCIATED CONDITIONS

- Frontal sinus fractures may disrupt the frontonasal duct.
- Intracranial injuries are present in 12–17% of patients with frontal sinus fractures.
- About 15% of patients with frontal sinus fractures have an associated CSF leak.
- Ocular injuries are present in up to 59%.

DIFFERENTIAL DIAGNOSIS

- Nasofrontoethmoid fractures, cribriform plate fractures, and facial fractures including the orbits, maxilla, nasal, and zygomatic bones
- Frontal fractures not involving the frontal sinus may have a similar presentation

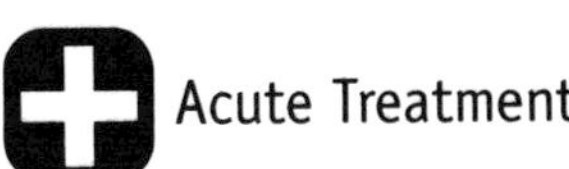

Acute Treatment

INITIAL STABILIZATION

- ABCs of trauma care, attend to the airway as the first priority
  - —RSI is the initial airway management of choice.
  - —Massive facial injuries may require a surgical airway if RSI is unsuccessful.
- If associated injuries are present, protect the cervical spine until cleared.
- Other major injuries and life-threats take precedence over the frontal sinus fracture.

ED TREATMENT

- If while irrigating a laceration overlying the frontal sinus the patient can taste the irrigating solution or notes the irrigating fluid in the nose, the frontal sinus is disrupted.
- If a simple anterior table fracture is noted, and posterior table fracture and intracranial injuries are ruled out, the presence of a frontonasal duct injury should be evaluated by instilling fluorescein into the frontal sinus. Lack of visualization of the fluorescein in the nose is indicative of disruption of the duct.
- Antibiotics are indicated in all patients with frontal sinus fractures. Intravenous antibiotics are indicated in patients with posterior table fractures or CSF leaks.
- Lacerations overlying frontal sinus fractures involving only the anterior table may be sutured in the ED. ENT or plastic surgery should evaluate lacerations associated with more complex sinus injuries.

MEDICATIONS

- Cefotaxime: adult: 2 g IV; peds: 50 mg/kg IV single dose
- Cephalexin: adult: 250–500 mg po qid; peds: 25–50 mg/kg/day div qid

HOSPITAL ADMISSION CRITERIA

- Patients with other significant associated trauma
- Patients with posterior table fractures (to neurosurgery or ENT)
- Patients with associated intracranial injuries (neurosurgery)
- Patients with CSF leak

HOSPITAL DISCHARGE CRITERIA

- Patients with frontal sinus fractures who may be discharged are those with isolated injuries only who have no involvement of the posterior table or evidence of an intracranial injury on CT. Oral antibiotics are indicated in these patients. Referral to ENT in 24–36 hours is appropriate.

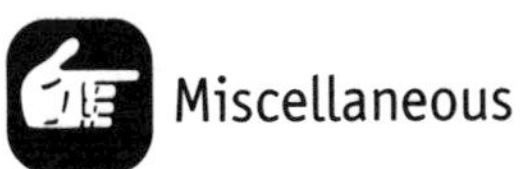

Miscellaneous

ICD-9 CODE

801.00

CORE CONTENT CODE

18.4.4.1

BIBLIOGRAPHY

Keefe SD, et al. Frontal sinus fractures. In: English GM, ed. *Otolaryngology*. Vol 4. Rev ed. Philadelphia: JB Lippincott, 1994: 342–364.

Manson PN. Maxillofacial injuries. *Emerg Med Clin North Am* 1984;2(4):761–82.

Rohrich RJ, et al. Management of frontal sinus fractures: Changing concepts. *Clin Plast Surg* 1992;19(1):219–32.

Authors: Mark L. Madenwald and David W. Munter

Fracture, Hamate: Hook, Body

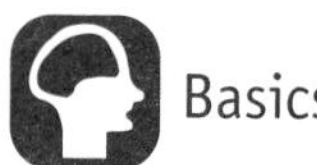

Basics

DEFINITION

- A fracture through the hook or the body of the hamate

INCIDENCE/PREVALENCE

Hook Fracture

- Hook of the hamate fractures account for <2% of all carpal bone fractures.
- Approximately 180 cases of hook of the hamate fracture are reported in the literature, a low number because routine x-rays usually are normal and symptoms are nonspecific.
- Average length of time from injury to correct diagnosis is 10 months.
- Fractures most commonly occur at the base of the hook.
- 98% of the fractures are in men, average age 33 years.

Body Fracture

Body of the hamate fractures are rare and much less common than hook fractures.

RISK FACTORS

Hook Fracture

- Sporting activities that involve a bat, club, or racket
- Golf is the sport that results in the most hook of the hamate fractures.

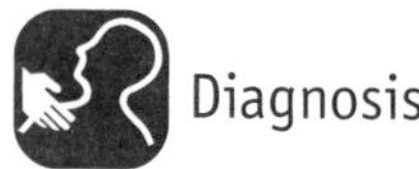

Diagnosis

DIFFERENTIAL DIAGNOSIS

- Flexor/extensor carpi ulnaris tendonitis/strain
- Metacarpal/carpal bone fracture or contusion
- Ulnocarpal ligament sprain
- Triangular fibrocartilaginous complex tear
- Ulnar artery thrombosis

HISTORY

Hook Fracture

- Hook of the hamate fractures occur in athletes who use equipment with a handle, e.g., golf clubs, baseball bats, and rackets.
- Athlete grips the handle of the club, bat, or racket over the distal ulnar aspect of the palm, placing the handle in close proximity to the hook of the hamate.
- In golf, the fracture often occurs when the club head accidentally strikes too much ground and a large divot is taken. In baseball, most fractures occur at the end of forceful check swings as opposed to swings that make contact with the ball.
- A less common mechanism of injury is a fall on an outstretched hand.

Body Fracture

Body fractures often result from punching a hard stationary object, such as a wall, with a closed fist. The fourth and fifth metacarpals are driven back into the hamate, leading to a fracture. Body fractures may accompany a boxer's fracture.

PHYSICAL EXAMINATION

- Point tenderness occurs in the palm over the hook of the hamate. The hook is located by projecting a line from the pisiform to the center of the head of the index metacarpal. Rarely, if the fracture is at the base of the hook, pain may be greater over the dorsal hamate than over the hook in the palm.
- Palpate the flexor/extensor carpi ulnaris tendons at their insertions and test flexion/extension strength in ulnar deviation to evaluate for tendon strain.
- Painful and weak grasp
- Check pulses. An Allen test will help to rule out ulnar artery thrombosis. Signs of partial or complete fourth/fifth flexor digitorum profundus (FDP) tendon rupture may be present. Pain with grip, decreased grip strength, crepitance with fourth/fifth finger motion, and, eventually, loss of active flexion at the fourth/fifth finger distal interphalangeal joints may indicate FDP injury; 14% of all hook fractures are correctly diagnosed only after FDP tendon rupture.
- Decreased sensation or weakness may be due to ulnar or median nerve injury. The fracture fragments may directly injure the nerves, or swelling and inflammation may indirectly injure them.

IMAGING

Hook Fracture

- The routine wrist series (anteroposterior [AP], lateral, and oblique views) usually are negative, often delaying diagnosis.
- Ring of the hook can be visualized on AP view; if it is not present, this may be a clue to a hook fracture.
- Carpal tunnel view often will aid in making the diagnosis. However, to obtain this view, the wrist must be forcefully hyperextended. During the acute phase of the injury, pain and limited range of motion may not allow proper positioning to make this x-ray possible.
- Another useful view is the radially deviated, thumb-abducted lateral view. The hook is seen in profile between the first and second metacarpals.
- Computed tomographic (CT) scanning is the gold standard for diagnosis but often is unnecessary if plain films show the fracture. CT scans are useful if plain films are negative and a fracture is highly suspected. CT scanning has the advantage of visualizing both hamates at the same time and can be used to evaluate the extremely rare case of a bipartite hamate, which usually is bilateral and is a normal variant. CT scan is performed with both hands in the praying position (palm to palm).

Body Fracture

- The routine wrist series (AP, lateral, and oblique views) are more useful for diagnosis of body fractures than for hook fractures. The oblique and lateral views are the most useful.
- CT scan may be needed to delineate further the exact fracture pattern and degree of fragment displacement. CT scan should be considered when routine films are negative but a fracture is highly suspected.

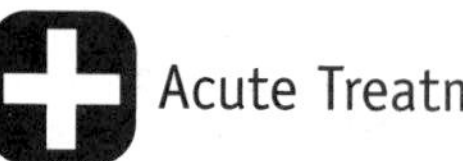

Acute Treatment

ACUTE TREATMENT (<2 WEEKS)

Hook Fracture

- One option is excision of the hook distal to the fracture. Most patients return to their previous level of functioning in their sport or occupation by 8 weeks. Excision has been the favored approach for both displaced and nondisplaced fractures.
- Conservative option for nondisplaced fractures is a short arm cast. The cast should immobilize the metacarpophalangeal joints of the fourth/fifth fingers and be a thumb spica to decrease micromotion at the hook. Cast should be worn for 6–8 weeks to prevent nonunion. If pain is still present after cast removal, then excision for nonunion is the treatment of choice.
- Decision between casting and surgery is based on the lifestyle demands of the patient. The athlete who does not want to risk having a nonunion after casting may opt for surgery to minimize the time away from sport. Similarly, a patient with a job that requires repetitive grabbing, gripping , or lifting may elect for excision to reduce the risk of an extended period of time away from work.

DELAYED TREATMENT (>2 WEEKS)

Hook Fracture

- Nonunion of the hook of the hamate is very common and not believed to be related to its blood supply, as it is in the scaphoid. Vessels enter the hook both proximally and distally, making avascular necrosis unlikely. Nonunion is related to micromotion from soft tissue attachments to the hook.
- Excision of the hook is the treatment of choice for nonunion injuries. The sooner the fragment is removed and the base smoothed, the less likely the chance for tendon rupture and/or neurovascular damage. Complete rupture of the FDP tendon is reported to occur in 15% to 20% of cases of nonunion. The FDP of the little finger ruptures more commonly than that of the ring finger. Excision is associated with a 3% complication rate; complications include ulnar/median nerve injury, ulnar palmar arch vessel injury, weakness, painful grip, altered sensation, flexor tendon adhesions, and scar tenderness.
- Alternative approach is open reduction and internal fixation (ORIF); the goal is to maintain maximal grip strength by preserving the pulley system for the fourth/fifth FDP tendons. Although this seems logical, the loss of grip strength associated with excision has been minimal, resulting in excision being the most popular surgical treatment method.

SPECIAL CONSIDERATIONS

Hook Fracture

Treatment for painless nonunion is excision to reduce the risk of tendon rupture and/or neurovascular injury.

TREATMENT

Body Fracture

- Oblique fractures are the most common and can be treated in a short arm cast for 4–6 weeks if the fragments are not displaced. Any displacement of the fracture fragments requires ORIF.
- Coronal fractures are less common and often are associated with dorsal dislocation of the fourth/fifth metacarpals. These should all be treated by ORIF.

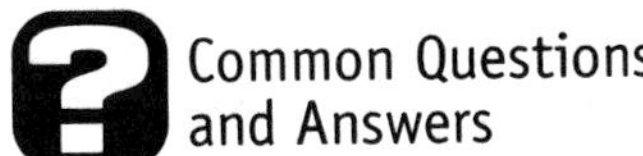

Common Questions and Answers

Physician responses to common patient questions:

Q: Which treatment option for hook fracture is most likely to get me back to my sport the quickest with the least amount of residual symptoms?

A: Excision of the hook of the hamate

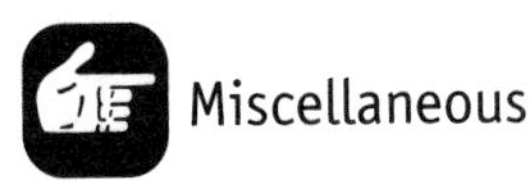

Miscellaneous

ICD-9 CODE

814.08 Closed hamate fracture

BIBLIOGRAPHY

Bhalla S, Higgs P, Gilula L. Utility of the radial-deviated, thumb-abducted lateral radiographic view for the diagnosis of hamate hook fractures: case report. *Radiology* 1998;209:203–207.

Binzer T, Carter P. Hook of the hamate fracture in athletes. *Op Tech Sports Med* 1996;4:242–247.

Bishop A, Beckenbaugh R. Fracture of the hamate hook. *J Hand Surg* 1988;13A: 135–139.

Boulas H, Milek M. Hook of the hamate fractures: diagnosis, treatment, and complications. *Orthop Rev* 1990;XIX: 518–529.

Carroll R, Lakin J. Fracture of the hook of the hamate: acute treatment. *J Trauma* 1993;34:803–805.

Chase J, Light T, Benson L. Coronal fracture of the hamate body. *Am J Orthop* 1997;26(8): 568–571.

Ebraheim N, Skie M, Savolaine E, Jackson W. Coronal fracture of the body of the hamate. *J Trauma* 1995;38:169–174.

Author: Mark Stovak

Fracture, Humeral Head

Basics

SIGNS AND SYMPTOMS

- Pain, swelling, and tenderness about the shoulder, especially around the greater tuberosity
- Difficulty in initiating active motion
- Position of patient is often with arm closely held against the chest.
- Crepitus may be present.
- Ecchymoses within 24–48 hours at area of fracture and may spread to chest wall, flank, and distal extremity
- Diminished peripheral pulses, or decreased sensation especially over the deltoid muscle (axillary nerve)

MECHANISM/DESCRIPTION

- Proximal humeral fractures involve fractures of the humeral head, lesser tuberosity, greater tuberosity, bicipital groove, and proximal humeral shaft.
- Mechanisms of injury
  —Fall onto an outstretched hand
  —High energy direct trauma
  —Excessive rotation of the arm in the abducted position
  —Electrical shock or seizure
  —Pathologic fracture from metastatic disease
- Typically seen in adults over the age of 45 years and the elderly
- Proximal humeral fractures account for 5% of all fractures.

CAUTIONS

- Excessive movement of the arm may produce further neurovascular injury.

CONTROVERSIES

- Pre-hospital reduction is not recommended as manipulation may induce neurovascular injury or displace a fracture.

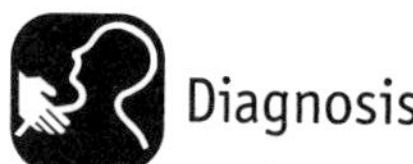

Diagnosis

ESSENTIAL WORKUP

- Careful history and physical examination to localize the injury and to rule out any other significant injuries
- Assessment of neurovascular status
  —Assess function of radial, median, ulnar, axillary (sensation to the lateral aspect of the shoulder), and musculocutaneous nerve (sensation to the extensor aspect of the forearm).
  —Presence of radial, ulnar, and brachial pulses, and good capillary refill in all digits
- Shoulder radiographs

IMAGING/SPECIAL TESTS

- Anteroposterior, lateral and axillary views or Transthoracic or 'y' view
  —The axillary view is necessary to assess tuberosity displacement, the glenoid articular surface, and the relationship of the humeral head to the glenoid.
  —CT scan can be useful in evaluating articular surfaces of glenoid and humeral head.

DIFFERENTIAL DIAGNOSIS

- Acute hemorrhagic bursitis
- Traumatic rotator cuff tear
- Dislocation
- Acromioclavicular separation
- Calcific tendinitis
- Pathologic fracture

PEDIATRIC CONSIDERATIONS

- In children, proximal humeral fractures consist of metaphyseal fractures and physeal separations. Three fracture patterns tend to be displayed depending on the age group.
- Children <5 years: Salter-Harris I fractures are seen
  —Neonatal fractures occur from obstetric trauma and pseudoparalysis are often seen.
  —Physeal separation in the infant may also be the result of physical abuse.
- Children 5–10 years: Metaphyseal fractures tend to occur in this age group because rapid growth causes thinning of the metaphyseal cortex. Most fractures are transverse or short oblique.
- Children >11 years: Salter-Harris II fractures tend to be seen in the adolescent

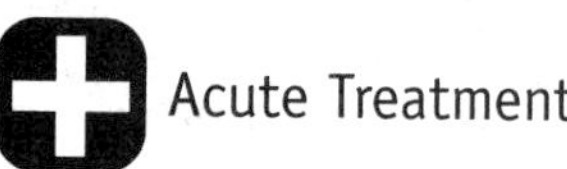

Acute Treatment

INITIAL STABILIZATION

- ABCs and secondary survey for associated injuries
- Immediate immobilization is important to prevent further fracture displacement or neurovascular injury.
  —Sling with arm supported at the side or in the Velpeau position
  —Axillary pad may also be used for comfort.
  —After immobilization perform another neurovascular exam.

ED TREATMENT

- Emergency Department treatment consists of proper immobilization, orthopedic consultation, and providing pain management.

- *Operative versus nonoperative treatment* is decided in conjunction with orthopedics.
- *Neer classification*: This system identifies the number of fragments and their location.
  - —The fractures consist of 2-part to 4-part fractures, and the locations include the anatomical neck, the surgical neck, the greater tuberosity, and the lesser tuberosity.
  - —Fracture-dislocation and humeral head splitting are also part of the Neer classification.
  - —In general, the higher the number of fragments in the fracture and the greater the degree of displacement, the more difficult it is to manage the patient with a closed reduction.
- *Nonoperative treatment*
  - —Initial immobilization and early motion: succeeds in many cases as most proximal humeral fractures are minimally displaced
  - —Use a sling, swathe, and axillary pad to immobilize.
  - —Closed reduction should be performed with consultation of an orthopedic surgeon.
  - —Conscious sedation should be used for all closed reductions.
  - —Following reduction, the stability of the fracture can be tested in different positions to ascertain that significant displacement requiring surgical intervention will not occur.
  - —1-part and 2-part fractures are often successfully treated with closed reduction, but 3-part and 4-part fractures are unstable and may need ORIF.

MEDICATIONS

- Pain medications are indicated for comfort.
- Conscious sedation should be used if attempting a closed reduction.

PEDIATRIC CONSIDERATIONS

- In children nearing skeletal maturity, determining the degree of displacement or separation of the proximal humeral epiphysis is essential as exact reduction is important to prevent later growth disturbance.

HOSPITAL ADMISSION CRITERIA

- Open fractures for operative management and parenteral antibiotic therapy
- Displaced fracture which cannot be treated through closed reduction and therefore requires operation
- Significant associated injuries which require admission and observation

HOSPITAL DISCHARGE CRITERIA

- Patients with either a nondisplaced fracture or a fracture that is successfully treated through closed reduction and who has no associated injuries

PEDIATRIC CONSIDERATIONS

- Pediatric patients are often less compliant with immobilization and less able to verbalize complaints and may benefit from admission to the hospital for observation and neurovascular checks.

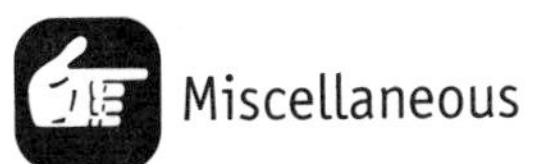

Miscellaneous

ICD-9 CODE

812.09

CORE CONTENT CODE

18.4.12.1.6

BIBLIOGRAPHY

Hawkins RJ, Angelo RL. Displaced proximal humeral fractures: Selecting treatment, avoiding pitfalls. *Orthop Clin North Am* 1987;18(3):421–431.

Morrissy RT, Weinstein SL. *Lovell and Winter's pediatric orthopaedics*. Vol. II. 4th ed. Philadelphia: Lippincott-Raven, 1996.

Neer CS. Displaced proximal humeral fractures: I. Classification and evaluation. *J Bone Joint Surg* 1970;52A:1077–1089.

Rasmussen S, Hvass I, Dalsgaard J, Christensen S, Holstad E. Displaced proximal humeral fractures: Results of conservative treatment. *Injury* 1992;23(1):41–42.

Rockwood CA, Green DP, Bucholz RW, Heckman JD. In: Rockwood CA, Green DP, eds. *Rockwood and Green's fractures in adults*. 4th ed. Philadelphia: Lippincott-Raven, 1996.

Authors: Nancy Kwon and Wallace Carter

Fracture, Humeral Shaft

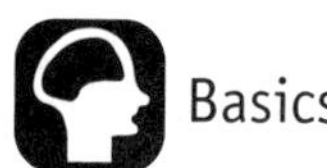

Basics

SIGNS AND SYMPTOMS

- Pain and swelling over the area of the humeral shaft
- Shortening, deformity, or decreased mobility
- Crepitus on gentle motion
- Possible weakness or numbness
  - —Associated nerve injury is the radial nerve

MECHANISM

- Most commonly direct trauma from a fall or direct blow to the upper arm
- Fall on elbow or outstretched arm
- Ball throwing

MECHANISM/DESCRIPTION

- Three types
  - —Nondisplaced
  - —Displaced or angulated
  - —Severely displaced or associated with neurovascular damage
- 3% of all fractures

PEDIATRIC CONSIDERATIONS

- Always consider child abuse especially with spiral fractures of the humerus which implies a rotational component to the injury.

CAUTIONS

- Immobilization with sling and swath and transport
- Rapid transport in presence of neurologic or vascular deficits

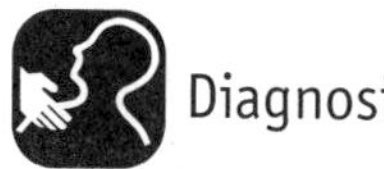

Diagnosis

ESSENTIAL WORKUP

- History and examination with special attention to a thorough neurovascular exam and skin integrity
- Consider associated injuries.
- Diagnosis is confirmed by x-ray.

IMAGING/SPECIAL TESTS

- AP and lateral views of the entire humerus are mandatory.
  - —Include shoulder and elbow views to exclude associated joint involvement.

DIFFERENTIAL DIAGNOSIS

- Contusion
- Tendon rupture
- Neuropraxia

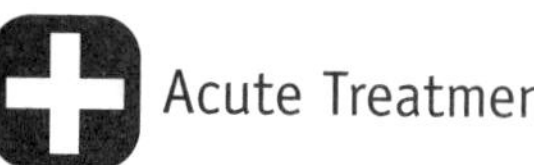

Acute Treatment

INITIAL STABILIZATION

- Pain control with NSAIDs or narcotic analgesics
- Immobilization with sling and swath or shoulder immobilizer pending definitive diagnosis
- Application of ice to limit swelling
- Open humerus fractures require covering with a sterile dressing, tetanus prophylaxis, and parenteral prophylactic antibiotics.

ED MANAGEMENT

- These fractures usually don't require elaborate reduction or immobilization.
- Nondisplaced fractures can be treated with a sugar-tong splint of the upper extremity.
- Grossly displaced or comminuted fractures require immobilization with a light hanging cast.
- Open fractures or fractures associated with neurovascular compromise require immediate orthopedic consultation.

HOSPITAL ADMISSION CRITERIA

- Open fractures or fractures associated with neurovascular compromise

HOSPITAL DISCHARGE CRITERIA

- Uncomplicated humeral shaft fractures should be referred to an orthopedic surgeon for follow-up.
- Orthopedic consultation in the ED is required for patients with grossly displaced or comminuted fractures.

Miscellaneous

- Always repeat the neurological examination after splint or cast application.
- Consider pathologic fractures with any humerus fracture produced by low energy mechanism as the humerus can be a common site of metastatic disease.

ICD-9-CM

812.21

CORE CONTENT CODE

18.4.12.1.6

BIBLIOGRAPHY

Magnusson AR. Humerus and elbow. In: Rosen P, et al., eds. *Emergency medicine: Concepts and clinical practice*. 4th ed. St. Louis: CV Mosby, 1998.

Simon R, Koenigskhecht S. *Emergency orthopedics, the extremities*. 3rd ed. Norwalk, CT: Appleton & Lange, 1993.

Zuckerman J, Koval K. Fractures of the shaft of the humerus. In: Rockwood CA, Green DP, eds. *Rockwood and Green Fractures in adults*. 4th ed. Philadelphia: Lippincott-Raven, 1996.

Authors: William Goldberg and Wallace Carter

Fracture, Lateral and Medial Malleoli

Basics

DEFINITION

- Any fracture involving the most distal portions of the fibula or tibia, commonly known as the lateral and medial malleoli, respectively

INCIDENCE/PREVALENCE

- Very common, especially with twisting injuries of the foot and ankle

SIGNS AND SYMPTOMS

- Local swelling
- Ecchymosis
- Deformity
- Tenderness to palpation over the medial or lateral malleolus
- Difficulty or inability to weight bear and/or ambulate

RISK FACTORS

- History of prior ankle injury(s)
- Inadequate rehabilitation of injury
- Skeletal immaturity
- Weakness in dynamic(muscles) and/or static(ligamentous) stabilizers of the ankle
- Abnormal gait and/or foot biomechanics
- Foot and ankle proprioceptive dysfunction (dysfunction in the ability of the foot and ankle to adapt to uneven terrain)

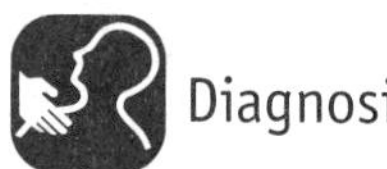

Diagnosis

DIFFERENTIAL DIAGNOSIS

- Contusion
- Ankle sprain (ligamentous injury)
- Tear of ankle retinacular structures
- Posttraumatic subluxation of peroneal tendon laterally or tibialis posterior tendon medially
- Syndesmosis injury ("high ankle sprain")

HISTORY

- Twisting injury of the foot and/or ankle
- May hear or feel a "pop"
- Occasionally caused by direct blow to the affected malleolus

PHYSICAL EXAMINATION

- Swelling and/or deformity over the affected malleolus
- Limited range of motion of the ankle
- Tender to palpation over the affected malleolus
- Antalgic gait or inability to bear weight
- May note instability of the ankle joint on examination

IMAGING

- Anteroposterior (AP), lateral, and mortise views (AP with foot in 15 degrees of adduction)
- On mortise film, the joint space between the talus and lateral malleolus, distal tibia, and medial malleolus should be equal around the entire talocrural joint. Inequality should raise suspicion of an unstable ankle injury
- Use Ottawa Ankle Rules when deciding whether to obtain x-rays.

POSTREDUCTION VIEWS

- Same as initial films

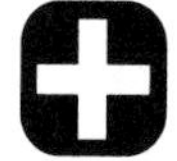

Acute Treatment

ANALGESIA

- Acetaminophen at recommended age- or weight-guided dosages every 6–8 hours as needed
- Consider nonsteroidal anti-inflammatory drugs.
- Narcotics as needed for severe pain only
- Cryotherapy (ice pack or frozen peas) applied 20–30 minutes every 2–4 hours for the first 24–48 hours after injury. Use caution to avoid thermal injury to the skin.

REDUCTION TECHNIQUES

- Isolated lateral malleolar fractures with <3 mm of displacement do not need reduction. Refer to orthopaedist for >3-mm displacement of lateral malleolus.
- Isolated medial malleolar fractures with any displacement, other than small avulsion injuries, should be referred to an orthopaedist. Do not attempt to reduce.

POSTREDUCTION EVALUATION

Check neurovascular status of foot.

IMMOBILIZATION

- Nonweight-bearing in stirrup or posterior splint, with ankle in neutral position, for 3–5 days.
- Isolated minimally displaced lateral malleolar fracture: short leg walking cast with ankle in a neutral position, or orthotic fracture boot, cam walker, for 4–6 weeks
- Isolated simple avulsion fracture of the medial malleolus: stirrup splint or cam walker can be used short term for comfort, typically 2–4 weeks.

SPECIAL CONSIDERATIONS

- Relative rest and elevation of affected limb for first 48–72 hours
- Check for radiographic healing in 2–4 weeks.
- Repeat x-ray every 2 weeks if not healing.
- Total healing time: 6–8 weeks. May take months to see complete radiographic healing.
- Athletes should cross-train while healing to maintain fitness.
- Proper rehabilitation of these injuries with a home instructional program or with formal physical therapy guidance is crucial to successful healing and return to full function.

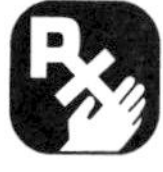

Long-Term Treatment

REHABILITATION

- After period of immobilization is complete, start standard ankle rehabilitation range of motion exercises, strengthening exercises, and proprioceptive training.
- The shorter the period of immobilization, the easier it should be for the patient to regain ankle motion and strength.
- Follow up every 2–3 weeks to assess progress of rehabilitation.

SURGERY

- See Referral/Disposition

REFERRAL/DISPOSITION

- Depends on the standard of care in the community. Some medical communities require all malleolar fractures, other than simple small avulsions, be seen by an orthopaedic surgeon.
- Unstable ankle joint (disrupted mortise)
- Fractures of both the lateral and medial malleoli (bimalleolar fracture) are unstable and should be referred.
- Trimalleolar fractures (bimalleolar fracture with fracture of posterior malleolus of the tibia) are unstable and require surgical fixation.
- Lateral malleolar fractures at the level of the fibular-tibial syndesmosis, or more proximal, should be referred because of the high incidence of deltoid ligament injury on the medial side.
- Fracture-dislocations of the ankle should be referred.
- Fracture of the posterior malleolus of the tibia involving >25% of the articular surface or displaced >2 mm should be internally fixed by an orthopaedic surgeon.
- Malleolar fracture on one side with complete ligament disruption on the opposite side is considered unstable, like a bimalleolar fracture.
- Medial malleolar fractures involving more than just the tip (avulsion) and those that are vertical or oblique should be seen by an orthopaedic surgeon even if not significantly displaced.

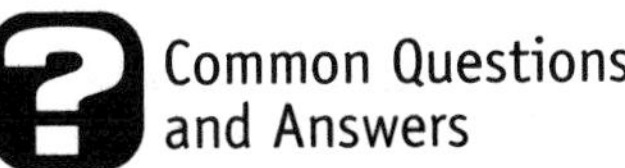

Common Questions and Answers

Physician responses to common patient questions:

Q: Will I need crutches?
A: Depending on the extent of the fracture, crutches with or without weight-bearing may be needed.
Q: What is the initial treatment?
A: Initial treatment should consist of protection, rest, ice, compression, and elevation of the ankle.

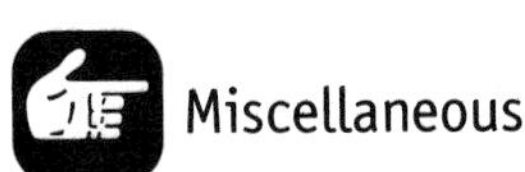

Miscellaneous

SYNONYMS

- Ankle fracture

ICD-9 CODE

824.2 Fracture, lateral malleolus, closed
824.8 Fracture, ankle not otherwise specified, closed

BIBLIOGRAPHY

Eiff MP, Hatch RL, Calmbach WL. *Fracture management for primary care.* Philadelphia: WB Saunders, 1998.

Port AM, McVie JL, Naylor G, et al. Comparison of two conservative methods of treating an isolated fracture of the lateal malleolus. *J Bone Joint Surg Br* 1996;78B:568–572.

Rockwood CA, Green DP, Bucholz RW, eds. *Rockwood and Green's fractures in adults.* Philadelphia: JB Lippincott, 1996.

Springfield DS, ed. *Instructional course lectures.* Rosemont, IL: American Academy of Orthopedic Surgeons, 1997.

Stiell IG, Greenberg GH, McDowell I, et al. Implementation of the Ottawa Ankle Rules. *JAMA* 1994;271:827–833.

Authors: Per Brolinson and Fred H. Brennan Jr.

Fracture, Le Fort

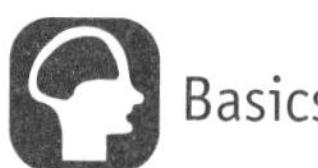

Basics

SIGNS AND SYMPTOMS

- Facial injury with massive swelling and ecchymosis
- Airway obstruction may be present.
- Dyspnea (especially when supine), malocclusion, vision disturbance (diplopia)
- Facial lengthening or flattening, periorbital ecchymosis (raccoon's eyes)
- CSF rhinorrhea, facial hemorrhage/epistaxis
- Facial anesthesia, midface mobility upon traction, open bite
- Frequently associated with multisystem injury (especially head and C-spine)

MECHANISM/DESCRIPTION

- Maxillofacial fractures caused by high-energy blunt trauma to the midface
  —The most common causes include motor vehicle accidents, physical assault, and domestic violence.
- Upon traction of the maxillary arch/hard palate you should find
  —Le Fort I: Movement of the hard palate and maxillary dentition only
  —Le Fort II: Movement of the hard palate, maxillary dentition, and the nose
  —Le Fort III: Movement of the entire midface including orbital rims (inferior and lateral aspects)

PEDIATRIC CONSIDERATIONS

- Maxillofacial fractures occur less frequently in children.
  —Because of the smaller facial skeleton there is a higher incidence of skull fractures and head trauma compared to midface injuries.
  —Le Fort fractures are particularly uncommon in young children. By ages 10–12, as facial morphology becomes adultlike, more mid- and lower facial fractures are seen.
  —Be suspicious of child abuse or family violence as possible causes of midfacial injuries, especially in children under 6.

CAUTIONS

- Airway management
  —Airway compromise is common.
  —Bag valve mask (BVM) ventilation may be difficult.
  —Avoid nasotracheal intubation.
- Strict cervical spine precautions
- Multisystem injury is likely with high-energy trauma.

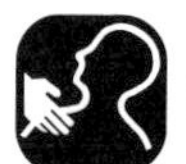

Diagnosis

ESSENTIAL WORKUP

- Evaluate the patency of the airway and need for immediate airway control.
- Le Fort fractures can be diagnosed by careful intraoral examination and the pattern of facial movement.
  —If fracture fragments are impacted, there may be little or no midface mobility.
  —Carefully evaluate the patient for CSF rhinorrhea and malocclusion.

IMAGING/SPECIAL TESTS

- Facial imaging may be delayed for 24–72 hours in patients requiring care of other life-threatening conditions.
- *Computed tomography* is the diagnostic standard for defining midface fractures.
- *Conventional radiographs* may be used as a screening test. The occipitomental (Waters) and lateral views of the skull may reveal bony fracture/asymmetry, subcutaneous emphysema, or layering of blood in the maxillary sinuses.

DIFFERENTIAL DIAGNOSIS

- Le Fort fracture classification
  —Le Fort I: transverse (horizontal) fracture/palate facial dysjunction
  —Le Fort II: pyramidal dysjunction
  —Le Fort III: craniofacial dysjunction
  —Le Fort IV: involves the frontal bone in addition to a Le Fort III maxillary fracture
- Different grade Le Fort fractures may be found on opposite sides of the face.

PEDIATRIC CONSIDERATIONS

- Young children are often frightened and in pain. Through kindness, patience, and distraction cooperation can be gained.
- Sedation may be required to perform a thorough exam after ruling out head injury.
- Incomplete (greenstick) fractures with minimal or no displacement can occur
- Be cognizant of possible child abuse and evaluate for prior nonaccidental trauma, if appropriate.

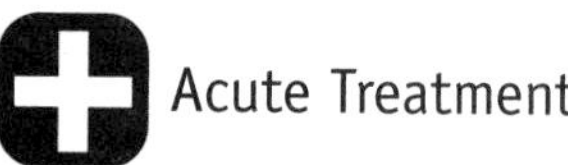

Acute Treatment

INITIAL STABILIZATION

- Aggressive airway control is paramount.
- Orally suction patients to minimize aspiration of blood, saliva, and stomach contents.
- Remove any foreign matter or teeth from the airway.
- After cervical spine clearance, stable and alert patients may be allowed to sit up and suction themselves.

- When airway management is needed, *rapid sequence induction* is recommended to maximize airway control and minimize rise of ICP in patients with head injuries.
  —If there is concern that paralysis will result in loss of airway tone and inability to intubate because of subsequent distortion of airway anatomy in patients with severe facial injuries, oral intubation under sedation with midazolam, etomidate, droperidol, or ketamine is an option.
- *Emergency cricothyroidotomy* may be necessary if orotracheal intubation is unsuccessful. Recall that BVM ventilation may be difficult due to loss of bony support and altered anatomy.
- *Nasotracheal intubation* is not recommended in patients with midface trauma because of the lack of success and danger of intracranial placement.

ED TREATMENT

- *Cervical spine*: Due to the risk of cervical spine injury in patients with head and maxillofacial trauma, it is imperative that radiographic clearance of the cervical spine is obtained.
- *Hemorrhage control*: Direct pressure should be applied to areas of bleeding and nasal packing (anterior and posterior) may be necessary for epistaxis. In some cases, manual reduction of the midface may be required to control intractable hemorrhage. Although blood loss from facial bleeding may be significant, it is rarely a primary cause of hemorrhagic shock.
- Early consultation with oral maxillofacial or plastic surgeon
- Analgesics, antibiotics, and tetanus prophylaxis

PEDIATRIC CONSIDERATIONS

- Surgical cricothyroidotomy should not be considered in children under age 10.
  —Needle cricothyroidotomy with jet ventilation may be attempted if intubation attempts fail.
- There is a higher incidence of multiple injuries in children, especially head trauma, skull fractures, and orthopedic injuries.
- Cervical spine injuries tend to involve upper levels more commonly in children. Also, spinal cord injury without radiographic abnormality (SCIWORA syndrome) may be seen.
- Definitive repair of pediatric facial fractures should not be delayed for more than 3–4 days. The facial bones heal rapidly and delayed repair may result in malunion and cosmetic deformity.

HOSPITAL ADMISSION CRITERIA

- All patients are admitted for ORIF of maxillofacial injuries.
- Patients should be admitted to an intensive care unit setting.

HOSPITAL DISCHARGE CRITERIA

N/A

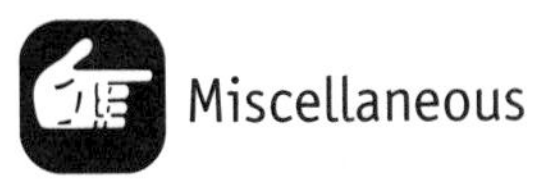

Miscellaneous

ICD-9-CM

802.4

CORE CONTENT CODE

18.4.4.3

BIBLIOGRAPHY

Colucciello SA, Sternbach G, Walker SB. The treacherous and complex spectrum of maxillofacial trauma: Etiologies, evaluation, and emergency stabilization. *Emerg Med Rep* 1995;16;7:59–69.

Hehmann RJ, Sargent LA. Maxillary fractures. *Trauma Q* 1992;9:67–75.

Hunter JG. Pediatric maxillofacial trauma. *Pediatr Clin North Am* 1992;39:1127–1143.

Le Fort R. Experimental study of fractures of the upper jaw. *Rev Chir de Paris* 1901;23:208, 360, 479. Reprinted in *Plast Reconstr Surg* 1972;50:497, 600.

Author: Raymond A. Viducich

Medications

	Adult Dose (mg/kg IV)	Pediatric Dose (mg/kg IV)
*Sedative/Analgesics**		
Diazepam	0.1–0.2	0.1–0.2
Droperidol	2.5 mg aliquots	1–1.5 mg aliquots
Etomidate	0.2–0.3	0.2–0.3
Fentanyl	2–10 μgm	2–3 μgm
Ketamine	2	1–2
Meperidine	1–2	1–2
Midazolam	0.1	0.15
Morphine sulfate	0.1–0.2	0.1–0.2
Defasciculating Drug		
Vecuronium	0.01	0.01
Paralytic Agents		
Pancuronium	0.1–0.15	0.1–0.15
Rocuronium	0.6	0.6
Succinylcholine	1.5	1.5–2
Vecuronium	0.1–0.3	0.1–0.3

*All of these sedatives/analgesics should be titrated to effect

Fracture, Lisfranc

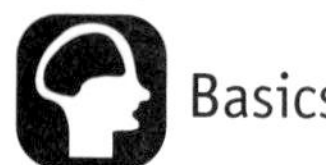

Basics

DEFINITION

- Injury occurs from direct or indirect mechanisms.
- Direct injury occurs with crush injury to the tarsometatarsal joint.
- Indirect injury occurs
  —when the hindfoot is placed in a fixed position and the forefoot is forcefully abducted, producing lateral displacement of the metatarsals, with associated fracture of the second metatarsal base
  —from an axially applied force to a plantar flexed foot ("tip-toe" position) causing disruption of the dorsal ligament complex
  —from a force applied to the heel in the axis of the foot with the toes in a fixed plantar position

INCIDENCE/PREVALENCE

- One in 50,000–60,000 orthopaedic injuries per year; 67% occur in motor vehicle accidents
- 0.2% of all fractures per year
- Rare in athletic population
- Second tarsometatarsal joint is most frequently injured.

SIGNS AND SYMPTOMS

- Midfoot pain and swelling
- Pain with weight-bearing on involved foot or inability to bear weight
- Plantar ecchymosis

RISK FACTORS

- Slips, falls, motor vehicle accidents

ASSOCIATED INJURIES AND COMPLICATIONS

- Cuneiform and cuboid fracture-dislocation
- Compartment syndrome of the foot
- Late recognition and treatment: posttraumatic arthritis with resulting pes planus and forefoot abduction, which may require tarsometatarsal arthrodesis

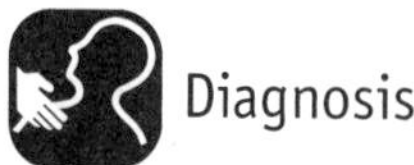

Diagnosis

DIFFERENTIAL DIAGNOSIS

- Lisfranc fracture-dislocation
- Tarsometatarsal sprain

HISTORY

Q: Is there midfoot pain?
A: High index of suspicion for these injuries needed. Up to 20% of subtle injuries may be missed on initial examination.
Q: Was the injury associated with low- or high-velocity trauma?
A: High-velocity trauma usually will have obvious deformity. Low-velocity trauma may cause only minor discomfort in midfoot.

PHYSICAL EXAMINATION

- Evaluate integrity of soft tissue and perform neurovascular examination. Marked swelling and deformity may indicate complete dislocation and risk for compartment syndrome.
- Palpate each articulation for tenderness and swelling. Medial cuneiform-first metatarsal joint is most frequent site of pain and swelling.
- Stress second metatarsal joint by elevating and depressing the second metatarsal head relative to first metatarsal head. Elicits pain in Lisfranc joint.
- Compression of midfoot from side to side reproduces pain in the interval between the bases of first and second metatarsals.

IMAGING

- Standard anteroposterior (AP) view: Medial shaft of second metatarsal should be aligned with medial aspect of middle cuneiform. Any malalignment indicates Lisfranc dislocation. Small fractures in and around Lisfranc joint should cause suspicion of significant injury in this area. "Fleck sign" avulsion fracture in medial cuneiform-second metatarsal space represents rupture of Lisfranc ligament. Compression fracture of cuboid ("nutcracker" injury) may be apparent.
- 30-degree oblique view: Medial shaft of fourth metatarsal should align with the medial aspect of cuboid. Any malalignment indicates disruption of the joint. Malalignment of first metatarsal joint frequently seen.
- Lateral view: Dorsal or plantar displacement of the metatarsals relative to the tarsal bones
- Weight-bearing lateral (both feet): flattening of longitudinal arch. Seen with subtle Lisfranc injuries.
- Weight-bearing AP (both feet): Diastasis >1–2 mm between first and second metatarsal bases indicates rupture of Lisfranc ligament.
- Stress views: Valgus stress can be applied to accentuate the injury.
- Computed tomographic scanning may be helpful in defining the extent of injury.

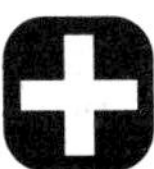

Acute Treatment

IMMOBILIZATION

- Bulky posterior splint for fracture with or without dislocation

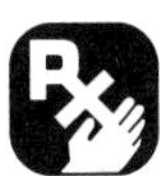

Long-Term Treatment

SURGERY

Any diastasis (>1 mm) or fracture requires operative reduction and screw fixation.

REFERRAL/DISPOSITION

- Early orthopaedic referral indicated for any fracture, dislocation, or instability of the Lisfranc joint

Common Questions and Answers

Physician responses to common patient questions:
Q: How long will I be in a cast?
A: Generally, surgically repaired injuries initially are immobilized in a nonweight-bearing cast for 6 weeks, followed by progressive weight-bearing in a cast or range of motion boot for another 3–6 weeks.
Q: How long before I can return to sports?
A: Athletes typically can return to sports at 4–5 months after injury.

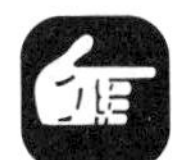

Miscellaneous

SYNONYMS

- Lisfranc fracture
- Tarsometatarsal fracture
- First-second metatarsal-cuneiform fracture

ICD-9 CODE

825.24 Fracture of other tarsal and metatarsal bones, closed. Cuneiform, foot
825.25 Fracture of other tarsal and metatarsal bones, closed. Metatarsal bone

BIBLIOGRAPHY

Clanton TO, Porter TA. Primary care of foot and ankle injuries in the athelete. *Clin Sports Med* 1997;16:435–466.

Mantas JP, Burks RT. Lisfranc injuries in the athlete. *Clin Sports Med* 1994;13:719–730.

Myerson MS, Thordarson DB, eds. *Foot and ankle disorders.* Philadelphia: WB Saunders, 2000.

Shapiro MS, Wascher DC. Rupture of Lisfranc's ligament in athletes. *Am J Sports Med* 1994;22:687–691.

Authors: Robin Merket and Kenneth Bielak

Fracture, Lunate/Kienbock Disease

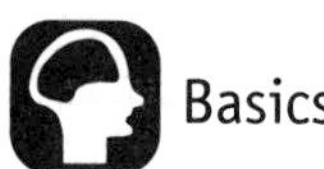

Basics

DEFINITION

Kienbock (pronounced Kine-bock) disease, or lunatomalacia, is a painful disorder of the wrist in which there are histologic and radiologic changes showing avascular necrosis of the lunate.

INCIDENCE/PREVALENCE

- Most commonly seen between ages 20 and 40 years
- Predilection for the right hand in manual laborers
- Bilateral changes occur less frequently than unilateral

SIGNS AND SYMPTOMS

- Painful, stiff, and often swollen wrist joint
- Usually >1 month of pain at presentation
- Pain most often mild to moderate in severity

RISK FACTORS

- Previous wrist trauma including lunate fracture
- Negative ulnar variance
- Repetitive trauma (manual labor)
- Anatomical and biomechanical features, including vulnerable blood supply or fixed position of the wrist (loss of range of motion)

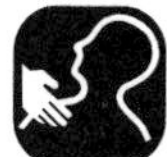

Diagnosis

DIFFERENTIAL DIAGNOSIS

- Physical examination
  —Triangular fibrocartilage complex tear (more lateral)
  —Scapholunate ligament instability
  —Distal radioulnar joint complex ligament instability
  —Monoarticular arthritides (multiple)
- X-ray
  —Lunate fracture
  —Degenerative joint disease carpals

HISTORY

Q: How long have you had the pain?
A: Longer duration increases probability.
Q: Was there an inciting traumatic event or repetitive trauma?
A: Both have been linked with occurrence of Kienbock disease.

PHYSICAL EXAMINATION

- Look for swelling, erythema, and calor at the radioulnar joint. Erythema and calor not associated with Kienbock disease.
- Evaluate range of motion; decreased in Kienbock disease, especially dorsiflexion.

IMAGING

X-ray and Tomography

- Standard anteroposterior (AP) and lateral views
- Initially the lunate may have normal architecture and density.
- Subsequently, increasing density of the lunate, then altered shape and diminished size
- Adjacent arthritic changes and carpal row collapse
- Tomography may be useful to detect early changes, including fracture lines.

Magnetic Resonance Imaging

- T1-weighted images show loss of signal intensity (corresponding to osteonecrosis).
- T2-weighted images initially may show hyperintensity (early signs of osteonecrosis).
- If negative, can rule out Kienbock disease in a patient with wrist symptoms; may show alternative diagnosis better than plain films.

CLASSIFICATION/STAGING OF DISEASE

- Lichtman classification of staging for Kienbock disease (via x-ray)
  —Stage I: normal architecture and bone density; may be either a linear or a compression fracture
  —Stage II: definite density changes, but size, shape, and anatomical relationship of the bones not altered. Later in this stage, AP view shows loss of height on radial side of lunate.
  —Stage III: entire lunate collapsed with associated proximal migration of the capitate and disruption of the carpal architecture. On lateral view, a dorsivolar ribbon-like elongation of the lunate is seen.
  —Stage IV: in addition to stage III changes, generalized degenerative changes in carpus

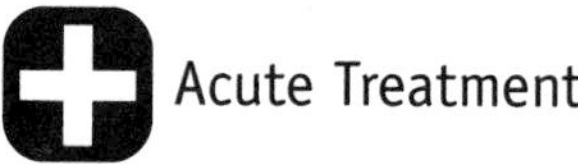

Acute Treatment

IMMOBILIZATION

In early stages, immobilization for 7 days is a reasonable first step because synovitis and tenosynovitis usually is resolved and examination may become more focused.

SPECIAL CONSIDERATIONS

Over time, it has become evident that immobilization will not prevent long-term collapse of the lunate. Some studies showed similar pain relief in conservative versus surgical treatment.

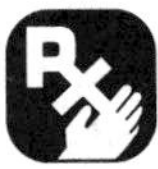

Long-Term Treatment

SURGERY

- If the patient still has pain after conservative measures, there are a few other options.
- If negative ulnar variance is present, radial shortening or ulnar lengthening
- Radial shortening is easier to perform and there is a lower rate of complications.
- Other surgical procedures include
  —excision of the lunate with insertion of a tendinous mass
  —proximal row carpectomy
  —wrist arthrodesis
- Silicone arthroplasty is no longer performed because of poor long-term results.

REFERRAL/DISPOSITION

- Prompt referral to an orthopaedist after detection to evaluate, accurately stage, and discuss with the patient available current treatments

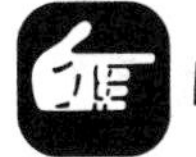

Miscellaneous

SYNONYMS

- Lunatomalacia
- Lunate avascular necrosis

ICD-9 CODE

723.3 Kienbock disease
732.8 Adult

BIBLIOGRAPHY

Alexander AH, Lichtman DM. Kienbock's disease. *Orthop Clin North Am* 1986;17:461–472.

Beckenbaugh RD, Shives TC, Dobyns JH, et al. Kienbock's disease: the natural history of Kienbock's disease and consideration of lunate fractures. *Clin Orthop* 1980;149:98–106.

Gelberman RH, Szabo RM. Kienbock's disease. *Orthop Clin North Am* 1984;15:355–367.

Jackson MD, Barry DT, Geiringer SR. Magnetic resonance imaging of the avascular necrosis of the lunate. *Arch Phys Med Rehab* 1990;71:510–513.

Kienbock R. Uber traumatische Malazie des Mondbeins und ihre Folgezustande: Entartungsformen und Kompressionsfra. *Fortschr Gebiete Roentgenstrahlen* 1910;16:78–103. Peltier LF, translator.

Kuschner SH, Brien WM, Bindiger A, et al. Review of treatment results for Kienbock's disease. *Orthop Rev* 1992;21:717–728.

Lichtman DM, Mack GR, MacDonald RI, et al. Kienbock's disease: the role of silicone replacement arthroplasty. *J Bone Joint Surg* 1977;59A:899–908.

Author: Kevin Burroughs

Fracture, Mandibular

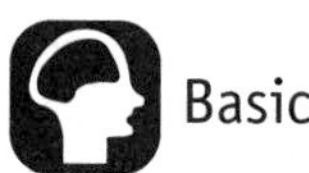

Basics

SIGNS AND SYMPTOMS

- Patient complaints include
  - —Facial asymmetry, deformity, dysphagia, and mandibular pain
  - —Malocclusion, decreased range of motion of the temporomandibular joint, or a grating sound conducted to the ear with movement of the mandible

MECHANISM/DESCRIPTION

- Fracture of the mandible is usually due to a direct force.
- The most common area to be fractured is the angle, followed by the condyle, molar, and mental regions.
- Because of its thickness the mandibular symphysis is rarely fractured.

ETIOLOGY

- The mandible is the third most common facial fracture following nasal and zygomatic fractures.
- Fractures usually result from a direct force applied to the mandible by motor vehicle accidents, personal violence, contact sports, or industrial accidents.
- Patients are often intoxicated and unable to give a clear history of events.

CAUTIONS

- First priority is to protect the airway as severe fractures of facial structures may result in airway obstruction from lack of glossal supporting structures, blood clots, loose teeth, dentures, or bony fragments.
- Protect the C-spine.

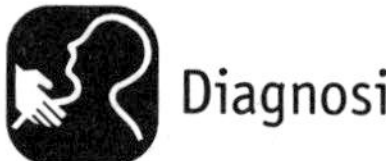

Diagnosis

ESSENTIAL WORKUP

Physical Examination

- Inspect the maxillofacial area for obvious deformity including areas of ecchymosis or swelling.
- Loose, fractured, or missing teeth, gross malalignment of teeth, separation of tooth interspaces, and ecchymosis or hematoma of the floor of the mouth
- Step-off, bony disruption, or point tenderness with palpation along the entire length of the mandible
- Protrusion or lateral excursion of the jaw. Interference with normal mandibular function including decreased range of motion or deviation of the mandible with opening
  - —The examiner should be able to insert three fingers between the mandible and maxilla.
  - —Mandible fracture is also suggested by inability of the patient to break a tongue depressor placed between the teeth and forced downward.
- Paresthesia of the lower lip or gums strongly indicates a mandibular fracture with secondary damage to the inferior alveolar nerve.
- Inability of the examiner to note motion of the mandibular condyles when palpated through the external ear canals with motion of the jaw is highly suggestive of a mandibular fracture.

IMAGING/SPECIAL TESTS

- Plain films including an AP, bilateral obliques, and a Townes view should be obtained.
  - —Mandibular views are best for evaluating the condyles and neck of mandible.
- Dental panoramic view should be obtained.
  - —Panorex best evaluates the symphysis and body.
- If condylar fracture is still suspect and not noted on initial radiographs, obtain CT of the condyles in the coronal plane.
- Multiple fractures are noted in greater than 50% because of the ringlike structure of the mandible.

DIFFERENTIAL DIAGNOSIS

- Contusions
- Dislocation of the mandible may also result from blunt trauma. If a single condyle is dislocated, the jaw will deviate away from the side of the dislocation. If fractured, the jaw will deviate towards the fractured side.
- Isolated dental trauma may have a similar presentation.

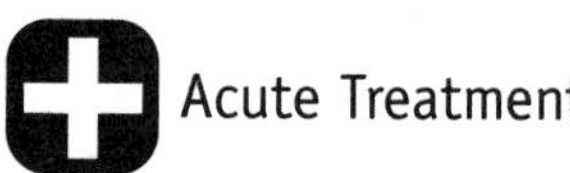

Acute Treatment

INITIAL STABILIZATION

- 20–40% of patients with mandibular fractures have associated injuries and emergency treatment is directed towards immediate, potentially lethal injuries such as airway obstruction, aspiration, major hemorrhage, cervical spine or cord injury, and intracranial injury.

- Airway must be protected as intraoral edema and hematoma, bony fragments, loose teeth, broken dentures, and loss of tongue support may compromise the airway.
- C-spine precautions must be maintained.
- If intubation is to be performed, an oral tracheal tube should be placed.
- If oral intubation cannot be performed secondary to extent of injuries, a blind nasotracheal intubation should be performed unless associated facial injuries are present, in which case cricothyrotomy is indicated.

ED TREATMENT

- With the exception of condylar fractures many mandibular fractures are associated with mucosal, gingival, or tooth socket disruption, and should be considered open fractures.
  - —Patients should receive antibiotics such as penicillin or erythromycin to cover intra-oral anaerobic pathogens.
- Tetanus prophylaxis if appropriate
- Definitive care usually consists of reduction and fixation by wiring upper and lower teeth in occlusion for 4–6 weeks.
  - —This may not be possible initially due to patient instability or local edema.
  - —Linear, nondisplaced or greenstick fractures may be treated with soft diet without wiring.
- If *mandible dislocation* is present, bilateral downward pressure while the jaw is open is placed on the occlusal surface of the posterior lower teeth while grasping the mandible.
  - —The goal is to free the condyle from its anterior position to the eminence.
  - —Reduction is facilitated by muscle relaxants (diazepam or midazolam), or anesthetic injection of mastication muscles.
  - —A bite block should be used or examiner's fingers should be wrapped in gauze to prevent injury.

MEDICATIONS

- Diazepam: adult: 10 mg IV; peds: 0.1–0.2 mg/kg/dose IV
- Midazolam: adult: 2–5 mg IV; peds: safety not established but 0.02–0.05 mg/kg/dose have been used
- Penicillin: adult: 500 mg po qid; peds: 25–30 mg/kg/24 hrs divided q 6 hrs po
- Erythromycin: adult: 500 mg po qid; peds: 30–50 mg/kg/24 hrs divided q 6–8 hrs po

PEDIATRIC CONSIDERATIONS

- Mandibular fractures are uncommon in children <6 years of age. When they do occur, they are usually greenstick fractures and can be managed with soft diet alone. The parents should be informed that because any fracture of the mandible has the potential to damage permanent teeth and cause facial asymmetry, long-term follow-up with a specialty consultant is advisable.

HOSPITAL ADMISSION CRITERIA

- Those fractures in which there is significant displacement or associated dental trauma, or those fractures that are thought to be open, require urgent specialty consultation for admission.
- The severity of associated trauma may indicate admission.
- Any patient with the potential for airway compromise, including oropharyngeal edema or bilateral mandibular body fractures, should be admitted.
- An unreliable patient with nondisplaced fractures should be admitted for definitive fixation.
- In the pediatric population, if the mechanism of injury is not appropriate to the injuries seen, pediatric or child protective services consultation should be obtained.

HOSPITAL DISCHARGE CRITERIA

- Relatively asymptomatic patients with nondisplaced, closed fractures may be discharged on analgesics and a soft diet. They should be referred to an otorhinolaryngologist or an oral maxillofacial surgeon within 1–2 days.

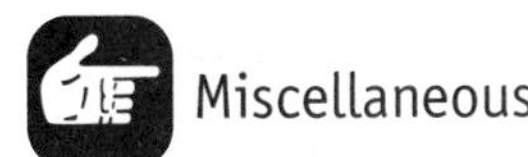

Miscellaneous

ICD-9-CM

802.20

CORE CONTENT CODE

18.4.4.2

BIBLIOGRAPHY

Alonso LL, Purcell TB. Accuracy of the tongue blade test in patients with suspected mandibular fracture. *J Emerg Med* 1995;13: 297–304.

Busuito MJ, Smith DJ, Robson MC. Mandibular fractures in an urban trauma center. *J Trauma* 1986;26:826–829.

Luyk NH, Ferguson JW. The diagnosis and initial management of the fractured mandible. *Am J Emerg Med* 1991;9:352–359.

Shepherd, S. Maxillofacial trauma: Evaluation and management by the emergency physician. *Emerg Med Clin North Am* 1987;5(2):371–392.

Authors: Anthony J. Musielewicz and David W. Munter

Fracture, Metacarpal Base/Shaft: I–V

Basics

DEFINITION

- Metacarpal shaft and base fractures are defined by their location, pattern, and displacement.
- Metacarpal fractures involving the first metacarpal (thumb) are considered separately from those involving the second to fifth metacarpals.
- Two intra-articular fractures of the thumb deserve special mention
  - —Bennett's fracture: fracture combined with a subluxation or dislocation of the metacarpal joint
  - —Rolando fracture: T- or Y-shaped fracture involving the joint surface

INCIDENCE/PREVALENCE

- Metacarpal fractures account for one-third of all hand fractures.
- Small finger is the most commonly injured, followed by the thumb, index, long finger, and ring finger.

SIGNS AND SYMPTOMS

- Tenderness and swelling over the dorsal hand
- Pain with motion
- Inability to make a fist

RISK FACTORS

- Gymnastics, contact sports, racquet sports

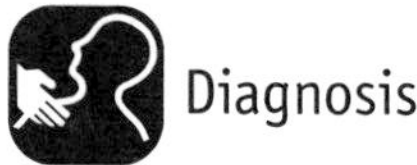

Diagnosis

DIFFERENTIAL DIAGNOSIS

- Metacarpal head and neck fractures
- Metacarpophalangeal collateral ligament injuries
- Carpometacarpal fracture dislocation

HISTORY

Q: Direct blow versus indirect blow with rotational torque?
A: Rotational torque often leads to spiral fractures.
Q: Was there a crush injury?
A: Nerve injury or damage to the extensor tendon frequently is associated with crush injuries

PHYSICAL EXAMINATION

- All patients require a thorough neurovascular examination distal to the fracture site. Fourth and fifth metacarpal base fractures may cause injury to the motor branch of the ulnar nerve resulting in paralysis of the intrinsic hand muscles.
- Evaluate for rotational malalignment
  - —All the fingers of a closed fist should point to the scaphoid tubercle.
  - —No crowding or digital overlap should be present when the digits are fully flexed.
  - —Plane of the fingernails should be parallel on the injured and normal hand.
- Function of the flexor and extensor tendons must be documented.

IMAGING

- Radiographic evaluation with three views is mandatory because many fractures are overlooked or misinterpreted.
- Standard anteroposterior and lateral views: Pronation of 10 to 30 degrees in lateral view facilitates view of the second and third metacarpals; supination of 10 to 30 degrees aids in viewing the ring and small fingers.
- Oblique views allow better visualization of intra-articular fractures, spiral fractures, and epiphyseal plate injuries.
- Tomograms or computed axial tomographic scans help define carpometacarpal relationships.
- Malrotation should be suspected if there is metacarpal shortening or a discrepancy in the shaft diameter.

POSTREDUCTION VIEWS

- Same as for Imaging

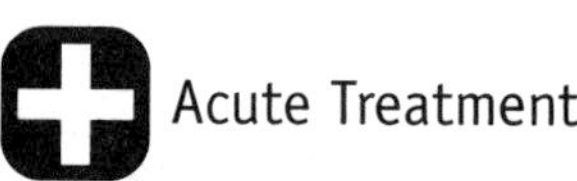

Acute Treatment

ANALGESIA

Once complete neurovascular examination is complete, wrist or hematoma block may facilitate reduction.

REDUCTION TECHNIQUES

Fractures amenable to closed manipulative reduction are transverse fractures, isolated spiral/oblique fractures with <5 mm of shortening, and extra-articular fractures of the thumb.

POSTREDUCTION EVALUATION

- Postreduction films are mandatory. Limits of angular deformity depends on mobility of different metacarpals at base: <10 degrees for second and third metacarpals; <20 degrees for fourth and fifth metacarpals; <25 degrees of both angulation and rotation are acceptable for the thumb.
- Orthopaedic referral is required if satisfactory reduction cannot be performed or maintained.
- Radiographs should be repeated 1 week after injury to reevaluate for angulation, rotation, and shortening.

IMMOBILIZATION

- Dorsal and volar splints must include all metacarpal shafts and wrist while avoiding immobilization of the MP. joint for 3–4 weeks.
- Functional brace (Galveston) if fracture requires significant reduction
- Thumb spica cast for extra-articular fractures of the thumb for 4–6 weeks
- Bulky compressive dressing for unstable fractures

SPECIAL CONSIDERATIONS

- Field management: Splint immobilization provides comfort and minimizes soft tissue injury.
- Ice packs should be used proximal to the metacarpals to prevent digital injuries.

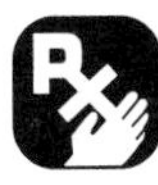

Long-Term Treatment

REHABILITATION

- Active motion as soon as 3–4 weeks for fractures treated with immobilization and closed reduction
- Buddy taping may provide stability when mobilization begins.
- Clinical union is manifest by absence of tenderness at the fracture site with palpation and range of motion. Radiographic union will lag behind clinical union by several weeks.

SURGERY

Open reduction internal fixation or closed reduction with percutaneous pinning is advocated for patients with malunion or unstable fractures (Bennett, Rolando, comminuted, intra-articular, spiral/oblique with shortening and rotation).

REFERRAL/DISPOSITION

- All surgical cases, including special situations such as multiple fractures, nerve or tendon injury, and open fractures
- Refer early if manipulative reduction is necessary; operative fixation may be needed.

Common Questions and Answers

Physician responses to common patient questions:
Q: What is a boxer's fracture?
A: Metacarpal neck fractures involving the small finger
Q: When can I return to play?
A: Return to play needs to individualized depending on the type of fracture, mobility, and clinical healing.

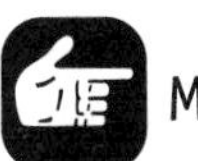

Miscellaneous

ICD-9 CODE

815.03 Metacarpal shaft fractures
815.02 Metacarpal base fractures
815.09 Multiple metacarpal fractures
815.01 First metacarpal fractures (thumb)

BIBLIOGRAPHY

Capo JT, Hastings H. Metacarpal and phalangeal fractures in athletes. *Clin Sports Med* 1998;17:491–511.

Harrison BP, Hilliard MW. Emergency department evaluation and treatment of hand injuries. *Emerg Med Clin North Am* 1999;17:793–822.

Matery RD, Weiss AP, Akelman E. Primary care of hand and wrist athletic injuries. *Clin Sports Med* 1997;16:705–724.

Simon RR, Koenigsknecht SJ, eds. *Emergency orthopedics.* Stamford, CT: Appleton Lange, 1996.

Author: Suraj Achar

Fracture, Metacarpal Neck: I–V

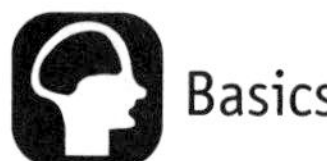

Basics

DEFINITION

- The metacarpal neck is the most proximal aspect of the metacarpal shaft immediately underneath the metacarpal head.
- Fractures about the metacarpal neck must be scrutinized for malrotation and angulation.
- As second and third metacarpals are necessary for handgrip power, much less angulation is tolerated in these injuries.

INCIDENCE/PREVALENCE

- Fifth metacarpal neck fractures (boxer's fractures) are the most common hand fracture.
- Fractures of the first metacarpal neck are uncommon.

SIGNS AND SYMPTOMS

- Swelling and tenderness on the dorsum of the hand, often accompanied by metacarpophalangeal (MCP) joint depression
- Extreme angulation may lead to pseudo-crawling, i.e., hyperextension of the MCP joint along with flexion of the proximal interphalangeal (PIP) joint as the patient attempts to extend the finger.

RISK FACTORS

Out-of-control tempers: Boxer's fractures usually are due to striking an opponent or a wall with a clenched fist.

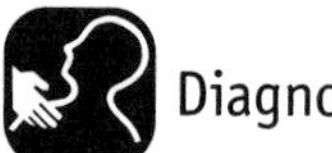

Diagnosis

DIFFERENTIAL DIAGNOSIS

- Metacarpal head fracture
- Metacarpal shaft fracture
- Open fracture
- MCP joint dislocation
- MCP joint sprain

HISTORY

- Axial load or direct trauma, often to clenched fist or dorsum of the hand
- Immediate pain and swelling noted

PHYSICAL EXAMINATION

- Tenderness and swelling about the dorsal aspect of the distal metacarpals. Examine skin closely for teeth marks or other injuries.
- Evaluate the digits for malrotation, which occurs more in fourth and fifth metacarpal neck fractures. Have the patient bring all the fingernails into the palm and compare with the noninjured hand. All the nails should point toward the base of the first metacarpal. If the injured finger is out of this alignment, strongly suspect significant fracture malrotation.

IMAGING

- Anteroposterior, oblique, and true lateral views of the hand usually are sufficient.
- Normally, the metacarpal neck is situated with 15 degrees of volar angulation. Ensure adequate visualization on the lateral view to evaluate the degree of fracture angulation.
- A conservative rule for limits of acceptable angulation of the second through fifth digits is 10-10-20-30. Thus, the second digit can only tolerate 10 degrees of angulation (in addition to the baseline 15 degrees); the fifth metacarpal can accept 30 degrees above the baseline. Many other experts will tolerate a greater degree of angulation of the fifth metacarpal; this decision often is influenced by the particular activity or sport of the patient.

POSTREDUCTION VIEWS

- Required after reduction of fourth or fifth metacarpal fractures with significant angulation

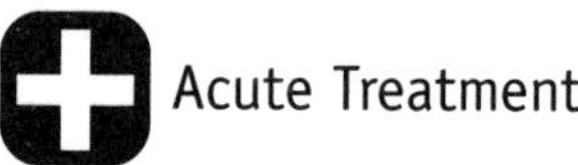

Acute Treatment

ANALGESIA

- Nonsteroidal anti-inflammatory drugs can be used along with ice for immediate analgesia.
- Narcotic analgesics may be necessary for sleep during the first few nights after the injury.

REDUCTION TECHNIQUES

- Closed reduction is considered in cases of significant angulation of fourth (>20 degrees) and fifth (>30 degrees) metacarpal neck fractures.
- Anesthesia can be obtained by hematoma block or ulnar nerve block. Flex the MCP, PIP, and distal interphalangeal (DIP) joints all to 90 degrees. Simultaneously apply dorsal pressure over the flexed middle phalanx and volar pressure over the fracture segment.
- Immediately immobilize the hand in an ulnar gutter splint with 30 degrees of wrist extension, MCP at 90 degrees, and IP joints in full extension.

POSTREDUCTION EVALUATION

Obtain a postreduction lateral view of the hand to ensure adequate reduction and immobilization.

IMMOBILIZATION

- Nondisplaced fractures of the second or third metacarpals can be immobilized in a radial gutter splint with the wrist in 30 degrees extension, MCP at 70–90 degrees, and PIP/DIP near full extension.
- Mildly angulated fourth (<30 degrees) and fifth (<40 degrees) metacarpal neck fractures can be immobilized in ulnar gutter splints with the same positions.
- Elevate the hand and apply ice for 20-minute intervals on a regular basis over the first 24–48 hours after injury.
- Splints should be applied to injuries requiring orthopaedic referral (see below) unless that consultant is immediately available.

INDICATIONS FOR ORTHOPAEDIC REFERRAL

- Open reduction and internal fixation is indicated for
  —Significant angulation of second (>10 degrees) and third (>10–20 degrees) metacarpal neck fractures, or those with any displacement
  —Any metacarpal neck fracture with significant malrotation or comminution
  —Any potential open fracture
  —Degree of residual angulation that is unacceptable to the patient
  —Inability to hold reduction position
  —Athlete who desires immediate return to play in cast orthosis

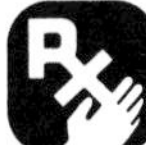

Long-Term Treatment

REHABILITATION

- Once the splints are removed, begin range of motion work with emphasis on handgrip and manipulation strength. Key to prevent stiffness of the MCP joint.
- Conservative guideline for return to contact sports with splint/orthotic protection is after 2–4 weeks of immobilization. Some experts may allow immediate return to play with a protective cast or splint.
- The protective orthosis should be used during contact sports for 8–10 weeks after the initial injury.
- Cosmetic deformity without functional loss still may ensue.

LENGTH OF IMMOBILIZATION

- Fractures should remain splinted for a minimum of 3–4 weeks, with follow-up every 2–4 weeks and reimaging at least once during the healing process.
- Clinical healing is defined as no tenderness with palpation of the fracture site.

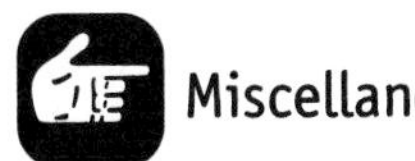

Miscellaneous

SYNONYMS

- Boxer's fracture: fifth metacarpal neck fracture

ICD-9 CODE

815.00 Metacarpal fracture of one hand

BIBLIOGRAPHY

Dimeff RJ. In: Salis RE, Massimino F, eds. *ACSM's essentials of sports medicine.* St. Louis: Mosby, 1996.

Eiff MP, Hatch RL, Calmbach WL. *Fracture management for primary care.* Philadelphia: WB Saunders, 1998.

Lillegard WA. Finger injuries. Presented at the 1997 AAFP Sport Medicine In-Depth Review Course, Dallas, Texas.

Author: Chris Koutures

Fracture, Middle Phalanx

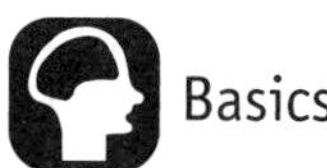

Basics

INCIDENCE/PREVALENCE

- Least common phalangeal fracture
- Most occur in the narrow shaft
- Subsequent disability depends on degree of initial injury and proper treatment
- Most can be treated closed, but knowledge of deformities common to specific injuries leads to selection of appropriate treatment

SIGNS AND SYMPTOMS

- Mechanisms of injury include direct blow (most common), axial load, axial traction, twisting/torque, and "grabbing a jersey"
- Pain, swelling, bruising, tenderness, loss of motion, and function are typical findings.
- Gross deformity in some cases
- Open (compound) fractures usually are obvious and require emergent care.
- May be mistaken for proximal interphalangeal (PIP) or distal interphalangeal (DIP) dislocation
- Malrotation less common than proximal phalanx fractures but if present must be detected and corrected early

ANATOMY

- Flexor digitorum superficialis (FDS) splits and inserts over a broad area of the volar surface of the middle phalanx.
- This volar FDS insertion is the predominant deforming force in middle phalanx fractures, resulting in apex volar angulation for distal shaft and neck fractures.
- Extensor central slip inserts dorsally onto the base of the middle phalanx, resulting in apex dorsal angulation for proximal fractures.
- Fractures of the middle two-thirds of the shaft may angulate in either direction.
- Thick cartilaginous volar plate between proximal and middle phalanges may complicate intra-articular (PIP) fractures of the base.
- PIP and DIP joint collateral ligaments can result in intra-articular avulsion fractures.

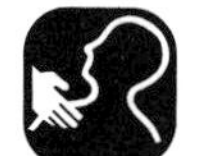

Diagnosis

DIFFERENTIAL DIAGNOSIS

- PIP dislocation
- DIP joint dislocation
- Tendon rupture
- Volar plate disruption
- Bone contusion
- Soft tissue contusion

HISTORY

- Determine mechanism of injury
- Assess function and degree of disability
- Develop an "index of suspicion"
- Review treatment rendered
- See Signs and Symptoms

PHYSICAL EXAMINATION

- Inspection/observation: location and degree of deformity, swelling, and ecchymosis
- Range of motion (ROM): usually decreased. Compare with contralateral side
- Rotational malalignment: With metacarpophalangeal (MCP) and PIP joints flexed to 90 degrees, all fingers should point toward the scaphoid. When viewed "end on," the plane of all fingernails should be symmetrical.
- Palpation: Feel for crepitus. Determine point of maximal tenderness.
- Provocation: Axial loading or distraction often results in pain at the fracture site.
- Adjacent structures: PIP and DIP joints, tendon function, and soft tissues
- Neurocirculatory function: sensation, capillary refill, skin color, and temperature

IMAGING

- Anteroposterior (AP), true lateral, and oblique views are diagnostic.
- Describe type, location, and displacement of fracture.
- Describe rotation of fragments, angulation, intra-articular versus extra-articular, and percentage of joint involved.
- Any differences in diameter of fragments suggest rotation.

POSTREDUCTION VIEWS

- AP, true lateral, and oblique views to confirm reduction
- Unacceptable, unstable, or unsure alignment: Early consultation with ortho/hand specialist advised.

ASSOCIATED INJURIES

- Digital nerve injury: contusion, transection (rare)
- Digital artery injury: open or closed fracture; usually does not require treatment
- Volar plate disruption: not uncommon with "jammed finger"; results in swan-neck deformity if detached from middle phalanx
- Tendon injury: complete or partial rupture, extensor central slip avulsion
- Joint instability: frank tear or bony avulsion of collateral ligament; detectable with thorough physical examination

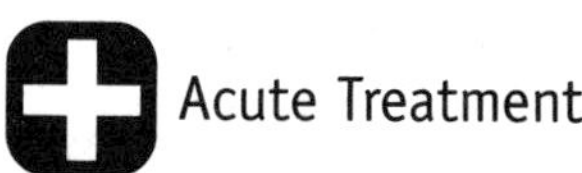

Acute Treatment

GENERAL PRINCIPLES

- Open (compound) fractures: sterile wet dressing, ice, elevate, splint, refer to ortho/hand, intravenous/intramuscular cephalosporin, or PCN/aminoglycoside for contaminated wounds, tetanus toxoid and/or immune globulin if indicated
- Significant displacement, angulation, intra-articular component, or any degree of rotational malalignment necessitates an ortho/hand consultation.

IMMOBILIZATION

- Closed fractures: Most can be managed with dynamic splinting ("buddy taping") for 10–14 days; 6–8 weeks longer for athletic activity.
- When necessary (see below), a radial or ulnar gutter splint may be used with the hand in a "position of function" = 70–90 degrees flexion at MCP, slight flexion at PIP, DIP.

- Dynamic splinting: Taping injured digit to adjacent uninjured digit allows maximal function with early mobilization and prevents stiffness. Only indicated for stable, nondisplaced, nonimpacted, nontransverse fracture (*not* indicated for oblique rotated, angulated, displaced fracture).
- Immobilization >3 weeks significantly increases the likelihood of impaired finger function.

ANALGESIA

- Metacarpal or digital block with plain 1% lidocaine or 0.5% bupivacaine provides quick relief and allows for reduction if necessary.
- Oral narcotics may be needed.

SPECIFIC FRACTURES

Spiral

- Very unstable
- Immobilize, ice, ortho/hand referral for surgical fixation

Displaced or Angulated Transverse

- Unstable
- Anesthesia
- Gentle longitudinal traction in conjunction with flexion and manipulation of the distal fragment
- Postreduction radiographs: if unstable with slight extension, open reduction internal fixation needed; if stable, immobilize in gutter splint in position of function for 4–6 weeks.
- Ortho/hand referral advised.

Nondisplaced Transverse

- Dynamic splinting or gutter splint for 10–14 days
- Repeat x-ray

Volar Plate Avulsion

- Intra-articular volar fractures due to PIP hyperextension or dorsal dislocation
- If >40% joint space involved or MP remains subluxed after reduction with axial traction and PIP flexion, refer to ortho/hand.
- Small avulsions: buddy taping or dorsal extension block splint with slight PIP flexion to prevent swan-neck deformity

Dorsal Avulsion

- Associated with extensor central slip rupture
- Large fragments with volar subluxation of MP: refer to ortho/hand.
- Small avulsions (or pure tendon injury): splint PIP in extension for 6 weeks, then nightly for 3–4 weeks to prevent boutonniere deformity.

Lateral Avulsion

- Large fragments, displacement >2–3 mm or >30% joint involvement: refer to ortho/hand
- Small nondisplaced fractures: continuous dynamic splinting for 3 weeks +3–4 weeks athletic activities

Basilar, Condylar

- Nondisplaced: dynamic splinting, early ROM
- Displaced or comminuted: splint; refer to ortho/hand.

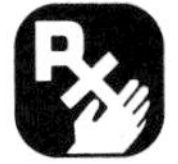

Long-Term Treatment

FOLLOW-UP CARE

- Restoration and maintenance of normal finger function requires careful attention to clinical and radiographic healing.
- Early ROM exercises for most (stable) fractures reduce stiffness and restore normal function.
- Formal occupational/hand therapy may be indicated.
- Athlete's return-to-play varies greatly with type of fracture and its stability and stage of healing; goal is life-long use and proper function of the hand.

DISPOSITION

- Swan-neck and boutonniere deformities can be prevented by careful early diagnosis and appropriate treatment.
- Scarring of the extensor or flexor mechanisms with decreased ROM are common complications of MP fractures.
- Fusiform swelling, cold intolerance, joint stiffness, and tenderness are common complications of intra-articular MP fractures.

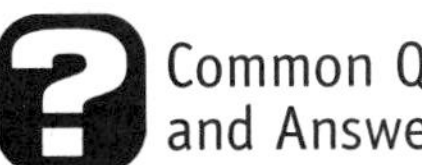

Common Questions and Answers

Physician responses to common patient questions:

Q: When can I return to play?

A: Many patients present with a sense of urgency about return-to-play decisions. They need to understand that several variables (stability, current clinical and radiographic healing status, and specific demands of sport/position) all direct such decisions. In general, most of those with stable fractures are able to return 1–2 weeks after the injury or even sooner. For unstable fractures, healing is much more important than participation. In some cases, early surgical intervention is desirable for earlier return.

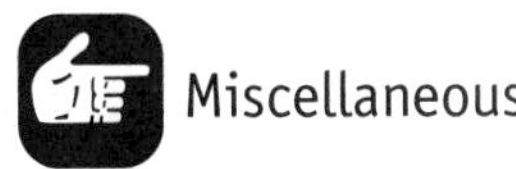

Miscellaneous

ICD-9 CODE

816.0 Fracture, closed phalanx

BIBLIOGRAPHY

Connolly JF. *Fractures and dislocations: closed management.* Philadelphia: WB Saunders, 1995.

Eiff MP, Hatch RL, Calmbach WL. *Fracture management for primary care.* Philadelphia: WB Saunders, 1998.

Simon RR, Koenigsknecht SJ. *Emergency orthopedics: the extremities.* Stamford, CT: Appleton and Lange, 1996.

Author: James E. Sturmi

Fracture, Nasal

Basics

ANATOMY

- The upper one-third of the nose is a bony tripod formed by a pair of nasal bones that meet in the midline, with the thin perpendicular plate of the ethmoid as a weak center strut.
- A pair of upper and lower lateral cartilages supported by the central quadrangular septal cartilage make up the lower two-thirds.

INCIDENCE/PREVALENCE

- Most frequently injured and fractured facial structure due to its prominence
- Most fractures occur in the lower half of the nasal bones where they are thinner and broader.

SIGNS AND SYMPTOMS

- Nasal deformity
- Epistaxis
- Nasal airway obstruction
- Periorbital swelling and ecchymosis

ASSOCIATED INJURIES AND COMPLICATIONS

- Septal hematoma
- Septal dislocation
- Cribriform plate injury with leakage of cerebrospinal fluid
- Laceration
- Orbital fracture
- Concussion

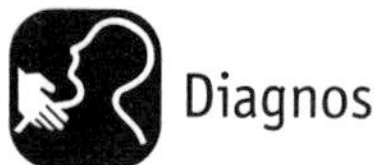

Diagnosis

HISTORY

- Force: Low-velocity trauma such as a blow from an elbow usually causes a simple fracture pattern. High-velocity trauma from a stick or fast moving ball/puck more likely causes a complex comminuted fracture as well as associated injuries to the face, head, and cervical spine.
- Direction of blow: Lateral is most common and can cause fracture displacement and dislocation of the septum. Direct blows can lead to nasal obstruction. Inferior blows can disrupt the septal cartilage and nasal tip.

PHYSICAL EXAMINATION

- Best if done either immediately after the injury or 3–5 days later when swelling will not interfere with assessment.
- Palpate nasal bones for deformity and crepitus.
- Ring test to rule out cerebrospinal fluid (CSF) leak by collecting fluid from the nose onto gauze to see if a clear ring of CSF diffuses out beyond the central area of blood.
- Intranasal examination must be performed on each side to evaluate for a bulging septal hematoma or septal dislocation. Use suction and a topical decongestant to control bleeding, then a nasal speculum or an otoscope along with a light source for adequate visualization.

IMAGING

- Diagnosis is clinical, as radiographs have not been shown to be helpful for diagnosis or management.
- X-rays for documentation can be obtained if there are potential legal issues.

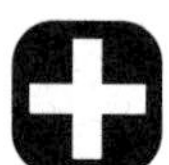

Acute Treatment

CONTROL BLEEDING

- Head-up position; lean forward to aid expectoration of blood
- Direct pressure, ice
- Topical decongestant
- Cautery of visible bleeding sites in Kiesselbach plexus using silver nitrate sticks
- For refractory epistaxis, may have to pack both sides of the anterior nose with a tampon or antibiotic-soaked petrolatum gauze
- Posterior epistaxis can require inflation of a Foley bulb within the nasal fossa in addition to anterior packing to achieve hemostasis.

INITIAL FRACTURE CARE

- Can consider immediate closed reduction before swelling develops if the nose is severely displaced and health provider is well trained.
- In most cases, simply provide analgesics and reexamine in 2–5 days.
- Adults with nondisplaced fractures that cause minimal deformity may not require reduction.

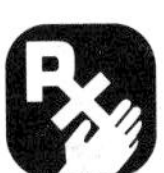

Long-Term Treatment

CLOSED REDUCTION

- For uncomplicated fractures, should be done within 5–10 days of the injury, before significant bone healing occurs.
- Local anesthesia using topical cocaine and lidocaine injection with or without sedation or general anesthesia for younger patients
- Blunt probe is placed within the nose and used to elevate the depressed nasal bone. Forceps are used to reduce septal deformity.
- External splint and packing for 1–2 weeks

OPEN REDUCTION

- For complicated fractures and those with persistent cosmetic deformity or functional problem such as airway obstruction

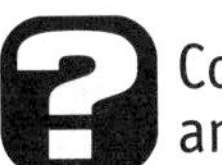

Common Questions and Answers

Physician responses to common patient questions:
Q: When can I return to play after a broken nose?
A: It can take 6 weeks for a nasal fracture to completely heal. An athlete should be advised that returning to competition before complete healing means that even minor contact could disrupt a minimally displaced or previously reduced fracture and require additional intervention. A general guideline is no contact for 1–2 weeks followed by return to play while wearing a nasal protective device for another 2–4 weeks.

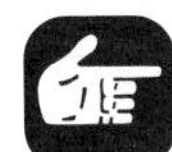

Miscellaneous

ICD-9 CODE

802.0 Fracture of nasal bones, closed
802.1 Fracture of nasal bones, open

CPT CODE

21310 Nasal bone fracture, closed treatment without manipulation
21315 Nasal bone fracture, closed treatment without stabilization
21320 Nasal bone fracture, closed treatment with stabilization
21325 Nasal bone fracture, open treatment of uncomplicated fracture
21337 Septal fracture, closed treatment with or without stabilization

See also: Septal hematoma

BIBLIOGRAPHY

Guyette RF. Facial injuries in basketball players. *Clin Sports Med* 1993;12:247–256.

Rubinstein B, Strong EB. Management of nasal fractures. *Arch Fam Med* 2000;9:738–742.

Author: Daryl A. Rosenbaum

Fracture, Olecranon

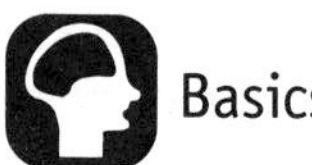

Basics

DEFINITION

- The olecranon is the curved process extending from the posterior proximal surface of the ulna. It forms a large portion of the articulating surface between the ulna and the trochlea of the humerus.
- For a fracture of the olecranon to be considered nondisplaced and stable, it must be displaced <2 mm, must not change in position with flexion to 90 degrees, and must not change in position with extension against gravity.

INCIDENCE/PREVALENCE

One of the more common fractures of the elbow. Together with fractures of the radial head, they account for more than half of the fractures at the elbow.

SIGNS AND SYMPTOMS

- Pain and swelling over the posterior elbow
- Elbow effusion, due to the intra-articular component of the fracture
- Painful and limited motion at the elbow

RISK FACTORS

- Direct trauma: most often associated with isolated injuries
- Fracture-dislocation also is possible with a high-energy mechanism of injury.

ASSOCIATED INJURIES AND COMPLICATIONS

- Ulnar nerve injury
- Discontinuity of the triceps mechanism
- Fracture-dislocation of the elbow
- Open fracture
- Can lead to chronic pain and arthritis

MANAGEMENT CONSIDERATIONS

Issue of fundamental concern when evaluating fractures of the olecranon is determining whether the fracture is displaced or nondisplaced. Nondisplaced fractures can be managed with casting; displaced fractures must be referred to an orthopaedic surgeon for fixation.

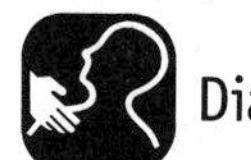

Diagnosis

DIFFERENTIAL DIAGNOSIS

- Radial head fracture
- Coronoid process fracture
- Olecranon bursitis

HISTORY

Q: Mechanism?
A: Higher-energy mechanisms of injury increase the likelihood of fracture-dislocation.

PHYSICAL EXAMINATION

- Determine if patient can extend the elbow against gravity. Inability to extend suggests either discontinuity of the triceps mechanism or a mechanical block. Either problem merits surgical consultation.
- Perform distal neurovascular examination. The ulnar nerve may be injured; more common in comminuted fractures.

IMAGING

- Standard radiographs: anteroposterior (AP) and lateral
- A true lateral view is necessary to evaluate for fracture displacement and articular disruption; slightly obliqued views are inadequate substitutes for a true lateral.
- Fat pad signs: Collection of intra-articular fluid, e.g., caused by intra-articular fracture, causes displacement and hence visualization of the fat pads around the elbow. The anterior fat pad sometimes may be visible in the normal elbow; the posterior fat pad usually is not visible on a normal lateral radiograph and may be the only radiographic evidence of occult fracture.
- Children: often helpful to obtain AP and lateral radiographs of the contralateral elbow for comparison

POSTREDUCTION VIEWS

Repeat radiographs are mandatory after reduction of fracture-dislocations involving the elbow, as either incomplete reduction or displacement of a previously nondisplaced olecranon fracture requires surgical referral.

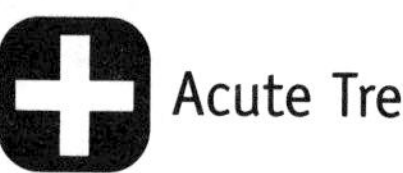

Acute Treatment

REDUCTION TECHNIQUES

- Undisplaced fractures: unnecessary
- Displaced fractures: surgical
- Fracture-dislocation: see Elbow Dislocation chapter

POSTREDUCTION EVALUATION

Undisplaced fractures: Repeat standard x-rays weekly until evidence of healing to ensure that there is no displacement requiring surgical referral.

IMMOBILIZATION

- Undisplaced fractures: Traditionally, all undisplaced fractures were once treated in a long arm cast for 3 weeks.
- To avoid elbow stiffness, a reliable patient can be treated symptomatically with immobilization for about 1 week in either a long arm cast or a sling.
- After 7 days, the patient can start pronation and supination.
- At 2–3 weeks, limited flexion and extension exercises can begin.
- Flexion past 90 degrees can occur when radiographs show complete bone healing.

SPECIAL CONSIDERATIONS

- Splinting: If there is a delay until casting can be accomplished, then temporary splinting may be done for patient comfort and protection. Undisplaced fractures should be splinted with the elbow flexed at 90 degrees. Displaced fractures should be splinted in a comfortable position with the elbow between 45 and 90 degrees and prompt orthopaedic consultation obtained.
- Elderly patients with undisplaced fractures: Because of their propensity to develop stiffness at the elbow, elderly patients should spend much less time immobilized. A sling can be used initially, and range of motion can begin once the patient is comfortable a few days later.
- Ice and oral analgesics are useful in the prehospital setting. Oral analgesics may be required for several days after casting.

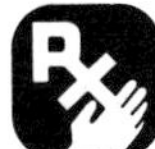

Long-Term Treatment

REHABILITATION

- Undisplaced fractures: protected range of motion advanced as described above. If the patient still has stiffness, then dynamic splinting and physical therapy referral for elbow range of motion may be of benefit.
- Displaced fractures: range of motion to be initiated as determined by the consulting surgeon

SURGERY

Referral is required for all displaced fractures, including avulsion fractures, transverse fractures, comminuted fractures, and fracture/dislocations.

REFERRAL/DISPOSITION

- Undisplaced fractures: Can be released to home in a splint or cast with follow-up x-rays in 1 week.
- Displaced fractures: disposition determined in consultation with a consulting surgeon

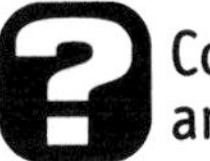

Common Questions and Answers

Physician responses to common patient questions:

Q: How long do I need to wear this cast/sling?

A: Undisplaced fractures: In the case of stable fractures, immobilization is for comfort and can be discontinued after initial pain and swelling have resolved in 3–7 days. If the patient is at particular risk for displacing an otherwise stable fracture, immobilization in a long arm cast for up to 3 weeks may be required. Displaced fractures: depends on the extent of injury and type of repair required.

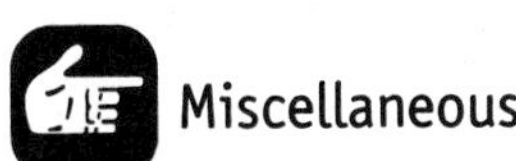

Miscellaneous

ICD-9 CODE

813.01 Fracture of olecranon process of ulna, closed

813.11 Fracture of olecranon process of ulna, open

BIBLIOGRAPHY

Rockwood C, Green D, Bucholz R, et al., eds. *Rockwood and Green's fractures in adults,* 4th ed. Philadelphia: Lippincott-Raven Publishers, 1996.

Schippinger G, Seibert FJ, et al. Management of single elbow dislocations. *Arch Surg* 1999;384(3):294–297.

Author: Greg Nakamoto

Fracture, Orbital

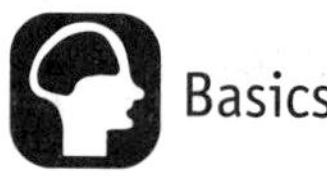

Basics

DEFINITION

- The orbit consists of the roof, floor, and medial and lateral walls. The medial wall is the thinnest, followed by the orbital floor. The orbital floor is the most commonly fractured area of the orbit.
- Orbital fractures are commonly due to blunt trauma; the floor is the most commonly fractured area of the orbit.
- Orbital blow-out fractures are those of the orbital floor not involving the orbital rim.
- The floor is formed by the maxillary, zygomatic, and palatine bones.
- The roof is formed by the frontal bone and lesser wing of the sphenoid.
- The lateral wall is formed by the zygomatic bone and the greater wing of the sphenoid.
- The medial wall is formed by the ethmoid, maxillary, lacrimal, and sphenoid bones.

INCIDENCE/PREVALENCE

- Approximately one-third of orbital blow-out fractures are sustained during sport. Other causes include traffic-related accidents and falls.
- Any sport with the potential for high-energy blows by ball, puck, stick, racquet, or opponent's finger, fist, elbow, knee, or foot makes one susceptible to orbital fracture.
- Athletes commonly involved in, but not limited to, soccer, basketball, hockey, racquet sports, football, baseball, rugby, skiing, and cycling.
- In the United States, >2 million eye injuries occur annually, with >40,000 resulting in some form of permanent visual impairment. One-third of all childhood blindness results from ocular trauma.
- Males are at higher risk of eye injuries because of increased incidence of trauma.
- For all eye injuries, there are two peaks: those aged 10–40 years and those older than 70 years.

SIGNS AND SYMPTOMS

- Orbital rim disruption as evidenced by bony step-off abnormalities
- Dysesthesia of the ipsilateral cheek and upper lip, which results from disruption of the infraorbital nerve as it traverses the orbital floor
- Subcutaneous crepitus in periocular region
- Ophthalmoplegia
- Subjective diplopia
- Enophthalmos
- Nosebleeds

RISK FACTORS

Floor fractures are common when objects larger than the orbital opening, such as a ball, a fist, or the dashboard of an automobile, impact the orbit, particularly the inferior lateral orbit.

ASSOCIATED INJURIES AND COMPLICATIONS

- Orbital emphysema
- Visual loss
- Central retinal artery occlusion from secondary optic nerve compression, i.e., orbital compartment syndrome, which can be characterized by visual loss, sluggish pupillary reaction and afferent pupillary defect
- Retrobulbar hemorrhage characterized by pain, tense ecchymotic lids, bloody chemosis and proptosis, restricted ocular motility, and evidence of compressive optic neuropathy
- Orbital roof fractures may be associated with pneumocephalus, intracranial injury, and cerebrospinal fluid leak and may be complicated by infection, leading to complications involving meningitis and abscess formation.

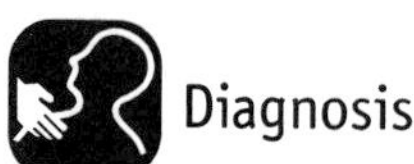

Diagnosis

DIFFERENTIAL DIAGNOSIS

- Other problems to be considered: contusion, globe injury (rupture, hyphema, or traumatic iritis), vitreous hemorrhage, ciliary body tear or bruise, lens dislocation, ocular muscle entrapment, scleral tear or retinal detachment

HISTORY

- Describe symptoms referable to the injured eye (e.g., pain, blurred vision, photophobia, double vision).
- Determine timing of injury and delineate the mechanism of trauma, including the source and size of projectile objects or particles.
- Ask whether safety glasses were worn at the time of injury.
- Ask about baseline visual acuity, a history of "lazy eye" in childhood, and past eye conditions, surgeries, and trauma.
- Past medical history, including medications and allergies

PHYSICAL EXAMINATION

- External features noting periocular abnormalities. Note the location, depth, and size of all lacerations, periocular ecchymosis, and edema. Evaluate for symmetry of facial sensation and stability of facial skeleton.
- Evaluate pupils for size, shape, symmetry, and response to light.
- Assess extraocular motility, paying special attention to impaired upward gaze seen with orbital floor fractures. Impairment of downward gaze is an indication of inferior rectus or oblique muscle entrapment.
- Examine the anterior segment with penlight, direct ophthalmoscope, or slit-lamp biomicroscope, looking at the conjunctiva, cornea, iris, lens, and anterior chamber.
- Examine the posterior segment with direct ophthalmoscope, paying special attention to the optic nerve, retinal vasculature, vitreous, and retina.
- Visual acuity with patient wearing spectacle correction
- Assess visual field.
- Palpate gently for crepitus or irregularity of the rim.
- Measure intraocular pressure using tactile tonometry (i.e., light pressure on the globes through closed eyelids), Schiotz tonometry, or slit lamp.

IMAGING

- Computed tomographic (CT) scan of the orbits with axial and coronal views is the study of choice.
- If CT is not readily available, a Waters view plain film projection may be reasonable for screening. Waters view best displays inferior orbital rims, nasoethmoidal bones, and maxillary sinuses. If patient is upright when film is taken, physician often can see an air-fluid level in the maxillary sinus, which may indicate fracture of the maxillary sinus (orbital floor).

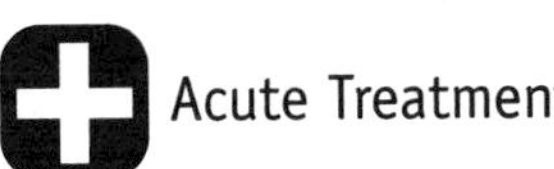

Acute Treatment

MANAGEMENT

- Airway, breathing, and circulation are the first priorities.
- Cervical spine evaluation.
- Control active bleeding with direct pressure.
- If an open globe injury is present or suspected, cover it with a protective shield and refer to ophthalmologist immediately.
- No nose blowing, as this can cause a sudden rise in paranasal sinus pressure and worsen orbital emphysema if present.
- Coughing episodes should be treated with antitussives for above reasons.
- Immediate referral to ophthalmology for open globe injury, facial fracture, symptomatic orbital emphysema, orbital compartment syndrome, retrobulbar hemorrhage, optic neuropathy, and to rule out other ophthalmologic injuries.
- Medications for pain control include acetaminophen, nonsteroidal anti-inflammatory drugs, narcotics, and local anesthetics. Avoid aspirin.
- Tetanus toxoid for open wounds if patient is not current on vaccinations.
- Nasal decongestant spray two times daily for the first 10 days for treatment of orbital emphysema to minimize edema.
- Ice packs for the first 24–48 hours.
- Consider intravenous or oral steroids to minimize edema and damage from a secondary compartment syndrome.
- Consider oral antibiotics, especially if orbital emphysema is present.
- Immediate surgical repair is recommended for motility disturbance due to extraocular muscle entrapment. Otherwise, surgical repair is recommended for persistent diplopia at 2 weeks, cosmetically significant enophthalmos, and large fractures.
- Neurosurgery evaluation for orbital roof fractures
- Controversy exists regarding the selection of patients requiring orbital fracture repair, as well as the timing of repair.

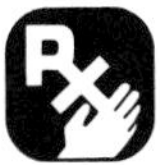

Long-Term Treatment

SURGERY

- Surgical repair as above.
- Surgical repair of medial wall fractures is reserved for enophthalmos and medial rectus entrapment.
- Surgical repair of roof fractures is indicated if there is bony displacement leading to impaired motility, vision loss, or globe malposition.

Common Questions and Answers

Physician responses to common patient questions:

Q: When can I return to work or play?
A: After clearance from ophthalmologist. Use of protective eyewear meeting the American Society for Testing and Materials (ASTM) standards will help reduce the risk for future eye injury.
Q: What symptoms should I look out for?
A: Any visual problems.

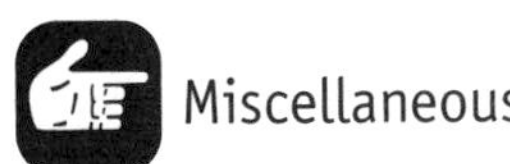

Miscellaneous

SYNONYMS

- Orbital blow-out fracture

ICD-9 CODE

802.6 Orbital floor (blow-out) fracture, closed
802.7 Orbital floor (blow-out) fracture, open
802.8 Orbital fracture not otherwise specified, excluding roof or floor
801.0–801.9 Orbital roof fracture

MEDICAL/LEGAL PITFALLS

- Failure to diagnose orbital fracture and/or associated intracranial or cervical spine injuries

BIBLIOGRAPHY

Beaver H, Lee A. Trauma emergencies in ophthalmology. *Hosp Med* 1998;34: 41–44,47–50.

Cantalano R. *Ocular emergencies.* Philadelphia: WB Saunders, 1992.

Jones NP. Orbital blowout fractures in sport. *Br J Sports Med* 1994;28:272–275.

Kerrison JB, Iliff NT. Orbital trauma. In: MacCumber M, ed. *Management of ocular injuries and emergencies.* Philadelphia: Lippincott-Raven Publishers, 1998.

Widell T. Orbital fractures. *http://www.emedicine.com/emerg/topic202.htm*

Authors: Tod Sweeney and William W. Dexter

Fracture, Patella

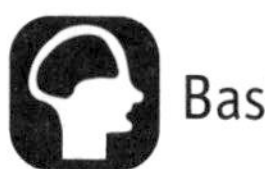

Basics

INCIDENCE/PREVALENCE

- Male-to-female ratio of 2:1
- 1% of all fractures
- Usually 20–50 years old

SIGNS AND SYMPTOMS

- Tenderness to palpation and pain with passive motion of the patella
- Crepitus or a palpable step-off
- Hemarthrosis, often with an effusion or diffuse swelling of the knee
- Limited range of active leg extension due to disruption of soft tissues

MECHANISMS OF INJURY

- Direct trauma: often comminuted, but minimally displaced. Associated with fractures of the tibia, femur, and hip as well as posterior hip dislocation
- Indirect trauma: exertional loading of the extensor mechanism beyond the tensile strength of the patella. Often with unexpected knee flexion; frequently transverse with significant displacement and disruption of the extensor retinaculum
- Patellar subluxation or dislocation: usually in adolescents. Associated with osteochondral fractures

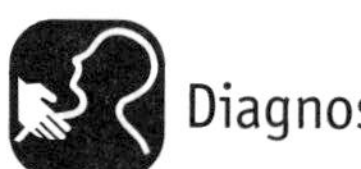

Diagnosis

DIFFERENTIAL DIAGNOSIS

- Bipartite patella: usually bilateral and not associated with point tenderness, with rounded edges at the proximal lateral corners of the patellae
- Anterior cruciate ligament tears may present with hemarthrosis, although often more tense with less extra-articular swelling.
- Fractures of the proximal tibia or distal femur should be ruled out radiographically.

HISTORY

- Activity (partial fall, exertional strain, etc.)
- Trauma (object, direction, force)
- Subluxation or dislocation
- Popping or snapping
- Locking or joint instability
- Speed and extent of swelling
- Characterization of pain
- Constitutional symptoms, especially with delayed presentation or evidence of infection
- Previous knee injuries
- Past medical and surgical history
- Medications and allergies

PHYSICAL EXAMINATION

- Pain and tenderness
- Pain with passive motion
- Crepitus or palpable defects
- Effusion or soft tissue swelling
- Full range of active knee extension implies preservation of extensor mechanism
- Distal neurovascular status: rule out associated injuries, especially hip, femur, leg, and ankle)
- Soft tissue injuries, contamination, or signs of infection
- Stress testing of ligaments should be delayed until after radiographic evaluation if there are concerns of growth plate injury in children.
- Open fractures should be ruled out due to risk of osteomyelitis and septic arthritis; saline may be injected intra-articularly after aspiration of hemarthrosis to test for suspected communication with soft tissue injuries.

IMAGING

- Anteroposterior and lateral radiographs: used to evaluate patella, distal femur, proximal tibia, and soft tissues
- Axial (sunrise, merchant) views: help identify osteochondral and other longitudinal fractures
- Computed tomography: used to detect suspected occult fractures
- Bone scan: used to evaluate stress fractures and osteomyelitis
- Magnetic resonance imaging: used to evaluate suspected soft tissue injuries

CLASSIFICATION

- Transverse (50% to 80%): usually displaced, of the middle and lower thirds.
- Often result from a strong quadriceps contraction, such as in a partial fall or in jumping sports; also with associated trauma.
- Stellate (30%): usually comminuted and nondisplaced. Often secondary to high-impact direct trauma in sport or motor vehicle accidents.
- Longitudinal (12% to 25%): either due to trauma (especially of the lateral facet) or subluxation/dislocation of the patella (often in adolescents, with resultant (osteo)chondral fragments)
- Sleeve fractures: primarily in 8- to 12-year-olds, especially after subluxation/dislocation, with significant articular cartilage and a small bony fragment avulsed from the distal pole. Often difficult to see on plain films; may have an ipsilateral patella alta (patella height to patellar ligament length ratio <0.8).
- Stress fractures: usually elderly, osteopenic patients with anterior knee pain after minor trauma

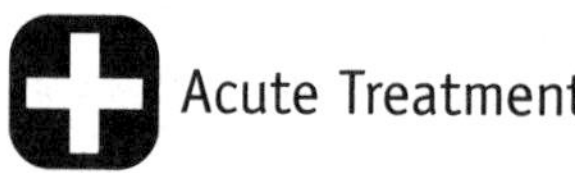

Acute Treatment

ANALGESIA

- Aspiration of hemarthrosis may be followed by injection of local anesthesia to facilitate assessment of the extensor mechanism.
- Consider aspiration of tense anterior hematomas.
- Ice and elevation to control swelling (avoiding prolonged, direct application)

IMMOBILIZATION

- Splinting and support in position of comfort (usually slight flexion) to minimize quadriceps contraction and fracture distraction

SPECIAL CONSIDERATIONS

- Open fractures: intravenous antibiotics and emergent referral for extensive irrigation and debridement, usually followed by internal fixation

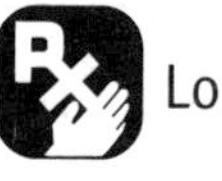

Long-Term Treatment

REHABILITATION

- Immobilization: long leg cast (ankle to groin) for nonoperative treatment and for 3–6 weeks after partial or total patellectomy. Early range of motion is recommended after stable internal fixation.
- Weight-bearing as tolerated in a cast or locked splint: reduces quadriceps contraction and fragment distraction
- Isometric exercises and straight leg raises: started within days of cast application or surgical fixation
- Range of motion exercises such as continuous passive motion may be started immediately after stable internal fixation, with a delay of 3–6 weeks for immobilization in nonoperative treatment and after unstable fracture repair. Exercises should be delayed no more than 6 weeks to reduce pain and improve range of motion.

- Resistance exercises may be added after radiographic evidence of healing is present (usually about 6 weeks). Several months of physical therapy may be required to achieve full strength and range of motion.

SURGERY

- Indications: displacement of 3 mm in any plane or of 2 mm of the articular surface, as well as with extensor mechanism insufficiency
- Timing: delayed with extensive or contaminated soft tissue injury
- Open reduction with internal fixation: modified tension band wiring with either circumferential wire loops or infrafragmentary wires or screws (depending on fragment configuration) in conjunction with repair of medial and lateral retinaculum. A small arthrotomy may be used to confirm reduction of the articular surface.
- Partial patellectomy: indicated with severe patellar comminution or inability to restore a smooth articular surface. Involves repair of retinaculum and reinsertion of patellar or quadriceps tendon to remaining patellar fragment near its articular surface.
- Total patellectomy: reserved for severe comminution precluding retention of any significant (>25%) patellar fragments. Involves soft tissue repair with shortening of the quadriceps tendon. Loss of knee extension strength is frequently reported.
- Osteochondral fractures: difficult to detect on plain films. Usually heal if nondisplaced, but require arthroscopic removal or screw fixation if displaced. Associated patellar instability may be surgically corrected at the same time.

REFERRAL/DISPOSITION

- Orthopaedic referral whenever criteria for nonoperative treatment are not met
- Emergent referral with evidence of an open fracture

NONOPERATIVE TREATMENT

- Displacement of <3 mm in any plane and <2 mm of the articular surface as well as full range of active knee extension
- Compressive dressings and aspiration of hemarthrosis (if present) before cast application may help control edema and discomfort.
- Immobilization in full extension in a long leg cast with weight-bearing as tolerated for 3–6 weeks
- Fracture alignment and healing should be monitored radiographically.

COMPLICATIONS

- Patellofemoral arthritis is the most common complication. Risk factors include incongruence of the articular surface and damage to articular cartilage. Treatment includes anti-inflammatory medications and physical therapy, with patellectomy and tibial tubercle elevation reserved for severe cases.
- A slight decrease in flexion is common but not usually clinically significant. Early postoperative motion and physical therapy help maintain range of motion, with manipulation under anesthesia and arthroscopic lysis of adhesions required if unsuccessful.
- Painful hardware: common complication. Managed by removal after fracture union (minimum 6 months) or tendon healing (minimum 3 months)
- Infection: local care for superficial infections. Osteomyelitis or septic osteoarthritis may require intravenous antibiotics with surgical irrigation and debridement, removal of loose hardware, and delayed closure.
- Radiographic evidence of avascular necrosis consists of a sclerotic area evident 1–2 months after injury, usually of the proximal fragment. Mostly asymptomatic, resolving spontaneously.
- Loss of fixation: often due to unrecognized comminution. Requires surgery if fragments are significantly displaced.
- Nonunion: very uncommon. Repeat surgery indicated if symptomatic.

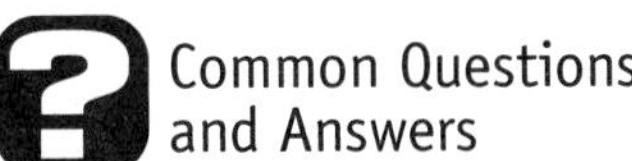

Common Questions and Answers

Physician responses to common patient questions:

Q: Will I be able to play again?
A: Most athletes with patella fractures return to play the following season (3–6 months) with little residual deficit. Return of function is more limited with comminuted, high-impact mechanisms of injury. Strength of terminal knee extension will be reduced by approximately 15% to 30% if patellectomy is required.

Q: How good are the outcomes for nonoperative management of patellar fractures?
A: If criteria for nonoperative treatment are met, studies have shown a failure rate of <5% for fractures managed nonoperatively.

Q: How successful are these surgeries?
A: Many patients have some residual complaints, but most report good-to-excellent results overall after open reduction internal fixation. Slightly fewer achieve this level of satisfaction after partial patellectomy, and fewer still after total patellectomy.

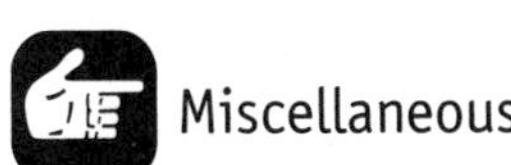

Miscellaneous

ICD-9 CODE

822.0 Patella fracture, closed
822.1 Patella fracture, open

BIBLIOGRAPHY

Carpenter JE, Kasman R, Matthews LS. Fractures of the patella. *Instructional Course Lectures* 1994;43:97–108.

Cohl SL, Sotta RP, Bergfeld JA. Fractures about the knee in sports. *Clin Sports Med* 1990;9:121–139.

Sanders R, Gregory PR. Patella fractures and extensor mechanism injuries. In: Browner BD, Jupiter JB, Levine AM, et al., eds. *Skeletal trauma,* 2nd ed. Philadelphia: WB Saunders, 1998:2081–2113.

Scheinberg RR, Bucholz RW. Fractures of the patella. In: Norman Scott W, ed. *The knee.* St. Louis: Mosby-Year Book, 1994:1393–1403.

Author: David Wallis

Fracture, Pelvic

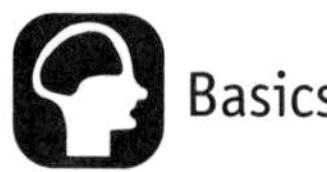

Basics

SIGNS AND SYMPTOMS

- Localized pain, swelling, ecchymoses, tenderness over hips, groin, and lower back
- Pain on hip movement, ambulation, sitting, standing, defecation
- Tenderness on lateral compression of pelvis, palpation of symphysis pubis or sacroiliac (SI) joints
- Often presents with other traumatic injuries including neurologic, intra-abdominal, genitourinary, perineal, rectal, vaginal, and vascular injury
- Gross pelvic instability, deformity, asymmetry in lower extremity
- Evidence of hemorrhagic shock
- Inability to actively or passively perform range of motion of involved hip

MECHANISM/DESCRIPTION

Key-Conwell Classification System

Type I Fractures

- Fracture of individual pelvic bone with no break in ring continuity
- Isolated rami fractures: commonly seen in falls in the elderly
- Avulsion fractures
  - —Three types: anterior superior, inferior iliac spine, and ischial tuberosity
  - —Result of sudden forceful muscle contraction or stretch
- Iliac wing fractures (Duverney's fractures) due to direct trauma or lateral compression
- Sacral fractures
- Coccygeal fractures

Type II Fractures

- Single break in pelvic ring continuity
- Two ipsilateral ischiopubic rami fractures; most common Type II fracture
- Symphysis pubis fracture: often associated with genitourinary injury
- Sacroiliac joint fracture or subluxation

Type III Fractures

- Multiple breaks in pelvic ring continuity
- High risk for associated injuries and pelvic hemorrhage
- Malgaigne fracture
- Anterior and posterior break in the ring on the same side
- Straddle fracture
  - —Fractures of all 4 pubic rami or ipsilateral fracture of 2 pubic rami with dislocation of symphysis pubis
  - —Due to lateral compression or straddle injury (i.e., fall on object)
- Open book fracture
  - —Wide separation of symphysis pubis (often >2.5 cm) associated with sacroiliac joint disruption from anterior/posterior pelvic compression
- Severe multiple fractures
  - —Crush injuries or falls resulting in multiple fractures and gross instability

Type IV Fractures

- Fractures involving the acetabulum

ETIOLOGY

- 60% of pelvic fractures occur from motor vehicle accidents, most commonly pedestrians struck by automobiles.
- 30% are due to falls from heights.
- Mortality rate from pelvic fractures reported is 6%–19%.
- Increases to nearly 50% with hemorrhagic shock
- Significant pelvic hemorrhage can occur in unstable pelvic fractures, particularly Type III fractures.
  - —Bleeding most commonly arises from the venous plexuses.
  - —Significant hemorrhage results in retroperitoneal hematoma formation that may tamponade in the enclosed pelvic space.

PEDIATRIC CONSIDERATIONS

- Children can have proportionately greater hemorrhage.
- Nonaccidental trauma is a concern.

CAUTIONS

- Pneumatic antishock garment (PASG) is an option, particularly when faced with a prolonged transport time or hemodynamically instability.
- Aggressive fluid resuscitation must occur before deflation of the PASG.

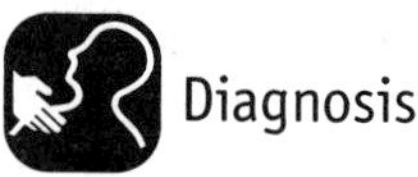

Diagnosis

ESSENTIAL WORKUP

- Pelvic radiology is the most valuable initial diagnostic test.
- A single AP view of the pelvis should be obtained as early as possible.
  - —Most significant unstable pelvic fractures will be seen on the single AP view.
  - —Other views include
    - —Inlet projection: 30° caudal view, allows visualization of posterior arch
    - —Outlet projection: 30° cephalic angulation, allows visualization of sacrum
    - —Judet oblique views (internal and external): allows evaluation of acetabulum

LABORATORY

- Type and crossmatch
- Hemoglobin/hematocrit, platelet count, and coagulation studies (PT/PTT)

IMAGING/SPECIAL TESTS

- CT scan may further delineate pelvic fracture(s) and retroperitoneal hematoma.
- MRI is indicated when there is evidence of neurologic injury.
- Abdominal ultrasound (US) or diagnostic peritoneal lavage (DPL) are rapid bedside evaluations for intraperitoneal hemorrhage.
  - —There is a high mortality rate in victims with pelvic fractures who undergo celiotomy; caution must be exercised to avoid false positive results.
  - —In the setting of pelvic fracture, the supraumbilical open approach for DPL should be used.

DIFFERENTIAL DIAGNOSIS

- Normal variants (i.e., os acetabuli epiphyseal line can mimic Type I fracture on x-ray)
- Ligamentous injury
- Spinal injury
- Intra-abdominal injury and hemorrhage

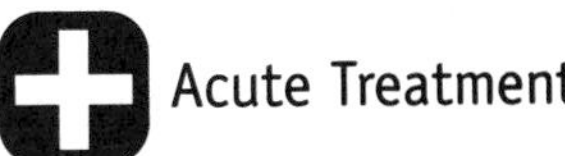

Acute Treatment

INITIAL STABILIZATION

- ABCs of trauma care
  —Avoid using lower extremity IV sites.
  —Aggressive resuscitation with blood or crystalloid, 0-negative or type-specific blood if hemodynamically unstable
  —Immobilize the pelvis to prevent further injury and decrease bleeding.
  —PASG: use in ED is controversial but allows rapid pelvic immobilization and pelvic compression to slow bleeding
  —External fixator requires more time to place than PASG but "splints" pelvis in a similar manner; contraindicated in severely comminuted pelvic fracture
  —Placement of a stabilization device should not interfere with further workup and care (DPL, etc.).

ED TREATMENT

- Determine which pelvic fractures are stable and unstable.
- Type I and II fractures are generally stable.
- Type III fractures are unstable.

Type I Fractures

- Treated conservatively with bed rest, analgesics, and comfort measures.

Type II Fractures

- Treated conservatively but management decisions should be made in conjunction with orthopedics.
- Insure there is no other break in the pelvic ring.

Type III Fractures

- Immediate orthopedics consultation; patient should remain NPO
- May require ED pelvic stabilization measures
- Assess for pelvic hemorrhage (see below).

Type IV Fractures

- Orthopedics consultation; patient to remain NPO

Pelvic Hemorrhage

- Angiography and selective vessel embolization
- Direct operative control of pelvic bleeding.

Prioritization of Studies: CT, Angiography, or Surgery

- In the hemodynamically *unstable* patient, a rapidly performed DPL or US can determine treatment course.
  —If the DPL or US is positive, the patient should go for celiotomy with external pelvic fixation followed by selective angiography.
  —If the DPL or US is negative, the patient should go to angiography.
  —In the hemodynamically stable patient, the patient can go to CT scan for evaluation of the abdomen, pelvis, and retroperitoneum.

MEDICATIONS

- Crystalloid fluids: NS or LR, IV bolus 2 L; peds: 20 cc/kg
- Blood products: crossmatched, type-specific, or 0-negative 4–6 IU; peds: 10 cc/kg

HOSPITAL ADMISSION CRITERIA

- Hemodynamic instability, and pelvic hemorrhage to the ICU
- Type III or IV pelvic fracture
- Other related injuries (genitourinary, intraabdominal, neurologic, etc.)
- Intractable pain

HOSPITAL DISCHARGE CRITERIA

- Type I or II fractures; hemodynamically stable with no evidence of other injuries

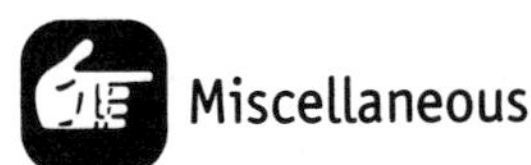

Miscellaneous

ICD-9-CM

808.8

CORE CONTENT CODE

18.4.15

BIBLIOGRAPHY

Berger JJ, Britt LD. Pelvic fracture hemorrhage: Current strategies in diagnosis and management. *Surg Annu* 1995;27: 107–112.

Cryer H, Miller F, Evers B. Pelvic fracture classification: correlation with hemorrhage. *J Trauma* 1988;28:973–980.

Cwinn AA. Pelvis and hip. In: Rosen P, et al., eds. *Emergency medicine: Concepts and clinical practice*. 4th ed. St. Louis: CV Mosby, 1998:739–762.

Jerrard DA. Pelvic fractures. *Emerg Med Clin North Am* 1993;11(1):147–163.

Author: Theodore C. Chan

Fracture, Posterior Malleolus

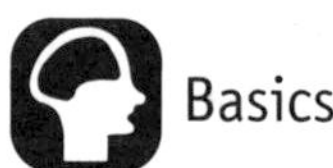

Basics

DEFINITION

- Ankle fracture involving the posterior malleolus
- Isolated posterior malleolus fractures result from vertical loading or anterior displacement of the tibia when the foot is planted, resulting in fracture of the posterior portion of the distal tibia.

INCIDENCE/PREVALENCE

Isolated posterior malleolus fractures are very uncommon, approximately 1% of all ankle fractures.

SIGNS AND SYMPTOMS

- Abduction or external rotation, posterior displacement of the talus, vertical loading, or combinations of these forces cause fractures of the posterior malleolus. X-ray is needed to confirm the diagnosis.
- Consider a fracture if patient is unable to bear weight or has significant swelling or ecchymosis or a "sprain" that persists in being painful but is not unstable.

RISK FACTORS

- Osteoporosis
- Repetitive vertical loading
- Associated injuries/complications
- Bimalleolar or trimalleolar (posterior malleolus fractures in conjunction with lateral malleolus fractures, medial malleolus fractures, or both)

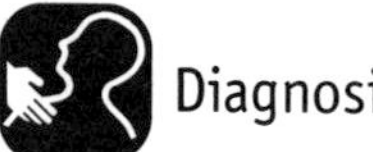

Diagnosis

DIFFERENTIAL DIAGNOSIS

- Grade 3 ankle sprain
- Other malleolus fractures
- Os trigonum syndrome
- Achilles' tendon injury
- Peroneal tendon subluxation and dislocation

HISTORY

- Very important to obtain exact mechanism of injury. Posterior malleolus fracture has been described as associated with external rotation-abduction injuries.
- History should address chronic versus acute.

PHYSICAL EXAMINATION

- Observe for obvious deformity, palpate for pain starting away from area of maximal tenderness, compare to uninvolved foot, and observe for ecchymosis and swelling.
- Check for ligamentous laxity.
- Assess neurovascular status.
- Assess ability to bear weight.
- Observe gait if able to bear weight.

IMAGING

- Anteroposterior (AP), lateral, and mortise views should be obtained.
- Use of stress views remains controversial because there are no standard techniques for anesthesia, positioning, or force used to elicit instability.
- External-rotation lateral view of the ankle can be helpful.
- Computed tomography (CT) and magnetic resonance imaging sometimes are used to evaluate complex ankle fractures.

POSTREDUCTION VIEWS

- Same as above

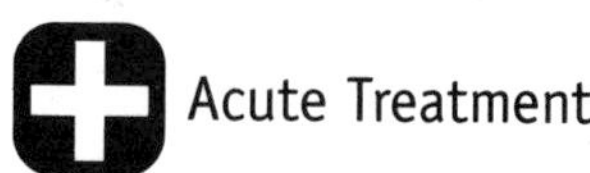

Acute Treatment

ANALGESIA

- Posterior splint, crutches, nonweight-bearing, and ice. Follow-up in 1 week.
- Nonsteroidal anti-inflammatory drugs, ice, and compression/immobilization

REDUCTION TECHNIQUES

- If >25% of the articular surface is involved or if the fracture is displaced >2 mm, then open reduction internal fixation (ORIF) is recommended.
- If ORIF is not chosen, closed reduction still is needed.

POSTREDUCTION EVALUATION

Oblique plain films, in addition to AP, lateral, and mortise views, as well as CT scan may be indicated.

IMMOBILIZATION

- Nonweight-bearing posterior splint for 1 week, then cast for total of 6 weeks
- If fracture is displaced, then surgical repair using plate and screws (ORIF)

SPECIAL CONSIDERATIONS

Posterior malleolus fracture is seen most often in a trimalleolar fracture, less likely isolated.

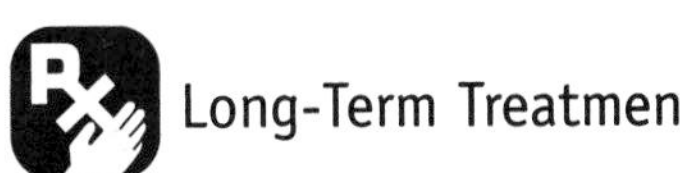

Long-Term Treatment

REHABILITATION

Range of motion, strengthening, and regaining proprioception are important.

SURGERY

If >25% of the articular surface is involved or if the fracture is displaced >2 mm, then ORIF is recommended.

REFERRAL/DISPOSITION

Orthopaedic referral should be considered for any isolated fractures of the posterior malleolus because they often are complicated by other injuries.

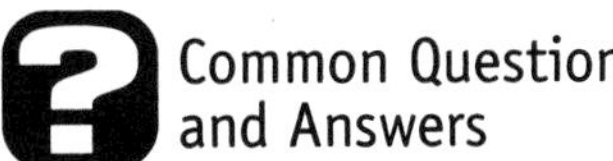

Common Questions and Answers

Physician responses to common patient questions:

It is important to discuss that ankle sprains and fractures often are difficult to differentiate and that many different outcomes exist depending on the severity and type of ankle fracture.

Miscellaneous

ICD-9 CODE

824.8 Fracture malleous, closed

BIBLIOGRAPHY

Canale ST. *Campbell's operative orthopaedics,* 9th ed. St. Louis: Mosby, 1998:2043–2066.

Clanton TO. Primary care of foot and ankle injuries in the athlete. *Clin Sports Med* 1997;16:435–466.

Leddy JJ. Prospective evaluation of the Ottawa Ankle Rules in a university sports medicine center. With a modification to increase specificity for identifying malleolar fractures. *Am J Sports Med* 1998;26: 158–165.

Prokuski LJ. Challenging fractures of the foot and ankle. *Radiol Clin North Am* 1997;35(3): 655–670.

Rockwood CA, Green DP, eds. *Rockwood and Green's fractures in adults,* 4th ed. Philadelphia: Lippincott-Raven Publishers, 1996:2234–2236.

Wedmore IS. Emergency department evaluation and treatment of ankle and foot injuries. *Emerg Med Clin North Am* 2000;18: 85–113,vi.

Authors: Thomas Trojian and Scott Mitchell

Fracture, Proximal Phalanx

Basics

INCIDENCE/PREVALENCE

- Second most common phalangeal fracture
- Subsequent disability depends on degree of initial injury and proper treatment

SIGNS AND SYMPTOMS

- Mechanisms of injury include direct blow, axial load, axial traction, twisting/torque, and "grabbing a jersey"
- Pain, swelling, bruising, tenderness, loss of motion, and function are typical findings.
- Gross deformity in some cases
- Open (compound) fractures usually are obvious and require emergent care.
- May be mistaken for metacarpophalangeal (MCP) or proximal interphalangeal (PIP) joint dislocation
- Malrotation is common with spiral and oblique shaft fractures and must be detected and corrected early.

ANATOMY

- No tendons attach directly to the proximal phalanx
- Most axial force applied to the finger is absorbed by the proximal phalanx.
- Intrinsic muscles of the hand (dorsal interossei) insert into the extensor expansion on the dorsum of the proximal phalanx.
- Thick cartilaginous volar plate between distal aspect of proximal phalanx and proximal aspect of middle phalanx
- PIP joint collateral ligaments can result in intra-articular avulsion fractures.
- MCP and PIP joint collateral ligaments are taut in flexion and lax in extension.

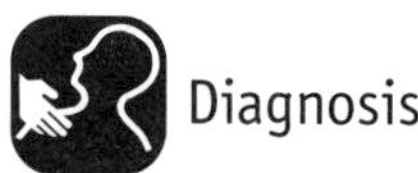

Diagnosis

DIFFERENTIAL DIAGNOSIS

- MCP joint dislocation
- PIP dislocation
- Tendon rupture
- Soft tissue contusion

HISTORY

- Determine mechanism of injury.
- Assess function and degree of disability.
- Develop an "index of suspicion."
- Review treatment rendered.
- See Signs and Symptoms.

PHYSICAL EXAMINATION

- Inspection/observation: location and degree of deformity, swelling, and ecchymosis
- Range of motion (ROM): usually decreased. Compare with contralateral side.
- Rotational malalignment: With MCP and PIP flexed to 90 degrees, all fingers should point toward the scaphoid. When viewed "end on," the plane of all fingernails should be symmetrical.
- Palpation: Feel for crepitus. Determine point of maximal tenderness.
- Provocation: Axial loading or distraction often results in pain at the fracture site.
- Adjacent structures: MCP and PIP joints, tendon function, and soft tissues
- Neurocirculatory function: sensation, capillary refill, skin color, and temperature

IMAGING

- Anteroposterior (AP), true lateral, and oblique views are diagnostic.
- Describe type, location, and displacement of fracture.
- Describe rotation of fragments, angulation, and intra-articular versus extra-articular.
- Any differences in diameter of fragments suggest rotation.

POSTREDUCTION VIEWS

- AP, true lateral, oblique to confirm reduction
- Unacceptable, unstable, or unsure alignment: Early consultation with orthopedic surgeon advised.

ASSOCIATED INJURIES

- Digital nerve injury: contusion, transection
- Digital artery injury: open or closed fracture; usually does not require treatment
- Tendon injury: complete or partial rupture; infrequent with proximal phalangeal fracture
- Joint instability: frank tear or bony avulsion of collateral ligament; detectable with thorough physical examination

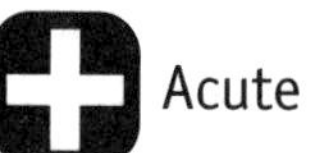

Acute Treatment

GENERAL PRINCIPLES

- Open (compound) fractures: sterile wet dressing, ice, elevate, splint, refer to orthopedic surgeon, intravenous/intramuscular cephalosporin, or PCN/aminoglycoside for contaminated wounds, tetanus toxoid and/or immune globulin if indicated
- Closed fractures: Most can be managed with dynamic splinting ("buddy taping") for 10–14 days. Immobilization for >3 weeks significantly increases the likelihood of impaired finger function.
- Fingers should *never* be immobilized in full extension.
- When necessary (see below), a radial or ulnar gutter splint may be used with the hand in a "position of function" = 70–90 degrees flexion at MCP, slight flexion at PIP, distal interphalangeal
- Significant displacement, angulation, intra-articular component, or any degree of rotational malalignment necessitates an orthopedic surgeon consultation.
- Dynamic splinting: Taping injured digit to adjacent uninjured digit allows maximal function with early mobilization and prevents stiffness. Only indicated for stable, nondisplaced, nonimpacted, nontransverse fractions (*not* indicated for articular, oblique rotated, unstable fractions)

SPECIFIC FRACTURES

Greenstick (Longitudinal Shaft)

- Stable due to intact periosteum
- Dynamic splinting, early ROM exercises, recheck x-ray in 7–10 days

Nondisplaced, Nonangulated, Comminuted Midshaft

- Usually stable
- Dynamic splinting, early ROM exercises

Nondisplaced Intra-articular Marginal (Base)

- Usually stable
- Dynamic splinting, early ROM exercises

Nondisplaced, Nonangulated, Transverse Midshaft

- Potentially unstable if periosteum not intact
- Dynamic splinting, early ROM exercises, recheck x-ray in 5–7 days; *or*
- Gutter splint 10–14 days, recheck x-ray in 10–14 days, dynamic splint if fragments remain in healing position

Displaced or Angulated Transverse Midshaft

- Volar angulation common, generally unstable, with variable response to closed reduction
- Technique
  —Metacarpal or digital block
  —Flex MCP joint to 90 degrees with axial traction
  —Flex PIP joint to 90 degrees with manual realignment of fracture fragments
  —If reduction achieved/maintained, apply gutter or Burkhalter splint; if not, refer to ortho/hand.

Impacted, Displaced Fractures of the Base

- Significant volar angulation requires reduction.
- Technique
  —Metacarpal or digital block
  —With axial traction, flex MCP joint to 90 degrees and correct volar angulation with direct pressure.
  —If reduction achieved/maintained, apply gutter or Burkhalter splint; if not, refer to ortho/hand.

Angulated Neck, Oblique/Spiral Shaft, Condylar (Distal), Displaced Marginal (Base), Large Displaced Avulsion Fractures

- Refer to ortho/hand for pin fixation or open reduction internal fixation (ORIF)

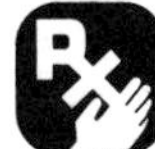

Long-Term Treatment

FOLLOW-UP CARE

Stable Fractures

- Dynamic splinting for 3 weeks; x-ray at 7–10 days to check alignment and stability
- Daily ROM exercises after 1 week
- Continued dynamic splinting for athletic activities for another 4–6 weeks

Stable Fractures after Closed Reduction

- Maintain reduction with gutter or Burkhalter splint; x-ray at 5 and 10 days in splint
- If reduction maintained, continue splint for 3–4 weeks; if reduction fails, refer to ortho/hand for ORIF or percutaneous fixation

Unstable Fractures

- Require ORIF or percutaneous fixation for optimal outcome

Athlete's Return to Play

- Varies greatly from physician to physician
- Goal is life-long use and proper function of the hand.

COMPLICATIONS

- Joint stiffness and subsequent functional disability. Adhesions between extensor mechanism and periosteum may result in loss of motion requiring surgical intervention. Adhesions between flexor superficialis and flexor profundus may follow prolonged immobilization and require surgical intervention to restore function.
- Arthritis can result from intra-articular fractures.
- Nonunion is rare except for improperly immobilized or open fractures.

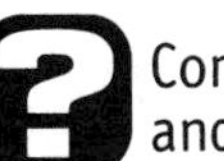

Common Questions and Answers

Physician responses to common patient questions:
Q: When can I return to play?
A: Decision based on stability, current clinical and radiographic healing status, and specific demands of sport. In general, most athletes with stable fractures are able to return 1-2 weeks after the injury or even sooner. For unstable fractures, early surgical intervention may be desirable for better outcome and earlier return.

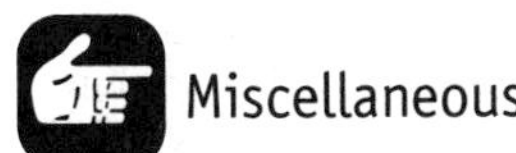

Miscellaneous

ICD-9 CODE

816.01 Fracture: phalanges, hand, middle/proximal, closed

BIBLIOGRAPHY

Connolly JF. *Fractures and dislocations: closed management.* Philadelphia: WB Saunders, 1995.

Eiff MP, Hatch RL, Calmbach WL. *Fracture management for primary care.* Philadelphia: WB Saunders, 1998.

Simon RR, Koenigsknecht SJ. *Emergency orthopedics: the extremities.* Stamford, CT: Appleton and Lange, 1996.

Author: James E. Sturmi

Fracture, Proximal Tibia

Basics

DEFINITION

- Fracture, consisting of any combination, that includes the articular surface of the medial or lateral tibial condyles
- Also known as tibial plateau fracture

INCIDENCE/PREVALENCE

- Tibial plateau fractures account for approximately 1% of all fractures and 8% of fractures in the elderly.
- Lateral tibial plateau fractures account for 55% to 70%, bilateral plateau fractures 11% to 31%, and medial plateau fractures 10% to 23%.

SIGNS AND SYMPTOMS

- Pain and swelling about the knee possibly associated with varus or valgus knee deformity may be seen.
- Tenderness to palpation is noted over the medial and/or lateral tibial plateau.
- Associated ligamentous injuries may show tenderness to palpation and instability of the collateral or cruciate ligaments.
- A large hemarthrosis usually is present.

MECHANISM OF INJURY

- Tibial plateau fractures occur as a result of
  —Force directed either medially (valgus deformity) or laterally (varus deformity)
  —Axial compressive force
  —Combination of both
- First coined a "fender fracture" by Cotton in 1929, 40% to 60% of tibial plateau fractures involve an automobile, usually auto versus pedestrian. Fracture results from a medially directed (valgus deforming) force.
- An axial compressive force, as with a fall from a height landing on an extended knee, usually results in a bicondylar type of fracture.
- Associated ligamentous injuries have been postulated to occur due to continued deforming force after the fracture has been sustained.

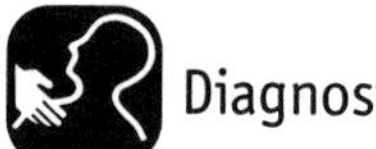

Diagnosis

DIFFERENTIAL DIAGNOSIS

- Intercondylar eminence fracture
- Collateral ligament avulsion
- Tibial tubercle avulsion
- Proximal fibular fracture
- Patella fracture

HISTORY

An accurate history will help to determine the direction of the force, velocity (high vs. low), and initial deformity produced.

PHYSICAL EXAMINATION

- Most accurate way to evaluate the extent of the soft tissue injuries
- Allows for evaluation of the vascular and neurologic status of the extremity
- Gives insight into any associated ligamentous injuries and subsequent stability of the extremity

IMAGING

Standard Radiographs in Anteroposterior (AP), Lateral, and Two Oblique Views

- Provide information allowing for accurate assessment of the fracture pattern
- Internal oblique view allows assessment of the lateral plateau, external oblique, and medial plateau.
- Initial x-rays may miss a small tibial plateau fracture.
- High index of suspicion must be maintained.

Tomography in the AP and Lateral Planes

- Reveals extent and position of the fracture lines
- Allows visualization of areas of depression

Computed Tomography (CT)

- Provides cross-sectional and sagittal assessment of the fracture pattern
- If necessary, three-dimensional reconstructions can be provided to enhance the understanding of the fracture.

Arteriography

- Should be considered in any tibial plateau fracture where the stability of the joint is in question
- Medial plateau fractures have a high incidence of vascular insult, and arteriography should seriously be considered.
- Presence of a palpable pulse does not exclude the possibility of an intimal tear that may lead to intraoperative occlusive thrombosis that could jeopardize the extremity.

Magnetic Resonance Imaging

- Allows for assessment of associated ligamentous injuries
- CT is preferred for bony evaluation.

ANCILLARY STUDIES

If diagnosis is in question after negative routine x-rays, an aspirate may help reveal the presence of fat globules.

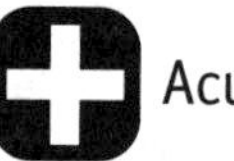

Acute Treatment

MANAGEMENT

- The goals of treating an intraarticular fracture of the tibia are to preserve pain free joint mobility, stability, axial alignment, and articular cartilage congruity, and avoid posttraumatic osteoarthritis. This is best accomplished by anatomical reduction of the joint surface and restoration of axial alignment.
- Intra-articular fractures, regardless of open or closed treatment, must be mobilized quickly to achieve the best range of motion.
- Only percutaneous or open reduction and stabile fixation allow early motion without loss of articular cartilage.
- Fractures initially treated by closed reduction often will show persistent displacement of articular cartilage fragments.
- If open reduction cannot be achieved due to mitigating circumstances, then treatment should consist of skeletal traction and early mobilization.

- Nonoperative treatment is possible with fracture bracing and strict nonweight-bearing if under adequate sedation there is no varus/valgus instability through a full arc of motion. This is best evaluated under anesthesia and C-arm visualization.
- Absolute indications for surgery include
  —Open fractures
  —Tibial plateau fractures with associated
    —Compartment syndrome
    —Acute vascular injury

TIMING OF SURGERY

- Open fractures, associated compartment syndrome, and fractures with associated vascular injuries should undergo surgical intervention immediately.
- Careful evaluation of fractures with tomography or CT is recommended.
- Delay of 24–48 hours will not compromise the outcome.
- Evaluation of soft tissue injury is important.
- Patients delayed >48 hours should be placed in skeletal traction.

POSTOPERATIVE MANAGEMENT

- Depends on the degree of stability achieved with fixation and the findings at surgery.
- If stable, early motion by continuous passive motion (CPM) is beneficial. Motion from full extension to 40–60 degrees the first night.
- CPM is increased to 90 degrees as quickly as possible.
- If CPM is not available, immobilization of the knee in 60–90 degrees of flexion is recommended for the first 48–72 hours, followed by active motion. Immobilization in flexion greatly affects postoperative motion.
- Nonweight-bearing ambulation is encouraged postoperatively.
- Stable type I–V fractures may start partial weight-bearing at 8 weeks. More comminuted fractures should be held nonweight-bearing for 10–12 weeks.
- Early motion, nonweight-bearing, is the key to success.

COMPLICATIONS

- Infection
- Wound slough
- Compartment syndrome (preoperative and postoperative)
- Fixation failure
- Loss of articular reduction
- Malunion
- Nonunion (rare)

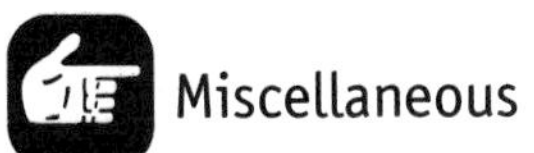

Miscellaneous

SYNONYMS

- Tibial plateau fracture

ICD-9 CODE

823.00

BIBLIOGRAPHY

Holh M, Johnson E, Wiss D. Fractures of the proximal tibia and fibula. In: Rockwood CA, Green DP, Bucholz RW, et al., eds. *Rockwood and Green's fractures in adults*, vol. 2, 4th ed. Philadelphia: JB Lippincott, 1991.

Moore T. Fracture dislocation of the knee. *Clin Orthop* 1981;156:128.

Schatzker J. Tibial plateau fractures. *Skeletal Trauma* 1992;1745–1769.

Schatzker J, McBroom R, Bruce D. The tibial plateau fracture. The Toronto experience. *Clin Orthop* 1979;138:94.

Author: John Tierney

Fracture, Radial Head

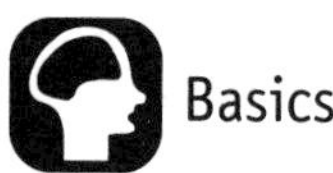

Basics

DEFINITION

- Fracture of the head of the radius, usually caused by direct longitudinal loading, as with a fall on outstretched hand (FOOSH) injury
- Any injury causing dislocation to the elbow may result in radial head fracture.

INCIDENCE/PREVALENCE

Radial head fractures account for about 30% of all elbow fractures in adults. Uncommon in children, accounting for only 1% of all fractures.

SIGNS AND SYMPTOMS

- Patient usually holds injured arm gently against the chest with elbow flexed.
- Typically there is pain and moderate swelling over the lateral side of the elbow.
- Any attempt to flex or extend the elbow or rotate the forearm may accentuate pain.

CLASSIFICATION OF FRACTURES

- Type I: nondisplaced or minimally displaced fracture of head or neck
  —Intra-articular displacement of the fracture <2 mm
  —Forearm rotation (pronation/supination limited only by acute pain and swelling
- Type II: displaced fracture of the head or neck
  —Fracture displaced >2 mm
  —Motion may be mechanically limited.
  —If fracture involves more than a marginal lip of the radial head and is not severely comminuted, repair by open reduction with internal fixation should be considered.
- Type III: severely comminuted fracture of the radial head and neck
  —Not reconstructible
  —Requires excision for movement
- Type IV (added to Mason's classifications by Johnston)
  —Radial head fracture with an associated elbow dislocation

ASSOCIATED INJURIES AND COMPLICATIONS

- Essex-Lopresti lesion: disruption of triangular fibrocartilage complex of the wrist and interosseous membrane of the forearm resulting in instability of the forearm and subluxation of the distal radioulnar joint
- Concomitant capitellar, olecranon, and coronoid fractures (often associated with elbow dislocation)
- Medial ligament tear
- Presence or absence of mechanical block with rotation. Examination achieved after aspiration of hematoma and intra-articular injection of anesthetic. Mechanical block associated with displaced fragment of radial head and affects surgical treatment.

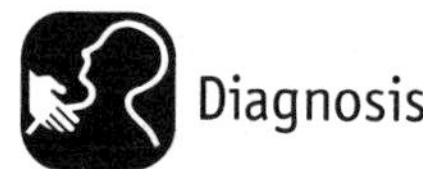

Diagnosis

DIFFERENTIAL DIAGNOSIS

- Other fractures of the elbow, including capitellar, olecranon, and coronoid
- Supracondylar fractures much more prevalent in children

HISTORY

Q: What is the mechanism of injury (FOOSH vs. direct trauma to elbow)?
A: This may help differentiate radial head fracture versus other fractures of the elbow.
Q: Is athlete a "high-demand" or "low-demand" user of the elbow?
A: This may affect choice of conservative versus more aggressive operative management.

PHYSICAL EXAMINATION

- Well-localized tenderness over the radial head (located just distal to the lateral epicondyle)
- Palpation of radial head with passive rotation of the forearm typically elicits pain and occasionally crepitation.
- Forearm and wrist always need to be palpated. Rule out associated injuries such as acute radioulnar dissociation and injury to the interosseous ligament of the forearm.
- Palpation of medial ligament necessary for signs of possible disruption
- Neurovascular status checked distally, especially with history of elbow dislocation

IMAGING

- Anteroposterior and lateral radiographs of the elbow usually sufficient
- If fat pad sign present (either anterior "sail sign" or posterior fat pad sign) and fracture not apparent, radiocapitellar views are helpful, taken with forearm in neutral rotation and x-ray beam angled 45 degrees cephalad.
- Computed tomographic scans helpful in estimating fracture size, degree of fragmentation, and displacement
- If wrist or forearm pain present, x-rays of the wrist in neutral rotation view should be taken.

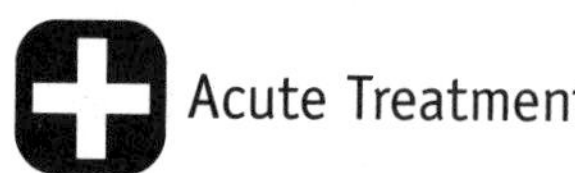

Acute Treatment

ANALGESIA

- Aspiration and injection of anesthetic may provide some pain relief.
- Type I
  —Treated nonoperatively
  —Sling for pain control no longer than 3–4 days
  —Active range of motion can begin as soon as pain permits. Flexion and extension of the elbow and supination and pronation of the forearm should be taken to the point where mild pain begins.
  —Ice therapy for 2–5 days
  —Nonsteroidal anti-inflammatory drugs and oral narcotics as necessary for pain control
- Type II
  —Without mechanical block: treated similarly to type I fractures, especially in the low-demand patient. Outcomes similar to that of type I fractures, but occasionally pain and arthritis may develop.
  —With mechanical block or associated injuries: for high-demand patient/athlete, strong consideration for open reduction with internal fixation. For the low-demand patient, complete excision may be considered.
- Type III
  —Early excision (within 48 hours) is preferred.
- Type IV
  —Treated as above, with obvious attention paid to reduction of dislocation and surgical repair of both fractures and associated ligamentous injuries.

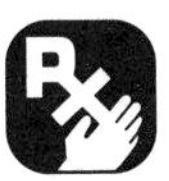

Long-Term Treatment

REHABILITATION

- Initiate range of motion exercises early.
- More aggressive strength and flexibility exercises added progressively as tolerated
- If range of motion does not improve on a weekly basis, supervised physical therapy may be required.

REFERRAL/DISPOSITION

Early orthopaedic input is essential in all but type I fractures due to potential need for surgical correction and controversy surrounding treatment.

LONG-TERM COMPLICATIONS

- Contractures and loss of motion may develop if early active range of motion is not initiated.
- Increased sensitivity to cold, which may persist for up to 1 year
- Long-term pain is rarely a complication.
- Nerve injuries in the form of partial ulnar nerve and posterior interosseus nerve injury have been documented, mainly associated with surgical exploration.

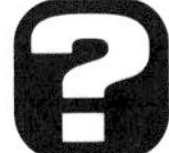

Common Questions and Answers

Physician responses to common patient questions:

Q: When can the athlete return to play?

A: In type I fractures, typically athletes can return to play as early as 6–8 weeks, depending on pain, range of motion, and strength. Protection of the elbow may be needed if returning to contact sports. In type II–IV fractures, return to play is based on extent of associated injuries and surgical correction.

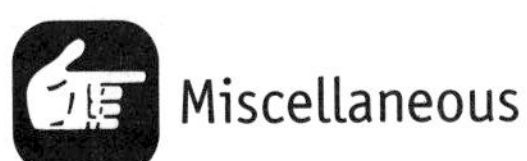

Miscellaneous

ICD-9 CODE

813.05

BIBLIOGRAPHY

Gutierrez G. Management of radial head fractures. *Am Fam Physician* 1997; 55:2213–2216.

Hotchkiss RN. Fractures and dislocations of the elbow. In: Rockwood CA, Green DP, Bucholz RW, et al., eds. *Rockwood and Green's fractures in adults,* 4th ed. Philadelphia: Lippincott-Raven Publishers, 1996, 997–1014.

Kuntz DG, Baratz ME. Elbow trauma and reconstruction: fractures of the elbow. *Orthop Clin North Am* 1999;30:37–61.

O'Connor FG, Ollivierre CO, Nirschl RP. Elbow and forearm injuries. In: Lillegard WA, Butcher JD, Rucker KS, eds. *Handbook of sports medicine: a symptom-oriented approach,* 2nd ed. Boston: Butterworth-Heinemann, 1999, 141–157.

Authors: Keith Stuessi and Thomas A. Balcom

Fracture, Rib

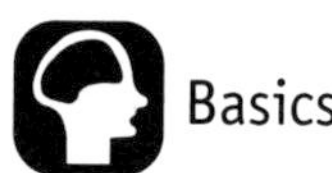

Basics

DEFINITION

- Acute chest trauma, especially in contact sports, as well as chronic overuse of the upper body can lead to rib fractures.
- Fractures may be complete, incomplete, or stress related.
- Often associated with other fractures, soft tissue injuries, and deep organ trauma

INCIDENCE/PREVALENCE

Isolated fractures of the upper four ribs are rare because they are well protected by the shoulder complex. When injury occurs, trauma can be significant enough to fracture other bones of the shoulder. Injury to other deep organs such as lungs, heart, bronchus, blood vessels, and/or esophagus must be considered.

- Blunt trauma to the lower eight ribs commonly results in fractures, most commonly related to blunt trauma of contact sports, such as football, hockey, and rugby.
- Forceful contraction, usually against a significant amount of resistance, of muscles with an attachment to the ribs may result in incomplete, complete, or avulsion fractures of the ribs.
- Chronic stress of upper body muscles, which attach to the ribs, can result in stress fractures of the ribs. Commonly seen in rowing, tennis, golf, gymnastics, and baseball.
- First rib fractures have been reported as a result of falling on an outstretched arm, as well as direct trauma. First rib stress fractures also reported in the literature.
- Avulsion fractures of the lower three floating ribs often occur at the attachment of the external oblique muscles. Known to occur in baseball pitchers and batters.
- Multiple rib fractures occur in high-impact trauma, such as automobile, motorcycle, and bicycle racing.
- Rib fractures more common in adults compared to children due to the relative inelasticity of the adult chest wall

SIGNS AND SYMPTOMS

- Localized pain over the involved rib(s)
- Sensation of crepitus over the fracture site(s)
- Pain generally exacerbated by deep inspiration, resulting in shallow, rapid breathing
- Pain aggravated by coughing and sneezing
- Other symptoms, such as increasing shortness of breath, increasing pain, cyanosis, and subcutaneous emphysema, may indicate serious life-threatening conditions requiring emergent attention.
- Palpable deformity may be present in complete displaced fracture.
- Swelling and ecchymosis may be present in the area of rib fractures.
- In athletes involved in sports with heavy upper extremity activity, stress fractures may present as gradual-onset localized rib pain with or without deformity. Pain may radiate backward.

RISK FACTORS

- Rib fractures most likely occur in contact and collision sports, such as football, hockey, boxing, wrestling, rugby, and soccer.
- As with any trauma, injuries can be more severe in athletes unprepared either from lack of conditioning or contact from the back or blind side.
- Stress fractures of the ribs more likely occur in sports with increased upper body demands, such as golf, rowing, gymnastics, baseball, tennis, racquet sports, and weight-lifting. Overuse and poor technique can contribute to rib stress fractures.
- Other predisposing factors include a history of bone or joint disease, poor nutrition, and calcium deficiency.

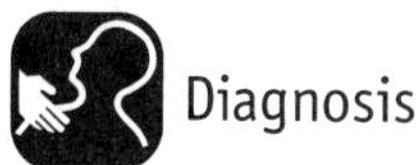

Diagnosis

DIFFERENTIAL DIAGNOSIS

- Rib contusion
- Muscle strain
- Rupture of pectoralis major
- Costochondral separation
- Sternoclavicular separation
- Costochondral sprain
- Sternal fracture (anterior)
- Intervertebral joint sprain
- Intervertebral disc injury
- Apophyseal joint sprain
- Paraspinal muscle strain
- Costovertebral joint sprain
- Scheuermann disease (posterior)
- Other causes of chest pain, such as cardiac causes, peptic ulcer disease, gastroesophageal reflux disorder, pneumothorax, pulmonary embolism, asthma, pleurisy, herpes zoster

HISTORY

- Acute rib fracture usually presents after chest trauma. Can result from a fall on an outstretched arm.
- Athlete may experience the sensation of having "the wind being knocked out."
- Athlete may recall feeling a "pop" when the trauma occurred.
- Athlete may complain of abdominal pain if the lower (11th and 12th) ribs are involved.
- Stress fractures usually occur in elite athletes who train intensely. These fractures tend to be more gradual in onset.

PHYSICAL EXAMINATION

- Localized rib tenderness is the cardinal finding.
- Obvious deformity or crepitation at the fracture site may be present.
- Palpable swelling with or without ecchymosis may be present at the fracture site.
- Subcutaneous emphysema may be present, especially with associated pneumothorax.
- With significant chest trauma, a thorough cardiopulmonary examination must be performed to rule out complications or associated injuries.
- If trauma occurred to the upper chest, special attention should be given to the neck, shoulders, and major vessels.
- If trauma occurred to the lower chest, a thorough abdominal examination should be performed to rule out injury to the liver, spleen, gastrointestinal tract, and kidneys.

IMAGING

- Chest radiographs should be taken after chest trauma to rule out complications such as pneumothorax and hemothorax.
- Rib series radiographs are not necessary for suspected isolated fractures of ribs 5–9.
- Rib series radiographs are indicated if ribs 1–2 or ribs 9–12 are involved.
- Rib series radiographs should be performed if there are suspected multiple rib fractures or pathologic fracture, the athlete is elderly, or there is preexisting pulmonary disease.
- With upper thoracic rib fractures, arteriography is indicated if there is evidence of vascular insufficiency, hemorrhage, or concomitant brachial plexus injury; marked displacement of the rib fragments; fractures of the scapula, vertebrae, or sternum; widening of the mediastinum; left apical cupping; or downward displacement of the left mainstem bronchus.
- Electrocardiogram, echocardiogram, or stress testing if cardiac complications are considered
- Intravenous pyelogram if renal complications are suspected

- Abdominal computed tomographic scan may be necessary if hepatic or splenic injury is suspected.

POSTREDUCTION VIEWS

- Most rib fractures heal without need for reduction or immobilization; thus, postreduction films are not required.
- Healing first rib fractures may compromise the vasculature to the upper extremity.
- Repeat films may be performed to monitor this complication during healing.

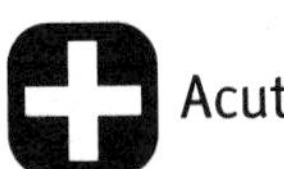

Acute Treatment

ANALGESIA

- Pain control is the cornerstone of treatment for rib fractures. Pain control may be required up to 3–6 after injury.
- Ice and nonsteroidal anti-inflammatory drugs may control symptoms, but stronger oral pain medications often are required.
- Local intercostal nerve blocks remain an option if other pain control techniques fail.

IMMOBILIZATION

- Strapping or a chest binder has been advocated to help with pain. These immobilization techniques can result in inhibition of deep breathing, leading to atelectasis and possibly pneumonia.
- If immobilization is deemed necessary for comfort, its use should be minimized.

SPECIAL CONSIDERATIONS

- Flail chest occurs when $\geq$3 ribs are fractured in two locations.
- Nonunion of rib fractures is rare but has been reported.

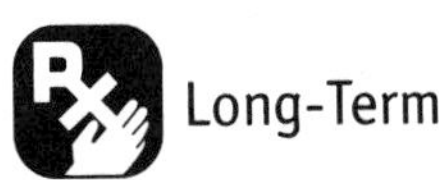

Long-Term Treatment

REHABILITATION

- Rib stress fractures may respond well to rehabilitation exercises, such as pushups, serratus press, upper extremity step-ups, and serratus rhythmic stabilization.
- Biomechanics of throwing, rowing, batting, or weight-lifting should be evaluated and corrected if necessary.

SURGERY

- Need for surgery is rare in cases of isolated rib fractures
- Exception is in the case of flail chest. ORIF may be required.
- Suspected internal injuries associated with rib fractures should be referred for possible surgical repair.
- Chronic pain due to recurrent stress fracture, nonunion, or recurrent dislocation or subluxation may improve with surgical excision of the involved rib.

REFERRAL/DISPOSITION

- The athlete should be encouraged to continue activities as tolerated, except for contact sports.
- Contact should be limited for the first 3 weeks following injury. Consider rib protection in contact sports after return.
- Monitor regularly for signs of delayed complications.

Common Questions and Answers

Physician responses to common patient questions:
Q: What should I do for the pain?
A: Start with icing. Your doctor will give you medication for pain. Sometimes pushing against and supporting the injured rib, especially with coughing or sneezing, will decrease pain. If necessary, a binder may be used for a very limited time.
Q: Do I need to have rib x-rays?
A: In most cases of isolated rib fractures, simple chest films are all that are required. If the first or the bottom couple of ribs are involved, other x-rays may be ordered.
Q: In what activity can I safely participate?
A: You should continue to be as active as you can tolerate. Do not hesitate to take the medication prescribed for pain. You should avoid collision or contact sports until your doctor has determined you are safe to return, usually in 3 weeks.
Q: How likely is it I may experience a stress fracture again?
A: It is important not only to allow the stress fracture to heal, but also determine what might have contributed to it. Your doctor may need to evaluate your training, technique, and nutritional status, and may conduct other laboratory tests. Once contributing factors are identified and corrected, you should be able to return to your previous level of activity.

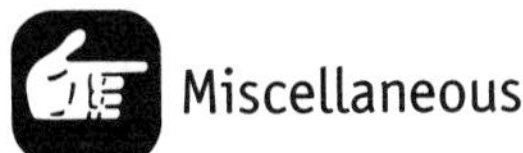

Miscellaneous

SYNONYMS

- Double fractures of the chest: steering wheel injury, flail chest, stove-in chest

ICD-9 CODE

- 807.0 Fracture, rib(s) closed. Note: fifth digit indicates number of ribs involved
- 0 = unspecified; 1 = one rib; 2 = two ribs... 8 = eight or more ribs, 9 = multiple ribs, unspecified
- 807.1 Fracture, rib(s) open
- 807.4 Fracture, rib(s) with flail chest
- Stress fracture code as Pathological fracture, specified site NEC 733.15

BIBLIOGRAPHY

Barrett GR, Shelton WR, Miles JW. First rib fractures in football players: a case report and literature review. *Am J Sports Med* 1988;16:674–676.

Brukner P, Karim K. *Clinical sports medicine.* New York: McGraw-Hill, 1997.

DePalma AF. *DePalma's the management of fractures and dislocations.* Philadelphia: WB Saunders, 1981.

George RB, Light RW, Matthay RA, eds. *Chest medicine: essentials of pulmonary and critical care medicine.* Baltimore: Williams & Wilkins, 1995.

Lord MJ, Ha KI, Song KS. Stress fractures of the ribs in golfers. *Am J Sports Med* 1996;24:118–122.

Miles JW, Barrett GR. Rib fractures in athletes. *Sports Med* 1991;12:66–69.

O'Kane J, O'Kane E, Marquet J. Delayed complication of a rib fracture. *Physician Sportsmed* 1998;26:69–77.

Proffer DS, Patton JJ, Jackson DW. Nonunion of a first rib fracture in a gymnast. *Am J Sports Med* 1991;19(2):198–201.

Rosen P, Barkin R, Danzl D, eds. *Emergency medicine: concepts and clinical practice.* St. Louis: Mosby-Year Book 1998.

Author: Robert Baker

Fracture, Sacral

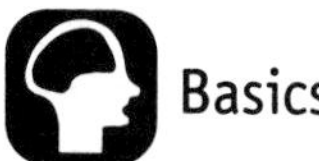

Basics

SIGNS AND SYMPTOMS

- Pain in buttocks, perirectal area, and posterior thigh
- Swelling and ecchymosis over the sacral prominence
- Possible sacral nerve dysfunction
  —Absence or diminished anal sphincter tone is an important finding.
  —Bowel or bladder incontinence

MECHANISM/DESCRIPTION

- Sacral fractures are rarely isolated injuries (<5%).
- They are frequently associated with pelvic fractures.
- They are defined by the orientation of the fracture line.
- Axial compression
- Direct posterior trauma
- Massive crush injury

PRE-HOSPITAL

- Sacral fractures are frequently associated with other spine and intra-abdominal injuries.
- Immobilize with backboard and C-spine collar

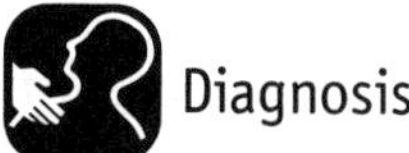

Diagnosis

ESSENTIAL WORKUP

- History and examination with attention to loss of anal sphincter tone, sensation in the perineum, and bowel and bladder sphincter control
- Sacral fractures rarely occur in isolation, look for associated injuries.
- Rectal exam will elicit pain in the sacrum.
- Displacement can be assessed with bimanual rectal exam.

IMAGING/SPECIAL TESTS

- Only 30% of sacral fractures detected on x-ray.
- Rostrally and caudally angulated AP views and coned down views of the lumbosacral junction may help.
- CT scan may better delineate the fracture and associated injuries.

DIFFERENTIAL DIAGNOSIS

- Contusion

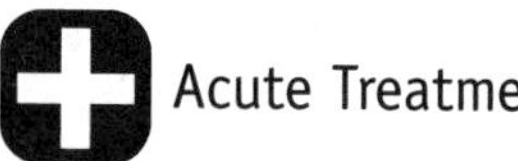

Acute Treatment

INITIAL STABILIZATION

- ABCs of trauma care
- Early immobilization in unstable pelvis or spine fractures
- Pain control with NSAIDs or narcotic analgesics

ED TREATMENT

- Vertical unstable fractures require a rapid and thorough assessment for life-threatening injuries and orthopedic consultation (see topic Fracture, Pelvic).
- Nondisplaced isolated sacral fractures are treated symptomatically with bedrest.
- Surgery may be required for fractures associated with neurological injury.
- Early orthopedic referral

Fracture Classification

Direction	Subtype	Associated Findings	Neurologic Exam
Transverse	*High Sacral*: fall from height	Transverse process fracture, alar fracture, (+) kyphosis	Rare motor weakness, (+) cauda equina syndrome
	Low Sacral: direct blow	Rectal tears, CSF leaks	Rare motor weakness, (+) cauda equina syndrome
Vertical	*Alar* (Zone I)	Sciatica, L5 root injury	Neurologic deficit *infrequent*
	Foraminal (Zone II)	Bowel/bladder dysfunction, L5, S1, S2 root injury, sciatica, foot drop	Neurologic deficit *frequent*
	Canal (Zone III)	Bowel/bladder dysfunction, sexual dysfunction, sciatica, L5, S1 root injury	Neurologic deficit *very frequent*

HOSPITAL ADMISSION CRITERIA

- Critically injured trauma patient with unstable pelvic fracture
- Neurologic impairment

HOSPITAL DISCHARGE CRITERIA

- All other types of isolated sacral fractures
- Consider intermediate care for elderly patients

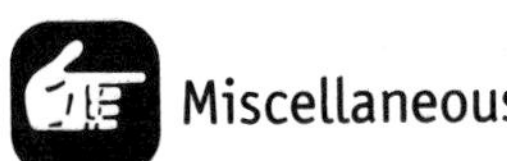

Miscellaneous

ICD-9-CM

805.6

CORE CONTENT CODE

18.4.3.1.4

BIBLIOGRAPHY

Cwinn AA. Pelvis and hip. In: Rosen P, et al., eds. *Emergency medicine: Concepts and clinical practice*. 4th ed. St. Louis: CV Mosby, 1998:739–762.

Pollack C. Pelvic trauma. In: Harwood-Nuss A, et al., eds. *The clinical practice of emergency medicine*. 2d ed. Philadelphia: Lippincott-Raven, 1996.

Simon R, Koenigsknecht S. Traumatic conditions of the hip. In: Simon R, et al., eds. *Emergency Orthopedics: The extremities*. 3rd ed. Norwalk CT, Appleton & Lange, 1993:425–427.

Authors: Jaime B. Rivas and Teresa Carlin

Fracture, Scaphoid

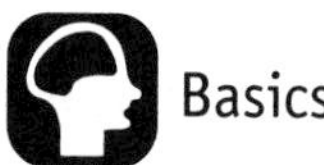

Basics

DEFINITION

- Fracture of the scaphoid bone is the most common carpal bone fracture.
- Injury occurs when the patient falls on the extended wrist.

INCIDENCE/PREVALENCE

- Fractures of the carpal bones account for 6% of all fractures.
- Fractures of the scaphoid bone account for 70% of all carpal fractures.

SIGNS AND SYMPTOMS

- Symptoms: Patient reports wrist pain after falling on the extended wrist.
- Signs: tender in the anatomical snuffbox (waist fracture or distal pole fracture) or just distal to Lister tubercle on distal radius (proximal pole fracture)
- Usually minimal swelling, unless fracture-dislocation is present

RISK FACTORS

- Young adult males are the most common patient (children: distal radial physis fails before scaphoid fracture; older adults: distal radial metaphysis fails before scaphoid fracture).
- Usually associated with falls, athletic injuries, or motor vehicle injuries

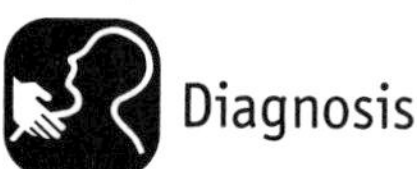

Diagnosis

DIFFERENTIAL DIAGNOSIS

- Scapholunate dissociation
- Distal radius fracture
- Wrist sprain

HISTORY

- Patient reports falling on the extended wrist
- Pain at the wrist, near base of the first metacarpal

PHYSICAL EXAMINATION

- Tender in anatomical snuffbox (between abductor pollicis longus and extensor pollicis brevis radially, and the extensor pollicis longus dorsally)
- Examiner places thumb or index finger in anatomical snuffbox and passively ulnarly deviates wrist to palpate scaphoid
- Early diagnosis usually based on clinical examination because initial radiographs usually negative

IMAGING

Radiographs

- Three views of the wrist: posteroanterior (PA), lateral, and "scaphoid" view, i.e., anteroposterior (AP) view of wrist with 30 degrees supination and ulnar deviation
- May request additional views: radial oblique, ulnar oblique, and PA wrist with clenched fist in radial and ulnar deviation
- Plain radiographs often negative immediately after injury
- Fracture may become apparent 10–14 days after injury (immobilization allows demineralization of the fracture line).
- Examine radiographs for evidence of the "Terry Thomas" sign (i.e., widening of the scapholunate distance).

Bone Scan

- May be necessary for patients with persistent snuffbox tenderness but negative plain radiographs
- Positive scan shows increased uptake at the scaphoid.

Computed Tomography/Magnetic Resonance Imaging

- Used to confirm scaphoid fracture
- May indicate early avascular necrosis

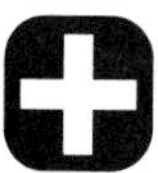

Acute Treatment

- Immobilize in long arm cast: elbow at 90 degrees flexion, forearm in neutral pronation/supination, wrist in slight extension (so-called position of function)
- Duration of immobilization depends on location of fracture: "waist" fracture 12 weeks; distal fracture 8 weeks; proximal pole fracture 16–20 weeks

ANALGESIA

- NSAIDs
- Narcotic analgesic

REDUCTION TECHNIQUES

- Surgical fixation

IMMOBILIZATION

- Long arm cast for 4–6 weeks, followed by short arm thumb spica cast for 8–10 weeks

SPECIAL CONSIDERATIONS

- Associated injuries include fracture of the distal radius, radial head, and lunate; soft tissue ligamentous injury leading to scapholunate dissociation; and possible injury to the median nerve

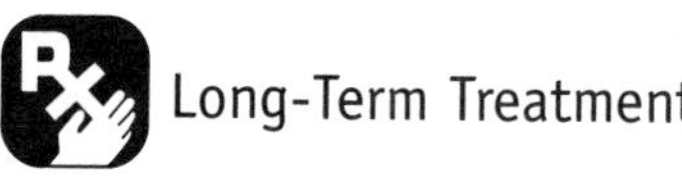

Long-Term Treatment

REHABILITATION

- Post-operative or post-casting hand therapy

SURGERY

- Acute injury: displaced fracture (>2 mm displaced)
- Subacute/chronic injury: development of avascular necrosis

REFERRAL/DISPOSITION

- Nondisplaced waist or distal pole fracture can be treated closed by primary care physician
- Refer patient with displaced scaphoid fracture
- Consider referring patient with proximal pole fracture (prone to nonunion and avascular necrosis)

COMPLICATIONS

- Avascular necrosis of the proximal fracture fragment, leading to wrist dysfunction and early osteoarthritis
- High incidence of fibrous nonunion at the fracture site (8% to 10%)
- Frequent malunion
- Carpal instability
- Posttraumatic arthritis

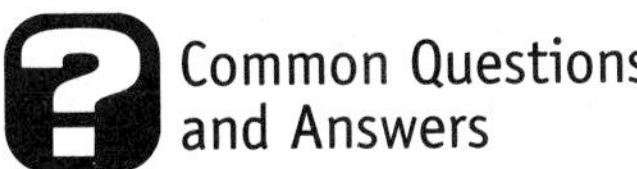

Common Questions and Answers

Physician responses to common patient questions:
Q: How do I make the diagnosis of scaphoid fracture?
A: History of a fall on the extended wrist, coupled with tenderness in the anatomical snuffbox
Q: What should I do if the patient has negative radiographs at the time of examination?
A: If the patient has the typical mechanism of injury and is tender in the anatomical snuffbox, the patient should be immobilized for 10–14 days and then reevaluated with repeat radiographs.
Q: What is the best form of immobilization?
A: For patients with the typical mechanism of injury and definite tenderness in the anatomical snuffbox, initial immobilization with a long arm thumb spica cast is recommended. For patients in whom the diagnosis is in doubt but tenderness in the anatomical snuffbox is present, immobilization in a short arm thumb spica cast or even a thumb spica splint is recommended.
Q: What should I do if the patient is still tender in the anatomical snuffbox after 10–14 days of immobilization, but repeat radiographs are negative?
A: Some physicians continue immobilization for another 2 weeks, then repeat radiographs. Most physicians recommend scintigraphy (bone scan) to confirm or deny the diagnosis.
Q: Is this a fracture that primary care physicians can safely treat?
A: The rate of serious complications, such as avascular necrosis or fibrous nonunion, among patients with scaphoid fractures is fairly high. Physicians who do not feel comfortable treating patients with this type of fracture should refer them to an experienced hand surgeon.

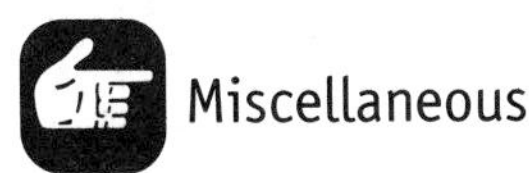

Miscellaneous

SYNONYMS

Fracture, carpal navicular

ICD-9 CODE

814.01 Fracture, scaphoid, wrist: closed
814.11 Fracture, scaphoid, wrist: open

BIBLIOGRAPHY

Cooney WP III, Linscheid RL, Dobyns JH. Fractures and dislocations of the wrist. In: Rockwood CA Jr, Green DP, Bucholz RW, eds. *Rockwood and Green's fractures in adults,* 3rd ed. Philadelphia: JB Lippincott, 1991: 563–678.

Author: Walter L. Calmbach

Fracture, Spinous and Transverse Processes

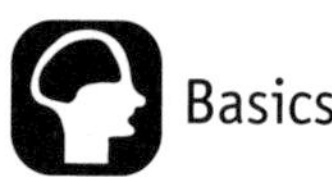

Basics

DEFINITION

- Transverse and spinous process fractures are considered minor spine injuries and usually are stable and benign. Both types can be markers of considerable trauma and should encourage the physician to look for additional injury.
- Fractures of the spinous process typically occur at C-7 or any of the lower cervical or upper thoracic vertebrae. They are commonly avulsion-type injuries resulting from contraction of the trapezius, rhomboid minor, and/or serratus posterior.
- Traditionally referred to as "clay shoveler's' injuries" but now are found mostly after sudden deceleration in motor vehicle accidents or forced flexion of the neck, often in football players and weight-lifters.

INCIDENCE/PREVALENCE

- Spinous process fractures are relatively rare since mechanization replaced clay shovelers.
- "Sentinel spinous process fractures" are associated with fractures of lamina and facets, which can lead to instability.
- Up to 21% of transverse process fractures resulting from high-energy trauma (e.g., motor vehicle accidents) are associated with visceral injuries (most commonly to the spleen and liver).
- Up to 11% have other spine injuries not detected by plain radiographs but identified on computed tomographic (CT) scanning.
- Transverse process fractures resulting from low-energy trauma (e.g., playing footballs) do not generally have associated spinal, nerve root, or visceral injuries.

SIGNS AND SYMPTOMS

- Localized pain over injured area without radiation
- Pain increased with neck flexion (lower cervical spinous process fracture) or hip flexion (lumbar transverse process fracture)

RISK FACTORS

- Growth spurts, training errors, improper technique, and repetitive trauma predispose the athlete to spine fractures.

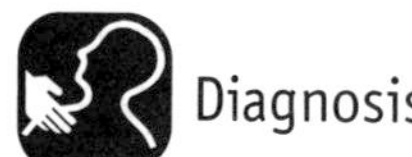

Diagnosis

DIFFERENTIAL DIAGNOSIS

- "Burst" fracture
- Lumbar strain
- Disc herniation
- Spondylolysis and/or spondylolisthesis

HISTORY

Q: What was the mechanism of injury?
A: Forceful hyperflexion of the neck (e.g., spearing in football) is associated with lower cervical spinous process fractures. Lumbar transverse process fractures usually result from direct trauma
Q: What makes the pain worse?
A: Pain with hip flexion indicates possible lumbar transverse process fracture. Pain with neck flexion suggests cervical spinous process fracture.

PHYSICAL EXAMINATION

- Careful neurologic examination for weakness, reflex changes, or sensory changes in a dermatomal distribution. As neurologic injuries are not commonly associated with minor fractures, abnormal results should raise suspicion of additional spinal injury.
- Pain worse with hip flexion (site of iliopsoas origin) seen in lumbar transverse process fractures
- Benign abdominal examination does not exclude coexistent intra-abdominal injury.

IMAGING

Cervical Lateral Radiograph

- Very important to visualize C-7 spinous process, which often is obscured by the shoulders
- Obtain "swimmers view" if necessary to visualize C7-T1 junction.
- Anteroposterior (AP) radiograph may show double shadow of spinous process due to avulsion.
- Flexion-extension films to rule out ligamentous instability and lamina or facet injury

Thoracolumbar AP Radiograph

- May show double shadow of spinous process due to avulsion
- Hematoma may obscure evidence of transverse process fracture. Loss of normal psoas shadow may be most prominent finding.
- Oblique radiograph to rule out defects in pars interarticularis

ADDITIONAL IMAGING

- CT scan: superior to plain films to evaluate extent of spinal fractures and rule out serious spine injury, but has limited field of view and high radiation dose
- Magnetic resonance imaging: only necessary if neurologic symptoms are present to evaluate extrinsic spinal cord compression or intrinsic cord injury

FOLLOW-UP RADIOGRAPHS

Radiographic appearance often lags behind clinical healing and should not be used as the primary criterion for return to play.

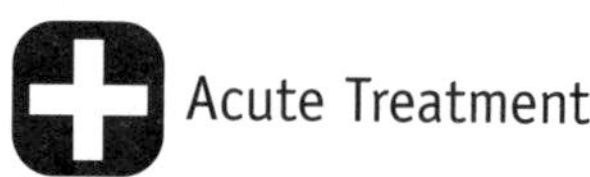

Acute Treatment

ANALGESIA

- Rest is often the most effective treatment for isolated injury.
- Cryotherapy repeated frequently within initial 36–48 hours may help prevent muscle spasm.
- Nonsteroidal anti-inflammatory drugs and gentle exercises may be helpful.

IMMOBILIZATION

In all cases of suspected spine injury, immobilization with a backboard and rigid cervical collar is mandatory until the patient can be cleared radiographically.

SPECIAL CONSIDERATIONS

If transverse process fractures result from high-energy trauma, there should be a high index of suspicion for associated visceral injuries. Urinalysis should be performed; if >8 red blood cells per high-power field are seen, perform cystogram and intravenous pyelogram to evaluate for possible urinary tract injury.

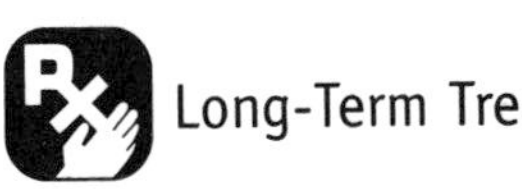

Long-Term Treatment

REHABILITATION

- With cervical injury, protection against flexion with an orthosis should be provided for 6–8 weeks.
- Isolated lumbar transverse process fractures can be treated with a corset for symptomatic relief. If there is associated spinal injury, a rigid orthosis or longer bracing is needed. The patient should be limited to isometric exercises with restricted upper extremity exercises until full range of motion and no tenderness to palpation are present.
- Isolated fractures of the transverse process usually cause disability for a few weeks and carry a very low likelihood of long-term sequelae.
- Contiguous transverse process fractures should be observed carefully for development of pseudoarthrosis or myositis ossificans.

SURGERY

Nonunion of fractured fragments is common in both injuries, but most authors advocate avoiding excision of fragments unless pain persists beyond the period of immobilization.

REFERRAL/DISPOSITION

Patients with isolated fractures do not need orthopaedic or neurosurgical referral.

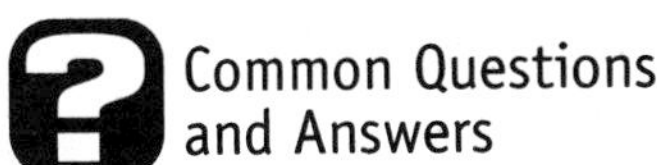

Common Questions and Answers

Physician responses to common patient questions:
Q: When can I play again?
A: The average time lost from sports reported in an NFL study was 25 days for lumbar transverse process fractures but varies from case to case, depending on the number of vertebral levels involved and any associated injury.
Q: Do I need protective equipment?
A: Athletes involved in contact sports may feel more comfortable in a flak jacket, although there is no evidence that they prevent reinjury or accelerate return to competition.

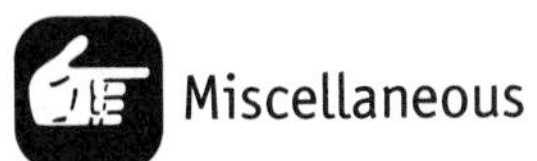

Miscellaneous

SYNONYMS

- Minor spinal fracture

ICD-9 CODE

805.0 Cervical fracture, closed
805.2 Thoracic fracture, closed
805.4 Lumbar fracture, closed

BIBLIOGRAPHY

Krueger M, Green D, Hoyt D, et al. Overlooked spine injuries associated with lumbar transverse process fractures. *Clin Orthop Rel Research* 1996;327:191–195.

Nicholas J, Nuber G, eds. *The lower extremity and spine in sports medicine.* St. Louis: Mosby, 1995.

Sturm J, Perry J. Injuries associated with fractures of the transverse processes of the thoracic and lumbar vertebrae. *J Trauma* 1984;24:597–599.

Tewes DP, Fisher D, Quick D, et al. Lumbar transverse process fractures in professional football players. *Am J Sports Med* 1995;23:507–509.

Authors: David Bazzo and Jason Bryant

Fracture, Sternum

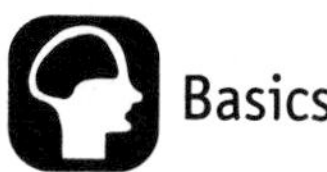

Basics

DEFINITION

- Fracture of the sternum
- Direct
  - —Results from direct force applied to the sternum, most often from a blow to the body of the sternum in the lower part; usually from a motor vehicle accident
  - —Fracture typically occurs near manubrium.
- Indirect
  - —Results from an indirect flexion-compression injury of the cervicothoracic spine, usually a forced flexion of the cervical spine that causes the upper two ribs to pull the manubrium posteriorly (downward and posterior force on the manubrium and upper two ribs)
  - —May be exacerbated by chin striking the manubrium
  - —Always involves the upper two segments of the sternum
- Muscular
  - —Results from violent muscular action that causes fracture through opposing muscle groups, i.e., tetanus
  - —Extremely rare

INCIDENCE/PREVALENCE

- Very rare, especially in children and adolescents, due to elasticity of sternum and costal cartilage
- Most commonly related to automobile accidents, typically from a direct mechanism, such as striking the steering wheel or dashboard.

SIGNS AND SYMPTOMS

- Pain
- Tenderness
- Bruising
- Swelling
- Deformity
- Possible dyspnea

RISK FACTORS

- Participation in activities with potential for high-impact thoracic injury

ASSOCIATED INJURIES AND COMPLICATIONS

- Vertebral fracture: especially from indirect mechanism. Most commonly thoracic vertebrae, but also may occur in lower cervical or upper lumbar vertebrae.
- Rib fracture: most often associated with a direct mechanism. Can cause flail chest.
- Trauma to heart, mediastinum, great vessels, tracheobronchial tree, lung parenchyma, or liver: mediastinal injury much less common with an indirect mechanism. Always consider cardiac contusion, especially with double or comminuted fracture and in fracture involving the sternal angle.
- Pneumothorax
- Tamponade

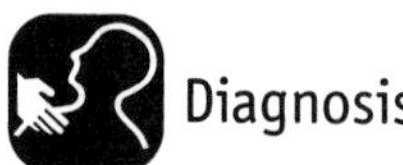

Diagnosis

DIFFERENTIAL DIAGNOSIS

- Costochondral dislocation
- Sternoclavicular dislocation
- Sternal contusion
- Costochondritis
- Cardiac contusion
- Cardiac ischemia

HISTORY

- Direct blow to chest wall
- Forced flexion of cervical spine (heavy blow to back of head or fall onto head)
- Pain with inspiration
- Crepitus with respiratory excursion
- Dyspnea, usually transient. If persistent, consider more severe underlying injury.

PHYSICAL EXAMINATION

- Localized tenderness
- Palpable or visible step-off (deformity present with displaced fracture)
- Palpable crepitus with respirations (more rare)
- Edema, ecchymosis
- Screen for associated rib fracture, clinical evidence of pulmonary contusion, vascular injury, pneumothorax, and pericardial friction rub

IMAGING

- Care must be taken not to confuse nonossified intrasternal cartilage in young patients with fractures.
- Chest posteroanterior (PA) and lateral radiographs (fracture missed in >80% of AP views): possible pneumothorax or mediastinal injury. Widened mediastinum should not be attributed to hematoma, but instead to underlying vascular injury until ruled out. Sternal fracture displacement and sternal dislocation occur in the sagittal plane.
- Electrocardiogram (ECG): May see ECG changes in >50%, especially if from a direct mechanism. No single test is consistently reliable for diagnosis of myocardial contusion. If initial ECG is normal, consider repeat in 24 hours. May see ST or T-wave abnormalities or bundle branch block. May see major arrhythmia in first 24 hours (rare).
- Cervical, thoracic, lumbar spine radiographs: especially if from an indirect mechanism.
- Consider other modalities (echocardiogram, computed tomography, aortography, serial creatine phosphokinase levels) if underlying injury is suspected.

POSTREDUCTION VIEWS

- Chest PA and lateral radiographs

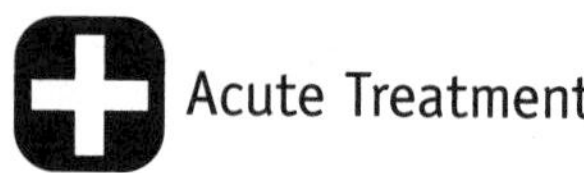

Acute Treatment

ANALGESIA

- Narcotics appropriate once associated injuries are ruled out.
- Consider hematoma block if reduction is necessary.

REDUCTION TECHNIQUES

- Most nondisplaced fractures are treated conservatively with rest and analgesia until symptoms subside.
- Some displaced fractures can be reduced by having the patient lay supine and hyperextending the thoracic spine by placing a sandbag transversely under the shoulders, slightly below the level of the spines of the scapulae. Extension can be maintained by bracing or bed rest.
- For simple displaced fractures, some authors recommend having the patient lay supine and simultaneously lifting the head and the extended lower extremities, thus separating the upper and lower part of the sternum. Use thumb to place pressure on the anteriorly displaced fragment (should infiltrate with local anesthetic first).
- Open reduction internal fixation: Primary indication is pain with respiration that limits respiratory excursion; also flail chest. If not stabilized, can have pseudoarthrosis that can be source of ongoing pain or instability.

POSTREDUCTION EVALUATION

Consider 24-hour inpatient observation and monitoring due to the relatively high likelihood of associated underlying injuries.

IMMOBILIZATION

- Immobilization typically is not necessary with nondisplaced fractures.
- Short-term immobilization may be necessary after surgical repair.

SPECIAL CONSIDERATIONS

Consider cardiac monitoring while performing reduction if available.

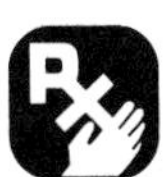

Long-Term Treatment

REHABILITATION

- Avoid aggravating activities and contact sports.
- May start general conditioning within the limits of discomfort.

SURGERY

- Surgical treatment for displaced fractures as above.
- Consider surgical repair if nonunion (rare).

REFERRAL/DISPOSITION

- Usually heals without any sequelae.
- Consider early orthopaedic referral if displaced fracture, open fracture, or flail chest.
- Early consultation as appropriate if there are associated underlying thoracic injuries (pneumothorax, cardiac contusion, etc.).

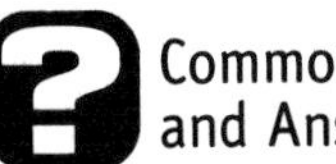

Common Questions and Answers

Physician responses to common patient questions:
Q: When can I return to play?
A: Contact sports should be avoided until symptoms subside, typically 6–12 weeks.
Q: When may I resume conditioning?
A: May do general conditioning or training program within the limits of discomfort posed by the injury.
Q: Is any special equipment necessary when returning to play?
A: Should consider chest protector if likelihood of reinjury.

Miscellaneous

ICD-9 CODE

807.2 Fracture of sternum, closed
807.3 Fracture of sternum, open
807.4 Fracture of sternum, open with flail chest

CPT CODE

21820 Fracture of sternum, closed treatment
21825 Fracture of sternum, open treatment

BIBLIOGRAPHY

Buckman R, Trooskin SZ, Flancbaum L, et al. The significance of stable patients with sternal fractures. *Surg Gynecol Obstet* 1987;164:261–265.

Jones HK, McBride GG, Mumby RC. Sternal fractures associated with sternal injury. *J Trauma* 1989;29:360–364.

Kitchens J, Richardson JD. Open fixation of sternal fractures. *Surg Gynecol Obstet* 1993;177:423–424.

Lyons FR, Rockwood CA. *Orthopaedic sports medicine: principles and practice.* Philadelphia: WB Saunders, 1994.

Mayba II. Sternal injuries. *Orthop Rev* 1986;XV:35–43.

Santos GH. Treatment of displaced fractures of the sternum. *Surg Gynecol Obstet* 1988;166:273–274.

Authors: Timothy J. Linker and Thomas L. Pommering

Fracture, Stress: Metatarsal, Navicular

 Basics

DEFINITION

- Overload, repetitive stress injury to bone
- Manifest as fatigue fractures to otherwise normal bone

INCIDENCE/PREVALENCE

- Stress fractures account for 0.7% to 15.6% of athletic injuries.
- Metatarsal fractures are second most common stress fractures; most frequent in track, running, and dance.
- Tarsal navicular stress fractures are rare but underappreciated; 73% occur in track.

SIGNS AND SYMPTOMS

- Metatarsals: forefoot pain that progressively worsens with activity
- Tarsal navicular: vague, dorsal midfoot pain sometimes radiating along the medial arch or into the ankle

RISK FACTORS

- Training errors: number, frequency, intensity, and duration of strain cycles
- Impact attenuation: muscle fatigue, training surfaces, footwear
- Gait mechanics: foot type, lower extremity alignment, altered gait
- Bone health: nutrition, genetics, hormones, bone disease

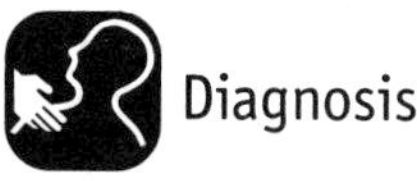 Diagnosis

DIFFERENTIAL DIAGNOSIS

- Tendinitis
- Tendon rupture, partial or complete
- Metatarsalgia
- Symptomatic accessory ossicle

HISTORY

Q: Pain onset acute or insidious?
A: Site of fracture.
Q: Pain location?
A: Usually insidious.
Q: Associated findings?
A: There is minimal or no swelling with stress fractures.
Q: Does pain improve or worsen during the activity?
A: Tendinitis pain often improves as the injured tissue warms up, but stress fracture pain persists or worsens during the activity.

PHYSICAL EXAMINATION

Metatarsal Stress Fracture

- Minimal or no forefoot swelling
- Tenderness at the base, head, or midshaft of the metatarsal
- Axial load applied to head of the metatarsal causes pain at the fracture site and distant to the examination site.
- Examine callous patterns, which may clue the examiner to excessive loads to individual metatarsals.

Navicular Stress Fracture

- Tender over the dorsum of the navicular at the "N" spot in the space between the anterior tibial tendon and the extensor hallucis longus tendon
- Biomechanical examination, joint range of motion, strength, and flexibility to assess predisposing conditions

IMAGING

Radiographs

- Metatarsals: Anteroposterior and lateral radiographs initially are normal, followed 2–3 weeks by periosteal thickening and sometimes a radiolucent line.
- Tarsal navicular: Plain radiographs often are normal throughout the course of a navicular stress fracture.

Bone Scan

- Metatarsals: very sensitive, but necessary only if a diagnosis is needed quickly, as with a competitive athlete. Not specific and must be correlated with clinical history and examination.
- Navicular: characteristically show radioactive uptake throughout the entire navicular.

Computed Tomographic Scan

- Metatarsals: not helpful
- Navicular: Thin sliced cuts in the plane of the talonavicular joint reveal the curvilinear fracture extending from the dorsal cortex surrounded by exuberant bony sclerosis. Computed tomography is helpful to determine an incomplete fracture versus a complete dorsoplantar transection of the navicular.

Magnetic Resonance Imaging

- Not generally necessary

POSTREDUCTION VIEWS

- NA

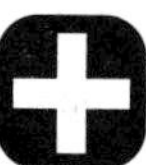 Acute Treatment

Metatarsals

- Cease sporting activities
- Nonweight-bearing only needed for pain control
- Rest period, average 6 weeks

Navicular

- Nonweight-bearing on crutches with below-the-knee cast or removable brace for 4–6 weeks. High failure rate with weight-bearing rest.
- Follow-up clinical assessment for tenderness at the "N" spot. Radiographic assessment not helpful. Continued tenderness should extend nonweight-bearing another 2–3 weeks.

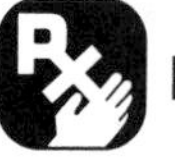 Long-Term Treatment

REHABILITATION

Metatarsals

- Nonweight-bearing aerobic training by swimming and pool running during the rest period
- Advance to biking and stair climbing before running
- Return to progressive gradual training only after pain-free walking and no local tenderness at the fracture site
- Consider biomechanical control with custom orthotic to address excessive lesser metatarsal loading

Navicular

- First 2 weeks following cast removal: activities of daily living, swimming, water running
- Second two weeks: Assess "N" spot; if nontender, then 5 minutes jogging on grass every other day. Gradually increase to 10 minutes per session.
- Third two weeks: Assess "N" spot; if nontender, then faster running for short distances, i.e., 50 meters on alternate days. Gradual speed increase.
- Fourth two weeks: Assess "N" spot; if nontender, then gradual return to full training over several weeks. Average time to return to sport is 5–6 months from diagnosis.
- Attention throughout the rehabilitation time to soft tissue massage and joint mobilization to the talocrural, subtalar, and midtarsal joints.
- Strength training to reverse the atrophy acquired during immobilization

SURGERY

Metatarsals

Surgery is rarely required for metatarsal stress fractures.

Navicular

- $\leq$10% of navicular stress fractures cannot be managed with nonweight-bearing cast.
- Surgical fixation with internal screw, bone grafting, or both is necessary for fractures not clinically healed by nonoperative means.

REFERRAL/DISPOSITION

- Metatarsal stress fractures not healing in a reasonably expected period of time should be referred to orthopaedic surgery or podiatry. Consider referring for biomechanical evaluation for recurrent stress fractures.
- Navicular: Refer the persistently symptomatic navicular stress fracture that does not heal by the above outlined protocol.

Common Questions and Answers

Physician responses to common patient questions:
Q: How did I get this stress fracture?
A: Risk factors for stress fractures include overuse or training errors, biomechanical factors, choice or age of shoe, nutrition, and menstrual issues for women.
Q: Will I be at risk of stress fracture recurrence?
A: Careful attention to the risk factors, particularly training errors, will minimize the risk of reinjury.
Q: Will I need surgery?
A: Surgery is rarely indicated for metatarsal and tarsal navicular stress fractures.

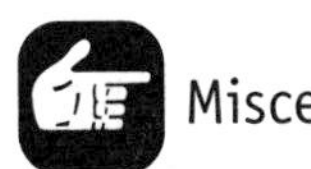

Miscellaneous

ICD-9 CODE

825.25 Metatarsals
825.29 Navicular (tarsals)

BIBLIOGRAPHY

Brukner P, Bennell K, Matheson G, eds. *Stress fractures*. Champaign, IL: Human Kinetics, 1999.

Khan KM, Brukner PD, Kearney C, et al. Tarsal navicular stress fracture in athletes. *Sports Med* 1994;17:65–76.

Quirk R. President's guest lecture: stress fractures of the foot. *Ankle Int* 1998;19: 494–496.

Wienfeld SB, Haddad SL, Myerson MS. Metatarsal stress fractures. *Clin Sports Med* 1994;16:319–338.

Author: Stephen Simons

Fracture, Talus

Basics

DEFINITION

- Relatively uncommon fracture usually involving the talar neck, lateral process, or osteochondral fracture of talar dome
- Talar neck fractures account for 50% of talar fractures; talar body fractures 40%, and talar head fracture 5% to 10%.
- Osteochondral fractures (a subset of talar body fractures) can occur in up to 6.5% of acute ankle sprains.
- Shepard fracture (posterior tubercle fractures) represents the largest single group of talar body fractures.
- "Snowboarder's ankle," a lateral process fracture, is the second most common type of talar body fracture.

INCIDENCE/PREVALENCE

Talar fractures constitute 3% to 6% of all foot fractures.

SIGNS AND SYMPTOMS

- Talar head fractures cause swelling and tenderness at the talonavicular joint.
- Talar neck fractures present with swelling and tenderness of the proximal dorsal foot. With displaced fractures, the normal ankle contours will be changed.
- Acute inversion injuries of the ankle that remain painful after conservative treatment should make the clinician suspicious for osteochondral lesion of the talus or a lateral process fracture.

RISK FACTORS

Snowboarding is associated with acute dorsiflexion/inversion injuries to the ankle, which can cause lateral process fractures.

ANATOMY

- Sixty percent to 70% of the talar surface consists of cartilage, accommodating seven different articulations
- The talus has no muscular insertions or origins and is held in place by its osseous neighbors and constraining ligamentous attachments.
- The tibiotalar articulation is responsible for hindfoot motion in the plantar/dorsiflexion plane, the subtalar joint provides hindfoot inversion/eversion motion, and the talus transmits axial force.

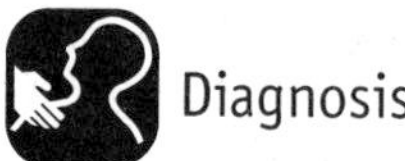

Diagnosis

DIFFERENTIAL DIAGNOSIS

Conditions that can mimic osteochondral fractures of the talar dome include osteochondritis desiccans and/or loose bodies.

HISTORY

- Fractures of the talar head and neck usually are found after high-velocity trauma, e.g., motorcycle accidents.
- Anterolateral osteochondral fractures are associated with an inversion-dorsiflexion injury of the ankle.
- Posterolateral osteochondral fractures are associated with plantar flexion, inversion, and external rotation of the ankle.
- Chronic osteochondral fractures present with pain following an adequate healing time for ligamentous injury, complaints of ankle "giving out," catching, or locking up.

PHYSICAL EXAMINATION

- Lateral talar process fractures have the same symptoms as an acute sprain of the anterior talofibular ligament. Findings may include tenderness inferior and anterior to the tip of the lateral malleolus, associated with pain on active and passive range of motion of the ankle and subtalar joints.
- Acute osteochondral fractures present with edema, ecchymosis, range of motion limited by guarding, and pain to palpation.

IMAGING

- Initial radiographic workup of most talar fractures should include ankle mortise views with routine anteroposterior and lateral views.
- To best view lateral osteochondral lesions with plain x-rays, films should be obtained with 10 to 35 degrees of internal rotation and maximal plantar flexion.
- Lateral osteochondral fractures have a thin, wafer-like appearance; medial osteochondral lesions have a deep, cup-shaped appearance.
- If plain x-rays show abnormalities of the talar dome, computed tomographic scan should be performed to determine size and nature of lesion, essential in preoperative planning.
- Bone scan is indicated if history and physical are suspicious for osteochondral fracture but x-rays are negative.

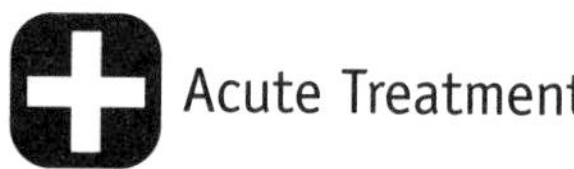

Acute Treatment

ANALGESIA

Intra-articular corticosteroid injections may offer temporary relief of osteochondral fractures, but have no beneficial effect on healing and are not generally recommended.

REDUCTION TECHNIQUES

- Displaced talar fractures require anatomical reduction to prevent arthrosis and avascular necrosis, and usually require surgical correction.
- Reduction of a displaced talar neck fracture can be attempted by plantar flexion of the foot, bringing the head and body into line.

POSTREDUCTION EVALUATION

Clinical signs and symptoms correlated with repeated radiographic examination are important during conservative treatment to assure proper healing.

IMMOBILIZATION

- Nondisplaced acute talar fractures may be treated in a short leg cast, nonweight-bearing for 6–12 weeks. There should be evidence of healing before weight-bearing is resumed.
- Subacute nondisplaced osteochondral fractures can be treated initially with cast immobilization and limited weight-bearing, with follow-up radiographs in 4–6 weeks.

SPECIAL CONSIDERATIONS

- Fifty percent of talar neck fractures go on to avascular necrosis, as well as do 25% to 50% of talar body fractures.
- Talar head fracture complications include midtarsal instability, talonavicular arthritis, and avascular necrosis of the talar head.

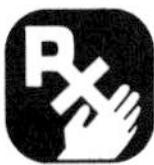

Long-Term Treatment

REHABILITATION

Standard range of motion, strengthening, and proprioceptive rehabilitation are appropriate after the fracture has healed.

SURGERY

- Any talar fracture that is displaced, even minimally, requires surgical treatment, given the risks of avascular necrosis and future arthrosis.
- Nondisplaced osteochondral fractures can be managed conservatively for up to 12 months without compromising subsequent surgical outcomes.
- Any loose body associated with a fracture may require arthroscopic removal.

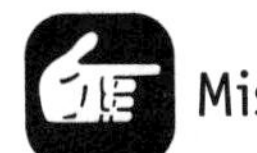

Miscellaneous

ICD-9 CODE

825.21 Closed talar fracture
825.31 Open talar fracture

BIBLIOGRAPHY

Boon AJ, Smith J, Laskowski ER. Snowboarding injuries. *Physician Sportsmed* 1999;27:94–104.

Higgins TF, Baumgaertner MR. Diagnosis and treatment of fractures of the talus: a comprehensive review of the literature. *Foot Ankle Int* 1999;20:595–605.

Mandracchia VJ, Buddecke DE Jr, Giesking JL. Osteochondral lesions of the talar dome. *Clin Podiatr Med Surg* 1999;16:725–742.

Mayer D. Isolated talus fractures: description of a new clinical sign. *Am J Emerg Med* 1997;15:412–414.

Shea DJ, Feder JM, Boylan JP. Fractures of the lateral process of the talus: two case reports and a comprehensive literature review. *Foot Ankle Int* 1998;19:1646.

Shea MP, Manoli A II. Recognizing talar dome lesions. *Physician Sportsmed* 1993;21:109–121.

Authors: James Bray and Karl B. Fields

Fracture, Tibial Plateau

Basics

SIGNS AND SYMPTOMS

- Painful, swollen knee
- Inability to bear weight on the injured leg
- Knee effusion (hemarthrosis)
- Decreased (both active and passive) range of motion of the knee
- Tenderness along the proximal tibia
- Possible varus or valgus deformity of the knee
- Possible joint instability due to associated ligamentous injury

MECHANISM/DESCRIPTION

- Fracture or depression of the proximal tibial articulating surface
- Also referred to as *tibial condylar fractures*
- Valgus or varus force applied in combination with axial loading
  —The pedestrian struck by an auto (fender fracture where the bumper of a vehicle strikes the lateral aspect of the proximal tibia) is the most common mechanism of injury.
    —This usually results in splitting or depression of the *lateral* plateau.
    —The younger the patient the more resistant the plateau is to depression.
    —Elderly patients present more often with depression type fractures.
  —Fall from a height causing femoral condyles to impact on tibial surface
  —Violent twisting force, e.g., skiing
- *Medial* plateau fractures are much less common and require significant force to occur.
  —Associated injuries include ligamentous damage (lateral collateral, posterior cruciate, and medial meniscus) and neurovascular injury (peroneal nerve and popliteal vessels) to that knee.

PEDIATRIC CONSIDERATIONS

- Tibial plateau fractures are rare in children because of the dense cancellous bone of the tibial plateau.

SCHATZKER CLASSIFICATION SYSTEM

- *Type 1* is a split-off fracture of the *lateral* tibial plateau without compression of the plateau.
  —Occurs in younger patients where the plateau resists depression
  —Usually occurs from a valgus force to the knee in combination with axial load
- *Type 2* is a combination of a split fracture and depression of all or a portion of the remaining *lateral* plateau.
  —The mechanism is similar to the above but these patients tend to be older and have weaker bones; the plateau can be depressed by the femoral condyle.
- *Type 3* is a local depression of the articulating surface of the *lateral* plateau.
- *Type 4* is a fracture/depression of the *Medial* plateau.
  —It requires much more force for this injury to occur.
  —Be suspicious for other injuries
  —Damage to the popliteal artery, peroneal nerve, lateral collateral ligament, medial meniscus, and cruciate ligaments must be suspected.
- *Type 5* is a bicondylar fracture.
  —High-impact injury associated with popliteal vessel injury, peroneal nerve injury, and development of compartment syndrome
- *Type 6* is a bicondylar, grossly comminuted fracture involving both the plateau and the metaphysis.
  —Occurs from a violent force, usually a fall from a height, with associated neurovascular compromise and compartment syndrome

CAUTIONS

- In high-energy mechanisms, associated major life-threatening injuries take precedence.
- Immobilize to prevent further neurologic or vascular injury

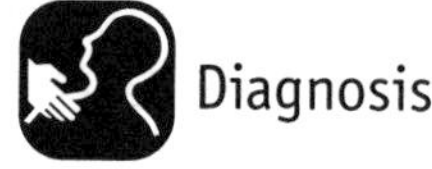

Diagnosis

ESSENTIAL WORKUP

- Neurovascular examination
  —High-energy mechanism (medial plateau or bicondylar fractures) carries risk of neurovascular damage and compartment syndrome
  —Check popliteal, posterior tibial, and dorsalis pedis arterial pulses.
  —Check integrity of peroneal nerve; ankle and toe dorsiflexion and sensation in webspace between great and second toes
- Plain radiography
  —Anteroposterior and lateral views of the knee and proximal tibia
  —Cross-table lateral view may demonstrate lipohemarthrosis (fat-fluid level).
  —Pay attention to areas of ligamentous attachment where avulsion fractures may take place; i.e., medial and lateral femoral condyles, intercondylar eminence, and fibular head.

IMAGING/SPECIAL TESTS

- Oblique views may identify fracture not apparent on other films.
- Tibial plateau view-AP view with the knee in 10–15° flexion helps visualize depressions
- Arthrocentesis to look for fat globules if mechanism strongly suggests fracture and effusion present without x-ray findings
- MRI can be used to better elucidate soft tissue injuries.
- Angiography indicated if
  —High-energy mechanism
  —Schatzker type 4, 5, or 6 fracture
  —Alteration in distal pulses
  —Expanding hematoma
  —Bruit
  —Injury to anatomically related nerves
- Compartment pressures if suspected compartment syndrome
  —Pain not over fracture site
  —Pain on passive stretch
  —Paresthesias
  —Abnormality of pulses
  —Pressures greater than 30 mm Hg are an indication for fasciotomy.

DIFFERENTIAL DIAGNOSIS

- Knee dislocation
- Cruciate ligament tears
- Meniscal tears

PEDIATRIC CONSIDERATIONS

- Include oblique views as part of routine radiography.

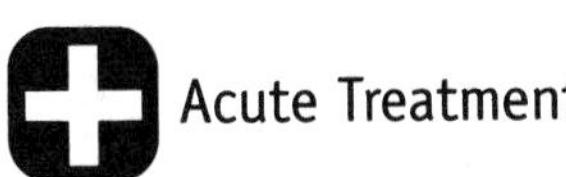

Acute Treatment

INITIAL STABILIZATION

- ABCs/ATLS protocol in multiple trauma victim
- Long-leg splint
- Ice
- Elevation

ED TREATMENT

- Nonweight-bearing
- Pain control
- Nondisplaced fractures or minimally displaced *lateral* plateau fractures without ligamentous injury
  —Aspiration of hemarthrosis and injection of local anesthetic
  —Examination for ligamentous instability
  —If knee is stable
    —Compressive dressing
    —Ice and elevation for 48 hours
    —Nonweight-bearing/crutches
  —Early orthopedic follow-up if knee not stable
- Open fractures
  —Remove contaminants.
  —Apply moist sterile dressing.
  —Assess tetanus immunity.
  —Antibiotics
  —Emergent orthopedic consultation

MEDICATIONS

- For open fractures
  —Cefazolin: 2 g IV loading dose (50 mg/kg in children)
  —Gentamycin: 1.5–2 mg/kg IV loading dose (2.5 mg/kg pediatric dose) *if* Gustilo-Anderson type III
  —Vancomycin: 1 g IV loading dose (10 mg/kg in children) *if* penicillin allergy

HOSPITAL ADMISSION CRITERIA

- Open fractures for débridement, irrigation, and intravenous antibiotics
- Comminuted, bicondylar fractures for traction
- High-energy mechanism for observation of neurovascular status
- Pain control

HOSPITAL DISCHARGE CRITERIA

- Nondisplaced fractures
- Minimally displaced, stable fractures of the *lateral* plateau

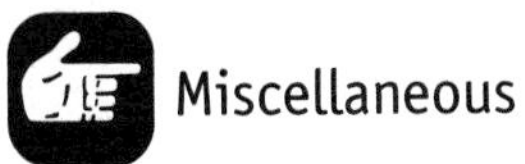

Miscellaneous

ICD-9-CM

823.00

CORE CONTENT CODE

18.4.13.1.5.1

BIBLIOGRAPHY

Rang M. *Children's fractures*. 2d ed. Philadelphia: JB Lippincott, 1984.

Simon RR, Koenigsknecht SJ. The proximal tibia and fibula. In: Simon RR, Koenigsknecht eds. *Emergency Orthopedics*. Norwalk CT, Appleton and Lange, 1996;273–286.

Torrey SB. Lower extremity and pelvis trauma. In: Barkin ed. *Pediatric Emergency Medicine*. St. Louis: CV Mosby 1992:357–365.

Wiss DA, Watson JT, Johnson EE. Fractures of the knee. In: Rockwood CA, Green DP, Bucholz RW, Heckman JD, eds. *Rockwood and Green's fractures in adults*. 4th ed. Philadelphia: Lippincott-Raven, 1996:1593–1652.

Author: Stacy Nunberg

Fracture, Volkmann: Posterolateral Tibiofibular Ligament Avulsion

Basics

DEFINITION

- Ankle fracture involving avulsion of the posterior lip of the tibia at its articular surface (Volkmann tubercle)
- Fracture occurs via a force through the posterior inferior tibiofibular ligament (PITFL) at its tibial attachment.

INCIDENCE/PREVALENCE

- Few data exist regarding incidence or prevalence of isolated posterior malleolar fracture.
- Volkmann fracture generally occurs concurrently with other injuries and results from the specific injury patterns discussed below.

ANATOMY

- Volkmann tubercle is part of the posterior malleolus of the ankle.
- The PITFL's attachment to the posterior malleolus resists posterior translation of the talus.
- The PITFL is one of four syndesmotic ligaments that maintain integrity between the tibia and fibula. Also referred to as the posterior tibiofibular ligament (PTFL).

MECHANISM

General

- Usually occurs with external rotation or abduction.
- Given that the PITFL is markedly stronger than the anterior inferior tibiofibular ligament (AITFL), the torsional/rotational forces rupture the AITFL but avulse the posterior tibial tubercle through an intact PITFL.

Classification

- The Lauge-Hansen (L-H), Danis-Weber, and AO systems have been used to describe ankle injury patterns.
- The L-H system can aid in closed reduction maneuvers.
- Volkmann fracture is classified by the L-H system as supination external rotation (SER) stage III, pronation external rotation (PER) stage IV, and pronation abduction (PA) stage II.
- In SER injuries, AITFL rupture and spiral fracture of the fibula precede Volkmann fracture.
- In PER injuries, deltoid ligament rupture, medial malleolar fracture, AITLF disruption, and oblique fibular fracture may precede Volkmann fracture.
- In PA injuries, deltoid ligament rupture or avulsion of the medial malleolus may occur first.

PEDIATRICS AND ADOLESCENTS

- Volkmann fracture is a rare injury in these age groups given the relative weak physis of the tibia.
- Salter-Harris fractures occur during external rotation and abduction injuries, which only occasionally involve the posterior tubercle. The fracture fragment usually is contiguous with the medial malleolar fragment.

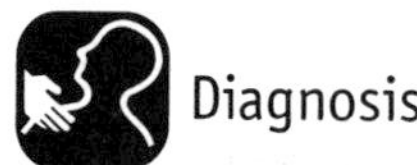

Diagnosis

HISTORY

- Ankle injury involving a Volkmann fracture is rarely subtle given typical concomitant fractures and ligament tears.
- The mechanism of injury reported and the presence of associated injuries should evoke suspicion.
- Any floor or field sport, particularly those with contact, can result in posterior malleolar fracture.
- Patients should be questioned for elapsed time since injury, mechanism, associated sounds such as "pops" or "cracks," and weight-bearing status.

PHYSICAL EXAMINATION

Emergent

- Should focus on neurovascular compromise secondary to joint dislocation or calf compartment syndrome
- Doppler ultrasound should be used if pulses are nonpalpable, and a detailed sensorimotor examination of the foot should be done.
- Concern for early compartment syndrome should prompt measurement of calf compartment pressures.

Nonemergent

- Systematic ankle, foot, leg, and knee examination should be performed.
- Observation, palpation, and range of motion should be done, followed by stability testing.
- Possible findings include an increased posterior drawer test, increased internal rotation, and, with associated syndesmotic instability, a positive squeeze and Cotton test.
- Examination sensitivity is increased by comparison with the unaffected limb.

IMAGING

Plain Radiographs

- Anteroposterior, lateral, and mortise views are standard.
- Lateral films generally show the posterior malleolar fracture, but do not reliably estimate the size of the avulsion or the articular surface involvement. Some authors recommend an external rotation lateral view (45–50 degrees) to estimate fragment size.
- Standard views will diagnose associated injuries that are almost always present.
- Stress radiographs are controversial and not routinely indicated.

Computed Tomographic Scan

If Volkmann fracture is seen on plain film evaluation, computed tomography (CT) is recommended to elucidate the extent of articular involvement and size of the fragment, which are instrumental in determining treatment.

Magnetic Resonance Imaging

Reserved for evaluation of soft tissues and generally not indicated unless CT films are inadequate

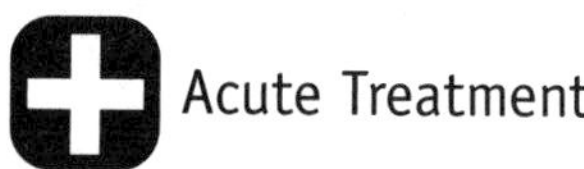

Acute Treatment

PRINCIPLES

- Complicated ankle fractures require immediate assessment of the neurovascular status of the foot.
- If compromised, reduction of dislocation or deformity should be accomplished immediately by closed reduction using the L-H classification to reverse order of injury.

CLOSED REDUCTION

- Generally not indicated
- Fracture of posterior malleolus usually is accompanied by fracture of lateral and/or medial malleoli and involves significant articular surface or fibular displacement.
- Small (<25% of distal tibia), nondisplaced incomplete fractures can be considered for a short leg walking cast with appropriate orthopaedic consultation.

PREOPERATIVE CARE

- Use of a modified Jones compression dressing and posterior splint is important to reduce swelling, which can increase risk of poor surgical outcome.
- Compression dressing with frequent icing and elevation can allow for operative intervention in the first 2–3 days.

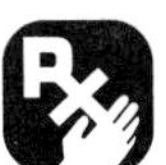

Long-Term Treatment

OPEN REDUCTION INTERNAL FIXATION

- Controversy exists as to whether all posterior malleolar fractures need to be internally fixated.
- Volkmann tubercle often reduces spontaneously with reduction of the fibula and/or medial malleolus.
- Size of the fragment and its proportion of the articular surface are predominant factors in determining the need for internal fixation.
- Some authors showed good results without fixation if the proportion of the articular margin involved was <25% to 40%.
- Most recommend internal fixation if 25% to 35% of the articular surface is fractured.
- If factors such as displacement of malleoli >2–3 mm, talar subluxation, plafond articular incongruity, or syndesmotic instability exist, internal fixation is recommended.

PROGNOSIS

- Posterior tubercle fractures adversely affect the prognosis of ankle fractures compared to single or bimalleolar fractures.
- These fractures have an increased risk of joint dislocation and osteoarthritis.
- Postoperative arthritis varies with the size of the fragment, but those requiring internal fixation have ≥35% likelihood of osteoarthritis.

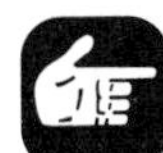

Miscellaneous

ICD-9 CODE

824.8 Fracture tibia distal end or epiphysis closed

BIBLIOGRAPHY

Dias LS. Fractures of the tibia and fibula. In: Rockwood CA Jr, Wilkins KA, King RE, eds. *Fractures in children, vol. 3,* 3rd ed. Philadelphia: JB Lippincott, 1991:1271–1381.

Ebraheim NA, Mekhail AO, Haman SP. External rotation-lateral view of the ankle in the assessment of the posterior malleolus. *Foot Ankle Int* 1999;20:379–382.

England SP, Sundberg S. Management of common orthopedic problems. *Pediatr Clin North Am* 1996;43:991–1012.

Mandracchia DM, Mandracchia VJ, Buddecke DE Jr. Malleolar fractures of the ankle: a comprehensive review. *Clin Podiatr Med Surg* 1999;16:679–723.

Michelson JD. Fractures about the ankle. *J Bone Joint Surg* 1995;77A:142–152.

Prokuski LJ, Saltzman CL. Challenging fractures of the foot and ankle. *Radiol Clin North Am* 1997;35:655–657.

Renstrom AFH, Kannus P. Injuries of the foot and ankle. In: DeLee JC, Drez D Jr, eds. *Orthopaedic sports medicine: principles and practice, vol. 2.* Philadelphia: WB Saunders, 1994:1705–1733.

Stanitski CL. Pediatric and adolescent sports injuries. *Clin Sport Med* 1997;16:613–633.

Vander Griend R, Michelson JD, Bone LB. Fractures of the ankle and the distal part of the tibia. *Instructional Course Lectures* 1997;46:311–321.

Vander Griend RA, Savoie FH, Hughes JL. Fractures of the ankle. In: Rockwood CA Jr, Green DP, Bucholz RW, eds. *Rockwood and Green's fractures in adults, vol. 2,* 3rd ed. Philadelphia: JB Lippincott, 1991:1983–2039.

Authors: Matt DesJardins and Guy Monteleone

Fracture, Zygoma

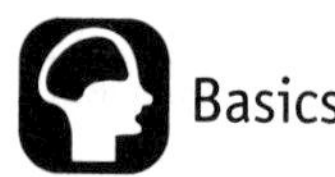

Basics

SIGNS AND SYMPTOMS

- Malar edema or flattening
- Periorbital ecchymosis, drooping lateral canthus
- Lateral subconjunctival hemorrhage, diplopia
- Infraorbital anesthesia, trismus/open bite

MECHANISM/DESCRIPTION

- Fractures of the zygoma result from blunt trauma to the side of the face.
- The most common mechanisms include motor vehicle accidents, falls, and physical assault.
- The direction and magnitude of force will determine the fracture type and degree of displacement
  —A blow to the side of the face directed posteriorly and medially will produce a zygomatic body (tripod) fracture
  —A lateral blow often results in an isolated zygomatic arch fracture

PEDIATRIC CONSIDERATIONS

- Maxillofacial fractures are rarely seen in the pediatric population.
  —Only 1% of all facial fractures is seen in children under age 6.
  —Children have a comparatively larger cranium than facial skeleton leading to a higher incidence of head trauma.
  —Falls and motor vehicle accidents account for the majority of facial trauma in children.
  —Consider nonaccidental trauma, particularly in children under age 6

CAUTIONS

- Airway compromise may occur with severe maxillofacial injuries.
- Assume that the patient with face or head injury has also sustained a C-spine injury until proven otherwise.

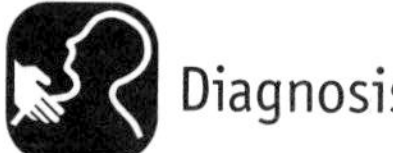

Diagnosis

ESSENTIAL WORKUP

- If a high velocity or severe blunt force mechanism is suspected, a thorough evaluation for associated injuries (C-spine, head, globe, other maxillofacial bones, etc.) is imperative.

Clinical Examination

- Intraoral palpation of the zygomatic body and arch for bony step deformity
- Assess sensation of the inferior orbital area (cheek, upper lip, and gingiva)
- Examine the globe and orbit carefully
  —Periorbital ecchymosis and lateral subconjunctival hemorrhages are common
  —Assess visual acuity, pupillary function, and extraocular movements
  —Inferior displacement of the globe may lead to diplopia and enophthalmos. Carefully evaluate extraocular movements.
- Mandibular movement may be restricted.
  —Trismus may be seen if there is impingement of the mandibular coronoid process by displacement of the zygomatic body.
  —Zygomatic arch fractures may impede the temporalis muscle or coronoid process.
  —Lastly, temporalis muscle contusion or TMJ effusion may cause pain that limits range of motion.
- Unilateral epistaxis may be present and typically resolves spontaneously

Radiographs

- The submental vertex (jug-handle) view is used to diagnose fractures of the zygomatic arch.
- Plain films are not as useful in the evaluation of zygomatic body fractures.
- The Waters' (occipitomental) view shows the inferior orbital rims and possibly layering of blood in the maxillary sinus.
- The articulation between the zygoma and frontal bone can be evaluated on the Caldwell view.

IMAGING/SPECIAL TESTS

- Computed tomography is the diagnostic standard for evaluation of zygomatic body fractures.
  —CT is not usually needed for isolated fractures of the zygomatic arch.

DIFFERENTIAL DIAGNOSIS

- Facial contusions
- La Forte fractures

PEDIATRIC CONSIDERATIONS

- Sedation may be required to properly examine some children.
- If a head injury is suspected, sedation is not recommended.
- If circumstances or injuries raise suspicions of child abuse, a comprehensive investigation for previous nonaccidental trauma is essential.

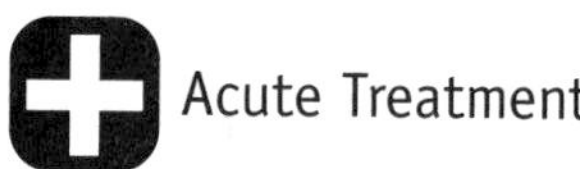

Acute Treatment

INITIAL STABILIZATION

- Airway management is particularly important if there are associated maxillofacial or mandibular injuries causing airway compromise.
  —Isolated zygoma fractures do not typically require aggressive airway intervention.
- Life-threatening conditions should be treated first, follow ABCs of trauma care.

ED TREATMENT

- Assume that the patient with head and maxillofacial trauma has a cervical spine injury.
  —The neck should be immobilized until radiographic clearance is obtained.
- Do not blindly clamp bleeding vessels as this may cause inadvertent damage to the facial nerve, parotid duct, etc.
- Early consultation with oral maxillofacial or plastic surgeon
- Analgesics, antibiotics, and tetanus prophylaxis if open injury

PEDIATRIC CONSIDERATIONS

- Multiple injuries are often seen in children including head trauma, skull fracture, and orthopedic injuries.
- Definitive repair of facial fractures should not be delayed beyond 3 or 4 days.
  —The facial bones heal rapidly in children and delays of more than 3 to 4 days may result in malunion and cosmetic deformity.

HOSPITAL ADMISSION CRITERIA

- Displaced or comminuted zygomatic body fractures require open reduction internal fixation.
- Associated head, neck, or other traumatic injuries requiring admission

HOSPITAL DISCHARGE CRITERIA

- Nondisplaced tripod fracture can be treated conservatively as an outpatient with close follow-up.
  —Delayed fracture displacement, poor cosmetic outcome, and difficulty with mandibular movement are indications for ORIF.
  —Isolated arch fractures are amenable to outpatient treatment. These typically require open reduction of fracture fragments. If the reduction is unstable, internal fixation is then performed.

PEDIATRIC CONSIDERATIONS

- Consult social services and local child welfare agency if needed.

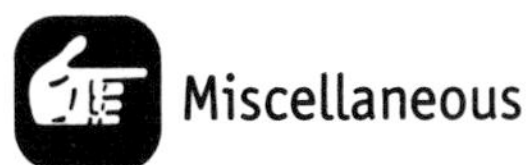

ICD-9-CM

802.4

CORE CONTENT CODE

18.4.4.7

BIBLIOGRAPHY

Colucciello SA, Sternbach G, Walker SB. The treacherous and complex spectrum of maxillofacial trauma: Etiologies, evaluation, and emergency stabilization. *Emerg Med Rep* 1995;16;7:59–69.

Covington DS, Wainwright DJ, Teichgraeber JF, et al. Changing patterns in the epidemiology and treatment of zygoma fractures: 10-year review. *J Trauma* 1994;37:243–248.

Hunter JG. Pediatric maxillofacial trauma. *Pediatr Clin North Am* 1992;39:1127–1143.

Rumsey C, Sargent LA. Zygomatic fractures. *Trauma Q* 1992;9:76–85.

Author: Raymond A. Viducich

Medications

Sedative/Analgesics*	Adult Dose (mg/kg IV)	Pediatric Dose (mg/kg IV)
Diazepam	0.1–0.2	0.1–0.2
Fentanyl	2–10 (mcg/kg)	2–3 (mcg/kg)
Ketamine	2	1–2
Meperidine	1–2	1–2
Midazolam	0.1	0.15
Morphine sulfate	0.1–0.2	0.1–0.2

*All of these sedative/analgesics should be titrated to effect.

Freiberg's Disease

Basics

DEFINITION

- Osteonecrosis of the superior portion of the metatarsal head of unknown etiology
- Fourth most common osteochondrosis
- Affects women more commonly than men

INCIDENCE/PREVALENCE

- Incidence unknown
- Male:female ratio 1:5
- Peak onset around 11–17 years, but may happen up into thirties
- Most common involvement is the second metatarsal head
- Second most common involvement is the third metatarsal head
- Usually affects the longest metatarsal
- Occasionally seen in sports requiring sprinting and jumping

RISK FACTORS

- No known risk factors
- May be related to repetitive microtrauma versus vascular deficiency or both

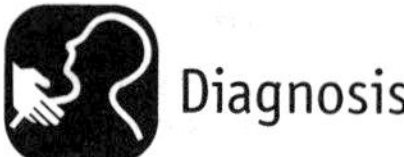

Diagnosis

DIFFERENTIAL DIAGNOSIS

- Fracture
- Septic joint
- Gout

HISTORY

- Slow development of significant pain over affected metatarsal head
- Patient may notice loss of motion.
- Pain increases with activity and motion.
- Pain worsens with weight bearing.
- Pain often relieved by rest

PHYSICAL EXAM

- Surrounding soft tissue swelling and warmth
- Tenderness over metatarsal head
- May be painful with motion
- As disease progresses, osteophytes may be palpable.
- May be limited motion of metatarsophalangeal joint
- Palpable crepitus in advanced disease

IMAGING

Radiography

- Normal in early stages
- As the disease progresses, osteonecrotic changes are seen on the superior/central head.
- Eventually the superior/central head collapses and flattens.
- Medial and lateral dorsal osteophytes develop.
- Osteophytes may break free, becoming loose bodies, best seen on the oblique.
- Cystic changes may be seen in the head.
- The inferior portion of the metatarsal head is usually not involved.

Bone Scan

- Hot spot over metatarsal head

MRI

- Classic osteonecrotic changes seen
- May be useful in early detection prior to radiographic changes

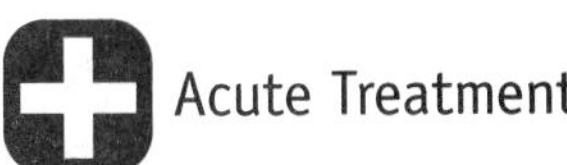

Acute Treatment

NONOPERATIVE TREATMENT

- Symptomatic relief for early stages of disease prior to collapse and loose body formation
- Goal is to restrict weight-bearing a sufficient time to allow healing to take place.
- Immediate cessation of sports
- Use of crutches to restrict weight bearing
- As symptoms subside, may progressively bear weight with use of metatarsal pads or a custom orthosis
- Occasionally may need a short leg walking cast with a toe plate
- By restricting weight bearing, the lesion may heal over a period of 6–12 weeks.
- Return to sports when asymptomatic with custom foot orthosis

OPERATIVE TREATMENT

- Indicated if nonoperative treatment fails or if disease is advanced
- Joint debridement with dorsal osteophyte excision, synovectomy, and loose body excision
- Other operative options include dorsiflexion osteotomy or metatarsal head excision in an older less demanding patient

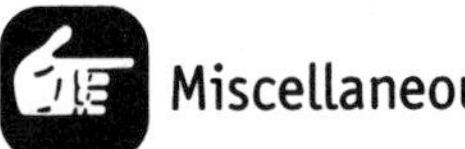

Miscellaneous

SYNONYMS

- Freiberg's infraction
- Eggshell fracture
- Koehler's second disease
- Peculiar metatarsal disease
- Malakopathy

ICD-9 CODE

732.9 Osteochondropathy not otherwise specified

BIBLIOGRAPHY

Helal B, Gibb P. Freiberg's disease: a suggested pattern of management. *Foot Ankle* 1987;8:94–102.

Katcherian DA. Treatment of Freiberg's disease. *Orthop Clin North Am* 1994;25:69–80.

Sproul J, Klaaren H, Mannarino F. Surgical treatment of Freiberg's infraction in athletes. *Am J Sports Med* 1993;21:381–384.

Authors: Angelo J. Colosimo and Robert S. Heidt Jr.

Glenohumeral Dislocation, Anterior

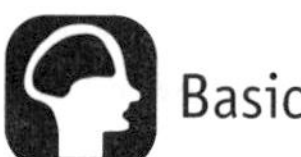

Basics

DEFINITION

Humeral head is displaced anteriorly out of the glenoid fossa due to some combination of hyperextension, external rotation, and abduction of the shoulder. Sometimes (less commonly) caused by anterior blow to the shoulder.

INCIDENCE/PREVALENCE

- Common, 45% of all dislocations are of the shoulder
- 2% lifetime incidence between 18 and 70 years of age
- 96% of glenohumeral dislocations are anterior

SIGNS AND SYMPTOMS

- Anterior fullness of the shoulder
- Forearm of affected arm often cradled with shoulder in externally rotated, partially abducted position
- Patient usually guarding and very uncomfortable
- Sulcus sign (depression in the skin below the acromion)

RISK FACTORS

- History of previous dislocation
- Generalized ligamentous laxity
- Sports such as wrestling, football, rugby, skiing, and skateboarding

ASSOCIATED INJURIES AND COMPLICATIONS

- Bankart lesions: detachment of inferior glenohumeral ligament–labral complex from anterior glenoid rim. Very common in younger patients. Strongly associated with dislocation recurrence.
- Rotator cuff tears: seen mainly in older dislocators. Often the subscapularis muscle with anterior dislocation.
- Fractures: humeral head and neck (significant displacement may be a contraindication to closed reduction), glenoid rim, and greater tuberosity avulsions. Seen especially with traumatic etiology.
- Hill-Sachs lesion: depression fracture of posterolateral humeral head.
- Neurologic injury: most commonly axillary nerve, brachial plexus or musculocutaneous nerve.
- Recurrence in young (athletic) primary dislocators extremely common without intervention.

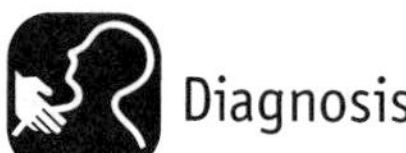

Diagnosis

DIFFERENTIAL DIAGNOSIS

- Acute subluxation
- Acromioclavicular joint separation
- Fractures
- Rotator cuff injury
- Posterior dislocation

HISTORY

- Often occurs after a fall on the outstretched arm or with reaching (making a tackle)
- First time event versus recurrence (may affect ease of reduction and affect long-term treatment plan)
- Amount of trauma involved (traumatic vs. atraumatic) can give clues to whether there is component of instability
- Duration shoulder has been dislocated (helps in decision concerning analgesia)

PHYSICAL EXAM

- Anterior fullness of shoulder with the "sulcus sign" under the acromion
- Perform neurovascular exam both before and after reduction to check for previously mentioned nerve injuries.
- Check deltoid muscle strength and lateral shoulder sensation to assess axillary nerve function (former probably not practical prior to reduction of dislocated shoulder).
- Check proximal and distal muscle function and range of motion before and after relocation.
- No crepitus should be felt or heard during relocation.

IMAGING

- At least two views orthogonal to each other required
- Standard anteroposterior (AP): head of humerus displaced medially on glenoid; difficult to distinguish anterior from posterior dislocations
- True lateral (transcapular, Y) view: humeral head displaced toward coracoid process
- Axillary view: allows easier visualization of associated injuries, but requires movement of an already uncomfortable patient

POSTREDUCTION VIEWS

- Westpoint (reverse axillary lateral) helps in showing bony Bankart lesions.
- Styker notch (AP internal rotation of humerus) good to demonstrate Hill-Sachs deformity

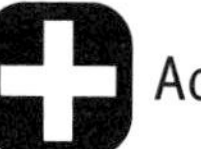

Acute Treatment

ANALGESIA

- Often not needed if reduction is performed immediately after dislocation
- Verbal coaching to relax the patient is helpful.
- Narcotic and benzodiazepine medications may be required, if reductions are not performed early, to relax spasm and ease relocation.
- Some sources recommend local glenohumeral joint anesthesia using 10–20 mL of 1% lidocaine.

REDUCTION TECHNIQUES

- Traction methods: Stimson (prone traction with weight applied to arm hanging down); supine traction/countertraction (gentle traction at 45 degrees of abduction while countertraction applied with folded sheet under axilla)
- Leverage techniques: Hennipen or Modified Kocher maneuver (with patient supine, externally rotate arm to 90 degrees; slowly abduct arm until dislocation reduced)
- Axilla pressure by assistant's hand may help guide the humeral head over the glenoid.
- Scapular manipulation: patient prone with arm hanging down, apply medially directed force to inferolateral border of scapula; may also do when patient is supine to assist with other techniques
- Combinations
- Experience, familiarity, and available resources (time and help) are important considerations when deciding which technique to use.

POSTREDUCTION CONSIDERATIONS

- Recheck neurovascular exam and rotator cuff; postreduction radiographs as previously mentioned
- Immobilization in sling and swathe: up to 3 weeks in younger patients, and only up to 10 days in in older patients (>40 years old) because of high rate of adhesive capsulitis
- Immobilization theoretically allows time for "scarring" of injured anterior structures and healing of pathologic lesions.

CONTRAINDICATIONS TO CLOSED REDUCTION

- Humeral head and neck fractures
- Significantly displaced (<1 cm) greater tuberosity fractures
- Severe scapula fractures
- Intrathoracic humeral head fractures

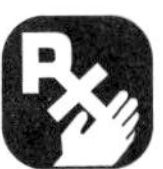

Long-Term Treatment

REHABILITATION

- Early range of motion in older patients to prevent adhesive capsulitis
- Strengthening of rotator cuff muscles and scapular stabilizers help in maintaining dynamic stability.
- Most helpful in nontraumatic dislocations in patients who have multidirectional instability or generalized ligamentous laxity.
- Immobilization and postimmobilization rehabilitation have not been shown to be effective in preventing recurrence in young, traumatic, first-time dislocators.

REFERRAL/SURGICAL FOLLOW-UP

- Increasing evidence for early arthroscopic Bankart repair in young, active, first-time dislocators with traumatic etiology
- Elective surgical stabilization typically indicated after three or more dislocations
- Patients with multidirectional instability should be treated with traditional methods, although surgical repair is often necessary with recurrences.
- Early orthopedic referral indicated for all except uncomplicated, recurrent anterior dislocations
- Orthopedic referred with humeral head or neck fractures and irreducible dislocations

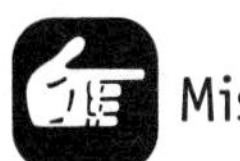

Miscellaneous

ICD-9 CODE

831.01

See also: Shoulder Instability

BIBLIOGRAPHY

Arciero RA, et al. Acute shoulder dislocation: indications and techniques for operative management. *Clin Sports Med* 1995;14:937–953.

Gleeson AP. Anterior glenohumeral dislocations: what to do and how to do it. *J Accident Emerg Med* 1998;15:7–12.

Wen DY. Current concepts in the treatment of anterior shoulder dislocations. *Am J Emerg Med* 1999;17:401–407.

Authors: Sourav Poddar and Allen Richburg

Glenohumeral Dislocation, Posterior

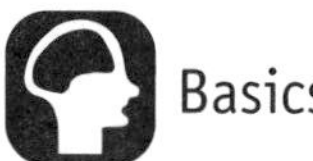

Basics

DEFINITION

A posterior glenohumeral dislocation occurs when the humeral head disarticulates from the glenoid and rests posteriorly to its normally seated position on the glenoid. Glenohumeral instability is classified by (a) mechanism (traumatic vs. atraumatic), (b) direction (anterior, posterior, superior, or inferior), (c) circumstance (acute, chronic, or recurrent), and (d) degree (subluxation vs. dislocation).

INCIDENCE/PREVALENCE

- The shoulder is the most commonly dislocated joint in the human body.
- Anterior dislocations are much more common than posterior dislocations.
- Posterior shoulder dislocations account for only 1%–3.8% of all shoulder dislocations.
- Posterior dislocations occur most often as a result of a seizure or electrical shock injury.
- Injury can occur in athletes with a fall upon a flexed elbow and adducted arm or by a direct axial load to the humerus.
- Extremely rare in pediatrics because force necessary to cause a dislocation will instead cause a proximal humerus fracture
- A posterior shoulder dislocation is the most commonly missed shoulder pathology. Approximately 60%–80% of these dislocations are inappropriately diagnosed at initial presentation.

SIGNS AND SYMPTOMS

- Severe shoulder pain that increases with movement
- Cardinal sign: an arm held in internal rotation and adduction with inability to externally rotate or abduct the arm
- Mild flattening of the anterior shoulder and loss of normal deltoid contour may be present.
- There may be prominence of the acromion and the corocoid process.
- The humeral head may be visible or palpable posteriorly.

RISK FACTORS

- History of seizure disorder
- History of posterior shoulder dislocation or instability
- Disorders such as Charcot shoulder and Ehlers-Danlos syndrome have been associated.
- Congenital anomalies such as scapular aplasia increase the risk of dislocation.
- A sports-specific risk factor for axial loading of the humerus would be offensive lineman.

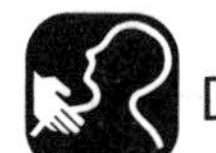

Diagnosis

DIFFERENTIAL DIAGNOSIS

- Acute subluxation
- Fractures (clavicle, scapula, and humerus)
- Rotator cuff pathology (strain, partial or complete tear)
- Acromioclavicular joint pathology
- Intraarticular pathology (labral, glenoid, or ligamentous)

HISTORY

- Mechanism of injury?
- Acute versus chronic in nature?
- History of previous injury or pain in affected shoulder?
- Previous or present description of pain, including location, intensity, and duration?
- Previous or present history of tingling, weakness, catching, locking?
- Any aggravating or alleviating factors?

PHYSICAL EXAM

- Routine observation, gentle palpation, range of motion, and strength of the affected extremity should be performed.
- It is of utmost importance to monitor the neurovascular status of the affected arm. Injury to the axillary vessels is rare but potentially catastrophic.
- Examine axillary nerve function by testing active contraction of the deltoid as well as sensation over the lateral aspect of the shoulder. Neurologic involvment is often in the form of a neuropraxia.

IMAGING

- Plain radiographs for a suspected posterior shoulder dislocation should include: (a) an anteroposterior view, (b) a trans-scapular lateral view (Y view), and (c) an axillary lateral view.
- The normal lateral projection of the greater tuberosity is lost in a posterior shoulder dislocation.
- With disarticulation of the humeral head posteriorly, the anterior rim of the glenoid is void of the humeral head, which is displaced medial to the glenoid convexity.
- A reverse Hill-Sachs lesion may be visible as an indentation of the anterior articular surface of the humeral head caused by the posterior rim of the glenoid.
- Advanced imaging (CT, MRI, or arthrography) should be reserved for evaluating the extent of associated humeral head fractures, glenoid fractures, rotator cuff, and labral pathologies.

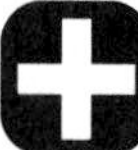

Acute Treatment

ANALGESIA

- Multiple factors influence the choice of anesthesia (i.e., analgesia for an on-the-field chronic and recurrent dislocator is very different from an electrical shock injury).
- Whenever possible, an analgesic and muscle relaxant should be administered prior to any reduction attempt.
- Conscious sedation or general anesthesia may be necessary if a gentle and atraumatic reduction cannot be obtained.

REDUCTION TECHNIQUES

- Early attempts at reduction should be performed in all cases except ones with associated fractures of the anatomic or surgical neck of the humerus.
- With the patient supine, gentle longitudinal traction is applied to the affected arm while the elbow is flexed at 90 degrees.
- While traction is applied, gentle internal rotation of the arm often unlocks the humeral head from the rim of the glenoid.
- It may be necessary to also use direct anterolateral pressure on the humeral head to unlock it from the glenoid rim.
- If an atraumatic reduction cannot be achieved, reduction in the operating room under general anesthesia should be considered.
- If this dislocation is seen hours or even days after occurring, it may be impossible to reduce nonsurgically.
- Associated fractures also may require operative intervention, and open reduction may be necessary.

POSTREDUCTION EVALUATION

- Confirm intact neurovascular status after any reduction attempt.
- Obtain postreduction radiographs to confirm reduction and to evaluate humeral or glenoid fractures.
- Consider repeat physical exam, taking care not to cause repeat dislocation.

IMMOBILIZATION

- Immobilization should not include the use of a sling and swathe because internal rotation should be avoided.
- A shoulder spica cast or commercial brace for posterior shoulder dislocation; arm held in 20 degrees of external rotation and 0–20 degrees of abduction
- Duration of immobilization depends on age, chronicity, associated fractures, and operative intervention

- For first-time uncomplicated dislocations, 7–14 days of immobilization for patients >45 years of age to avoid shoulder stiffness. Younger patients are immobilized 3–6 weeks to allow capsular scarring to occur.

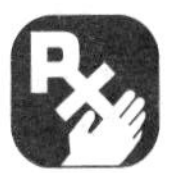

Long-Term Treatment

REHABILITATION

- Independent of the duration of immobilization, aggressive physical therapy should be completed.
- Initiate range of motion early, and follow with program for muscular strengthening.
- Recovery and maintenance of full strength of the external rotators may aid in preventing future dislocations.
- Advanced rehabilitation program for athletes concentrating on sport-specific activities and proprioception
- Return to athletics for first-time nonoperative dislocators in approximately 6–12 weeks to reduce likelihood of future dislocations
- Repeat nonoperative dislocators may return to activity once pain free and full strength has been recovered. These patients are very likely to have recurrent dislocations.

SURGICAL TREATMENT

- A conservative nonoperative trial of physical therapy may allow an individual with an uncomplicated dislocation to resume pain-free daily activities.
- Athletes (specifically overhead athletes) may continue to have disability which is not amendable to an extended conservative trial of rehabilitation (3–6 months). In these patients operative intervention should be considered following the initial dislocation.
- Surgical intervention is indicated with associated injuries such as fractures, rotator cuff tears and suspected labral pathology after an initial dislocation.
- Surgical intervention should also be considered in an individual with chronic dislocations.
- Operative interventions often include examination under anesthesia, diagnostic arthroscopy, and arthroscopic or open stabilization procedures.
- Open stabilization procedures (such as the Bankhart repair, Putti-Platt, and Neer capsular shift) have historically had superior results to arthroscopic stabilization.
- Recent advances in arthroscopic stabilization procedures have documented recurrence rates at approximately 5%. Long-term results are still unavailable on arthroscopic stabilizations.
- Trends to explore the use of thermally assisted arthroscopic capsular shifts in shoulder instability is currently underway.

REFERRAL

Orthopaedic referral should be considered for all posterior shoulder dislocations. Potential associated injuries of fractures, rotator cuff tears, and labral pathology require evaluation.

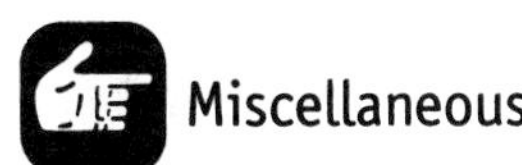

Miscellaneous

SYNONYMS

- Posterior shoulder dislocation
- Shoulder instability

ICD-9 CODE

831.02

BIBLIOGRAPHY

Andrews JR, Wilk KE. *The athlete's shoulder.* New York: Churchill Livingstone, 1994.

Canale TS. *Campbell's operative orthopaedics.* St. Louis: CV Mosby, 1998.

Dee R, Mango E, Hurst LC. *Principles of orthopaedic practice*. New York: McGraw-Hill, 1989.

Author: Shannon M. Urton

Glenoid Labral Tears/SLAP Lesions

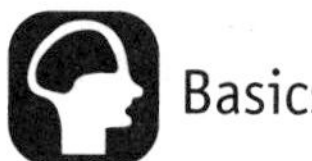

Basics

DEFINITION

- A Bankart lesion is an avulsion of the labrum from the bony attachment on the glenoid.
- A SLAP lesion is a tear of both the anterior and posterior aspects of the superior portion of the labrum. The acronym *SLAP* is an abbreviation for superior labrum anterior and posterior.

ANATOMY

- The glenoid labrum is the cartilagenous band that lies on the edge of the glenoid fossa. It stabilizes the articulation of the humeral head with the glenoid fossa.
- The labrum can be damaged acutely with a shoulder dislocation/subluxation or damaged due to chronic, repetitive stress at the attachment of the long head of the biceps tendon on the labrum.

INCIDENCE/PREVALENCE

One study demonstrated a 97% incidence of labrum tears after acute shoulder dislocations. The incidence of labrum damage from overuse injuries is unknown.

SIGNS AND SYMPTOMS

- Painful clicking, usually reproducible by the patient
- Locking symptoms may be present.
- Pain with overhead and across-the-chest arm movements
- May be difficult to distinguish from impingement syndrome

MECHANISMS

- Labrum injuries can occur with the throwing motion. It has been proposed that traction of the long head of the biceps on its attachment to the glenoid labrum during either the acceleration or deceleration phase of the throwing motion can cause a SLAP lesion.
- Traumatic dislocation of the humeral head frequently damages the labrum.
- Chronic stretching of the shoulder capsule, as occurs in swimming, may produce shoulder instability or subluxation, which also can result in damage to the labrum.

RISK FACTORS

- Throwing sports
- Swimming
- History of shoulder dislocation or instability
- A fall on an outstretched arm (shearing force placed on the labrum during upward motion of the humeral head)

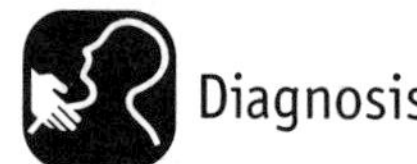

Diagnosis

DIFFERENTIAL DIAGNOSIS

- Rotator cuff tendinitis
- Instability of the glenohumeral joint
- Bicipital tendinitis (long head)
- Referred pain from the neck or thorax

HISTORY

- Acute trauma to the shoulder, especially shoulder dislocation
- Repetitive motions of the shoulder, especially throwing motions or swimming
- Typically, the symptoms are gradual in onset and chronic at the time of presentation.

PHYSICAL EXAM

- Repetitive, reproducible, usually painful click with specific shoulder movements (typically throwing type movements)
- Pain with traction on the long head of the biceps as with resisted flexion of the elbow or resisted supination of the wrist
- Reproduction of pain when the humeral head is pushed in a superior direction and rotated by the examiner in an attempt to entrap the torn labrum between the humeral head and the glenoid
- Physical exam findings can be subtle and inconsistent, making the clinical diagnosis difficult
- Physical exam findings are also frequently confused with rotator cuff tendinitis because the provocative testing may cause pain with both types of problems

IMAGING

- Plain radiographs do not show the labrum, which is a soft tissue structure, but they are useful to help rule out other pathology such as fractures, calcific tendinitis, and degenerative changes.
- CT arthrotomogram, MRI, or MRI with contrast are helpful if positive, but there is a high false-negative rate (30% in some studies).
- Accuracy of the MRI improves if contrast is used.
- It is likely that the sensitivity and specificity of MRI will improve as MRI technology progresses.
- Diagnostic arthroscopy: definitive diagnosis may require surgical evaluation (usually arthroscopic).

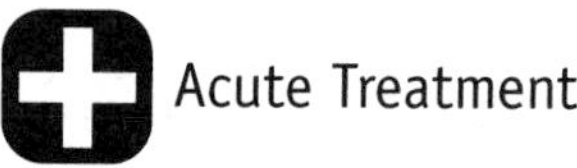

Acute Treatment

ACUTE INJURIES

With an acute shoulder dislocation there is often an associated labrum tear and the shoulder should be immobilized in internal rotation for a period of 3 weeks. If the labrum is torn at its attachment to the bone, there is a possibility it may heal back down into place.

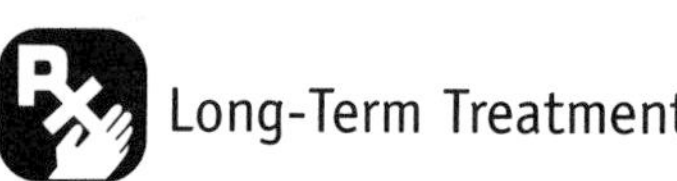

Long-Term Treatment

REHABILITATION

- Some patients choose to "live with the pain" if it is mild and intermittent.
- Shoulder strengthening exercises are of limited value, but are worth trying.

SURGICAL TREATMENT

- Surgical repair or debridement of the torn labrum is the definitive treatment.
- Arthroscopic stapling, suturing, or debridement are the procedures of choice in most instances.
- Open surgical repair (Bankart repair) is occasionally necessary.

REFERRAL/DISPOSITION

Decisions about the long-term management of the labrum tear are similar to those faced in the care of a meniscal cartilage tear in the knee. If the tear does not heal initially, it is unlikely to heal over time. Exercises are not usually effective. Ultimately, patients must decide if they are willing to live with the pain, which may be very episodic and specific to certain movements, or wish to proceed with surgery.

Common Questions and Answers

Physician responses to common patient questions:

Q: Will exercises fix the problem?
A: No, if the labrum did not heal after the initial injury, it is unlikely to heal as the result of shoulder exercises. Exercises can help to improve the biomechanics of the shoulder, which may reduce the stress on the labrum. This can help to reduce symptoms. Some exercises, however, may actually aggravate the injury and should be avoided. An exercise program should be individualized for each patient. Typically, overhead or "bench press" type shoulder exercises tend to be problematic.

Q: Will there be any long-term consequences if I decide not to have surgery?
A: Glenoid labrum problems are similar to meniscus tears in the knee. The catching or locking symptoms may be intermittent. If the symptoms are not too bad and the injury does not interfere with athletic performance, nonsurgical management is an option. The risk of this strategy is that continued stress to the damaged labrum may extend the tear.

Miscellaneous

ICD-9 CODE

718.01 Cartilage derangement, shoulder, old
718.31 Cartilage derangement, shoulder, recurrent

BIBLIOGRAPHY

Burkhardt SS, Morgan CD, Kibler WB. Shoulder injuries in overhead athletes. *Clin Sports Med* 2000;19:125–128.

Gartsman GM, Hammerman SM. Superior labrum, anterior and posterior lesions. *Clin Sports Med* 2000;19:115–124.

Rames RD, Karzel RP. Injuries to the glenoid labrum, including SLAP lesions. *Orthop Clin North Am* 1993;24:45–53.

Taylor DC, Arciero RA. Pathologic changes associated with shoulder dislocation. *Am J Sports Med* 1997;25:306–311.

Authors: Michael J. Henehan, Gregory A. Whitley, and W. Mark Peluso

Haglund's Deformity (Pump Bump)

Basics

DEFINITION

Haglund's deformity is an abnormal prominence of the posterosuperior surface of the calcaneus. It can give rise to Haglund's disease, which consists of retrocalcaneal bursitis, Achilles' tendinitis, and pre-Achilles' bursitis or superficial bursitis. These occur due to compression of the distal Achilles' tendon and the surrounding soft tissues, between the os calcis and the posterior shoe counter.

INCIDENCE/PREVALENCE

- More common in females who start wearing high heels and shoes with restrictive heel counters

SIGNS AND SYMPTOMS

- Dull, achy, exertional posterior heel pain
- Tenderness and thickening of the overlying skin at the Achilles' tendon attachment
- Palpable swelling anterior to or posterior to the Achilles' tendon
- Active or passive dorsiflexion of the ankle intensifies the pain.

RISK FACTORS

- Heel varus
- Rigid or poorly shaped heel counters
- Cavus foot
- Rigid plantarly flexed first ray

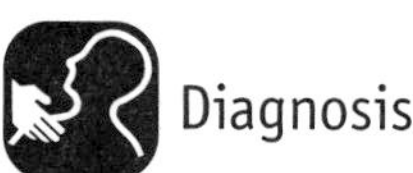

Diagnosis

DIFFERENTIAL DIAGNOSIS

- Pre-Achilles' bursitis
- Achilles' tendinitis/tendinosis
- Retrocalcaneal bursitis
- Calcaneal stress fracture
- Ankle impingement
- Tibiotalar degenerative joint disease

HISTORY

- Increase in training program, specifically number of miles run
- Change in shoe wear (shoes with rigid heel counters can irritate the subcutaneous tissues, and can inflame the underlying bursae)

PHYSICAL EXAM

- Prominent-appearing posterosuperior portion of the calcaneus
- Careful, discreet palpation to differentiate between swelling in the Achilles' tendon and swelling in the retrocalcaneal bursa
- Palpation medially as well as laterally within the retrocalcaneal bursa

IMAGING

- Increased angle on lateral radiographs between two lines as follows
  —Posterior calcaneal angle: line reaching prominent point of bursal surface, line of the most inferior projection of the calcaneus, prominent bump if the intersection angle is greater than 75 degrees
  —Parallel pitch lines: Base line, medial tuberosity and anterior tuberosity, parallel line, posterior lip of talar articular facet, abnormal if the prominence extends above the parallel line
- MRI ordered to evaluate the integrity of the Achilles' tendon and the retrocalcaneal bursa

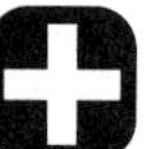

Acute Treatment

- Shoe modification
- Achilles' stretching program
- U-shaped pad
- Heel pad
- Soft tissue modalities (i.e., ice, ultrasonography, iontophoresis)
- Decrease in mileage and hill work
- Minimization of hard-surface running
- Nonsteroidal antiinflammatories
- Immobilization with a short-leg walking cast
- Aspiration and injection with corticosteroids

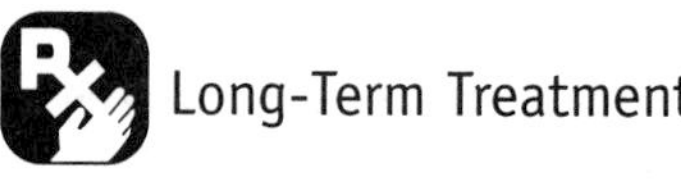

Long-Term Treatment

REHABILITATION

- Achilles' stretching program
- Soft tissue modalities (i.e., ice, ultrasonography, iontophoresis)

SURGICAL TREATMENT

- Partial calcaneal osteotomy: complete resection of the bursal projection
- Postoperative course: short leg walking cast provided for 8 weeks, 2 weeks partial weight-bearing, full weight-bearing over succeeding 6 weeks, until cast removal
- Rehabilitation program consisting of conditioning exercises and functional retraining

REFERRAL/DISPOSITION

- Surgery as indicated above

Common Questions and Answers

Physician responses to common patient questions:

Q: When can I return to play?

A: The time to return to play is dependent on the severity and number of associated conditions involved. Return to play after conservative treatment ranges from 4 to 12 weeks, whereas surgery and postoperative course limits and prevents strenuous activity for 4 to 6 months. Athletes may return to strenuous activity when local symptoms have resolved at this time.

Miscellaneous

SYNONYMS

- Haglund's disease
- Haglund's syndrome
- Pump bump

ICD-9 CODE

727.3 Bursitis not otherwise specified

See also: Achilles' tendinitis, heel bruise

BIBLIOGRAPHY

Stephens MM. Haglund's deformity and retrocalcaneal bursitis. *Orthop Clin North Am* 1974;25:41–46.

Stephens MM. Heel pain: shoes, exertion, and Haglund's deformity. *Phys Sportsmed* 1992;20:87–95.

Vega MR, Cavolo DJ, Green RM, et al. Haglund's deformity. *J Am Podiatry* 1984;74:129–135.

Authors: Dan Somogyi and Ian Shrier

Hallux Valgus (Bunions)

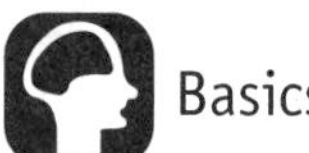

Basics

DEFINITION

Hallux valgus refers to a subluxation of the first metatarsophalangeal (MTP) joint with lateral or valgus deviation of the great toe and medial or varus deviation of the first metatarsal, leading to a bony prominence at the medial aspect of the joint (medial eminence or bunion).

INCIDENCE/PREVALENCE

- More common in females (female:male ratio approximately 10:1)
- Familial tendency

SIGNS AND SYMPTOMS

- Pain and swelling over the medial eminence are the principal complaints.
- Symptoms are aggravated by tight or poorly fitting shoe wear.
- Repetitive athletic activities may cause blisters or an inflamed adventitious bursa overlying the medial eminence.
- Diminished weight-bearing capacity of the first metatarsal leads to increased pressure on the lesser metatarsals (mostly the second metatarsal) with the development of pain and a plantar keratosis (callus) beneath the metatarsal head.
- With severe deformities, pronation or rotation of the great toe may cause callus formation on the medial aspect of the interphalangeal (IP) joint.
- Impingement of the dorsal medial sensory nerve to the hallux may cause numbness or tingling on the medial aspect of the great toe.
- Occasionally patients present with a stress fracture of the second metatarsal.

RISK FACTORS

Extrinsic Factors

- Hallux valgus occurs almost exclusively in shoe-wearing societies.
- Higher incidence in females is thought to be related to constricting footwear.

Intrinsic Factors

- Pes planus and forefoot pronation lead to increased pressure on the medial aspect of the great toe and attenuation of the medial capsular structures at the first MTP joint.
- A rounded MTP articulation is more prone to lateral subluxation then a flat articulation.
- Metatarsus primus varus and an increased 1st and 2nd intermetatarsal angle is often implicated in juvenile or adolescent hallux valgus.
- Cystic degeneration of the medial capsule of the first MTP joint, Achilles' tendon contracture, collagen-deficient diseases with hyperelasticity, and neuromuscular disorders (i.e., cerebral palsy) are also associated with hallux valgus.

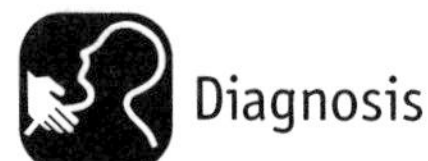

Diagnosis

DIFFERENTIAL DIAGNOSIS

- Hallux rigidus (degenerative arthritis of the great toe MTP joint with dorsal bunion)
- Hallux interphalangeus (valgus at the IP joint, not the MTP joint)
- Gout

HISTORY

- Pain over the medial eminence aggravated by tight or rigid footwear is the most common complaint.
- Pain under the second metatarsal head with a plantar keratosis is also common.
- Blisters, swelling, or callus formation over the medial eminence may occur with athletic activities.
- Numbness or tingling of the medial aspect of the great toe may occur from pressure on the medial sensory nerve to the hallux.
- Callus formation on the medial aspect of the great toe IP joint occurs from hallux pronation.

PHYSICAL EXAM

- Note the severity of hallux valgus and rotational deformity of the great toe in both the standing and non-weight-bearing positions.
- Assess for pes planus.
- Check active and passive range of motion at the first MTP joint (normal extension = 70 degrees).
- Evaluate sensation of the great toe.
- Examine lesser toes for associated deformities such as metatarsalgia, plantar keratosis, hammer toe, overriding second toe, and bunionette (prominence of the lateral aspect of the fifth metatarsal head and medial deviation of the fifth toe joint).
- Evaluation for Achilles' tendon contracture, hyperelasticity associated with collagen-deficient disorders, and neuromuscular disorders.

IMAGING

- Weight-bearing anteroposterior and lateral radiographs of the foot are used to grade the severity of the deformity.
- The hallux valgus angle is the angle subtended by the axis of the proximal phalanx and the first metatarsal (normal <15 degrees, mild to moderate <30 degrees, severe <40 degrees).
- The 1st and 2nd intermetatarsal angle is measured by lines bisecting the axis of the first and second metatarsals (normal <9 degrees, mild to moderate <14 degrees, severe >14 degrees).
- Radiographs also assess MTP joint congruity or subluxation, lateral sesamoid subluxation, the shape of the metatarsal head, and degenerative changes of the MTP joint.
- Lateral radiographs are helpful for evaluating arthritic changes of the MTP joint and identifying hallux rigidus.

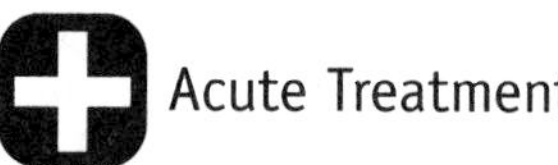

Acute Treatment

- Initial treatment consists of shoe wear modification and patient education.
- Wider footwear with a roomy toe box will help decrease pressure and friction on the medial eminence.
- Shoes with flexible and nonconstricting stitching over the medial eminence are recommended (shoes can be professionally stretched to provide additional room).
- High-heeled shoes (which place increased pressure on the forefoot) should be avoided.
- Medial longitudinal arch support may decrease pressure on the first metatarsal, especially in patients with pes planus.
- Activity modification in joggers and runners (substituting bicycling or other nonimpact activities) may significantly decrease symptoms and stress on the forefoot.

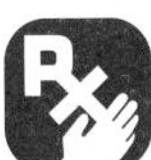

Long-Term Treatment

SURGICAL TREATMENT

- Numerous surgical procedures have been developed to correct hallux valgus.
- The procedure chosen should address the presence and severity of the enlarged medial eminence, increased hallux valgus and intermetatarsal angles, pronation (rotation) of the great toe, and lateral sesamoid subluxation.
- Operative procedures include medial eminence resection, proximal phalangeal osteotomy, distal metatarsal osteotomy, medial capsular reefing, lateral capsular and adductor hallucis release, and joint fusion or replacement.

REFERRAL/DISPOSITION

Patients should be referred for surgical consideration when nonoperative treatment including footwear and activity modification have not adequately relieved symptoms.

SPECIAL CONSIDERATIONS

- Treatment of an athlete with hallux valgus should be nonoperative until pain and symptoms are significantly affecting athletic performance.
- Stiffness, decreased range of motion, pain, and reduced function of the MTP joint are potential risks of surgery and may hamper athletic performance (particularly in sprinters and dancers who require MTP motion for strength in toe push-off).

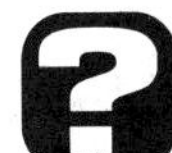

Common Questions and Answers

Physician responses to common patient questions:

Q: Will my bunion get worse as I age?

A: Hallux valgus is likely to progress without appropriate management. With activity modification, proper footwear, and selective use of orthotic arch supports, symptoms and complications can largely be controlled.

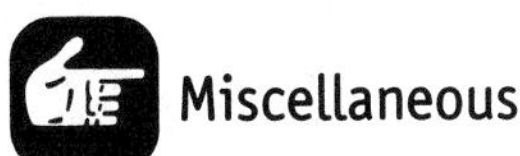

Miscellaneous

SYNONYMS

- Hallux valgus
- Bunion
- Metatarsus primus varus

ICD-9 CODE

735.0 Hallux valgus, acquired
755.66 Hallux valgus, congenital

BIBLIOGRAPHY

DeLee JC, Drez D. *Orthopaedic sports medicine*. Philadelphia: WB Saunders, 1994.

Donley BG, Tisdel CL, Sferra JJ, et al. Diagnosing and treating hallux valgus: a conservative approach for a common problem. *Clev Clin J Med* 1997;64:469–474.

Snider RK, ed. *Essentials of musculoskeletal care*. Chicago: American Academy of Orthopaedic Surgeons, 1997.

Author: Jonathan Drezner

Hammer/Claw/Mallet Toe

Basics

DEFINITION

- Hammer toe is a plantar flexion contracture of the proximal interphalangeal (PIP) joint. Passive extension of the metatarsophalangeal (MTP) joint is common. The distal interphalangeal (DIP) joint is neutral or slightly extended. The second toe is most commonly affected.
- Claw toe is an extension contracture of the MTP joint with a flexion contracture of the PIP joint and sometimes the DIP joint. Claw toe usually results from weakness in the intrinsic muscles of the foot secondary to a neurologic condition and commonly affects multiple toes.
- Mallet toe is a flexion contracture of the DIP joint with normal alignment of the MTP and PIP joints. The second toe is most commonly affected.

SPECIAL CONSIDERATION

The distinction between hammer toe and claw toe deformities can be difficult (both have flexion contractures of the PIP joint). However, in claw toe, deformities of multiple toes are involved and there is always an extension deformity of the MTP joint and often a flexion contracture of the DIP joint.

INCIDENCE/PREVALENCE

- Hammer, claw, and mallet toes are the most common deformities of the lesser toes.
- Incidence increases with age.
- More common in females (female:male ratio of approximately 9:1 in ages 15–30).

SIGNS AND SYMPTOMS

Hammer Toe

- Painful callus over the dorsal aspect of the PIP joint (from rubbing against the undersurface of the shoe) is most common.
- Secondary metatarsalgia with plantar keratosis (callus) under the metatarsal head may occur if MTP joint subluxation is present.

CLAW TOE

- Painful callus formation over the dorsal PIP joint, beneath the metatarsal head, or on the end of the toe

MALLET TOE

- Painful callus at the tip of the toe

COMPLICATIONS

Complications of lesser toe deformities include MTP joint subluxation or dislocation, metatarsalgia, intractable keratosis, adventitious bursa formation, ulceration of callus, infection, and osteomyelitis.

RISK FACTORS

- Hammer and mallet toe deformities are usually the result of long-term poorly fitting and constricting footwear.
- Abnormally long ray or digital length
- Pressure or deforming force from adjacent digits (i.e., hallux valgus)
- Inflammatory joint disease
- Pes cavus may indicate an associated neuromuscular disorder.
- Claw toes are found in associated neurologic conditions such as peripheral neuropathies (diabetes and alcoholism), Charcot-Marie-Tooth disease, cerebral palsy, muscular dystrophy, and spinal cord tumors.

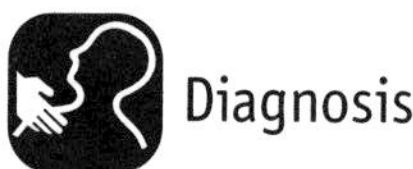

Diagnosis

DIFFERENTIAL DIAGNOSIS

- Hammer toe (flexion of the PIP joint)
- Claw toe (extension of the MTP joint and flexion of the PIP and DIP joints)
- Mallet toe (flexion of the DIP joint)
- Hard corn (keratosis over the lateral aspect of the fifth toe)
- Interdigital (soft) corn (keratosis and maceration resulting from pressure between two adjacent toes)

HISTORY

Painful callus formation and difficulty with shoe wear are the principal complaints in lesser toe deformities.

PHYSICAL EXAM

- Patients should be evaluated both standing and non-weight bearing. (In hammer toe deformities, extension of the MTP joint is common in the standing position but may largely resolve when non-weight bearing).
- Toes should be passively stretched to determine if the deformity is flexible (reducible to neutral position), semirigid (partially reducible), or rigid (nonreducible).
- Inspection for the presence of calluses, ulcers, adventitious bursa, infection, and interdigital maceration
- Calluses are common on the dorsum of the PIP joint and under the metatarsal head (hammer and claw toes) or on the tip of the toe (hammer, claw, and mallet toes).
- Dorsal dislocation of the proximal phalanx onto the metatarsal head may occur in advanced cases.
- A cross-over deformity of the second toe resting on top of the great toe may exist with medial subluxation of the second MTP joint.

IMAGING

- Weight-bearing anteroposterior radiographs are helpful to assess for the presence of MTP joint subluxation or dislocation.
- Lateral radiographs best confirm the deformity.
- Advanced imaging (bone scan or MRI) may be indicated when ulceration is present and osteomyelitis is suspected.
- Electromyography and nerve conduction studies may be useful to evaluate for peripheral neuropathies in claw toe deformities.

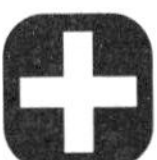

Acute Treatment

- Shoes with a roomy toe box are recommended to accommodate the deformity (an elevated toe box may eliminate dorsal pressure on the PIP joint).
- High-heeled shoes should be avoided.
- Passive manual stretching and strengthening exercises for the intrinsic foot muscles (laying a towel flat on the floor and using the toes to crumple it beneath the foot) may be helpful for flexible deformities.
- Debridement of hyperkeratotic lesions and home use of a pumice stone may reduce painful calluses.
- Foam pads used over the callosity or a cushioned toe cap to protect the end of the toe may reduce symptoms.
- Metatarsal pads placed proximal to the MTP joint may reduce pressure on the metatarsal heads.
- Taping the toe in a corrected position may stabilize a subluxed MTP joint.
- Nonsteroidal anti-inflammatory medications may be appropriate to relieve pain and inflammation.

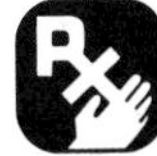

Long-Term Treatment

SURGICAL TREATMENT

- Surgery is indicated when nonoperative treatment is unsuccessful in relieving symptoms.
- Flexible deformities of the interphalangeal (IP) joints may be repaired with flexor tendon transfer or tenotomy.
- Rigid deformities of the IP joints are treated with arthroplasty (joint resection) or arthrodesis (joint fusion).
- Extension deformities of the MTP joint are corrected with a capsular release but may require bony resection when severe subluxation or dislocation is present.

REFERRAL/DISPOSITION

Referral for surgical consideration is recommended when conservative treatment has not adequately relieved symptoms.

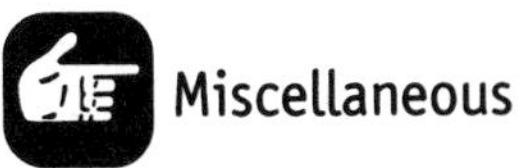

Miscellaneous

ICD-9 CODE

735.4 Hammer toe, acquired
755.66 Hammer toe, congenital
735.5 Claw toe, acquired
754.71 Claw toe, congenital
No ICD-9 code is designated for mallet toe; use of hammer toe codes is conventional.

BIBLIOGRAPHY

DeLee JC, Drez D. *Orthopaedic sports medicine*. Philadelphia: WB Saunders, 1994.

Schuberth JM. Hammer toe syndrome. *J Foot Ankle Surg* 1999;38:166–178.

Snider RK, ed. *Essentials of musculoskeletal care*. Chicago: American Academy of Orthopaedic Surgeons, 1997.

Author: Jonathan Drezner

Hamstring Strain

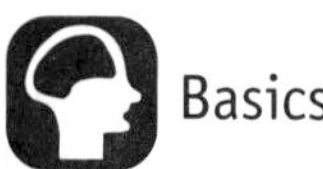

Basics

DEFINITION

This injury occurs when there is excessive stretching of the musculotendinous unit within the hamstring muscle group, which is composed of the biceps femoris (long and short heads), semitendinosus, and semimembranosus. Typically the injury occurs during running or jumping activities after the muscle experiences an excessive load during a single eccentric muscle contraction (the muscle develops tension while lengthening at the same time). Most commonly, injury to the musculotendinous unit occurs at the point of bony origin of the muscle, the musculo-tendinous junction, the muscle belly, or the bony insertion of the tendon.

INCIDENCE/PREVALENCE

- Hamstring injuries are among the most common strain injuries in runners, particularly sprinters.
- Hamstring injuries often recur and become chronic, which emphasizes the importance of adequate healing and rehabilitation.

SIGNS AND SYMPTOMS

- Signs and symptoms depend on the severity of the injury and its location (myotendinous junction, muscle belly, or tendon itself).
- Muscle strain injuries have traditionally been classified into first, second, and third degrees of severity.
- A first-degree strain is a mild strain in which there is only disruption of a few muscle fibers so that only minor amounts of swelling and pain are present; there is minimal or no loss of range of motion and strength.
- A second-degree strain, like the first-degree strain, is a partial tear. However, a moderate strain involves greater damage to the muscle, which results in a loss of strength.
- A third-degree strain is a complete rupture of the musculotendinous unit, and in hamstring strains this usually occurs at the insertion near the ischial tuberosity. There is a significant loss in range of motion and strength, and often a palpable defect in the musculotendinous unit.

RISK FACTORS

As cited by Agre (1985) in *Sports Medicine*:

- Insufficient flexibility of the hamstring muscles
- Physiologic shortening of the hamstring muscles due to fatigue, resulting in a loss of flexibility
- Poor strength and/or endurance of the hamstring muscles
- Inequality of the strength of the right and left hamstrings
- Strength imbalance between quadriceps and hamstring muscles
- Inadequate warm-up and stretching prior to activity
- Dys-synergic contraction of the hamstrings during running
- Poor running style, placing greater strain on the hamstring muscles
- Return to physical activity too quickly following injury and prior to full rehabilitation, leading to recurrent injury

ASSOCIATED INJURIES AND COMPLICATIONS

- Acute and old bony avulsions of the ischial tuberosity
- Stress fracture of the pelvis
- Traction apophysitis
- Ectopic muscle calcification/myositis ossificans

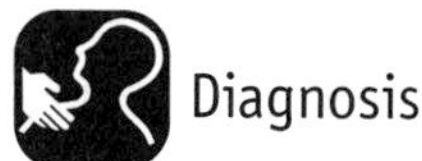

Diagnosis

DIFFERENTIAL DIAGNOSIS

Along with the associated injuries outlined above, other clinical entities should be considered in the diagnosis of hamstring strain injury.

- Piriformis syndrome
- Gluteus medius insertion tendinitis
- Posterior trochanteric bursitis
- Ischiogluteal bursitis
- Tight iliotibial tract
- Pain from the low back origin
- Sacroileitis
- Exertional posterior thigh compartment/hamstring syndrome

HISTORY

- Acute versus chronic?
- Initial versus recurrent?
- An acute initial hamstring strain injury will enter the treatment protocol for hamstring strain at a different phase than a recurrent, chronic injury (see treatment protocol section).
- Did the patient hear an audible "pop"? A positive response increases the likelihood of a higher grade injury.
- Was the patient able to continue his activities? How about ambulation? A negative response increases a suspicion of a high-grade injury.
- What position was the patient's lower extremity when he felt a "pull" or heard the "pop"? If the hip is in the extreme of hip flexion with the knee in full extension, there is an increased chance of a bony avulsion.

PHYSICAL EXAM

- Inspection for observation of swelling and ecchymosis
- Palpation to determine maximum site of tenderness and possible defect in musculotendinous unit
- Most common injury site is biceps femoris, long head.
- May increase the index of suspicion for avulsion and radiographic workup
- Active range of motion examination to assess strength and flexibility deficit
- Passive range of motion examination of the hamstring group via passive straight leg raising or knee extension with hip at neutral to assess severity of injury
- Manual resistance testing to determine severity of injury
- Perform neurovascular exam to ensure acute posterior thigh compartment syndrome has not developed subsequent to inflammation and hematoma formation

IMAGING

- Radiographs of anteroposterior view of pelvis may be helpful if avulsion fracture is suspected.
- Ultrasonography, MRI, and CT scan have been used as research tools but are rarely used in the clinical situation unless rehabilitation is not progressing and the diagnosis is in question.
- MRI may help determine the prognosis of hamstring injuries.

PROGNOSIS

- Longer recovery time (>6 weeks) is usually associated with those who have complete tendinous or myotendinous junction ruptures, hemorrhage, >50% cross-sectional muscle involvement, distal tendinous or myotendinous lesions, and localized peritendinous fluid collections.
- Shorter recovery time (<5 weeks) is seen with superficial muscle injuries and muscle belly injuries involving small cross-sectional area of muscle.

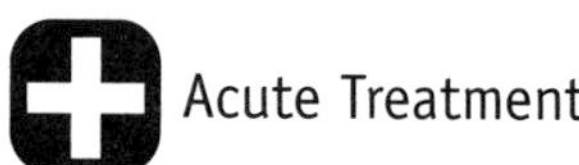

Acute Treatment

As advocated by Clanton and Coupe (1998), and similarly by Worrell (1994), the treatment protocol for hamstring strain is as follows.

PHASE I: ACUTE

- 3 to 5 days. Goal: control pain and edema. Treatment: rest, ice, compression, elevation.
- 1 to 5 days. Goal: limit hemorrhage and inflammation. Treatment: immobilization in extension, nonsteroidal antiinflammatory drugs (NSAIDs).

- After 1 to 5 days. Goal: prevent muscle fiber adhesions. Treatment: pain-free passive range of motion (PROM) (gentle stretching), active-assisted range of motion (AAROM).
- Up to 1 week. Goal: normal gait. Treatment: ambulatory aids.

PHASE II: SUBACUTE (DAY 3 TO >3 WEEKS)

- Goal: control pain. Treatment: ice, compression, and electrical stimulation.
- Goal: full active range of motion (AROM). Treatment: pain-free pool activities.
- Goal: alignment of collagen. Treatment: pain-free PROM, AAROM.
- Goal: increase collagen strength. Treatment: pain-free submaximal isometrics, stationary bike.
- Goal: maintain cardiovascular conditioning. Treatment: well-leg stationary bike, swimming with pull buoys, upper body exercise.

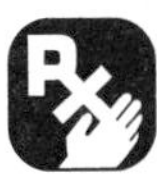

Long-Term Treatment

PHASE III: REMODELING (1–6 WEEKS)

- Goal: achieve phase II goals. Treatment: ice and compression.
- Goal: control pain and edema. Treatment: ice and electrical stimulation.
- Goal: increase collagen strength. Treatment: prone concentric isotonic exercises, isokinetic exercise.
- Goal: increase hamstring flexibility. Treatment: moist heat or exercise prior to pelvic-tilt hamstring stretching.
- Goal: increase eccentric loading. Treatment: prone eccentric exercises, jump rope, unilateral eccentric exercise (e.g., standing catch).

PHASE IV: FUNCTIONAL (2 WEEKS TO 6 MONTHS)

- Goal: return to sport without reinjury. Treatment: walk/jog, jog/sprint, sport-specific skills and drills.
- Goal: increase hamstring flexibility. Treatment: pelvic-tilt hamstring stretching.
- Goal: increase hamstring strength. Treatment: prone concentric and eccentric exercises, unilateral eccentric exercise (e.g., standing catch)
- Goal: control pain. Treatment: heat, ice, and modalities; NSAIDs as needed.

PHASE V: RETURN TO COMPETITION (3 WEEKS TO 6 MONTHS)

- Goal: avoid reinjury. Treatment: maintenance stretching, and strengthening.

INDICATIONS FOR RETURN TO ACTIVITY

- Free from pain
- Flexibility, strength, power, endurance, coordination, and athletic agility should have returned to normal levels.
- Any sensation of tightness or pain in the hamstrings warrants concern, and the athlete should be cautioned about the risk of reinjury if return to activity is attempted too soon.
- Isokinetic testing may be used as an adjunctive measure to determine readiness for return to activity.
- Most clinicians recommend the hamstring-quadriceps ratio to be between 50% and 60%.
- Restoration of the injured leg's strength to be within 10% of the uninjured leg

REFERRAL/DISPOSITION

- Surgical indications: complete rupture at or near the origin from the ischial tuberosity or distally at its insertion, soft tissue avulsion with a large defect, or bony avulsion with displacement by 2 cm

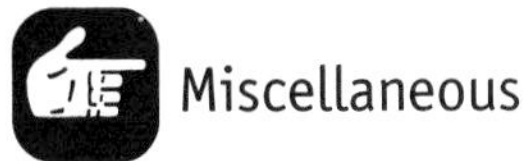

Miscellaneous

BIBLIOGRAPHY

Agre JC. Hamstring injuries: proposed aetiological factors, prevention, and treatment. *Sports Med* 1985;2:21–23.

Brandser EA, El-Khoury GY, Kathol MH, et al. Hamstring injuries: radiographic, conventional tomographic, CT, and MR imaging characteristics. *Radiology* 1995;197:257–262.

Clanton TO, Coupe KJ. Hamstring strains in athletes: diagnosis and treatment. *J Am Acad Orthop Surg* 1998;6:237–248.

Jonhagen S, Nemeth G, Eriksson E. Hamstring injuries in sprinters: the role of concentric and eccentric hamstring muscle strength and flexibility. *Am J Sports Med* 1994;22:262–266.

Kujala UM, Orava S, Jarvinen M. Hamstring injuries: current trends in treatment and prevention. *Sports Med* 1997;23:397–404.

Pomeranz SJ, Heidt RS. MR imaging in the prognostication of hamstring injury: work in progress. *Musculoskel Radiol* 1993;189:897–900.

Worrell TW. Factors associate with hamstring injuries: an approach to treatment and preventative measures. *Sports Med* 1994;17:338–345.

Authors: Alex Lai and Aurelia Nattiv

Heel Bruise/Heel Fat Pad Syndrome

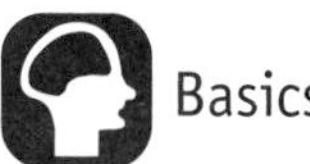

Basics

DEFINITION

- The heel pad is divided into small compartments containing fat and surrounded by fibrous connective tissue that is attached to the skin.
- The encapsulated fat acts in a hydraulic fashion to absorb shock by resisting compressive loads.
- Degeneration or trauma may cause local loss of the heel pad or rupture of the fibrous tissue septa, which may result in loss of the heel pad compressibility.
- Cause is often multifactorial.
- The syndrome may result from a direct blow to the bottom of the heel, resulting in a bruise and loss of heel pad elasticity.
- Displacement, loss, or atrophy of fat pads causes pain from excessive pressure.

INCIDENCE/PREVALENCE

- More common with increasing age, obesity, and diabetes
- Relationship with athletic overuse injuries (stress-related pathogenesis)
- More common with occupations requiring prolonged standing or walking on hard surfaces

SIGNS AND SYMPTOMS

- Pain primarily with weight bearing and relieved with rest.
- Pain is usually nonspecific and occurs over the heel pad.

RISK FACTORS

- Advanced age
- Obesity
- Occupations requiring prolonged standing or walking
- Repetitive trauma, such as in distance runners, hurdlers, long jumpers, and triple jumpers

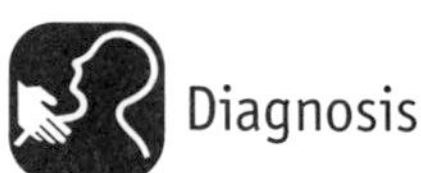

Diagnosis

DIFFERENTIAL DIAGNOSIS

- Calcaneal spurs
- Local inflammatory conditions (plantar fasciitis, subcalcaneal bursitis, periostitis, tenosynovitis, Sever's disease, blister)
- Systemic inflammatory conditions (ankylosing spondylitis, Reiter's syndrome, psoriatic arthritis, rheumatoid arthritis, sarcoidosis, gout, and pseudogout)
- Calcaneal fracture or stress fracture
- Entrapment (tarsal tunnel syndrome, entrapment of nerve to abductor digiti quinti or medial calcaneal nerve)
- Infectious (osteomyelitis, tuberculosis)
- Tumors (glomus tumor of heel pad, osteoid osteoma, osteoblastoma, chondromyxoid fibroma, chondrosarcoma, simple and aneurysmal cysts)
- Neuropathy (diabetes mellitus, alcoholism, reflex sympathetic dystrophy)
- Metabolic (osteomalacia, Paget's disease)

HISTORY

- Gradual onset of plantar heel pain, which may be unilateral or bilateral
- May have a history of local trauma
- Pain may radiate into the arch or proximally to the medial heel area.
- If pain is severe enough, a patient may walk on the ball or lateral aspect of the foot.

PHYSICAL EXAM

- Thorough examination of the lower extremity, including neurovascular exam, is recommended.
- Exam is facilitated by having the patient lay prone.
- Tenderness directly over the weight-bearing part of the calcaneus rather than on the distal tuberosity
- May have palpable absence or diminution of a compressible pad
- In prolonged cases, the underlying bone can be felt underneath the skin due to significant fat pad atrophy.

IMAGING

- Anteroposterior, lateral, and oblique plain radiographs
- Radiographs may reveal calcaneal spurs or calcifications, fractures, tumors, arthrosis, or other unusual causes of heel pain
- Consider bone scan, MRI if stress fracture is suspected.

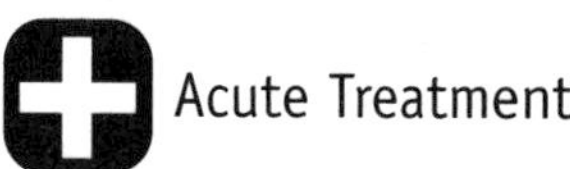

Acute Treatment

ANALGESIA

- Nonsteroidal antiinflammatory drugs of choice
- Modified weight-bearing activities
- Injections of local anesthetics/steroids (caution should be exercised with repeated injections or improper technique due to the risk of irreversible damage to the heel pad by mechanical disruption of the heel septae and by steroid-induced fat necrosis)

IMMOBILIZATION

- Rarely necessary; symptom-directed
- Treat other associated conditions (e.g., night splints in plantar fasciitis)

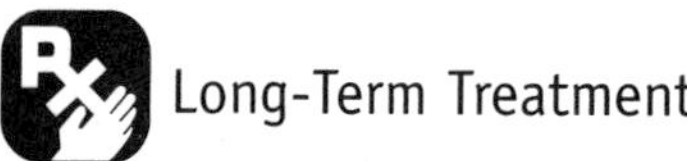

Long-Term Treatment

REHABILITATION

Various methods for altering the biomechanical forces on the heel have been advocated:

- Weight control
- A well-fitted heel cup cushions the heel and prevents the heel pad from splaying, thereby improving the intrinsic cushioning of the calcaneus. There is no consensus as to which type of orthosis is best. Regardless of whether over-the-counter heel cups or custom orthoses are used, consistent features should be support of the arch, presence of adequate cushioning material, recess for area of pain beneath the heel, and slight medial elevation.
- Shoes with softer mid-soles, which provide more cushioning of the fat pad
- Raising the heel may thereby transfer the weight-bearing anteriorly with heel strike and in mid-stance.
- Medial heel wedge to relieve the pressure on the medial tuberosity, causing more lateral pressure
- Physical therapy may be useful for patients not adequately responding to other conservative modalities.

SURGICAL TREATMENT

- Surgery reserved for patients when conservative treatment fails to provide adequate pain relief
- Some experts advocate that symptoms be present for more than 1 year despite appropriate conservative treatment before surgery is considered.
- Surgical options are directed toward the cause of heel pain and include spur resection, wide release of plantar fascia, drilling decompression, and neurolysis.
- It is important to have an exact diagnosis of the pain before surgical intervention, due to the multifactorial and often recurrent nature of plantar heel pain.

DISPOSITION

- Responds very well to conservative treatment and is usually self-limited

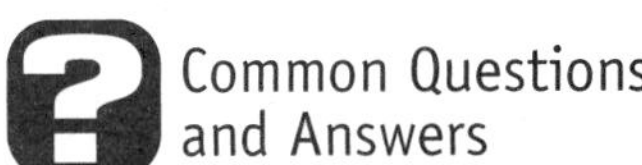

Common Questions and Answers

Physician responses to common patient questions:

Q: Should I use a soft heel cup or a more rigid one?

A: Each type has been used with some success. The hard cups are intended to encompass the heel pad beneath the calcaneus, helping to restore some of its compressibility. The softer cups are designed primarily to cushion the fat pad. Athletes who run a lot in their sport often prefer softer heel cups or orthotics.

Q: What can an athlete do to help prevent heel fat pad syndrome?

A: Training errors should be identified and corrected. The athlete should be certain to wear proper shoes with an energy-absorbing heel cushion, avoiding excessive wear of the shoes. Mileage should be increased gradually, and running on steep hills should be avoided. Training on safe and shock-absorbing surfaces is essential (e.g., running on an all-weather track or on a surface softer than concrete or asphalt).

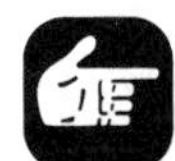

Miscellaneous

SYNONYMS

- Calcaneodynia
- Heel pain syndrome
- Calcaneal neuritis
- Policeman's heel
- Runner's heel
- Tennis heel
- Stone bruise
- Tuber calcanei pain
- Subcalcaneobursitis

ICD-9 CODE

924.20 Heel contusion
825.0 Fracture of calcaneus, closed
728.71 Plantar fasciitis
733.19 Stress fracture not otherwise specified
726.91 Heel spur (exostosis)

BIBLIOGRAPHY

Bateman JE. *Disorders of the foot and ankle, medical and surgical management*. Philadelphia: WB Saunders, 1991.

Bordelon RL. *Orthopedic sports medicine, principles and practice*. Philadelphia: WB Saunders, 1994.

Cailliet R, ed. *Foot and ankle pain*. Philadelphia: FA Davis, 1997.

Karr SD. Subcalcaneal heel pain. *Orthop Clin North Am* 1994;25:161–175.

Simons SM. Foot injuries of the recreational athlete. *Phys Sports Med* 1999;27:57–70.

Turgut A, Gokturk E, Kose N, et al. The relationship of heel pad elasticity and plantar heel pain. *Clin Orthop Rel Res* 1999;360:191–196.

Authors: Thomas L. Pommering and Timothy J. Linker

Hematomas, Epidural and Subdural

Basics

DEFINITION

- In epidural hematoma (EDH), blood is confined to the space between the inner table of the calvaria and the dura mater. In subdural hematoma (SDH), localized bleeding occurs below the dura mater, directly adjacent to brain parenchyma, and can be acute or chronic (this chapter focuses on acute SDH).
- EDH and SDH are neurosurgical emergencies. With prompt appropriate treatment, a patient with an EDH can often achieve complete neurologic recovery, whereas a missed diagnosis may result in death within hours. Mortality for patients with acute SDH is much higher (50%–90%), presumably due to greater underlying injury to the brain tissue itself.

INCIDENCE/PREVALENCE

- EDH: incidence is about 1% of head trauma admissions; most commonly presents in young adults; 85% arise from arterial bleeding, usually of the middle meningeal artery, as a result of a temporal skull fracture.
- Acute SDH: incidence is about 2% of head trauma admissions; occurs either secondary to a parenchymal laceration (which implies a severe underlying brain tissue injury) or due to disruption of a surface or bridging vessel (in which case underlying brain injury may be less severe). This mechanism is more common in older individuals and in athletes such as boxers. It is the most common athletic injury resulting in death.

SIGNS AND SYMPTOMS

- EDH: classic presentation involves brief posttraumatic loss of consciousness followed by a complete recovery period lasting several hours (lucid interval), often with headache, followed by rapid deterioration; classic presentation occurs in up to 25% of patients.
- SDH: typically presents with immediate loss of consciousness followed by only incomplete recovery of mental status, then deterioration; incomplete recovery due to underlying brain parenchymal damage; slower course due to slower accumulation of venous blood

RISK FACTORS

- High-energy trauma is a risk factor for both EDH and SDH.
- SDH: bridging veins can also be torn during acceleration-deceleration injuries without actual head impact.

ASSOCIATED INJURIES AND COMPLICATIONS

- EDH: associated temporal or other skull fracture
- SDH: underlying brain parenchymal injury
- Both: sequelae of increased intracranial pressure, including obtundation, Cushing's reflex, respiratory distress, and death

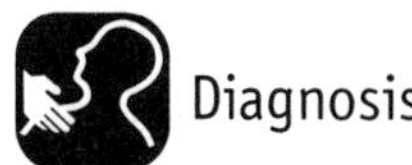

Diagnosis

DIFFERENTIAL DIAGNOSIS

- Concussion
- Uncomplicated skull fracture
- Intracerebral hemorrhage/cerebrovascular accident
- Subarachnoid hemorrhage
- Second impact syndrome

HISTORY

- Mechanism? Higher energy trauma resulting in skull fracture is a risk factor for EDH; alternatively, acute SDH due to high-energy trauma implies more underlying brain tissue damage.
- Lucid interval? Presence of a lucid interval is more common with EDH.
- Deterioration in mental status? Regardless of mechanism or level of recovery after initial unconsciousness, any patient with a deterioration of mental status after a head trauma should be evaluated for a possible neurosurgical emergency.

PHYSICAL EXAM

- EDH: skull exam to look for fracture
- Both: complete neurologic exam initially followed by serial exams to assess for herniation (ipsilateral pupillary dilatation, contralateral hemiparesis) and signs of increased intracranial pressure (obtundation, hypertension, bradycardia, respiratory depression)

IMAGING

- Skull films do not show acute blood and so not useful for ruling out either EDH or SDH. Moreover, plain x-rays in 40% of patients with EDH show no fracture.
- EDH and SDH are most readily diagnosed by CT. In EDH, hematoma is hyperdense (acute blood), biconvex, sharply demarcated, and adjacent to the skull; mass effect is common. Hematoma in SDH can be slightly less dense than in EDH (from mixing with cerebrospinal fluid), concave, and conforming to the underlying brain; accompanying parenchymal injury and edema may be seen; may become isodense with brain parenchyma as early as 4 days.

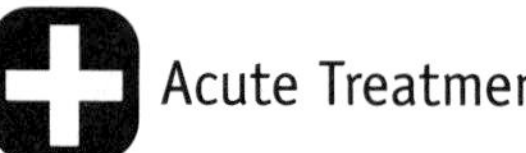

Acute Treatment

INITIAL MANAGEMENT CONSIDERATIONS

- Stabilization of vital signs
- Rapid neurosurgical consultation for any symptomatic EDH or SDH, or for any asymptomatic EDH or SDH over 1 cm at its thickest measurement (or >5 mm in pediatric patients)
- EDH: steroids started acutely then tapered over several days to decrease intracranial pressure are optional.
- SDH: delay of surgery over 4 hours associated with significantly increased mortality
- Both: institution of medical interventions to control elevated intracranial pressure is important but should not delay definitive neurosurgical treatment.
- Both: for asymptomatic hematomas less than 1 cm, admission in a monitored bed for observation, with repeat imaging or neurosurgical consultation if there is any deterioration.
- If there is a high index of suspicion of EDH or SDH but a negative CT scan, such patients should be admitted for 24 hours observation because EDH and SDH can evolve slowly. If headache or other symptoms persist, repeat CT or MRI before considering discharge.

SPECIAL CONSIDERATIONS

Delayed EDH (hematoma not present on initial CT, but found on follow-up scan) comprises up to 10% of cases in most series. Theoretical risk factors include rapidly correcting shock, lowering intracranial pressure (either medically or surgically, including evacuating a contralateral hematoma), and coagulopathies. A high index of suspicion is necessary to make the diagnosis.

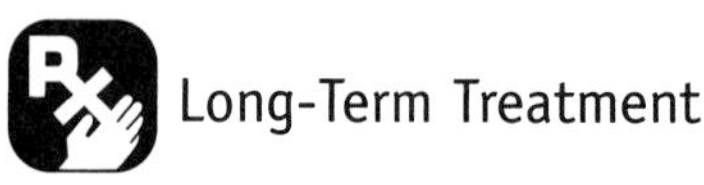

Long-Term Treatment

REHABILITATION

- Physical therapy or occupational therapy as determined by the particular neurological deficit

SURGICAL TREATMENT

- Acute neurosurgical referral as described above
- Any patient with known EDH or SDH who is initially stable but later develops new symptoms suggestive of mass effect, herniation, or increased intracranial pressure should be referred for emergent neurosurgical evaluation.

REFERRAL/DISPOSITION

- Neurosurgical referral for either EDH or SDH as described above
- EDH: in the case of nonsurgical EDH, may be discharged if neurologically stable after 24 hours of observation. Follow-up CT scan in 1 week if stable, then again in 1 to 3 months until documented resolution.
- SDH: because of underlying brain injury, period of observation required before determination of clinical stability may be longer than for EDH. Furthermore, more likely to need rehabilitation or temporary/permanent skilled nursing care.

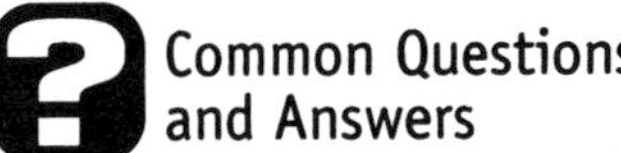

Common Questions and Answers

Physician responses to common patient questions:

Q: What is the mortality rate of EDH and SDH?

A: About 12% for EDH in the era of CT diagnosis, as low as 5% if treated optimally within a few hours. The mortality rate is twice as high if there was no lucid interval, presumably because of associated brain parenchyma injury. SDH has a mortality rate of 50% to 90%. In one series, the mortality rate was as low as 30% if surgery was undertaken within 4 hours of injury, compared with 90% when surgery was delayed for more than 4 hours.

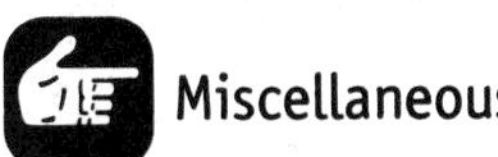

Miscellaneous

SYNONYMS

- For SDH: subdural hemorrhage
- For EDH: epidural hemorrhage, extradural hematoma, extradural hemorrhage

ICD-9 CODE

852.2 Subdural hemorrhage following injury without mention of open intracranial wound
852.3 Subdural hemorrhage following injury with open intracranial wound
852.4 Extradural hemorrhage following injury without mention of open intracranial wound (EDH following injury)
852.5 Extradural hemorrhage following injury with open intracranial wound
Fifth-digit subclassification: 0, unspecified state of consciousness; 1, with no loss of consciousness; 2, with brief (<1 hour) loss of consciousness; 3, with moderate (1–24 hours) loss of consciousness; 4, with prolonged (>24 hours) loss of consciousness and return to preexisting conscious level; 5, with prolonged (>24 hours) loss of consciousness without return to preexisting conscious level; 6, with loss of consciousness of unspecified duration; 9, with concussion, unspecified.

BIBLIOGRAPHY

Domenicucci M, Signorini P, Strzelecke J, et al. Delayed post-traumatic epidural hematoma: a review. *Neurosurg Rev* 1995;18:109–122.

Greenberg M, ed. *Handbook of neurosurgery*, 4th ed. Vols. 1 and 2. Lakeland, FL: Greenberg Graphics, 1997.

Stieg P, Kase C. Intracranial hemorrhage: diagnosis and emergency management. *Neurol Clin* 1998;16:373–390.

Author: Greg Nakamoto

Herniated Nucleus Pulposis

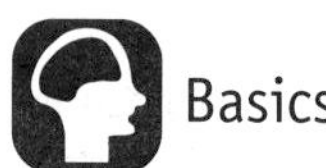

Basics

DEFINITION

Loss of the central content of the intervertebral disc through tears in the surrounding annular fibers by excessive forces or structural degeneration.

ANATOMY

- The intervertebral disc functions as a "shock absorber" to help disseminate flexion, rotational, and compressive forces throughout the spine.
- The nucleus pulposis is composed of an elastic mucopolysaccharide matrix and occupies the central portion of the disc.
- The annulus fibrosis consists of a network of collagen fibers that encircle the outer portion of the disc.
- The outer one third of the annulus contains unmyelinated nerve fibers, whereas the nucleus and inner two thirds of the annulus are essentially anneural.
- Radial or circumferential tears can occur within the annulus, allowing the nucleus pulposis to herniate out from its central position to encroach upon the supportive longitudinal ligaments of the spine, or to enter the central or lateral vertebral foramen.
- In the cervical spine, disc herniation most frequently occurs at the C5–6 and C6–7 levels. In the lumbar spine, L5–S1 and L4–5 levels are most common.
- Discogenic pain can be caused by the compression of nociceptive outer annular fibers or the precipitation of inflammatory peptides within the nucleus.
- Radicular pain can be caused by the impingement of discogenic material against exiting spinal nerves, with weakness or pain presenting in specific dermatomal and myotomal distributions.

INCIDENCE/PREVALENCE

Discogenic pathology has been reported often among athletes, although its actual incidence may be similar to that in the general population.

SIGNS AND SYMPTOMS

- Neck or low back pain with localized paraspinal muscular tenderness or "spasm"
- Radiating pain or paresthesias down the buttock, posterior thigh, and below the level of the knee may indicate a radiculopathy caused by discogenic pathology in the lumbar spine.
- Pain or paresthesias referred from the neck toward the scapular region, shoulder, or distal upper extremities may indicate a radiculopathy in the cervical spine.
- Pain that increases with prolonged sitting, standing, or walking and is relieved in the supine position
- Precipitation of symptoms with coughing, sneezing, or the Valsalva maneuver
- Loss of normal range of motion in the cervical or lumbar spine by muscular guarding
- Weakness in extremity muscles of specific myotomal distributions may indicate nerve root compression by discogenic material. Atrophy present in these muscles suggests significant loss of neural axons.

RISK FACTORS

- Traumatic forces produced by excessive flexion, compression, or rotation of the spine
- Sports such as American football, crew, bowling, baseball, hockey, tennis, diving, wrestling, gymnastics, and weight lifting all contain loading components that can potentially cause disc herniation in the cervical/lumbar spine.

ASSOCIATED INJURIES AND COMPLICATIONS

- Stingers: Transient neuropraxic or axonotmetic injury commonly seen in contact sports such as American football and wrestling
- Burners: Symptoms of unilateral shoulder or arm pain with "burning dysesthesias" often accompanied by arm weakness, which occurs immediately following traumatic contact to the cervical spine
- Cauda equina syndrome: Loss of bowel or bladder function can result in rare cases of large lumbar disc herniations in which multiple, usually bilateral nerve roots of the cauda equina are compressed. Characteristic neurologic deficits of multiple lumbosacral nerve root pathology may be seen along with loss of sphincter tone and saddle anesthesia. Emergent surgical decompression is indicated to minimize nerve root damage.
- Cervical myelopathy: Rarely a cervical disc can herniate posteriorally enough to compress the spinal cord and cause a symptomatic myelopathy. The athlete may complain of leg dysesthesias and weakness in addition to neck symptoms. This is also a surgical emergency.

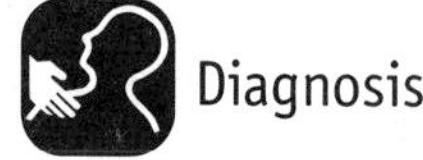

Diagnosis

DIFFERENTIAL DIAGNOSIS

- Cervical/lumbosacral strain: Neck or low back pain of paraspinal musculature or posterior ligamentous origin
- Facet syndrome: Posterior spinal element pain caused by excessive loading of the facet joint capsule or degeneration
- Discitis: Infection within the disc; consider in children presenting with back pain
- Peripheral nerve entrapment or plexus level lesion
- Spondylolysis/stress fracture of the pars intraarticularis: Common in gymnasts and dancers

HISTORY

- Describe your activity the moment you began to experience symptoms.
- Are symptoms worsened by a forward bent posture or prolonged sitting?
- Which positions relieve the symptoms?
- Does the pain radiate into your arms or below your knees?
- Do you have numbness in your buttock region or have you noticed any change in your bowel/bladder functioning?

PHYSICAL EXAM

- Observe gait for compensatory shifting of the trunk to minimize pain with ambulation.
- Palpate paraspinal muscles for tenderness, lateral shift, or spasm. Observe for range of motion restrictions in the cervical/lumbar spine.
- Check for asymmetry or loss of muscle stretch reflexes to the biceps, triceps, brachioradialis, quadriceps, and gastrocnemius muscles. Test sensation of extremity dermatomal patterns and manual muscle strength.
- Neural tension testing of the lower lumbosacral spine can be achieved by utilizing the straight leg raising (SLR) test with the patient in the supine and seated position. A positive SLR test result will usually reproduce radicular symptoms while the leg is raised 20 to 70 degrees above the plane of the table. Localized pain in the posterior thigh produced above 70 degrees may be the result of stretch on tightened hamstring muscles.
- Neural compression testing in the cervical spine can be achieved by using the Spurling's test. This checks for foramenal encroachment upon an inflamed nerve root, and can be performed by extending, laterally flexing, and rotating the cervical spine while performing downward compression upon the head. A positive test result will reproduce symptoms of paresthesias, pain, and numbness distal to the shoulder and arm of the side on which the neck is being laterally flexed.
- Always examine for possible upper motor neuron pathology by checking Babinski's sign, and testing for ankle and upper extremity clonus.

IMAGING

- MRI, because of its resolution in visualizing soft tissue structures, has become the imaging study of choice in detecting intervertebral disc pathology.
- Plain roentgenograms are useful in screening for vertebral body or posterior spinal element pathology, and may occasionally show intervertebral disc space narrowing in cases of discogenic pathology.
- Degenerative changes on radiography and MRI may be found in a high percentage of asymptomatic individuals and does not correlate with pain.
- Electrodiagnostic studies: Needle EMG may be useful in detecting axon loss in radiculopathy caused by disc herniation.
- Discography: Injection of contrast material into the intervertebral disc can show extrusion of content into the spinal canal, identifying tears.

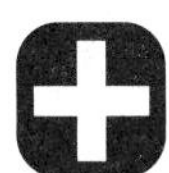

Acute Treatment

MODALITIES

- Ice applied to the cervical or lumbar paraspinal muscles has an analgesic effect and may inhibit reflex muscular spasm.
- Physical medicine modalities such as electrical stimulation, ultrasonography, and hot packs may provide symptomatic relief of pain, but probably do not alter the long-term outcome.

MEDICATIONS

- Nonsteroidal antiinflammatory medications can be used acutely in athletes with discogenic pain to provide analgesia.
- Opiate-based medications may be necessary in the short-term management of severe pain.
- Oral steroids such as prednisone or medrol dosepak have been advocated by many clinicians to help with back pain and inflammation. However, side effects of oral steroids and the lack of controlled studies showing their benefit make this practice controversial.

MANIPULATION/MANUAL MEDICINE

- Frequently used to correct muscle imbalances and spinal segment dysfunctions, may provide symptomatic relief of pain

SPINAL INJECTION

Epidural or selective nerve root injections using a steroid/local anesthetic mixture are frequently used to deliver a small concentration of medication to the site of discogenic pathology to relieve symptoms.

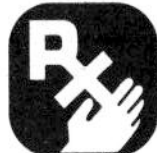

Long-Term Treatment

REHABILITATION

Lumbosacral stabilization exercises or McKenzie exercises are frequently used in cases of discogenic low back pain to strengthen spinal and abdominal musculature and to prevent the spine from moving into "vulnerable" positions that may precipitate symptoms.

SURGICAL TREATMENT

Surgical management of discogenic pathology may be acutely indicated in cases involving progressive neurologic deterioration and in cauda equina syndrome and cervical myelopathy.

Common Questions and Answers

Physician responses to common patient questions:

Q: Should an athlete who sustains frequent "stingers" be precluded from participation in contact sports?

A: Without the presence of "spear tackler's spine," there is no clear evidence to support preclusion from contact sports. However, frequent stingers should warrant a thorough workup for this condition. Technical aspects of the athlete's tackling/contact and other preventive measures should be addressed.

Q: In an athlete who sustains an acute lumber disc herniation, how long should he or she wait before returning to sport?

A: The medical literature is vague on this point. In most cases, the rehabilitation for an acute lumbar disc herniation can begin days following injury. A neurologic examination should be performed frequently following injury, and those with progressive deficits should be referred to a spine surgeon. Those with lower extremity weakness as a result of nerve root injury without progressive deficits should participate in a strengthening program and can return once strength has returned and activity-induced pain has resolved. Exact timing for return to play has to be individualized and depends on neurologic deficits, tolerance of pain, and the risk:benefit ratio of returning.

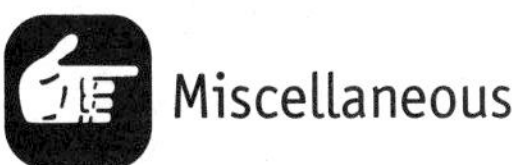

Miscellaneous

ICD-9 CODE

722.0–722.9 Discogenic disease/disc herniation syndrome

BIBLIOGRAPHY

Calliet R. *Low back pain syndrome*. Philadelphia: FA Davis, 1988.

Cannon DT, Aprill CN. Lumbosacral epidural steroid injections. *Arch Phys Med Rehabil* 2000;81(suppl 1):87–99.

Healy JF, Healy BB, Wong WH. Cervical and lumbar MRI in asymptomatic older male. *J Comput Assist Tomogr* 1996;20:107–112.

Authors: Ryan O'Connor and Michael T. Andary

Hip Injury

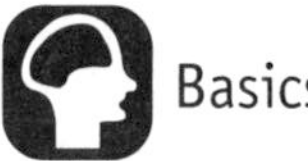

Basics

SIGNS AND SYMPTOMS

- Groin pain, medial knee pain, pain with ambulation/weight-bearing
- History of chronic bone loss or high-impact trauma
- Obvious signs of trauma
  —Deformity or angulation, swelling, open fracture, or missile entrance wound
- Lower extremity held in position of comfort
  —Hip fracture: flexion, abduction, external rotation of hip
  —Posterior hip dislocation: flexion, *adduction, internal rotation* of hip, flexion of knee, hip totally immobile
  —Anterior hip dislocation: flexion, *abduction, external rotation* of hip, thigh shortening due to spasm, hip totally immobile

MECHANISM/DESCRIPTION

- Hip fracture = fracture of proximal femur; classified by
  —Location
  —Displacement and angulation
  —Open or closed, and degree of comminution
  —Arrangement of fracture lines and fragments
- Hip dislocation = disarticulation of femoral head from acetabulum
  —Often coexists with fracture
- Femoral head/neck fracture (intracapsular)
  —Usually elderly patients with bone loss
  —Trauma often minor
  —Patient may or may not be ambulatory.
- Intertrochanteric fracture (extracapsular)
  —Usually elderly patients with bone loss
  —Nonambulatory with significant pain
  —Often due to fall
  —Extremity often shortened
- Subtrochanteric fracture
  —Usually due to direct trauma
  —Common site for pathologic fracture
  —Occasional site of stress fracture in runners and military recruits
  —Extremity may be shortened with noticeable displacement of the proximal fragment.
- Posterior dislocation
  —Often due to MVA in which the knees strike the dashboard
  —Much more common than anterior
- Anterior dislocation
  —Often due to fall or trauma resulting in sudden abduction of thigh

PEDIATRIC CONSIDERATIONS

- Fracture usually requires high-impact trauma.
- Must suspect nonaccidental trauma
- Must consider pathologic fracture if trauma is minor

PRE-HOSPITAL

- Neurovascular exam is essential

CAUTIONS

- DO NOT apply traction
- Monitor closely for development of hemorrhagic shock

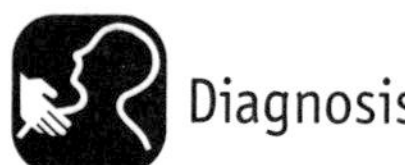

Diagnosis

ESSENTIAL WORKUP

- Radiographs as outlined below
  —Remove splints and clothing prior to taking films
  —A patient with a worrisome exam and negative standard films has a hip fracture until proven otherwise
- Assess distal pulses, palpate compartments, evaluate sensation and motor function
- If pulses are not equal or palpable, bedside Doppler may be necessary
- Search for associated injuries
- In suspected child abuse, obtain skeletal survey or bone scan

LABORATORY

- CBC, type, and screen

IMAGING/SPECIAL TESTS

- Standard films—AP pelvis and true lateral of hip
- AP pelvis with hip internally rotated 15-20° will optimally image the femoral neck
- Pelvic inlet and outlet views may identify associated or symptomatic pubic ramus or acetabular fractures.
- Judet views (oblique films of the hip) aid in the evaluation of the acetabulum.
- CT, MRI, or bone scan if fracture not identified; MRI is preferred
- Joint aspiration +/− arthrogram under fluoroscope if suspect a septic joint, foreign body, or hemarthrosis, especially in GSW to hip

DIFFERENTIAL DIAGNOSIS

- Pubic ramus fracture
- Acetabular fracture
- Septic joint
- Isolated fractures of the greater or lesser trochanters
- Thigh, knee, ankle, or foot injury
- Trochanteric bursitis
- Ileotibial band tendinitis
- Hip contusion

PEDIATRIC CONSIDERATIONS

- Pediatric fracture patterns are different because of the developing cartilaginous components; fracture classification and management are also different.
- Suspect nonaccidental trauma in the absence of an obvious mechanism.
- Be concerned about hip pain that may be due to a separate process (limb-length discrepancy, neuromuscular disorders, neoplastic invasion of bone).

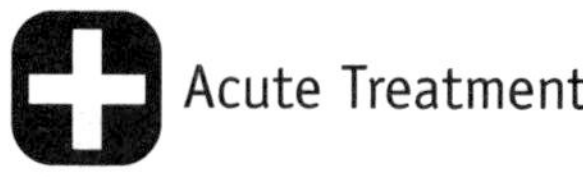

Acute Treatment

INITIAL STABILIZATION

- ABCs of trauma care
- Monitor blood pressure continuously; the thigh can contain 4–6 units of blood.

ED TREATMENT

- Remove splint and clothing; maintain pelvis and hip stability.
- Pain control is essential; parenteral analgesia acceptable in isolated hip injuries.
  —A femoral nerve block can be performed in multiple trauma patients or pediatric patients.
- Orthopedic consultation is necessary for all hip fractures and is emergent in cases of fracture with neurovascular compromise.
- For closed fractures that require internal fixation, give cefazolin within 24 hours prior to operation.
- Open fractures must go directly to the OR for irrigation and debridement.
  —For open fractures with a laceration of >1 cm, extensive soft-tissue injury, or obvious contamination, give cefazolin and gentamicin or tobramycin in the ED, as well as tetanus booster if indicated.
- For injuries with highly contaminated wounds add penicillin G to cover Clostridial species.
- For gunshot wounds to the femur, culture the missile track and cover with an iodine dressing.

Hip Dislocation

- In a true orthopedic emergency, incidence of posttraumatic arthritis increases linearly with time.
- Perform reduction in ED
- Often requires deep sedation or neuromuscular blockade to reduce
- Patients with prior hip arthroplasty may be reduced in the ED with conscious sedation.

MEDICATIONS

- Cefazolin: adult: 2 g IM/IV; peds: 20 mg/kg IM/KG
- Gentamicin/tobramycin: 1.5 mg/kg IV
- Penicillin G: adults: 2 million IU IV; peds: 25,000 IU/kg/day IV divided q 8 hrs

PEDIATRIC CONSIDERATIONS

- Assess markers for nonaccidental trauma
  - —Delay in presentation; history of mechanism inconsistent with the injury
  - —Isolated trauma to the thigh, associated burns, bruises, or linear abrasions
  - —Assess for dislocation of the femoral capital epiphysis

HOSPITAL ADMISSION CRITERIA

- All hip fractures or dislocations
- Septic joint
- Suspicion of occult fracture
- Suspicion of nonaccidental trauma in children

HOSPITAL DISCHARGE CRITERIA

- Hip pain attributable to other cause
- Fracture ruled out (negative radiographs *plus* negative clinical exam)
- Patient with successful reduction of dislocated hip arthroplasty may be considered for discharge in consultation with orthopedics and with appropriate follow-up arranged.

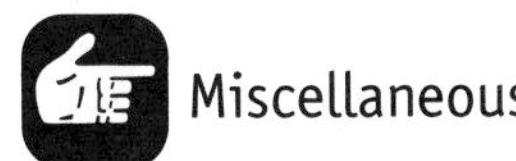

Miscellaneous

ICD-9-CM

959.6

CORE CONTENT CODE

18.4.13.1.8

BIBLIOGRAPHY

Hughes L, Beaty J. Fractures of the head and neck of the femur in children. *J Bone Joint Surg* 1994;76A(2):283–292.

Long W, et al. Management of civilian gunshot injuries to the hip. *Orthop Clin North Am* 1995;26(1):123–131.

Lyons R. Clinical outcomes and treatment of hip fractures. *Am J Med* 1997;103(2A): 51S–64S.

Zuckerman J. Hip fracture. *N Engl J Med* 1996;334(23):1519–1525.

Author: Chris Ho

Hip Pointer

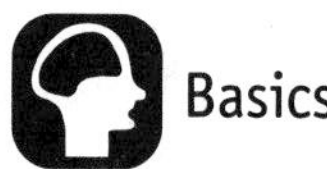

Basics

DEFINITION

- Contusion to the iliac crest

INCIDENCE/PREVALENCE

- Most common in contact/collision sports such as football, wrestling, soccer, and lacrosse

SIGNS AND SYMPTOMS

- Acute, severe pain at the site of contusion
- Athlete usually not able to continue activity
- Posture often flexed to side of injury

RISK FACTORS

- Collision sports
- Inadequate iliac crest protection

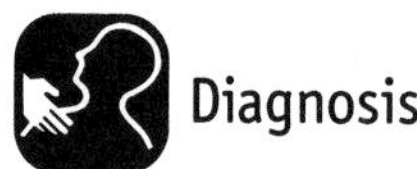

Diagnosis

DIFFERENTIAL DIAGNOSIS

- Compression fracture to iliac crest
- Avulsion fracture of anterior superior iliac spine
- Intraabdominal injury

HISTORY

- Direct blow to the iliac crest

PHYSICAL EXAM

- Inspect for swelling, deformity, or ecchymosis
- Tenderness to palpation over iliac crest
- Abdominal exam may reveal muscle spasm but should not be tender to palpation.
- Weakness and pain with active abdominal muscle and/or hip flexor contraction

IMAGING

- Plain radiographs to rule out fracture
- Oblique views may be helpful.

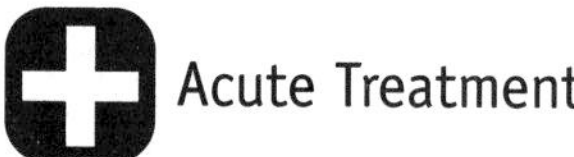

Acute Treatment

ANALGESIA

- Narcotics such as codeine may be appropriate for first 48 to 72 hours.
- Nonsteroidal antiinflammatory drugs indicated at onset until resolution
- Some clinicians prefer to give corticosteroid burst to decrease symptoms.
- Modalities per certified athletic trainer or physical therapist in acute phase
- Ice three to four times daily in acute phase

SPECIAL CONSIDERATIONS

- Crutches for partial or non-weight bearing may be necessary for first few days of treatment.
- Some clinicians prefer to inject with local anesthetic and corticosteroid to decrease symptoms and speed recovery; increases risk of infection and bleeding

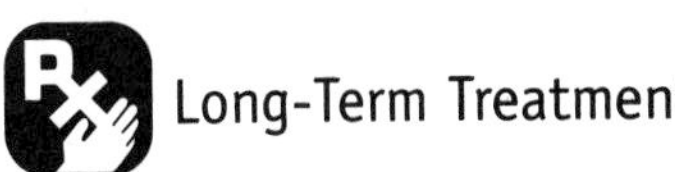

Long-Term Treatment

REHABILITATION

- Gentle abdominal and hip stretching when tolerated
- Gradual abdominal and hip strengthening
- Progressive functional activity
- Protection with padding upon return to play

REFERRAL/DISPOSITION

- For evidence of intraabdominal trauma or displaced iliac crest fracture

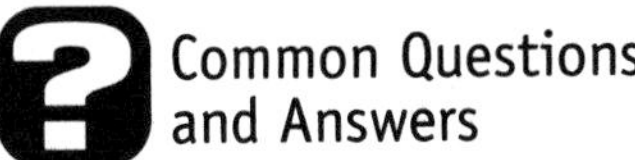

Common Questions and Answers

Physician responses to common patient questions:

Q: When can the athlete play?

A: Return to play can take place when there is minimal to no tenderness at the contusion site, near normal or normal abdominal and hip muscle strength, and adequate protection/padding.

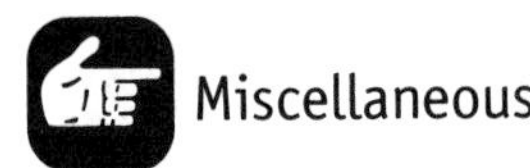

Miscellaneous

SYNONYMS

- Bruised hip or contusion

ICD-9 CODE

924.01

BIBLIOGRAPHY

Garrick JG, Webb DR. *Sports injuries diagnosis and treatment*. Philadelphia: WB Saunders, 1999.

Mellion MB, ed. *Sports medicine secrets*. Philadelphia: Hanley & Belfus, 1999.

Author: Andrew Tucker

Iliotibial Band Friction Syndrome

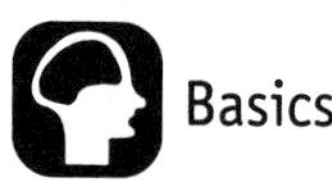

Basics

DEFINITION

- Iliotibial band friction syndrome (ITBFS) is an overuse tendinitis or bursitis that occurs when the posterior edge of the ITB impinges against the lateral epicondyle.
- Pain occurs after foot strike in the gait cycle, usually at about 30 degrees of knee flexion.
- Leads to inflammation in the tendon and/or the bursa that lies between the tendon and lateral epicondyle

INCIDENCE/PREVALENCE

- Incidence as high as 12% of all running-related overuse injuries
- Second most common running injury to patellofemoral syndrome

SIGNS AND SYMPTOMS

- Lateral knee pain made worse with running
- Pain with ascending and descending stairs
- Stiff-legged walking in advanced cases

RISK FACTORS

- Extrinsic: runners with less experience, higher mileage, off-cambered courses, improper training, downhill running
- Intrinsic: over-pronators, lean individuals with less fat and connective tissue between the band and femoral condyle, genu/tibial varum, leg length differences

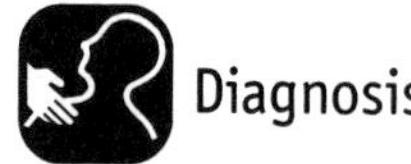

Diagnosis

DIFFERENTIAL DIAGNOSIS

- Patellofemoral syndrome
- Lateral meniscal damage
- Degenerative joint disease
- Lateral collateral ligament sprain
- Popliteal or biceps femoris tendinitis
- Peroneal nerve injury
- Gout and other metabolic arthritides
- Referred pain

HISTORY

- What sports are you involved in? Sports that require continuous running or repetitive knee flexion (i.e., bicycling) predispose to ITBFS.
- Did the pain start suddenly? Pain from ITBFS usually starts as a minor discomfort and becomes progressively worse.
- Was there trauma involved? ITBFS is usually an overuse injury not associated with trauma.
- When does the pain start? Often the patient starts exercising without pain, which then develops at a predictable distance.
- Have you changed your training recently? Large increases in distance and increased running on cambered surfaces or hills increase the likelihood of ITBFS.

PHYSICAL EXAM

- Extensive musculoskeletal exam with particular attention to the lower extremities
- Evaluate iliac crests and leg length. Discrepancies of leg length cause tightening ITB, causing more friction.
- Evaluate femur/tibia angles. Genu varum tightens the ITB, predisposing to ITBFS.
- Feet and footwear should be closely evaluated. Excessive pronation and cavus feet cause internal rotation of the tibia and predispose to ITBFS. Footwear can give clues as to pronation pattern.
- Flex the knee to 30 degrees and palpate over the lateral femoral condyle. Palpation will cause pain especially over the lateral joint line, lateral femoral condyle, Gerde's tibial tubercle, and occasionally over the head of the fibula.
- Perform Obers test. Position patient on unaffected side with the involved knee in 90 degrees of flexion. The leg is abducted at the hip and the examiner then grasps the ankle allowing the knee to return to an adducted position. A person with ITBFS remains abducted due to a contracture of the ITB.
- Perform Malacrea's test. As the patient lies on the unaffected side with the involved leg abducted, varus stress is applied to the ankle as the knee is flexed from 0 to 45 degrees. A positive test result reproduces the ITBFS pain.

IMAGING

- Generally not needed except to rule out other disease processes

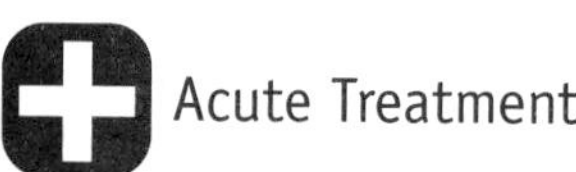

Acute Treatment

ANALGESIA

- Appropriate doses of nonsteroidal antiinflammatory drugs along with modalities including ice, ultrasonography, and electrical stimulation

IMMOBILIZATION

Relative rest is very important, but no forms of immobilization are used.

SPECIAL CONSIDERATIONS

Steroid injections can be considered after appropriate interventions are used.

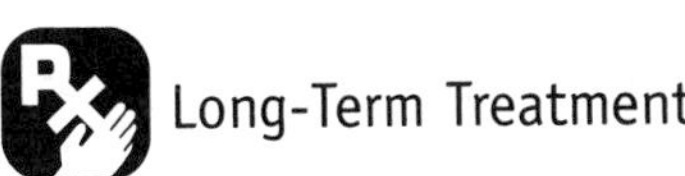

Long-Term Treatment

REHABILITATION

- Physical therapy with the use of modalities may improve symptoms.
- An aggressive stretching and strengthening program targeting the ITB and the muscles attached
- Goals are to restore range of motion and improve flexibility while increasing strength.

SURGICAL TREATMENT

- Only after exhaustive nonoperative therapy
- Procedures involve decreasing impingement on the femoral condyle by a release of a portion of the posterior ITB.

REFERRAL/DISPOSITION

If no improvement is seen after extensive therapy and training modification, then referral to an orthopedic surgeon is warranted.

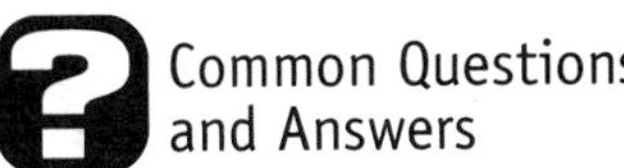

Common Questions and Answers

Physician responses to common patient questions:
Q: When can I return to sport/activity?
A: An attempt to return too early with pain can result in significant delay. Activity can be resumed when symptoms have improved nearly 100% or have resolved. Earlier return can be accomplished using non-weight-bearing activities such as swimming or running in the deep end of a pool. Return should be gradual with gentle buildup on level ground progressing in distance/resistance and elevation.
Q: How long will I have pain?
A: Most patients recover in about 6 weeks and are able to resume full activity at that time.
Q: How can I prevent ITBFS?
A: Maintain flexibility with adequate warmup periods and stretching before and after exercise.

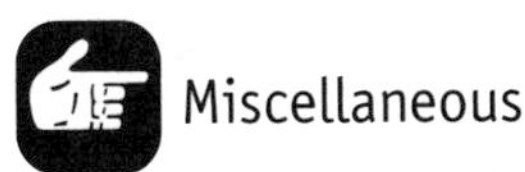

Miscellaneous

SYNONYMS

- Iliotibial band tendinitis

ICD-9 CODE

728.89 Iliotibial band friction syndrome

BIBLIOGRAPHY

Fredericson M, Guillet M, DeBenedictis L. Quick solutions for iliotibial band syndrome. *Phys Sports Med* 2000;28:120–122.

Orchard J, Fricker P, Abud A, et al. Biomechanics of iliotibial band friction syndrome in runners. *Am J Sports Med* 1996;24:375–379.

Reid D. *Sports injury assessment and rehabilitation*. New York: Churchill Livingstone, 1992.

Author: Andrew Dahlgren

Impingement, Subacromial Bursitis and Rotator Cuff Tendinitis

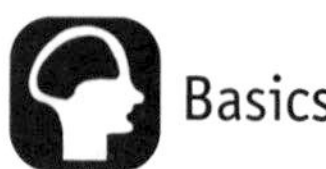

Basics

DEFINITION

Repetitive shoulder activity causes breakdown in the cuff muscles from tensile overload and results in tendinitis. Weakness in the rotator cuff muscles (supraspinatus, infraspinatus, teres minor, or subscapularis) results in loss of effective dynamic glenohumeral movement. This causes impingement of the cuff muscles under the acromion, enhancing the pain and inflammation.

INCIDENCE/PREVALENCE

- Very common in athletes, especially in those with repetitive motion of the arms (i.e., throwing, racquet sports, swimming, weight lifting)
- In individuals under 25 years of age, impingement is usually related to laxity caused by instability.
- In those 25 to 40 years of age, impingement is usually due to overuse of the rotator cuff.
- In those over 40 years of age, impingement is caused by use of the cuff muscles over threshold. This may result in partial or full-thickness tears, in addition to impingement.

SIGNS AND SYMPTOMS

- Shoulder pain with overhead activity
- Weakness in the shoulder musculature
- Crepitations
- Numbness/paresthesias (usually between the lateral neck to the elbow)
- Night pain
- Pain at rest (usually in more severe cases)

RISK FACTORS

- Weight lifting (olympic-style)
- Throwing or racquet sports
- Swimming
- "Industrial" athletics (repetitive, overhead motion)
- Shoulder instability
- Previous shoulder surgery or trauma
- Individuals with more "hooked" acromiums (type III > type II > type I)

ASSOCIATED INJURIES AND COMPLICATIONS

- Rotator cuff tear (partial or full)
- Adhesive capsulitis
- Thoracic outlet syndrome
- Brachial plexus injury
- Axillary nerve entrapment
- Pancoast tumor

Diagnosis

DIFFERENTIAL DIAGNOSIS

- Rotator cuff tear (partial- or full-thickness)
- Adhesive capsulitis
- Acromioclavicular sprain/injury
- Labral tear
- Bicipital tendonitis
- Thoracic outlet syndrome
- Brachial plexus injury
- Fracture: clavicle, humerus, scapula
- Subluxation of glenohumeral joint
- Axillary nerve entrapment
- Pancoast tumor
- Bankhart lesion (avulsion fracture of glenoid)
- Hill-Sacks lesion (impact fracture of humeral head)

HISTORY

- First rule out cervical spine disease, neck pain.
- Symptoms: weakness, crepitation, numbness, "slipped out," night pain, dead arm
- Exacerbation: pain presents more at rest or with activity
- Duration: chronic (overuse) versus acute (traumatic)
- Activation: right or left handed, type of job, sports, hobby
- History of previous trauma or surgery

PHYSICAL EXAM

Observation

- How the athlete carries arm/shoulder (i.e., recent dislocation, guarding)
- Deltoid atrophy (i.e., C5 plexus injury)
- Scapular winging (i.e., long thoracic nerve palsy)
- Infraspinatus fossa scalloping (inferior branch of the suprascapular nerve)

Palpation

- Cervical spinous process: rule out cervical neck pathology as cause of shoulder pain
- Subacromial bursa: distal to acromion
- Biceps tendon (long head)/bicipital groove
- Insertion of the deltoid on the humerus: pain at site but no pain with palpation; axillary nerve pain referral site
- Coracoid process: pain referral site for impingement

Range of Motion (ROM)

1. Abduction (0–180 degrees)
2. Adduction (0–50 degrees)
3. Flexion: forward (0–180 degrees) and horizontal (0–130 degrees)
4. Extension (0–90 degrees)
5. Internal rotation (0–100 degrees) (adduction and internal rotation: "bra strap")
6. External rotation (0-60 degrees) (abduction and external rotation:"shampoo hair")

Manual Muscle Testing

- Deltoid: full abduction, resist at 90 degrees
- Supraspinatus: abduction to 90 degrees, 30 degrees forward flexion, resist downward pressure
- Infraspinatus and teres minor: arm at side, 90 degrees at elbow, resist external rotation (i.e. "opening the door")
- Subscapularis: hand behind back, push-off; Gerber's lift-off test

Special Tests

- Hawkin's test: 90 degrees of forward flexion at the shoulder and elbow, support elbow, pain with internal rotation of arm
- Neer's test: arm straight, thumb down, passive forward flexion (pain at 60–120 degrees).
- Arc test: shoulder abduction, gets "stuck" or painful at 60–120 degrees
- Impingement test: inject subacromial bursa with lidocaine, helps differentiate between impingement and tear; after injection, pain, ROM, and strength should improve if impingement and not a tear
- Drop arm test: patient cannot hold arm at 90 degrees of abduction, indicates cuff tear
- Speed's test: arm straight, forward flexion to 90 degrees, palm up, resisted downward pressure, palpate the bicipital tendon at groove; pain indicates bicipital tendonitis
- Yergason's test: elbow at 90 degrees, forearm pronated, hold patient's wrist and direct patient to actively supinate/flex against resistance; picks up subluxing long head of biceps tendon out of groove

IMAGING

Imaging is often not needed in light of good history and physical exam and a straightforward case.

Radiography

- Anteroposterior (AP) view and axillary (trans-scapular) views bare minimum to order. Radiographs helpful for acute injuries to rule out fractures, dislocations. With impingement, may be helpful to get additional views.
- Internal and external AP rotational views help visualize humerus (i.e., Hill-Sacks lesions).
- Stryker notch view helps visualize posterolateral humeral head deformity (i.e., Hill-Sacks lesions).
- West Point (modified axillary) view allows visualization of the anterior/inferior glenoid (i.e., Bankhart lesions).

- Outlet or Alexander view allows for visualization of subacromial space; helpful in elderly patients with severe impingement.
- Calcification on the tendon is associated with bicipital tendonitis or severe impingement.

MRI

In severe or confusing cases, MRI is helpful in diagnosis of rotator cuff tears, labrum tears, biceps tendon rupture. An MRI arthrogram is often useful to further displace a torn labrum, thus improving visualization of the anatomy.

Arthrography

Arthrography is used in adhesive capsulitis to show decreased volume, and is helpful in diagnosing labral tears. It is often an uncomfortable procedure for the patient.

Electromyography/Nerve Conduction Study

- Helpful if there is weakness in addition to an altered neurologic exam (sensation, reflexes) etc.; has the highest sensitivity when symptoms have persisted >3 weeks

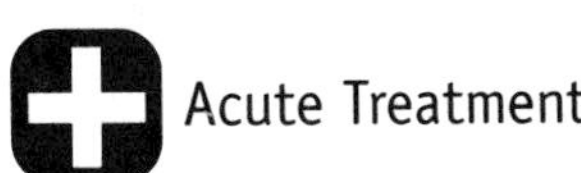

Acute Treatment

ANALGESIA

- Nonsteroidal antiinflammatory drugs, acetaminophen; in severe cases, short-term pain relief with narcotics
- Prednisone, oral: short-course of 40 mg daily for 5 days
- Subacromial bursa injection (5–10 mL 1:1:1 mixture of lidocaine/marcaine/corticosteroid; use a 22- to 25-gauge, 1.5-inch long needle)

MANAGEMENT

- Relative rest: decrease use of affected shoulder
- Home exercise program (HEP): exercise done daily, three sets per exercise
- ROM: Dangling arm circles, finger wall-walking, broom-handle exercises
- Strengthening: Sword-from-sheath exercises, posterior dumbbell raises, proprioceptive neuromuscular facilitation, scapular stabilizing exercises using light weights or flexible elastic cords.

SPECIAL CONSIDERATIONS

- In the younger athlete, impingement is often due to another underlying problem (i.e., instability).
- Certain athletes (i.e., mentally challenged, unmotivated, etc.) may need assistance of formal physical therapy without a trial of HEP.

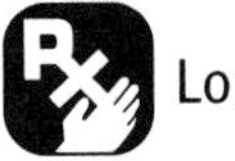

Long-Term Treatment

REHABILITATION

- Formal physical therapy: pain relief via contrast baths, hydroculator, ultrasonography, ice, mobilization/manipulation
- ROM strengthening: deltoid, rotator cuff musculature, scapular stabilizers, biceps
- ROM flexibility: biceps, triceps, glenohumeral joint
- Trans-membrane corticosteroid: (i.e., phonophoresis, iontophoresis)
- Return to normal function
- Sports-specific retraining

SURGICAL TREATMENT

- Anterior acromioplasty: the acromium is "shaved" to allow more space for the rotator cuff. It is used only if conservative measures fail. There is a less favorable outcome in younger (50% success rate) than older athletes.
- Surgical debridement of rotator cuff: often accompanies an anterior acromioplasty

REFERRAL/DISPOSITION

- Presence of a fever and a tense joint capsule (i.e., a potentially septic joint)
- Severe disease that is refractory to physical therapy, modalities and steroid injections
- Rotator cuff tear, full-thickness
- Extra cervical rib, causing shoulder symptoms

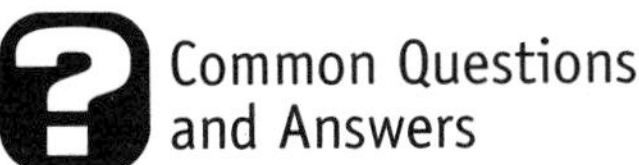

Common Questions and Answers

Physician responses to common patient questions:

Q: Will I ever be able to return to my sport?
A: If caught early with no other shoulder pathology and treated with aggressive conservative therapy, many athletes are able to return to their prior level of competition.
Q: How soon will my shoulder stop hurting after a cortisone injection?
A: Often pain relief is immediate, due to the analgesia. This will wear off.
Q: Because my shoulder impingement is severe, will I need surgery?
A: If no other shoulder pathology is present, and treated with aggressive conservative therapy, most athletes respond and avoid surgery.

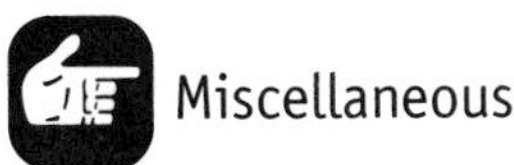

Miscellaneous

SYNONYMS

- Calcific tendonitis of the shoulder
- Subacromial bursitis
- Shoulder impingement syndrome

ICD-9 CODE

726.10 Rotator cuff syndrome (not otherwise specified)
726.11 Calcifying tendonitis, shoulder
726.20 Impingement, shoulder
726.12 Bicipital tenosynovitis

BIBLIOGRAPHY

Arroyo JS, Hershon SJ, Bigliani LU. Special considerations in the athletic throwing shoulder. *Orthop Clin North Am* 1997;28:69–78.

DeLee JC, Drez D, eds. *Orthopedic sports medicine, principles and practice*. Philadelphia: WB Saunders, 1994.

Norberg FB, Field LD, Savoie FH. Repair of the rotator cuff: mini-open and arthroscopic repairs. *Clin Sports Med* 1994;19:77–100.

Sigman SA, Richmond JC. Diagnosing shoulder injuries. *Phys Sports Med* 2000;23:25–34.

Staheli L, ed. *Fundamentals of pediatric orthopedics*, 2nd ed. Philadelphia: Lippincott-Raven, 1998.

Tucker AM. Approach to the athlete with shoulder problems. Personal communication, 1997.

Author: Mark Lavallee

Instability, Anterior

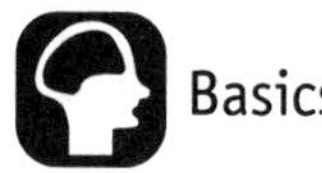

Basics

DEFINITION

- A recurrent symptomatic anteroinferior subluxation or dislocation of the glenohumeral (GH) joint

INCIDENCE/PREVALENCE

- The most dislocated joint in the body. In a study of 8,056 dislocations 45% involved the GH joint.
- Anterior dislocations are the most common. In a study of 394 shoulder dislocations and separations, 84% were anterior GH dislocations.
- Recurrence rate for athletes under age 25 is over 85%.

SIGNS AND SYMPTOMS

Patients complain of pain and the feeling of impending dislocation with the arm in a provocative position.

RISK FACTORS

- History of previous dislocation
- Younger patients
- Athletes participating in repetitive overhead activities such as throwing or volleyball

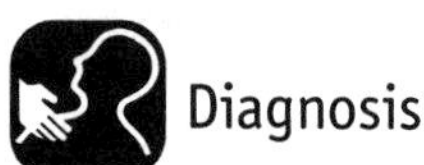

Diagnosis

DIFFERENTIAL DIAGNOSIS

- Diagnoses that can mimic anterior instability include multidirectional instability, acromioclavicular instability, superior labral anterior posterior (SLAP) lesions, biceps tendon subluxation, and subscapularis tear.
- One should always rule out referred pain from the cervical spine.

HISTORY

- Patients usually give a history of prior dislocation or subluxation. The symptoms will be reported to occur when the arm is placed in the provocative position of extreme abduction and external rotation.
- Patients also may complain of a "dead arm" that occurs with subluxation.

PHYSICAL EXAM

- A thorough exam of the cervical spine, proximal humerus, and scapula should be performed when evaluating anyone with shoulder pain. If multidirectional instability is suspected an assessment of ligamentous laxity should addressed. A complete neurologic exam should be performed to identify any central or peripheral neuropathy.
- Apprehension test: Arm is placed at 90 degrees abduction and 90 degrees external rotation. Patient is asked to rotate the arm internally. A feeling of pain or subluxation is a positive test result.
- Relocation Test: With the patient supine, the apprehension test is repeated. A posteriorly directed force is applied to the humerus. If symptoms abate, the test result is positive.
- Sulcus sign: Patient is seated while a caudal traction force is applied to the arm. A subacromial sulcus of more than 2 cm or contralateral asymmetry is a positive test result for inferior instability.
- Load and shift test: The patient is seated while the examiner loads the humerus into the glenoid and then attempts to sublux the head anteriorly.

IMAGING

- Imaging studies should be used only as a supplement. The diagnosis of instability is made by the history and physical exam.
- Radiography: The initial series includes an anteroposterior (AP), true AP (best to evaluate articular surfaces), axillary lateral (best to identify articular incongruity), and scapular Y. Additional views include the Westpoint view (good for identifying a bony Bankart/anteroinferior glenoid rim fracture) and Stryker notch view (good for identifying a Hill-Sachs lesion/ posterolateral humeral head compression fracture).
- MRI: This test is usually noncontributory. Because of the normal variation of the labrum and GH ligaments, most studies overestimate the frequency of labral tears. MRI can identify rotator cuff tears, biceps abnormalities, and occasionally lesions associated with humeral avulsion of the GH ligament.
- Postreduction views are necessary for the acute treatment of a shoulder dislocation.

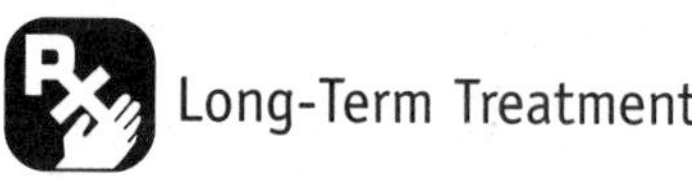

Long-Term Treatment

REHABILITATION

- Early treatment consists of brief immobilization followed by early range of motion and strengthening.
- Rotator cuff strengthening: Initial strengthening should begin in the plane of the scapula. Internal and external rotation exercises are begun at the side. When apprehension subsides, overhead strengthening begins.
- Scapular stabilization: Exercises include rowing, push-ups with maximal protraction, scaption (elevation of the humerus in external rotation in the scapular plane), and press-ups.

SURGICAL TREATMENT

- Absolute indications for surgery include more than three dislocations per year, dislocation at rest, or failed nonoperative therapy.
- Relative indications for surgery include first-time dislocations in young (<30 years) athletes or laborers.
- Surgical technique: Repair the traumatic lesion by reattaching the torn labrum and GH ligaments. Avoid restriction of motion by not overtightening the capsule.
- Arthroscopic stabilization: Has advantage of easier postoperative rehabilitation and less restriction of motion secondary to scarring. Has disadvantage of a higher recurrence rate of 12%. To reduce rate of recurrence, capsular laxity must be addressed with either capsular imbrication or thermal capsulorrhaphy.
- Open stabilization (Bankart procedure): Has more successful outcome, with recurrence rates of less than 5%. Has the disadvantage of slowed rehabilitation secondary to injury to the subscapularis tendon.

REFERRAL/DISPOSITION

Any recurrent dislocator or young, athletic, first-time dislocator should be sent to an orthopedic surgeon for evaluation. Any patient failing nonoperative modalities should also be referred.

Common Questions and Answers

Physician responses to common questions:
Q: Do I need surgery?
A: In general, surgery is required only when physical therapy has failed. Most young patients (<30 years) require surgical intervention.
Q: Is arthroscopic surgery better than an open procedure?
A: In the hands of a good arthroscopist with experience in shoulder stabilizations, the success rates have probably improved beyond previously reported rates of 85%. The open procedure is still the gold standard with a success rate of 95%.

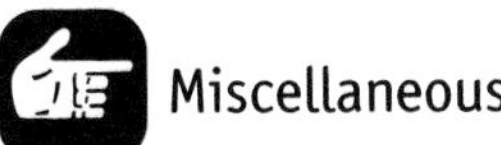

Miscellaneous

SYNONYMS

- Glenohumeral dislocation
- Glenohumeral subluxation
- Dead-arm syndrome

ICD-9 CODE

718.81 Instability
831.0 Dislocation

BIBLIOGRAPHY

Bankart AS. Recurrent or habitual dislocation of the shoulder. *BMJ* 1923;2:1132–1133.

Cave EF, Burke JF, Boyd RJ. *Trauma management*. Chicago: Year Book Medical, 1974.

Jobe FW, ed. *Operative techniques in upper extremity sports injury*. St. Louis: Mosby Year Book, 1996.

Kazar B, Relovszky E. Prognosis of primary dislocation of the shoulder. *Acta Orthop Scand* 1969;40:216–224.

Matthews LS, Pavlovich LJ. *Disorders of the shoulder: diagnosis and management*. Philadelphia: Lippincott Williams & Wilkins, 1999.

Nevaiser RJ, Nevaiser TJ, Nevaiser JS. Anterior dislocation of the shoulder and rotator cuff. *Clin Orthop* 1993;291:103–106.

Rowe CR, Patel D, Southmayd WW. The Bankart procedure. *J Bone Joint Surg [Am]* 1978;60:1–16.

Authors: Andrew R. Curran, Arnold D. Scheller Jr., and Glen Ross

Instability, Multidirectional

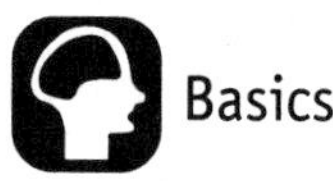

Basics

DEFINITION

- Multidirectional instability (MDI) is the increase of glenohumeral translation in more than one direction causing either dislocation (complete loss of glenohumeral articulation) or subluxation (partial loss) anteriorly, inferiorly or posteriorly.
- Laxity objectively describes the extent to which the humeral head can be translated on the glenoid without symptoms.
- Hallmark pathology of MDI is a large, patulous inferior capsular.

INCIDENCE/PREVALENCE

- Multidirectional instability is much more common than previously realized, but still represents less than 5% of all shoulder instability.
- Most patients are in their third decade of life, but range in age from teenagers to middle age.

SIGNS AND SYMPTOMS

- Most common complaint is vague pain often radiating to the deltoid insertion, initially occurring after activity and progressing to pain at rest, and in late stages may develop to night pain
- May complain of transient neurologic symptoms, such as numbness ("dead arm") or tingling due to transient subluxation
- May also complain of rotator cuff weakness or that shoulder "slips out" of joint
- Inferior instability: pain while carrying briefcase or heavy suitcase
- Posterior instability: pain while arm in forward flexed, internally rotated position (e.g., pushing open a heavy door or during pull-through phase of rowing stroke)
- Anterior instability: pain with arm in overhead, abducted, externally rotated position (e.g., during wind-up or early acceleration of a throw)

RISK FACTORS

- Repetitive microtrauma (especially overhead motion): butterfly and backstroke swimmers, gymnasts, baseball pitchers, and weight lifters
- Generalized ligamentous hyperlaxity

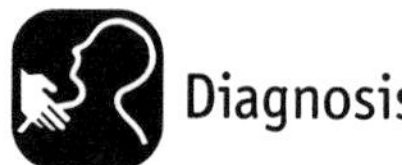

Diagnosis

DIFFERENTIAL DIAGNOSIS

- Unilateral instability (anterior or posterior)
- Acute dislocation or subluxation
- Primary impingement (especially in a young patient)
- Cervical disc disease
- Brachial plexitis
- Thoracic outlet syndrome
- Voluntary dislocator

HISTORY

- Low- versus high energy trauma? MDI is associated with recurrent or trivial trauma.
- Unilateral versus bilateral shoulder problems? 30% to 70% of patients with MDI have symptoms in the opposite shoulder.
- Did the shoulder go back in place on its own or was it put back in place? With MDI after an acute dislocation the shoulder usually reduces spontaneously or is self-reduced.
- Previous shoulder surgery? Previous unsuccessful repair for presumed unilateral instability may indicate MDI.
- Can you dislocate the shoulder voluntarily? Patients with emotional problems who purposely cause repeated dislocation will not benefit from surgery until their emotional problems are resolved. But patients who dislocate voluntarily and do not have emotional problems could benefit from surgery.

PHYSICAL EXAM

- Often general ligamentous laxity is present (e.g., thumb to forearm), elbow hyperextension, metacarpo-phalangeal joint hyperextension, genu recurvatum, patellofemoral subluxation (40%–70%)
- Sulcus test involves inferior traction on the arm while at the side. Inferior translation of at least 1 to 2 cm causing anterior soft tissue dimple (positive sulcus sign) indicates inferior instability and is highly suggestive of MDI.
- Anterior and posterior load and shift and/or drawer tests usually result in anterior and posterior displacement without popping.
- Cervical range of motion, upper extremity strength, sensory function (including axillary nerve), and reflexes should be evaluated.
- Muscle guarding may make the examination difficult, and multiple repeat exams are often necessary.

IMAGING

- MDI is a clinical diagnosis based on the history and physical exam, but plain films at 90 degrees to one another should be obtained to document uncommon bony lesions such as Bankhart and Hill-Sachs lesions and glenoid dysplasia.
- Anteroposterior in internal rotation (Styker notch): humeral head shifted medially on glenoid; generally normal but may show Bankhart lesion or reactive bone
- Axillary view: good to rule out posterior dislocation, also better visualization of Bankhart and Hill-Sachs lesions and glenoid and humeral neck fractures; requires some glenohumeral manipulation
- West Point (reverse axillary lateral): good to evaluate anterior instability because it provides good visualization of the glenoid rim.
- Weight-bearing traction films should show inferior laxity
- Sophisticated imagery is usually not necessary, but if the diagnosis is in doubt, double-contrast CT arthrography may show increased capsular volume. MRI is expensive and cannot diagnose MDI but can rule out other pathology.

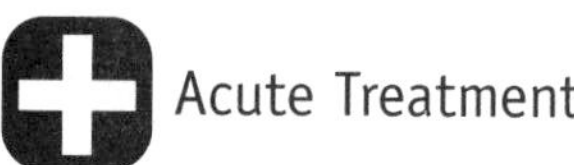

Acute Treatment

ANALGESIA

Nonsteroidal antiinflammatory drugs can decrease pain and inflammation, but analgesic usually is not necessary.

REDUCTION TECHNIQUES

Usually spontaneously reduce or self reduce; see anterior and posterior shoulder dislocation for specific reduction techniques

IMMOBILIZATION

- Usually immobilize with a sling for 3 weeks for acute, first-time dislocator, although there is no demonstrated association between length of immobilization and recurrence.
- Immobilization for recurrent dislocators is of less value, although some authorities suggest immobilization for each occurrence.
- Use caution in immobilizing older patients who are more likely to develop joint stiffness.

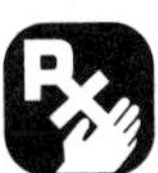

Long-Term Treatment

REHABILITATION

- First-line treatment is prolonged course of physical therapy with emphasis on strengthening deltoid and rotator cuff muscles for at least 6 months and probably up to 1 year. Symptomatic relief is gradual.
- If patient is pain free after 6 months, prior activity may be resumed.
- May develop secondary impingement syndrome, which can be relieved by a subacromial injection of a steroid preparation if necessary to allow continuation of physical therapy
- May need to change prior activity (i.e., a butterfly stroke swimmer may need to choose a different stroke or a pitcher may need to change his delivery)

SURGICAL TREATMENT

- Surgery is indicated only for symptomatic, painful shoulders after the patient fails aggressive, prolonged physical therapy (usually at least 6 months).
- Laxity alone is not an indication for surgery.
- Some authorities advocate earlier surgery if there is a documented glenohumeral ligament avulsion on double-contrast CT or MRI.
- Neer et al. described the open inferior capsular shift repair technique with good success in 1974, and it is now the standard surgical intervention for MDI.
- Recently, there have been reports of glenoid osteotomy and arthroscopic inferior capsular shift repairs, both with comparable success rates, but to date the literature is sparse. Also capsular shrinkage procedures have gained popularity, but again data are lacking.

REFERRAL/DISPOSITION

- Most patients with MDI should be referred for physical therapy. Those patients who fail physical therapy can be referred to an orthopedist for consideration of surgical treatment.
- Asymptomatic, pain-free voluntary dislocators with emotional problems who purposely dislocate their shoulder repeatedly for shock value do not benefit from surgery and may need a psychiatric referral.

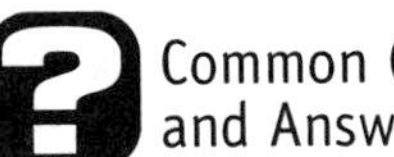

Common Questions and Answers

Physician responses to common patient questions:
Q: When can I play again?
A: Regardless of whether the treatment is conservative physical therapy or surgery, the time until resumption of full sports is generally 6 months. If surgery is required, then postoperative immobilization with a sling is typically for 3 to 6 weeks, with early supervised range of motion exercises. Light sports and throwing can start at about 4 months postsurgery if strength is at least 90% and full range of motion is achieved.
Q: Will I need surgery on my other shoulder?
A: About 10% to 13% of patients require bilateral surgical repair.

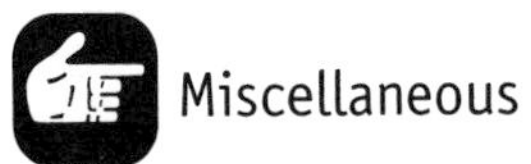

Miscellaneous

ICD-9 CODE

726.19 Shoulder, ligament or muscle instability
718.81 Shoulder, joint instability

BIBLIOGRAPHY

Foster CR. Multidirectional instability of the shoulder in the athlete. *Clin Sports Med* 1983;2:355–367.

Mahaffey BL, Smith PA. Shoulder instability in young athletes. *Am Family Physician* 1999;59:2773–2782.

Schenck TJ, Brems JJ. Multidirectional instability of the shoulder: pathophysiology, diagnosis, and management. *J Am Acad Orthop Surg* 1998;6:65–73.

Yamaguchi K, Flatow EL. Management of multidirectional instability. *Clin Sports Med* 1995;14:885–903.

Authors: David Bazzo and Jason Bryant

Intermetatarsal (Morton's) Neuroma

Basics

DEFINITION

Intermetatarsal or interdigital (Morton's) neuroma is characterized by perineural fibrosis of the common digital nerve as it passes between the metatarsal heads. A neuroma is a benign neoplasm of the nerve secondary to abnormal pressure or repetitive trauma.

INCIDENCE/PREVALENCE

- This condition has a female:male ratio of 5:1.
- It is most common between the second and third intermetatarsal spaces of athletes.
- Neuromas in the first or fourth intermetatarsal spaces are rare, but they can occur.

SIGNS AND SYMPTOMS

- Plantar pain in the forefoot is the most common presenting complaint.
- Some athletes complain of severe burning pain accentuated by activity.
- Other athletes state that it feels like the sock is wadded up in the shoe, causing them to take the shoe off and rub the foot so that the burning, numbness, and "pins and needles" will go away.
- Night pain is rare.
- Symptoms are aggravated by wearing high heels and tight-fitting shoes.

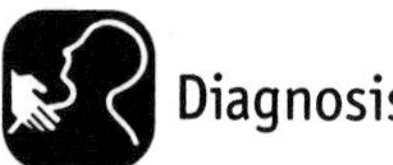

Diagnosis

DIFFERENTIAL DIAGNOSIS

- Hammer toe
- Metatarsalgia
- Stress fracture
- Metatarsophalangeal synovitis
- Bursitis
- Tendinitis

PHYSICAL EXAM

- Exquisite tenderness on digital pressure between the metatarsal heads will be elicited where the neuroma is located.
- Compression of the webspace reproduces the pain, and a "click" (Mulder's click) may be felt. Firmly squeezing the metatarsal heads together also elicits severe pain localized to the affected interspace.
- A fullness or small induration may be felt in the affected interspace consistent with a plantar mass.
- Palpate dorsally along the metatarsal shafts and heads to assess for metatarsalgia or stress fractures.
- Assess mid-foot motion and digital (toes) motion to assess for arthritis or synovitis.

IMAGING

- Radiographs of the foot are normal.
- MRI or ultrasonography may detect a neuroma, but are unreliable and are rarely, if ever, indicated.

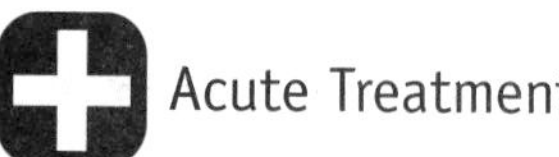

Acute Treatment

CONSERVATIVE MEASURES

- Patients should be advised to wear soft-soled shoes with a wide toe box.
- Patients should avoid wearing high heels.
- Pain also may be relieved by placing a metatarsal pad or bar to elevate and spread the metatarsal heads.
- Activity modification may be necessary, depending on the severity of the symptoms.
- Nonsteroidal antiinflammatory agents are useful for short-term treatment of pain.

CORTICOSTEROID INJECTION

- Corticosteroid injections can significantly reduce symptoms
- A mixture of long- and short-acting corticosteroids and a local anesthetic can be used. One can mix 1 to 2 mL of lidocaine (without epinephrine) and about 1 mL of both prednisolone (4 mg) and dexamethasone (4 mg) and inject the mixture just proximal to the metatarsal heads. Sometimes more than one treatment (once weekly for 3 weeks) is needed. The success rate with this treatment is approximately 70%

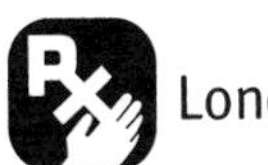

Long-Term Treatment

SURGICAL TREATMENT

- Persistence of symptoms after conservative therapies warrants surgical excision of the neuroma.
- Excision is usually performed under local anesthesia, and is an outpatient procedure.

REFERRAL/DISPOSITION

Persistence of pain despite conservative efforts and injection therapy indicate the need for further evaluation.

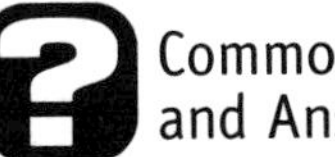

Common Questions and Answers

Physician responses to common patient questions:
Q: What are the adverse outcomes of this condition?
A: Adverse outcomes include chronic, intermittent pain and the need for activity modification.
Q: What are the complications of surgery?
A: Symptoms may become worse if a painful stump of nerve develops after surgical excision. There may be permanent loss of sensation on the plantar aspect of the foot where the surgery was performed.
Q: Will the neuroma come back?
A: There is a 5% to 10% recurrence rate of neuromas after excision and steroid injection.

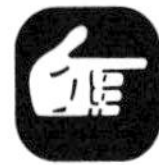

Miscellaneous

SYNONYMS

- Interdigital neuroma

ICD-9 CODE

355.6

BIBLIOGRAPHY

Mercier LR. *Practical orthopedics.* St. Louis: Mosby-Year Book, 1995.

Scuderi GR, McCann PD, Bruno PJ. *Sports medicine: principles of primary care.* St. Louis: Mosby-Year Book, 1997.

Snider RK, ed. *Essentials of musculoskeletal care.* Rosemont, IL: American Academy of Orthopaedic Surgeons, 1998.

Subotnik SI. *Sports medicine of the lower extremity.* New York: Churchill Livingstone, 1989.

Author: James Fambro

Interphalangeal Collateral Ligament Sprain

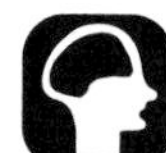

Basics

DEFINITION

- Injury to a collateral ligament at the interphalangeal joint of the finger, usually the proximal interphalangeal joint (PIP)
- 1st degree: pain, but no laxity with stress
- 2nd degree: pain and laxity, but firm end point with stress
- 3rd degree: pain and loss of firm end point with stress

INCIDENCE/PREVALENCE

- 1st- and 2nd-degree sprain much more common than 3rd-degree sprain
- Index finger most often affected
- Radial collateral ligament (RCL) more often affected than ulnar collateral ligament (UCL)

SIGNS AND SYMPTOMS

- Pain and swelling over lateral aspects of PIP joint
- Decreased range of motion (ROM) secondary to pain and swelling
- Instability in more severe injuries

MECHANISMS

- Abduction or adduction force applied to the finger, usually while extended

RISK FACTORS

- Contact and ball-handling sports: football, wrestling, basketball, baseball
- Prior injury or dislocation of PIP joint

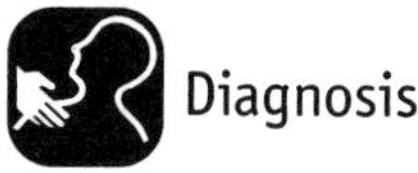

Diagnosis

DIFFERENTIAL DIAGNOSIS

- Phalangeal fracture
- IP dislocation
- Central slip injury
- Volar plate injury
- Often associated with one or more of above

HISTORY

- Finger struck by player or ball during play
- Often dislocated with relocation on playing field
- Usually presents acutely in first few weeks, but may become chronic

PHYSICAL EXAM

- Assure that maximum tenderness is over lateral aspects and not dorsal (suggestive of central slip injury, which can have significant consequences if missed)
- Test for stability in extension and with 20 to 30 degrees of flexion
- Use gentle force to avoid overstressing joint and extending partial tear into a complete one
- Instability with lateral stress (opening beyond 20 degrees) suggests loss of integrity
- Loss of active ROM may be due to either pain or volar plate/central slip injury, so digital block may be necessary to test active ROM
- Assess function of flexor and extensor tendons at MCP, PIP, and DIP joints to rule out tendon injury

IMAGING

- Posteroanterior, true lateral, and oblique radiographs of involved fingers

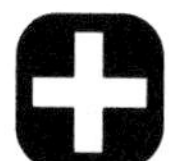

Acute Treatment

IMMOBILIZATION

- Treatment guided by which finger is involved, level of activity, and degree of pain and disability
- 1st degree: buddy tape continuously for 10 to 14 days then during physical activity for an additional 2 to 4 weeks
- 2nd degree: splint in 30 degrees of flexion acutely; buddy tape or splint in 30 degrees of flexion continuously for 2 to 3 weeks, then buddy tape during physical activity for an additional 4 to 6 weeks
- 3rd degree: some treat as severe 2nd degree, but surgery may be warranted if "unstressed instability," tissue interposition limiting joint motion, or lack of joint congruity is observed on radiographs

SPECIAL CONSIDERATIONS

- Displaced intraarticular and large avulsion fractures with displacement may require open reduction and internal fixation (ORIF).
- Central tenderness over the dorsal PIP suggests central slip injury, which can lead to a chronic boutonniere deformity.
- Central tenderness over the volar aspect suggests possible volar plate injury.

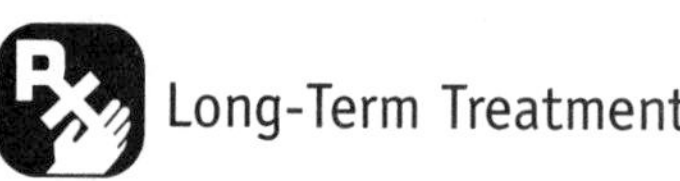

Long-Term Treatment

REHABILITATION

Depending on severity, begin passive ROM exercises in 1st week and active ROM after 1 to 2 weeks, later for more severe injuries.

SURGICAL TREATMENT

- Generally necessary if instability with active ROM, tissue interposition limiting joint motion, or lack of joint congruity are observed on radiographs
- Routine surgical repair for all complete tears is controversial
- Pro: helps ensure stability of pinch (especially in radial collateral ligament of index finger), shorter duration of disability
- Con: most complete tears heal well with conservative treatment, operative trauma may limit joint motion.

REFERRAL/DISPOSITION

- Follow up in 1 to 2 weeks for reevaluation.
- Refer significant fractures for possible ORIF.
- If uncertain of possible central slip/volar plate injury, refer to hand or follow up in 7 to 10 days and reevaluate.
- Chronic disability may be seen in athletes with delayed presentation or multiple dislocations.
- Chronic symptoms may respond to extended splinting and buddy taping with protected ROM exercises for several weeks to months.
- Surgical repair may be indicated if disability and instability persist after a sufficient trial of conservative treatment.

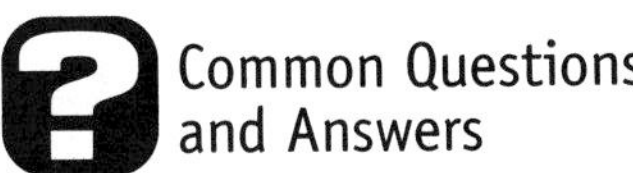

Common Questions and Answers

Physician responses to common patient questions:
Q: When can I return to play?
A: Depending on circumstances, immediate return to play with buddy taping with or without splinting may be appropriate, particularly for less important fingers, although not without some risk of further injury. More importantly, return to play is possible when disability no longer interferes with performance.
Q: How long until there is full recovery (no residual soreness)?
A: Several months to a year is not uncommon.
Q: Will the swelling resolve completely?
A: Some permanent joint enlargement from scar tissue is expected, with or without surgery.

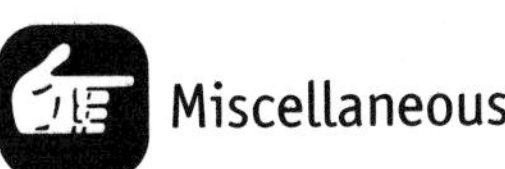

Miscellaneous

SYNONYMS

- Mild injuries: "jammed finger"

ICD-9 CODE

842.13 Interphalangeal sprain

BIBLIOGRAPHY

Alexy C, De Carlo M. Rehabilitation and use of protective devices in hand and wrist injuries. *Clin Sports Med* 1998;17:635–655.

Palmer RE. Joint injuries of the hand in athletes. *Clin Sports Med* 1998;17:513–531.

Posner MA, Nicholas JA, Hershman EB, eds. *The upper extremity in sports medicine.* St. Louis: CV Mosby, 1995.

Rockwood CA Jr, ed. *Rockwood & Green's fractures in adults,* 4th ed. Philadelphia: Lippincott-Raven, 1996.

Author: Michael Mikus

Intersection Syndrome

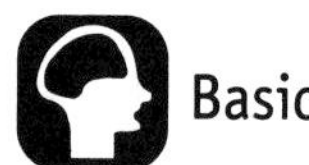

Basics

DEFINITION

- Intersection syndrome is an inflammatory condition located at the crossing of the first extensor compartment over the second compartment.
- The abductor pollicis longus (APL) and extensor pollicis brevis (EPB) comprise the first compartment.
- The extensor carpi radialis longus (ECRL) and brevis (ECRB) comprise the second compartment.
- Friction occurs between muscle bellies of the APL and EPB with the tendon sheath containing the ECRL and ECRB.
- Pain usually occurs 4 to 6 cm proximal to the radial styloid.
- Common in rowers, weight lifters, skiers, and racquetball players from repetitive wrist flexion/extension
- Patient usually presents with pain, crepitus, and squeaky sensation in the dorsal aspect of the wrist.

INCIDENCE/PREVALENCE

- The syndrome is most common in rowers who "feather" the oar during the recovery phase of the rowing stroke.
- Feathering the blade occurs during the recovery phase when the rower rotates the thin part of the blade parallel to the water and swings forward to begin another stroke.

SIGNS AND SYMPTOMS

- Pain in the radial dorsal aspect of the wrist
- Palpable and/or audible crepitus
- Swelling proximal to the radial styloid
- Squeaky sensation

RISK FACTORS

- Overuse, repetitive activities
- Rowing
- Weight lifting

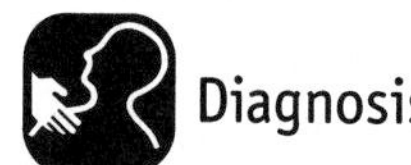

Diagnosis

DIFFERENTIAL DIAGNOSIS

- deQuervain's tenosynovitis
- Radial styloid fracture
- Scaphoid fracture
- Flexor tendonitis
- Extensor pollicis longus tenosynovitis

HISTORY

- Commonly misdiagnosed as deQuervain's
- Finkelstein's test is used to assess for pathology within the first compartment.
- Usually history of increase in activity that requires repetitive wrist flexion/extension

PHYSICAL EXAM

- Swelling proximal to the radial styloid
- Crepitus on palpation
- Pain exacerbated by ulnar deviation of the hand
- Finkelstein's test causes pain, but not at radial styloid.
- Overlying area can be warm to the touch but usually no erythema is noted.
- Vascular exam is normal.
- Neurologic exam is intact.

IMAGING

Wrist and forearm radiographs usually show normal views with occasional soft tissue swelling.

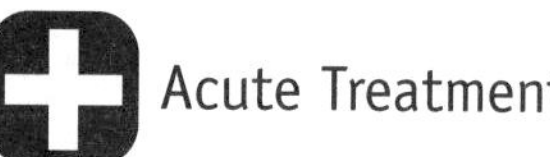

Acute Treatment

ANALGESIA

- Rest
- Ice
- Nonsteroidal antiinflammatory drugs (NSAIDs)
- Splints
- Immobilization
- Thumb spica splint or wrist splint in slight extension

SPECIAL CONSIDERATIONS

- Injection is usually reserved after no resolution with 2 to 3 weeks of splinting.
- The injection is given adjacent to area of maximal swelling.
- Recovery is usually achieved after splinting at 20 degrees wrist extension for 2 to 3 weeks
- 60% recovery response to conservative therapy
- Occupational therapy may be beneficial.
- Surgery for nonresponders

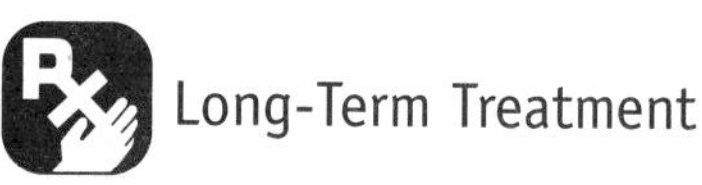

Long-Term Treatment

REHABILITATION

- Treat intersection syndrome similar to overuse injuries.
- Conservative therapy using ice, rest, NSAIDs, and splints

SURGICAL TREATMENT

Surgery is indicated for patients who have failed conservative therapy and splints.

REFERRAL/DISPOSITION

- If no improvement after adequate, conservative therapy, surgical referral is advised.
- Most cases resolve with splinting after 2 to 3 weeks.

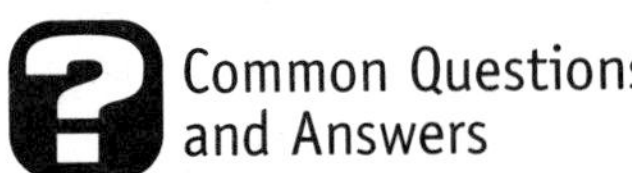

Common Questions and Answers

Physician responses to common patient questions:
Q: What did I do wrong to cause this?
A: The athlete could have started a new activity and overused the wrist extensors or could have done too much of a common activity.
Q: How can I avoid this recurrence?
A: Careful attention should be directed to technique, rehabilitation exercises, and gradual training resumption when pain free.

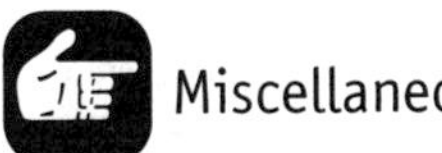

Miscellaneous

SYNONYMS

- Oarsman syndrome
- Crossover syndrome
- Peritendonitis crepitans

ICD-9 CODE

727.05 Other tenosynovitis of the hand and wrist

BIBLIOGRAPHY

Fulcher SM, Kiefhaber TR, Stern PJ. Upper-extremity tendinitis and overuse syndromes in the athlete. *Clin Sports Med* 1998;17(3):433–448.

Hanlon DP, Luellen JR. Intersection syndrome: a case report and review of the literature. *J Emerg Med* 1999;17(6):969–971.

Nguyen DT, McCue FC III, Urch SE. Evaluation of the injured wrist on the field and in the office. *Clin Sports Med* 1998;17(3):421–432.

Verdon ME. Overuse syndromes in the hand and wrist. *Prim Care Clin Office Practice* 1996;23(2):305–319.

Werner SL, Plancher KD. Biomechanics of wrist injuries in sports. *Clin Sports Med* 1998;17(3):407–420.

Author: Paul Johnson

Knee Dislocation

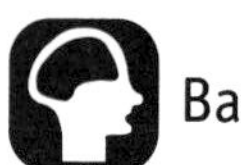

Basics

SIGNS AND SYMPTOMS

- Vascular injury to popliteal artery is the primary concern in this injury
- Grossly deformed knee
- Grossly unstable knee in anterior/posterior plane, or on varus/valgus stress
  —Anterior and posterior cruciate ligament, and collateral ligament injury
- Lack of distal pulses
- Signs of distal ischemia
  —Pallor, paresthesias, pain, paralysis
- Unequal temperature of lower extremities

ETIOLOGY

- High energy injuries such as MVA, auto versus pedestrian, and athletic injuries
  —Football most common

MECHANISM/DESCRIPTION

- Defined by the position of the tibia in relationship to the distal femur
- *Anterior dislocation*
  —Most common dislocation; accounts for 60%
  —Hyperextension of the knee
  —Rupture of the posterior capsule at 30°
  —Rupture of the posterior cruciate ligament (PCL) and popliteal artery (PA) occurs at 50°.
- *Posterior dislocation*
  —Direct blow to the anterior tibia with the knee flexed at 90°
  —Anterior cruciate ligament (ACL) is usually spared.
- *Medial dislocation*
  —Varus stress causing tear to ACL, PCL and lateral collateral ligament (LCL)
- *Lateral dislocation*
  —Valgus stress causing tear to ACL, PCL and medial collateral ligament (MCL)
- *Popliteal artery injury*
  —PA injury occurs in 33% of dislocations.
  —If vascular injury is not reversed within 6–8 hours, amputation rate approaches 90%.
  —Anterior dislocations place traction on the PA and cause contusion or intimal injury which may result in delayed thrombosis.
  —Posterior dislocations cause direct intimal fracture or transection of the artery with immediate thrombosis.
- *Peroneal nerve injury*
  —Less common than arterial injury
    —If present, must rule out concomitant arterial insult
  —Characterized by hypesthesia at first web space and lack of dorsiflexion of the foot
  —Poor prognosis for recovery
  —Medial dislocations cause injury by traction to the nerve.
  —Rotatory injuries have a high incidence of traction and transection.

CAUTIONS

- Documentation of pulses and motor response is essential.
- Splint in slight flexion to prevent traction or compression of the popliteal artery

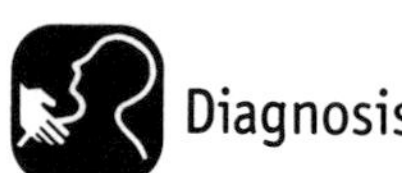

Diagnosis

ESSENTIAL WORKUP

- Complete and careful physical exam including
  —*Pulses*: by palpation, Doppler, ankle-brachial pressure indexes, and distal perfusion
  —*Neurologic*: sensation to the first web space and great toe, movement of the toes, dorsiflexion of the foot
- Knee x-rays
- Repeat examination if any closed reduction is attempted.
- Arterial imaging if any signs of limb ischemia exist

IMAGING/SPECIAL TESTS

- AP and lateral plain X-rays
- Angiogram is indicated for any patient with poor distal perfusion, pulse return after reduction, abnormal pulses, signs of peroneal nerve injury, and ischemic symptoms despite normal pulse.

DIFFERENTIAL DIAGNOSIS

- Tibial plateau fracture
- Supracondylar femoral fracture

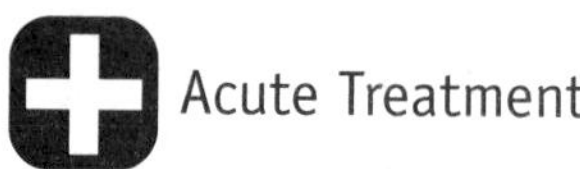

Acute Treatment

INITIAL STABILIZATION

- ABCs especially since this occurs most frequently in the multiply injured patient
- Fluid resuscitation as hypotension may alter distal pulses and perfusion.
- Closed reduction must be performed immediately for any limb ischemia.
- Early surgical consultation in an open injury or a high suspicion of arterial injury

ED TREATMENT

- Closed reduction by longitudinal traction and lifting femur into normal alignment without placing pressure on the popliteal artery
- Posterior leg splint in 15° of flexion at knee
- IV analgesia for patient comfort
- Vascular and orthopedic surgical consultation for open injury, evidence of popliteal artery injury, or unable to reduce dislocation

HOSPITAL ADMISSION CRITERIA

- All patients with knee dislocation require admission for either arterial injury repair or observation of limb perfusion.

HOSPITAL DISCHARGE CRITERIA

- N/A

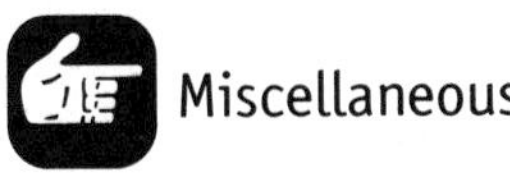

Miscellaneous

ICD-9-CM

836.50

CORE CONTENT CODE

18.4.13.2.4

BIBLIOGRAPHY

Ghalambor N, Vangsness CT. Traumatic dislocation of the knee: A review of the literature. *Bull Hosp J Dis* 1995;54(1):19–24

Kendell RW, Taylor DC, Salvian AJ, et al. The role of arteriography in assessing vascular injuries associated with dislocations of the knee. *J Trauma* 1993;35(6):875–878.

Stewart C. Knee injuries: Diagnosis and repair. *EM Med Reports* 1997;18(1):1–12.

Treiman GS, Yellin AE, Weaver FA, et al. Examination of the patient with a knee dislocation: The case for selective arteriography. *Arch Surg* 1992;127(9): 1056–1062.

Authors: Kelly Anne Foley and Francis Counselman

Lateral Collateral Ligament Tear

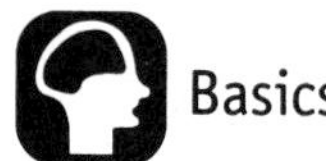

Basics

DEFINITION

- Partial or complete sprain of the lateral collateral ligament (LCL) due to an acute force

INCIDENCE/PREVALENCE

- Least commonly injured knee ligament
- Wrestling the most likely associated sport
- May be associated with injury to other ligaments [anterior collateral ligament (ACL) or posterior collateral ligament (PCL)], or structures of the posterolateral corner (popliteus, biceps femoris, iliotibial band, popliteofibular ligament)

SIGNS AND SYMPTOMS

- Acute lateral knee pain associated with a mechanism of varus stress with knee in slight flexion
- Patient may feel or hear a pop
- Swelling variable, effusion not common with low-grade injuries; associated ligamentous injuries may cause significant effusion
- Instability symptoms in high-grade injury or with associated underlying varus knee
- Possible peroneal nerve symptoms

RISK FACTORS

- Unclear if previous LCL injuries predispose to recurrent injury
- Varus knee, otherwise normal, does not seem to be predisposed to LCL injury.

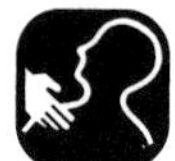

Diagnosis

DIFFERENTIAL DIAGNOSIS

- Proximal fibula avulsion fracture
- Biceps femoris strain
- Iliotibial band strain
- Popliteus strain/tear
- Associated cruciate injury
- Lateral meniscus tear
- Lateral compartment chondral/osteochondral injury
- Peroneal nerve injury

HISTORY

- Varus stress to partially flexed knee from direct force or indirect stress (e.g., stepping into a hole)
- Acute lateral knee pain
- Possible pop
- Mild disability with low-grade injury; difficult weight bearing with high-grade injury/associated injuries
- Instability with high-grade injury or moderate injury in underlying varus knee
- Possible peroneal nerve symptoms

PHYSICAL EXAM

- Local swelling over ligament
- Tender to palpation over ligament
- Palpation in figure-of-4 position: normally a pencil like structure, but less distinct with partial tears (grade II) or complete tears (grade III)
- Varus stress testing: grade I sprain, no increased laxity; grade II sprain, increase in laxity at 20 to 30 degrees; grade III sprain, increase in laxity at full extension
- Careful assessment of ACL (Lachman's test) and PCL (posterior drawer), posterolateral structures (external rotation recurvatum test, external rotation roll-out test at 90 and 30 degrees, posterolateral drawer sign)
- Peroneal nerve sensory and motor function

IMAGING

- Plain films to rule out avulsion fracture of fibula
- MRI if needed to assess other structures (ACL, PCL, posterolateral corner)

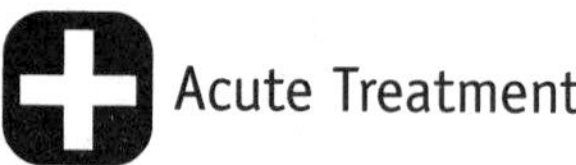

Acute Treatment

ANALGESIA

- Ice and compression in acute setting
- Nonsteroidal antiinflammatory drugs until acute pain subsides
- Narcotics appropriate for 48 to 72 hours for grade II or III injuries or combined ligamentous injuries

IMMOBILIZATION

- Grade I injury: no immobilization needed
- Grade II or III: short-term use of knee immobilizer (up to 1 week) followed by hinged brace
- Bracing for activities of daily living until gait normal and ligament nontender
- Bracing continues for contact or collision sport for the remainder of that season.

SPECIAL CONSIDERATIONS

Consider more prolonged immobilization and bracing in varus knee, which increases stress on the injured ligament.

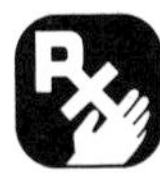

Long-Term Treatment

REHABILITATION

- In acute setting, start isometric quadriceps exercises and straight leg lifts.
- Range of motion exercises may begin immediately.
- Stationary bike as soon as motion allows
- When gait is normal, begin jogging and resistance exercises.
- Progress to half sprints, full sprints, and cutting.

SURGICAL TREATMENT

Surgery is considered for grade III/combined ligamentous injuries.

REFERRAL/DISPOSITION

- Referral to orthopedic surgery for avulsion fracture or suspicion for grade III and/or combined injury

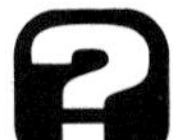

Common Questions and Answers

Physician responses to common patient questions:
Q: When can I play?
A: Average return to play for grade I injury is 1 to 2 weeks; grade II, 4 to 6 weeks. Return to play is greatly dependent on the type of activity.
Q: Am I more likely to injure it again?
A: Once healed, there are no data to suggest that the ligament is more predisposed to recurrent injury.

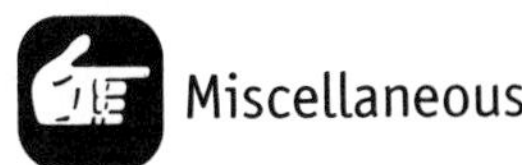

Miscellaneous

ICD-9 CODE

844.0

BIBLIOGRAPHY

Garrick JG, Webb DR. *Sports injuries: diagnosis and treatment*. Philadelphia: WB Saunders, 1999.

Safran MR, McKeag DB, Van Camp SP, eds. *Manual of sports medicine*. Philadelphia: Lippincott-Raven, 1998.

Scuderi GR, McCann PD, Bruno PJ, eds. *Sports medicine: principles of primary care*. St. Louis: CV Mosby, 1997.

Author: Andrew Tucker

Lateral Epicondylitis

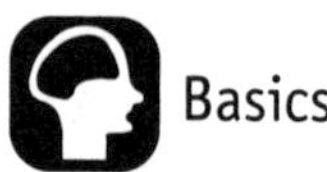

Basics

DEFINITION

- Lateral epicondylitis is an overuse injury of the forearm and wrist extensor muscles, which causes pain at the lateral elbow.

INCIDENCE/PREVALENCE

- Accounts for approximately 90% of elbow epicondylitis.
- Precipitated by tennis and other sports that require repetitive forearm dorsiflexion, radial deviation, and supination.
- Occurs in dominant arm 75% of time.

SIGNS AND SYMPTOMS

- Pain at lateral elbow
- Pain with wrist and forearm motions
- Pain with gripping objects

RISK FACTORS

- Age 40 to 60 years
- Improper equipment (wrong size grip, overstrung racquet, wrong weight racquet)
- Poor technique (especially backhand and overhead serve)
- Playing tennis for more than 2 hours per week

ASSOCIATED INJURIES AND COMPLICATIONS

Posterior interosseous nerve entrapment (radial tunnel syndrome) may coexist in up to 15% of cases.

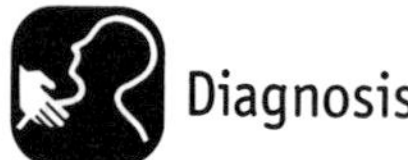

Diagnosis

DIFFERENTIAL DIAGNOSIS

- Posterior interosseous nerve entrapment (radial tunnel syndrome)
- Osteoarthritis (especially radial capitellar)
- C7 radiculopathy
- Musculocutaneous nerve entrapment
- Chronic compartment syndrome of anconeus muscle

HISTORY

- Pain pattern? Pain initially subsides with use, but returns with continued use or after use suggests an overuse injury.
- Numbness or tingling? Radicular symptoms suggest nerve entrapment or radiculopathy.
- Two-handed backhand? Most tennis players with lateral epicondylitis use a one-handed backhand.
- Equipment used, location, and frequency of play? Many cases of lateral epicondylitis are associated with improper equipment, old tennis balls, and fast surfaces.

PHYSICAL EXAM

- Localized tenderness over lateral epicondyle
- Tenderness with resisted wrist extension
- Tenderness with resisted middle finger extension

IMAGING

- Not usually needed for initial treatment
- Standard elbow radiography series (anteroposterior and lateral) should be obtained if other potential injuries are suspected (e.g., fracture or tumor) or if injury is not responding to appropriate treatment.
- Up to 25% of cases have associated calcification in extensor aponeurosis; however, presence of these deposits does not affect initial treatment.

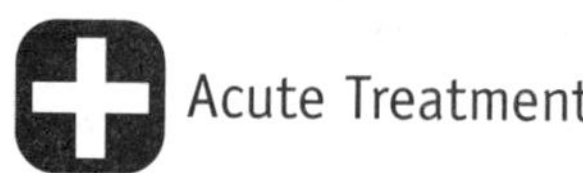

Acute Treatment

ACTIVITY MODIFICATION

- Relative rest: decreasing drills, particularly if activities are painful. Change from singles to doubles.
- Equipment modifications: decrease racquet string tension; use only new, dry tennis balls; play on grass court if available.

ANTIINFLAMMATORY TREATMENT

- Ice after activity
- Antiinflammatory medications: consider nonsteroidal antiinflammatory drugs, usually used before injected corticosteroids.
- Modalities: consider the use of ultrasonography, phonophoresis, or iontophoresis. Some studies have shown them to be useful in returning an athlete to activity sooner, but they show no long-term benefit.

OTHER TREATMENTS

- Forearm stretching and strengthening program
- A forearm counterforce brace during activities may help some patients; the use of a night wrist splint is particularly useful in patients with morning pain.

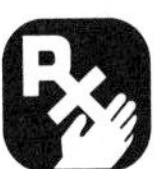

Long-Term Treatment

REHABILITATION

- Technique modification: lessons from a professional instructor or coach about proper serving and backhand techniques
- Equipment: ensure athlete is using properly sized, weighted, and strung racquet.
- Stretching and strengthening: ensure athlete is on appropriate conditioning program, preactivity warm-up, and postactivity cool-down programs.

SURGICAL TREATMENT/REFERRAL

Consider referral for surgical debridement for individuals whose symptoms do not respond to conservative treatment.

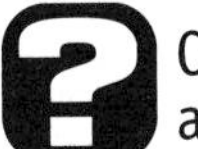

Common Questions and Answers

Physician responses to common patient questions:
Q: If the problem is my forearm and wrist, why does my elbow hurt?
A: The lateral elbow serves as the origin of the forearm muscles.

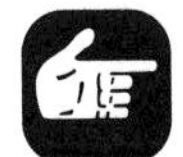

Miscellaneous

SYNONYMS

- Tennis elbow

ICD-9 CODE

726.32

BIBLIOGRAPHY

Kraushaar BS, Nirschl RP. Tendinosis of the elbow (tennis elbow). *J Bone Joint Surg [Am]* 1999;81:259–278.

Plancher K, Halbrecht J, Lourie G. Medial and lateral epicondylitis in the athlete. *Clin Sports Med* 1996;15:283–305.

Thurston AJ. Conservative and surgical treatment of tennis elbow. *Aust N Z J Surg* 1998;68:568–572.

Author: Craig C. Young

Low Back Pain

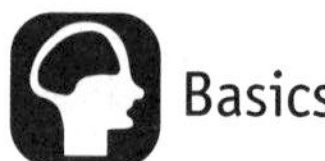

Basics

DEFINITION

- Acute low back pain is pain of less than 3 months' duration localized below the costal margin but above the inferior gluteal folds with or without leg pain.

INCIDENCE/PREVALENCE

- Approximately 70% of people in developed countries will experience low back pain at some time in their lives.
- Annual prevalence in the U.S. population is 15% to 20%.
- Approximately 1% of the U.S. population is chronically disabled because of back problems, and another 1% temporarily disabled.
- Most common between the ages of 35 and 55

SIGNS AND SYMPTOMS

- Pain located below the costal margin but above the inferior gluteal folds
- Possible radiation of pain to buttocks and lower extremity
- Pain aggravated by movement and alleviated by rest
- Limited range of motion of back
- Paraspinal muscular spasm is common.

RISK FACTORS

- Age
- Activity
- Occupation
- Obesity
- Smoking
- Sedentary life-style
- Psychosocial factors

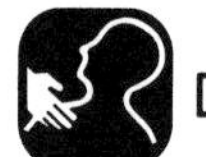

Diagnosis

DIFFERENTIAL DIAGNOSIS

- Herniated disc
- Musculoskeletal sprains and strains
- Degenerative joint disease
- Posterior facet syndrome
- Spondylolisthesis
- Spinal stenosis
- Osteoporosis
- Ankylosing spondylitis
- Referred pain
- Tumor
- Infection
- Fracture
- Genitourinary
- Gynecologic
- Psychogenic

HISTORY

- Initial history should focus on the patient's age and pain characteristics (onset, duration, severity, quality, radiation, aggravating factors, alleviating factors).
- Question patient about mechanism of injury and occupation.
- Determine if serious underlying conditions (red flags) are responsible for the back pain: fracture (steroid use, trauma, menopausal status); infection (fever, intravenous drug use, adenopathy, immunosuppression); cancer (weight loss, adenopathy, previous cancer); cauda equina syndrome (bowel or bladder incontinence, saddle anesthesia, major limb motor weakness).
- Assess psychological and socioeconomic problems.

PHYSICAL EXAM

- Assess severity of pain by observing the patient's gait, posture, and demeanor.
- Prior to examining the back, check the temperature, weight, skin, abdomen, pelvis, groin, peripheral pulses, and lymph nodes for pathology that may mimic spinal disease. A rectal exam should be performed to assess sphincter tone.
- With the patient standing, assess stance, spinal curvature, range of motion, heel-walk, toe-walk, and squat. Locate area of maximal pain.
- With patient sitting, assess deep tendon reflexes of the knee and ankle.
- With the patient supine, assess the straight leg raise, ankle and great toe dorsiflexion, hip range of motion, sacroiliac joint stability, muscle strength testing, and sensory testing.
- With the patient in the prone position, assess buttock symmetry and perform femoral stretch test.

IMAGING

- In the absence of red flag symptoms, imaging can usually be delayed until 30 days after the initial assessment. This approach allows 90% of patients to recover spontaneously and avoids unneeded procedures.
- If symptoms persist greater than 30 days, consider plain radiographs, CT scan, MRI, and bone scan.

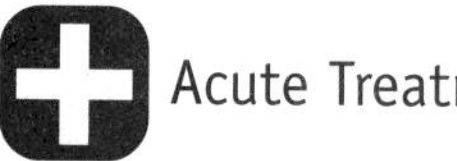

Acute Treatment

GENERAL

- Bed rest for 2 to 4 days may be required in patients with severe initial symptoms of sciatica. Prolonged bed rest (greater than 4 days) should be avoided.
- Patients should be advised to stay active because this speeds recovery and reduces time away from work. Begin with low-stress aerobic activity such as walking, riding a bicycle, swimming, and eventually jogging.
- After approximately 2 weeks of general activity, specific conditioning exercises for trunk muscles may be helpful.
- Physical therapy may be helpful during the first month of symptoms.

MEDICATIONS

- Nonsteroidal antiinflammatory drugs are the agents of choice to treat acute low back pain. Tylenol may be used as an alternative.
- Prolonged opioid use (>2 weeks) should be avoided.
- Muscle relaxants may be beneficial.

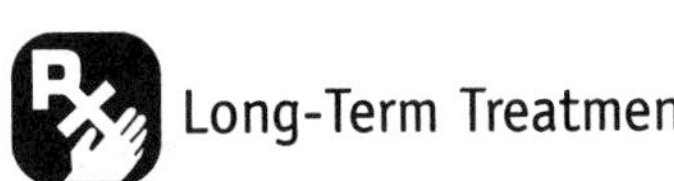

Long-Term Treatment

PREVENTION

Exercise programs, posture training, body mechanics training, and weight loss are advised.

SURGICAL TREATMENT

- Considered only when serious spinal pathology or nerve root dysfunction due to a herniated lumbar disc is detected
- Patients with acute low back pain alone, without findings of serious conditions or significant nerve root compression, rarely benefit from surgery.

REFERRAL

- Rapidly progressive neurologic deficits, symptoms of cauda equina syndrome or cord compression, acute vertebral collapse, suspicion of infection

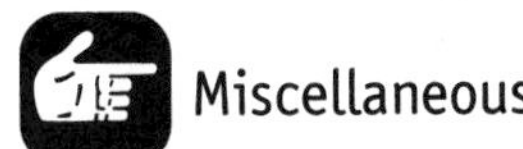

Miscellaneous

SYNONYMS

- Lumbar strain
- Lumbar sprain
- Lumbago
- Low back syndrome

ICD-9 CODE

722 Intervertebral disc disorders
724.2 Lumbago
724.5 Backache, unspecified

BIBLIOGRAPHY

Acute low back problems in adults. AHCPR Publication No. 95-0642, December 1994.

Rakel RR. *Essentials of family practice,* 2nd ed. Philadelphia: WB Saunders, 1998.

Taylor RB. *Manual of family practice: manual of family practice.* Boston: Little, Brown, 1996.

Authors: Thomas D. Armsey, Robert G. Hosey, and Steve Brook

Lower Back Pain and Lumbar Strains

Basics

DEFINITION

- Acute pain is felt in the low lumbar, lumbosacral, or sacroiliac region. It is often accompanied by sciatica, pain radiating down the distribution of the sciatic nerve.
- Chronic low back pain is the same unremitting pain that has been present for more than 3 months.

INCIDENCE/PREVALENCE

- 90% of people experience low back pain in their lifetime, and 5% to 10% will develop chronic back pain.
- The most common musculoskeletal reason for office visits to primary care providers

SIGNS AND SYMPTOMS

- Pain in low back is exacerbated by movement and is often accompanied by focal muscle spasm in the lumbar extensors.
- Patients prefer to stand in a semiflexed position and move slowly rather than sit motionless on the exam table.

RISK FACTORS

- Sedentary life-style
- Poor posture
- Chronic flexion injuries

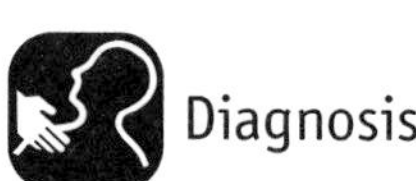

Diagnosis

DIFFERENTIAL DIAGNOSIS

- 85% mechanical back pain (MBP)
- 5% symptomatic herniated disc
- 4% compression fracture
- 4% spondylolysis/spondylolisthesis
- 2% tumor, infection, rheumatologic disease or referred pain

HISTORY

The patient should be assessed for the following red flags:

- Is patient under 20 or over 55 with no prior history of back pain? Most MBP occurs in patients 30 to 50 years of age.
- Known or previous cancer? Assume bone metastasis until otherwise proven.
- Intravenous drug abuse? Assume spinal abscess if tender.
- Is pain worse when you lie down? MBP is relieved by bed rest.
- Is pain associated with fever, chills, or weight loss? Look for infection or tumor.
- Loss of bowel or bladder control and/or caudal anesthesia? Look for cauda equina syndrome.

PHYSICAL EXAM

- Walk on heels (L4–5), then toes (S1–2).
- Back muscles uncoordinated or guarding (signs for spasm)
- Ankle and knee reflexes (objective data without reliance upon patients volition)
- Straight leg raising and crossed straight leg raising (possible acute disc herniation)

IMAGING

- If no red flags are identified in the history, then no imaging tests or laboratory tests are indicated.
- If a red flag is identified, then proceed with diagnostic testing as indicated.

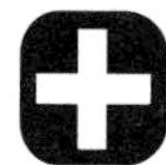

Acute Treatment

NATURAL HISTORY OF MBP

Regardless of treatment:

- 33% resolves within 1 week.
- 70% resolves by 3 weeks.
- 90% to 95% resolves in 3 months.

ANALGESIA

- Tylenol for 2 weeks [as effective as nonsteroidal antiinflammatory drugs (NSAIDS) if given on schedule]
- NSAIDS provide pain relief and allow early ambulation (caution for renal insufficiency, pregnancy, hypertension, gastrointestinal intolerance)
- Short-term nonopioid on a schedule basis (Ultram 50 mg three times daily)
- Short-term muscle relaxants or opioids to assist sleep (potential for dependence)

BEDREST

- Relative bedrest for approximately 2 days (longer bedrest delays recovery)

EXERCISE

- Begin walking as soon as possible.

MANIPULATIVE MEDICINE

- Manual therapy aimed at restoring maximal pain-free movement of the musculoskeletal system has significant proven benefit for acute low back pain.
- Passive therapy such as massage, physical therapy modalities, and traction have no proven benefit.

SYSTEMIC CORTICOSTEROIDS

- Contraindicated
- No proven benefit and significant potential harm (avascular necrosis of the hip)

INJECTION THERAPY

- No proven benefit for acute MBP

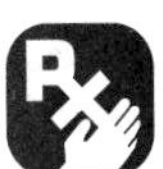

Long-Term Treatment

REHABILITATION

- Avoid debilitation—keep activity as normal as possible. It takes twice as long to regain conditioning as it does to lose it.
- Goal of therapy is increasing function, not absence of pain

SURGICAL TREATMENT

Surgery has not been proven to help back pain without radiculopathy.

REFERRAL/DISPOSITION

- Early osteopathic or chiropractic referral is often beneficial.
- Early orthopedic or physical therapy referral is rarely indicated.

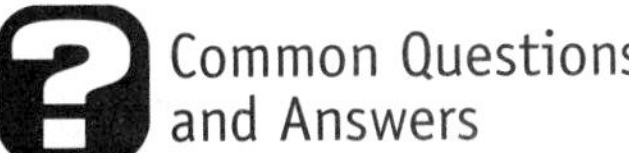

Common Questions and Answers

Physician responses to common patient questions:

Q: If I am having this much pain it must be serious, right?

A: We are pretty good at finding serious conditions and at this time we have no hint that anything bad is going on. Your symptoms should resolve in the next few weeks.

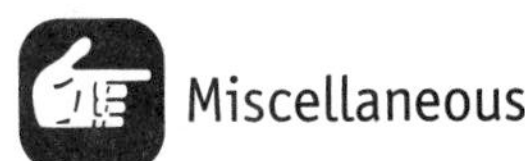

Miscellaneous

ICD-9 CODE

724.5 Back Pain

BIBLIOGRAPHY

Bigos S, et al. *Acute low back pain in adults.* Clinical practice guide No. 14, AHCPR publication No. 95-0642.

Malmivaara A, et al. The treatment of acute low back pain—bed rest, exercises or ordinary activity? *N Engl J Med* 1995;332:352–355.

Author: John Hill

Lunate Dissociation

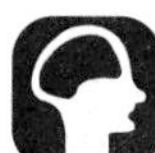

Basics

DEFINITION

- Injury typically occurs with a fall on the outstretched hand in forced axial loading or by the pushing of a heavy object with the wrist in the same position.
- The spectrum of this injury is from scapholunate sprain to full-blown scapholunate dissociation (SLD) with advanced collapse (SLAC) of the wrist.
- There are three main ligamentous structures that bind the scaphoid to the lunate: the volar radioscapholunate ligament (largest), scapholunate interosseous ligament, and radiocapitolunate ligament.
- At least two of the three ligaments connecting the scaphoid to the lunate must be torn, which subsequently results in painful intercarpal instability.
- Dissociation is classified by the pattern of carpal collapse, either dorsal or volar in nature.
- Scapholunate instability is the most common and most significant ligament injury of the wrist.

INCIDENCE/PREVALENCE

- More common in adolescents than in adults
- One study done at the Cleveland Clinic revealed that 14.8% of athletic participants under the age of 16 in the past 10 years sustained upper extremity injuries, and of these 9% involved the wrist.
- The incidence of lunate dissociation is uncommon, but failure to identify the injury results in long-term disability.
- SLD is more common in football than any other sport.

SIGNS AND SYMPTOMS

- Physicians have noted that 100% of their patients had dorsal wrist pain, 91% had decreased grip strength, and 71% had decreased range of motion.
- Patients can experience clicking with wrist motion.

RISK FACTORS

- Any injury involving excessive wrist extension and ulnar deviation with intracarpal supination, which typically occurs after a fall onto an outstretched pronated hand
- Patients with increased ulnar negative variance are at increased risk.

ASSOCIATED INJURIES AND COMPLICATIONS

- Because the mechanism of injury typically involves a fall on an outstretched hand, scaphoid fracture must be ruled out.
- If the diagnosis of lunate dissociation is missed, there is a risk of arthritic degeneration and development of SLAC wrist.

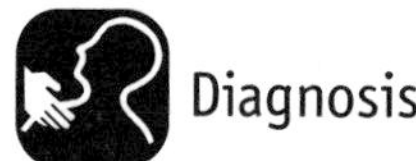

Diagnosis

DIFFERENTIAL DIAGNOSIS

- Scaphoid fracture
- Lunotriquetral injuries
- Colles fracture
- Scaphoid impaction syndrome
- Dorsal wrist ganglion cyst

HISTORY

- Obtain a detailed mechanism of injury to determine if SLD is a possible injury.
- Ask to localize pain. SLD is normally over the dorsal wrist above Lister's tubercle (distal radius).
- How long ago did the injury occur? Most patients present acutely.

PHYSICAL EXAM

- Observe for swelling, compare with opposite wrist, palpate over the lunate (distal to Lister's tubercle), as well as over the anatomic snuff box (to differentiate from scaphoid fracture).
- Check pulses and do neurologic exam.
- Finger extension test: hold wrist in flexion and test active finger extension against resistance; causes pain over lunate.
- Watson's scaphoid test may be positive. The examiner places the thumb on the scaphoid tubercle, and the four fingers wrap around the distal radius. While the wrist is in ulnar deviation, pressure is directed dorsally with the thumb at the volar scaphoid. The wrist is then radially deviated. Pain is the hallmark of a positive test result, although a dramatic "clunk" may be felt or heard.

IMAGING

- Posteroanterior (PA), lateral, and oblique views of the wrist; clenched fist view
- Look for "Terry Thomas" or "Dave Letterman" sign on PA view (a gapping of at least 3 mm between scaphoid and lunate).
- Scapholunate angle of more than 60 degrees on lateral view; clenched fist view accentuates injury

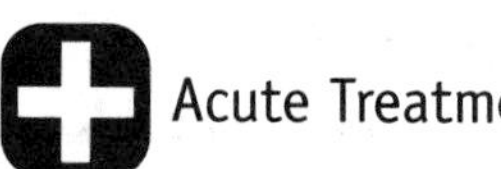

Acute Treatment

ANALGESIA

- NSAIDs, narcotics

REDUCTION TECHNIQUES

- Only for least severe injury "dynamic scapholunate instability" (no radiographic evidence of malalignment is present with the diagnosis established by dorsal scapholunate tenderness and positive Watson test result)
- Recommended for experienced providers only

IMMOBILIZATION

- Immobilize with splint in correct anatomic position. True dissociation of the scapholunate is best treated surgically.

SPECIAL CONSIDERATIONS

This should be considered a "season-ending" injury because prolonged immobilization after surgery is necessary to avoid severe degenerative arthritis.

REFERRAL

- Immediate referral to hand surgeon.

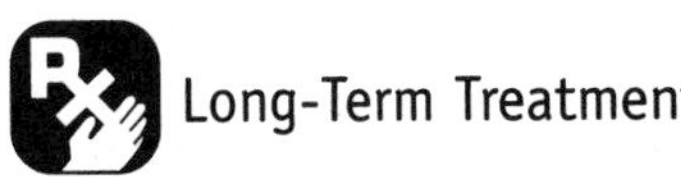

Long-Term Treatment

REHABILITATION

After prolonged immobilization to maintain carpal bone alignment, physical therapy for range of motion and strengthening is necessary.

SURGICAL TREATMENT

- Open reduction and internal fixation with or without capsulodesis

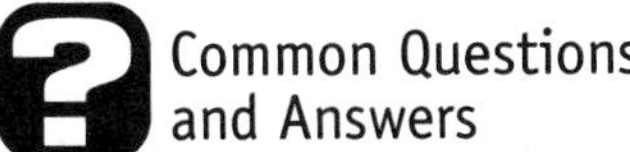

Common Questions and Answers

Physician responses to common patient questions:
Q: Will I ever play again?
A: The surgery results in approximately 35% loss of flexion and extension. This should still allow an athlete to return to activity in most cases.
Q: Why do I need surgery?
A: The ligament in your wrist has torn and the bones shifted so they cannot heal correctly without surgery.

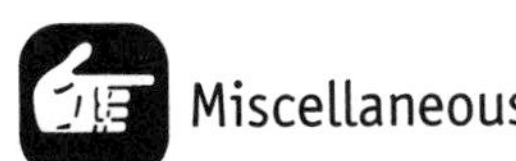

Miscellaneous

SYNONYMS

- Wrist sprain (caution not to misdiagnose SLD as wrist sprain due to long-term disability and poor outcome if not treated early)
- Scapholunate dissociation

ICD-9 CODE

824.01 Sprain, wrist, carpal (joint)

BIBLIOGRAPHY

Cohen MS. Ligamentous injuries of the wrist in the athlete. *Clin Sports Med* 1998;17: 533–552.

Mastey RD. Primary care of hand and wrist athletic injuries. *Clin Sports Med* 1997;16: 705–724.

Nguyen DT. Evaluation of the injured wrist on the field and in the office. *Clin Sports Med* 1998;17:421–432.

Rettig AC. Epidemiology of hand and wrist injuries in sports. *Clin Sports Med* 1998;17: 401–406.

Ritchie JV, Munter DW. Emergency department evaluation and treatment of wrist injuries. *Emerg Med Clin North Am* 1999;17:823–842.

Authors: Thomas Trojian and Scott Mitchell

MCP Collateral Ligament Sprain

 Basics

DEFINITION

- Injury to the collateral ligaments of the metacarpophalangeal (MCP) joints; most commonly the MCP joint of the thumb
- Mechanism of injury to the ulnar collateral ligament (UCL) of the MCP joint of the thumb is sudden, forced, radial deviation (abduction) and extension, resulting in partial or complete tear of the ligament
- Mechanism of injury to the radial collateral ligament (RCL) of the MCP joint of the thumb is forced adduction or twisting of the flexed joint

INCIDENCE/PREVALENCE

- Isolated injuries to collateral ligaments of the MCP joints are uncommon, except for those of the MCP joint of the thumb, which is the focus of this chapter
- UCL injuries of the MCP joint of the thumb (gamekeeper's thumb or skier's thumb) occur more often than RCL injuries
- UCL sprain is the second most common injury encountered by skiers and most common ligamentous injury to the thumb
- UCL sprain is frequently seen in football players, ball-handling athletes, and other contact sports

SIGNS AND SYMPTOMS

- Hallmark symptom of acute UCL injury is pain and swelling localized to the ulnar aspect of the MCP joint along the UCL.
- Weakness of thumb, weakness with pinch
- RCL injuries have pain and swelling localized to the radial aspect of the metacarpal head, and activities such as twisting open a jar lid can exacerbate the symptoms.

ASSOCIATED INJURIES AND COMPLICATIONS

- Complete rupture of the collateral ligament (proper and accessory) and volar plate
- Stener's lesion: adductor aponeurosis becomes interposed between the torn end of the UCL (thumb) and its insertion into the base of the proximal phalanx (not seen in RCL complete tears).
- Three types of avulsion fractures: small fragment at the base of the proximal phalanx; a large, intraarticular fracture that involves at least 25% of the articular surface of the base of the proximal phalanx; and an avulsion fracture involving the volar plate
- Dislocation of the thumb MCP joint

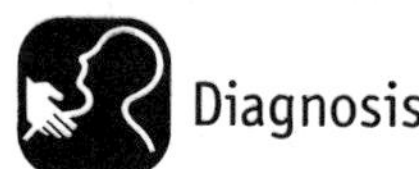

Diagnosis

DIFFERENTIAL DIAGNOSIS

- Complete tear of collateral ligament
- Dislocation of the thumb MCP joint
- Fracture

HISTORY

- Acute versus chronic? Prompt diagnosis leads to a better outcome.
- Mechanism of injury

PHYSICAL EXAM

- Important to differentiate a sprain from a complete tear
- Always compare with asymptomatic thumb.
- Examine the joint for swelling, ecchymosis, and areas of tenderness.
- Anteroposterior (AP) and lateral radiographs should be obtained prior to stressing the joint because a nondisplaced fracture can be displaced as a result of the stress.
- If radiographs negative, the stability of the ligament should be tested.
- Test the ligaments by applying radial stress (UCL) or ulnar stress (RCL) to the MCP joint in full extension and in 30 degrees flexion.
- Opening the joint line 15 degrees greater than the contralateral thumb or 30 degrees absolute indicates ligament rupture; less than 30 degrees laxity assumes partial tear.
- If unable to make a clear distinction on clinical exam, stress radiographs are indicated

IMAGING

- AP and lateral radiographs of the thumb prior to stressing the joint to evaluate for a fracture
- Stress radiographs in full extension and in 30 degrees flexion (always compare with the contralateral thumb)
- Additional radiographic signs that indicate a complete rupture are volar subluxation of the proximal phalanx seen on a lateral view and radial deviation of the proximal phalanx seen on an AP view.
- Stress films are contraindicated in children with Salter-Harris fractures.
- MRI has been used successfully for diagnosis (not cost effective).

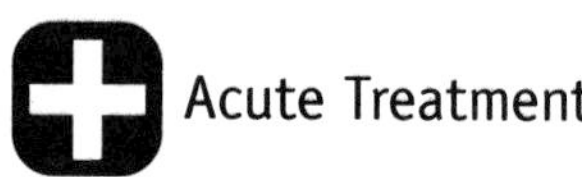

Acute Treatment

ANALGESIA

- Nonsteroidal antiinflammatory drugs, ice

OTHER TREATMENTS

- No detectable instability: immobilization (thumb spica splint) for 2 weeks
- Incomplete tear with stable joint: thumb spica cast for 3 to 6 weeks, depending on severity of the injury
- Thumb is immobilized in slight flexion in the spica cast; the interphalangeal joint is not immobilized to allow active motion and prevent scarring of the extension mechanism

- Complete tear (joint open >30 degrees under stress): repair surgically
- Avulsion fracture: small avulsions that are not intraarticular can be treated nonoperatively; large intraarticular fragments require surgical repair.
- Avulsion fracture: rotated or displaced more than 1 mm require surgical repair; if nondisplaced, thumb spica cast (application as above) for 4 to 6 weeks
- Symptoms may persist for months.
- Surgical repair is necessary for Stener's lesion; failure to recognize this injury or inadequate treatment can result in chronic instability.

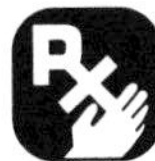

Long-Term Treatment

REHABILITATION

- When the cast is removed, range of motion exercises are performed several times a day; a removable splint is worn for an additional 2 to 3 weeks.
- Sports participation: protect the thumb for approximately 3 months either by buddy taping it in adduction to the index finger or by using a splint.

REFERRAL

Prompt referral to an orthopedist or hand surgeon is indicated for all but uncomplicated injuries and when a Stener's lesion cannot be ruled out on the basis of physical examination and standard radiographs.

Miscellaneous

ICD-9 CODE

842.12 Metacarpophalangeal joint sprains

BIBLIOGRAPHY

DeLee JC, Drez D Jr., eds. *Orthopaedic sports medicine: principles and practice.* Philadelphia: WB Saunders, 1994.

Fricker R, Hintermann B. Skier's thumb. Treatment, prevention and recommendations. *Sports Med* 1995;19: 73–79.

Garrick JG, Webb DR. *Sports injuries: diagnosis and management*, 2nd ed. Philadelphia: WB Saunders, 1999.

Green DP, Hotchkiss RN, Pederson WC, eds. *Green's operative hand surgery*, 4th ed. Philadelphia: Churchill Livingstone, 1999.

Husband JB, McPherson DA. Bony skier's thumb injuries. *Clin Orthop Rel Res* 1996;327:79–84.

Author: Kathleen Weber

MCP Dislocation

Basics

DEFINITION

- Dislocation of proximal phalanx over metacarpal
- Usually requires disruption of stabilizing ligament
- May occur dorsally (common), laterally (uncommon), or volarly (rare)
- Dorsal: may be "simple," in which articular surfaces are in partial contact, or "complex," in which the volar plate or other tissue is interposed between articular surfaces
- Lateral: results from injury to collateral ligament, usually the radial collateral ligament (RCL) of the index finger
- Volar: rare, but may result from severe or repetitive blows to knuckle, leading to rupture of dorsal capsule with subsequent volar displacement of the proximal phalanx

INCIDENCE/PREVALENCE

- Metacarpophalangeal (MCP) dislocations are much less common than proximal interphalangeal (PIP) dislocations because of support from surrounding structures and protected position.
- Usually occurs in outer digits (index and small fingers)
- Nearly always a single digit, but multiple digits may be involved

SIGNS AND SYMPTOMS

- Pain, loss of function, and generally obvious deformity

RISK FACTORS

- Contact and ball-handling sports
- Prior history of injury or dislocation

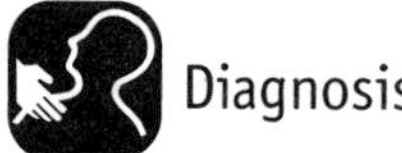

Diagnosis

DIFFERENTIAL DIAGNOSIS

- Fracture of phalanx or metacarpal
- Tendon rupture
- Disruption of volar plate

HISTORY

- Dorsal dislocation generally results from forced hyperextension of digit, as in striking the heel of an opponent while diving to make a tackle, or a fall on the outstretched hand.
- Lateral dislocation is usually caused by an ulnarly directed blow to the MCP joint.
- Volar dislocation may be seen with punching in boxing and martial arts.

PHYSICAL EXAM

- Dorsal simple: there is obvious deformity with the phalanx resting at 60 to 90 degrees of hyperextension over the head of the metatarsal.
- Dorsal complex: much more subtle deformity, with only slight hyperextension of the phalanx, but with pathognomonic dimpling or puckering of the palmar aspect of the finger where the volar plate is caught between the ends of the bones (proximal phalanx and head of metacarpal); slight lateral deviation also may be noted, distinguishing it from a simple dislocation.
- Lateral: obvious lateral deformity, and because it is accompanied by lateral collateral ligament injury, there is often lateral instability with active range of motion (ROM)
- Volar: obvious deformity of phalanx positioned palmar to metacarpal

IMAGING

- Anteroposterior (AP), lateral, and oblique views of involved digit generally show deformity and any accompanying fracture.
- Presence of a sesamoid in the widened joint space of the involved digit is pathognomonic for a complex dorsal dislocation.
- Postreduction views: AP, lateral, and oblique to evaluate for congruity and fracture

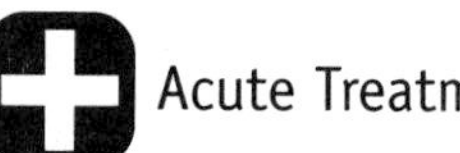

Acute Treatment

ANALGESIA

- Usually not necessary for simple dislocations, but wrist block may facilitate reduction and prevent false conclusion that dislocation is complex if patient prevents reduction due to pain
- For complex dislocations, digital block or general anesthesia in the operating room may be necessary if closed reduction is to be attempted.

REDUCTION TECHNIQUES

- Document neurovascular status before and after reduction.
- Dorsal simple: first, relax flexors by placing wrist and IP joints into flexion; next, accentuate dislocation slightly by hyperextending proximal phalanx to 90 degrees, and then push base of proximal phalanx into flexion, while maintaining contact with metacarpal head to prevent entrapment of the volar plate (thus converting a simple dislocation into a complex one).
- Dorsal complex: attempt at closed reduction is warranted but usually not successful; reduction technique is similar to that of a simple dislocation.
- Lateral: closed reduction is usually accomplished with gentle longitudinal traction, taking care not to interpose any soft tissue.
- Volar: generally is performed open because concomitant dorsal hood injury needs repair

POSTREDUCTION EVALUATION

- Evaluate and document neurovascular status.
- Evaluate tendon function.
- AP, lateral, and oblique radiographs to evaluate for congruity and fracture

IMMOBILIZATION

- Dorsal simple: splint in 50 to 70 degrees of flexion for 7 to 10 days if no evidence of significant instability; buddy taping also may be implemented.
- Dorsal complex: postoperative buddy taping for 4 to 6 weeks with or without splinting at the prerogative of the surgeon
- Lateral: splint in position of function (50 degrees) for 2 to 4 weeks.
- Volar: postoperative buddy taping for 4 to 6 weeks with or without splinting at the prerogative of the surgeon

SPECIAL CONSIDERATIONS

In dislocations of the thumb, assessment of the ulnar collateral ligament is essential.

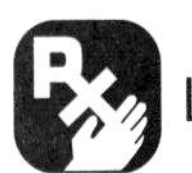

Long-Term Treatment

REHABILITATION

- Passive ROM in the first week, and active ROM after 2 to 3 weeks, depending on the severity of the injury
- Occupational therapy may be indicated in more severe injuries.

SURGICAL TREATMENT

Surgery is often necessary for reduction as discussed above, and may be indicated for repair of severely damaged structures.

REFERRAL/DISPOSITION

Other than simple dorsal dislocations with no instability or involvement of the volar plate, most MCP dislocations should be followed up with a hand surgeon within a week.

Common Questions and Answers

Physician responses to common patient questions:
Q: When can I return to play?
A: With adequate protection and splinting of uncomplicated dislocations, athletes may return to activities within 1 to 2 weeks, sooner for low-risk sports with minor injuries, longer for more serious injuries requiring surgery.

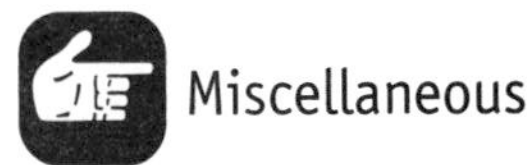

Miscellaneous

ICD-9 CODE

834.01 Metacarpophalangeal dislocation

BIBLIOGRAPHY

McCue FC III, Cabrera JM, Strickland JW, et al. *Hand injuries in athletes.* Philadelphia: WB Saunders, 1992.

Palmer RE. Joint injuries of the hand in athletes. *Clin Sports Med* 1998;17:513–531.

Rockwood CA Jr., ed. *Rockwood & Green's fractures in adults,* 4th ed. Philadelphia: Lippincott-Raven, 1996.

Authors: Michael Mikus and Bradford Stiles

Medial Collateral Ligament Tear

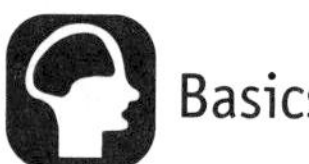

Basics

DEFINITION

- Tension injury to the medial collateral ligament (MCL) occurs most commonly with a valgus stress (i.e., a blow to the lateral knee).
- Classification is by clinical exam: grade I, MCL tenderness but no laxity; grade II, lax to valgus stress at 20 degrees of flexion, no laxity in extension; grade III, lax with no end point on valgus stress at 20 degrees and lax in full extension

SIGNS AND SYMPTOMS

- Antalgic gait and a sense of the knee being "loose"
- Limited range of motion
- Pain over the MCL and medial aspect of the knee
- Swelling, either localized or intraarticular

ASSOCIATED INJURIES AND COMPLICATIONS

- Medial meniscus tear, commonly in the posterior horn
- Anterior cruciate ligament (ACL) tear
- Posterior oblique ligament injury; anteromedial rotatory instability
- Dislocation of the knee (rare)

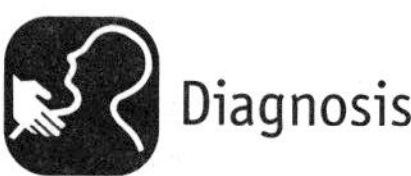

Diagnosis

DIFFERENTIAL DIAGNOSIS

- Medial meniscus tear
- Medial knee contusion
- Patellar instability, subluxation, or dislocation
- Fracture of the distal femoral physis

HISTORY

- During football, an acute blow to the lateral aspect of the knee when the foot is planted results in a valgus stress.
- The medial joint line is under tension and can open, producing "buckling" and an injury to the MCL (closed-chain injury).
- The injury may be seen in soccer players who are struck on the instep while passing the ball (open-chain injury).
- Overuse injuries to the MCL have been reported in breast-stroke swimmers.
- History of a "pop" should suggest associated meniscus or ACL injury.

PHYSICAL EXAM

- Observe for antalgic gait.
- Localized tenderness on palpation over MCL and medial joint line.
- Valgus stress at full extension should be performed to ensure the joint capsule and ACL are intact. Valgus stress at 20 degrees flexion relaxes the capsule and tests for MCL laxity. Always compare the exam to the unaffected knee.
- Determine the amount of joint line opening. If it is more than 10 mm, coexisting intraarticular pathology (torn ACL or meniscus) will be present 80% of the time.
- Posterior oblique ligament injury can lead to anteromedial rotatory instability and posterior horn medial meniscus tears. Anterior drawer testing with the foot in external rotation can assess anteromedial translation, but may be difficult to perform in acute injury.
- Lachmann's exam should be performed to evaluate a concomitant ACL tear.
- Ecchymosis and swelling in a young patient should prompt evaluation for physeal injury.
- Assess neurovascular status of the extremity. Popliteal nerve and artery injuries can be limb threatening and should not be missed.

IMAGING

- Routine knee radiographs of the knee are usually normal in isolated MCL injuries.
- Calcification of the MCL (Pelligrini-Steida lesion) is seen in chronic MCL injury.
- MRI: used if concomitant ACL or meniscus injury suspected
- Stress views: helpful in children to rule out Salter-Harris fractures. Note whether tenderness exists to palpation completely around physis, then stress views can be avoided.

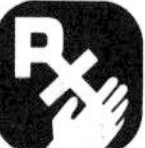

Long-Term Treatment

ISOLATED MCL INJURIES

- In grade I and II MCL injuries, PRICE (pressure, rest, ice, compression, elevation) and nonsteroidal antiinflammatory drugs are first line.
- Ice should be applied 20 minutes every 3 to 4 hours. More vigorous icing has led to common peroneal nerve palsies, due to cryoinjury of the nerve where it becomes superficial, approximately 10 cm below the fibular head.
- If the athlete walks with an antalgic gait, a neoprene sleeve or ACE wrap should be used with crutches until weight-bearing is tolerated.
- Early mobilization and a goal-oriented rehabilitation program should be prescribed: goal 1 is to achieve pain-free gait; goal 2 should be to regain flexion of the knee to 90 degrees. Once accomplished, stair climbing or raised-seat biking can be started. Goal 3 is full active knee motion. A program of quad strengthening, and gradual return to jogging and agility drills is instituted.
- When the patient can get through the entire protocol in one session and when the injured knee is 90% as strong as the unaffected leg, return to play is permitted.
- Early mobilization has been demonstrated to return patients to work and play faster, while giving similar long-term results.
- Isolated grade III injuries with tolerable symptoms can be rehabilitated similarly.
- Some clinicians immobilize patients with disabling symptoms for a short time (1 week) prior to rehabilitation.
- Surgical repair has been advocated.
- There is no difference in outcome for immobilization, early mobilization, and surgery, although patients treated with early rehabilitation were able to return to sport faster and were slightly more unstable at follow-up.

REFERRAL/DISPOSITION

- Referral is suggested when there is suspicion of ACL or meniscal injury.
- Some clinicians have suggested arthroscopy for all complete MCL injuries with more than 6 mm of joint opening.

COMBINED MCL/ACL INJURIES

- Early referral
- MRI is helpful to delineate pathology.
- Aggressive rehabilitation is undertaken to restore knee motion and get through the inflammatory phase of the injury. Then the ACL is usually reconstructed, and the MCL is permitted to scar down on its own. This approach has minimized postoperative arthrofibrosis.
- Rehabilitation protocols after surgery are similar to ACL protocols. If there is significant rotational instability, repair of the MCL is often performed as well.

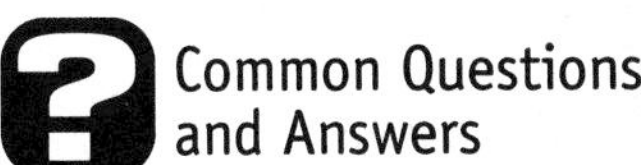

Common Questions and Answers

Physician responses to common patient questions:

Q: How long until I can return to play?
A: For most sports, athletes with grade I injuries return in an average of 10 days. Those with grade II sprains return in 2 to 3 weeks. Those with grade III sprains return in 3 to 4 weeks. Soccer players may require several more weeks because the use of the instep to kick and pass the ball exerts a valgus force that subjects the injured MCL to recurrent stress.

Q: Should I wear a brace?
A: Although many college players still wear braces, most epidemiologic studies demonstrate either no effect or only slightly decreased risk of injury while wearing the MCL brace.

Q: Will I get early arthritis?
A: A 10-year follow-up on isolated MCL injuries suggests that most patients have excellent function and no major radiographic evidence of arthritis.

Q: Will it always bother me?
A: After rehabilitation, most patients note minor aggravating symptoms, but these usually do not affect one's ability to participate in activities.

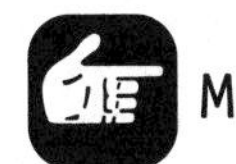

Miscellaneous

ICD-9 CODE

844.1 Sprain, medial collateral, knee
717.82 Old sprain, medial collateral, knee

BIBLIOGRAPHY

Albright JP, Powell JW, et al. Medial collateral ligament knee sprains in college football: effectiveness of preventive braces. *Am J Sports Med* 1994;22:12–18.

Ballmer PM, Jakob RP. The non-operative treatment of isolated complete tears of the MCL of the knee. *Arch Orthop Trauma Surg* 1988;107:273–276.

Fetto J, Marshall J. Medial collateral ligament injuries of the knee: a rationale for treatment. *Clin Orthop* 1978;132:206–218.

Reider B. Medial collateral ligament injuries in athletes. *Sports Med* 1996;21:147–156.

Reider B, Sathy MR, Talkington J, et al. Treatment of isolated medial collateral ligament injuries in athletes with early functional rehabilitation. *Am J Sports Med* 1993;22:470–477.

Shelbourne KD, et al. ACL/MCL injury. Nonoperative management of MCL tears with ACL reconstruction. *Am J Sports Med* 1991;20:283–286.

Authors: Delmas J. Bolin and David A. Stone

Medial Tibial Stress Syndrome

 Basics

DEFINITION

- Medial tibial stress syndrome is typically an overuse injury, a syndrome of pain over the posteromedial border of the middle to distal thirds of the tibia, at the periosteal/fascial junction. It is generally attributed to periostitis.

INCIDENCE/PREVALENCE

- Unknown, but extremely common

SIGNS AND SYMPTOMS

- Often insidious and progressive
- Temporally related to sudden increase in intensity/duration of activity, or change in playing/running surface
- Early in course: pain with onset of exertion, usually relieved by rest
- Sometimes relieved as activity continues
- Often worse with toe-off
- Late in course: pain after cessation of activity, possibly worse than the pain with activity
- As the condition progresses, pain may persist throughout the inciting activity.

RISK FACTORS

- Repetitive stress, especially running and jumping
- Foot overpronation or other lower extremity alignment abnormalities
- Increase in training intensity
- Change in running/playing surface

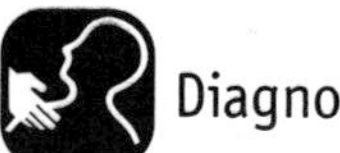

DIFFERENTIAL DIAGNOSIS

- Stress fracture
- Compartment syndrome
- Muscular strain
- Nerve entrapment
- Fascial defects
- Popliteal artery entrapment syndrome
- Effort-induced venous thrombosis

HISTORY

See Signs and Symptoms.

PHYSICAL EXAM

- Tenderness to palpation along the middle to distal thirds of the tibia, along the posteromedial border
- Foot/ankle examination to evaluate for excessive pronation or other alignment abnormalities
- Chronic cases: induration, soft tissue swelling, or nodularity

IMAGING

- Plain films of anteroposterior and lateral tibia are often normal; may show cortical hypertrophy or demineralization.
- Bone scan: diffuse uptake along the posteromedial border of the tibia, often seen better on delayed images
- MRI: effective diagnostically in cases where diagnosis unclear

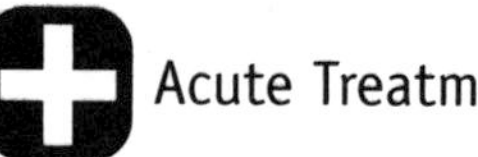

ANALGESIA

- Nonsteroidal antiinflammatory drugs most beneficial in acute stages

IMMOBILIZATION

- No benefit

ICE

- Most beneficial in acute stage

REST

- Complete rest if possible
- Otherwise, 20% to 50% reduction in mileage/inciting activity, with slow return to previous level of activity as symptoms resolve
- Cross-training with nonimpact activities: swimming, water running, bicycling

SPECIAL CONSIDERATIONS

- Special taping techniques by athletic trainers may improve symptoms.
- For very flat feet (pes planus), consider more supportive shoes or supportive inserts.
- For very high-arched feet (pes cavus), consider increased cushioning in shoes or shock-absorbing inserts.

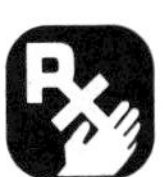

Long-Term Treatment

REHABILITATION

- Target-specific stretching and strengthening exercises
- Towel calf stretches
- Tracing alphabet with toes
- Alternate heel/toe walking

SURGICAL TREATMENT

Past attempts for severe/refractory cases had limited success.

CHANGES IN TRAINING TECHNIQUES

- Increase rest days.
- Add in cross-training days with non-weight-bearing activity such as swimming and biking.
- Slow increase in training intensity/duration, with no more than a 10% increase per week.

CUSTOM ORTHOTICS

- For foot overpronation or other inciting alignment abnormalities

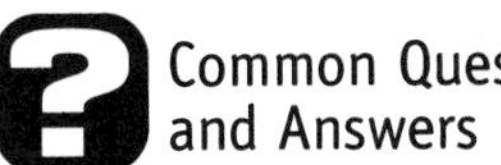

Common Questions and Answers

Physician responses to common patient questions:

Q: How long do I need to abstain from activity?
A: Until pain and tenderness resolve, followed by a slow, structured return to prior level of activity.
Q: Is there any benefit to special taping or an ACE bandage?
A: There is no good evidence that it will shorten recovery, but it may help to improve symptoms.
Q: I am involved in competitive sports, and I cannot take time off from training. What can I do?
A: Relative rest, with a 20% to 50% decrease in training intensity/duration. Work in cross-training days, with non-weight-bearing activity.
Q: What rehabilitation exercises can I do?
A: Exercises aimed at stretching and strengthening involved musculotendinous units. Use a towel to pull your foot toward you and stretch your calf. Trace the alphabet with your feet. Alternate walking on toes and heels.

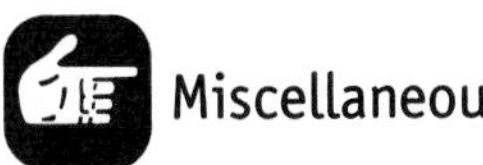

Miscellaneous

SYNONYMS

- Shin splints
- Medial tibial stress syndrome
- Tibialis posterior myofasciitis
- Soleus syndrome

BIBLIOGRAPHY

Abramowitz AJ, et al. The medial tibial stress syndrome. The role of surgery. *Orthop Rev* 1994;23:875–881.

Beck BR. Tibial stress injuries. An aetiological review for the purposes of guiding management. *Sports Med* 1998;26:265–279.

Kelly W, et al. *Textbook of rheumatology.* Vol. 1. Philadelphia: W.B. Saunders. 1997, 558–559.

Locke S. Exercise related chronic lower leg pain. *Aust Fam Physician* 1999;28:569–573.

Touliopolous S, Hershman EB. Lower leg pain. Diagnosis and treatment of compartment syndromes and other pain syndromes. *Sports Med* 1999;27:193–204.

Authors: Jason D. Johnson and Benjamin Hasan

Medial Tibial Stress Syndrome/Shin Splints

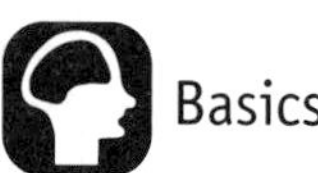

Basics

DEFINITION

- Overuse injury of the lower leg caused by a stress reaction involving fascia, bone, or periosteum at the posteromedial border of the middle and distal third of the tibia
- The cause of pain is unclear, but may occur due to a traction effect on the tibia by the soleus, crural fascia, tibialis posterior, or flexor digitorum longus
- Medial tibial stress syndrome (MTSS) is also known as periostalgia or shin splints.

INCIDENCE/PREVALENCE

- Difficult to measure due to lack of consistency in terminology and diagnostic criteria
- 10% to 15% of all running injuries are due to shin splints.
- 5% of all injuries in military trainees are from shin splints.
- Most common in runners; also in tennis, volleyball, basketball, long-jumping, gymnastics, and dancing

SIGNS AND SYMPTOMS

- Dull, aching pain along the middle to distal third of the posteromedial tibial border
- Pain may be sharp, penetrating, and severe in chronic cases

RISK FACTORS

- History of previous injury
- Recent changes in training pattern, including frequency, duration, or intensity
- Inappropriate or excessively worn footwear
- Increased maximum pronation and maximum pronation velocity, hindfoot and forefoot varus
- Menstrual dysfunction (see Menstrual Disorders topic)

CLASSIFICATION

- MTSS injuries can be graded similarly to other overuse injuries based on clinical assessment.
- Grade 1: symptoms that occur at the beginning of the activity and dissipate with continued activity, or develop at the end of the activity
- Grade 2: symptoms during activity with late onset
- Grade 3: symptoms during activity with early onset that persists throughout activity
- Grade 4: symptoms that limit the quality and/or quantity of training
- Grade 5: symptoms that prevent training

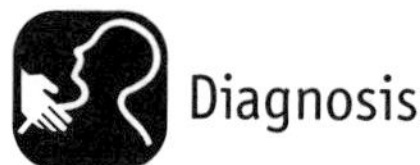

Diagnosis

DIFFERENTIAL DIAGNOSIS

- Tibial stress fracture
- Chronic exertional compartment syndrome
- Superficial peroneal nerve entrapment
- Deep vein thrombosis
- Rupture of the gastrocnemius muscle
- Fascial herniation
- Popliteal artery entrapment syndrome
- Bone neoplasm
- Peripheral vascular disease
- Delayed-onset muscle soreness
- Effort-induced venous thrombosis
- Referred pain

HISTORY

- Has the training regimen changed recently? An inappropriate increase in intensity, duration, or frequency without time for adequate recovery can lead to overuse injuries such as MTSS.
- Were the shoes properly fitted and are they in good condition? Shoes should be chosen with consideration for foot and ankle alignment and running biomechanics (e.g., heel striker vs. forefoot striker). Running shoes should be replaced every 300 to 500 miles.
- Are you having pain at night while sleeping? Night pain may indicate a bone tumor or stress fracture.
- Does the pain present during the activity and completely resolve with 10 to 15 minutes of rest? This is more consistent with chronic exertional compartment syndrome, which can also present with parasthesias. The physical exam in such cases is often normal.
- Any other recent injuries to your lower extremities or back? Leg pain can occur as a result of alterations in gait due to injury at other sites.

PHYSICAL EXAM

- Tenderness at the posteromedial border of the tibia is typically found. Pain is usually elicited from 4 cm proximal to the medial malleolus and continuing proximally for up to 12 cm.
- Pain may be provoked with passive ankle dorsiflexion, active plantarflexion against resistance, or one-legged hopping.
- Carefully evaluate for alignment problems such as pronation, pes planus, and hindfoot or forefoot varus.

IMAGING

- Plain radiographs are usually normal. Posterior cortical hypertrophy may be noted in chronic cases.
- Periosteal thickening, subperiosteal changes, or cortical defects suggest a stress fracture.
- Triple-phase bone scan reveals a diffuse, longitudinal uptake along the posteromedial tibia only on the delayed phase. A stress fracture, however, is usually positive in all three phases with a focal, fusiform uptake.

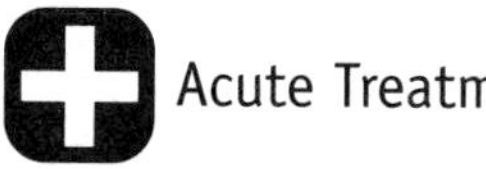

Acute Treatment

ANALGESIA

- Ice massage may be helpful for pain relief.
- Other modalities such as ultrasonography, phonophoresis, acupuncture, and electrical stimulation are used, but data on their effectiveness are limited.
- Nonsteroidal antiinflammatory drugs (NSAIDs) also may be helpful for pain relief.
- Because studies indicate that MTSS does not involve inflammation, the antiinflammatory effects of NSAIDs are not thought to play a significant role in treatment.
- A long pneumatic splint can he helpful for reducing pain with weight bearing in more severe cases.

ACTIVITY MODIFICATION

- Relative rest from impact loading activities is necessary.
- For those with mild symptoms (i.e., pain that occurs only with activity and does not impair performance), the inciting activity should be reduced.
- For those with severe symptoms (i.e., pain that impairs daily activities or performance), impact activities should be avoided until symptoms are controlled.
- Cross-training activities such as swimming, cycling, and water running with or without a floatation vest are important to maintain proper fitness.

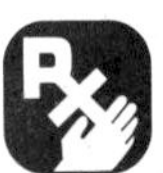

Long-Term Treatment

REHABILITATION

- A comprehensive flexibility program should be instituted before and after each training session.
- Attention is directed to the quadriceps, hamstrings, heel cord, and dorsiflexors.
- Strengthening of the deep and superficial posterior compartment musculature is important and should include both concentric and eccentric calf exercises.

MALALIGNMENT

- Prospective studies have yet to consistently demonstrate a cause-and-effect relationship between malalignment and MTSS.
- Consider the use of orthoses in those with marked malalignment or for those with mild malalignment who do not respond well to initial treatment.

RETURN TO ACTIVITY

- Light running or jogging can be initiated after the athlete is pain free for several days.
- Workouts should initially be confined to flat, soft surfaces.
- Training should progress in a gradual, stepwise fashion.
- Although individualization of the progression of training is necessary, training increases in increments of 10% per week are often used as a starting point.
- A preinjury training level is typically achieved in about 6 weeks.
- A long pneumatic splint may accelerate the recovery process.

REFERRAL/DISPOSITION

- Menstrual dysfunction should be evaluated and treated if present.
- If a thorough trial of conservative management is unsuccessful, the diagnosis should be reconsidered and a referral to a sports medicine specialist should be sought.
- In recalcitrant cases, posteromedial fasciotomy with midline release of the soleus fascia may be helpful.
- In chronic cases of MTSS, it is not unusual for recovery to be prolonged. In some cases recovery may be even longer than for a tibial stress fracture.

Common Questions and Answers

Physician responses to common patient questions:

Q: Why do I keep getting pain in my lower legs even though I usually rest for 1 or 2 days when it hurts?

A: This is not enough time to allow for adequate healing. In addition, evaluation of the training routine, shoes, foot posture, flexibility, and strength are needed to address potential causes of reinjury.

Q: How long before I can return to running the way I was before?

A: In mild cases the pain should resolve in 1 to 2 weeks, during which time a cross-training program is used to maintain fitness. Another 4 to 6 weeks is needed to gradually increase training to preinjury levels. If symptoms are more severe, these time frames may be significantly lengthened.

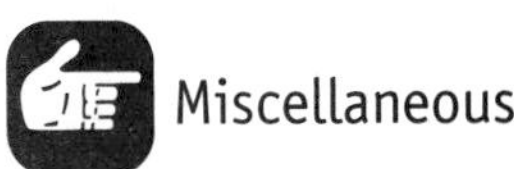

Miscellaneous

SYNONYMS

- Shin splints
- Periostitis
- Chronic periostalgia
- Soleus syndrome
- Tibial stress syndrome

ICD-9 CODE

844.9

BIBLIOGRAPHY

Batt ME. Shin splints: a review of terminology. *Clin J Sports Med* 1995;5:53–57.

DiFiori JP. Overuse injuries in children and adolescents. *Phys Sports Med* 1999;27:75–89.

Fredericson M, Bergman AG, Hoffman KL, et al. Tibial stress reaction in runners: correlation of clinical symptoms and scintigraphy with a new magnetic resonance imaging grading system. *Am J Sports Med* 23:472–481.

Kortbein PM, Kaufman KR, Basford JR, et al. Medial tibial stress syndrome. *Med Sci Sport Exerc* 32(suppl):27–33.

Authors: Joseph P. Luftman and John P. DiFiori

Meniscal Tears

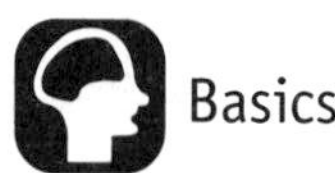

Basics

DEFINITION

- An injury to either the medial or lateral meniscus of the knee caused by twisting, shearing, or compressive forces from contact or noncontact mechanisms

INCIDENCE/PREVALENCE

- One of the most common knee problems
- Traumatic tears typically develop between the ages of 13 and 40 years.
- Degenerative tears typically develop in patients over 40.
- Posterior horn of medial meniscus is the most common location.

SIGNS AND SYMPTOMS

- Usually associated with a traumatic event, but can be insidious (degenerative tear)
- Pain directly over medial or lateral joint line of the knee
- Pain usually with weight bearing and twisting or turning of knee or squatting
- May be associated with slow onset of effusion over a couple of hours
- Catching, locking, or clicking sensation in many
- Giving way episodes possible
- Symptoms may get better with time, but typically recur with resumption of activities

RISK FACTORS

- Abnormal mechanical axis
- Ligament deficiency
- Degenerative joint disease
- Congenital anomalies (i.e., discoid meniscus)
- Poor quadriceps control

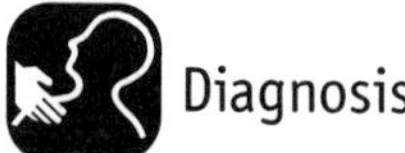

Diagnosis

DIFFERENTIAL DIAGNOSIS

- Capsulitis
- Intraarticular loose body
- Ligamentous injury
- Patellar subluxation
- Chondromalacia patellae; pain may occasionally radiate to joint line

HISTORY

- Joint line pain medial or lateral?
- Acute swelling? Suggestive of traumatic event such as meniscal tear, ligament tear, or osteochondral injury
- Catching/locking/clicking? Mechanical symptoms are suggestive of flap or bucket-handle meniscal tears, ligaments tears, or loose bodies.
- Recurrent pain and mild swelling? Suggestive of a chronic tear
- Giving way? Pain reflex inhibition of quadriceps

PHYSICAL EXAM

- Check for effusion/hemarthrosis, which is sign of meniscal, ligament, or osteochondral injury.
- Palpate the entire knee. Pain over the medial or lateral joint line is suggestive of meniscal injury and is the most important physical exam finding.
- Check range of motion (ROM). A locked knee, one that has new inability to come to full extension, is suggestive of a bucket-handle meniscal tear, ligament tear, or loose body.
- Check extensor mechanism function. Can the patient perform a straight leg raise? Are the quadriceps atrophic?
- Check stability to varus/valgus at 0 and 30 degrees of flexion.
- Check anterior and posterior drawer/Lachman/and Pivot shift to assess cruciate ligaments.
- Positive McMurray's test: Palpable click and pain over joint line are produced when meniscal fragment catches during test. Don't be fooled by crepitation from patellofemoral joint. Also, not all meniscal tears produce a positive McMurray's test result.

IMAGING

- Standard weight-bearing anteroposterior/lateral/Rosenberg and Merchant views to rule out any bony problems such as loose body, fracture, arthritis, or osteochondritis dissecans
- MRI is useful when history and physical exam are indeterminate or for operative planning.

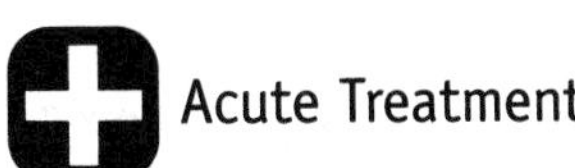

Acute Treatment

ANALGESIA

- Initial treatment is with ice (no more than 20 minutes per hour), nonsteroidal antiinflammatory drugs, gentle ROM exercises, and isometric quadriceps exercises.
- Physical therapy modalities, such as iontophoresis and electrical stimulation, can assist in the acute phase of pain control.

IMMOBILIZATION

- Do not immobilize unless suspecting a fracture, major ligamentous injury, or a large bucket-handle meniscus tear.
- May cause unnecessary stiffness
- If choosing to provide support, a hinged knee brace is a good option to help prevent stiffness associated with an immobilizer.

SPECIAL CONSIDERATIONS

A locked knee is a relative indication for urgent arthroscopic surgery, and orthopedic referral should be made immediately to assist in scheduling.

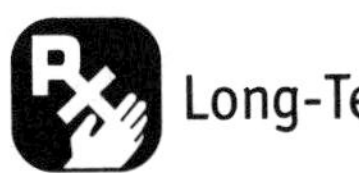

Long-Term Treatment

REHABILITATION

- Small, stable meniscal tears (<1 cm, peripheral) with no other pathologic conditions can usually be treated nonoperatively, and most spontaneously improve over 6 weeks to 3 months, regardless of treatment.
- A generalized rehabilitation program for the knee is a good option to help stimulate quadriceps and hamstring strength to protect the knee from further injuries.

SURGICAL TREATMENT

- Surgery is indicated for any locked knee, unstable meniscal tear, or for failure of nonoperative treatment.
- Surgery consists of outpatient arthroscopic partial meniscectomy or repair of the meniscal tear, depending on location of tear, type of tear, and patient health factors.

REFERRAL/DISPOSITION

- Surgery as indicated above
- Mechanical symptoms
- Any acutely locked knee
- Any associated ligamentous injury

Common Questions and Answers

Physician responses to common patient questions:

Q: Will I need surgery for this injury?

A: Most patients will eventually require arthroscopic surgery for a meniscus tear.

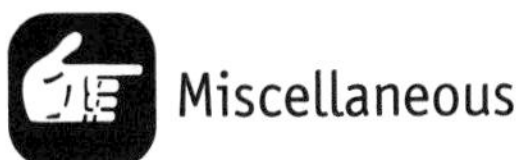

Miscellaneous

SYNONYMS

- Cartilage tear (common usage by patients for a meniscal tear)

ICD-9 CODE

836.2

BIBLIOGRAPHY

Belzer JP, Cannon WD Jr. Meniscus tears: treatment in the stable and unstable knee. *J Am Acad Orthop Surg* 1993;1:41–47.

Miller RH. *Knee injuries in Campbell's operative orthopaedics*. Chicago: CV Mosby, 1998.

Newman AP, Daniels AU, Burks RT. Principles and decision making in meniscal surgery. *Arthroscopy* 1993;9:33–51.

Silbey MF, Fu FH. *Knee injuries in sports injuries*. Philadelphia: Williams & Wilkins, 1994.

Authors: John Langland, Angelo J. Colosimo, and Robert S. Heidt Jr.

Olecranon Bursitis

Basics

DEFINITION

- Inflammation of the superficial olecranon bursa

Acute

Direct trauma may be single or multiple traumatic episodes.

Chronic

- Results from multiple episodes of trauma during the resorptive phases of acute bursitis
- Bursal linings change to that of fibrosis

Septic

- Superimposed infection of acute or chronic olecranon bursitis
- Develops from skin wounds, dermatitis, or hematogenous

INCIDENCE/PREVALENCE

- Common

SIGNS AND SYMPTOMS

Acute

- Swelling and tenderness of the bursa after a direct blow
- Range of motion (ROM) usually normal

Chronic

- Bursal walls thick and fibrotic
- May have moveable subcutaneous nodules

Septic

- Pain over olecranon bursa with ROM
- Tender to palpation

RISK FACTORS

Acute

- Direct elbow trauma

Chronic

- Multiple episodes of elbow trauma

Septic

- History of elbow trauma
- Skin lesions

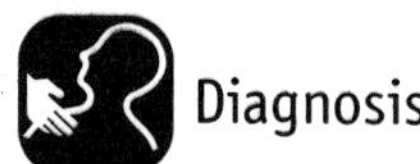

Diagnosis

DIFFERENTIAL DIAGNOSIS

- Cellulitis
- Fracture
- Arthritis
- Ligamentous injury
- Tendinitis
- Contusion

HISTORY

Acute

- History of elbow trauma

Chronic

- Multiple episodes of elbow trauma

Septic

- Painful, swollen, erythematous elbow with or without systemic symptoms

PHYSICAL EXAMINATION

Acute

- Swollen, fluctuant fluid collection of superficial olecranon bursa without joint findings
- ROM usually normal

Chronic

- Swollen, fluctuant fluid collection of superficial olecranon bursa without joint findings
- Fibrotic trabeculae and villi may form a subcutaneous mass.
- ROM usually normal

Septic

- Swollen, fluctuant fluid collection of superficial olecranon bursa
- Often tender along olecranon bursa with or without movement
- Overlying skin abrasions and erythema often present

IMAGING

- Plain x-rays negative

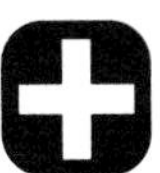

Acute Treatment

PREVENTION

- High-quality elbow pads
- Softer playing surfaces (natural turf)

PROCEDURES

- Ice
- Nonsteroidal anti-inflammatory drugs
- Monitor
- Aspiration
  - —Perform when distension causes significant discomfort and loss of motion
  - —Aseptic fluid typically straw colored
  - —Painful bursa should be aspirated and fluid analyzed for cell count, crystals, and gram stain.
  - —*Staphylococcus A* most common organism in septic bursa
- Steroid injections
  - —Used by some clinicians with mixed results
  - —Contraindicated if infection suspected
- Incision and drainage
  - —Most recommended for septic bursa
- Surgery
  - —For refractory cases that limit activity

MEDICATION

- Antibiotics
  - —Intravenous antibiotics if systemic symptoms present
  - —Oral antibiotics if no systemic signs present
  - —Treat *Staphylococcus Aureus*

Miscellaneous

SYNONYMS

- Miner's elbow
- Student's elbow

ICD-9 CODE

726.33

BIBLIOGRAPHY

Brukner P, Kahn K. *Clinical sports medicine.* Sydney: McGraw-Hill, 1994.

DeLee JC, Drez D. *Orthopaedic sports medicine.* Philadelphia: WB Saunders, 1994.

Salter RB. *Textbook of disorders and injuries of the musculoskeletal system.* Baltimore: Williams & Wilkins, 1983.

Author: Dan Ostlie

Onychocryptosis

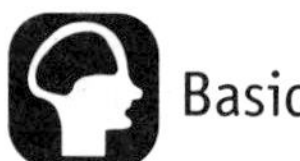

Basics

DEFINITION

- Alteration in the proper fit of the nail plate into the lateral or medial nail groove
- Improper fit leads to callous formation, edema, and perforation in the nail groove as a result of the rubbing of the nail plate against the nail groove.
- Three stages
  - —Stage 1: erythema, slight edema, and pain when pressure is applied to the lateral nail groove
  - —Stage 2: increased stage 1 symptoms, drainage, and infection
  - —Stage 3: worsening stage 1 symptoms, presence of granulation tissue, and lateral wall hypertrophy

INCIDENCE/PREVALENCE

- 26% of pathologic nail conditions
- Majority of cases occur in males in their second and third decades
- 2:1 male-to-female ratio <30 years old and 1:1 >30 years old

SIGNS AND SYMPTOMS

- Pain, swelling, and limitation of activities
- Cardinal signs of inflammation (redness, warmth, tenderness, and edema)
- In-curvated nail margin

RISK FACTORS

- Shoes with tight-fitting toe box
- Improper nail-trimming techniques
- Improper fitting cleats
- Senior athletes
- Diabetes
- Trauma, acute and repetitive
- Hyperhidrosis
- Obesity
- Poor stance and gait
- Skeletal abnormalities
- Subungual neoplasms
- Family history of in-curvated nails
- Arthritis
- Immune deficiency
- Congenital and acquired nail disorders
- Onychomycosis

ASSOCIATED INJURIES AND COMPLICATIONS

- Paronychia
- Cellulitis
- Osteomyelitis

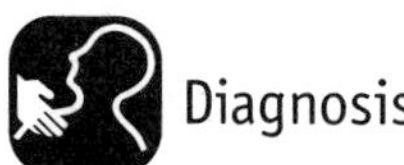

Diagnosis

DIFFERENTIAL DIAGNOSIS

- Foreign body
- Tumor

HISTORY

- Ask about tight-fitting shoes: small toe boxes predispose to onychocryptosis.
- Cardinal signs of infection: may have superimposed bacterial infection requiring antibiotics.
- Ask about recurrence and previous treatment: may impact on treatment choice.
- History of immune deficiency or abnormal wound healing: increased chance for severe infection.

PHYSICAL EXAMINATION

- Inspect for foreign bodies
- Cardinal signs of ascending infection
- Presence of excess medial or lateral wall tissue

IMAGING

Plain films and/or bone scan may be required for severely infected toe if osteomyelitis is suspected.

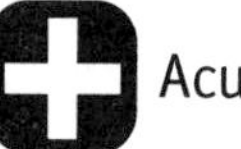

Acute Treatment

ANALGESIA

- Depends on planned treatment option and patient discomfort level
- Recommend performing local anesthesia or a digital block with 1% to 2% lidocaine without epinephrine before manipulation
- Ibuprofen or acetaminophen for postsurgical pain control

IMMOBILIZATION

- Patients may be full weight-bearing after nonsurgical treatments.
- Partial weight-bearing for 24–48 hours after surgery may be needed, but generally weight-bearing is well tolerated.

NONSURGICAL TREATMENT

- Patients should be instructed in maintenance of proper foot hygiene, avoidance of wearing shoes with tight-fitting toe box, soaking the feet, properly trimming nails (cutting the nail straight across), and avoidance of repetitive trauma.
- Cure rates can be as high as 75% with good patient compliance for stage 1 lesions.
- If infection is suspected, it is important to remove the source of the infection and treat with antibiotics directed against gram-positive bacteria.

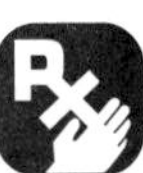

Long-Term Treatment

SURGERY

- May be recommended for recurrent stage 1 lesions as below for stage 2 lesions
  - —Stage 2: remove with a wedge excision the distal outer nail edge without matricectomy
  - —Stage 2 or 3: partial removal of the medial or lateral nail with matricectomy (medial/lateral nail avulsion) with or without electrosurgical or phenol cauterization
  - —Stage 3: in addition to above, ablation of the medial or lateral wall tissue to promote normalization of the medial/lateral nail fold
- Major contraindications include disorders causing digital ischemia, e.g., diabetes, peripheral vascular, and collagen diseases.

REFERRAL/DISPOSITION

Immunocompromised individuals with a severe infection may require hospitalization for administration of intravenous antibiotics.

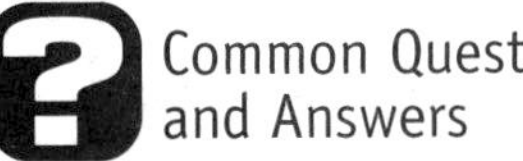

Common Questions and Answers

Physician responses to common patient questions:
Q: How long before return to activity after surgical treatment?
A: Impact activities should be avoided until patient is pain-free and clear of infection.
Q: What is the frequency of symptomatic nail regrowth following distal nail wedge resection, nail avulsion, phenol, and electrosurgical cauterization?
A: Distal nail wedge resection 70%; nail avulsion 50% to 80%; phenol cauterization 4% to 25%; electrosurgical cauterization <5%.

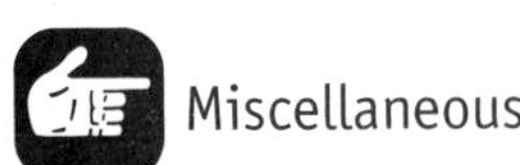

Miscellaneous

SYNONYMS

- Ingrown toenail
- Unguis incarnatus
- In-fleshed toenail
- Embedded toenail

ICD-9 CODE

703.0 Ingrown toenail

CPT CODE

11730 Nail removal, partial or complete
11750 Permanent nail removal (matricectomy), partial or complete

BIBLIOGRAPHY

Ikard RW. Onychocryptosis. *J Am Coll Surg* 1998;187:96–102.

Mann JL, Coughlin MJ. *Surgery of the foot and ankle.* St. Louis: Mosby-Year Book, 1993.

Pfenninger JL, Fowler GC. *Procedures for primary care physicians.* St. Louis: Mosby-Year Book, 1994.

Zuber TJ, Pfenninger JL. Management of ingrown toenails. *Am Fam Physician* 1995;52:181–188.

Authors: Jamie Edwards and Suzanne Hecht

Onychomycosis

Basics

DEFINITION

- Fungal infection of the fingernails or toenails

INCIDENCE/PREVALENCE

- 22–130 cases/1,000 population
- Found in 20% of U.S. population between ages 40 and 60 years
- Incidence of infection increasing worldwide
- Predominant age/sex varies with type of infection, but all are rare before puberty.
- Seen in 40% of patients with fungal infections at other locations

CAUSES

- Onychomycosis can be divided into fungal infections caused by
  —Dermatophytes: *Trichophyton rubrum, T. mentagrophytes, Epidermophyton floccosum*
  —Yeast: *Candida albicans, C. parapsilosis, C. tropicalis*
  —Nondermatophyte molds: *Scopulariopsis brevicollis, Hendersonula toruloidea, Alternaria tenuis*

SIGNS AND SYMPTOMS

Dermatophytes

- 80% involve the toenails, with the hallux most commonly affected
- Fungi invade the nail by growing into either the ventral edge or the distal lateral nail groove.
- Initially, a small area of onycholysis develops at the distal nail tip.
- Soft yellow keratin accumulates in this area and further nail lifting occurs.
- Eventually, the nail appears thickened with hyperkeratotic debris and a yellow-brown discoloration.
- Pain usually is absent.
- Three clinical forms occur depending on the location of the organism: distal subungual onychomycosis, proximal subungual onychomycosis, and superficial white onychomycosis.

Yeast

- 70% of cases involve the hand, with the dominant hand most commonly affected
- Initial cuticle detachment is followed by yellow-brown discoloration of the lateral nail.
- Secondary changes to the nail can occur and include irregular borders, rough surfaces, and striations.
- Pain usually is mild and exacerbated by prolonged contact with water.

Molds

- Most common in patients >60 years old
- Usually affects the hallux

RISK FACTORS

Dermatophytes

- Immunosuppression
- Hyperhidrosis
- Diabetes mellitus
- Peripheral vascular disease
- Tight-fitting or rubber shoes
- Warm, moist environment

Yeast

- Immunosuppression
- Hyperhidrosis
- Diabetes mellitus
- Malnutrition
- Damage to cuticle
- Malignancies
- Direct contamination

Molds

- Peripheral vascular disease
- Soil contamination

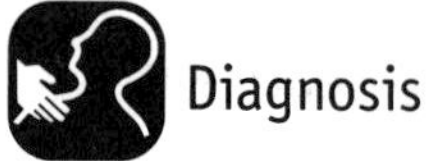

Diagnosis

DIFFERENTIAL DIAGNOSIS

- 50% of thick nails are caused by conditions other than onychomycosis.
- Psoriasis
- Trauma
- Herpetic whitlow
- Endocrine disease
- Black nail paronychia
- Eczema
- Scleroderma
- Dermatomyositis
- Lichen planus
- Tumor
- Trophic changes
- Medications
- Yellow nail syndrome

HISTORY

- Description of location, duration, and associated symptoms
- History of any nail trauma
- Detailed history of footwear and barefoot activities
- Determine if tinea infections are present at other sites, e.g., tinea cruris, tinea capitis
- History of onychomycosis
- Determine risk factors, such as diabetes mellitus, peripheral vascular disease, and immunosuppression

PHYSICAL EXAMINATION

- Examine all nails; note areas of involvement, discoloration, and deformity.
- Examine nails for signs of trauma.
- Carefully examine surrounding tissue for signs of secondary infection.
- Examine skin for other fungal infections.
- Assess peripheral pulses.

LABORATORY

- Diagnosis should be established with both a potassium hydroxide (KOH) examination and culture.
- Topical antifungal medications should not be applied for 2 days before KOH examination and culture.
- KOH examination
  —Remove crumbling debris from several nails using a 1-mm curette.
  —Add 5% KOH and heat gently.
  —100% sensitivity if hyphae observed in >2 preparations examined.
- Culture
  —Clean nail with alcohol to remove bacteria.
  —Obtain crumbling debris with 1-mm curette as described above.
  —Inoculate onto Sabouraud's medium with and without antibiotics to identify the fungal species.
  —Cultures are negative in 30% of cases.

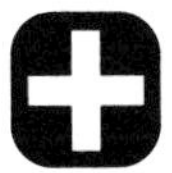

Acute Treatment

TREATMENT

- Council patients about medications.
- Discuss cost, side effects, and continuous versus pulse dosing.
- Patients should be made aware that nails might not appear normal until several months after completion of treatment.
- Antimycotic agents should not be used in patients with preexisting liver dysfunction.
- Before initiating medications, the nail should be debrided. Remove as much of the crumbling hyperkeratotic debris as possible.
- Terbinafine: 80% to 100% cure rate
  —Fingernails: 250 mg q.d. for 6 weeks or 500 mg q.d. for 1 week/month for 2 months
  —Toenails: 250 mg q.d. for 12 weeks or 500 mg q.d. for 1 week/month for 3 months
  —Liver function tests (LFTs) should be checked if patients use terbinafine for >6 weeks.
- Itraconazole: 80% cure rate
  —Fingernails: 200 mg q.d. for 6 weeks or 200 mg b.i.d. for 1 week/month for 3 months
  —Toenails: 200 mg q.d. for 12 weeks or 200 mg b.i.d. for 1 week/month for 3 months
  —LFTs should be checked periodically if continuous therapy is >1 month.
  —LFTs are not required for itraconazole pulse therapy.
- Griseofulvin: 40% to 60% cure rate
  —Fingernails: 333 mg b.i.d for 6 months
  —Toenails: 333 mg b.i.d. for 12 months
  —LFTs should be checked periodically.
- Topical treatments for onychomycosis generally are not effective, but may result in a more rapid cure when used in conjunction with oral agents.
- In persistent onychomycosis, surgical or chemical (40% urea) nail avulsion may be required in combination with oral therapy.

PREVENTION

- Avoid going barefoot in public places, such as public showers, swimming pools, hotel rooms, health clubs/facilities, and locker rooms.
- Keep feet dry and cool.
- Wear absorbent cotton socks.
- Apply topical antifungal cream, spray, or powder to feet and toenails regularly.
- Discard old shoes that may harbor fungi.
- Apply an antifungal powder or spray to the inside of shoes at least once a week.

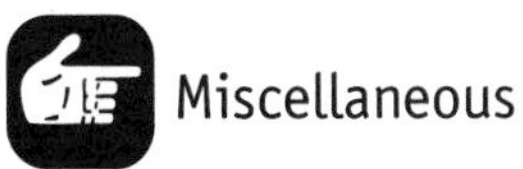

Miscellaneous

SYNONYMS

- Nail ringworm
- Tinea unguium

ICD-9 CODE

110.1 Dermatophytosis of nail
112.3 Candidiasis of skin and nails

BIBLIOGRAPHY

Habif TP. *Clinical dermatology: a color guide to diagnosis and therapy*. St. Louis: Mosby, 1995.

Jaffe R. Onychomycosis: recognition, diagnosis, and management. *Arch Fam Med* 1998;7:587.

Sams WM, Lynch PJ, eds. *Principles and practice of dermatology*, 2nd ed. New York: Churchill Livingstone, 1996.

Authors: Thomas D. Armsey and Steve Brook

Osteitis Pubis

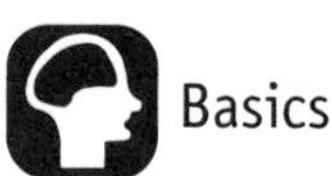

Basics

DEFINITION

- Chronic pelvic/groin pain caused by repetitive stress at the symphysis pubis
- Inflammation at the symphysis pubis

SIGNS AND SYMPTOMS

- Severe groin pain with the athlete being unable to stand on one leg, or a dull ache in the groin
- Pain exacerbated with adduction with resistance (difficulty kicking the ball)
- May develop pain in the sacroiliac joint on the same side
- Difficulty making cutting movements
- Coach or athlete may notice a change in athlete's technique (e.g., in soccer).

RISK FACTORS

- Athlete between 20 and 30 years old (more motion at the symphysis pubis before age 30, when it reaches adult maturity)
- Muscle imbalances around the pelvis; in general, the athlete will have much stronger hip flexors and adductors than abductors and hip extensors
- Decreased range of motion of the hip joint
- Hard training
- Frequent competition
- Uneven, poorly maintained playing surfaces

ETIOLOGY

- Tendinosis of the adductor and gracilis muscle at their origins along the inferior pubic ramus
- True etiology unknown; possibly secondary to muscular traction on pelvis, causing excessive motion at the symphysis and resulting in inflammation
- Avascular necrosis of the pubis may occur.
- Subluxations of the symphysis pubis may result in traumatic arthritis.

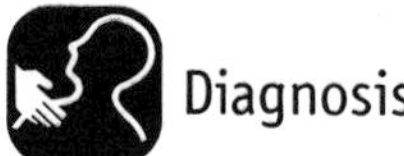

Diagnosis

DIFFERENTIAL DIAGNOSIS

- Adductor/gracilis tendonitis
- Inguinal hernia
- Prostatitis
- Femoral neck stress fracture
- Genitourinary (GU) infection
- GU neoplasm
- Urolithiasis
- Ankylosing spondylitis of the pubic symphysis
- "Sports hernia" (any athlete presenting with a prolonged history of groin pain, the "sports hernia/Gilmore groin" must be at the top of the differential. Probable association between the two problems. Both have a similar mechanism of injury. Think of the two injuries on a continuum.)

PHYSICAL EXAMINATION

- Tenderness over symphysis pubis and adductor tendons
- Loss of integrity of the fascia of the anterior abdominal wall at the insertion on the pubis
- Pain on resisted elevation of the leg in the supine position
- Pain with contraction of the adductor or low abdominal muscles
- Tenderness and "relaxation" of the inguinal canal
- Pain reproduced with one-legged stance
- Waddling gait

IMAGING

- Standard anteroposterior pelvis
- Rispoli radiographic changes
  - —Stage 1: osteolysis of the os pubis at the origin of the gracilis, adductor longus, or adductor brevis
  - —Stage 2: asymmetry and widespread erosions of the symphysis pubis
  - —Stage 3: arthrosis of symphysis pubis developing with deformity
  - —Stage 4: myositis of adjacent muscles and calcifications of tissues around symphysis
- "Flamingo" views: stress views, with patient standing on one leg, looking for shifting at the pubic symphysis (>3 mm)
- Bone scan: increased bone metabolic activity in the area of the symphysis
- Computed tomographic scan: helpful in early stages; may see hematomas, soft tissue swelling, and small avulsion.

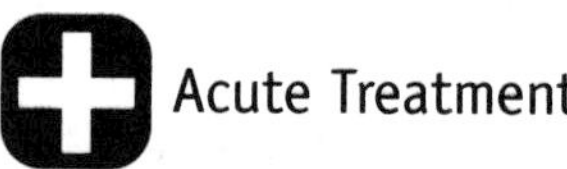

Acute Treatment

INITIAL TREATMENT

- Rest, ice, and nonsteroidal anti-inflammatory drugs
- Work on the biomechanical weakness, hip range of motion, abdominal strengthening, and pelvic stabilizers
- Corticosteroid injection into the symphysis pubis and surrounding tissue can be beneficial.
- Functional progress back to sport
- General return to sport in 4–8 weeks

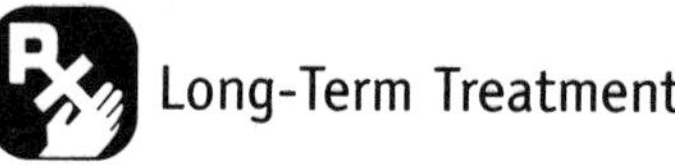

Long-Term Treatment

REHABILITATION

- Range of motion of hip
- Abdominal strengthening
- Pelvic stabilizer strengthening
- Look for pelvic asymmetry/sacroiliac dysfunction

SURGERY

- Reserved for recalcitrant cases only. Procedures include
  - —Nescovic technique (reefing the abdominal muscles to the pubis and Poupart ligament)
  - —Arthrodesis of the symphysis
  - —Tenotomy of the gracilis/removal of bony ossicles

REFERRAL/DISPOSITION

- Refer when not responding to conservative management, i.e., rest and gradual return over 2–3 months
- Consider corticosteroid injection

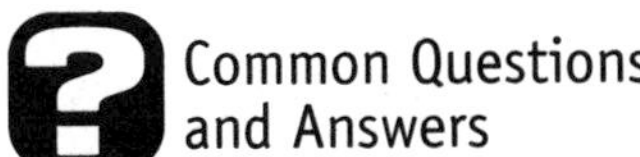

Common Questions and Answers

Physician responses to common patient questions:
Q: When can I return to play?
A: Usual time frame is 6–10 weeks, depending on how long symptoms were present before starting treatment.
Q: What can I do to prevent this from happening?
A: Work hard to strengthen the hip abductors, pelvic stabilizers, and abdominal muscles. Also work on a good flexibility program for the hip flexors, extensors, and adductors.
Q: If I have surgery, how long am I out of sports/activity?
A: Depends on the surgeon, but generally it is recommended no activity for 8 weeks and then gradual return.

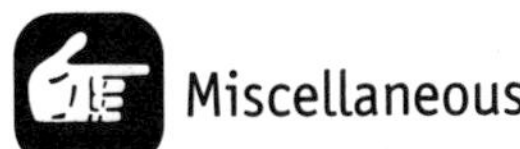

Miscellaneous

SYNONYMS

- Osteochondritis of the symphysis pubis
- Pubic symphysitis
- Gracilis syndrome
- Osteochondritis of the pubis
- Pubalgia
- Osteitis necroticans pubis
- Rectus adductor syndrome
- Traumatic inguinal leg syndrome
- Peterson syndrome

ICD-9 CODE

733.5 Osteitis pubis
843.8 Sprain/strain hip pelvis
739.4 Sacroiliac dysfunction

BIBLIOGRAPHY

DeLee JC, Drez D. *Orthopedic sports medicine.* Philadelphia: WB Saunders, 1994.

Gilmore J. Groin pain in soccer players. *Clin Sports Med* 1998;17:787–794.

Nicholas JA, Hershman EB. *The lower extremity and spine in sports medicine.* St. Louis: Mosby, 1995.

Author: Eric Jenkinson

Osteochondritis Dissecans

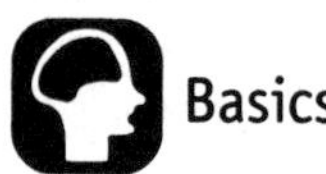

Basics

DEFINITION

- Osteochondritis dissecans (OCD) is an acquired defect in the articular cartilage and underlying bone.
- Previously classified into juvenile and adult forms
- Often affects the femoral condyles, talar dome, and humeral capitellum, but can occur in all large joints

INCIDENCE/PREVALENCE

Incidence estimated to be 15–30 cases per 100,000 persons.

SIGNS AND SYMPTOMS

- Vague joint pain
- Locking
- Restricted range of motion
- Pain with activity or weight-bearing

RISK FACTORS

- Repetitive microtrauma or overuse
- Familial predisposition
- OCD in one joint is risk factor for contralateral involvement; 20% to 30% of patients with OCD of the knee have bilateral involvement.
- Throwing sports and gymnastics are specific risk factors for OCD of the elbow.

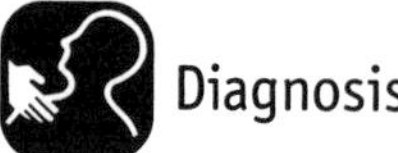

Diagnosis

DIFFERENTIAL DIAGNOSIS

- Meniscal or ligamentous injury
- Tendinitis
- Patellofemoral pain syndrome
- Osteoarthritis
- Posttraumatic osteochondral defect
- Spontaneous osteonecrosis of the knee
- Crystal-induced arthropathies

HISTORY

- Insidious onset of symptoms
- Preceding injury to joint surface seen in <50% of patients
- Stiffness after periods of rest

PHYSICAL EXAMINATION

- Effusion and/or crepitus may be present.
- Decreased or painful range of motion
- Poorly localized joint line tenderness

IMAGING

- X-ray is standard for diagnosis.
- Bone scan occasionally is useful for diagnosis if onset is acute and x-rays are negative.
- Ultrasound is unreliable.
- Magnetic resonance imaging (MRI) is gold standard for staging after diagnosis.

MRI STAGING CLASSIFICATION

- Stage I: subchondral lesion of low signal intensity
- Stage II: hypointense rim on images indicating demarcation but not separation of lesion
- Stage III: high signal intensity and underlying cystic changes indicative of instability
- Stage IV: partial or complete dislocation of osteochondral fragment into the joint space

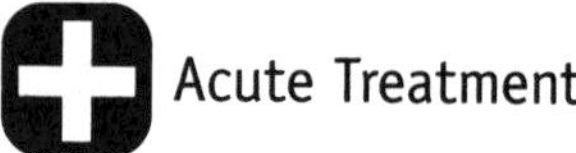

Acute Treatment

IMMOBILIZATION

- Stage I OCD is treated nonoperatively with either activity restriction or immobilization. Weight-bearing is restricted for 6–8 weeks
- Stage II OCD is treated nonoperatively in juveniles with open joint physis. Treatment of adults is controversial and may depend on the size of the lesion.
- Stage III–IV and those who fail nonoperative therapy should be referred for surgical management.

SPECIAL CONSIDERATIONS

- Progression of symptoms to joint stiffness or locking necessitates arthroscopy to evaluate and treat for possible loose bodies.
- Nonsteroidal anti-inflammatory drugs are useful adjunctive therapy.

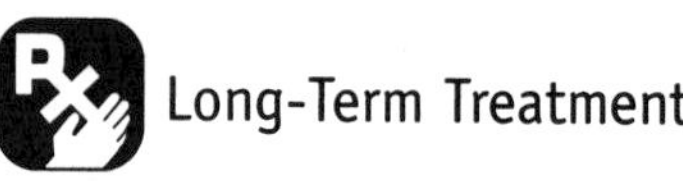

Long-Term Treatment

REHABILITATION

- Physical therapy may be initiated for conservatively managed patients. Stretching, range of motion exercises, conditioning exercises, and quadriceps strengthening are beneficial
- Postsurgical physical therapy can be tailored to the procedure.

SURGERY

- Arthroscopy has better outcomes compared to open procedures.
- Comparing excision, curettage, and drilling, the highest success rates were seen when all three therapies were used together.

REFERRAL/DISPOSITION

Orthopaedic referral is indicated for all patients with unstable OCD or those who fail conservative treatment.

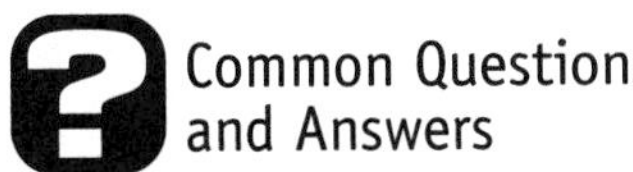

Common Questions and Answers

Physician responses to common patient questions:

Q: How fast can I return to competitive sports?

A: Stable lesions require break from competitive sports for at least 6–8 weeks. Patients must be pain-free before return to sports. MRI and/or bone scan may be useful to evaluate healing.

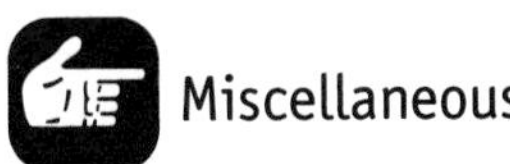

Miscellaneous

ICD-9 CODE

732.7

BIBLIOGRAPHY

Bohndorf K. Osteochondritis dissecans: a review and new MRI classification. *Eur Radiol* 19987;8:103–112.

Hixon AL, Gibbs LM. Osteochondritis dissecans: a diagnosis not to miss. *Am Fam Physician* 2000;61:151–158.

Stabler A, Glaser C, Reiser M. Musculoskeletal MR: knee. *Eur Radiol* 2000;10:230–241.

Tol JL, Struijs PA, Bossnyt PM, Verhagen RA, van Dijk CN, et al. Treatment strategies in osteochondral defects of the talar dome: a systematic review. *Foot Ankle Int* 2000;21:119–126.

Authors: Suraj Achar and Jeff Taylor

Patellar Dislocation and Instability

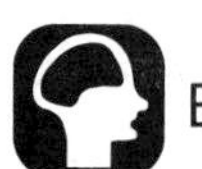

Basics

DEFINITION

- Patellar instability is defined as hypermobility of the patella in either the medial or lateral direction.
- Medial instability is extremely rare.
- Complete dislocation and subluxation represent variations in severity of instability.
- Acute dislocation typically occurs with a twisting injury and strong contraction of the quadriceps; rarely it is due to direct trauma to the medial aspect of the patella.

SIGNS AND SYMPTOMS

- Athlete often describes tearing or ripping noise, which may be heard by other players.
- Most often, athlete reports spontaneous reduction as knee is brought from flexion into extension.
- Rapid swelling due to formation of large hemarthrosis
- Usually athlete is instantly disabled, unwilling or unable to move the knee and bear weight.
- Severe pain to knee acutely after injury
- Symptoms after acute subluxation usually are less severe than after complete dislocation.

RISK FACTORS

- Prior history of subluxed or dislocated patella
- Recurrence rate 15% to 50% after initial dislocation
- Adolescent females
- Patella alta ("high riding patella")
- Excessive genu valgum
- Weak vastus medialis
- Excessive tibial torsion

ASSOCIATED INJURIES AND COMPLICATIONS

- Avulsion fracture of the superomedial pole of the patella
- Osteochondral fractures of the lateral femoral condyle or posterior patellar articular surface
- Tear of the medial patellofemoral ligament
- Concomitant major ligamentous or meniscal injury

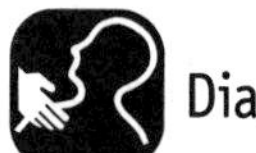

Diagnosis

DIFFERENTIAL DIAGNOSIS

- Subluxation versus dislocation
- Although history of patellar dislocation is fairly classic, consider other entities that cause early effusions, e.g., anterior cruciate ligament (ACL) tear, meniscal tear, and fractures.

HISTORY

Q: Initial or recurrent?
A: This will directly impact your treatment and potential referral.
Q: History of previous knee injury or patellofemoral pain syndrome (PFPS)?
A: Risk factors for patellar instability similar to PFPS and knee injuries typically lead to weak quadriceps.

PHYSICAL EXAMINATION

- Immediately after dislocation, may show patella dislocated laterally and prominence medially due to uncovered medial femoral condyle
- Obvious effusion
- Tenderness most apparent over the medial retinaculum and vastus medialis
- Limited range of motion with knee in extended position
- Fear of redislocation when knee is flexed
- Positive apprehension sign with movement of patella laterally
- Check ACL and menisci, as up to 12% of patellar dislocations have associated major ligamentous or meniscal injury.

IMAGING

- Standard anteroposterior, lateral, and notch views
- Sunrise view mandatory. Rule out presence of associated osteochondral fractures. Avulsion fracture or calcification along the medial edge of the patella is considered pathognomonic for patellar dislocation

POSTREDUCTION VIEWS

- Similar to prereduction films

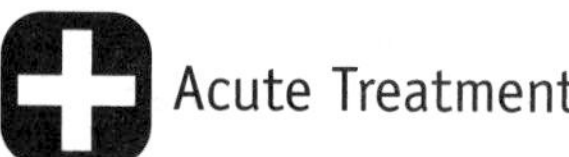

Acute Treatment

ANALGESIA

- If not reduced spontaneously, may require conscious sedation for pain control and muscle relaxation.
- Alternatively, arthrocentesis performed with instillation of 10–15 mL of lidocaine and/or bupivacaine.

REDUCTION TECHNIQUES

- Extension of the leg with hip flexed (reduces tension of quadriceps tendon)
- Gentle pressure on patella directed lateral to medial

POSTREDUCTION EVALUATION

- Postreduction radiographs to confirm reduction and rule out fractures
- Examine anterior ACL and medial and lateral menisci to rule out accompanying tears.
- After reduction, rest, ice, focal compression, and elevation are indicated for the first 24–48 hours.

IMMOBILIZATION

- Knee immobilization is maintained for approximately 2–3 weeks, although early passive range of motion in terminal extension is allowed to minimize disuse atrophy.
- Hinged brace may be substituted for knee immobilizer as early as 1 week.

SPECIAL CONSIDERATIONS

A significant number of patients develop large hemarthrosis. Aspiration may be considered after 48–72 hours both to relieve pain and to check for fat globules, which might help diagnose an occult osteochondral fracture.

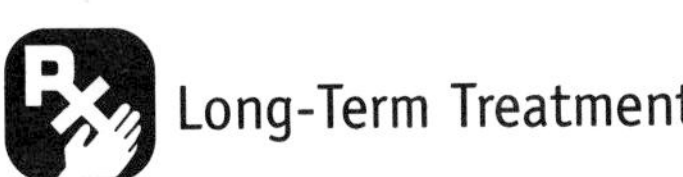

Long-Term Treatment

REHABILITATION

- Isometric quadriceps exercises are begun as soon as possible, although it is often difficult and painful for the athlete to produce a contraction that involves the vastus medialis.
- Active range of motion exercises are started at 1 week and physical therapy consultation given for medial quadriceps strengthening.
- Knee immobilizer or hinged brace is used for ambulation until 100 degrees of painless flexion is present, there is no effusion, and a normal heel-to-toe gait is possible.
- Immobilizer or hinged brace ultimately is replaced with a neoprene sleeve with a lateral buttress until normal, painless activities of daily living are possible.

SURGERY

- Typically patients who fail a conservative trial of approximately 6 months become surgical candidates.
- Surgical management includes lateral retinacular release alone, proximal extensor mechanism realignment alone, or combined proximal and distal realignment.

REFERRAL

- Orthopaedic referral indicated if
  —Osteochondral fracture noted on either plain radiographs or magnetic resonance imaging
  —Recurrent patellar dislocations despite adequate rehabilitation, especially in younger patients (<14 years old) in whom recurrence rates can reach 60%
  —Evidence of joint locking
  —High-risk athlete participates in activities involving pivoting, who is at increased risk of recurrent patellar dislocation

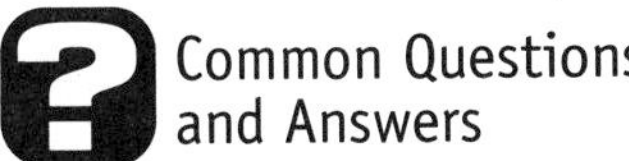

Common Questions and Answers

Physician responses to common patient questions:

Q: How long before I can return to sports?

A: Evidence of adequate healing (absence of sensations of instability, lack of effusion, and absence of pain on patellofemoral compression) and adequate function (able to perform rotational movements such as pivoting, cutting, and twisting without evidence of instability). Athlete may need McConnell taping or patellar stabilizing braces to accomplish this.

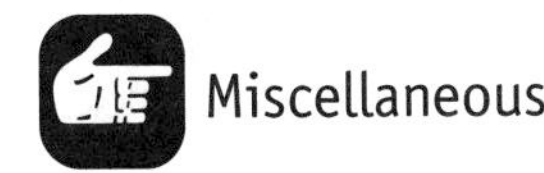

Miscellaneous

ICD-9 CODE

836.3

BIBLIOGRAPHY

Drez D, Delee JC, eds. *Orthopaedic sports medicine: principles and practices.* Philadelphia: WB Saunders, 1994.

Garth WP, Pomphry M Jr, Merrill K. Functional treatment of patellar dislocation in an athletic population. *Am J Sports Med* 1996;24:785–791.

Iobst CA, Stinitski CL. Pediatric and adolescent sports injuries: acute knee injuries. *Clin Sports Med* 2000;19:621–635.

Kilgore KP. The knee: patellar dislocation. In: Ruiz E, Cicero JJ, eds. *Emergency management of skeletal injuries,* 1st ed. St. Louis: Mosby-Year Book, 1995.

Roberts DM, Stallard TC. Emergency department evaluation and treatment of knee and leg injuries. *Emerg Med Clin North Am* 2000;18:67–84.

Author: Keith Stuessi

Patellar/Quadriceps Tendinitis

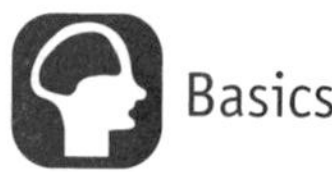

Basics

DEFINITION

- Symptomatic degeneration of the patella/quadriceps tendon with vascular disruption and an inflammatory repair response
- Often triggered by overuse and repetitive overload of the tissues

SIGNS AND SYMPTOMS

- Tenderness at the proximal or distal pole of the patella, primarily with loading activities such as landing from a jump, running up or down a hill, or weighted leg extensions

RISK FACTORS

- Poor flexibility of hamstrings and quadriceps muscles
- Repetitive overload activities
- Jumping/landing sports
- "Too much, too soon"

BLAZINA'S CLASSIFICATION OF "JUMPER'S KNEE"

- Phase I: pain only after practice/participation
- Phase II: pain during activity but not sufficient to interfere
- Phase III: pain during and after activity that interferes with ability to play
- Phase IV: complete tendon disruption

ASSOCIATED INJURIES AND COMPLICATIONS

Tendinitis can progress to noninflammatory degenerative tendinosis or tendon rupture.

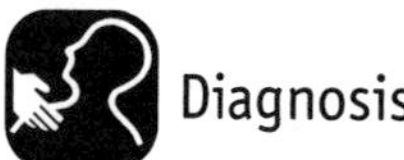

Diagnosis

DIFFERENTIAL DIAGNOSIS

- Tendinitis
- Sinding-Larsen-Johansson (SLJ) disease (if skeletally immature)
- Partial tear of tendon

HISTORY

Q: Chronic or acute?
A: Acute may be more likely to be a tear
Q: What activities cause the most discomfort?
A: Jumping and running activities are commonly involved.
Q: Swelling or associated injury?
A: Often means separate injury rather than tendinitis
Q: Do nonsteroidal anti-inflammatory drugs (NSAIDs) help?
A: May help more with acute process
Q: Change in technique, training regimen, or equipment?
A: Usually the common culprits in overuse injuries

PHYSICAL EXAMINATION

- Point tender on quadriceps tendon insertion on patella or at the inferior pole of the patella
- Often have very tight quadriceps and hamstrings, which puts more tension on the patella tendon
- With the leg in extension and relaxed, tilt the patella up by pushing down on the superior pole of the patella and palpate under the distal pole. This is often a more positive test than just palpation of the distal pole with the knee flexed or hanging off the table.
- Check for ability to perform a straight-leg raise. Athlete will not be able to do if an acute tendon rupture.
- Check for intra-articular effusion, which most likely represents other pathology than tendinitis, such as a meniscus tear.

IMAGING

- Usually not necessary unless an acute injury (look for fracture or avulsion), skeletally immature (SLJ), or chronic injury (look for calcification)
- Magnetic resonance imaging (MRI) can show the degree of degeneration, tear, or intrasubstance debris.

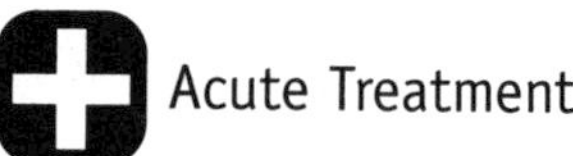

Acute Treatment

PHASES I AND II

- Control inflammation with ice and NSAIDs, with or without modalities
- Adequate warmup (with or without neoprene sleeve)
- Ensure hamstring and quadriceps flexibility
- Activity modification to reduce repetitive load of deceleration/jumping
- Progressive eccentric rehabilitation program
- Possible patella tendon strap

PHASE III

- Initial rest versus severe activity modification
- Rehabilitate as for phases I and II
- If fail, evaluate for tendinosis/partial tear with MRI
- If MRI positive, then surgical debridement may be necessary.

PHASE IV

- Acute surgical repair

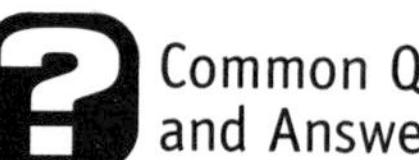

Common Questions and Answers

Physician responses to common patient questions:
Q: How do I stretch my quadriceps?
A: Lunge stretch and lying supine with one leg hanging off the table both allow the quadriceps to be stretched without excessive tension at the patella tendon. For this reason, pulling the foot to the buttock is not as recommended.
Q: Would a cortisone injection help?
A: This should be avoided due to the high risk of intratendon injection and subsequent tendon rupture.

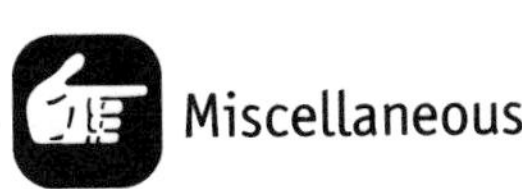

Miscellaneous

SYNONYMS

- Jumper's knee

ICD-9 CODE

726.64

BIBLIOGRAPHY

Blazina ME. Jumper's knee. *Orthop Clin North Am* 1973;4:665–678.

Buckwalter J. Loading of healing bone, fibrous tissue, and muscle: implications for orthopaedic practice. *J Am Acad Orthop Surg* 1999;7:291.

Fyfe I, Stanish WD. The use of eccentric training and stretching in the treatment and prevention of tendon injuries. *Clin Sports Med* 1992;11:601.

Kelly DW, Carter VS, Jobe FW, Kerlan RK. Patellar and quadriceps tendon rupture: jumper's knee. *Am J Sports Med* 1984; 12:375.

Rice EL, Anderson KL III. Volleyball. In: Fu FH, Stone DA, eds. *Sports Injuries.* Baltimore: Williams & Wilkins, 1994:689–700.

Authors: Paul Stricker and Kurt Spindler

Patellar/Quadriceps Tendon Rupture

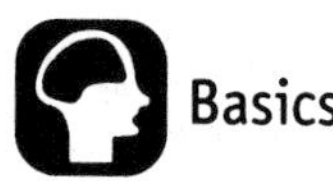

Basics

DEFINITION

- Extensor mechanism disruption of the knee can occur with a variety of injuries to the lower extremity.
- Injuries include patellar fractures, quadriceps tendon ruptures, and patellar tendon ruptures
- Quadriceps tendon ruptures can occur when there is an avulsion fracture of the superior pole of the patella.
- Patellar tendon ruptures can occur when there is an avulsion fracture of the inferior pole of the patella or the tibial tuberosity.
- Both tendon ruptures can occur within the midsubstance of the tendon or through a diseased portion of the tendon.

INCIDENCE/PREVALENCE

- Patellar/quadriceps tendon ruptures occur most often in the third or fourth decade of life.
- Extensor mechanism disruptions occur most often as a result of a comminuted or transverse patella fracture.
- Second leading cause of extensor mechanism disruptions is patellar or quadriceps tendon ruptures.
- Patella fracture or tendon rupture can occur after anterior cruciate ligament reconstruction, which uses the patella tendon as a graft.

SIGNS AND SYMPTOMS

- Knee pain
- Edema
- Ecchymosis
- Hemarthrosis possible
- Focal deformity
- Inability to extend the leg

RISK FACTORS

- Trauma
- History of tendinitis
- Steroid use
- Systemic lupus erythematosus
- Rheumatoid arthritis
- Diabetes mellitus
- Quinolone use
- Previous surgery

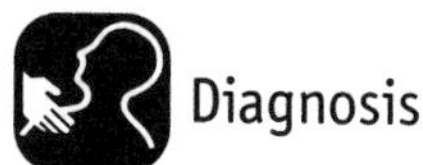

Diagnosis

DIFFERENTIAL DIAGNOSIS

- Fracture
- Muscular strain (grade I or II)
- Patellar subluxation/dislocation
- Meniscal or ligamentous pathologies
- Osgood-Schlatter disease
- Sinding-Larsen-Johansson syndrome

HISTORY

- Acute onset with or without direct trauma
- Knee pain or injury
- Mechanism of injury, specifically, jumping, stumbling, or slipping
- Acute onset of swelling
- Pop heard or felt
- Can continue with activity
- Can bear weight after injury
- Steroid injection or other risk factors

PHYSICAL EXAMINATION

- Effusion or edema usually present
- Pain over anterior knee at patella or tibial tuberosity
- Inability to actively extend the affected knee to terminal extension
- Passive extension relatively pain-free
- Pain with knee flexion
- Altered gait if able to bear weight
- Palpable defect may be present.

IMAGING

- Standard radiographs of the knee often are very helpful.
- Anteroposterior and lateral views should be obtained.
- Patellar view is helpful.
- Comparison views of the contralateral knee often are helpful.
- Radiographs may show avulsion fractures of superior or inferior patellar poles, or the tibial tuberosity.
- Patellar migration in either superior or inferior direction without patellar fractures is conclusive for rupture.

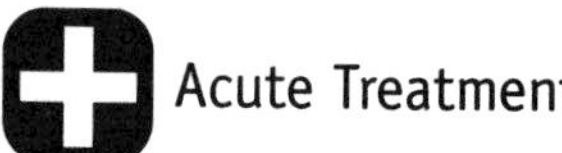

Acute Treatment

IMMOBILIZATION

Immobilization of the knee with a straight-leg immobilizer or bulky dressing should be continued until surgical intervention is completed.

SPECIAL CONSIDERATIONS

Rest, ice, compression, elevation, and crutch-assisted ambulation should be continued until surgical fixation is achieved.

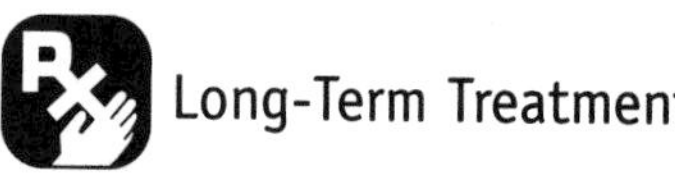

Long-Term Treatment

SURGERY

- Surgical intervention is necessary to restore the extensor mechanism of the knee.
- Exact surgical intervention will depend on which portion of the extensor mechanism was disrupted.
- Immediate repair within 2–6 weeks of injury is ideal.
- Late repair will be technically more difficult.
- Operative interventions may vary, but a primary repair is ideal.
- Supplemental reinforcement of the primary repair may necessitate semitendinosus tendon grafting, cerclage fixation, and/or use of synthetic grafts.

REFERRAL/DISPOSITION

- All extensor mechanism ruptures should be referred for orthopaedic evaluation.
- Best results are achieved with early surgical repair.

POSTOPERATIVE REHABILITATION

- Based on quality of tissue and extent of repair
- Traditionally, a straight-leg cast was in place for 6 weeks despite repair technique. Postoperative knee braces with motion control and extension locks are now favored for immobilization.
- Weight-bearing to tolerance is permitted.
- Considerable debate about initiation and progression of range of motion program
- Ambulation without assistance can be initiated when motion and strength have returned.
- Comprehensive physical therapy program should be completed before return to athletics.

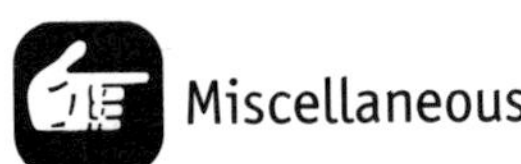

Miscellaneous

SYNONYMS

- Extensor mechanism disruption

ICD-9 CODE

727.65 Quadriceps tendon rupture
727.66 Patellar tendon rupture

BIBLIOGRAPHY

Canale ST, ed. *Campbell's operative orthopaedics*. St. Louis: Mosby, 1998.

Enad JG. Patellar tendon ruptures. *South Med J* 1999;92:563–566.

Griffin LY, ed. *Sports medicine*. Rosemont, IL: American Academy of Orthopaedic Surgery, 1994.

Matava MJ. Patellar tendon ruptures. *J Am Acad Orthop Surg* 1996;4:287–296.

Authors: Angelo J. Colosimo and Shannon M. Urton

Patellofemoral Pain Syndrome (PPS)

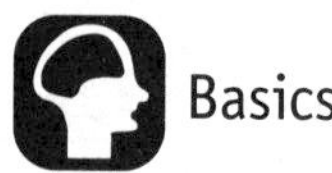

Basics

DEFINITION

- Overuse injury with pain in the anterior knee (patellar/peripatellar area)
- Thought to be caused by subtle malalignment of the patella
- Pain usually under the patella

INCIDENCE/PREVALENCE

- Anterior knee pain represents 20% to 40% of all knee problems.
- Most common running injury, i.e., "runner's knee"
- Patella tracking problem resulting from increased Q-angle more common in women

SIGNS AND SYMPTOMS

- Insidious onset of anterior knee pain with activity
- Frequently poorly localized and positional
- Often associated with ambulating stairs
- "Giving way" of the knee from lancinating pain if severe
- Anterior knee "grinding" or "swelling"

RISK FACTORS

- Family history of patellofemoral or anterior knee pain
- Malalignment of bony anatomy, such as increased Q-angle >12 degrees in males or >15 degrees in females
- "Miserable malalignment syndrome," i.e., increased femoral anteversion, inward looking patella, external tibial torsion, pronated feet, and bayonet sign
- Valgus deformity of the leg
- Vastus medialis oblique (VMO) muscle dysplasia or atrophy
- Varus position of the subtalar joint
- Thigh and leg muscles tight

ASSOCIATED INJURIES AND COMPLICATIONS

- Chondral injury, especially with history of blunt trauma
- Increased residual laxity or tearing of the medial patellar stabilizers with lateral dislocation of the patella

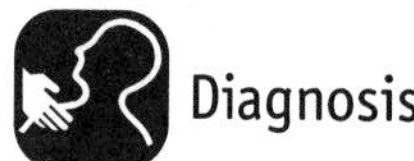

Diagnosis

DIFFERENTIAL DIAGNOSIS

- Patellar or quadriceps tendinitis
- Patellar instability with subluxation or dislocation
- Osteochondral defect of the trochlear or patellar surface resulting in chondromalacia
- Iliotibial band syndrome
- Anterior fat pad inflammation
- Synovial plica
- Retinacular strain
- Osgood-Schlatter disease
- Sinding-Larsen-Johansson disease
- Referred pain from the hip, often affecting the anterior distal thigh and knee
- Multiple other sources of knee pain and arthritis, e.g., gout, infection, reflex sympathetic dystrophy, neuroma, or sickle cell disease

HISTORY

- Past effusion, if knee now swollen
- Subluxation versus dislocation episodes and/or history of direct trauma
- Crepitation (relates to prognosis)
- Bilaterality (relates to prognosis)
- Prior treatments, including nonsteroidal anti-inflammatory drugs, taping, physical therapy, orthotics, injections, or surgery

PHYSICAL EXAMINATION

- Gait and overall limb alignment (see Risk Factors)
- Ask patient to point exactly where the pain originates
- Examine skin for scars.
- Note atrophy of the lower extremity, especially VMO.
- Knee range of motion, noting crepitation and angle of onset of crepitation
- Presence or absence of J-sign (abrupt lateral motion of patella with full extension) on dynamic evaluation of patella
- Squinting patella or "grasshopper eyes"
- Patella alta or patella baja
- Effusion
- Test for ligamentous instability and meniscal pathology
- Rule out patellar tendinitis and quadriceps tendinitis
- Evaluate for prepatellar, infrapatellar, and pes anserine bursae
- Tenderness over lateral retinaculum present in 90% of patients with malalignment
- Examine for patellar facet tenderness
- Patellar glide and apprehension
  - —Divide patella into quadrants.
  - —If moves one quadrant or less medially, then a tight lateral retinaculum is present.
  - —If >3 quadrants laterally, then a loose medial retinaculum is present.
  - —If >4 quadrants laterally, dislocatable patella is present.
- Passive patellar tilt test: with knee in full or 30 degrees of flexion, if cannot get the lateral border of patella to horizontal with posterior pressure on medial edge, a tight lateral retinaculum is present.

IMAGING

Plain Films

- Anteroposterior bilateral standing: shows early joint space narrowing; may show varus or valgus orientation of femur/knee/tibia
- Lateral of affected knee: evaluate for patella alta (patella length to patellar tendon length <0.8) or patella baja (patella length to patellar tendon length >1.2) with Insall method.
- Merchant view of bilateral patellofemoral joints
  - —Does not distort the trochlea/patella, as with Hughston or sunrise view taken with x-ray beam at angle to cassette
  - —Evaluate for femoral condyle dysplasia
  - —Lateral condyle typically is 1 cm higher than the medial condyle
  - —Congruence angle (measures subluxation) normal at -8 ± 6
  - —Sulcus angle (a shallow angle correlates well with instability) typically 137 ± 6
  - —Tilt angle 2 ± 2 in normals; 12 ± 2 in abnormals (measures tilt); other measures exist but can become cumbersome.
- Tunnel view if osteochondral deficit lesion suspected.

Computed Tomography

- Useful to evaluate patellofemoral relationships (e.g., tilt and subluxation), especially in patients with suspected subluxation at <30–45 degrees of flexion that cannot be visualized well on plain film
- Useful to evaluate intraosseous lesions
- Useful to plan selective surgical realignment procedures

Magnetic Resonance Imaging

- Provides information similar to computed tomography
- May add evaluation of articular cartilage (stage III and IV chondromalacia can be evaluated reliably with accuracy of 89%), quadriceps muscle, tendon and fat pad, medial and lateral patellar retinacula

Bone Scintigraphy

- Increased uptake at patella and distal femur believed to indicate poor prognosis with prolonged pain (average 6–9 months).
- Positive bone scan correlates with chondromalacia with positive predictive value of 72%.

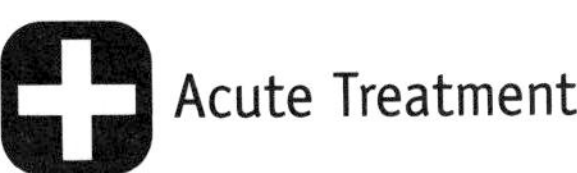

Acute Treatment

- Activity modification is difficult for most patients.
- Adequate trial of nonsteroidal anti-inflammatory drugs offered significant relief to 55% to 63% of patients within 5 days in one study.
- Stretching of hamstrings, quadriceps, and iliotibial band
- Rehabilitation includes heat/cold, ultrasound, and iontophoresis
- Assess for worn or inadequate shoes
- Orthotics for significant forefoot or hindfoot motion problems (full-length orthotic for athlete)
- Trial of taping with McConnell tape: patients who report good pain relief with this method may respond to an active brace that pulls the patella medially, such as the On-Track (San Diego, CA), Palumbo (Vienna, VA), or Tru-Pull (DePuy Orthotec, Warsaw, IN).
- Simple elastic knee sleeves with passive patellar restraints (silicone patellar ring) (Genutrain knee brace, Bauerfeind, Germany) or with a patellar cutout not shown to be helpful in one randomized controlled study with 59 participants. These braces may be helpful in patients with patella alta and no significant tilt.
- Protonics Brace (Inverse Technology Corp., Lincoln, NE) provides a high volume of submaximal concentric contractions to the quadriceps and hamstrings, facilitating proper alignment of the patella in the femoral groove and reducing the congruence angle and subsequently pain. Shown to be effective in one randomized controlled study with 100 patients, with congruence angle improving by 17% and pain decreasing by 47% after 4 weeks.
- Injections considered of limited value, except in ruling out other entities in the differential diagnosis, e.g., in iliotibial band tendinitis, if an injection in the knee removes the pain, the disorder is in the knee and pain is not being transmitted to the knee.

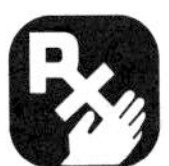

Long-Term Treatment

REHABILITATION

- 80% of patients respond to nonoperative therapy
- Stretching of the hamstring, quadriceps, and iliotibial band
- Regain full motion at the knee and hip, i.e., hip flexion contracture is present
- May perform biofeedback and surface electromyography (EMG) to determine onset and amplitude of individual muscle activation. This may improve exercise performance for rehabilitation.
- Mainstay of maintenance therapy is quadriceps strengthening exercises, performed in either open or closed chain fashion.
  —Controversial whether the VMO muscle can be isolated from the other quadriceps muscles and selectively strengthened.
  —Straight-leg raises performed with the leg fully extended and externally rotated to the 2 or 10 o'clock position for the right and left leg, respectively, may be performed if the patient cannot do wall slides because of pain.
  —Alternatively, patients may begin with straight-leg raises with the Muncie method.
- Muncie method
  —Incorporates more hip adductor muscle function, which increases EMG activity of the VMO muscle compared to other straight-leg raising methods
  —Uninjured knee is bent up with the heel of the foot 2 inches proximal to the joint line of the injured knee for beginners, at the joint line of the injured knee for intermediates, or 2 inches distal to the joint line of the injured knee for advanced.
  —Patient sits forward, hugs the bent knee, and externally rotates the affected leg to maintain the big toe at the 10 or the 2 o'clock position.
  —Foot on the injured leg is dorsiflexed as much as possible and the quadriceps of the straight leg contracted until the heel lifts off the ground.
  —Patient lifts leg 1 inch and holds this position for 5 seconds.
  —Foot is lowered slowly to the floor, relaxing the heel and then the quadriceps.

—Two sets of 10 repetitions should be performed with both legs each day.
—Shown in one prospective, randomized controlled trial to be more beneficial than traditional straight-leg raises or a course of physical therapy in a group of 64 patients

- Closed chain exercises, such as 4- to 6-inch lateral step-ups or wall slides, are started when patients can perform straight-leg raises without pain.
  —Wall slide exercises are performed with knee motion from 5 to 60 degrees of flexion. Easier to perform with a small stability or Swiss ball in the small of the back.
  —We feel that closed chain exercises more closely simulate real-life activities and provide more joint proprioception and should be used, if tolerated.
  —Closed chain exercises exert less peak patellofemoral joint force and may improve patellofemoral congruence.

SURGERY

- After 6 months of nonoperative therapy performed in a conscientious manner, surgery may be considered.
- We typically follow the recommendations of Fulkerson and Stutter. Surgical options depend on whether the patient is skeletally mature and whether significant subluxation or tilt is present. Degree of chondromalacia also affects decision making.
- In skeletally immature patients, proximal soft tissue procedures are recommended, such as semitendinosus tenodesis or lateral retinacular release.
- In skeletally mature patients, surgery depends on the amount of abnormal congruence (signifying subluxation) or tilt.
- In patients with only abnormal tilt, lateral release procedures typically are performed.
- In patients with Q-angles >20 degrees and abnormal congruence angles, a distal realignment procedure typically is performed, such as an anterior medial tibial tubercle transfer (Fulkerson).
- In patients with abnormal congruence angles and/or Q-angles >20 degrees with associated tilt, anterior medial tibial tubercle transfer (Fulkerson) with combined lateral release and/or proximal reconstruction may be performed. Elmslie-Trillat and Hughston techniques have been used successfully.
- Dislocators are operated on if symptoms of patellofemoral instability were present before their dislocation.
- Patellectomy and derotational osteotomies are last resorts.

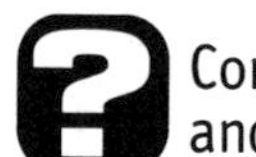

Common Questions and Answers

Physician responses to common patient questions:

Q: Must I stop running completely?
A: 80% of patients respond to a nonoperative therapy, most within 4 weeks. Pain should be your guide when returning to activity. Achiness is anticipated, but sharp, intense pain is harmful.
Q: How long until I get better?
A: Studies show that in athletes with patellofemoral pain followed for 5–7 years, 27% to 75% were pain-free at 6–8 months, and approximately 50% had a significant decrease in pain at 6–8 months; 70% of patients remained pain-free at 7 years in 1 study.
A: How can I predict if I will get better?
Q: Correlates of improvement at 7 years in one study included maintenance of quadriceps strength and function, young age, short stature, negative findings of patellar pain and crepitation, and nonappearance of bilateral symptoms during the follow-up period.
Q: Will I get arthritis in my knee?
A: Most patients (65%) with patellofemoral pain do not get patellofemoral osteoarthritis.

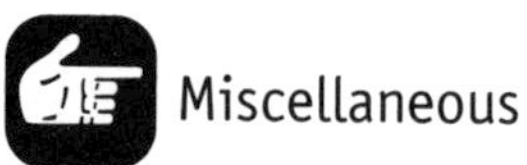

Miscellaneous

SYNONYMS

- Patellofemoral pain syndrome
- Chondromalacia patella

ICD-9 CODE

719.46 Knee pain
717.7 Chondromalacia patella

BIBLIOGRAPHY

Arroll B, et al. Patellofemoral pain syndrome: a critical review of the clinical trials on nonoperative therapy. *Am J Sports Med* 1997;25:207–212.

Bellemans J, et al. Anteromedial tibial tubercle transfer in patients with chronic anterior knee pain and a subluxation-type patellar malalignment. *Am J Sports Med* 1997;25:375–382.

Blnd L, Hansen L. Patellofemoral pain syndrome in athletes: a 5.7-year retrospective follow-up study of 250 athletes. *Acta Orthop Belg* 1998;64:393–400.

Dahl M. Limb length discrepancy. *Pediatr Clin North Am* 1996;43:849–866.

Davis W, Fulkerson J. Initial evaluation of the athlete with anterior knee pain. *Op Tech Sports Med* 1999;7:55–58.

Dye S, et al. The mosaic of pathophysiology causing patellofemoral pain: therapeutic implications. *Op Tech Sports Med* 1999;7:46–54.

Grelsamer R. The nonsurgical treatment of patellofemoral disorders. *Op Tech Sports Med* 1999;7:65–68.

Hartig D, Henderson J. Increasing hamstring flexibility decreases lower extremity overuse injuries in military basic trainees. *Am J Sports Med* 1999;27:173–176.

Kannus P, et al. An outcome study of chronic patellofemoral pain syndrome. *J Bone Joint Surg* 1999;81A:355–363.

Kaufman K, et al. The effect of foot structure and range of motion on musculoskeletal overuse injuries. *Am J Sports Med* 1999;27:585–593.

Kelly M. Proximal realignment and medial tibial tubercle transfer. *Op Tech Sports Med* 1999;7:76–80.

Merchant A. Radiography of the patellofemoral joint. *Op Tech Sports Med* 1999;7:59–64.

Natri A, Kannus P, Jarvinen M. Which factors predict the long-term outcome in chronic patellofemoral pain syndrome? A 7 year prospective follow-up study. *Med Sci Sports Exerc* 1998;30:1572–1577.

Nigg B, et al. Shoe inserts and orthotics for sport and physical activities. *Med Sci Sports Exerc* 1999;31[7 Suppl]:S421–S428.

Papagelopoulos P, Sim F. Patellofemoral pain syndrome: diagnosis and management. *Orthopedics* 1997;20:148–157.

Powers C, et al. The effects of patellar taping on stride characteristics and joint motion in subjects with patellofemoral pain. *JOSPT* 1997;26:286–291.

Roush M, et al. Anterior knee pain: a clinical comparison of rehabilitation methods. *Clin J Sports Med* 2000;10:22–28.

Schreiber S. Arthroscopic surgery and the lateral release for patellofemoral disorders. *Op Tech Sports Med* 1999;7:69–75.

Stiene H, et al. A comparison of closed kinetic chain and isokinetic joint isolation exercise in patients with patellofemoral dysfunction. *JOSPT* 1996;24:136–141.

Timm K. Randomized controlled trial of protonics on patellar pain, position, and function. *Med Sci Sports Exerc* 1998;30: 665–670.

Way M. Effects of a thermoplastic foot orthosis on patellofemoral pain in a collegiate athlete: a single-subject design. *JOSPT* 1999;29:331–338.

Witvrouw E, et al. Reflex response times of vastus medialis oblique and vastus lateralis in normal subjects and in subjects with patellofemoral pain syndrome. *JOSPT* 1996;24:160–165.

Authors: Edward Snell and David Crane

Peroneal Tendon Dislocation/Subluxation

Basics

DEFINITION

- Elevation of the posterior periosteal attachment of the superior peroneal retinaculum off the fibula, which allows the peroneal brevis tendon to subluxate forward over the posterior ridge of the fibula
- Traumatic injury results in elevation by forceful contraction of the peroneal muscles, usually with the ankle in forced dorsiflexion.
- Congenital dislocation
- Acquired dislocation as seen in disorders of severe muscular contraction

INCIDENCE/PREVALENCE

- Generally a rare injury in most sports
- Congenital dislocation found in 3.3% of neonates.

SIGNS AND SYMPTOMS

- Swelling over the posterolateral malleolus
- Pain over the posterolateral malleolus
- Ankle instability

RISK FACTORS

- Forced dorsiflexion of the ankle, as in sudden deceleration
- Likely sports include downhill skiing, ice skating, soccer, basketball, rugby, and gymnastics.
- Small study revealed possible pes planus as a risk.

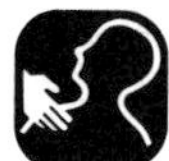

Diagnosis

DIFFERENTIAL DIAGNOSIS

- Ankle sprain
- Fibular fracture

HISTORY

Q: Is this a first time injury or a recurrent injury?
A: Important in determining operative versus nonoperative treatment
Q: Did you hear any snapping or popping at the time of the injury?
A: This injury usually occurs with a snapping sensation in the posterolateral ankle.
Q: Did you experience immediate pain?
A: This injury is associated with intense pain and if examined early possibly localized over the posterolateral ankle rather than the anterolateral ankle as seen in lateral ankle sprains.
Q: Has your pain subsided?
A: Pain usually subsides and the patient is left with instability.
Q: Do you have continued popping or snapping during activity?
A: May have popping or snapping during activity, unlike a lateral ankle sprain.

PHYSICAL EXAMINATION

Acute Injury

- Very difficult to distinguish from ankle sprain especially, because of the swelling and pain
- Tenderness and swelling over the posterolateral region of the superior peroneal retinaculum (vs. tenderness over the anterior talofibular ligament in ankle sprain)
- Pain elicited with active eversion with the foot held in dorsiflexion

Chronic Injury

- Examiner may be able to reproduce subluxation with dorsiflexion and eversion against resistance.
- Possible tenderness or swelling over the lateral malleolus
- Chronic instability

IMAGING

- Anteroposterior ankle but best seen on mortise view (15–20 degrees of internal rotation)
- Pathognomonic is a thin rim of avulsed cortical bone from the lateral aspect of the lateral malleolus.
- Some success with high-resolution ultrasound

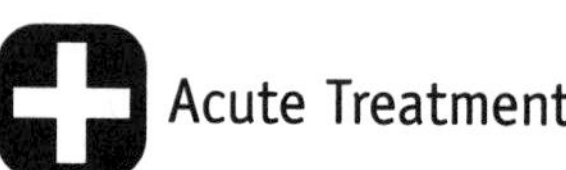

Acute Treatment

- Analgesia
- Ice
- Nonsteroidal anti-inflammatory drugs

IMMOBILIZATION

- Acute nonsurgical treatment is not well established.
- Main problem is persistent pain, instability, and redislocation.
- Options include nonweight-bearing cast for 5–6 weeks with the ankle in midplantar flexion (to relax the tendons), strapping the ankle, or compression bandages.

SPECIAL CONSIDERATIONS

- Surgery should be considered in all cases secondary to the high incidence of recurrence with nonoperative treatment.
- Repeated dislocations cause bone changes that further exacerbate recurrent instability.
- Surgery allows a quick return to normal lifestyle and athletics with no instability.
- Surgical procedure has very low morbidity.

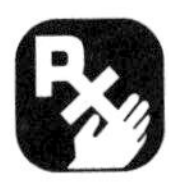

Long-Term Treatment

SURGERY

- Surgery should be considered in all patients with acute injury and is the only appropriate management in congenital, acquired, and chronic injury.
- Many techniques exist but all attach the superior peroneal retinaculum and the periosteum back to the bone when repositioning the peroneal tendon.
- Postoperative below-the-knee cast in relaxed plantar flexion and slight eversion for 6 weeks

REFERRAL/DISPOSITION

Immediate referral for surgical evaluation is appropriate for most patients.

CONSERVATIVE TREATMENT

- J-shaped pad with compression and lateral heel wedge occasionally useful
- Some chronic cases are minimally symptomatic and do not significantly alter athletic performance.

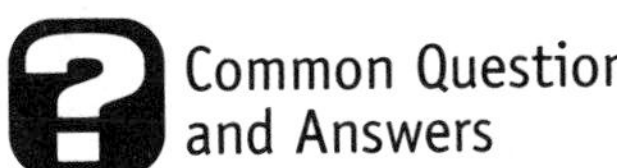

Common Questions and Answers

Physician responses to common patient questions:

Q: What is my chance of recurrent dislocation without surgery?

A: High recurrence rate of 50% to 75%.

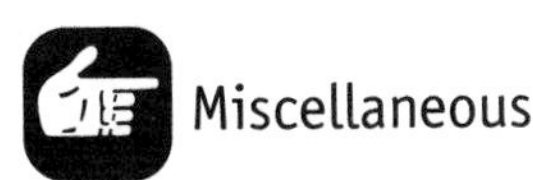

Miscellaneous

ICD-9 CODE

959.7 Injury, ankle

BIBLIOGRAPHY

Mason RB, Henerson JP. Traumatic peroneal tendon instability. *Am J Sports Med* 1996;24:652–658.

Safran MR, O'Malley D Jr, Fu FH. Peroneal tendon subluxation in athletes: new exam technique, case reports, and review. *Med Sci Sports Exerc* 1999;31[7 Suppl]:S487–S492

Author: Andrea Clarke

Phalangeal Injuries

Basics

SIGNS AND SYMPTOMS

- Pain, swelling, and ecchymosis are common findings
- Subungual hematoma frequently encountered with tuft fracture

MECHANISM/DESCRIPTION

- Typically results from direct trauma (e.g., sledgehammer or falling object) or stubbed toe
- Dislocation of interphalangeal joint are common with axial load injury (kicking an immovable object)

CAUTIONS

- It is frequently difficult to distinguish fracture from dislocation; therefore, reduction of a suspected dislocation should not be attempted in the pre-hospital setting unless there is obvious neurologic or vascular compromise

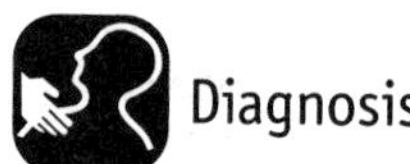

Diagnosis

ESSENTIAL WORKUP

- X-ray of involved digit

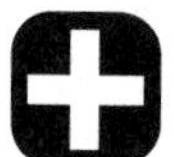

Acute Treatment

NONDISPLACED FRACTURES

- Buddy tape nondisplaced fractures (remember to place absorptive padding between toes)
- Hard-sole shoe
- Weight-bearing as tolerated with crutches or cane
- Oral analgesics
- Pain improves over 2–3 weeks

DISPLACED INTRA-ARTICULAR FRACTURES OF INTERPHALANGEAL JOINT

- Closed reduction with longitudinal traction
- Short leg-walking cast with toe platform
- If unstable after closed reduction, then open reduction internal fixation (ORIF) is required

INTERPHALANGEAL JOINT DISLOCATIONS

- Digital block anesthesia
- Longitudinal traction with gentle downward pressure on distal phalanx to reduce dislocation
- Buddy tape to next toe for 2–3 weeks
- Rarely sesamoid bone block attempts at reduction
- Unstable reductions require operative management

DISTAL TUFT FRACTURE

- Hard soled shoe
- Oral analgesics
- Drain subungual hematoma if present
- Weight-bearing as tolerated

HOSPITAL ADMISSION CRITERIA

- Unstable or blocked dislocations and unstable fractures of great toe require ORIF

HOSPITAL DISCHARGE CRITERIA

All other fractures may be discharged with follow-up in 2–3 weeks to evaluate healing

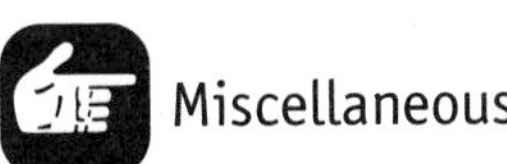

Miscellaneous

ICD-9-CM

959.7

CORE CONTENT CODE

18.4.13.1.1

BIBLIOGRAPHY

Heckman JD. Fractures and dislocations of the foot. In: Rockwood CA, Green DP, Bucholz RW, Heckman JD, eds. *Rockwood and Green's fractures in adults*. 4th ed. New York: Lippincott-Raven, 1996:2267–2405.

Simon RS, Koeningsknecht SJ. Metatarsal fractures. In: Simon RS, Koeningsknecht SJ, eds. *Emergency orthopedics: The extremities*. 2d ed. Norwalk, CT: Appleton & Lange, 1987:288–291.

Author: Kevin Reilly

PIP Joint Dislocations

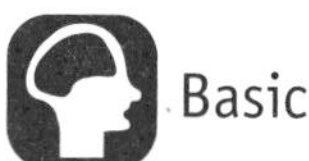

Basics

DEFINITION

- Dislocation of the proximal interphalangeal (PIP) joint
- Hinge joint allowing flexion and extension with little lateral movement, as collateral ligaments are tight through entire range of motion
- Dislocations may be dorsal (most common), ventral, or rotary subluxation, where the twisting injury to the finger causes buttonholing of the head of the proximal phalanx through a tear in the central slip and lateral band.

INCIDENCE/PREVALENCE

- Most commonly injured joint in the hand

SIGNS AND SYMPTOMS

- Swelling and deformity if not already reduced by coach or friend

RISK FACTORS

- Playing sports

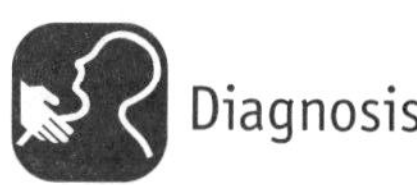

Diagnosis

DIFFERENTIAL DIAGNOSIS

- Fracture-dislocation: Large dorsal fracture-dislocations can be missed, with the volar fracture involving >75% of joint surface with dorsal subluxation of the remaining portion of the middle phalanx.
- Central extensor tendon rupture (boutonniere injury) rupture of central slip allows lateral bands to slip below PIP joint and cause PIP flexion with distal interphalangeal (DIP) extension.

HISTORY

- Ascertain the direction of dislocation if already reduced
- Determine mechanism: "jammed" finger may be due to longitudinal or hyperextension mechanism.

PHYSICAL EXAMINATION

- Deformity will indicate direction of dislocation.
- Careful palpation about the joint to locate the most tender area can help differentiate between injuries.
  —Volar tenderness: volar plate
  —Lateral joint line tenderness: collateral ligaments
  —Dorsal tenderness: central slip injury
- Neurologic examination before and after reduction: check sensation in distal finger
- Check extensor tendon function
  —Have patient actively extend PIP and DIP joints.
- If able to extend DIP but not PIP joint, consider central slip rupture, which may lead to a boutonierre deformity.
  —Extended DIP and flexed PIP with late loss of DIP flexion is the most disabling problem.
- Check flexion
  —Have patient actively flex PIP joint with other fingers held in extension
  —Check DIP flexion with PIP held in extension
  —If unable to flex DIP, consider flexor digitorum profundus rupture, which requires surgical consultation.
- Check collateral ligaments
  —Apply radial and ulnar stress with PIP joint in full extension and 30 degrees of flexion
  —Look for increased laxity
- Check volar plate
  —Excessive hyperextension is consistent with volar plate injury.
  —If volar plate unstable and not treated properly, will lead to hyperextension of the PIP and flexion of DIP, a swan-neck deformity.

IMAGING

- X-rays: two views, including anteroposterior and lateral before reduction if possible
- Oblique view if initial x-rays are negative but high suspicion of fracture
- Ensure joint congruity to rule out fracture dislocation
- May see small volar avulsion fracture
- With rotary subluxation will see true lateral view of middle phalanx with oblique view of proximal phalanx, or vice versa

POSTREDUCTION VIEWS

- No need to obtain postreduction views

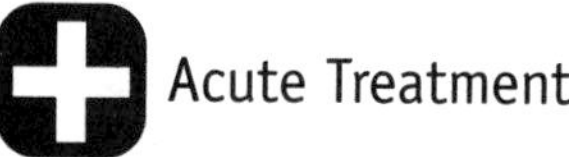

Acute Treatment

DORSAL DISLOCATION

Reduction

- If reduced before onset of swelling, reduction is easier.
- Reduce with longitudinal traction and gentle pressure to the dorsal aspect of the mid phalanx.

Postreduction Evaluation

- X-rays: two views if not already obtained
- Rule out dorsal fracture-dislocation.
- Check collateral ligament stability after reduction.

Immobilization

- Stable: splint for 1–2 weeks in 15–20 degrees of flexion (also may use extension block splint) until pain-free. Often have volar plate injury; if so, consider splint in flexion for 4–5 weeks.
- Splint should include only PIP joint; may be dorsal or volar.
- Buddy tape additional 3–4 weeks
- Can treat with buddy taping alone for 3–6 wks if no volar plate injury

VOLAR DISLOCATION

Reduction

- Same as for dorsal dislocation
- Closed treatment if minimally displaced avulsion fracture
- Avulsion fracture reduces with full extension.

Postreduction Evaluation

- X-rays: two views
- Check collateral ligament stability after reduction.

Immobilization

- Splint PIP joint in full extension for 6 weeks (dorsal or volar splint) as central slip often involved, DIP and metacarpophalangeal joints free
- Need to actively and passively flex DIP joint
- Night splint for additional 3–4 weeks
- Splint until full active extension of PIP joint and active flexion of DIP joint

ROTARY SUBLUXATION

Reduction

- Sometimes difficult to reduce closed
- Closed reduction
  - —Digital block
  - —Gentle traction with metacarpal phalangeal and PIP joint at 90 degrees of flexion
  - —Dorsiflex wrist (relaxes extensor mechanism)
  - —Apply gentle rotatory and traction force

Postreduction Evaluation

- X-rays: two views
- Check collateral ligament stability after reduction.

Immobilization

- Buddy tape after closed reduction.

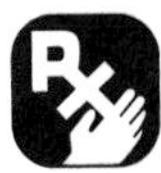

Long-Term Treatment

REHABILITATION

- Dorsal dislocation: work on range of motion when out of splint
- Volar dislocation: work on range of motion of DIP and MP joints while in splint
- Rotary subluxation: start active and passive range of motion (ROM) when out of splint; add resisted ROM when pain-free active and passive ROM

SURGERY

- Unable to reduce closed
- Dorsal fracture-dislocation carries significant risk of long-term disability if improperly treated
- Volar dislocation with significant avulsion fracture or fracture does not reduce with extension and carries high risk of disability if treated improperly.

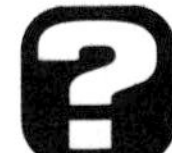

Common Questions and Answers

Physician responses to common patient questions:
Q: When can I return to play?
A: Immediately with buddy taping or if able to play in splint
Q: Dorsal fracture dislocations?
A: Volar lip fracture involves >20% to 70% of articular surface. Joint is unstable after reduction and requires referral.
Q: Recurrent dorsal dislocations?
A: Can occasionally see pseudo-boutonniere deformity. Treat with dynamic splinting.

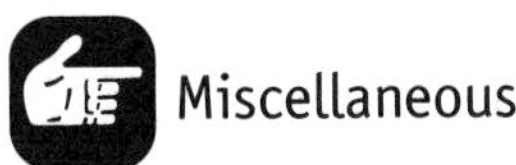

Miscellaneous

SYNONYMS

- Jammed finger

ICD-9 CODE

834.02

BIBLIOGRAPHY

Eiff MP, Hatch RL, Calmbach WL. Finger fractures. In: *Fracture management for primary care.* Philadelphia: WB Saunders, 1998.

Green DP, Butler TE. Fractures and dislocations in the hand. In: Rockwood CA, Green DP, Bucholz RW, Heckman JD, eds. *Rockwood and Green's fractures in adults, vol. 1,* 4th ed. Philadelphia: Lippincott-Raven Publishers, 1996.

Green DP, Strickland JW. The hand. In: Delee JC, Drez D, eds. *Orthopaedic sports medicine: principles and practice.* Philadelphia: WB Saunders, 1994, 945–1017.

Palmer RE. Joint injuries of the hand in athletes. *Clin Sports Med* 1998;17:513–531.

Authors: Mark Snowise and William W. Dexter

Piriformis Syndrome

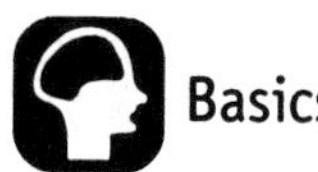

Basics

DEFINITION

- Sciatic nerve irritation as it courses underneath or through the piriformis muscle causing buttock pain with or without radiation into the leg
- Etiology unknown, but thought to involve piriformis muscle spasm or hypertrophy
- Direct irritation on the sciatic nerve may be caused by inflammatory agents released from an injured piriformis muscle.

INCIDENCE/PREVALENCE

- 6 per 100 cases of sciatica
- 6:1 female-to-male ratio

SIGNS AND SYMPTOMS

- Cramping or aching pain in the buttock with or without pain radiating into the hamstrings
- Sensation of "tight hamstrings"
- Point tenderness to deep palpation over any part of the piriformis muscle
- Pain increased with sitting

RISK FACTORS

- In roughly 20% of the population, the sciatic nerve passes through the piriformis muscle, which may irritate the nerve and cause pain.
- Leg length discrepancy

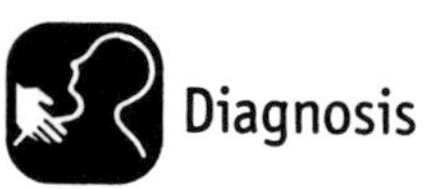

Diagnosis

DIFFERENTIAL DIAGNOSIS

- Herniated lumbar nucleus pulposus
- Cord tumor
- Spinal stenosis
- Posterior facet syndrome
- Spondylolisthesis
- Vertebral lumbar fracture
- Aneurysm of the inferior or superior gluteal artery
- Fibrotic band around the sciatic nerve
- Hematoma
- Gluteal abscess
- Pelvic tumor
- Endometriosis and other pelvic diseases
- Bursitis: obturator internus, trochanteric or ischial

HISTORY

- Trauma to the gluteal region seen in <50% of cases
- Sitting on hard surfaces exacerbates pain.
- Location of referred pain; not likely piriformis syndrome if below the knee
- Complaint of pain with movements that cause external hip rotation
- Women may complain of dyspareunia.

PHYSICAL EXAMINATION

- Buttock pain with or without radiation to hamstrings produced by combination of hip flexion, adduction, and internal rotation. This maneuver stretches the piriformis muscle.
- Pace sign: weakness in resisted abduction and external rotation
- Tenderness to palpation over the piriformis muscle
- Sciatic notch tenderness
- Usually normal neurologic examination
- Pelvic and/or digital rectal examination elicits pain ipsilaterally proximal to the ischial tuberosity.

IMAGING

- Diagnostic imaging is rarely helpful in confirming the diagnosis.
- Clinical history and physical examination are key to diagnosing piriformis syndrome.
- Further diagnostic tests may be needed to rule out other potential diagnoses.
- Magnetic resonance imaging (MRI) and computed tomography (CT) can be used if history and physical examination not conclusive.
- Atrophy or fibrous tissue replacement of the piriformis muscle on MRI or CT supports the diagnosis.

OTHER TESTS

Electromyographic (EMG) findings of peroneal and/or tibial H reflex prolongation in the adducted, internally rotated, flexed hip strongly supports the diagnosis.

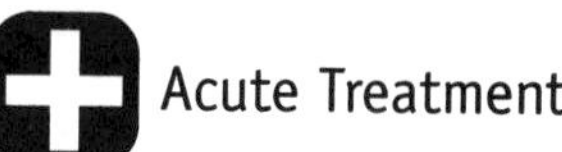

Acute Treatment

ANALGESIA

- Nonsteroidal anti-inflammatory drugs for 10–14 days
- Short course of analgesics and/or muscle relaxants may be beneficial.
- Ice
- Acetaminophen

IMMOBILIZATION

- Relative rest for short period, but should begin piriformis stretch and physical therapy as soon as possible

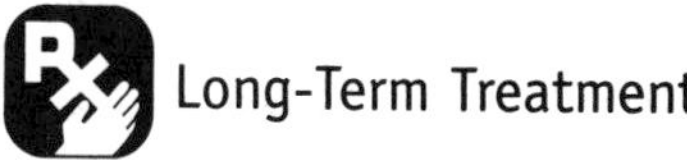

Long-Term Treatment

REHABILITATION

- Physical therapy incorporating stretching and strengthening of the piriformis muscle. Also should incorporate correction of pelvic obliquities and leg length discrepancies.
- Deep muscle massage with ultrasound

INJECTIONS

With no improvement after conservative therapy, consider local injection of anesthetic (1% to 2% lidocaine hydrochloride with or without bupivacaine 4–6 mL) directly into the tender area within the piriformis muscle, which may confirm the diagnosis.

SURGERY

- If conservative treatment fails, surgical release of the piriformis muscle around the sciatic nerve should be used as a last resort.
- Patients with documented EMG nerve impairment have the best outcome after surgical release.

REFERRAL/DISPOSITION

- Surgery as indicated above for recalcitrant cases of piriformis syndrome

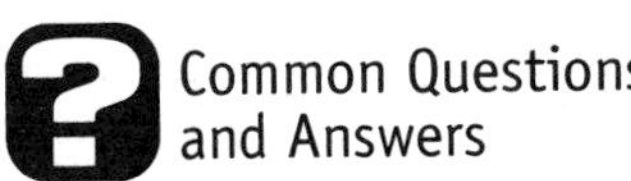

Common Questions and Answers

Physician responses to common patient questions:

Q: What activities should I avoid if I have piriformis syndrome?

A: Any activities that involve prolonged sitting (i.e., biking).

Q: How long after surgery before returning back to activity?

A: Weight-bearing as tolerated 5–10 days after surgery with gradual return to full activity. Avoidance of prolonged sitting for 4–6 weeks after surgery is recommended.

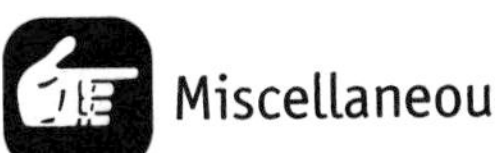

Miscellaneous

SYNONYMS

- Pyriformis syndrome
- Sciatica
- Sciatic neuritis
- "Hip pocket neuropathy"
- "Wallet neuritis"

ICD-9 CODE

724.3 Sciatica

CPT CODE

90782 Intramuscular injection: diagnostic, prophylactic, or therapeutic.

BIBLIOGRAPHY

Parziale JR, Hudgins TH, Fishman LM. The piriformis syndrome. *Am J Orthop* 1996;25:819–823.

Silver JK, Leadbetter WB. Piriformis syndrome: assessment of current practice and literature review. *Orthopedics* 1998;21:1133–1135.

Steiner C, Staubs C, Ganon M, et al. Piriformis syndrome: pathogenesis, diagnosis and treatment. *JAOA* 1987;87:318–323.

Authors: Jamie Edwards and Suzanne Hecht

Plantar Fasciitis

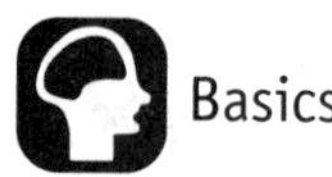

Basics

DEFINITION

- Typically inflammation of the plantar fascia insertion at the medial calcaneus on the anteromedial side of the heel

INCIDENCE/PREVALENCE

In the running population, plantar fasciitis accounts for 10% of running injuries.

SIGNS AND SYMPTOMS

- Pain at the anteromedial aspect of the heel
- Worsens with activity such as running or walking
- Worst pain with first few steps in the morning
- Pain intensity increases with prolonged weight-bearing, especially while walking barefoot and in dress shoes.
- Pain can radiate across the medial side of the heel and less so to the lateral aspect.

RISK FACTORS

- Excessive torsion and hyperpronation with poor supporting footwear
- Poor shock dissipation with cavus foot
- Hindfoot valgus with pronation deformity
- Increasing age and weight

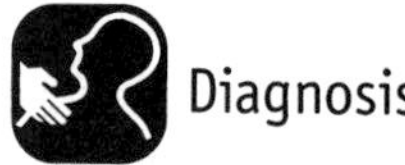

Diagnosis

DIFFERENTIAL DIAGNOSIS

- Stress fracture to calcaneus
- Intrinsic muscle strain (abductor hallucis, flexor digitorum brevis, quadratus plantae)
- Plantar fibromatosis
- Entrapment of branches of the posterior tibial nerve usually at or after passage through the posterior tarsal tunnel: medial plantar nerve, lateral plantar nerve, or medial calcaneal nerve
- Radicular symptoms of L-4 to S-1 (sciatic nerve)

HISTORY

- Typically an insidious and progressive process
- Rarely an acute problem secondary to trauma
- Worst with first few steps out of bed in the morning and abates quickly
- Worsens with activity late in the day

PHYSICAL EXAMINATION

- Pain localized to anteromedial aspect of the heel with palpation
- Tight Achilles' heel cord
- Pes planus
- Passive range of motion: hypermobility of subtalar joint, midtarsal joint, and first ray
- Gait evaluation: calcaneus everted at heel lift

IMAGING

Rarely needed, but plain radiographs and/or bone scan may be helpful to rule out stress fracture.

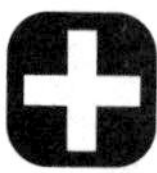

Acute Treatment

ANALGESIA

- Nonsteroidal anti-inflammatory drugs of choice for analgesic effect
- Early morning stretching of heel cord as well as throughout the day
- Ice massage and deep friction massage of the arch and insertion
- Soft heel pads (Silastic)
- Arch taping during athletic activities
- Custom orthotic and medial heel wedge
- Motion control shoes with rigid heel counters
- Night splints
- Supination strap
- Judicious use of long-acting steroid injections for the in-season athlete (1–3/year)

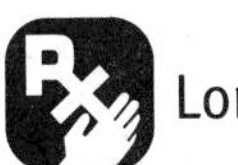

Long-Term Treatment

REHABILITATION

- Conservative therapy may last 4–12 months or more
- Postoperative therapy includes splint for 2 weeks, mild stretching and ambulation with crutches and walking boot, pool running for 3 weeks, and return to activity in 3–4 months

SURGERY

Surgery can be considered after failure of extensive conservative therapy, even up to 2 years: operative release of proximal fascia of deep abductor fascia

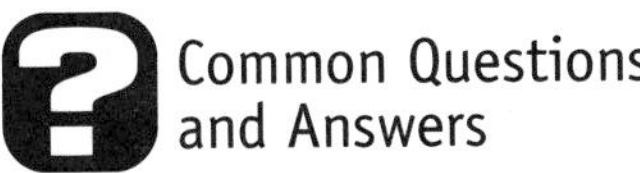

Common Questions and Answers

Physician responses to common patient questions:
Q: When should I consider surgery?
A: After exhaustive conservative treatment of at least 6 months to 1 year has failed.

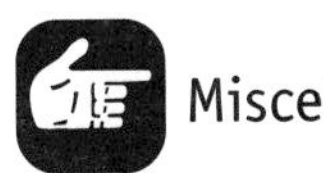

Miscellaneous

SYNONYMS

- Enthesopathy of plantar fascia

ICD-9 CODE

728.71 Plantar fasciitis (also plantar fascial fibromatosis and traumatic plantar fasciitis)

BIBLIOGRAPHY

Clanton TO, Porter DA. Primary care of foot and ankle injuries in the athlete. *Clin Sports Med* 1997;16:453–466.

Author: Kenneth Bielak

Posterior Cruciate Ligament (PCL) Tear

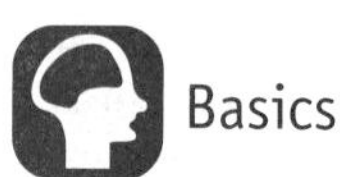

Basics

DEFINITION

- Rupture of any or all parts of the posterior cruciate ligament (PCL) of the knee (anterolateral portion, posteromedial portion, anterior meniscofemoral ligament, and posterior meniscofemoral ligament)

INCIDENCE/PREVALENCE

- Proportion of all knee injuries in general population 3%; trauma patients 37%; athletes unknown
- Most PCL tears occur traumatically with dashboard injuries where there is posterior translation of the proximal tibia in the flexed knee during a motor vehicle accident and usually accompanied by other ligament injuries.
- Injuries incurred during an athletic event usually caused by hyperflexion or hyperextension of the knee and are isolated injuries.

SIGNS AND SYMPTOMS

- Pain and swelling in the knee
- May walk with a slight limp
- May experience instability with twisting or walking down inclines
- Discomfort felt with flexion
- Anterior patellar contusions may be seen.
- Posterior knee or popliteal ecchymosis may be found.

RISK FACTORS

- Contact sports, especially American football

ASSOCIATED INJURIES AND COMPLICATIONS

- Anterior cruciate ligament (ACL) tear
- Lateral or medial collateral ligament tears
- Meniscal derangement
- Tibial plateau fractures
- Boney avulsions at the insertions of the cruciate ligament
- Avulsion fracture at the tibial tubercle
- Fibular head fracture
- Posterior knee subluxation or dislocation caused by hamstring force in the PCL-deficient knee
- Chondrosis

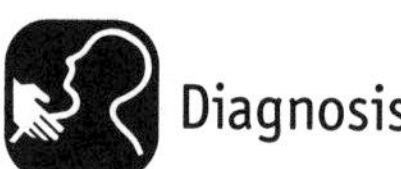

Diagnosis

DIFFERENTIAL DIAGNOSIS

- ACL tear
- Tibia or fibular fracture
- Medial or lateral collateral ligament tear
- Meniscal derangement

HISTORY

Q: Mechanism of injury?
A: To understand direction of applied forces and determine single versus multiple ligament involvement.
Q: Age of injury?
A: Acute versus chronic.
Q: Knee swelling?
A: Immediate (within 3–4 hours) in cruciate tears, fractures, and dislocations; remote (between 12 and 24 hours) in meniscal derangement.
Q: Associated knee instability and direction of instability?
A: Differentiate between other ligament pathology.
Q: Joint locking or clicking?
A: Evaluate associated meniscal pathology.

PHYSICAL EXAMINATION

Neurovascular Examination

- Perform neurovascular examination before other provocative tests
- Important to determine and document associated nerve damage or vascular injury

Comprehensive Knee Examination

- Rule out other ligament or meniscal injury

Posterior Drawer Test

- Perform with the knee flexed at 90 degrees and hip flexed at 45 degrees
- Force is applied to elicit abnormal posterior tibial translation.
- 90% sensitive and 99% specific for diagnosing PCL tears
- Posterior translation of 0–5 mm (grade 1), 5–10 mm (grade 2), and >10 mm (grade 3)

Observe Medial Tibial Plateau Anterior to Medial Femoral Condyle

- Perform with knee flexed at 90 degrees; normally 1-cm step-off
- Absence should raise suspicion for PCL tear.

Posterior Sag Test

- Supine patient flexes both hips and knees to 90 degrees with examiner supporting both heals.
- Posterior tibial translation is consistent with PCL deficiency.

Prone Drawer Test

- Perform with foot in various degrees of rotation
- PCL injuries may lead to rotatory instability.

Quadriceps Active Test

- With knee flexed 60 degrees and patient supine, foot is secured to examination table while patient attempts isometrically to extend knee.
- In PCL-deficient knee, subluxed tibia will translate anteriorly to recreate the tibial plateau step-off.

Dynamic Posterior Shift Test

- Slow extension of knee from 90 degrees to full extension while patient is supine and hips flexed at 90 degrees
- With PCL tear there will be "clunk" near full extension caused when subluxed tibia is reduced.

Posteromedial Instability Test

- Tibia suddenly shifts anteriorly as knee is brought from 45 to 20 degrees of flexion while varus force, compression, and internal rotation is placed on the tibia.
- Posteromedial instability occurs with PCL, medial collateral ligament, and posterior oblique ligament tears.

External Rotation Recurvatum Test

- Lift great toes of supine patient
- Posterolateral instability caused by PCL tear is determined when the injured knee drops into varus angulation with hyperextension and the tibia externally rotates.

Reversed Pivot Shift Test

- Valgus force is applied and external rotation of foot while knee is brought from 90 degrees of flexion to full extension.
- Subluxed tibia will shift into anterior reduction at 20–30 degrees.

Measurement of Tibial External Rotation

- Measure medial border of foot while knee is in 30 or 90 degrees of flexion
- Evaluate posterolateral corner pathology

IMAGING

- Anteroposterior, lateral, and oblique radiographs; important to rule out boney avulsions or other fractures
- Flexion weight-bearing posteroanterior and patellar radiographs: can distinguish chondrosis from chronic PCL deficiencies
- Stress radiographs: 8 mm or more posterior tibial translation indicative of complete PCL tear
- Radionuclide bone scans: able to distinguish early chondrosis from chronic PCL deficiencies
- Magnetic resonance imaging: reported to be up to 100% sensitive and specific in evaluating PCL rupture. Also can evaluate other soft tissue pathology of the affected knee.

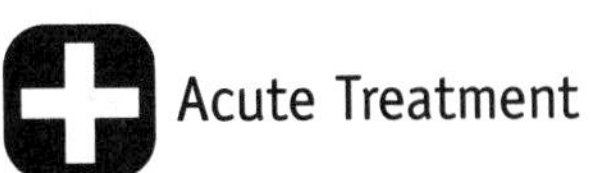

Acute Treatment

ANALGESIA

- Ice
- Nonsteroidal anti-inflammatory drugs
- Compression
- Elevation

IMMOBILIZATION

- Partial weight-bearing
- Possible immobilization in full extension for grade 3 lesions

SPECIAL CONSIDERATIONS

- Early surgical repair indicated for patients with associated avulsion fractures or other ligament involvement

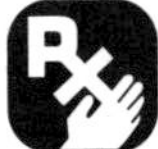

Long-Term Treatment

REHABILITATION

Grade 1 and 2 Lesions

- Early range of motion
- Aggressive quadriceps rehabilitation
- Partial weight-bearing
- Protection of knees against posterior sag
- PCL brace may be useful but not proven effective.

Grade 3 Lesions

- 2–4 weeks of immobilization in full extension to protect posterolateral structures from posterior tibial translation
- Quadriceps sets and straight-leg raise exercises
- Partial weight-bearing

SURGERY

- Indications include bony avulsion fractures, persistent pain in grade 3 patients, combined ligament injuries, and chronic symptomatic severe PCL laxity

REFERRAL/DISPOSITION

- Surgery as indicated above
- Early orthopaedic referral for all except uncomplicated grade 1 and 2 lesions
- Early physical therapy referral may be beneficial, as loss of proprioception and sprint speed is a major problem with return to play.

Common Questions and Answers

Physician responses to common patient questions:
Q: How long before athlete can return to play?
A: In grade 1 and 2, uncomplicated patients expect return to play within 2–4 weeks depending on sport. In grade 3, uncomplicated patients expect 3 months before return to play.

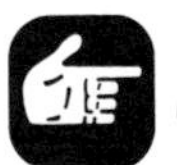

Miscellaneous

ICD-9 CODE

717.84

BIBLIOGRAPHY

Harner CD, Hoher J. Evaluation and treatment of posterior cruciate ligament injuries. *Am J Sports Med* 1998;26:471–482.

Miller MD, Bergfeld JA, Fowler PJ, et al. The posterior cruciate ligament injured knee: principles of evaluation and treatment. *Instructional Course Lectures* 1999;48:199–207.

St. Pierre P, Miller MD. Posterior cruciate ligament injuries. *Clin Sports Med* 1999;18:199–221.

Author: J.C. Buller

Posterior Interosseous Nerve Syndrome

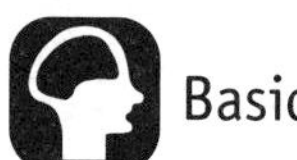

Basics

DEFINITION

- Posterior interosseous nerve, a major motor branch of the radial nerve, is trapped after passing under the extensor carpi radialis longus and causes pain on the deep extensor muscles mass and inability to extend the hand

SIGNS AND SYMPTOMS

- Dull or sharp pain in the deep extensor muscle group distal to the radial head
- No objective sensory findings
- Inability to extend wrist and fingers

RISK FACTORS

- Soft tissue masses, such as a thick arcade of Frohse
- Rarely other soft tissue masses such as lipoma, neuroma, or fibroma
- Tight arm bands, e.g., holding a rifle sling wrapped around the forearm for prolonged periods, as seen in military recruits

ASSOCIATED INJURIES AND COMPLICATIONS

- Direct trauma to the nerve, as with laceration

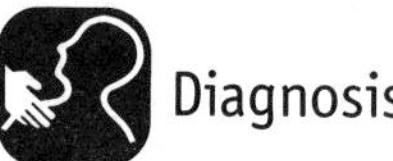

Diagnosis

DIFFERENTIAL DIAGNOSIS

- Other radial nerve injuries

HISTORY

- Pain in the deep exterior muscle group

PHYSICAL EXAMINATION

- Sensation intact
- Radial deviation of the hand upon wrist extension due to paralysis of extensor carpi ulnaris muscle
- Intact extensor carpi radialis longus and brevis, which are innervated distal to the posterior interosseous nerve
- Unable to extend digits at the metacarpophalangeal joint
- Tenderness on deep palpation along proximal radius

ELECTRODIAGNOSTIC TESTING

- Normal sensory nerve action potentials
- Drop in compound muscle action potential amplitude or conduction when stimulated between brachialis and brachioradialis muscles and recorded proximal to extensor indicus proprius
- Needle examination reveals membrane instability in muscles distal to supinator muscle.
- Triceps, brachioradialis, and extensor carpi radialis longus and brevis are spared.
- Supinator muscle may or may not be affected.

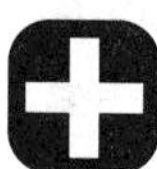

Acute Treatment

SPECIAL CONSIDERATIONS

- Conservative treatment in the first 3 months with splinting.
- If severe, a dynamic splint is needed to hold the fingers in extension. Occupational therapy consult.

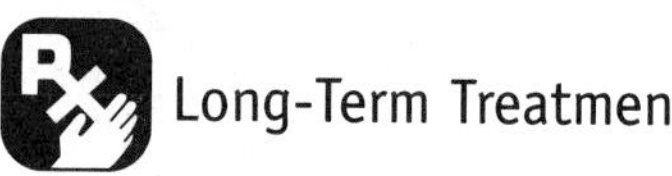

Long-Term Treatment

REHABILITATION

- Surgical referral if symptoms not improved after 3 months

SURGERY

Surgical decompression may be necessary in refractory cases.

REFERRAL/DISPOSITION

- Will need range of motion to prevent flexion contracture of elbow after surgery

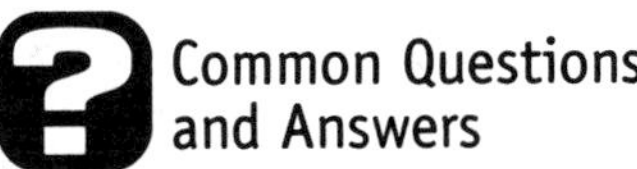

Common Questions and Answers

Physician responses to common patient questions:
Q: When will function return?
A: Function usually returns with conservative therapy in a few weeks. Surgery is rarely necessary.

Miscellaneous

ICD-9 CODE

354.3 Radial nerve lesion

BIBLIOGRAPHY

O'Connor FG, Ollivierre CO, Nirschl RP. Elbow and forearm injuries. In: Lillegard WA, Butcher JD, and Rucker KS, eds. *Handbook of sports medicine* 2nd ed. Boston: Butterworth Heinemann, 1999, 150–151.

Authors: Ahmed Khalifa and Ayse Dural

Posterolateral Capsular Tear

Basics

DEFINITION

- Posterolateral corner (PLC) of the knee is composed of a series of anatomical layers.
- The deepest layer, which is variable among patients, includes the popliteus tendon, fabellofibular ligament, and popliteofibular ligament.
- When some or all of these structures are attenuated or torn, a pathologic state of ligamentous laxity occurs.
- In this state, an external rotation force applied to the knee causes the tibial plateau to sublux posteriorly to the lateral femoral condyle.

INCIDENCE/PREVALENCE

- Injury to the PLC is infrequent but must always be suspected in any knee injury.
- May occur in conjunction with cruciate or lateral collateral ligament injury or any multiligamentous knee injury
- High association of chronic PLC insufficiency in the setting of failed cruciate ligament reconstruction

SIGNS AND SYMPTOMS

Acute Injury

- Pain located in the posterolateral aspect of the knee
- Mechanism of injury may be an anteromedially directed blow or noncontact hyperextension and external rotation force to the knee.
- In these cases, associated cruciate ligament or peroneal nerve injury may be present.

Chronic Injury

- Instability of the knee in full extension necessitating ambulation on a semiflexed knee
- Varus thrust during gait

RISK FACTORS

- Any collision sport or recreation where running and cutting activities may cause an anteromedially directed blow or a noncontact hyperextension external rotation force to the knee

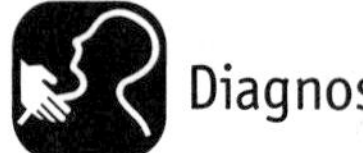

Diagnosis

DIFFERENTIAL DIAGNOSIS

- Lateral collateral ligament injury
- Knee dislocation
- Tibial plateau fracture

HISTORY

Q: Have you ever injured your knee?
A: Patient may describe a recent or remote contact or noncontact injury to the knee.
Q: What type of pain is in your knee?
A: Patient may complain of acute pain with a more recent injury or a dull, less intense pain in the chronic setting.
Q: Does your knee give out after your anterior crucicate ligament reconstruction?
A: Knee instability indicates persistent ligamentous dysfunction. Patients who present with a failed ligamentous reconstruction of the knee must be carefully evaluated for PLC insufficiency.

PHYSICAL EXAMINATION

- Comprehensive knee examination must be performed in any patient with a knee injury.
- Assess the vascular and neurologic status of the leg and foot. Diminished pulses may indicate a vascular injury.
- Inspect the leg. In acute PLC injury, anteromedial abrasion or contusion implies a posterolaterally directed force.
- Assess alignment and gait. Inspection standing may reveal asymmetrical varus involvement on the affected side. In chronic injury, varus thrust in the stance phase of gait may be present and formal gait analysis indicated.
- Perform a complete ligamentous examination. Cruciate and collateral ligaments must be evaluated to rule out a multiple ligamentous injury and knee dislocation.
- Test anterior and posterior translation with the knee in 30 degrees of flexion (Lachman examination) and 90 degrees of flexion (Drawer test).
- Test varus and valgus laxity with the knee fully extended at 30 degrees of flexion.
- If a knee dislocation is suspected, an arteriogram may be warranted.
- Assess and document peroneal nerve function. In varus laxity, the peroneal nerve may be acutely injured or chronically irritated. Perform the two tests that specifically address the PLC.
  —Tibial external rotation test (external rotation dial test) is the most helpful.
  —With the patient in the prone position, the foot is passively externally rotated and compared to the contralateral limb.
  —Amount of rotation is measured with the thigh-foot angle.
  —Test should be performed with the knee in both 30 and 90 degrees of flexion.
  —>10-degree increase in external rotation with the affected knee in 30 degrees of flexion represents a pathologic state.
  —Reverse pivot shift test addresses tibial plateau subluxation.
  —With the patient supine, a valgus force is applied to the 90-degree flexed knee.
  —If PLC is insufficient, the lateral tibial plateau will be subluxed posteriorly relative to the lateral femoral condyle.
  —Knee is slowly extended.
  —Visible shift or clunk near 30 degrees of flexion implies reduction of the subluxation.

IMAGING

- Plain radiographs are helpful in ruling out associated injuries.
  —Lateral capsular avulsion fracture, or Segond sign, represents an ACL injury and may be associated with injury to the lateral and posterolateral structures.
  —Avulsion fracture of the fibular head indicates lateral collateral ligament (LCL) injury.
- Magnetic resonance imaging (MRI)
  —Most effective way to visualize the PLC
  —Useful in detecting acute tears
  —Allows assessment of associated ligamentous and cartilaginous injuries
  —In the chronic setting, long-standing radiographs allow assessment of alignment and need for osteotomy before reconstruction.

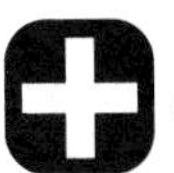

Acute Treatment

ANALGESIA

- Management of acute injury involves recognition that a serious knee injury has occurred.
- Plain radiographs and MRI assist in confirming the diagnosis.
- Acute PLC injuries are amenable to surgical repair if treated early.

IMMOBILIZATION

Immobilization with pain and swelling control comprise initial treatment.

SPECIAL CONSIDERATIONS

- Acute PLC injuries are amenable to surgical repair if treated early.
- If surgical intervention is delayed >2–3 weeks, the tissues are not suitable for repair and reconstruction may be required.

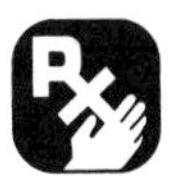

Long-Term Treatment

REHABILITATION

- There is no specific rehabilitation for posterolateral instability.
- Best results are achieved with early diagnosis and intervention.
- As these injuries often occur in conjunction with other ligamentous injuries, ensure that the patient has satisfactory range of motion before operating.
- Patients who developed excessive knee hyperextension or varus thrust during gait may benefit from gait retraining before reconstruction.

SURGERY

Management of chronic PLC instability is more difficult than management of the acute problem.

Acute PLC Injury

- Repair or reconstruction of anatomical structures is indicated along with other associated ligamentous reconstructions (usually ACL or PCL).
- Specific structures to be addressed include the LCL, popliteus tendon, fabellofibular ligament, and popliteofibular ligament.
- Depending on the extent of injury, options for treatment include primary repair, advancement, augmentation, or reconstruction.

Chronic Posterolateral Rotatory Instability

- Primary repair of structures usually is impossible.
- Assessment of both gait and lower extremity alignment is important.
- Patient with preexisting varus malalignment and varus thrust during gait will not have a successful reconstruction because the lateral structures will be attenuated and nonfunctional.
- In this setting, proximal tibial osteotomy may be indicated before ligamentous reconstruction. The most critical structures to reconstruct are the popliteofibular ligament, popliteus, and LCL.
- Anatomical reconstructions, favored over nonanatomical reconstructions (biceps tenodesis), may be performed with a patellar tendon autograft or a split Achilles' tendon allograft.
  —Graft with a bone plug is secured to the isometric point on the femur, usually in close proximity to the femoral epicondyle and LCL origin.
  —Graft is passed through a drill hole in the fibular head and secured to itself.
  —When indicated, a separate limb of the graft may be passed through the proximal tibia and secured to the bone.
  —Advancement or recession of the LCL or popliteus may be indicated, depending on the amount of laxity present.

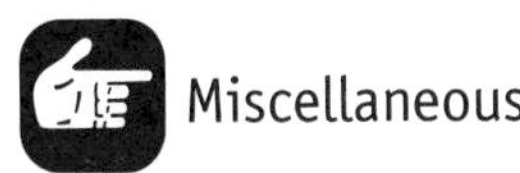

BIBLIOGRAPHY

Albright JP, Brown AW. Management of chronic posterolateral rotatory instability of the knee: surgical technique for the posterolateral corner sling procedure. In: Cannon WD, ed. *Instructional course lectures.* Rosemont, IL: American Academy of Orthopedic Surgeons, 1998;47:369–378.

Ferrari JD, Jach BR. Posterolateral instability of the knee diagnosis. *Sports Med Arthrop Rev* 7:273–288.

Veltri DM, Warren RF. Posterolateral instability of the knee. In: *Instructional course lectures.* Rosemont, IL: American Academy of Orthopedic Surgeons, 1995:441–453.

Authors: Paul Favorito, Angelo J. Colosimo, and Robert S. Heidt Jr.

Pronator Syndrome

Basics

DEFINITION

- Median nerve entrapment within the ligament of Struthers, a tendinous band of the pronator teres muscle or lacertus fibrosis, or the proximal arch of the flexor digitorum superficialis

INCIDENCE/PREVALENCE

- Not common, but should be considered in any patient with carpal tunnel symptoms or hand numbness

RISK FACTORS

- Repetitive occupational pronation/ supination
- Acute forceful pronation or wrist flexion
- Weightlifters with hypertrophied pronator-flexor mass

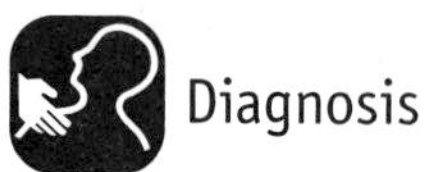

Diagnosis

DIFFERENTIAL DIAGNOSIS

- Median neuropathy at the wrist (carpal tunnel syndrome) (common)
- C-6 or C-7 radiculopathy (common)
- Anterior interosseous syndrome (Kiloh-Nevin syndrome) (uncommon)
- Thoracic outlet syndrome (rare)
- Neuralgic amyotrophy (brachial neuritis, Parsonage-Tuner syndrome) (rare)

HISTORY

- Typically causes an aching pain in proximal forearm, occasional hand pain, and dysesthesias of the radial three and a half digits
- Often exercise or activity induced
- Motor and sensory symptoms can be poorly defined.

PHYSICAL EXAMINATION

- Thickened or hypertrophied pronator muscle mass
- Tenderness or Tinel sign in the proximal anterior forearm with radiation to the palm and/or radial three and a half digits
- May have weakness or atrophy of the hand intrinsic innervated by the median nerve (LOAF muscles): *l*umbricals (first two on radial side of hand), *o*pponens pollicis, *a*bductor pollicis brevis, and *f*lexor pollicis brevis
- May have weakness of the extrinsic finger flexors, wrist flexors, and pronator quadratus
- Tests of Spinner can determine location of median nerve entrapment.
  —Resisted elbow flexion causes pain: lacertus entrapment of median nerve
  —Resisted pronation causes pain: pronator entrapment of median nerve
  —Resisted PIP flexion causes pain: flexor digitorum superficialis entrapment of median nerve

IMAGING

Plain radiographs of the elbow rule out bone involvement such as a supracondyloid process (exostosis that attaches to ligament of Struthers).

ELECTRODIAGNOSTIC MEDICINE

- Most valuable diagnostic test
- Needle electromyography (EMG) is the most helpful to identify evidence of denervation.
- Symptoms often must persist for minimum 4–6 weeks before positive findings on EMG.

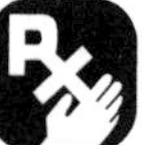

Long-Term Treatment

REHABILITATION

- "APORIM"
  —Activity modification: avoidance of provocative activities
  —Protection from external compression
  —Orthoses: night splints to prevent excessive elbow flexion
  —Rehabilitation: assess proximal and distal kinetic chain (shoulder girdle and wrist) for strength, flexibility, and movement
  —Injections can be considered at point of compression, but exercise caution to avoid direct injection into nerve bundle.
  —Nonsteroidal anti-inflammatory medications

SURGERY

- Consider exploration of the elbow and release of the median nerve from the ligament of Struthers to the flexor digitorum superficialis arch

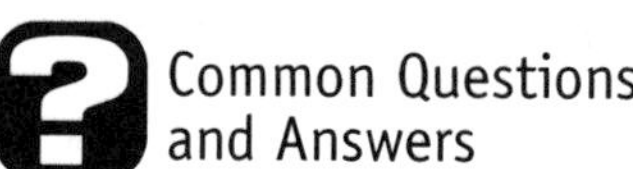

Common Questions and Answers

Physician responses to common patient questions:
Q: What is the prognosis?
A: Prognosis usually depends on the severity of median neuropathy. Worse prognosis with extensive axon loss and atrophy. Expect some reinnervation of distal musculature once the median nerve is free from compromising structures.

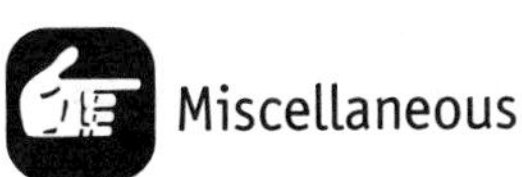

Miscellaneous

SYNONYMS

- Lacertus fibrosis syndrome
- Pronator teres syndrome
- Sublimis bridge syndrome

ICD-9 CODE

354.1

BIBLIOGRAPHY

Dumitru D. *Electrodiagnostic medicine.* Philadelphia: Hanley & Belfus, 1994:856–867.

Dawson DM, Hallett M, Wilbourn AJ, eds. *Median nerve entrapment in entrapment neuropathies.* Philadelphia: Lippincott-Raven Publishers, 1999:99–111.

Hartz CR, Linscheid RL, Gramse RR, et al. Pronator teres syndrome: compressive neuropathy of the median nerve. *J Bone Joint Surg* 1981;63A:885–890.

Kopell HP, Thompson WAL. Pronator syndrome: a confirmed case and its diagnosis. *N Engl J Med* 1958;259:713–715.

Authors: Larry Chou, Joel M. Press, and Venu Akuthota

Quadriceps

Basics

DEFINITION

- Spectrum of injuries ranging from functional, overuse insertional tendinopathy to partial and complete tendon rupture
- Tendon rupture occurs from indirect trauma when the quadriceps contracts rapidly with body weight on the affected lower extremity, which is held in slight flexion, engaging the patella within the femoral condyles.

INCIDENCE/PREVALENCE

- Quadriceps tendinitis is common among high and long jumpers, and among volleyball and basketball players
- Quadriceps tendinitis is a subcategory of "jumper's knee," comprising approximately 25% of such cases.
- Complete quadriceps tendon rupture is rare but occurs three times more often than patellar tendon rupture.

SIGNS AND SYMPTOMS

- Athletes with quadriceps tendinitis may report painful clicking at the superior pole of the patella with stress of the extensor mechanism.
- Tenderness and bogginess may be noted superior to the patella on examination of those with tendinitis.
- With tendon rupture, severe knee pain, swelling, and perceived instability often are noted immediately and prevent weight-bearing.
- Athletes with tendon rupture may give prior history of chronic low-level pain from "jumper's knee."
- More severe tendon ruptures may be associated with gross distal displacement of the patella (patella baja).

STAGING

- Stage 1: pain after practice or game
- Stage 2: pain at beginning of activity, disappearing after warmup and recurring after activity
- Stage 3: pain remains during and after activity
- Stage 4: complete tendon rupture

RISK FACTORS

- Primary risk factor for quadriceps tendinitis is functional overload from repetitive stress on the extensor mechanism of the knee during jumping.
- Quadriceps tendinitis typically develops after age 15 years, before which various types of traction apophysitis about the knee predominate with overuse.
- Participation in sports on hard surfaces may increase the risk of quadriceps tendinitis.
- Large majority of quadriceps tendon ruptures occur after age 40.
- Male-to-female ratio for quadriceps tendon rupture is 6:1
- Ruptures frequently occur in the setting of preexisting tendinitis.

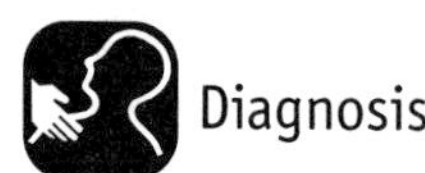

Diagnosis

DIFFERENTIAL DIAGNOSIS

- Rectus femoris strain
- Patellar tendinitis
- Patellar tendon rupture
- Patellar dislocation
- Bipartite patella
- Patellofemoral arthritis
- Osgood-Schlatter disease
- Sinding-Larsen-Johansson disease
- Distal femoral physeal injuries

HISTORY

Q: Stumbled prior to injury or felt a pop?
A: Athletes with quadriceps tendon ruptures typically recall stumbling just before loading the affected leg and often recall a pop upon injury.

PHYSICAL EXAMINATION

- Examine extensor mechanism of all acutely injured knees
  —Quadriceps tendon rupture frequently is misdiagnosed (38% in one study).
  —Misdiagnosis occurs because physicians fail to test the extensor mechanism of acutely injured knees.
  —Delay may result in negative outcomes (described below).
- Examine patient in seated position
  —Seated postioning optimizes palpation for a defect often present in acute ruptures.
  —With delayed presentations, the defect may be masked by the large hematoma and later scar formation that it causes.
- Test active extension and ability to maintain complete extension against gravity
  —With complete ruptures including the retinaculi, active extension is limited.
  —Ruptures with intact retinaculi are marked by inability to maintain complete extension against gravity but may have intact active extension.
- Examine contralateral knee
  —Systemic disorders associated with bilateral quadriceps tendon rupture include rheumatoid arthritis, gout, systemic lupus erythematosus, chronic renal failure, secondary hyperparathyroidism, diabetes mellitus, and peripheral vascular disease.

IMAGING

- Lateral radiographs may reveal distal displacement of the patella (patella baja).
- Comparison with the contralateral side may be helpful.
- Magnetic resonance imaging typically is not necessary but may be helpful in evaluating difficult diagnostic cases, including partial tears or late presentations.

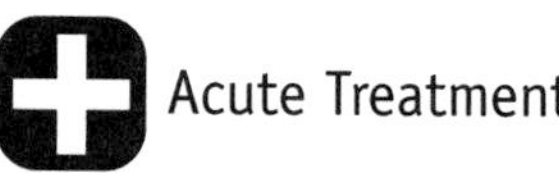

Acute Treatment

CONSERVATIVE MEASURES

- Stage 1 and 2 quadriceps tendinitis
  —Best managed conservatively
  —Relative rest from jumping and sports participation
  —Physical therapy for stretching and strengthening of the quadriceps group
  —Ultrasound
  —Postexertional icing
  —Stepwise return to jumping and participation
- Stage 3 tendinitis
  —Managed as stages 1 and 2
  —May require prolonged rest from the inciting activity and/or reduction in training frequency
- Partial tears of the quadriceps tendon
  —Treated as stages 1 to 3
  —Addition of crutches initially to reduce weight-bearing on the affected leg

SURGERY

- Acute rupture of the quadriceps tendon (stage 4) requires prompt surgical repair
- Time from injury to repair is the greatest determinant of outcome in athletes with quadriceps tendon ruptures. Repair within 1–2 weeks yields significantly better outcomes.
- End-to end repairs and tendon-to-bone repairs are used depending on the level of the rupture.

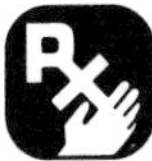

Long-Term Treatment

DELAYED PRESENTATION TENDON RUPTURE

Late repair of ruptures with a variety of surgical techniques reduces disability, but outcomes are suboptimal compared with timely repair.

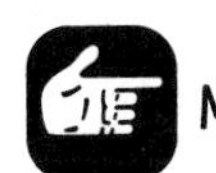

Miscellaneous

ICD-9 CODE

726.9 Tendonitis
844.8 Quadriceps tendon rupture

BIBLIOGRAPHY

Ferretti A, Ippolito E, Mariani P, et al. Jumper's knee. *Am J Sports Med* 1983;11:58–62.

Ferretti A, Puddu G, Mariani P, et al. The natural history of jumper's knee. *Int Orthop* 1985;8:239–242.

Roels J , Martens M, Burssens A. Patellar tendinitis (jumper's knee). *Am J Sports Med* 1978;6:362–368.

Rougraff BT, Reeck CC, Essenmacher J. Complete quadriceps tendon ruptures. *Orthopedics* 1996;19:509–514.

Authors: Andrew Concoff and Gary A. Green

Quadriceps Contusion

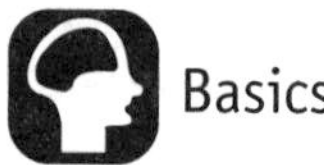

Basics

DEFINITION

Quadriceps Contusion

External blow to the anterior, medial, or lateral thigh in the area of the muscle belly of the quadriceps femoris

Myositis Ossificans Traumatica

Formation of heterotopic bone and cartilage in soft tissue as a result of physical trauma

INCIDENCE/PREVALENCE

- 1% to 2% of football players in 1 year will get a quadriceps contusion
- Most common mechanism is a knee or helmet to the anterior thigh

SIGNS AND SYMPTOMS

- Pain and swelling in the anterior thigh
- Decreased knee range of motion
- Patients with a hematoma may have a palpable anterior thigh mass.

RISK FACTORS

- More prevalent in contact sports (rugby, judo, football)
- Prior quadriceps contusion predisposes to more severe injury.
- Coagulation disorders predispose to hematoma formation.
- Delay in onset of therapy leads to a higher percentage of complications and delay in recovery.

ASSOCIATED INJURIES AND COMPLICATIONS

- Myositis ossificans traumatica (MOT)
- Compartment syndrome of the anterior thigh
- Traumatic pseudoaneurysm

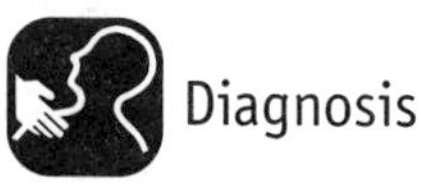

Diagnosis

DIFFERENTIAL DIAGNOSIS

- Quadriceps strain
- Active arterial bleeding
- Quadriceps tendon rupture
- Iliacus rupture

HISTORY

- Trauma and subsequent pain, swelling, and decreased range of motion
- Important questions to ask:

Q: Is this an initial or a repeat injury?
A: Repeat injuries are more likely to go on to develop MOT.
Q: When did it happen?
A: Delay in therapy increases time to recovery and risk of MOT.
Q: Are you getting better?
A: If athletes are not improving or are regressing in therapy, MOT and other complications are more likely.
Q: Are you anticoagulated or do you have a bleeding disorder?
A: This predisposes to more severe bleeding.

PHYSICAL EXAMINATION

- Knee range of motion: the more limited the range of motion, the higher the complication rate.
- Severe pain at rest or with mild passive stretch: Pain seemingly out of proportion to the injury and a tense anterior thigh suggest compartment syndrome.
- Early masses suggest a hematoma; late masses suggest MOT; pulsatile masses suggest pseudoaneurysm.
- Patients with severe quadriceps contusions often get knee effusions without intra-articular pathology.
- Thigh circumference should be measured at regular intervals to assess when expansion of edema and hematoma have stopped.

IMAGING

Plain Radiographs

- Reveal MOT 2–5 weeks after the initial injury
- Advantages
  —Inexpensive
  —Well-described progress of events
- Disadvantage
  —Takes 2–5 weeks to become positive

Ultrasound

- Can differentiate among rupture, contusion, MOT, and pseudoaneurysm
- Advantages
  —No radiation
  —Noninvasive
  —Will show rare complications
  —May show MOT before plain films
- Disadvantages
  —Operator dependent
  —Not as well described or as easily available as plain films

Triple-Phase Bone Scan

- Shows increased uptake at the site of MOT
- Advantages
  —Will often reveal MOT before plain radiographs
  —Shows maturity of the lesion
- Disadvantages
  —Expensive
  —Radiation exposure
  —Nonspecific information

Computed Tomography

- Accurately shows size, density, and location of MOT lesion
- Advantages
  —Precise measurement of MOT
  —Differentiates MOT from osteosarcoma
- Disadvantages
  —Expensive
  —Radiation
  —No time advantage over plain films

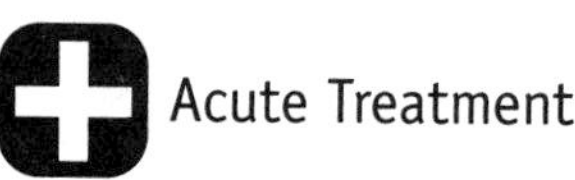

Acute Treatment

ANALGESIA

Do not use nonsteroidal anti-inflammatory drugs for the first 48 hours as they may increase the risk of bleeding.

IMMOBILIZATION

- Limit hemorrhage and edema with rest, ice, compression, and elevation
- Maximally flex the knee for additional thigh compression

ON THE FIELD

- Assume the injury is worse than it looks.
- Removing the athlete from contact is the best way to prevent further injury.
- Athletes definitely should not return to play if they
  —Have severe pain
  —Have decreased range of motion
  —Are unable to run or perform the demands of their sport
  —Have significant thigh swelling

Long-Term Treatment

REHABILITATION

- After athlete is pain-free at rest and thigh girth has stabilized, should begin range of motion exercises.
- May bear weight as tolerated
- May stop using crutches when can attain 90 degrees of motion and no limp
- Functional rehabilitation may begin when the patient has >120 degrees of motion, including isometric, kinetic chain, and endurance exercises.
- May participate in noncontact exercises at this time
- When full strength, motion, and coordination are achieved, athlete may resume contact sports wearing a thigh pad for the next 3–6 months.

SURGERY

- Simple contusions and hematomas do not require surgery.
- Athletes with MOT who have persistent pain and limited motion may have the heterotopic bone removed when it has matured, usually 6–12 months after the initial injury. Bone scan or plain films determine maturity of the tumor.
- Severe anterior compartment syndrome requires fasciotomy.
- Traumatic pseudoaneurysm requires surgery.

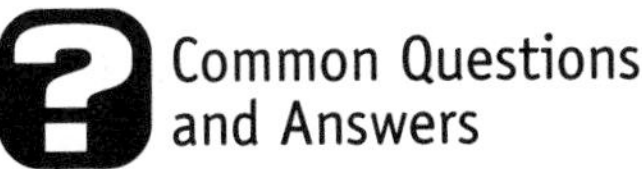

Common Questions and Answers

Physician responses to common trainer or patient questions:
Q: Should I try to aspirate a quadriceps hematoma?
A: No. By the time you attempt to aspirate it, it has already coagulated. Also, aspiration attempts increase the risks of infection and could make the bleeding worse.
Q: Are there any drugs that prevent MOT?
A: Proteolytic enzymes, intralesional hyaluronidase, and corticosteroids have all been tried; none have proven more effective than good physical therapy.
Q: Are there any modalities that prevent MOT?
A: Ultrasound, radiation therapy, and iontophoresis have been tried with variable success, but none have been studied systematically. Massage and heat can be harmful.

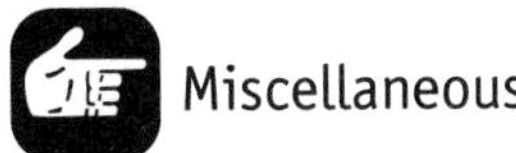

Miscellaneous

SYNONYMS

- Charlie horse
- Myositis ossificans
- Quadriceps hematoma

ICD-9 CODE

924.00 Quadriceps contusion or quadriceps hematoma
728.12 Myositis ossificans traumatica

BIBLIOGRAPHY

Annenberg A, Vaccaro P, Zuelzer W. Traumatic pseudoaneurysm in a wrestler. *Ann Vasc Surg* 1990;4:69–71.

Futani H, Itahara S, Maruo S, Tateishi H. A report on 2 cases of myositis ossificans in childhood. *Acta Orthop Scand* 1998;69:642–645.

Jackson D, Feagin J. Quadriceps contusion in young athletes. *J Bone Joint Surg* 1973;55A:95–105.

Kirkpatrick J, Koman L, Rovere G. The role of ultrasound in the early diagnosis of myositis ossificans. *Am J Sports Med* 1987;15:179–181.

Lipscomb A, Thomas E, Johnson R. Treatment of myositis ossificans in athletes. *Am J Sports Med* 1976;4:111–120.

Mellerowicz H, Stelling E, Kefenbaum A. Diagnostic ultrasound in the athlete's locomotor system. *Br J Sports Med* 1990;24:31–39.

Robinson D, On E, Halperin N. Anterior compartment syndrome of the thigh in athletes: indications for conservative treatment. *J Trauma* 1992;32:183–186.

Rooser B, Bengtson S, Hagglund G. Acute compartment syndrome from anterior thigh muscle contusion: a report of eight cases. *J Orthop Trauma* 1991;5:57–59.

Rothwell A. Quadriceps hematoma: a prospective clinical study. *Clin Orthop* 1982;171:97–103.

Ryan J, Wheeler J, Hopkinson W, Arlieri R, Kulakewski W. Quadriceps contusion: West Point update. *Am J Sports Med* 1991;19:299–304.

Walton M, Rothwell A. Reactions of thigh tissues of sheep to blunt trauma. *Clin Orthop* 1983;176:273–281.

Wang S, Lomasney L, Demos T, Hopkinson W. Diagnosis: traumatic myositis ossificans. *Orthopedics* 1999;22:991–995.

Young J, Laskowski E, Rock M. Thigh injuries in athletes. *Mayo Clinic Procs* 68:1099–1106.

Authors: Michael J. Henehan and Gregory A. Whitley

Redundant Plica

 Basics

DEFINITION

Plica is a redundant fold of embryonic synovium adjacent to the patella.

INCIDENCE/PREVALENCE

- Occurs more often in females than males
- Occurs more often in growing adolescents

SIGNS AND SYMPTOMS

- Episodes of anterior knee pain
- May be associated with swelling of the knee
- Patient may describe a feeling of knee instability, "catching," "buckling," or "giving way" with episodes of pain.

RISK FACTORS

- Congenital presence of plica
- Extensor mechanism malalignment, e.g., quadriceps/vastus medialis oblique [VMO] weakness, increased Q-angle
- Repetitive flexing and extending of the knee, e.g., running, jumping

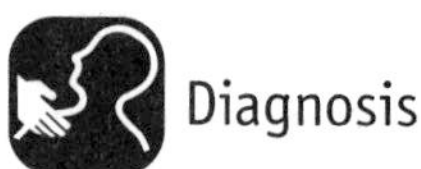

Diagnosis

DIFFERENTIAL DIAGNOSIS

- Other painful patellofemoral conditions, e.g., chondromalacia patella, osteochondritis dissecans of the medial femoral condyle
- Medial meniscus tear

HISTORY

- Complaint of anterior knee pain
- Pain over suprapatellar or medial peripatellar region
- Pain worse after long periods of knee flexion (e.g., sitting), especially when accompanied by a distinct snap or pop when knee is extended
- May have a history of overuse or direct trauma
- Painful catching episodes over medial patellofemoral joint
- May describe feeling of instability with episodes of pain

PHYSICAL EXAMINATION

- Palpation over the medial patellofemoral joint may demonstrate a tender thickened band in the anterior synovium
- Often difficult to palpate; best done while passively flexing and extending the knee while holding the tibia in internal rotation
- May find other problems associated with extensor mechanism malalignment, e.g., chondromalacia patella, patellar subluxation
- Assess hamstring and heel cord tightness, as these conditions tend to aggravate the problem

IMAGING

- X-ray studies do not usually show any bony abnormality.
- Patellar views (e.g., sunrise, Merchant view, Hughston patellar view) may demonstrate a lateral patellar tilt consistent with weakness of the vastus medialis or an increased Q-angle
- Magnetic resonance imaging may demonstrate inflammation and thickening of the anteromedial synovium of the knee in extreme chronic cases.
- Ultrasound imaging may have limited use in evaluating thickening of the synovial plica, but is very dependent on operator experience and expertise.

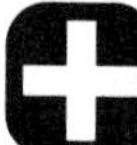

Acute Treatment

ANALGESIA

- Nonsteroidal anti-inflammatory drugs
- Ice

PROTECTION

- Activity modification
- Consider external patellar support

REST

- Relative rest to reduce repetitive flexion of the knee
- May consider short-term immobilization (1–3 days) if pain is severe

ICE

- Ice 20 minutes 3–4 times daily to reduce inflammation until swelling and pain have resolved

COMPRESSION

- Elastic bandage can be used for comfortable level of compression during the acute phase to help to reduce swelling.
- Consider using an open patellar knee brace with a patellar support to reduce patellar mobility and recurrent "pinching" of the plica

ELEVATION

Elevating the knee above the level of the heart as possible may help reduce swelling within the plica.

SUPPORT

- Open patellar knee brace with a patellar support to reduce patellar mobility may help reduce the chance of recurrent trauma to the plica when the patient returns to activity.
- McConnell taping (a physical therapy taping technique using strong supportive tape surrounding the patella) may be used for short-term improvement in patellar alignment and reduction in patellar hypermobility.

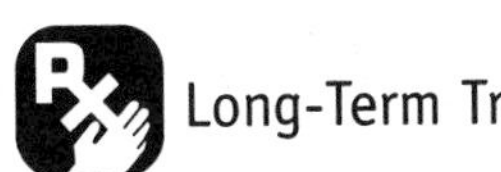

Long-Term Treatment

REHABILITATION

- VMO strengthening (quad sets, straight-leg raises, terminal arc extensions of the knee)
- Hamstring stretching
- Heel cord stretching
- Ice for ~20 minutes after exercise
- Consider phonophoresis

INJECTION

- Intra-articular corticosteroid injection into the knee often produces a decrease in inflammation of the plica and associated symptoms and may be considered if initial conservative treatment has failed.
- Corticosteroid injection may help to resolve the problem and negate the need for arthroscopic intervention.

SURGERY

- If plica is fibrotic and symptoms persist, arthroscopic removal of the plica is indicated.
- For chronic painful plica, arthroscopic removal often provides good relief of symptoms and return to normal function.
- Surgery should be combined with rehabilitative strengthening of the VMO to reduce the chance of recurrence.

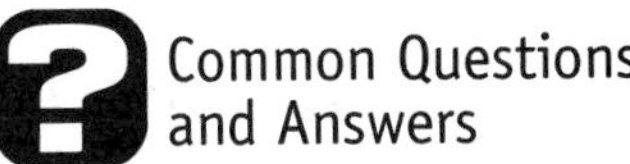

Common Questions and Answers

Physician responses to common patient questions:

Q: How did I get a plica?

A: A plica usually occurs after chronic and repetitive pinching of the lining of the knee caused by weakness of the quadriceps (vastus medialis) muscle or a larger than normal angle from the hip to the knee pulling the kneecap more sideways (commonly seen in growing, adolescent females), or after an acute trauma to the front of the knee.

Q: Will a "plica" go away without surgery?

A: Unless the inflammation has been present for a long time and scar tissue has formed, an inflamed plica often will resolve with ice, anti-inflammatory drugs, and rehabilitative exercises.

Q: Why does a "plica" only hurt some of the time?

A: Pain that occurs with plica irritation usually occurs only after the plica becomes inflamed, often from being pinched between the kneecap and thigh bone from such activities as running, jumping, going up and down stairs, or sitting with the knee flexed for an extended period of time.

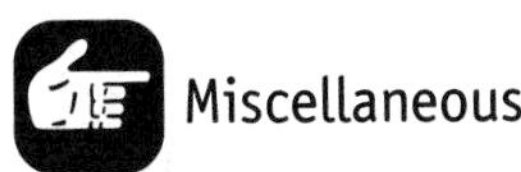

Miscellaneous

SYNONYMS

- Patellofemoral syndrome
- Synovitis of the knee

ICD-9 CODE

727.83 Plica syndrome of the knee

BIBLIOGRAPHY

Baker MM, Juhn MS. Patellofemoral pain syndrome in the female athlete. *Clin Sports Med* 2000;19:315–329.

Dupont J. Synovial plicae of the knee. *Clin Sports Med* 1997;16:88–123.

Tindel NL, Nisonson B. The plica syndrome. *Orthop Clin North Am* 1992;23:613–618.

Author: Douglas Browning

Reflex Sympathetic Dystrophy

Basics

DEFINITION

- Exaggerated response to injury manifested by four characteristics:
  - —Intense or unduly prolonged pain
  - —Vasomotor disturbances
  - —Delayed functional recovery
  - —Various associated trophic changes

SIGNS AND SYMPTOMS

- Pain out of proportion to the precipitating injury, often burning and nondermatomal in nature, due to sympathetic dysfunction
- Significant pain with light touch or cold exposure may occur.
- Temperature usually decreased but may be increased
- Skin may appear mottled, erythematous (in early stages), or pale (later stages).

RISK FACTORS

- Prior noxious event
  - —Usually preceded by an event such as a fracture or surgery
  - —In children, usually a history of a sprain or minor injury
- Constitutional or psychiatric predisposition
  - —Suspected by some
  - —"Sympathetic hyperreactors" described as those with a history of increased sweating in the palms, poor cold tolerance, and emotional lability

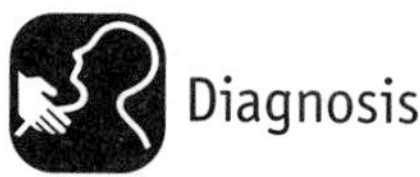

Diagnosis

DIFFERENTIAL DIAGNOSIS

- Causalgia, presenting similar signs and symptoms to reflex sympathetic dystrophy (RSD) but associated with an actual nerve lesion
- Fracture/stress fracture, ruled out with appropriate imaging studies
- Infection
- Tumor
- After other possible causes of pain have been excluded, diagnosis of RSD can be made clinically or on the basis of pain relief with sympathetic blockade.

HISTORY

- Often follows trivial or minor trauma, such as a sprain in children.
- Chronic exaggerated pain occurs in association with neuropathic changes and sympathetic dysfunction.
- Female-to-male ratio 1:1 in adults; approximately 6:1 in children
- Average age in patients <18 years is 10–13 years.
- Lower extremity preponderance in pediatric patients and upper extremity preponderance in adults

PHYSICAL EXAMINATION

- Allodynia
- Edema
- Cold or warm extremity
- Mottling or cyanosis
- Joint contractures and atrophy
- Hyperhidrosis

IMAGING

Plain X-ray

- May demonstrate osteoporosis as early as 2–4 weeks after injury
- Spotty osteoporosis is seen in early stages and is more diffuse and homogeneous in late stages.
- Findings are less consistently positive in pediatric/adolescent cases.

Bone Scan

- Increased uptake in 2/3 of adult patients with RSD
- Findings less reliable in pediatric patients
  - —1/3 exhibit increased uptake (usually in late stages of disease).
  - —1/3 exhibit normal findings.
  - —1/3 exhibit decreased uptake (usually in early stages).
- Often more helpful to rule out other disorders, such as stress fractures or tumor, causing pain

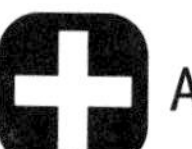

Acute Treatment

IMMOBILIZATION

- Often used but not recommended for treatment of RSD, except in rare cases
- Should be coordinated with an orthopaedic surgeon

PAIN MANAGEMENT

- Pain center referral is generally appropriate, but the facility should be familiar with RSD patients.
- Pain center may help coordinate the necessary multidisciplinary treatment and assist with medications and nerve blocks.

PHYSICAL THERAPY

- Mainstay of RSD treatment
- Tactile desensitization is most effective if used early.
- Joint mobilization, progressive weight-bearing, strengthening, and return to daily activities are important aspects of care directed by physical therapy.
- Transcutaneous electrical nerve stimulation can be beneficial.
- Early referral to physical therapy is key.

MEDICATIONS

- Nonsteroidal anti-inflammatory drugs, often of variable effect
- Tricyclic antidepressants, especially helpful if the patient has sleep disturbances, decreased energy, and decreased appetite
- Oral steroids of questionable benefit

PSYCHIATRIC EVALUATION

- Behavioral management
- Relaxation techniques
- Stress management

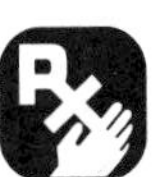

Long-Term Treatment

REHABILITATION

- Physical therapy is the mainstay of treatment.
- Therapy is continued to help restore function in patients.

SYMPATHETIC BLOCK

- Timing of sympathetic blocks is variable according to different authors.
- Often performed if the patient continues to have symptoms despite conservative treatment.
- Usually provides substantial improvement if not complete resolution
- Should be coordinated with ongoing physical therapy

SYMPATHECTOMY (OPERATIVE OR CHEMICAL)

- Only considered in the most recalcitrant cases and where vascular dysfunction affects the integrity of the limb involved

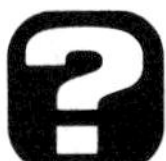

Common Questions and Answers

Physician responses to common patient questions:

Q: What is the time course of the disease?

A: RSD has an extremely variable prognosis. It may resolve in a few weeks or over several years, but may result in an even more prolonged disability.

Q: Will this condition resolve?

A: The course is extremely variable. In general, the prognosis is more favorable in younger patients, but in one series of 70 patients, 54% still had some symptoms at 2–8 years (mean 3) of follow-up.

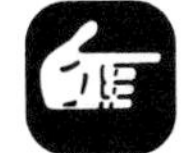

Miscellaneous

SYNONYMS

- Complex regional pain syndrome type I
- Causalgia: complex regional pain syndrome type II
- Shoulder-hand syndrome
- Sudeck atrophy
- Neurovascular dystrophy
- Pain dysfunction syndrome

ICD-9 CODE

337.20
337.21 Upper extremity
337.22 Lower extremity

BIBLIOGRAPHY

Barbier O, Allington N, Rombouts JJ. Reflex sympathetic dystrophy in children: review. *Acta Orthop Belg* 1999;65:91–97.

Dietz FR, Matthews KD, Montgomery WJ. Reflex sympathetic dystrophy in children. *Clin Orthop* 1990;258:225–231.

Stanton RP, Malcolm JR, Wedsock KA, et al. Reflex sympathetic dystrophy in children. *Orthopedics* 1993;16:773–779.

Wilder RT, Berde CB, Wolohan M, et al. Reflex sympathetic dystrophy in children. *J Bone Joint Surg* 1992;74A:910–919.

Authors: Thomas Kim, Lyle J. Micheli, and Thomas A. Balcom

Rotator Cuff Tears

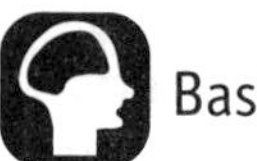

Basics

DEFINITION

- Partial or complete tears or disruption of any one or combination of the four rotator cuff muscles of the glenohumeral joint
- Supraspinatus and infraspinatus muscle/tendon complexes are the most common tears.
- Rotator cuff muscles are the supraspinatus, infraspinatus, teres minor, and subscapularis muscles.

INCIDENCE/PREVALENCE

- Rare in young athletes
- More common in athletes >40 years, especially those with a history of many years of repetitive overhead sports

SIGNS AND SYMPTOMS

- Pain and weakness with abduction from 80–120 degrees, or with internal or external rotation with shoulder at 90 degrees of abduction
- Chronic overuse presents with gradual onset of pain with activities of daily living, nocturnal pain, and upper extremity exertional activities.

RISK FACTORS

- Over-40 weekend warrior with years of repetitive overhead use (e.g., swimming, tennis, volleyball, gymnastics, weight-lifting, and throwing sports)
- Previous trauma
- Sports with potential fall risk, such as equestrian, skiing, and body surfing

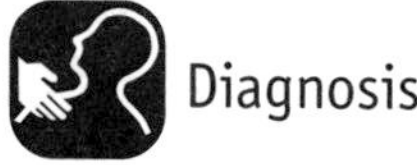

Diagnosis

DIFFERENTIAL DIAGNOSIS

- Rotator cuff strains
- Glenoid labrum tear
- Subluxation or unstable shoulder
- Subacromial impingement
- Isolated bicipital tendonitis
- Acromioclavicular joint disorders
- Glenohumeral arthritis
- Rare subacromial abscess or tumors

HISTORY

- Mechanism of injury
  —Acute traumatic events such as a fall, direct blow, or forceful boxing punch
  —Traumatic hyperextension of abducted arm
  —Traumatic external or internal rotation of abducted arm
  —Anterior dislocation
- Chronic overhead arm use may present insidiously.

PHYSICAL EXAMINATION

- Diminished range of motion
- Pain with arm abduction, especially at 80–120 degrees of arc
- Loss of strength
- Atrophy of cuff muscles
- Crepitus of supraspinatus muscle during abduction
- Drop-arm test is positive.
  —Arm is passively abducted to 90 degrees
  —Patient is instructed to slowly return the arm to the side
  —Severe pain or inability to do so is positive test for a torn rotator cuff complex.
- Empty-can test is positive.
  —Resistance applied to arm abducted 90 degrees, angled 30 degrees anteriorly with a medially rotated forearm (thumbs down/"empty can")
  —Test is positive for inability to do so or severe pain, indicating a tear of the supraspinatus tendon.
- Test external rotation strength
  —Perform test with elbow flexed 90 degrees at the side
  —Pinpoints infraspinatus and teres minor involvement
- Lift-off test for subscapularis is positive.
  —Inability to lift the dorsum of the hand off the back hip
  —Significant pain with internal rotation can preclude an accurate test.
- Poor scapular stability
- Anterior glenoid-humeral laxity
- Subacromial bursa injection (10 mL of 1% lidocaine) may distinguish bursal pathology and minor impingement from distinct tears of the rotator cuff tears (no pain relief or strength improvement from the injection).
- Comprehensive testing of active and passive range of motion, strength testing, and adequate neurovascular testing

IMAGING

- Plain radiographs may show calcifications along the tendons of the rotator cuff muscles; subacromial osteophytes; or superior or anterior migration of the humeral head.
- Magnetic resonance imaging is helpful to identify tears.
- Ultrasound, computed tomographic arthrography, and arthrograms can be helpful.

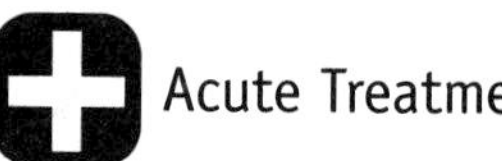

Acute Treatment

ANALGESIA

- Nonsteroidal anti-inflammatory drugs of choice initially
- More potent analgesics may be temporarily necessary to relieve nocturnal symptoms.

IMMOBILIZATION

Sling may provide some relief for the acutely injured shoulder.

Long-Term Treatment

REHABILITATION

- Prolonged rehabilitation emphasizing increased range of motion and strengthening is indicated for the partial tear.
- Normalizing scapulothoracic stabilization and posterior capsular flexibility with 1:1 strength ratio for rotator cuff to anterior/middle cuff deltoid muscles.

SURGERY

- For complete tears, surgery may be warranted in the active athlete.
- Early operative repair provides the best chance for functional recovery.

REFERRAL/DISPOSITION

- Acute full-thickness tears should be referred early on.
- Partial tears after failed conservative therapy

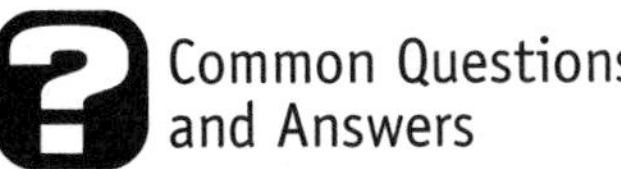

Common Questions and Answers

Physician responses to common patient questions:
Q: When should I consider surgery?
A: Surgery is an option, especially for the young and/or active athlete, and should be considered early on for diagnosis of complete tears of the rotator cuff.
Q: How long will rehabilitation take?
A: Rehabilitation of a partial tear of the rotator cuff is a prolonged process that may take months to return to preinjury status.

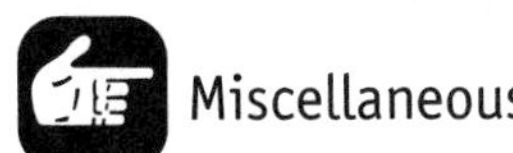

Miscellaneous

SYNONYMS

- Tear of the supraspinatus
- Tear of the infraspinatus
- Tear of the teres minor
- Tear of the subscapularis muscle

ICD-9 CODE

727.61 Complete atraumatic tear of rotator cuff
726.1 Rotator cuff syndrome
726.10 Rotator cuff bursa or tendon inflammation
726.11 Calcifications of rotator cuff tendons
840.4 Rotator cuff tear traumatic
840.6 Supraspinatus tear

BIBLIOGRAPHY

Breazeale NM, Craig EV. Partial-thickness rotator cuff tears. *Orthop Clin North Am* 1997;28:145–155.

Hulstyn MJ, Fadale PD. Shoulder injuries in the athlete. *Clin Sports Med* 1997;16: 663–679.

Author: Kenneth Bielak

Scapholunate Dissociation

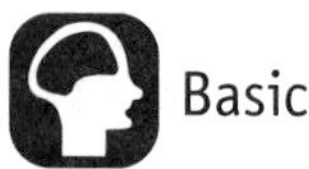

Basics

DEFINITION

- Carpal instability between the scaphoid and the lunate that develops after disruption of at least 2 of the 3 scapholunate ligaments

INCIDENCE/PREVALENCE

- Most common form of carpal instability
- More precise epidemiologic data lacking

SIGNS AND SYMPTOMS

- Dorsal- and radial-sided wrist pain with loss of motion and weakness of grasp, usually after a traumatic wrist injury

RISK FACTORS

- Active individuals who have negative ulnar variance (relatively shortened distal ulna compared with radius recognized on a posteroanterior radiograph of the wrist)

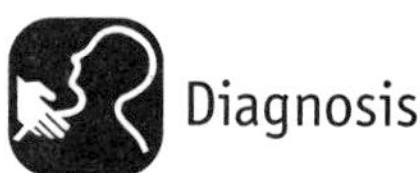

Diagnosis

DIFFERENTIAL DIAGNOSIS

- Scaphoid or lunate fracture
- Ligament sprain/partial tear
- Lunotriquetral injury
- Perilunate dislocation
- Kienbock disease (osteochondroses of the lunate)
- Extensor carpi radialis tendonitis
- Dorsal ganglion cyst

HISTORY

Mechanism of injury usually involves a fall or direct blow onto an outstretched, pronated hand causing hyperextension of the wrist and ulnar deviation.

PHYSICAL EXAMINATION

- Tenderness and swelling most commonly localized to the scapholunate interval, palpated just distal and slightly ulnar to Lister tubercle of the distal radius
- Perform diagnostic maneuver, such as scaphoid shift or Watson test
  —Examiner stabilizes the scaphoid by placing forefingers on the distal radius and thumb on the distal pole of the scaphoid volarly while holding the wrist in ulnar deviation.
  —Patient's wrist is brought into radial deviation as the thumb of the examiner applies pressure to the distal pole of the scaphoid.
- When the scaphoid is unstable, this maneuver will force the distal pole to sublux dorsally or skid, which is palpable by the examiner; patient's pain also reproduced.

IMAGING

Anteroposterior (AP) and Lateral Radiographs

- Imperative to obtain
- Findings can be subtle.
- Views should be compared with the uninjured wrist.
- Key findings on AP view include
  —Gap in the scapholunate interval >2 mm (Terry Thomas sign)
  —Scaphoid has foreshortened appearance because it is subluxed into a more vertical position.
  —Distal pole of the scaphoid is seen on end (cortical ring sign)
- Key findings on the lateral view include
  —Pattern in which the lunate lies volar to the capitate but is flexed dorsally (also known as dorsal intercalated segment instability)
  —Scapholunate angle >70 degrees (normal 30–60)
- Many scapholunate dissociations, particularly those that are acute, present as dynamic instabilities. When there is clinical evidence without demonstration on routine x-rays, radiographs should be obtained in a "clenched fist" position.
- Cineradiography (dynamic arthrogram) can be helpful to demonstrate instability, but most special radiographic studies are not helpful or warranted.

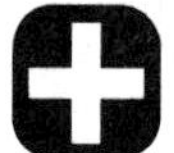

Acute Treatment

ANALGESIA

- Ice plus acetaminophen, nonsteroidal anti-inflammatory drugs, or opioids

REDUCTION TECHNIQUES

- Open reduction and internal fixation with direct ligamentous repair is the procedure of choice.
- Dorsal capsular augmentation (capsulodesis) is commonly added to provide a secondary restraint to hold the scaphoid in a reduced position.
- Within the first 3–4 weeks of injury, closed reduction and percutaneous pinning of the scapholunate dissociation under cineradiographic control may be successful.

IMMOBILIZATION

- Wrist is immobilized in a neutral or slightly dorsiflexed position in a thumb spica cast for 8 weeks, then the pins are removed.
- Often followed by a short-arm cast for 4 weeks.
- Patient is fitted with a protective splint and a rehabilitation program is begun.

SPECIAL CONSIDERATIONS

- Surgical techniques described above mainly reserved for acute injury (defined as 3–8 weeks after injury), after which the ligaments are believed to heal poorly and no longer amenable to repair by direct suture.
- Repair sometimes successful long after acute disruption if there are no degenerative joint changes and an adequate ligament is present, as determined at surgery.

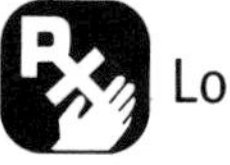

Long-Term Treatment

REHABILITATION

Supervised rehabilitation program working with range of motion and strengthening exercises usually is necessary for 1–2 months.

SURGERY

- More complex surgery often needed when a scapholunate dissociation is treated late and there is no longer adequate ligament remaining for direct suture
- When there are no arthritic changes at the radioscaphoid joint, a partial wrist arthrodesis is most commonly performed (scaphoid-trapezium-trapezoid or scaphoid-capitate fusion).
- Once degenerative arthritis is present, the wrist can be treated with only more formal salvage-type procedures, i.e., excision of the scaphoid with fusion of the midcarpal joint or a proximal row carpectomy.

DISPOSITION

- Decisions about return to play must be individualized based on sport-specific demands.
- In general, an athlete may return after demonstrating progression in strength and range of motion in a supervised rehabilitation program.
- An orthosis such as silicone or synthetic fiberglass cast should be used for protection during participation in sports for about 6 months and then can be removed if maximum strength and range of motion have returned.

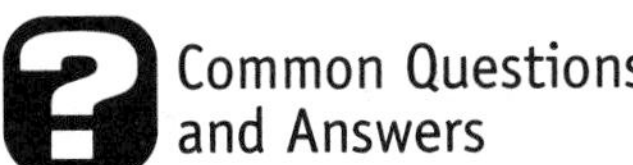

Common Questions and Answers

Physician responses to common patient questions:

Q: Am I at risk for long-term disability because of this injury?
A: Surgical correction during the acute phase of injury yields the best results with minimal potential for long-term disability.
If there is a delay in diagnosis or treatment (>8 weeks after injury), arthritic changes usually develop at the radial styloid articulation. Subsequently, a progressive arthritic pattern can occur which is termed scapholunate dissociation with advanced collapse (SLAC) wrist. At this stage, even with surgical reconstruction, there will be a loss of motion.

Q: What limitations am I going to have after surgery?
A: Following open reduction and internal fixation with direct ligamentous repair and a dorsal capsulodesis, there is an expected loss of 15–20 degrees of wrist flexion.

An STT or SC fusion results in approximately 35% loss of wrist motion in the flexion- extension plane, which still permits high-demand sport activities.

If a formal salvage-type of procedure is needed, approximately 50% loss of motion in the flexion-extension plane and 20% loss of grip strength can be expected, which is acceptable for most sport-related activities.

Q: When can I return to athletic competition?
A: See Disposition above.

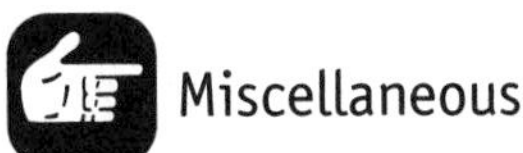

Miscellaneous

SYNONYMS

- Rotary subluxation of the scaphoid
- Scapholunate instability

ICD-9 CODE

833.00

BIBLIOGRAPHY

Cohen M. *Clinics in sports medicine.* Philadelphia: WB Saunders, 1998.

DeLee JC, Drez D. *Orthopaedic sports medicine.* Philadelphia: WB Saunders, 1994.

Halikis MN, Taleisnik J. *Clinics in sports medicine.* Philadelphia: WB Saunders, 1996.

Lister G. *The hand: diagnosis and indications.* Edinburgh: Churchill Livingstone, 1993.

Pappas AM. *Upper extremities injuries in the athlete.* Edinburgh: Churchill Livingstone, 1995.

Watson HK, Hempton RF. Limited wrist arthrodesis. *J Hand Surg* 1980;5:320–327.

Authors: Joseph Armen and Robert L. Jones

Sciatica

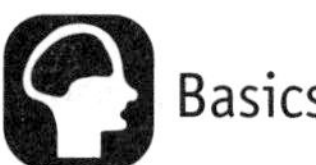

Basics

DEFINITION

- Radicular pain in the distribution of a sciatic nerve root (L-4, L-5, S-1, S-2, or S-3), usually producing symptoms along the posterior or lateral aspect of the lower extremity extending to the ankle or foot
- May include pain in the distribution of that root, dermatomal sensory disturbances, weakness of the muscles innervated by that root, and hypoactive stretch reflexes

INCIDENCE/PREVALENCE

- Lower back pain (LBP) extremely common in the general population and seen in a number of sports, e.g., football, gymnastics, tennis

LBP

- General population: 5% annual occurrence; 60% to 90% lifetime incidence
  —Men and women equally affected
  —Second most common reason to visit primary care physician

Sciatica

- Accounts for only 2% to 3% percent of all patients with LBP
- Peaks in the fourth to fifth decades of life

ETIOLOGY

- Compression or trauma of the sciatic nerve or its roots, i.e., herniation of the nucleus pulposus, spondylolisthesis
- Inflammation of the sciatic nerve resulting from metabolic or infectious disorders

SIGNS AND SYMPTOMS

- Sharp or "electrical" pain, radiating along the sciatic nerve dermatomal distribution (most commonly L-4, L-5, S-1), usually to the ankle or foot
- Often associated with dermatomal sensory disturbances, motor weakness, and hypoactive reflexes
- Onset of pain is immediate, within a few hours, or days after the inciting incident.
- May complain of radicular symptoms and not localized back pain
- 95% involve the L-5 or S-1 nerve root
- Aggravating factors are trunk flexion or rotation, prolonged sitting or standing, coughing, and sneezing.
- Muscle atrophy reflects long-standing condition.

RISK FACTORS

- Occupations or activities that require repetitive lifting or movement in the forward bent-and-twisted position
- Osteoporosis

ASSOCIATED INJURIES AND COMPLICATIONS

- Cauda equina syndrome
- Herniation of the nucleus pulposus (most common)
- Spinal stenosis
- Spondylolisthesis

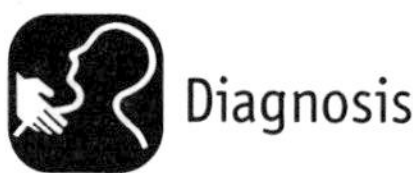

Diagnosis

DIFFERENTIAL DIAGNOSIS

- Ankylosing spondylitis
- Cauda equina syndrome
- Extrinsic nerve compression, e.g., from wallet or prolonged cycling
- Pathologic, traumatic, or osteoporotic compression fracture
- Herniation of the nucleus pulposus
- Infection, e.g., osteomyelitis, epidural abscess
- Neoplasm, primary or metastatic
- Osteoarthritis
- Paget disease
- Piriformis syndrome
- Spinal stenosis
- Spondylolisthesis
- Synovial cyst
- Trauma, e.g., hematoma, musculoligamentous strain, fracture
- Nonspinal causes, e.g., abdominal aortic aneurysm, herpes zoster, hip arthritis, psychogenic, vascular claudication

HISTORY

- Determine any red flags. Warning signs to increase your clinical suspicion as cited by the Agency for Health Care Policy and Research:
  —Age <20 years or >50 years
  —History, or signs and symptoms, of infection or malignancy
  —Unexplained weight loss
  —Immunosuppression
  —Severe or atypical pain
  —Trauma
  —Fracture
  —Intravenous drug use
  —Abdominal pain
  —Significant neurologic deficit
  —Bowel/bladder dysfunction
  —Saddle anesthesia
- Evaluate and manage any positive red flags.
- Determine constitutional signs.
- Mechanism of injury or inciting incident
- Length of symptoms
- Psychosocial issues that may add to symptoms and prolong pain

PHYSICAL EXAMINATION

- Detailed neurologic (motor, sensory, and reflexes) and vascular examination include rectal tone and anal sensation
- Criterion for abnormal findings is reproduction of pain in radicular distribution, rather than reproducing LBP
- Straight-leg raise (SLR) of involved leg: performed in supine position; reproduces sciatic-type pain between 30 and 60 degrees
- Crossed SLR: raise contralateral leg; results in reproduction of pain on the affected side
- Sitting knee extension: performed while patient is sitting; passive extension of the knee reproduces pain (modification of SLR)
- Ankle dorsiflexion or chin to the chest: performed either with SLR or crossed SLR; exacerbates the pain.

- Test specific nerves
  —Sensory loss
  L-4: anteromedial leg, medial malleolus
  L-5: lateral lower leg, web space between the great and second toe
  S-1: back of lower leg, lateral aspect of foot
  —Motor weakness
  L-4: knee extension (quads)
  L-5: extensor hallucis longus (great toe)
  S-1: foot plantar flexion (toe raises)
  —Reflex (hypoactive)
  L-4: patellar
  L-5: none
  S-1: Achilles'

IMAGING

- Anteroposterior and lateral radiographs of lumbar sacral spine usually not indicated unless
  —Red flags are present (see History)
  —Unresolved back pain >4–6 weeks
  —Back pain with constitutional symptoms, history of intravenous drug abuse, cancer, or diabetes
- Magnetic resonance imaging (MRI; preferred study) or computed tomographic (CT) myelography (used primarily when MRI is contraindicated, i.e., hardware, pacemaker) indicated for
  —Suspected cauda equina syndrome
  —Abscess
  —Neoplasm
  —6 weeks' failed conservative therapy for sciatica
- CT is study of choice for identifying bony vertebral injuries.
- Abdominal ultrasound or CT to evaluate for abdominal aortic aneurysm

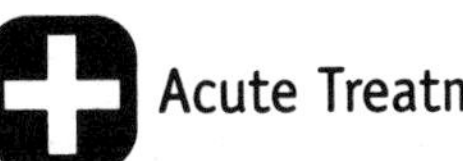

Acute Treatment

TREATMENT

- Nonsteroidal anti-inflammatory drugs, acetaminophen
- Symptomatic relief with ice or heat
- Short course of bed rest (in severe cases)
- Avoid activities that aggravate symptoms while gradually increasing activity level
- Physical therapy
- Epidural steroid injection
- Surgery referral for any suspicion of cord compression, bilateral sciatica, significant or progressive neurologic deficit, or disabling sciatica

PROGNOSIS

- Acute pain is almost always self-limited.
- Majority resolve with time
- Estimated recovery time: 90% within 4–6 weeks

REHABILITATION

- Physical therapy directed to restore motor or strength deficits

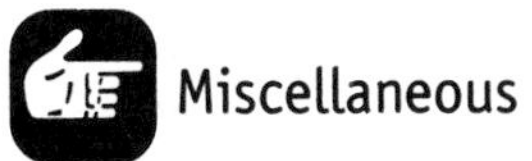

Miscellaneous

ICD-9 CODE

724.3 Sciatica

BIBLIOGRAPHY

Clinical practice guideline number 14: acute low back problems in adults. Rockville, MD: US Department of Health and Human Services, Agency for Health Care Policy and Research, 1994; AHCPR Publication No. 95-0642.

Bridwell KH, DeWald RL, et al., eds. *The textbook of spinal surgery,* 2nd ed. Philadelphia: Lippincott-Raven Publishers, 1997.

Connelly C. A rational approach to low back pain. *Patient Care* 2000;34:23–48.

Deyo RA, Rainville J, Kent DL. What can the history and physical examination tell. *JAMA* 1992;268:760–765.

Frymoyer JW. Back pain and sciatica. *N Engl J Med* 1988;318:291–300.

Young JL, Press JM, Herring SA. The disc at risk in athletes: perspectives on operative and nonoperative care. *Med Sci Sports Exerc* 1997;29[Suppl]:222–232.

Author: Kathleen Weber

Scoliosis

Basics

DEFINITION

- Lateral curvature of the spine exceeding 10 degrees (with rotation of the spine) in children older than 10 years of age. Considered idiopathic only after other causes have been excluded.

POSSIBLE CAUSES

- By definition, unknown; listed are some theories, none proven in isolation.
- Genetic
  —Positive familial history for scoliosis in 30% (not predictive for severity).
- Connective tissue disorder
  —Platelet calmodulin levels may be predictive of curve progression.
- Neurological (Equilibrium system)
  —Most widely supported theory
  —Abnormalities noted in vestibular, ocular, proprioceptive, and vibratory functions.
- Hormonal
  —Lower levels of melatonin secreted from pineal body in those with AIS.
  —Growth stimulating hormone: more of an influential factor than etiologic factor studies.

PATHOLOGY

- Lateral curvature of the spine with rotation

EPIDEMIOLOGY

- Prevalence
  —Generally considered 1.9% to 3% for curves exceeding 10 degrees.
  —0.3% for curves exceeding 20%
- Female:Male ratios
  —1.4:1 for curves 11 degrees to 20 degrees
  —5:1 for curves more than 20 degrees

GENETICS

- Positive familial history for idiopathic scoliosis in 30% (not predictive for severity)

COMPLICATIONS (NATURAL HISTORY)

- Reduced pulmonary function for patients with thoracic curves over 60 degrees.
- Progression of lumbar curves over 50 degrees in adult life with degenerative disc disease and pain.
- Cosmetic and emotional factors.

PROGNOSIS

- Risk of curve progression is related to patient's maturity (Risser sign, menarcheal status) and to the size of the curve.
- Curves less than 20° to 25° have a low risk of progression, even if patient is Risser 0 or Risser I
- Curves 25° to 45° have higher risk of progression, particularly in the immature
- Curves more than 45° to 50° have much higher risk of progression regardless of maturity

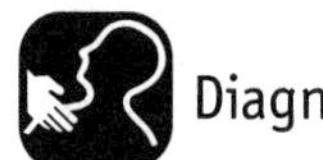

Diagnosis

- Juvenile idiopathic scoliosis onset between 3 and 10 years of age
- Infantile idiopathic scoliosis onset younger than 3 years of age
- Congenital scoliosis
- Scoliosis associated with neurofibromatosis
- Scoliosis associated with tumors (osteoid osteoma, other)
- Neuromuscular scoliosis
- Postural scoliosis (from leg length discrepancy for example)
  —No rib hump or rotation
  —Disappears with forward bending
  —Long curve
  —No progression

DATA GATHERING

History

Question: Onset?
Significance: Consider when first noted, by whom, rate of worsening, previous treatment, associated signs or symptoms, familial history, etc.
Question: Pain?
Significance: Patients with idiopathic scoliosis should not have pain.
Question: Night pain?
Significance: If pain, consider tumor such as osteoid osteoma or other tumor.
Question: Other signs or symptoms?
Significance: Review of systems (especially neurological).

PHYSICAL EXAMINATION

Finding: General inspection to look for skin changes such as:

- Café au lait, pigmentation or other signs of neurofibromatosis for example, dysraphic signs (hairy patches, etc.).
- Assess for maturity, hyperelasticity, contracture, congenital anomalies.
- Assess for deformity, symmetry of spine, shoulders and trunk, including decompensation, abnormalities of thoracic kyphosis or cervical or lumbar lordosis.
- The Adam forward bending test is used to look for rib or paraspinous elevations.
- Assess for leg length discrepancy, congenital anomalies and neurological abnormalities (including abdominal reflex).

Special Questions

Finding: Crankshaft phenomenon
Significance: Progression of curve size and rotation following posterior spinal fusion, due to continued anterior spinal growth.
Finding: Patient is Risser 0, open triradiate cartilages, less than 10 years old, and is prior to the occurrence of peak height velocity (the time of maximum spinal growth).
Significance: Consider anterior fusion in addition to posterior fusion.

Physical Examination Tricks

Finding: Scoliometer
Significance: To measure rib rotation.
Finding: Abnormal abdominal reflex
Significance: May suggest intraspinal pathology including syrinx.

LABORATORY AIDS

- Usually not helpful unless to rule out associated metabolic conditions.
- Pulmonary function testing are useful preoperatively.

IMAGING STAGES

- Plain standing PA and lateral scoliosis films on a long 3 foot x-ray cassette.
- Risser classification of iliac apophysis ossification is an indicator of maturity
- MRI is not routinely necessary
- 7% prevalence of abnormalities found in left thoracic curves
- Curve patterns are classified according to the King classification.
- Renal ultrasound or IVP are for evaluation of patient with congenital scoliosis.

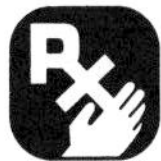

Long-Term Treatment

- Treatment
  —Concepts for treatment are based on the severity of the deformity present and on the likelihood of progression
- Observation
  —Curves less than 25°
    —Immature patients (Risser 0, 1, 2) should be re-evaluated in 4 to 6 months.
    —Skeletally mature patients (Risser 4 or 5) usually do not require follow up unless special circumstances
  —Curves 25° to 45°
    —Risser 4 or 5 patients usually re-evaluated in 1 year

BRACE TREATMENT

- Curves 25° to 45° (Risser 0, 1): brace on initial evaluation; 30° to 45° (Risser 2 or 3): brace on initial evaluation.
- Curves 25° or greater (in Risser 0–3 patient) that have demonstrated more than 10° progression during the period of observation.
- Continue brace treatment until maturity (2 years post-menarchal and Risser 4 in females, Risser 5 in males).

OPERATIVE MANAGEMENT

- Recommended when curves exceed 45° to 50°
  —Exception: Balanced thoracic and lumbar curves less than 55° may be observed for progression
- Thoracic curves and double major curves
  —Posterior segmental fixation instrumentation remains current state-of-art (TSRH, Isola, CD-Horizon, etc.)
  —Newer techniques of anterior spinal instrumentation for the thoracic spine
  —Thorascopic technique for those who need anterior thoracic fusion to prevent the crankshaft phenomenon
  —Thoracolumbar and lumbar curves
- Anterior spinal fusion using solid rod segmental constructs

GENERAL TREATMENT MODALITIES

- Brace types
  —Thoracolumbosacral orthosis (TLSO): Success reported with use more than 16 hours daily.
  —Milwaukee: Significantly improved outcome when compared to natural history.

DRUGS

- Post-operative continuous epidural infusion helpful for pain control

SIGNS TO WATCH FOR

- Back pain associated with idiopathic scoliosis.
- Present in 23% at time of initial evaluation (additional 9% during follow up).
- Of those with back pain, only 9% found to have identifiable cause such as spondylolysis, Scheuermann, syrinx, disc herniation, tumor, tether cord.

PROGNOSIS

- Overall, good prognosis for the majority of patients

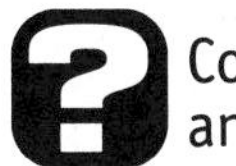

Common Questions and Answers

Q: How long do you observe a patient with spinal asymmetry before ordering an X-ray?
A: It depends on the presence or absence of abnormalities on the physical examination. If any of the signs mentioned here are seen in conjunction with significant back pain, an X-ray or referral is indicated. The scoliometer is also a useful tool in screening patients.
Q: If a child presents with scoliosis and back pain, which occurs especially at night and is relieved with asprin, what diagnosis is suggested?
A: Scoliosis associated with osteoid osteoma.

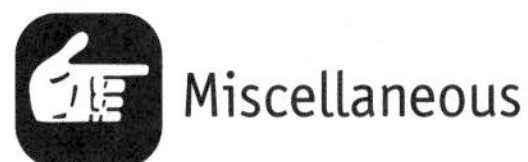

Miscellaneous

ICD-9-CM

737.30 Scoliosis idiopathic
737.32 Scoliosis infantile progressive

BIBLIOGRAPHY

Lonstein JE. Scoliosis. In: Morrissy RT, Weinstein SL, eds. *Lovell and Winter's pediatric orthopaedics*, 4th ed. Philadelphia: Lippincott-Raven, 1996:625–685.

Lonstein JE, Carlson JM. The prediction of curve progression in untreated idiopathic scoliosis during growth. *J Bone Joint Surg* 1984;66-A:1061–1071.

Author: John P. Dormans

Sesamoid Dysfunction

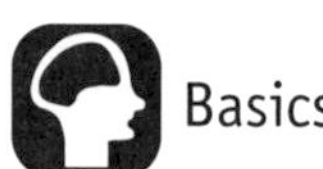

Basics

DEFINITION

Sesamoid Function

- Protect the tendon of the flexor hallucis longus
- Absorb a majority of the weight-bearing on the medial aspect of the forefoot
  —Sesamoid bones bear up to three times body weight during normal gait.
  —Medial or tibial sesamoid bears the majority of this weight.
- Increase the mechanical advantage of the intrinsic muscles of the great toe

Location

- Sesamoid bones are contained within the double tendon of the flexor hallucis brevis on the plantar surface of the foot.
- Sesamoids articulate dorsally with the plantar facets on the first metatarsal head.
- Sesamoid bones are connected by the intersesamoid ligament.
- Medial sesamoid is located just distal to the lateral sesamoid.

Size

- Medial sesamoid is larger than the lateral sesamoid and generally averages 9–11 mm wide and 12–15 mm long.
- Lateral sesamoid is generally 7–9 mm wide and 9–10 mm long.

Ossification of Hallucal Sesamoids

Ossification of the sesamoids occurs between 7 and 10 years of age.
Multiple ossification centers can be present in these bones, resulting in multipartite sesamoids.

Biomechanics

- In a standing position, the sesamoids are located just proximal to the first metatarsal head.
- When the first metatarsophalangeal (MTP) joint dorsiflexes, the sesamoids are pulled distally, covering and protecting the plantar surface of the first metatarsal head and absorbing the weight-bearing forces on the medial aspect of the forefoot.
- Flexor hallucis brevis provides the active plantar flexion force at the first MTP joint, but the sesamoid complex provides an increased mechanical advantage in plantar flexion.

Sesamoid Dysfunction

- Sesamoid dysfunction that restricts the range of motion of the MTP joint may lead to development of an abnormal gait pattern.
- Athlete typically everts the foot to decrease dorsiflexion excursion in the latter portion of the stance phase of gait or may toe-off prematurely to minimize dorsiflexion of the great toe during pushoff.

INCIDENCE/PREVALENCE

Sesamoiditis accounts for about 30% of all sesamoid injuries.

SIGNS AND SYMPTOMS

- Pain and discomfort during the toe-off stage of gait
- Restricted range of motion of the first MTP joint
- Pain on direct palpation over the first MTP joint, often localized over the lateral sesamoid
- Pain with motion over the first MTP joint
- Edema in the first MTP joint
- Diminished strength of plantar flexion or dorsiflexion
- MTP joint synovitis may be present.
- Plantar keratosis beneath the sesamoids may be present.

RISK FACTORS

- Sports or other activities that require repetitive push off the ball of the foot, rapid acceleration and deceleration, jumping, running, and frequent changes of direction
- Worn out shoes or shoes with inadequate forefoot cushion
- Sports that require no shoes or a very minimal shoe
- "At-risk" sports, e.g., tennis, ballet, gymnastics, basketball, and soccer
- Abnormal foot biomechanics, such as a hypermobile plantarflexed first ray

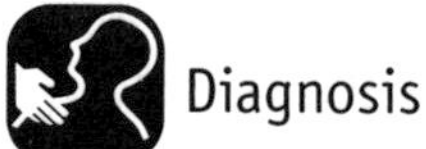

Diagnosis

DIFFERENTIAL DIAGNOSIS

- Sesamoid stress fracture
- Avascular necrosis
- Hallucis tendonitis
- Metatarsalgia
- Isolated synovitis or arthritis of the first MTP joint
- Acute sesamoid fracture
- Nonunion fracture of the sesamoid
- Entrapment neuropathies of the digital nerves

HISTORY

- Pain over the first MTP region with ballistic activities

PHYSICAL EXAMINATION

- Edema and erythema are present in the sesamoid region.
- Plantar fullness or fluid-filled bursal cyst may be palpated under the sesamoids.
- Passive dorsiflexion of the first MTP joint exacerbates the pain.
- Direct palpation and side-to-side pinch testing of the sesamoids produce pain.

IMAGING

- X-ray examination of the foot including anteroposterior, lateral, oblique, and axial views.
- Axial views should be completed with the toes in dorsiflexion, known as the "sesamoid view."
- Bone scan examination can differentiate a bipartite sesamoid from a fractured sesamoid, as the bipartite sesamoid will be cold.
- Computed tomographic scan and magnetic resonance imaging can be used if the diagnosis is in question, but generally are not necessary.

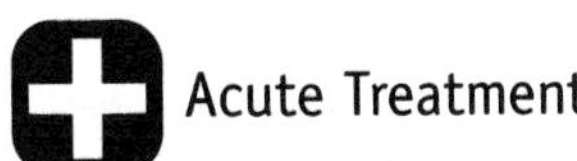

Acute Treatment

ANALGESIA

- Ice massage
- Relative reset
- Limitation of athletic activity
- Nonsteroidal anti-inflammatory drugs

IMMOBILIZATION

- Limit dorsiflexion and plantar flexion of the great toe by immobilizing it
- Immobilization accomplished by
  —Taping the first MTP joint
  —Wearing a stiff-soled shoe
  —Inserting a stiff forefoot plate under the insole of the athletic shoe to reduce motion at the MTP joint
  —Using a Camwalker

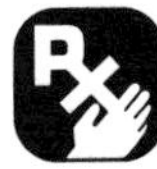

Long-Term Treatment

TREATMENT OPTIONS

- Custom orthotics with or without cutouts for the sesamoid bones
- Short-leg walking cast can be considered for recalcitrant cases.
- Corticosteroid injection into the sesamoid area

SURGERY

- Surgical excision used as a last resort, as many biomechanical changes result and may create problems that are worse in the long run

FOLLOW-UP

Periodic follow-up, after activities are modified and a treatment plan has been initiated, at approximately 4- to 8-week intervals until the patient is completely symptom-free.

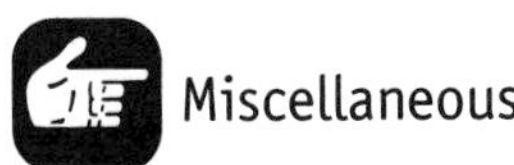

Miscellaneous

ICD-9 CODE

733.99

BIBLIOGRAPHY

Harries M, Williams C, et al. *Oxford textbook of sports medicine.* New York: Oxford University Press, 1994.

Hockenbury RT. Forefoot problems in athletes. *Med Sci Sports Exerc* 1999;31:448–458.

McDermott EP. Basketball injuries of the foot and ankle. *Clin Sports Med* 1993;12:381–382.

Omey ML, Micheli LJ. Foot and ankle problems in the young athlete. *Med Sci Sports Exerc* 1999;31:470–486.

Van Wyngarden T. The painful foot, part I: common forefoot deformities. *Am Fam Physician* 1997;55:1866–1876.

Authors: Per Brolinson and Kristen L. Bodine

Spinal Stenosis

Basics

DEFINITION

- Stenosis of the spinal canal defined by narrowing of the AP diameter of the spinal canal or loss of CSF fluid around the cord. The later has been defined as *functional spinal stenosis*.
- A general consensus defines spinal stenosis as an AP diameter of <13mm from C3 to C7.
- Spinal stenosis is also divided into congenital and acquired forms.

INCIDENCE AND PREVALENCE

- Most often occurs in the lumbar spine, but can also occur in the cervical spine
- Rarely occurs in the thoracic spine
- The absolute incidence or prevalence of spinal stenosis is unknown, however lumbar spinal stenosis is an increasing cause of disability in older patients.

SIGNS AND SYMPTOMS

- Back pain
- Leg pain, numbness, or fatigue; often bilateral
- Cervical spinal stenosis may present with bilateral radicular pain or weakness in the arms with or without involvement of the lower extremities.

RISK FACTORS

- Degenerative changes in the intervertebral discs, ligaments, and facet joints, as well as osteophyte formation surrounding the canal
- Older age
- Spondylitic disease of the spine may contribute to stenosis.

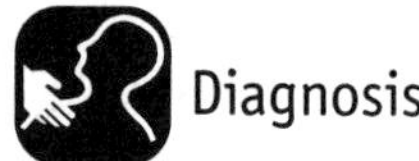

Diagnosis

DIFFERENTIAL DIAGNOSIS

- Vascular claudication
- Space occupying lesion such as a neoplasm
- Herniated disc
- Trauma, e.g., compression fracture
- Degenerative subluxation of the vertebrae (spondylolisthesis)
- Infectious process, e.g., diskitis or epidural abscess
- Spear tacklers spine
  —Developmental narrowing of the cervical spinal canal
  —Straightening or reversal of the normal cervical lordotic curve
  —Preexisting minor post-traumatic x-ray evidence of bony or ligamentous injury
  —Documentation of using spear-tackling techniques

HISTORY

- Typically the earliest complaint is back pain
- Bilateral leg pain often involving the buttocks and thighs and spreading toward the feet
- The pain may variably be described as burning, cramping, or dull fatigue.
- Classically, the symptoms of lumbar canal stenosis worsen with ambulation or standing and are relieved by sitting.
- In severe late-stage cases where the sacral roots are impinged, visceral disturbance may manifest with urinary incontinence.
- The history for cervical spinal stenosis should include transient quadriplegia after a tackle or just bilateral "stingers" (numbness and pain down both arms).

PHYSICAL EXAM

- The spine must be examined for abnormal curvature or limitation in range of motion.
- Commonly, flexion relieves symptoms and extension is painful.
- The back should be examined for tenderness, which may suggest a fracture, neoplasm, or infection.
- The straight-leg test should be done to rule out disc herniation. Generally, patients with lumbar spinal stenosis do not have a positive straight leg test.
- A femoral stretch test where the knee is flexed in a prone position may elicit pain in patients with spinal stenosis at L3–L4.
- The physical exam should also include an examination of the skin, nails, and distal pulses of the feet to evaluate for possible vascular claudication. Patients with vascular claudication will often have pallor, nail dystrophy, absence of hair, and distal pulses in their feet. Popliteal and femoral pulses need to be examined.
- Cervical spinal stenosis requires a careful active range of motion exam of the neck and upper extremity neurologic exam.

IMAGING

- Plain films are not diagnostic but may demonstrate degenerative spine disease or spondylolisthesis.
- In the C-spine, a vertebral canal/vertebral body ratio under 0.8 was defined by Torg as spinal stenosis. The "Torg" ratio is not commonly used by radiologists because it leads to many false positives.
- CT scans with or without intrathecal contrast injection (CT myelogram) may demonstrate encroachment of the canal by osteophytes, hypertrophied lamina, or other degenerative changes.
- MRI is currently the preferred method to establish a diagnosis and exclude other conditions. MRI is both noninvasive and visualizes the soft tissue structures that may be obstructing the canal.

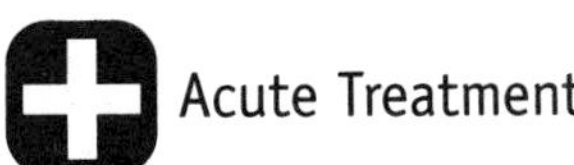

Acute Treatment

CONSERVATIVE MANAGEMENT

- Nonsurgical management of lumbar stenosis may be attempted initially in patients who do not have severe pain or significant weakness. Physicians with patients on warfarin sodium, or who have severe risks for complications with decompressive surgery, may not be candidates for invasive procedures.
- NSAIDS and exercises may provide some relief for patients with lumbar spinal stenosis. Flexion exercises that reduce lumbar lordosis are especially useful.
- Morbidly obese patients should be encouraged to lose weight.
- Nonsurgical management of lumbar spinal stenosis has not shown benefit on long-term follow-up.
- Management of acute symptomatic cervical spinal stenosis after trauma includes stabilization of the spine with a cervical collar and transport to an emergency setting.

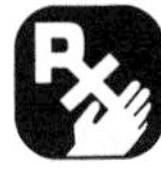

Long-Term Treatment

SURGERY

- Most patients benefit from decompression of the lumbar canal.
- Typically, multilevel decompressive laminectomies are needed because the canal stenosis often occurs at multiple levels.
- Multilevel laminotomies, foraminotomies, and even decompression of the lateral recesses may be alternative methods of treatment.
- Most patients with radiographic and clinical evidence of spinal stenosis get significant long-term relief with decompressive surgery.

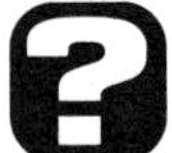

Common Questions and Answers

Physician responses to common patient questions:
Q: If I am diagnosed with cervical spinal stenosis, can I return to contact sports?
A: Experience with the National Center for Catastrophic Sports Injury Research suggests that athletes with significant cervical spinal stenosis are at increased risk of quadriplegia and should not participate in contact or collision sports. Referral to a spine specialist is indicated for competitive athletes wishing to return to play.
Q: What test can be ordered to evaluate a patient with surgical hardware for spinal stenosis?
A: CT mylogram

Miscellaneous

ICD-9 CODE

723.0 Spinal stenosis of cervical region
724.0 Spinal stenosis, unspecified region
724.01 Thoracic region
724.02 Lumbar region
Note: Use 724.00 only when a more specific code is not available

BIBLIOGRAPHY

Alvarez, JA. Hardy, R. Lumbar spine stenosis: a common cause of back and leg pain. *American Family Physician* 1998;57(8): 1825–1834.

Cantu RC. The cervical spinal stenosis controversy. *Clinics in Sports Medicine* 1998;17(1): 121–126.

Author: Suraj Achar

Spondylolysis and Spondylolisthesis

Basics

DEFINITION

From Greek, *spondylo* vertebra + *lysis* loosening, *listhesis* slippage

Spondylolysis

- Involves a defect in the pars interarticularis of the vertebral complex
- Defect ranges from a stress reaction to traumatic fracture.
- Defect may be an overuse stress reaction or a traumatic fracture.

Spondylolisthesis

- Results from anterior displacement of a vertebral body on the subjacent vertebra.
- Most common segment involved is the L-5–S-1 level, followed by L4–5. Most cases (80%) are bilateral.

INCIDENCE/PREVALENCE

- Incidence up to 11% in athletic populations; 2% to 5% in the general population
- Highest incidence in sports emphasizing extension activities, e.g., gymnastics, ballet, volleyball, weight-lifting, football, and wrestling
- Peak age of symptomatic onset is 10–15 years, although spondylolysis usually originates between ages 5–10 years.

ETIOLOGY

- Physical shear forces may account for the etiology of spondy.
- Shear forces on the normal lumbar lordosis are increased in extension and accentuated by combined extension and lateral side-bending.
- Genetic factors may play a role.
- High incidence (25% to 69%) demonstrated in studies on twins and first-degree relatives.
- Spondy may be either an overuse injury to the affected vertebral level or a traumatic fracture.

SIGNS AND SYMPTOMS

History

- Most patients asymptomatic
- Low back pain is the most common complaint of symptomatic patients.
- Pain may radiate into the buttocks or thigh, but patients rarely experience true radicular signs or symptoms.
- Pain is worse with activity, especially extension/lateral side-bending.

PHYSICAL EXAMINATION

- Symptomatic patient may be tender to palpation of the paraspinal musculature and possibly in the midline.
- Patient often may exhibit hamstring tightness or spasm that worsens lordosis at the spine.
- Some suggest performing the one-legged extension test.
  - —Pain when a patient stands on one leg and hyperextends the back may indicate spondy.
  - —This maneuver creates combined extension/lateral side-bending, which may produce pain.
- If significant listhesis is present (grade III or more, see below), may appreciate a step-off when palpating the spinous processes.
- Gait analysis may demonstrate a pelvic waddle in extreme cases.

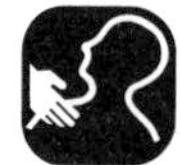

Diagnosis

CLASSIFICATION OF SPONDYLOLISTHESIS

Isthmic (Spondylolytic)

- Listhesis caused by breakdown of the pars interarticularis
- Most common cause of listhesis, representing up to 50% in some series

Dysplastic (Congenital)

- Failure of development of the superior facets
- Represents ~20% of all cases of listhesis
- Major slippage can occur.

Degenerative

- Degeneration of the superior facets or disc material
- Major cause of spinal stenosis

Traumatic

- Disruption of the posterior elements of the neural arch other than pars (pedicles or lamina)

Pathologic

- Due to osteoporosis, rheumatoid arthritis, tumor, or infection

GRADING OF SPONDYLOLISTHESIS

- Grading system proposed by Meyerding in 1932
  - —Grade I: L-5 vertebral body has slipped forward on the sacrum a distance of up to 25% of its length
  - —Grade II: L-5 vertebral body has slipped forward a distance of 25% to 50% of its length
  - —Grade III: L-5 vertebral body has slipped a distance of 50% to 75% of its length
  - —Grade IV: L-5 vertebral body has slipped a distance of >75% of its length.
- Some add grade V to include L-5 vertebral body that has slipped off the sacrum, also termed spondyloptosis.

IMAGING

Plain Films

- Usually diagnostic
- Typical x-ray series includes an erect anteroposterior (AP), lateral, and obliques ×2.
- Obliques are the diagnostic x-rays.
- Visualize the "scotty dog": will have a radiolucent line through its neck representing the defect through the pars interarticularis
- Standing lateral x-ray can help with grading of listhesis.
- Weight-bearing x-rays may worsen the apparent slip by up to 25%.
- On standing AP view, when a large slip has occurred (grade IV/V), an "inverted Napoleon's hat sign" can be seen, representing the radiographic appearance of spondyloptosis. Clinically, this puts the cauda equina at risk for compromise.

Triple-Phase Bone Scan

- Often necessary to evaluate the acuity of the injury
- Defect may be present on x-ray and not be the cause of symptoms.
- X-ray may be negative, while the bone scan demonstrates the defect.
- Bone scan can be positive as soon as 48–72 hours after injury.
- Test less helpful in older patients, especially those with significant osteoarthritis of the L-spine due to high-false positive rate.
- Not recommended in asymptomatic patients or in patients with symptoms >1 year.

Single-Photon Emission Computed Tomographic Scan

- Improves resolution of bone scans
- May be more helpful in demonstrating stress reactions at the pars

Computed Tomographic Scan

- Delineates bony pars defect or neural compression
- May detect osseus fragments near the pars defect

Magnetic Resonance Imaging

- Visualizes the entire lumbar spine in two orthogonal planes and assesses relationship of cauda equina to sacrum

DIFFERENTIAL DIAGNOSIS

- Infection
- Tumor
- Herniated nucleus pulposus
- Mechanical low back pain

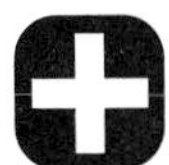

Acute Treatment

Initial Treatment

- PRICES: Protection (and Pain medications), Rest, Ice, Compression, Elevation, Support (and strengthening/stretching exercises)
- Anti-inflammatory drugs
  —Will help decrease symptoms
  —If one class of nonsteroidal anti-inflammatory drugs (NSAIDs) does not work, try a different class.
  —Allow adequate trial of NSAIDs (up to 7 days)

IMMOBILIZATION

Bracing

- Some advocate use of braces such as the thoracolumbar sacral orthosis.
- When to use these braces is not clear.
- Most suggest using the brace if initial attempts at relative rest, NSAIDs, and ice do not significantly improve pain.

Duration

- Reported duration of bracing is variable, ranging from 6 weeks to 6 months.
- Patients with positive x-ray and negative bone scan demonstrate a chronic injury that does not need to be braced.

SPECIAL CONSIDERATIONS

There is tremendous variation in the treatment of spondy.

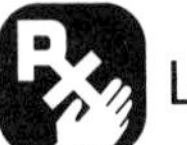

Long-Term Treatment

FOLLOW-UP

- Monitor symptoms, gait abnormalities, and radiographic progression
- Most patients with spondy eventually will have mild-to-no symptoms.
- X-rays: Data on the timing and frequency of follow-up x-rays are not clear. After skeletal maturity, progression is less likely.
- Risk factors to consider when assessing for slip progression of listhesis
  —Clinical factors: age (10–15 years), gender (female), recurrent symptoms, and postural deformity (gait disturbances)
  —Radiographic factors: type of slip (dysplastic spondy), degree of slip (grades III/IV), and increasing angle of slip

REHABILITATION

- After initial symptoms improve, the patient should begin some specific exercises.
- Typical rehabilitation includes stretching hamstrings and gluteals, while strengthening low back, leg, and abdominal musculature.

SURGERY

- Indications include
  —Slip progression
  —Persistent pain or gait abnormality despite treatment
  —Neurologic deficit
  —High amount of slip in the skeletally immature patient (grade III/IV or high slip angle >55 degrees)
- Surgical procedure
  —Most suggest *in situ* fusion, i.e., fusion of one level of vertebral body to another.
  —Postoperative casting/bracing is not generally indicated.
  —Return to noncontact sports permissible.

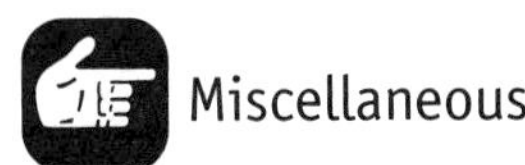

Miscellaneous

ICD-9 CODE

756.1

BIBLIOGRAPHY

Comstock CP, Carragee EJ. Spondylolisthesis in the young athlete. *Phys Sport Med* 1994;22:39–46.

Frymoyer JW. Degenerative spondylolisthesis: diagnosis and treatment. *J Am Acad Orthop Surg* 1994;2:9–15.

Hensinger RN. Current concepts review: spondylolysis and spondylolisthesis. *J Bone Joint Surg* 1989;71A:1098–1107.

Hilibrand AS, Urquhart AG, Graziano GP, et al. Acute spondylolytic spondylolisthesis: risk of progression and neurological complications. *J Bone Joint Surg* 1995;77A: 190–196.

Ikata T, Ryoji M, Katoh S, et al. Pathogenesis of sports-related spondylolisthesis. *Am J Sports Med* 1996;24:94–98.

Jimenez CE. Advantages of diagnostic nuclear medicine. *Phys Sports Med* 1999;27.

Johnson RJ. Low-back pain in sports: managing spondylolysis. *Phys Sports Med* 1993;21:53–68.

Muschik M, Hahnel H, Robinson PN, et al. Competitive sports and the progression of spondylolysis. *J Pediatr Orthop* 1996;16: 364–369.

Pizzutillo PD, Hummer CD. Nonoperative treatment for painful adolescent spondylolysis. *J Pediatr Orthop* 1989;9: 538–540.

Renshaw TS. Managing spondylolysis: when to immobilize. *Phys Sports Med* 1995;23:75–80.

Stinson JT. Spondylolysis and spondylolisthesis in the athlete. *Clin Sports Med* 1993;12:517–528.

Author: Guy Monteleone

Sternoclavicular Joint Injury

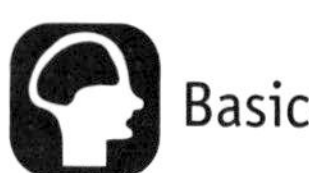

Basics

SIGNS AND SYMPTOMS

- Patient presents with the affected arm foreshortened and supported across the chest by opposite hand
- Inability to abduct or externally rotate the affected arm because of severe pain over sternoclavicular junction
- In *anterior dislocation*, medial end of the clavicle is visibly prominent, palpable, and may be fixed or mobile
- In *posterior dislocation*, loss of normal inner prominence of the clavicular head may be masked by significant local swelling
  —Head tilted toward injured side because of spasm of the sternocleidomastoid muscle
  —Venous congestion in the neck or upper extremities, diminished pulses on affected extremity, shortness of breath, hoarseness, dysphagia, or signs of shock may suggest life-threatening impingement of the posteriorly displaced clavicle upon vascular structures in the mediastinum

MECHANISM/DESCRIPTION

- The sternoclavicular joint (SCJ) can dislocate in the anterior or posterior direction
- It is among the least frequently dislocated joints in the body
- Due primarily to trauma from vehicular or athletic injuries; congenital dislocations are extremely rare
- *Anterior dislocation* is much more common
  —Caused by an anterolateral force compressing the shoulder followed by backward rolling
- *Posterior dislocation* is caused either from a direct anterior-to-posterior blow to the medial clavicle or from a posterolateral force compressing the shoulder followed by forward rolling
- *Posterior dislocation is a surgical emergency*
  —Compression of trachea, esophagus, and great vessels in the mediastinum demand immediate reduction

PEDIATRIC CONSIDERATIONS

- The medial physeal growth plates of the clavicles fuse between ages 22 and 25
- True dislocations of the SCJ are extremely rare in children because of the strong ligamentous attachments about the medial physis
- Fractures through the medial physis mimic SCJ dislocations
- In patients less than 25 years of age, SCJ dislocations are classified as Salter-Harris Type I or II fractures

CAUTIONS

- Vital signs and an initial neurovascular exam of the affected extremity are mandatory
- The affected arm should be splinted in the position of most comfort prior to transport to the hospital

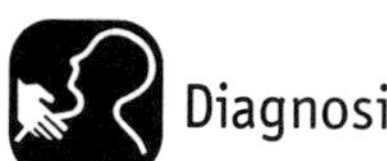

Diagnosis

ESSENTIAL WORKUP

- Careful history to elicit mechanism of injury, time from the injury, and initial symptoms
- Respiratory, neurologic, and vascular assessments mandatory
- Appropriate analgesia for patient comfort

IMAGING/SPECIAL TESTS

- Rockwood view: x-ray beam aimed at manubrium in a 40° caudal tilt
- Plain chest radiograph is needed to rule out possible pneumothorax in patients with posterior dislocation
- CT scan is the best study to evaluate the SCJ
  —Useful in the ED when plain films are inconclusive
  —Accurately differentiate fractures from dislocations
  —Demonstrates the position of the medial end of the clavicle in relation to the structures in the mediastinum
  —Shows detailed anatomy of the structures of the thoracic outlet and mediastinum

DIFFERENTIAL DIAGNOSIS

- Sternoclavicular sprain/subluxation
- Medial clavicle fracture
- Septic joint
- Osteoarthritis

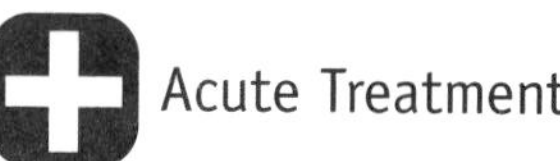

Acute Treatment

INITIAL STABILIZATION

- Patients in respiratory distress require endotracheal intubation and immediate reduction
- Emergent reduction is also needed in patients with hoarseness, dysphagia, or neurovascular compromise (upper extremity weakness, paresthesia, diminished pulses, signs of shock)
- *Patients with posterior dislocations represent true orthopedic and surgical emergencies* and appropriate consults should be obtained promptly
- Appropriate analgesia (e.g., narcotics or NSAIDs) necessary for pain control

ED TREATMENT

- *Anterior dislocations* may be reduced in the ED
- Conscious sedation is necessary for pain control and muscle relaxation
- A rolled towel is placed between the shoulder blades in the supine position
  —Longitudinal traction is applied to the ipsilateral arm in the extended position with the shoulder abducted at 90°
  —An assistant can maintain gentle inward pressure over the displaced medical end of the clavicle
  —After reduction, immobilization is achieved using a well-padded figure-eight dressing
  —Many anterior dislocations remain unstable after reduction; however, open reduction and internal fixation is rarely indicated as the deformity is mainly cosmetic without functional loss
  —*Posterior dislocations* require prompt reduction, best achieved in the OR under general anesthesia

—If an appropriate surgeon is not immediately available to reduce a posterior dislocation in the OR, reduction may be attempted in the ED to relieve serious airway, neurologic, or vascular compromise
—After adequate sedation, a small incision is made directly over the medial head of the clavicle
—A sterile towel clamp can carefully be used to encircle the medial clavicular head and gentle anterior traction applied to reduce the dislocation
—A surgical consultant should subsequently evaluate the patient

PEDIATRIC CONSIDERATIONS

- During childhood, the medial physeal growth plate of the clavicle provides 80% of longitudinal bone growth
- Fractures in the medial clavicle have tremendous capability for healing and remodeling
- Nonunion and significant malunion rarely occur
- Anteriorly displaced fractures of the medial clavicle that mimic SCJ dislocation can be placed in a figure-eight splint without reduction
- Posteriorly displaced fractures uniformly require reduction and should be considered a surgical and orthopedic emergency

MEDICATIONS

- Patients may require oral analgesics upon discharge
  —Acetaminophen: 500–1000 mg q 6 hrs PRN
  —Ibuprofen: 400–800 mg q hrs PRN with meals
  —Acetaminophen 300 mg with codeine: 30 mg q 6 hrs PRN

HOSPITAL ADMISSION CRITERIA

- All posterior dislocations of the SCJ require admission for prompt reduction in the operating room and evaluation for potential intrathoracic complications

HOSPITAL DISCHARGE CRITERIA

- Anterior dislocations of the SCJ that can be reduced and splinted, in the absence of neurovascular compromise, may be discharged with appropriate orthopedic follow-up

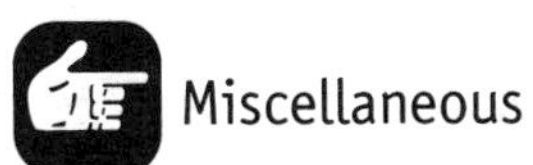

Miscellaneous

ICD-9-CM

810.01

CORE CONTENT CODE

18.4.10.5

BIBLIOGRAPHY

Cope R. Dislocations of the sternoclavicular joint. *Skeletal Radiol* 1993;22:233–238.

Cope R, Riddervold HO, Shore JL, et al. Dislocations of the sternoclavicular joint: Anatomic basis, etiologies, and radiologic diagnosis. *J Orthop Trauma* 1991;5(3): 379–384.

Gardner MH, Bidstrup BP. Intrathoracic great vessel injury resulting from blunt chest trauma associated with posterior dislocation of the sternoclavicular joint. *Aust N Z J Surg* 1983;53:427–430.

Lewonowski K, Bassett GS. Complete posterior sternoclavicular epiphyseal separation. *Clin Orthop* 1992;281:84–88.

Winter J, Sterner S, Maurer D, et al. Retrosternal epiphyseal disruption of medial clavicle: Case and review in children. *J Emerg Med* 1988;7:9–13.

Authors: Robert Chang and Wallace Carter

Subungual Exostosis and Hematoma

Basics

DEFINITION

Subungual Exostosis

Benign bony growth from the distal phalanx's terminal tuft commonly causing deformity of the nail

Subungual Hematoma

Acute, traumatic, subungual collection of blood, manifested by an area of black or blue discoloration, usually caused by a direct blunt impact or chronic, repetitive stresses to the nail unit

INCIDENCE/PREVALENCE

Subungual Exostosis

- Seen more commonly after the second and third decades of life
- Usually affects the great toe or rarely a finger

Subungual Hematoma

- Commonly seen in sport-specific patterns, e.g., "tennis toe" and "jogger's toe"
- Seen more commonly in sports that require frequent pivoting and abrupt stops that can lead to jamming of the toe into the front of the shoe, e.g., basketball, handball, and racquet sports
- Seen commonly in sports that require repeated kicking, e.g., soccer and football
- Trauma, e.g., fingertip slammed in a car door, hammer blow, or blunt trauma

SIGNS AND SYMPTOMS

Subungual Exostosis

- Pain and swelling over the exostosis can affect gait
- Pain associated with trauma is common because the tumor protrudes and is easily traumatized

Subungual Hematoma

- Collection of blood under the nail with or without edema/erythema
- Can be extremely painful with throbbing pain
- Minor trauma: hematoma may be painless and may not develop immediately.
- May have evidence of a callus on the skin distal to the affected nail

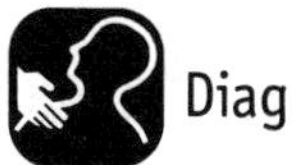

Diagnosis

DIFFERENTIAL DIAGNOSIS

Subungual Exostosis

- Subungual osteochondroma: can differentiate histologically because the exostosis has a fibrous cartilage cap over the bony growth and the osteochondroma has hyaline cartilage.
- Fibroma
- Subungual verruca vulgaris
- Multiple exostosis: consider an autosomal dominant multiple exostosis syndrome

Subungual Hematoma

- Subungual melanomas
- Glomus tumor (extremely painful nodule under the nail; pain worse when exposed to cold temperatures)

PHYSICAL EXAMINATION

Subungual Exostosis

- Presence of a firm mass noted at the distal portion of the terminal phalanx
- Nail plate can be elevated laterally by the tumor but is rarely injured.
- Pain on direct pressure

Subungual Hematoma

- Examine nail unit
- Toes most likely affected in sport-specific pattern are
  - —"Tennis toe": more commonly lateral nail of the hallux or second toe, depending on which is longer
  - —"Jogger's toe": second through fifth toes
  - —Kicking sports: second or third toe
- Observe for any extension of discoloration from under the nail plate into the proximal nailfold and nail matrix (Hutchinson melanotic whitlow sign); suspect subungual melanoma

IMAGING

Subungual Exostosis

- Radiograph mandatory if hard subungual mass noted on examination
- Outgrowth of bone projecting from the distal phalanx's tuft with a broad base and a radiolucent cartilaginous cap

Subungual Hematoma

- Anteroposterior, lateral, and oblique radiographs should be obtained when a hematoma involves >25% of the visible nail to assess for fracture.
- Less acute cases can be observed.

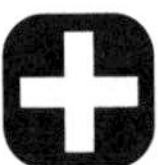

Acute Treatment

TREATMENT

Subungual Exostosis

- Excision of tumor

Subungual Hematoma

- Immediate elevation and application of ice or immersion in ice water may reduce pain and bleeding.
- Evacuation of hematoma can be done by puncturing the nail plate using thermal cautery or a drill (18-gauge needle).
- Nail removal if the normal architecture of the nail plate or its surrounding structures has been damaged. Wound repair if needed.

PREVENTION

Subungual Hematoma

- Well-fitted footwear with sturdy, high, wide toe boxes
- Keep nails trimmed.
- Orthotic devices
- Referral to a podiatrist may be necessary.

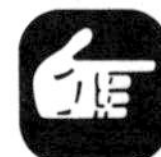

Miscellaneous

SYNONYMS

Subungual Hematoma

- Tennis toe
- Jogger's toe
- Sportsman's toe

ICD-9 CODE

726.91 Subungual exostosis
924.3 Subungual hematoma

BIBLIOGRAPHY

Adams BB. Running-related toenail abnormality. *Physician Sportsmed* 1999;27:85–87.

Carroll RE, Chance JT, Inan Y. Subungual exostosis in the hand. *J Hand Surg* 1992;17B:569–574.

Champion RH, Burton JL, Burns DA, et al., eds. *Rook/Wilkinson/Ebling textbook of dermatology,* 6th ed. Oxford: Blackwell Science, 1998.

Tanzi EL, Scher RK. Managing common nail disorders in active patients. *Physician Sportsmed* 1999;27:35–47.

Author: Kathleen Weber

Superficial Radial Nerve (Wartenberg Disease)

Basics

DEFINITION

- Compression mononeuropathy of the superficial branch of radial nerve in the distal forearm
- Radial nerve, arising from C5–8, provides motor function to the extensors of the forearm, wrist, fingers, and supinator, in addition to its sensory function.
- Superficial radial nerve (SRN) becomes susceptible to injury as it pierces deep fascia to become subcutaneous between the tendons of the extensor carpi radialis longus and brachioradialis muscles.

INCIDENCE/PREVALENCE

- Not known, but rare

SIGNS AND SYMPTOMS

- Symptoms primarily limited to the dorsoradial aspect of the distal forearm and hand (wrist, hand, dorsal thumb, and index finger)
- Paresthesias (numbness and tingling)
- Hyperesthesia
- Less commonly, pain or burning

RISK FACTORS

- Wrist compression, i.e., tight bands, tape, watches, archery guards, gloves, or straps of a racquetball racquet, cast, soft tissue mass
- Direct trauma in contact sports
- Laceration
- Sports involving repetitive pronation and supination at the wrist, e.g., batting, throwing, and rowing

ASSOCIATED INJURIES AND COMPLICATIONS

- de Quervain syndrome

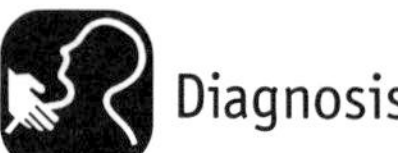

Diagnosis

DIFFERENTIAL DIAGNOSIS

- de Quervain syndrome
- Intersection syndrome
- Lateral antebrachial cutaneous neuropathy
- Thumb carpometacarpal arthritis
- C-6 radiculopathy

HISTORY

- Determine whether pain or sensory deficit is the primary symptom. If pain is the main complaint, then de Quervain disease may be the underlying disorder.
- Duration of symptoms helps to determine treatment options and prognosis.
- Location of symptoms

PHYSICAL EXAMINATION

- Positive Tinel sign along the radial aspect of the midforearm
- Wrist flexion, ulnar deviation, and pronation place traction on the nerve and increase symptoms.
- Sensation deficit on the dorsoradial aspect of the hand
- Finkelstein test typically negative. If positive, consider an associated de Quervain syndrome. With SRN injury, pain can be present with thumb abduction and adduction, differentiating this from de Quervain syndrome.

STUDIES

- Lidocaine test: Because the terminal branch of the lateral antebrachial cutaneous nerve often shares distribution with the SRN, its compression can mimic that involving the SRN.
- Diagnostic nerve block to the cutaneous nerve in the proximal forearm just distal to the cubital crease and adjacent to the cephalic vein may help define its contribution to any pathology.
- Nerve conduction study may be inconsistent, but helpful. Indicated if the symptoms are persistent, surgery is being considered, or if the diagnosis is in doubt.
- The most common technique records the sensory nerve action potentials from the web space between the thumb and index finger with stimulation originating in the distal forearm.
- Sensory action potential, conduction velocity, and amplitude are decreased.
- Motor testing is normal.

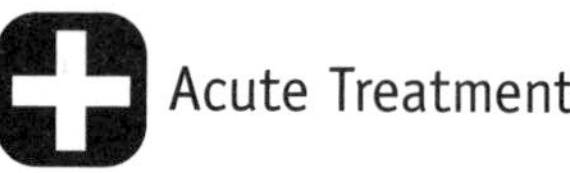

Acute Treatment

- Remove constricting bands/devices
- Avoid repetitive trauma to the area. Consider padding the area if this is not an option during the athletic season.
- Avoid repetitive pronation, wrist flexion, and ulnar deviation.
- Thumb spica splint in 20 degrees of wrist extension with the thumb in 45 degrees of metacarpal phalangeal flexion
- Nonsteroidal anti-inflammatory drugs
- Ice
- Steroid injection and anesthetic in the area of maximum pain can be helpful.
- Desensitization

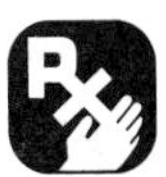

Long-Term Treatment

SURGERY

- Provides variable response

REFERRAL/DISPOSITION

If conservative treatment fails after about 6–12 months, then surgical exploration/decompression should be considered.

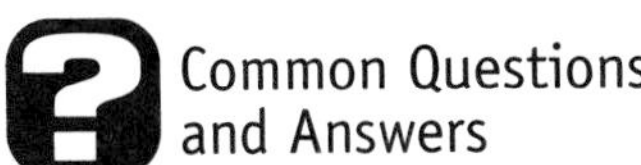

Common Questions and Answers

Physician responses to common patient questions:
Q: When can I expect the symptoms to resolve?
A: If present >3 days, the neurapraxic injury may require up to 3 months to reach maximum improvement.
Q: How long do I need to wear the splint?
A: Usually 2–4 weeks or until symptoms resolve.
Q: How long do I need to wear the protective padding?
A: Until symptoms resolve.

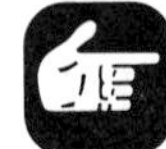

Miscellaneous

SYNONYMS

- Wartenberg syndrome entrapment
- Cheiralgia paresthetica
- Prisoner's palsy
- Handcuff disease
- Radial sensory nerve

ICD-9 CODE

955.3

See also: Peripheral nerve compression

BIBLIOGRAPHY

Anto C, Aradhya P. Clinical diagnosis of peripheral nerve compression in the upper extremity. *Orthop Clin North Am* 1996;27:227–236.

Plancher KD, Peterson RK, Steichen JB. Compressive neuropathies and tendonopathies in the athletic elbow and wrist. *Clin Sports Med* 1996;15:331–371.

Steinberg GG, Akins CM, Baran DT. *Orthopedics in primary care,* 2nd ed. Philadelphia: Lippincott, Williams & Wilkins, 1992:73.

Terrono AL, Millender LH. Management of work-related upper-extremity nerve entrapments. *Orthop Clin North Am* 1996;27:783–793.

Authors: Karl B. Fields, Coley Gatlin, and Dominic McKinley

Suprascapular Nerve Palsy

Basics

INCIDENCE/PREVALENCE

- Relatively uncommon; true incidence unknown
- May occur in up to 20% of high-level volleyball players
- Ganglion cyst found at spinoglenoid notch in 1% of cadavers in recent study
- Spinoglenoid ligament present in 50% to 60% of shoulders
- Suprascapular neuropathy in 7% of athletes with peripheral nerve injuries

SIGNS AND SYMPTOMS

- Depends on level of injury.
- If proximal, may have posterior/lateral shoulder pain along with weakness and atrophy of supraspinatus and infraspinatus.
- If lesion is distal to sensory branches at spinoglenoid notch, painless, isolated infraspinatus atrophy and weakness of external rotation may be seen.

RISK FACTORS

- More common in volleyball players and overhead throwing athletes, possibly due to traction injury or scar formation from overuse
- May be particularly associated with "floating serve" in volleyball, which requires intense eccentric contraction of infraspinatus to decelerate the arm and stabilize the shoulder. This can stretch the suprascapular nerve across the lateral edges of the scapular spine.
- Sudden downward depression of shoulder (traction injury to nerve near plexus origin)
- Compression by ganglion cyst, tumor, or ligament at scapular or spinoglenoid notch
- Direct trauma, e.g., scapular fracture

ANATOMY

- Suprascapular nerve arises from the upper trunk of the brachial plexus at Erb's point, carrying fibers from the C-5 and C-6 nerve roots, with variable contributions from C-4.
- It crosses the posterior triangle of the neck, runs deep to the trapezius, and passes under the transverse scapular ligament via the scapular notch.
- Crossing the supraspinatus fossa, it sends two branches to the supraspinatus and sensory branches to the acromioclavicular and glenohumeral joints.
- The nerve makes a sharp turn around the spinoglenoid notch and passes into the infraspinatus fossa, where its branches terminate.
- Three main sites of injury
  —Scapular notch
  —Spinoglenoid notch
  —Near origin from upper trunk of brachial plexus

COMPLICATIONS

- Ganglion cysts at the spinoglenoid notch may be secondary to labral injuries, especially superior labrum anterior and posterior lesions.
- Secondary impingement may develop due to loss of supraspinatus/infraspinatus function.

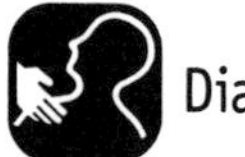

Diagnosis

DIFFERENTIAL DIAGNOSIS

- Cervical radiculopathy
- Brachial plexopathy/"stinger"
- Rotator cuff tendonitis/tear
- Labral pathology
- Turner-Parsonage syndrome/neuritis

HISTORY

Q: Traumatic versus atraumatic?
A: May yield clues to mechanism of injury; traction injury caused by blunt trauma has a good prognosis.
Q: Painful versus painless?
A: Painless weakness suggests distal lesion.
Q: Overhead throwing athlete?
A: If yes, may increase risk of suprascapular nerve lesion.

PHYSICAL EXAMINATION

- Inspection is key. Look for supraspinatus or (especially) infraspinatus atrophy.
- Evidence of cervical radiculopathy
- External rotation testing versus resistance to evaluate infraspinatus strength
- Jobe's test to evaluate supraspinatus strength
- Complete neurologic examination to determine type and extent of injury
- Thorough shoulder examination to evaluate for associated injury
- Tenderness to palpation at scapular notch present in up to 77% cases
- Cross-body adduction test (forward flexed arm externally rotated and adducted across body) puts tension on suprascapular nerve at spinoglenoid notch; may help differentiate from rotator cuff lesion.
- Injection into scapular notch may help determine source of pain, but is rarely necessary.

IMAGING

- Plain films of neck and shoulder to evaluate for bony abnormalities
- 30-degree cephalic tilt view helps visualize scapular notch; obtain especially if scapular fracture magnetic resonance imaging may be used to detect ganglion cysts, tumors, or associated labral injury.

NEURODIAGNOSTICS

- Electromyography of entire shoulder girdle
- Nerve conduction velocity studies from Erb's point to the supraspinatus, with comparison to unaffected side
- Wait minimum 3–4 weeks after onset of complaint before neurodiagnostics, as false-negatives may result if done earlier

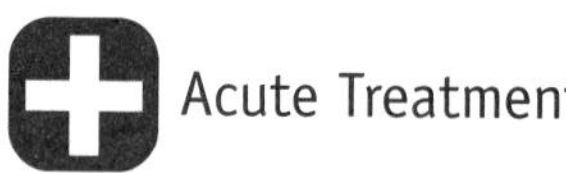

Acute Treatment

TREATMENT

- Unless there is a well-defined lesion causing suprascapular nerve compression, nonoperative therapy is recommended. This includes
  —Rest from overhead movements/throwing/exacerbating activities
  —Physical therapy to strengthen external rotation and stabilize scapula
  —Nonsteroidal anti-inflammatory drugs or analgesics if needed

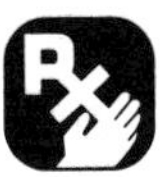

Long-Term Treatment

SURGERY

- If labral tear with associated ganglion cyst cause symptoms, repair/debridement of labral tear may allow cyst to resolve, thereby relieving pressure on the suprascapular nerve.
- If conservative management not beneficial after 3–6 months, refer for surgical exploration.

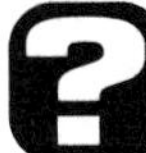

Common Questions and Answers

Physician responses to common patient questions:

Q: When can I return to play?

A: Depends on severity and cause of the neuropathy. As strength increases and atrophy and symptoms resolve, a gradual return to play may be initiated.

Q: Will I regain my normal strength and muscle shape?

A: Return of muscle strength usually occurs over time once the cause of the injury has been treated. However, especially with long-standing, severe lesions, muscle atrophy may not fully resolve.

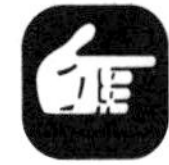

Miscellaneous

ICD-9 CODE

354.8

BIBLIOGRAPHY

Butters KP. Nerve lesions of the shoulder. In: DeLee JC, Drez D, eds. *Orthopaedic sports medicine: principles and practice.* Philadelphia: WB Saunders, 1994:657–663.

Chochole MH, Senker W, Meznik C, et al. Glenoid-labral cyst entrapping the suprascapular nerve: dissolution after arthroscopic debridement of an extended SLAP lesion. *Arthroscopy* 1997;13(6): 753–755.

Authors: Philip H. Cohen and James C. Puffer

Syndesmodial Injury of the Lower Leg

Basics

DEFINITION

- Injury occurs with sudden forceful external rotation of the ankle.
- The talus is pressed against the fibula, opening the distal tibiofibular articulation and rupturing the tibiofibular syndesmosis.
- Relevant injured structures include the interosseous membrane, anterior/posterior/inferior tibiofibular ligaments, and interosseous ligament.

INCIDENCE/PREVALENCE

- 1% of all ankle sprains

SIGNS AND SYMPTOMS

- Pain over anterior ankle and anterior syndesmosis
- Sense of tightness, but usually little swelling
- Inability to push off on the injured leg

RISK FACTORS

- Slalom skiing
- Football

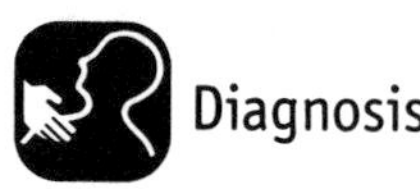

Diagnosis

DIFFERENTIAL DIAGNOSIS

- Rupture versus sprain of syndesmosis
- Lateral ankle sprain
- Medial ankle sprain
- Fracture of the distal fibula
- Fracture of the distal tibia
- Talar dome fracture

HISTORY

- Often incomplete
- Patients commonly report an inversion mechanism.
- Common injuries occur in soccer (player tackling ball), football (player prone, has foot stepped on), and skiing (slalom skiers, catch ski on gate).
- Focus history on mechanism of injury; raise index of suspicion with history of forceful external rotation, hyperdorsiflexion, or hyperplantarflexion.

PHYSICAL EXAMINATION

- Less swelling than anticipated with severe lateral ankle sprain
- Palpation of the tibia and fibula are helpful to rule out fracture.
- Anterior joint line and anterior syndesmosis often are tender.
- Squeeze test: Compression above midcalf produces distal pain in the anterior ankle joint (syndesmosis).
- External rotation test: Distal lower leg is stabilized while mediolateral force/external rotation of the foot is performed. Positive test is ≥3 mm difference relative to unaffected side.
- Pushoff test: Pushoff/heel raise on affected side may be weak or absent.
- Evaluate distal neurovascular status with any lower leg injury to rule out acute compartment syndrome.

IMAGING

- X-rays
  - —Standing mortise view to evaluate talocrural angle; any side-to-side difference >5 degrees is significant.
  - —Anteroposterior view to evaluate tibiofibular clear space; >4 mm is termed diastasis or incompetency of the syndesmotic ligaments.
  - —Varus and valgus ankle stress views are essential to assess instability.
- Bone scan is helpful if stress views not tolerated.
- Magnetic resonance imaging can clarify diagnosis and extent of soft tissue injury.
- Computed tomography can rule out talar dome injuries.

ASSOCIATED INJURIES AND COMPLICATIONS

- Deltoid ligament tear
- Fibular or medial malleolar fracture
- Heterotopic ossification or synchondrosis of the syndesmosis in 25% to 100% of cases
- Tibiofibular synostosis resulting in prolonged pain and chronic disability
- Longer healing time and more missed practices
- Missed talar dome fracture

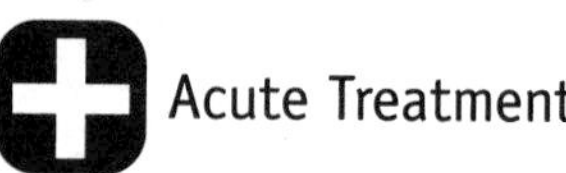

Acute Treatment

Syndesmosis Injuries without Fracture

- If frank diastasis (widening of syndesmosis), screw or K-wire fixation with repair of the deltoid ligaments, followed by casting for 8–12 weeks.
- If no diastasis, short-term immobilization in a nonweight-bearing cast or boot for 10 days to 2 weeks suggested, followed by aggressive rehabilitation for proprioception, range of motion, strength, flexibility, and agility.
- Return to play is variable, usually 3–4 weeks, but can be months.

Syndesmosis Injuries with Fracture

- Screw fixation followed by casting with or without weight-bearing for 6 weeks, followed by appropriate rehabilitation

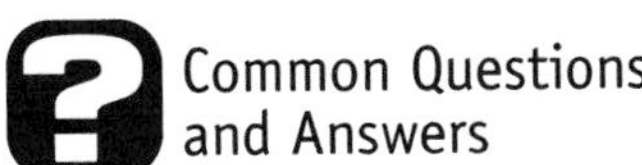

Common Questions and Answers

Physician responses to common patient questions:
Q: When can I go back to play?
A: In many sports communities, these injuries are immobilized for a variable period ranging from a few days in elite professional and collegiate athletes to 2 weeks for high school athletes. Then, aggressive rehabilitation to restore motion, strength and proprioception is done. Injuries usually result in 4 weeks away from sport.

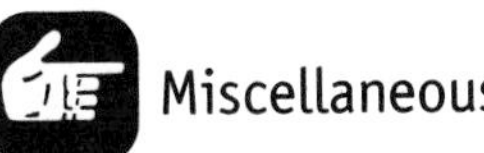

Miscellaneous

SYNONYMS

- High ankle sprain

ICD-9 CODE

845.00 Sprain, ankle and foot

BIBLIOGRAPHY

Boytim MJ, Fischer DA, Neurman L. Syndesmotic ankle sprains. *Am J Sports Med* 1991;19:294–298.

Hopkinson WJ, St. Pierre P, Ryan JB, et al. Syndesmosis sprains of the ankle. *Foot Ankle* 1990;10:325–330.

Wuest TK. Injuries to the distal lower extremity syndesmosis. *J Am Acad Ortho Surg* 1997;5:172–181.

Authors: Delmas J. Bolin and David A. Stone

Tarsal Tunnel Syndrome/Posterior Tibial Nerve Entrapment

Basics

DEFINITION

- Foot pain and paresthesias along the plantar aspect of the foot and toes resulting from posterior tibial nerve entrapment in the tarsal tunnel

ANATOMY

- Tarsal tunnel is a fixed anatomical space bordered by the calcaneus and talus superiorly, inferiorly, and laterally, and by the flexor retinaculum medially.
- Structures passing through the tunnel include the tibialis posterior, flexor digitorum longus, and flexor hallucis longus tendons. Posterior tibial artery, veins, and tibial nerve also course through the tunnel.
- Tibial nerve branches at various locations through the tunnel into the medial and lateral plantar nerves. Medial calcaneal nerve pierces through the flexor retinaculum to the medial side of the heel. Tarsal tunnel can be viewed as an upper tunnel or lower tunnel as different clinical entities based on nerve branching locations.
- Tarsal tunnel differs from carpal tunnel, with discrete individual septations forming tunnels encasing the tendons and neurovascular structures.

INCIDENCE/PREVALENCE

- Unknown; rare compared to other peripheral mononeuropathies

SIGNS AND SYMPTOMS

- Numbness/tingling that progresses to a burning sensation to the plantar aspect of the foot. Intermittent initially, can become constant.
- Plantar foot pain accentuated by walking and foot dorsiflexion
- Nocturnal pain often relieved with walking
- Pain worse at the end of the day
- Loss of two-point discrimination
- Positive Tinel sign over the tunnel
- Symptoms reproduced with venous tourniquet, inversion, and eversion.
- Occasional fusiform swelling over the nerve course
- Motor weakness or loss as late finding/poor prognosis
- Tenderness distal or proximal to area of entrapment (Valleix sign)

RISK FACTORS

- Local trauma
- Abnormal foot/ankle mechanics, i.e., excessive pronation
- Systemic disease
- Repetitive activity
- Weight gain
- Fluid retention
- Previous foot or ankle surgery
- Accessory muscles
- Space-occupying lesions

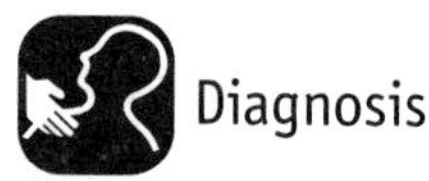

Diagnosis

DIFFERENTIAL DIAGNOSIS

- Plantar fasciitis
- Calcaneal bursitis
- Tendinitis
- Tenosynovitis
- S-1 radiculopathy
- Peripheral vascular disease, including popliteal artery entrapment
- Peripheral neuropathy
- Systemic disease, e.g., Reiter disease
- Bony abnormalities, e.g., degenerative changes, previous fractures

HISTORY

- Tarsal tunnel syndrome presents with a nonspecific, highly variable clinical picture.
- History of trauma or repetitive activity, e.g., running, is helpful.
- Patient describes numbness, tingling, and burning to the medial aspect and sole of the foot. Can include calf symptoms.
- Patients lack morning pain and particularly often lack heel pain more typical of plantar fasciitis.
- Nocturnal pain may awaken the patient.

PHYSICAL EXAMINATION

- Inspect for biomechanical abnormalities such as excessive varus or valgus heel
- Observe for swelling
- Palpate for soft tissue thickening or light touch-induced paresthesias
- Diminished two-point discrimination often occurs early
- Diminished pinprick sensation to plantar foot
- Intrinsic muscle weakness, although possibly present, is difficult to assess.
- Atrophy of abductor hallucis or abductor digiti minimi as a late finding
- Percussion sign (Tinel sign)
- Cuff sign (pain with pneumatic pressure device around leg)
- Pain with dorsiflexion or heel eversion

IMAGING

- Plain x-ray to rule out displaced fractures, accessory ossicles, and bony exostoses
- Electrodiagnostic studies if positive may be helpful, but frequently are insensitive and negative.
- Electromyography of leg and foot muscles
- Magnetic resonance imaging is test of choice to evaluate tunnel contents. Bony and soft tissue structures can be viewed, e.g., ganglion cysts, accessory or hypertrophied muscles, bone spurring.

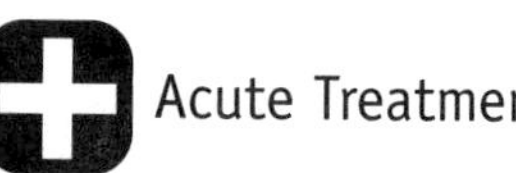

Acute Treatment

INITIAL MANAGEMENT

- Nonoperative measures should be tried first.
- Conservative efforts with nonsteroidal anti-inflammatory drugs, ice, relative rest, local steroid injection, flexibility, and strengthening exercises

IMMOBILIZATION

- Rigid ankle-foot orthosis
- Walking cast
- Medial longitudinal arch supports

SPECIAL CONSIDERATIONS

- Untreated patients risk nerve atrophy from continued pressure by space-occupying lesions

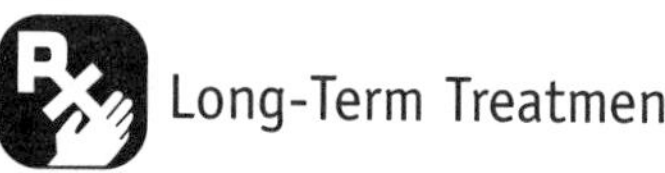

Long-Term Treatment

REHABILITATION

- Correct abnormal foot mechanics with shoe orthoses, especially in runners
- Well supportive shoes
- Physiotherapy to strengthen foot intrinsic and extrinsic muscles
- Weight loss for obese patients
- Stockings to decrease swelling and venous stasis

SURGERY

- Indicated for acute cases with space-occupying lesions and recalcitrant conservatively treated cases
- Flexor retinaculum release
- Dissection of lateral and medial plantar nerves beyond compression site
- Best surgical results in cases with tumor or coalition
- Poor surgical results in patients with idiopathic or postraumatic cases
- Long-term surgical benefits vary

REFERRAL/DISPOSITION

- Surgical referral for cases recalcitrant to conservative treatments

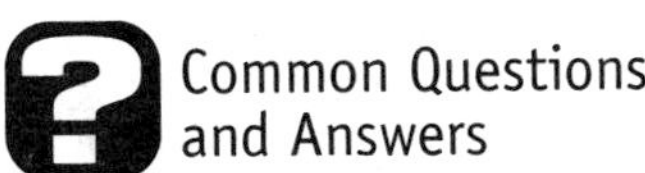

Common Questions and Answers

Physician responses to common patient questions:

Q: Is surgical treatment necessary?
A: Many cases of tarsal tunnel syndrome can be managed with relative rest from exercise, biomechanical control, and anti-inflammatory drugs.

Q: Can I do permanent damage if this is untreated?
A: Search for a surgically treatable cause is necessary to avoid permanent nerve compression, sensory deficits, and motor weakness.

Miscellaneous

SYNONYMS

- Posterior tibial nerve entrapment

ICD-9 CODE

355.5

BIBLIOGRAPHY

Bailie DS, Kelikian AS. Tarsal tunnel syndrome: diagnosis, surgical technique and functional outcome. *Foot Ankle Int* 1998;19:65–72.

Finkel JE. Tarsal tunnel syndrome. *Magn Reson Imaging Clin N Am* 1994;2:67–78.

Jackson DL, Haglund BL. Tarsal tunnel syndrome in runners. *Sports Med* 1992;13:146–149.

Jackson DL, Haglund BL. Tarsal tunnel syndrome in athletes: case reports and literature review. *Am J Sports Med* 1991;19:61–65.

Lau TC, Daniels TR. Tarsal tunnel syndrome: a review of the literature. *Foot Ankle Int* 1999;20:201–209.

Authors: Stephen Simons and David Pacholke

Temporomandibular Joint Injury

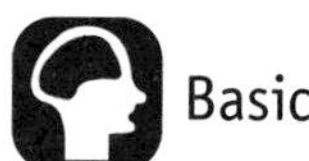

Basics

SIGNS AND SYMPTOMS

- Dull, aching unilateral jaw, ear, or head pain
  - —Exacerbated by opening the mouth
- A "popping" or "clicking" sensation may be noted with chewing
- Limited range of motion of the mandible
- Symptoms more conspicuous in the evening and less prominent upon awakening
- Pain may refer to a variety of locations on the ipsilateral hemicranium and supraclavicular region
- Dentoskeletal malocclusion
- Mandibular deviation with opening and closing of the mouth
- Temporomandibular joint (TMJ) capsule tenderness
- Tenderness over the muscles of mastication
- A palpable click can often be palpated with opening and closing of the mouth

MECHANISM/DESCRIPTION

- The cause of temporomandibular pain dysfunction syndrome (TMPDS) is unknown
- May be related to an abnormality in neuromuscular mechanics
  - —Trauma, dentoskeletal malocclusion, and bruxism are important contributors
- 10–20 million adults suffer TMPDS
- Patients present in fourth decade of life
- Females to male ratio of 2:1

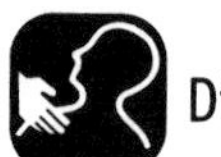

Diagnosis

ESSENTIAL WORKUP

- Diagnosis based on clinical presentation above
- Exclude other causes of unilateral facial or head pain

LABORATORY

- No specific laboratory tests are indicated

IMAGING/SPECIAL TESTS

- Plain radiographs are of little value
- Tomograms, bone scintigraphy, CT scan, and MRI are not necessary during the initial evaluation of TMPDS in the emergency department

DIFFERENTIAL DIAGNOSIS

- Myocardial ischemia
- Carotid or vertebral artery dissection
- Intracranial hemorrhage (subarachnoid hemorrhage)
- Temporal arteritis
- Multiple sclerosis may present with pain similar to trigeminal neuralgia
- Trigeminal or glossopharyngeal neuralgia
- Vascular headache
- Dental abnormalities
- Herpes zoster
- Salivary gland disorder, otitis media, external otitis, and sinusitis
- Elongated styloid process pain often precipitated by swallowing or turning the head

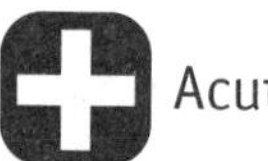

Acute Treatment

INITIAL STABILIZATION

N/A

ED TREATMENT

- Refer to dentist or oral-maxillofacial surgeon for occlusal splints
- Additional therapeutic options include
  - —Tricyclic antidepressants
  - —Vapocoolant spray with physiotherapy

—Behavior modification
—Intra-articular and local injections of anesthetics or steroids
- Treat as outpatients with pain medication, muscle relaxants and warm compresses

MEDICATIONS

- Oral or parenteral analgesics
- Muscle relaxants

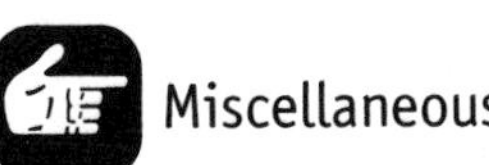

Miscellaneous

ICD-9-CM

524.60

CORE CONTENT CODE

6.3.14

BIBLIOGRAPHY

Marbach JJ. Temporomandibular pain dysfunction syndrome. History, physical examination and treatment. *Rheum Dis Clin North Am* 22(3):477–98.

Author: Timothy J. Mader

Thoracic Outlet Syndrome

Basics

DEFINITION

- Neurologic and/or vascular symptoms in the upper extremity due to pressure on the nerves and/or vessels in the thoracic outlet area

INCIDENCE/PREVALENCE

- More common in middle-aged women, workers involved in repetitive activity, and overhead athletes

SIGNS AND SYMPTOMS

- May see combination or individual signs of neurologic, arterial, and/or venous deficits

Neurologic

- Pain, paresthesias, and numbness
- Ulnar distribution (common)
- Sensory loss, motor weakness, and atrophy (late findings)
- Weak grip
- Difficulty with fine motor skills of the hand
- Cramping of forearm muscles

Arterial

- Ischemic pain
- Numbness
- Fatigue
- Paresthesias
- Coldness
- Painful throbbing
- Distal embolization
- Heavy arm feeling
- Pulsating lump above the clavicle

Venous

- Pain
- Edema
- Cyanosis
- Vein distension in hand

Other

- Ill-defined ache or burn
- Chronic headache
- Ulcerations
- Raynaud syndrome
- Thrombosis
- Aneurysm
- Chest pain
- Infrascapular pain

Selmonosky Triad

- Elevation of hands produces symptoms
- Supraclavicular tenderness
- Weakening of fourth and fifth fingers

RISK FACTORS

- Middle-aged female
- Repetitive work
- Overhead activity
- Poor posture

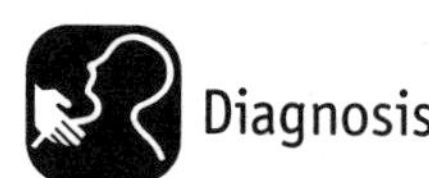

Diagnosis

DIFFERENTIAL DIAGNOSIS

- Subclavian steal
- Cervical disc
- Cervical spondylosis
- Pancoast tumor
- Carpal tunnel syndrome
- Ulnar entrapment
- Reflex sympathetic dystrophy
- Brachial neuritis
- Shoulder impingement
- Neurofibroma

HISTORY

- Early on, symptoms occur with certain postures only.
- Worsens with lifting heavy objects, overhead activity, and extension and lateral rotation of shoulder

PHYSICAL EXAMINATION

- Usually normal except for provocative maneuvers
- Auscultation: bruit in supraclavicular space
- Tinnels of supraclavicular area reproduces symptoms.
- EAST test: Abduct arm to 90 degrees, flex elbow to 90 degrees, extend arm. Have patient open and close hands for 3 minutes.
- Wright test: Hyperabduct the arm over the head, extend and rotate the neck, and have patient take a breath. Loss of radial pulse.
- Military brace test: Pull the arm down and back. Loss of pulse is positive sign.
- Provocative elevation test: Elevate both arms above 90 degrees. Open and close hands rapidly 15 times.
- Passive elevation of shoulder: When the patient has symptoms, grab patient's arms from behind and elevate the shoulder passively. Relief of symptoms is positive sign.
- Adson maneuver: Rotate the head toward the test arm, extend the neck, laterally rotate and extend the shoulder. Have patient take a breath. Loss of pulse is positive sign.
- Allen test: Flex elbow to 90 degrees, extend and laterally rotate the shoulder. Have patient rotate head away from test arm. Loss of pulse is positive sign.

IMAGING

- Chest, cervical spine, and shoulder x-rays
- Ultrasound of vascular structures
- Spiral computed tomography
- Myelogram, arteriogram, and venogram if needed
- Electromyography
- Nerve conduction test

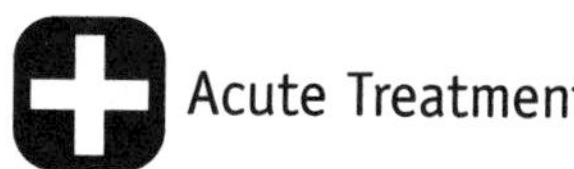

Acute Treatment

ANALGESIA

- Nonsteroidal anti-inflammatory drugs
- Muscle relaxer

IMMOBILIZATION

- Sling for comfort
- Maintain range of motion by stretching several times a day

SPECIAL CONSIDERATIONS

- Refer to surgery if severe neurologic or vascular signs
- Physical therapy for stretching and strengthening exercises
- Weight loss
- Posture correction

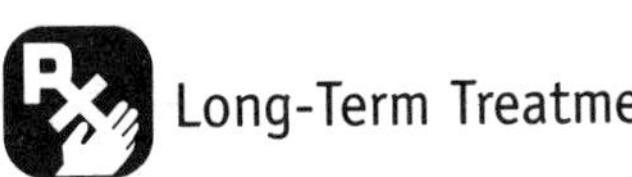

Long-Term Treatment

REHABILITATION

- Most patients will improve with conservative physical therapy.

SURGERY

- May include first rib resection, anterior scalene release, fascial release, or pectoralis minor release

REFERRAL/DISPOSITION

- Refer to vascular surgeon referral if signs of vascular compromise or if severe neurologic signs

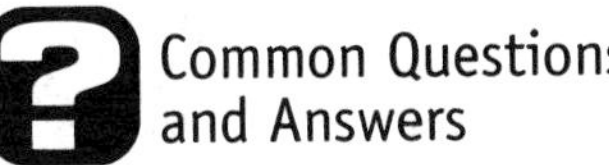

Common Questions and Answers

Physician responses to common patient questions:
Q: Do I need to stop playing my sport?
A: If the sport brings on symptoms, yes.
Q: When can I go back to play?
A: When you are asymptomatic in provocative moves or after surgical correction.
Q: Do I need surgery?
A: Only if severe symptoms or if no improvement occurs with physical therapy.

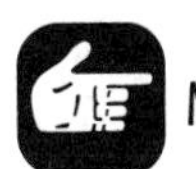

Miscellaneous

ICD-9 CODE

353.0

BIBLIOGRAPHY

Kibler WB, ed. *The team physicians handbook.* Philadelphia: Hanley & Belfus, 1990.

Magee DJ, ed. *Orthopedic physical assessment.* Philadelphia: WB Saunders, 1997.

Snider RD, ed. *Essentials of musculoskeletal medicine.* Rosemont, IL: American Academy of Orthopaedic Surgeons, 1997.

Author: Martha Pyron

Thoracic Spine Injury

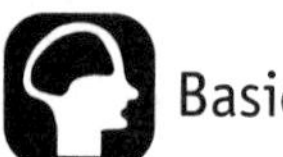

Basics

SIGNS AND SYMPTOMS

- Significant force is required to produce thoracic vertebral fractures, so other injuries may obscure those directly related to thoracic fractures
- Primary symptoms of thoracic vertebral fracture occur from pain at the fracture site or impingement of nearby structures by bone fragments
- Common signs and symptoms
  —Localized soft tissue defect
  —Pain or tenderness
    —Localized—pain and tenderness over spinous process
    —Referred—paraspinal, anterior chest or abdomen
  —Paraspinal muscle spasm
  —Paresthesia or dysesthesia
  —Weakness (focal or global)
  —Distal areflexia, flaccid plegia
  —Bowel or bladder incontinence
  —Priapism
  —Loss of temperature control
  —Spinal shock—hypotension with bradycardia

ETIOLOGY

- The thoracic spine is very rigid due to the rib cage and the costovertebral articulations. The spinal canal is narrowest in the thoracic spine
- Since traumatic thoracic spine fractures require enormous forces, motor vehicle accidents or falls from height account for the majority of fractures
  —A small percentage is caused by penetrating injuries and will be covered in a separate section
  —50% of all spinal fractures and 40% of all spinal cord injuries occur at the thoracolumbar junction (T11-L2)

MECHANISM/DESCRIPTION

- The following forces account for most thoracic fractures
  —Axial compression
  —Flexion-rotation
  —Shear
  —Flexion-distraction
  —Extension
- The spinal column can be divided into three anatomically distinct columns. If two of the three columns are disrupted, then the spinal column is unstable
  —Posterior column: posterior bony arch and interconnecting ligamentous structures
  —Middle column: posterior aspects of the vertebral bodies, posterior annulus fibrosis, and the posterior longitudinal ligament
  —Anterior column: anterior longitudinal ligament, anterior anulus fibrosis, and anterior vertebral body
- Major vs. minor fractures
  —Minor
    —Isolated articular fracture
    —Transverse process fracture
    —Spinous process fracture
    —Pars interarticularis fracture
  —Major
    —Compression fracture
    —Burst fracture
    —Seat belt injury
    —Fracture dislocation
- Compression fracture (anterior or lateral flexion)
  —Fracture of anterior portion of vertebral body with intact middle column of spine
  —May be posterior column disruption
  —Type A: fracture through both endplates
  —Type B: fracture through superior endplate
  —Type C: fracture through inferior endplate
  —Type D: both endplates intact
- Burst fracture (axial loading)
  —Fracture through middle column of spine
  —May have spreading of posterior elements and lamina fractures
  —Type A: fracture through both endplates
  —Type B: fracture through superior endplate
  —Type C: fracture through inferior endplate
  —Type D: burst in middle column with rotational injury leading to subluxation
  —Type E: burst in middle column with asymmetric compression of anterior column
- Seat belt injury (flexion distraction)
  —Distraction of posterior and middle columns with anterior column intact
  —Typically caused by lap belts used without shoulder harness
  —Type A: through bone
  —Type B: primarily ligamentous
  —Type C: disruption of bone through middle column
  —Type D: through ligaments and disk with no middle column fracture
- Fracture dislocations
  —Failure of all three columns following compression, tension, rotation, or shear forces
  —Type A: flexion rotation; fall from height
  —Type B: shear–violent force across long axis of trunk
  —Type C: flexion distraction; bilateral facet dislocation

CAUTIONS

- If the patient's positioning initially prevents placement of a long spinal board, then a short board should be placed until the patient is fully extricated
- Patients with neurologic deficit should be transported directly to a trauma center

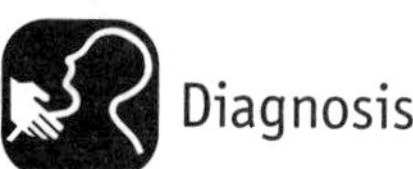

Diagnosis

ESSENTIAL WORKUP

- Rapid evaluation of airway, breathing and circulation
- Primary and secondary trauma survey
- Detailed neurologic exam with specific attention to evidence of spinal cord injury, including rectal tone
- Thorough spine exam noting any deformity or tenderness
- Any midline tenderness elicited on examination, distracting injury, or intoxication mandates plain film spine radiography
- If fracture is present, determine if it is stable or unstable, as defined by descriptions of columns above

IMAGING/SPECIAL TESTS

- Pain or tenderness, severe motor vehicle accident, or falls from height are indications for AP and lateral plain film views of the spine
- Thin-cut CT scanning is indicated in any patient with evidence of spinal fracture or ligamentous injury on plain films to assess spinal canal integrity or in patients with normal plain films and significant pain or tenderness and mechanism for severe injury

DIFFERENTIAL DIAGNOSIS

- Arthritis (degenerative and rheumatoid)
- Ankylosing spondylitis
- Spina bifida
- Congenital malformation
- Neoplasm
- Pathologic fracture

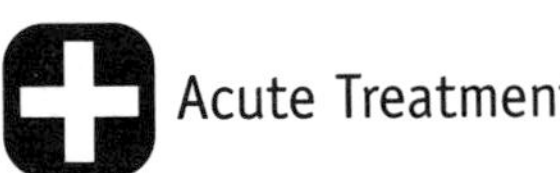

Acute Treatment

INITIAL STABILIZATION

- Follow the ABCs of trauma resuscitation
- Airway intervention should be done with inline cervical immobilization
- Preserve residual spinal cord function and prevent further injury by stabilizing the spine

ED TREATMENT

- Perform all needed resuscitation and diagnostic tests with the patient in full spinal immobilization
- If spinal cord injury is suspected, administer high dose steroids and consult a neurosurgeon
- If spinal fracture or ligamentous injury is suspected without neurologic impairment, arrange CT or MRI scanning while simultaneously consulting neurosurgery or orthopaedic surgery
- Pain control should be administered as soon as possible. NSAIDs, opiates, and benzodiazepines are the mainstays of treatment

MEDICATIONS

- High-dose steroid protocol
  —Solumedrol: 30 mg/kg IV bolus within 8 hours of injury, followed immediately by an infusion of 5.4 mg/kg/hr for the next 23 hours

HOSPITAL ADMISSION CRITERIA

- Patients with significant spinal cord or column injury should be treated in a regional trauma center
- Unstable spinal column injury
- Cord or root injury
- Ileus
- Pain control
- Concomitant traumatic injury

HOSPITAL DISCHARGE CRITERIA

- Stable minor fractures after orthopaedic or neurosurgical evaluation

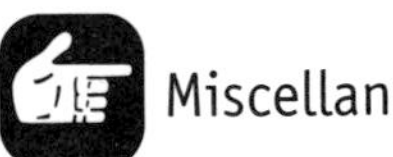

Miscellaneous

ICD-9-CM

952.10

CORE CONTENT CODE

18.4.3.1.2

BIBLIOGRAPHY

Block BE. Thoracic and lumbar spine injuries in children. *Contemporary orthopedics* 1994;29(4):253–60.

Chiles BW 3rd, Cooper PR. Acute spinal injury. *N Engl J Med* 1996;334(8):514–520.

El-Khoury GY, Whitten CG. Trauma to the upper thoracic spine: Anatomy, biomechanics, and unique imaging features. *Am J Roentgenol* 1993;160:95–102.

Kinashita H. Pathology of spinal cord injuries due to fracture-dislocations of the thoracic and lumbar spine. *Paraplegia* 1996;34(1): 1–7.

Author: Richard D. Zane

Thumb Ulnar Collateral Ligament Sprain (Skier's Thumb)

Basics

DEFINITION

Skier's Thumb (Gamekeeper Thumb)

- Sprain of the ulnar collateral ligament (UCL) of the first metacarpophalangeal (MCP) joint, with or without a bony avulsion from the insertion on the phalanx

Stener Lesion

- Proximal end of the ligament becomes trapped superficial to the adductor pollicis aponeurosis
- Surgery required to prevent permanent instability in 14% to 87% of all complete tears

INCIDENCE/PREVALENCE

- 5.6% to 6% of all skiing injuries

SIGNS AND SYMPTOMS

- Pain at the origin and insertion of the UCL
- Tenderness and swelling over the ulnar aspect of the first MCP joint
- Mild-to-complete instability on stress testing of UCL with MCP joint in flexion, depending on whether it is a first-, second-, or third-degree sprain

RISK FACTORS

Wrist straps used in skiing are no longer believed to increase the risk of injury.

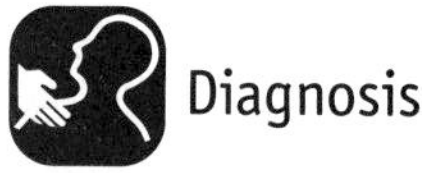

Diagnosis

HISTORY

- Stress to the thumb in extended and/or abducted position
- Usually in skiing, but often occurs in other sports such as football and judo

PHYSICAL EXAMINATION

- Pain at the origin and insertion of the UCL
- Tenderness and swelling over the ulnar aspect of the first MCP joint
- Mild-to-complete instability on stress testing of UCL with MCP joint in flexion, depending on whether it is a first-, second-, or third-degree sprain

IMAGING

X-rays (Posteroanterior/Lateral)

- Rule out bony avulsion or other fractures
- Stress x-rays to determine if the tear is partial (usually treated conservatively) or complete (often treated surgically)
- Because of associated muscle spasm, many clinicians advise local anesthetic infiltration before x-rays.

Ultrasound

- Research suggests that ultrasound eventually may be an inexpensive method of diagnosing a complete tear and presence of a Stener lesion.
- Results to date are too inconsistent for it to be recommended at this time.

Magnetic Resonance Imaging

- Ordered to diagnose whether there is a complete tear or if there is a Stener lesion present

Magnetic Resonance Arthrography

- Ordered to diagnose whether there is a complete tear or if there is a Stener lesion present
- Unclear whether arthrography provides additional benefit over simple magnetic resonance imaging (MRI)

GENERAL INFORMATION

- Diagnosis may be made based on physical examination if the examination is done within a couple of hours.
- Swelling and muscle spasm make clinical diagnosis of a complete tear difficult if the examination is performed later.
- Stress x-ray is recommended to make the diagnosis of complete UCL tear.
- Ultrasound or MRI may be helpful in assessing whether a Stener lesion is present.

ASSOCIATED LESIONS

- Avulsion of bony fragment at the insertion of UCL on the phalanx

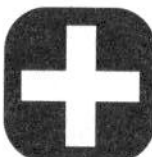

Acute Treatment

PARTIAL TEARS

- Treatment is nonsurgical.
- Protection with thumb spica splint (3–6 weeks), rest, ice, compression, and nonsteroidal anti-inflammatory drugs
- Rehabilitation therapy, including range of motion and strengthening. Start date depends on severity of injury.

COMPLETE TEARS

- If a Stener lesion can be ruled out with MRI or magnetic resonance arthrography, good results can be expected with conservative treatment (i.e., brace or cast).
- If a Stener lesion is present, treatment should be surgical.
- If presence of a Stener lesion cannot be determined, management is controversial. As early surgical repair yields superior results compared with conservative treatment, surgery is preferred by many clinicians. However, most late repairs are successful; therefore, some clinicians will treat patients with a trial of conservative treatment and reserve surgery for patients who continue to have symptoms.

AVULSION FRACTURES

If avulsion-type fracture is present, treatment is a thumb spica cast for 4–6 weeks.

COMPLICATIONS

- Most common complication is instability, resulting in difficulty pinching the second and first fingers together.
- Other complications are related to surgical interventions (local numbness, infection).

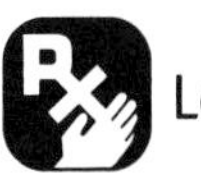

Long-Term Treatment

CHRONIC INSTABILITY

- Surgery is the preferred treatment.
- Conservative treatment is limited to bracing and strengthening exercises, but the majority of patients do not obtain satisfactory results.

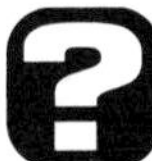

Common Questions and Answers

Physician responses to common patient questions:

Q: When can I return to play?

A: Depends on severity and whether surgery is performed. Incomplete tears usually are treated with splinting for 4–8 weeks, with range of motion exercises and strengthening beginning after 3 weeks. A protective splint should be worn for sports until range of motion and strength have returned to normal, usually within 6–8 weeks of injury. If surgery is performed, range of motion and strengthening exercises usually begin 6 weeks after surgery. A protective splint usually is prescribed until range of motion and strength have returned to normal.

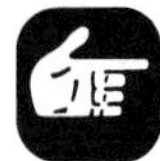

Miscellaneous

SYNONYMS

- Stener lesion
- Gamekeeper thumb
- Skier's thumb

ICD-9 CODE

841.1

BIBLIOGRAPHY

Ballas MT, Tytko J, Mannarino F. Commonly missed orthopedic problems. *Am Fam Physician* 1998;57:267–274.

Deibert MC, Aronsson DD, Johnson RJ, et al. Skiing injuries in children, adolescents, and adults. *J Bone Joint Surg Am* 1998;80A: 25–32.

Harper MT, Chandnani VP, Spaeth J, et al. Gamekeeper thumb: diagnosis of ulnar collateral ligament injury using magnetic resonance imaging, magnetic resonance arthrography and stress radiography. *J Magn Reson Imaging* 1996;6:322–328.

Husband JB. Bony skier's thumb injuries. *Clin Orthop* 1996;327:79–84.

Richard JR. Gamekeeper's thumb: ulnar collateral ligament injury. *Am Fam Physician* 1996;53:775–1780.

Authors: Ian Shrier and Dan Somogyi

Triceps Tendinitis

Basics

DEFINITION

- Inflammation of the triceps tendon at or above the insertion onto the olecranon
- Classically an overuse injury due to repetitive extension of the elbow
- May result from direct trauma

INCIDENCE/PREVALENCE

- Uncommon, but higher prevalence observed in certain groups (see Risk Factors)

SIGNS AND SYMPTOMS

- Pain in the posterior elbow
- Pain on full extension/flexion of the elbow
- Swelling at or above the tendinous insertion

RISK FACTORS

- Commonly associated with posterior impingement, presence of loose bodies, or classic tennis elbow
- Activities such as hammering, weight lifting, throwing (baseball), and platform diving

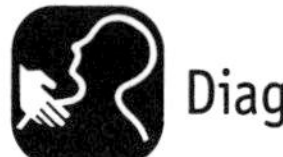

Diagnosis

DIFFERENTIAL DIAGNOSIS

- Olecranon fracture/stress fracture
- Subtendinous bursitis

HISTORY

- Increasing pain in the posterior elbow over several weeks that worsens over course of the day and associated with slight morning stiffness and some improvement over weekend in construction workers

PHYSICAL EXAM

- Tenderness at or above the triceps insertion onto the olecranon
- Swelling in the same area
- Increased pain with resisted extension of the elbow

IMAGING

Anteroposterior and lateral plain films are usually normal but may reveal degenerative calcification, hypertrophy of the ulna in the proximity of the triceps insertion, or a triceps traction spur.

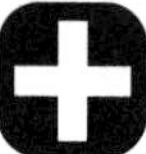

Acute Treatment

- PRICEMM: protection, rest, ice, compression, elevation, medications (NSAIDS), and modalities (strap as in classic tennis elbow to divert fulcrum pull from insertion)

SPECIAL CONSIDERATIONS

Limit ice to 20 minutes three or four times daily to avoid damage to the ulnar nerve in the cubital tunnel.

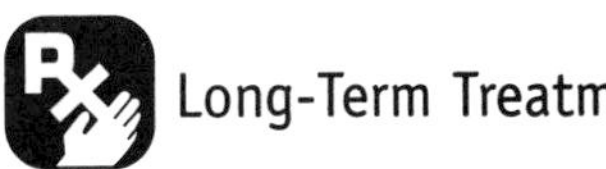

Long-Term Treatment

REHABILITATION

- Graduated stretching and strengthening following period of rest
- French stretch: (1) clasp fingers together with hands above head; (2) keep elbows close to head; (3) reach down behind head attempting to touch back; (4) hold, then repeat
- French press: as with stretch, except holding a dumbbell
- Towel stretch: (1) injured arm overhead with uninjured reaching behind back; (2) one end of towel in each hand; (3) pull, hold, and repeat

SURGICAL TREATMENT

- Rare, but operative treatment described with elliptical resection of diseased tissue

REFERRAL/DISPOSITION

- Return to sport/activity when no longer tender at or above tendon insertion, strength regained, and full range of motion

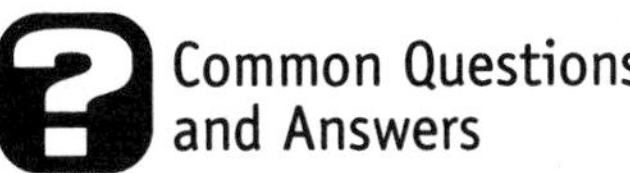

Common Questions and Answers

Physician responses to common patient questions:
Q: Can this entity be injected?
A: The literature mentions possible injection not recommended secondary to rupture risk with direct tendon injection.

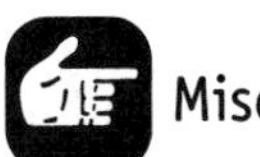

Miscellaneous

ICD-9 CODE

727.09 Elbow tenosynovitis

BIBLIOGRAPHY

Chumbley EM, O'Conner FG, Nirschl RP. Evaluation of overuse elbow injuries. *Am Fam Physician* 2000;61:691–700.

Mellion, Walsh, Shelton, eds. *Team physician's handbook*. Philadelphia: Hanley & Belfus, 1997.

Strauch RJ. Biceps and triceps injuries of the elbow. *Orthop Clin North Am* 1999;30: 95–107.

Authors: James Blount and Robert L. Jones

Triceps Tendon Rupture

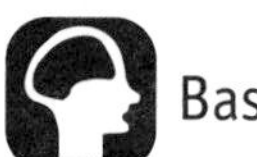

Basics

DEFINITION

- Triceps tendon ruptures are defined as a partial or complete tear of the triceps muscle or tendon at one of several sites, including the musculotendinous junction or the tendinous insertion into the bone. The latter scenario occasionally includes a piece of bone from the olecranon insertion. There also have been several cases of tears of the muscle belly.

INCIDENCE/PREVALENCE

- Triceps tendon ruptures are rare and have been described as the least common of all tendon injuries.
- This injury is more commonly seen in men and affects individuals in the age range of 7 to 70 years.

SIGNS AND SYMPTOMS

- The usual mechanism of injury involves a fall on an outstretched arm (causing a deceleration-type injury) or a direct blow to the posterior arm or elbow.
- Activities can be significantly limited, including those requiring pushing and reaching overhead.

RISK FACTORS

Several predisposing factors have been described, including hyperparathyroidism secondary to chronic renal failure, steroid use, and both local and systemic injection, the former possibly secondary to olecranon bursitis.

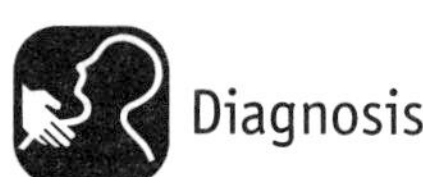

Diagnosis

DIFFERENTIAL DIAGNOSIS

- Olecranon fracture (intraarticular)
- Triceps tendonitis or strain
- Triceps contusion
- Avulsion fracture of the olecranon
- Radial head fracture
- Olecranon bursitis

HISTORY

- Patients usually present with pain and swelling of the posterior elbow.
- May have ecchymosis over area of triceps insertion
- Can also have decreased active elbow extension

PHYSICAL EXAM

- Patients have localized swelling at the posterior elbow.
- Tenderness in the area of the triceps tendon insertion
- Sometimes a palpable defect can be appreciated just proximal to the olecranon.
- Pain and weakness with resisted elbow extension
- Modified Thompson test can help determine the integrity of the musculotendinous unit. This test is best accomplished with the upper arm supported, the elbow flexed to 90 degrees, and the forearm and hand hanging relaxed. This can be done by allowing the forearm to hang over the side of a table or the back of a chair. Upon squeezing the triceps muscle belly, the elbow should reflexively extend if the tendon is intact. If there is a complete rupture of the tendon, the elbow will not extend.

IMAGING

- Radiographs occasionally show one or several bony flecks from the tip of the olecranon that have been avulsed with the tendon.
- Sometimes a larger fracture of the olecranon can be seen.
- Associated injuries and findings may include radial head or neck fractures, as well as wrist fractures (probably secondary to the common mechanism of injury, a fall on an outstretched hand).
- Ultrasonography can be used to diagnose triceps tendon ruptures but may be operator dependent.
- Magnetic resonance imaging can be helpful in the diagnosis and can differentiate between complete and partial tendon ruptures.

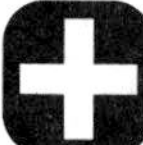

Acute Treatment

ANALGESIA

- Ice and nonsteroidal antiinflammatory drugs are the mainstay of acute therapy.
- If injury is associated with a larger olecranon fracture or radial head or wrist fracture, narcotic pain medication may be warranted.

IMMOBILIZATION

- If nonoperative repair is chosen, the elbow can be immobilized in a posterior splint in approximately 30 degrees of flexion for 4 to 6 weeks.
- Subsequent to immobilization, the patient is sent to physical therapy for rehabilitation.

SPECIAL CONSIDERATIONS

- When a triceps tendon rupture is diagnosed, it is imperative to determine whether the tear is partial or complete. This will determine whether operative or nonoperative therapy is appropriate.
- Loss of elbow motion and triceps strength (the inability to extend the elbow against even minor resistance) is consistent with a complete tendon rupture. The treatment for this is surgery.
- If there is some active elbow extension, particularly against resistance, the more likely diagnosis is a partial tendon rupture.
- Although some clinicians suggest surgical repair for both partial and complete tears because of its low morbidity and high success rate, others support nonsurgical treatment of partial tendon ruptures with close clinical observation.

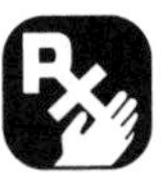

Long-Term Treatment

REHABILITATION

After a period of immobilization, patients should be sent to physical therapy for increased range of motion and progressive strength recovery.

SURGICAL TREATMENT

- Surgical repair can be more easily accomplished during the first 2 weeks after the injury.
- There are several methods of repairing triceps tendon ruptures that yield excellent results.
- A common repair technique reattaches the tendon with wire or suture through drill holes in the olecranon.
- For approximately 4 weeks postoperatively, the elbow is splinted in 30 degrees of flexion.

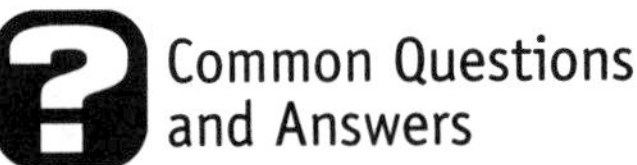

Common Questions and Answers

Physician responses to common patient questions:

Q: When can I resume my usual work/play activities?

A: Treatment for triceps tendon rupture commonly yields excellent return of motion and strength. Rehabilitation, after the period of immobilization, is the key to attaining full recovery and patients should be able to resume full activity in 2 to 4 months.

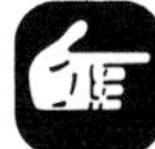

Miscellaneous

SYNONYMS

- Triceps tendon rupture
- Triceps tendon avulsion
- Triceps tendon tear
- Avulsion fracture of the olecranon
- Triceps muscle tear

ICD-9 CODE

727.60 Nontraumatic rupture of unspecified tendon
813.01 Olecranon fracture (closed)
729.5 Pain, extremity (upper)

BIBLIOGRAPHY

Aso K, Torisu T. Muscle belly tear of the triceps. *Am J Sports Med* 1984;12:485.

Bach RB, Warren RF, Wickiewicz TL. Triceps rupture: a case report and literature review. *Am J Sports Med* 1987;15:285.

Farrar EL, Lippert FG. Avulsion of the triceps tendon. *Clin Orthop Rel Res* 1981;161:242.

Kaempffe FA, Lerner RM. Ultrasound diagnosis of triceps tendon rupture. *Clin Orthop Rel Res* 1996;332:138.

Pantazopoulos TH, Exarchou E, Stavrou Z, et al. Avulsion of the triceps tendon. *J Trauma* 1975;15:827.

Stannard JP, Bucknell AL. Rupture of the triceps tendon associated with steroid injection. *Am J Sports Med* 1993;21:482.

Strauch RJ. Biceps and triceps injuries of the elbow. *Orthop Clin North Am* 1999;30:95.

Viegas SF. Avulsion of the triceps tendon. *Orthop Rev* 1990;19:533.

Waugh RL, Hathcock TA, Elliot JL. Ruptures of muscles and tendons. *Surgery* 1949;25:370.

Author: Robert L. Jones

Turf Toe

Basics

DEFINITION

- Hyperextension sprain of the first metatarsophalangeal (MTP) joint

INCIDENCE/PREVALENCE

- Marked increase in incidence since the introduction of artificial turf

SIGNS AND SYMPTOMS

- Grade 1 sprain: pain over plantar or medial aspect, no ecchymosis, minimal swelling, and limited pain with weight bearing
- Grade 2 sprain: more intense and diffuse pain of the MTP joint, pain with motion, and significant pain with weight bearing, causing a limp
- Grade 3 sprain: marked swelling, ecchymosis, severe pain with motion, and inability to bear weight

RISK FACTORS

- Playing on artificial turf, more flexible shoewear, decreased flexibility of first MTP joint (abnormal motion is <60 degrees of dorsiflexion)
- Running backs or offensive linemen are more susceptible.
- Decreased ankle range of motion, pes planus, and flattening of the first metatarsal head may be risk factors.

MECHANISMS

- Most common mechanism is a hyperextension injury to the MTP joint. This causes tearing of the joint capsule at the metatarsal neck.
- A hyperflexion injury can also cause symptoms of turf toe. This results in a sprain of the dorsal capsule.
- A valgus type injury can occur but is unusual and is associated with other injuries.

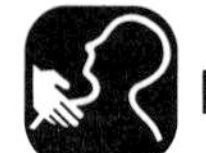

Diagnosis

DIFFERENTIAL DIAGNOSIS

- Fracture of the first metatarsal or proximal phalanx, sesamoiditis, strain of flexor hallucis

HISTORY

- Hyperextension or toeing off
- May be recurrent injury
- Can be very painful

PHYSICAL EXAM

- Restricted range of motion of the MTP joint with swelling and ecchymosis
- Difficulty weight bearing, especially with toe off
- May have laxity of the ligamentous capsule; degree and position depending on mechanism of injury

IMAGING

- Standard three views of foot; may need oblique views to rule out sesamoid fracture
- Bony pathology that can be seen: small capsular avulsions, fractures of the sesamoids, separation of bipartite sesamoid, or proximal migration of sesamoid
- Stress views can show gross instability of the joint.
- CT may show loose body or sesamoid fracture.

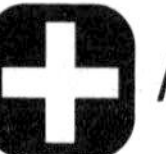

Acute Treatment

ANALGESIA

- Ice
- Nonsteroidal antiinflammatory drugs
- Rest

IMMOBILIZATION

- Immobilization of the first MTP joint may be needed for pain relief, but early controlled range of motion is crucial.
- Loss of motion of the first MTP is a common problem after this injury and may increase the risk for further injury.
- May need stiff shoe or steel shank to prevent further injury.

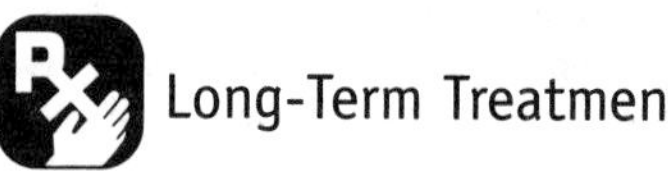

Long-Term Treatment

REHABILITATION

- Early range of motion is key.
- Using a steel shank insert for the shoe may allow the athlete to return to play sooner.
- The athlete should be evaluated for custom orthotics, especially if this is a chronic injury.

SURGICAL TREATMENT

Surgery for this type of injury is rarely needed. Possible indications for surgery would be a loose body in the first MTP joint, sesamoid fracture, separation or migration of the sesamoid, or gross instability of the first MTP joint.

REFERRAL/DISPOSITION

Referral should be considered if the athlete has not responded to conservative treatment. Depending on the degree of injury, this could be 2 weeks to 2 to 3 months.

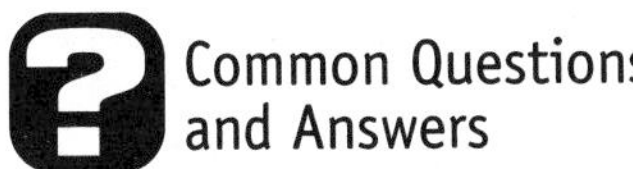

Common Questions and Answers

Physician responses to common patient questions:

Q: When can I go back to playing?

A: If the athlete can pass a typical functional progression for that sport and do so without pain or limp, then he or she can return to play. The functional progression should be undertaken using an orthotic apparatus or insert if needed.

Q: If I go back too early, will it cause further damage?

A: There are problems to going back too early. If the athlete cannot perform without limp, he or she is at risk for reinjury. Specifically for turf toe, the key is early range of motion. If this is not addressed, risk for reinjury is increased.

Q: Will a corticosteroid shot help me get back sooner?

A: Studies have not shown quicker return with the use of a corticosteroid injection.

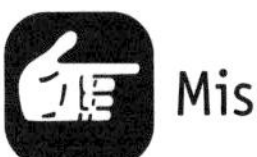

Miscellaneous

SYNONYMS

- Astroturf toe
- First MTP sprain

ICD-9 CODE

845.16 Sprain/strain, metatarsophalangeal joint
825.25 Fracture, metatarsophalangeal
827.0 Fracture, sesamoid
826.0 Fracture, phalanges, foot

BIBLIOGRAPHY

Clanton TO, Ford JJ. Turf toe injury. *Clin Sports Med* 1994;13:731–741.

DeLee JC, Drez DD. *Orthopedic sports medicine.* Philadelphia: WB Saunders, 1994.

Author: Eric Jenkinson

Ulnar Collateral Ligament Injuries of the Elbow

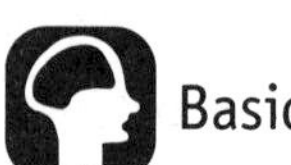

Basics

DEFINITION

- Pain and instability at the medial aspect of the elbow due to a sprain, attenuation, or rupture of the ulnar collateral ligament
- Incompetence of the ulnar collateral ligament is associated with medial elbow laxity.

ANATOMY

- Ulnar collateral ligament is made up of three bands: anterior, posterior, and transverse.
- The anterior band is taut in both flexion and extension of the elbow and is the primary stabilizer of the medial elbow. The anterior band itself is made up of anterior and posterior bundles, of which the posterior bundle is felt to be most important in providing medial elbow stability. Disruption of the anterior band leads to medial elbow instability.
- The posterior band is taut when the elbow is flexed beyond 90 degrees, but does not alter elbow stability if disrupted.
- The transverse band plays no role in joint stability because its origin and insertion is on the same bone.

INCIDENCE/PREVALENCE

- Common with sports requiring high-velocity throwing or overhead activities
- Most commonly seen in skeletally mature individuals 16 to 40 years of age
- Males affected more often than females

SIGNS AND SYMPTOMS

- Medial elbow pain, especially during the late cocking and/or acceleration phase of throwing
- Sensation of the elbow "opening" during throws
- Decreased velocity and/or distance of throws
- Lateral and posterior elbow pain, especially if throwing continues

MECHANISMS

- Valgus stress applied to the elbow acutely, but more often due to chronic valgus stress

RISK FACTORS

- Participation in sports requiring high-velocity throwing or overhead activity (i.e., baseball pitching, javelin throwing)

ASSOCIATED INJURIES AND COMPLICATIONS

- Ulnar nerve symptoms: Pain and paresthesias to the ulnar aspect of the forearm, hypothenar region of the hand, and fourth and fifth digits; secondary to an ulnar neuritis arising from compression, traction, inflammation, subluxation from the cubital tunnel, or abrasion on osteophytes of the ulnar nerve
- Valgus-extension overload syndrome: Posterior elbow pain during valgus stress from posteromedial olecranon impingement within the olecranon fossa due to ulnar collateral ligament incompetence
- Radiocapitellar overload syndrome: Lateral elbow pain during valgus stress as force across the radiocapitellar joint increases due to ulnar collateral ligament incompetence

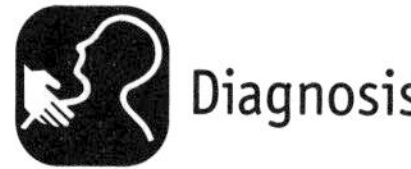

Diagnosis

DIFFERENTIAL DIAGNOSIS

- Medial epicondylitis
- Medial epicondylar apophysitis (in the skeletally immature athlete)
- Medial epicondylar physeal fracture (in the skeletally immature athlete)
- Flexor-pronator muscle tear
- Osteochondritis dissecans
- Ulnar neuritis
- Osteoarthritis
- Loose bodies
- Triceps tendonitis

HISTORY

- Classically, medial elbow pain acutely starts with a single "pop" or giving way of the elbow during a throw. It is often preceded by low-grade elbow pain before the single event. May indicate acute rupture of the ulnar collateral ligament.
- More often, low-grade medial elbow pain worsens with continued throwing without any history of a single throw as an initiating event. May indicate sprain or attenuation of the ulnar collateral ligament.

PHYSICAL EXAM

- Pain on palpation 2 cm distal to the medial epicondyle at the insertion of the ulnar collateral ligament on the ulna
- Pain worsened by valgus stress applied to the elbow
- Valgus stress test: To detect medial elbow instability, firmly lock the athlete's hand and wrist between the examiner's elbow and trunk. Bend the athlete's elbow 30 degrees to free the olecranon from the olecranon fossa. With the heel of the examiner's hand, gently apply valgus stress to the elbow. Palpate the medial joint line with a thumb or finger over the ulnar collateral ligament feeling for laxity at the medial joint line of the elbow. Compare the laxity to the contralateral elbow. Increased laxity or no firm end point indicates incompetence of the ulnar collateral ligament due to rupture or attenuation.
- Milking Maneuver: Flex the athlete's elbow to 90 degrees with forearm in supination. Apply traction on the athlete's thumb while palpating the medial joint line of the elbow, feeling for laxity in the ulnar collateral ligament. This maneuver effectively detects laxity in the important posterior bundle of the anterior band of the ulnar collateral ligament.
- Tinel's sign of the ulnar nerve

IMAGING

- Radiographs [anteroposterior (AP), lateral, oblique]: Radiographs can show calcification within the ulnar collateral ligament, indicating chronic stress and injury. Osteophytes seen at the olecranon and/or proximal ulna may be secondary signs of instability. In the skeletally immature athlete, comparison views of the contralateral elbow may need to be obtained to compare widths of the medial epicondyle apophyses. Medial epicondylar fractures displaced 5 mm or more warrant orthopedic consultation.
- Gravity valgus stress radiographs: Athlete is supine with shoulder abducted 90 degrees in full external rotation, forearm in full supination, and elbow in 30 degrees of flexion. The shoulder is supported by the edge of the x-ray table but the forearm is allowed to hang by gravity. AP radiographs of both elbows are taken in this position, and the distance of the medial joint space at the ulnohumeral articulation is measured. A larger measurement in the affected elbow suggests medial elbow laxity due to an incompetent ulnar collateral ligament.
- Manual stress radiographs: Valgus stress is manually applied to the elbow over the x-ray table in similar fashion as performing a valgus stress test. AP radiographs of both elbows are taken in this position, and the same measurements as in the gravity stress radiographs are taken to determine medial elbow laxity.
- MRI: Can show partial or full-thickness tears of the ulnar collateral ligament. False-negative readings may be encountered with ulnar collateral ligament attenuation.
- MR arthrography and CT arthrography: Valuable in determining partial undersurface tears of the ulnar collateral ligament.

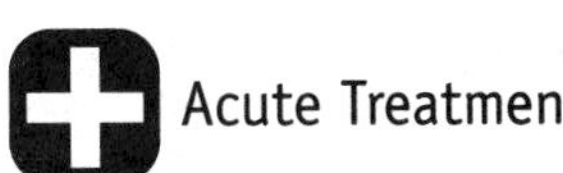

Acute Treatment

ANALGESIA

- Ice elbow 20 minutes three times daily as needed.
- Nonsteroidal antiinflammatory drugs as needed

IMMOBILIZATION

- Immobilization with sling as needed

ACTIVITY MODIFICATION

- No throwing or painful elbow activities until cleared by a physician

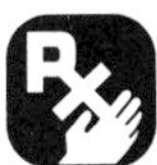

Long-Term Treatment

SURGICAL TREATMENT

- Surgical reconstruction is indicated for the complete rupture of the ulnar collateral ligament or failed nonsurgical treatment after 3 to 6 months in the athlete who desires a return to high-level competitive throwing or overhead sports.
- The gold standard for reconstruction of the ulnar collateral ligament is use of a free autogenous graft (palmaris longus tendon).
- Postoperative rehabilitation programs vary, but most incorporate hand and wrist motion exercises immediately with transfer from a posterior splint to a functional brace at 2 weeks. Wrist and elbow strengthening exercises are initiated, and full elbow range of motion is expected by about 6 weeks.
- Throwing generally can begin by 4 months with return to competitive throwing after 6 months to 1 year.

NONSURGICAL TREATMENT

- If evaluation reveals no complete tear of the ulnar collateral ligament, early nonsurgical treatment can be initiated.
- Complete rest for 2 to 4 weeks; active range of motion allowed when pain free
- Physical therapy modalities of ice, heat, phonophoresis, ionophoresis, and electrical stimulation can be used to aid healing.
- After pain-free rest of 2 to 4 weeks, begin wrist- and elbow-strengthening program.
- Begin throwing program at about 3 months if elbow has full range of motion and strength equal to the contralateral side.
- Start with short toss throws then slowly progress to stages of long toss, 50%, 75%, and 100% velocity throws.
- The number of throws at each stage and the time to full velocity must be coordinated with the athlete, physician, rehabilitation specialist/athletic trainer, and coach.
- Persistence of elbow pain and medial instability despite 3 to 6 months of nonsurgical treatment is an indication for surgical treatment.

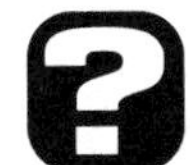

Common Questions and Answers

Physician responses to common patient questions:

Q: Do I need surgery?

A: Yes, for the athlete diagnosed with a complete rupture of the ulnar collateral ligament who desires to return to high-level throwing or overhead sports, surgery is indicated. If the ulnar collateral ligament is not torn, but instead sprained or attenuated, a trial of nonsurgical treatment is warranted with hopes that healing will take place. If there is no improvement (i.e., continued pain and instability symptoms) in 3 to 6 months, then surgical reconstruction should be considered.

Q: Will my completely ruptured ulnar collateral ligament heal by itself?

A: No, not to the degree that it allows the athlete to return to high-velocity throwing or overhead sports. Rest and rehabilitation allow for some scarring of a completely torn ulnar collateral ligament so that the majority of daily activities can be performed without pain. However, this type of healing usually will not fully restore a completely torn ulnar collateral ligament sufficiently to allow for effective return in throwing athletes.

Q: After surgery, will I be able to throw as well as I did before?

A: With current surgical techniques and rehabilitation protocols, return to an athlete's previous level of competition is about 68% after ulnar collateral ligament reconstruction. Whether or not the athlete returns with the same level of effectiveness using the same style of play is controversial, and determination is made on an individual basis.

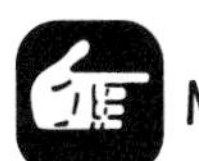

Miscellaneous

ICD-9 CODE

841.1 Ulnar collateral ligament sprain (including rupture)

BIBLIOGRAPHY

Ciccotti MG, Jobe FW. Medial collateral ligament instability and ulnar neuritis in the athlete's elbow. *Instr Course Lect* 1999;48:383–391.

Conway JE, Jobe FW, Glousman RE, Pink M. Medical instability of the elbow in throwing athletes. Treatment by repair or reconstruction of the ulnar collateral ligament. *J Bone Joint Surg Am* 1992;74(1): 67–83.

Fritz RC, Steinbach LS, Tirman PFJ, et al. MR imaging of the elbow: an update. *Radiol Clin North Am* 1997;35:117–114.

Safran MR. Elbow injuries in athletes. *Clin Orthop Rel Res* 1995;310:257–277.

Authors: Quincy Wang, Aaron L. Rubin, and Marc R. Safran

Ulnar Nerve Palsy

Basics

DEFINITION

- Any abnormal condition with inflammation and wasting of the ulnar nerve

ANATOMY

- The ulnar nerve arises from the medial cord of the brachial plexus and is composed of fibers from the C8 and T1 nerve roots.
- The nerve passes from the anterior to the posterior compartment of the arm, giving off no branches in the upper arm.
- It penetrates the arcade of Struthers, which is a fibrous raphe located 8 cm above the medial epicondyle and formed by the medial intramuscular septum, medial head of the triceps, and deep investing fascia of the arm and internal brachial ligament.
- The nerve passes behind the medial epicondyle into the cubital tunnel, whose boundaries are the ulnar collateral ligament of the elbow, medial edge of the trochlea, medial epicondylar groove, and arcuate ligament.
- The ulnar nerve then passes between the humeral and ulnar heads of the flexor carpi ulnaris.
- After coursing through the flexor carpi ulnaris, it exits by piercing the deep surface of the muscle to lie between the flexor carpi ulnaris and flexor digitorum profundus.
- The ulnar nerve enters the hand by passing through Guyon's canal, formed by the volar carpal ligament, the hamate, the pisiform, and the pisohamate ligament.

INNERVATION BY THE ULNAR NERVE

- Articular branch to the elbow joint
- Motor branches to the flexor carpi ulnaris and medial half of the flexor digitorum profundus
- Motor branches to intrinsic muscles of the hand and ulnar innervated muscles of the hypothenar eminence
- Sensory branches to the fifth digit and medial half of the fourth digit and medial aspects of the palmar and dorsal surfaces of the hand

SIGNS AND SYMPTOMS

- Point tenderness in the upper arm, elbow, or forearm, most often in the medial aspect
- Paresthesias (early) or sensory loss (late) of the ring and small fingers
- Feeling of clumsiness or incoordination in the hand, especially after overhead or throwing activities in the athlete
- Muscle wasting of the intrinsic muscles of the hand
- Hypothenar eminence atrophy
- Weakness of the flexor carpi ulnaris and flexor digitorum profundus is rarely seen

MECHANISMS

- Direct trauma
- Compression
- Entrapment
- Traction injury
- In the throwing athlete, the condition usually results from direct injury or as part of the lateral compression and medial tension forces involved in the act of throwing.
- In cyclists, ulnar nerve compression occurs more commonly at Guyon's canal from direct pressure from the handle bar.

RISK FACTORS

- Subluxing or hypermobile ulnar nerve
- Congenital cubitus valgus deformity
- Posttraumatic valgus deformity following an elbow fracture
- Several systemic and metabolic conditions (e.g., diabetes mellitus, hypothyroidism, multiple myeloma, hemophilia, renal disease, acromegaly)
- Occupational activities (e.g., keyboard operators, those who do excessive driving, repetitive heavy lifting)
- Lesions in the cubital tunnel or Guyon's canal (e.g., ganglia, osteophytes, osteoarthritis, tumors, synovial cysts, rheumatoid arthritis, anomalous muscles)
- Certain athletic activities (e.g., repetitive overhand throwing, cycling)

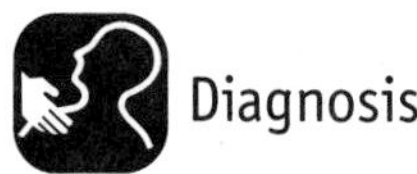

Diagnosis

DIFFERENTIAL DIAGNOSIS

- Cervical disc lesion
- Thoracic outlet syndrome
- Pancoast's tumor
- Metabolic problems causing diffuse peripheral neuropathies
- Multiple sclerosis and other myelopathies
- Carpal tunnel syndrome
- Medial epicondylitis

HISTORY

- Early in course, patients often report symptoms as being intermittent.
- Paresthesias and tingling of forearm and hand occur before motor weakness of the hand is experienced.
- Athletes may report a history of a feeling of clumsiness in the hand, especially with throwing.
- As condition progresses, the athlete may report a decrease in performance.
- Question about possible external sources of compression (e.g., leaning elbow on a desk or arm rest for long periods of time).
- Obtain any history of past or recent elbow injury.

PHYSICAL EXAM

- Inspect elbow for deformities (flexion contractures, varus and posttraumatic deformities).
- Examine muscles for atrophy (hypothenar eminence, intrinsic hand muscles, and forearm flexors).
- Observe the hand for any evidence of claw deformity.
- Examination of cervical spine, including range of motion and Spurling's test
- Thoracic outlet testing: Adson's test, Allen's maneuver, Wright's test
- Tinel's sign may be elicited by tapping over the course of the ulnar nerve and may help to localize site of compression.
- Elbow flexion test is performed by holding elbow in maximum flexion for 60 seconds and attempting to elicit distal symptoms.
- Examine the ulnar groove of the elbow for evidence of a dislocating ulnar nerve or one that may be manually subluxed.
- Evaluation of the wrist includes Allen's test and attempt to elicit Tinel's sign over carpal tunnel and Guyon's canal.
- Sensory evaluation includes two-point discrimination of fingers and palmar and dorsal surfaces of the hand.
- Motor examination includes muscle strength testing of flexor digitorum profundus (ring and small fingers compared with index finger) and intrinsic muscles of the hand (finger abduction and adduction).
- Pinch meter testing and grip testing may detect more subtle weaknesses.
- Froment's sign: Patient attempts to grasp a piece of paper between thumb and index finger. Result is positive if, when paper is pulled away, the distal phalanx of the thumb flexes, indicating weakness of the adductor pollicis.

IMAGING

Radiography

- Anteroposterior (AP) and lateral plain films of the elbow in addition to a cubital tunnel view (elbow is maximally flexed and the beam directed as an AP view of the distal humerus)

Electrodiagnostic Studies

- Electromyography
- Nerve conduction velocity
- Often helpful when positive, but negative studies do not rule out the diagnosis
- Useful in sorting out ulnar nerve compression at the wrist from a more proximal lesion

CLASSIFICATION BY SEVERITY OF SYMPTOMS

- McGowan grade I: only paresthesias and minor hypesthesia of ulnar nerve
- McGowan grade II: weakness of the interossei
- McGowan grade III: obvious sensory loss, muscle atrophy, occasional clawing of the ring and small fingers, and significant functional motor impairment

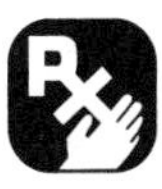

Long-Term Treatment

REHABILITATION

- Can attempt conservative treatment in patients with McGowan grade I
- Purpose is to minimize the pressure increases around the ulnar nerve with elbow flexion or direct pressure
- Avoidance of recurrent valgus stress and direct pressure
- Icing can help prevent edema and inflammation about the ulnar nerve
- Antiinflammatory medication
- For cubital tunnel syndrome, can use an anterior splint with the elbow positioned at 30 degrees of flexion for several weeks
- Local steroid injection for compression at elbow has not been found to be effective.
- When site of compression is Guyon's canal, try splinting the wrist in slight dorsiflexion. Local injection of corticosteroid may be effective at this site if patient fails activity modification and oral antiinflammatory medications.
- In the throwing athlete, prior to return to play (following surgery or conservative management), throwing biomechanics should be observed and appropriate changes made as indicated.

SURGICAL TREATMENT

- Indicated for patients with McGowan grade I compression who fail conservative treatment and for patients with McGowan grade II or III compression
- Decompression: indicated for localized compression of the nerve by the aponeurosis between the two heads of the flexor carpi ulnaris or by the muscle itself
- Anterior transposition of the ulnar nerve: nerve brought to new position anterior to the medial epicondyle, either in subcutaneous or submuscular position, depending on the procedure performed
- Medial epicondylectomy: not recommended for the athlete due to the vulnerability of the origin of the ulnar collateral ligament and anatomic changes that occur when reattaching the flexor pronator muscle mass
- For Guyon's canal syndrome, a surgical release of the canal is performed in combination with surgical release of the carpal tunnel.

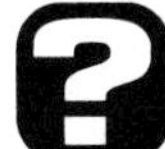

Common Questions and Answers

Physician responses to common patient questions:

Q: Will I get normal feeling and use of my hand and arm back?

A: Prognosis for this disorder is dependent on the severity of symptoms. There have been good results in getting athletes back to preoperative level of activity when surgery has been needed. However, as the degree of compression increases, the likelihood of full return of function decreases.

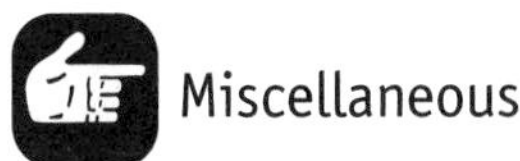

Miscellaneous

SYNONYMS

- Ulnar neuropathy
- Ulnar neuritis
- Ulnar nerve entrapment
- Ulnar nerve impingement
- Cubital tunnel syndrome
- Guyon's canal syndrome
- Handle bar palsy

ICD-9 CODE

354.2 Ulnar nerve neuropathy

BIBLIOGRAPHY

DeLee JC, Drez D Jr. *Orthopaedic sports medicine*. Philadelphia: WB Saunders, 1994.

Glousman RE. Ulnar nerve problems in the athlete's elbow. *Clin Sports Med* 1990;9: 365–377.

Halpern B, Herring SA, Altchek D, et al. *Imaging in musculoskeletal and sports medicine*. Malden, MA: Blackwell Science, 1997.

Magee DJ. *Orthopedic physical assessment*. Philadelphia: WB Saunders, 1997.

Norkus SA, Meyers MC. Ulnar neuropathy of the elbow. *Sports Med* 1994;17:189–199.

Author: Linda Mansfield

Vertebrobasilar Arterial Insufficiency

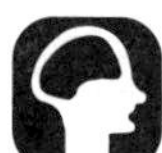

Basics

DEFINITION

- An interruption of blood flow to the vertebrobasilar (posterior) circulation, which constitutes the arterial supply to the brainstem, cerebellum, and occipital cortex
- Symptoms are dependent on which branch or branches of the vertebrobasilar circulation that have been compromised.
- The term *vertebrobasilar insufficiency* refers to all transient ischemic attack (TIA) syndromes of the posterior circulation.

INCIDENCE/PREVALENCE

- In the United States, approximately one fourth of strokes and TIAs occur in the vertebrobasilar distribution.
- Brainstem infarctions have been reported in autopsy series at a rate of 2 per 1,000 cases.
- One clinical study suggested that the disease occurs 25% as frequently as occlusion of the carotid artery and its branches.
- Embolic phenomena cause infarction in the vertebrobasilar territory in 9% to 40% of reported cases.
- Affects men twice as often as women
- More frequent in individuals over age 70

SIGNS AND SYMPTOMS

- Dizziness
- Vertigo
- Diplopia
- Visual field defects
- Nystagmus
- Dysphagia
- Limb ataxia
- Truncal ataxia (falling to side of lesion)
- Contralateral deficit in pain and temperature perception
- Ipsilateral limb and trunk numbness
- Ipsilateral loss of taste
- Cranial nerve palsies
- Bilateral limb weakness

RISK FACTORS

General

- Atherosclerosis is the most common cause; therefore, patients with cardiovascular risk factors such as age, hypertension, diabetes, smoking, and dyslipidemias are at higher risk.
- Infarction causes a vestibular syndrome that typically has an abrupt onset in patients with risk factors for stroke, such as hypertension, diabetes, smoking, known occlusive vascular disease, or myocardial abnormalities, including atrial fibrillation and valvular heart disease.
- Other disease processes that can impact arterial supply include fibromuscular dysplasia and vertebrobasilar aneurysms.

Sports Specific

- Any sport that predisposes the athlete to mechanical occlusion or stenosis of the vertebral artery at the C1–2 level; most often caused by lateral flexion (e.g., Bow hunter's stroke)
- Neck trauma leading to vertebral artery dissection

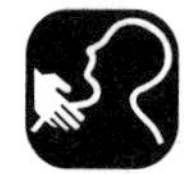

Diagnosis

DIFFERENTIAL DIAGNOSIS

- Benign positional vertigo
- Vertebral artery dissection
- Labyrinthitis
- Multiple sclerosis
- Stroke
- TIA
- Vestibular neuronitis
- Vertebrobasilar aneurysm
- Basilar artery dissection
- Basilar artery migraine
- Posterior fossa tumor
- Vasculitis

HISTORY

- A high degree of clinical suspicion is necessary in the young healthy athlete.
- Vertigo is the hallmark symptom and often described as a swimming or swaying sensation.
- Vertigo may be the only symptom in one third of patients.
- Disabling vertigo may remain for days; usually improves within the first week, and resolves within weeks to months
- Vertigo from a brainstem stroke is usually accompanied by other symptoms, including diplopia, reduced vision, dysarthria, dysphagia, and focal sensory or motor deficits
- These additional findings distinguish a brainstem stroke from vestibular neuritis.
- Infarction and hemorrhage of the inferior cerebellum, however, can cause vertigo, nystagmus, and postural instability, with few additional symptoms that distinguish this condition from vestibular neuritis.
- Abrupt onset of isolated vertigo lasting for minutes suggests a TIA.
- TIAs often last less than 30 minutes.
- Isolated transient vertigo may precede a stroke in the branches of the vertebrobasilar artery by weeks or months.

PHYSICAL EXAM

- The hallmark of posterior circulation stroke is crossed neurologic deficits (i.e., ipsilateral cranial nerve deficits with contralateral motor weakness).
- Infarction or hemorrhage of the brainstem or the cerebellum may cause nystagmus that changes its direction with a change in the direction of gaze (gaze-evoked nystagmus).
- In patients with cerebellar stroke, nystagmus may be present only when the patient is gazing in one direction, thereby appearing similar to a peripheral vestibular nystagmus.
- Purely vertical nystagmus or torsional nystagmus are almost always due to a central disorder, whereas horizontal and torsional components may occur simultaneously in patients with either peripheral or central disorders.
- Visual fixation may have little effect on the intensity of central vestibular nystagmus.
- Patients with acute cerebellar stroke are often unable to walk without falling, and with the Romberg test the direction of tilting or falling may be variable.
- The type of nystagmus and the severity of postural instability can help to differentiate a peripheral vestibular disorder from an inferior cerebellar stroke (the former produces nystagmus that remains in the same direction when the direction of gaze changes and is suppressed by visual fixation, whereas the latter causes other forms of nystagmus).
- A peripheral vestibular lesion produces unidirectional postural instability with preserved walking, whereas an inferior cerebellar stroke often causes severe postural instability and falling when walking is attempted.
- The presence of cranial nerve signs, motor weakness, prominent dysmetria (past pointing), sensory changes, or abnormal reflexes suggests a central process.
- The absence of additional neurologic findings does not exclude the possibility of a stroke limited to the inferior cerebellum.
- Dysmetria, a major finding of the cerebellar system, may be minimal or absent after an inferior cerebellar stroke.

IMAGING/LABORATORY STUDIES

- Immediate brain imaging is mandatory when a central process is likely, particularly to rule out an evolving cerebellar hematoma that would require emergency neurosurgical intervention.
- Brain imaging is recommended when the examination of a patient with the acute vestibular syndrome does not result in the findings that are typical of a peripheral vestibular disorder.
- Imaging is recommended if the onset of symptoms is sudden in a patient with risk factors for stroke or if there is a new, severe headache accompanying the acute vertigo.
- The decision whether to perform brain imaging can be deferred for 48 hours if the patient has isolated acute vertigo, peripheral vestibular nystagmus that is suppressed by visual fixation, and is unstable but can still walk.
- If there is marked improvement in 48 hours, the syndrome is consistent with a vestibular neuritis, and brain imaging is not necessary.
- When immediate brain imaging is indicated, MRI and angiography are preferred.
- During the first day of vertigo, routine MRI is a sensitive method for detecting an inferior cerebellar infarction, but may be less sensitive for identifying a hemorrhage (imaging sequences that maximize the identification of both infarction and hemorrhage in the posterior fossa should therefore be requested).
- If prompt MRI and angiography are not available, then CT of the brain should be performed, with fine cuts through the cerebellum and clear visualization of the fourth ventricle, to rule out a cerebellar hemorrhage.
- CT scans of the cerebellum are usually normal in the first hours after an infarction in the cerebellum, although asymmetry in the fourth ventricle may be an early sign of swelling.
- If immediate brain imaging is indicated and a normal CT scan is obtained on the first day of acute vertigo, then subsequent MRI and angiography are recommended.
- Other tests that may be helpful to limit the differential diagnoses and that would preclude such therapies as anticoagulants include chest radiography, complete blood count, electrolytes, blood urea nitrogen, serum glucose, erythrocyte sedimentation rate, urinalysis, thyroid function tests, Venereal Disease Research Laboratory test, coagulation profile, and electrocardiography.

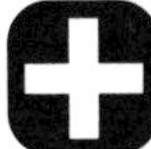

Acute Treatment

- As above
- Supportive measures such as securing the airway, maintaining breathing, and circulation
- Cautious control of blood pressure, because a precipitous decrease can impact cerebral perfusion pressure
- Consider antihypertensive medication only in cases of hypertensive emergencies with ongoing end-organ damage, a mean arterial pressure greater than 130 mm Hg, or systolic blood pressure greater than 220 mm Hg.
- Intravenous therapy to provide isotonic hydration and to avoid hyperglycemia, which appears to exacerbate neuronal injury in stroke.
- Treat vomiting with antiemetics to avoid aspiration.
- Consult the Neurology Department.
- Neurosurgery is indicated for surgical evacuation of cerebellar hemorrhages and to manage cerebellar infarction complicated by hydrocephalus.
- Consider interventional neuroradiology (i.e., intraarterial thrombolysis or percutaneous transluminal cerebral angioplasty).

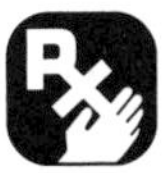

Long-Term Treatment

- Antiplatelet agents such as aspirin are the first line of treatment for patients with vertebrobasilar arterial thrombotic disease once hemorrhagic lesions have been excluded
- No randomized clinical trials have been conducted to determine antiplatelet therapy's efficacy in treating vertebrobasilar arterial thrombotic disease.
- No randomized clinical trials involving patients with vertebrobasilar TIAs have compared anticoagulants with antiplatelet therapy or placebos.
- A strong argument favoring the use of anticoagulants in vertebrobasilar arterial thrombotic disease would exist in settings where the embolic source of thrombi is known or suspected (i.e., atrial fibrillation).
- Use of low-molecular-weight heparins has shown no significant increase in outcome over conventional treatments.
- Patients who have had vertebrobasilar TIAs generally have a more favorable prognosis than those with carotid territory TIAs because there is less risk in developing a completed stroke. Collateral circulation may account for improved outcome in these patients.

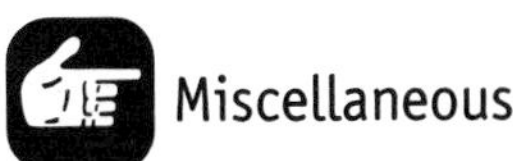

Miscellaneous

MEDICAL/LEGAL PITFALLS

- Failure to recognize etiology of vertigo in the elderly
- Failure to avoid excluding vertebrobasilar arterial thrombotic disease on the basis of a negative CT scan
- Failure to initiate therapy after hemorrhage has been reliably excluded
- Failure to initiate antiplatelet therapy when diagnosis of brainstem infarction is suspected may increase likelihood of permanent ischemic deficits.
- Failure to take precautions when feeding patients with brainstem infarction

ICD-9 CODE

435.3

BIBLIOGRAPHY

Hotson JR, Baloh RW. Acute vestibular syndrome. *N Engl J Med* 1998;339:680–685.

Lang E. Vertebrobasilar atherothrombotic disease. http://www/emedicine.com/emerg/topic834.htm.

Neurologic disorders. In: *Harrison's textbook of internal medicine*. 2330–2339.

Author: William W. Dexter

SECTION II

Population-Specific Musculoskeletal Injuries

Avascular Necrosis of the Proximal Femoral Epiphysis (Legg-Calve-Perthes Disease)

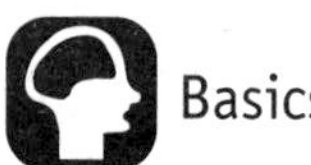

Basics

DEFINITION

- Juvenile idiopathic avascular necrosis of the femoral head
- Affects children 2 to 13 years of age, but is most common between ages 4 and 9 years, mean age 7
- More common among boys than girls (5:1)
- Most prevalent among whites and Chinese, rare in blacks and Native Americans
- Bilateral in 10%

INCIDENCE/PREVALENCE

- Incidence in general population 1 in 1,200 to 1 in 12,000
- Prevalence 75 in 100,000

SIGNS AND SYMPTOMS

- Painless limp; if painful, it is worse with activity and relieved by rest
- Referred pain to groin, anterior thigh, or knee
- Limited range of motion (ROM) and muscle atrophy

RISK FACTORS

- Low birth weight
- Short stature
- Delayed bone maturation
- Involved family member (after index sibling incidence 1 in 35)
- Familial thrombophilia and hypofibrinolysis (controversial)

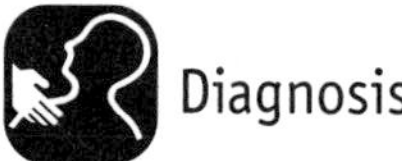

Diagnosis

DIFFERENTIAL DIAGNOSIS

- Inflammatory: septic arthritis, osteomyelitis, transient synovitis
- Trauma: fracture
- Neoplasm
- Congenital: limb abnormality
- Developmental: hip dysplasia, slipped capital femoral epiphysis

HISTORY

- Is there any pain?
- Does pain vary with activity?
- How long has the limp/pain been present? Inflammatory synovitis can mimic Legg-Calve-Perthes disease (LCPD) but usually resolves in 10 to 14 days. LCPD symptoms are present for about 6 weeks.

PHYSICAL EXAM

- Exam of the musculoskeletal system with a focus on the pelvis and lower extremities
- Include ROM testing; limited abduction and internal rotation; hip flexion contracture +/−
- Evaluate for muscle atrophy of the thigh, calf, and buttocks, which is seen in long-standing cases.
- Measure for possible leg length discrepancy, which indicates advanced involvement of the femoral head.
- Evaluate gait. Trendelenburg gait is observed with abductor weakness.
- Perform log roll test of extended leg on exam table; painful and reduced ROM is observed compared with the opposite side.

IMAGING

- Anteroposterior and frog-leg lateral views of pelvis; can appear normal early in course
- Femoral head appears smaller then opposite with a widened articular cartilage space.
- With disease progression, a crescent-shaped radiolucent line may be seen in the central portion of the femoral head, especially on the lateral view.
- Fracture, fragmentation, and resorption
- Extent of femoral head involvement determines severity of disease.
- Bone scan and MRI can be used to evaluate before radiographic changes are apparent.

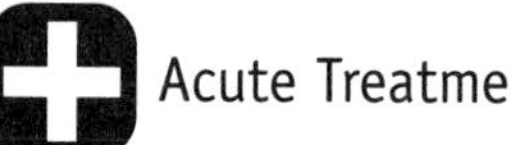

Acute Treatment

ANALGESIA

- Standard doses of nonsteroidal antiinflammatory drugs help reduce the synovitis.
- Nonpharmacologic: activity restriction, crutches for non-weight bearing, and bed rest

IMMOBILIZATION

- Abduction bracing/casting can be used for symptom relief and to hold the femoral head in the acetabulum.
- Casting/bracing may be discontinued when there is radiographic evidence of subchondral reossification, usually after 12 to 18 months.
- Nonsurgical treatment is controversial due to several recent studies showing no change in outcomes.

SPECIAL CONSIDERATIONS

Both surgical and nonsurgical treatments are aimed at symptom reduction, prevention of capital femoral epiphysis destruction, and attainment of a spherical femoral head at healing.

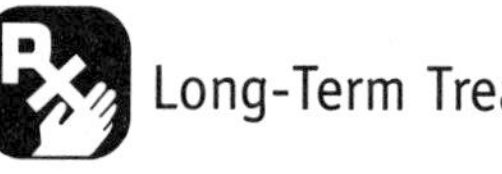

Long-Term Treatment

REHABILITATION

- Formal therapy program recommended during and after bracing due to extensive atrophy, contracture, and loss of motion
- Home stretching program encouraged to maintain ROM

SURGICAL TREATMENT

- Goal is containment of femoral head leading to round femoral head.
- Techniques vary depending on age of child and severity of femoral head involvement.
- Advantages include less time required in a brace and earlier return to activity.
- Disadvantages include necessity of two operations.

REFERRAL/DISPOSITION

All patients with suspected LCPD should be referred to an orthopedic surgeon immediately.

Avascular Necrosis of the Proximal Femoral Epiphysis (Legg-Calve-Perthes Disease)

Common Questions and Answers

Physician responses to common patient questions:

Q: Will my child get better?

A: LCPD is a self-limiting, self-healing disease lasting 2 to 4 years. The shape of the femoral head, age of onset, duration of disease, and ROM all factor into the prognosis.

Q: Will my child always limp? Can he or she play sports later in life?

A: During the disease the limp will likely persist. Children with LCPD are able to play sports once the disease has resolved and ROM and strength have returned. Depending on the degree of residual damage to the femoral head, high-impact contact sports are contraindicated

Q: What are the long-term consequences of LCPD?

A: If left untreated, 50% of patients will develop osteoarthritis by the fifth to sixth decade of life. The extent of femoral head deformity correlates with the degree of arthritic involvement. Osteochondritis dissecans occurs in about 5% of patients with LCPD.

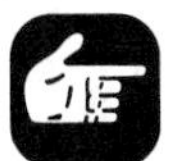

Miscellaneous

SYNONYMS

- Perthes disease

ICD-9 CODE

732.1 Juvenile osteochondrosis of hip and pelvis

BIBLIOGRAPHY

Koop S, Quanbeck D. Common orthopedic problems II. *Pediatr Clin North Am* 1996;43:1053–1066.

Roy D. Current concepts in Legg-Calve-Perthes disease. *Pediatr Ann* 1999;28:748–751.

Thompsin G, Scoles P. The hip. In: Behrman R, ed. *Nelson textbook of pediatrics*, 16th ed. Philadelphia: WB Saunders, 2000: 2077–2082.

Author: Andrew Dahlgren

Calcaneal Apophysitis (Sever's Disease)

Basics

DEFINITION

- Sever's disease, also known as calcaneal apophysitis, is an overuse syndrome causing adolescent heel pain. This traction apophysitis is the foot equivalent to Osgood-Schlatter disease.

ANATOMY

- The posterior calcaneus develops as a secondary ossification center.
- This secondary ossification center provides attachment for the tendoachilles.
- This secondary ossification site is not contiguous with a diarthrodial joint; therefore, this portion of bone is called an apophysis instead of an epiphysis.
- A physis (open growth plate) separates the apophysis from the body of the calcaneus.
- The calcaneal physis typically closes between ages 12 and 15.

INCIDENCE/PREVALENCE

- Typically occurs during an adolescent growth spurt
- Described most often between ages 9 and 12; most frequent at age 11 in girls and age 12 in boys
- Affects boys more frequently than girls

SIGNS AND SYMPTOMS

- Intermittent or continuous posterior heel pain during or following increased sport or play activity
- Pain can be bilateral or unilateral.
- Pain is usually absent in the morning.
- No swelling
- No ecchymoses or skin changes

RISK FACTORS

- Adolescent growth spurt
- Increased or excessive sport and play activity
- Tight gastrosoleus complex
- Weak ankle dorsiflexors
- Biomechanical factors such as genu varum and forefoot varus
- Poor quality or worn out athletic shoes
- Poorly cushioned or low-healed shoes such as soccer, baseball, track, or cycling cleats

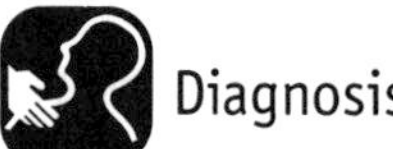

Diagnosis

DIFFERENTIAL DIAGNOSIS

- Calcaneal bursitis
- Insertional Achilles' tendonitis
- Fat pad syndrome
- Plantar fasciitis
- Calcaneal stress fracture
- Tarsal tunnel syndrome
- Tarsal coalition
- Calcaneal osteomyelitis

HISTORY

- Eight- to twelve-year-old child presents with heel pain worsened with increased activity.
- Recent growth spurt coinciding with vigorous sport or play activities
- Sports requiring a lot of running and jumping activities are particularly prone to cause this overuse syndrome.
- Pain can be unilateral or bilateral and relieved with rest.
- The pain may become severe enough to stop sport activity and even require crutch walking.

PHYSICAL EXAM

- Absence of swelling or erythema
- Tenderness just anterior to the Achilles insertion on the heel
- Tenderness with medial and lateral compression of the heel to the posterior one third of the calcaneus
- Pain aggravated by standing on tiptoe (Sever's sign)
- Heel cord inflexibility with sometimes less than 10 degrees of dorsiflexion
- Biomechanical contributors such as forefoot varus, hallux valgus, pes cavus, and pes planus

IMAGING

- Radiographs may show fragmentation, sclerosis, and increased density of the apophysis, but these radiographic changes can be normal.
- Imaging is not necessary to make this clinical diagnosis, but may be helpful to rule out other causes of heel pain.

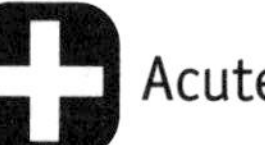

Acute Treatment

ANALGESIA

- Rest or reduce activity to a pain tolerance level.
- Ice
- Nonsteroidal medication for pain control
- Heel lifts
- Viscoelastic heel cups
- Short leg walking cast or boot walker for severe cases

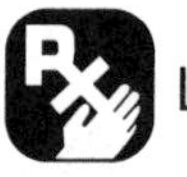

Long-Term Treatment

REHABILITATION

- Gastrosoleus stretching exercises; knee straight and knee flexed stretch with the heel maintained on the floor or ground
- Strengthening of the quadriceps and gastrosoleus to better equip these muscle groups to act as shock absorbers
- Strengthening of the foot dorsiflexors
- Custom shoe orthoses to correct significant biomechanical abnormalities
- Good quality shoe with adequate shock absorption and firm heel counter
- Time to symptom resolution varies, but abates totally with skeletal maturity
- No reports of long-term sequelae from Sever's disease

REFERRAL/DISPOSITION

- Necessary only when clinician is uncertain of diagnosis.

SURGICAL TREATMENT

- Not indicated

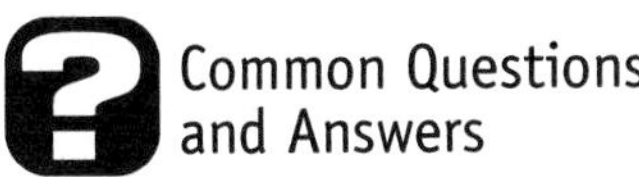

Common Questions and Answers

Physician responses to common patient questions:
Q: Can I continue playing sports?
A: Total rest may hasten the recovery from this heel pain, but may not be necessary. Reducing the amount of activity may allow sports participation without worsening the heel pain.
Q: Will there be long-range damage if I do not rest?
A: Current evidence does not suggest any long-term sequelae.

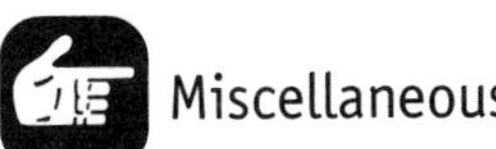

Miscellaneous

SYNONYMS

- Calcaneal apophysitis

ICD-9 CODE

732.5

BIBLIOGRAPHY

Madden CC, Mellion MB. Sever's disease and other causes of heel pain in adolescents. *Am Family Physician* 1996;54:1995–2000.

Stanitski CL. Pediatric and adolescent sports medicine. *Clin Sports Med* 1997;16:613–633.

Authors: Stephen Simons, Berent Krumm, and David Pacholke

Developmental Dysplasia of the Hip

Basics

DEFINITION

A range of congenital hip disorders: from mild acetabular dysplasia to dislocation of the femoral head from the acetabulum.

CAUSES

- Perinatal factors
  - —Breech presentation
  - —Ligamentous laxity
  - —Collagen vascular disorders
- Neonatal factors
  - —Hip positioned in extended, adducted fashion

PATHOLOGY

Due either to mechanical forces or to underlying laxity. Femoral head not positioned correctly within acetabulum, resulting in a shallow acetabulum, unable to contain the femoral head.

EPIDEMIOLOGY

Incidence of hip dysplasia is 0.5% to 2% of live births; however, true dislocation occurs in 0.1% to 0.2% of live births.

GENETICS

Most patients are first-born females, with familial history of affected first-degree relative.

COMPLICATIONS

- If left untreated, congenital hip dysplasia results in limp, pain, and accelerated degenerative disease of the hip.
- Rarely, there is avascular necrosis of the femoral head.

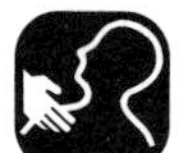

Diagnosis

- Infection
- Environmental
  - —Culture-associated neonatal swaddling
- Congenital
  - —Arthrogryposis
  - —Lumbosacral agenesis
  - —Spina bifida
  - —Neonatal Marfan syndrome
  - —Fetal hydantoin syndrome
  - —Larsen syndrome

DATA GATHERING

History

Question: Breech delivery?
Significance: Higher incidence of developmental dysplasia of the hip in breech delivery.
Question: Familial history of hip dysplasia?
Significance: 10% to 20% of patients have familial history.

PHYSICAL EXAMINATION

Gluteal and Thigh Skin-Fold Asymmetry

Finding: Ortolani test
Significance: Have infant supine, stabilize pelvis, abduct and externally rotate hip with examiner's middle finger over greater trochanter. Palpable click is positive sign produced by reduction of dislocated hip.
Finding: Barlow test
Significance: Passive dislocation of hip on adduction and internal rotation. Palpable click is positive sign as hip dislocates.

Physical Examination Tricks

Examination may be normal initially, in spite of the presence of hip dysplasia. Consequently, hip evaluation should be performed as part of neonatal physical examination through 4 months of age.

LABORATORY AIDS

Imaging

Test: X-ray studies
Significance: Not useful prior to 3 months, and may be normal because of difficulty determining hip/acetabulum relation in unossified femoral head.
Test: Ultrasound both static and dynamic imaging
Significance: Can determine hip joint spacial relationships. Ultrasound is useful in monitoring progress of therapy.

False Positives

Hip clicks will be present in 10% of infants; only a small percentage will have hip dysplasia.

Pitfalls

Overdiagnosis is a problem because avascular necrosis of femur can occur (rarely) as a result of therapeutic interventions.

Requirement for Testing

Ultrasonographer must be experienced in hip imaging.

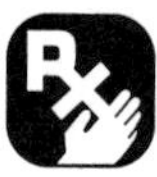

Long-Term Treatment

- Triple diaper: Not effective in moderate or severe dysplasia
- Pavlik harness: Effective if used prior to 6 months of age
- Complications include avascular necrosis of proximal femur, femoral nerve palsy, and medial knee instability.
- Closed or open reduction: If diagnosis/ therapy delayed beyond 6 months.
- Duration: If harness is used prior to 4 months of age, the average therapy takes 3 to 4 weeks.

WHEN TO EXPECT IMPROVEMENT

In children treated early (age <4 months), duration of splinting is 3 to 4 weeks, with subsequent weaning from splint.

SIGNS TO WATCH FOR

- Ultrasound or x-ray evidence of ongoing subluxation/dislocation

PROGNOSIS

If diagnosed early, prognosis is uniformly excellent.

PITFALLS

- Overdiagnosis early
- However, any infant with a hip click deserves an evaluation by an orthopedist.
- Missed early diagnosis can result in more complicated management and less favorable outcome.

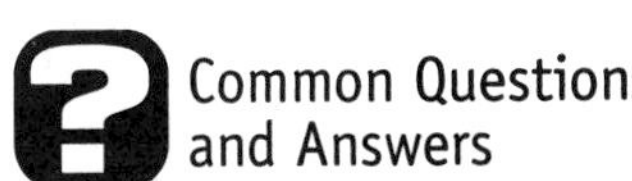

Common Questions and Answers

Q: If my patient has a hip click at birth demonstrating an unstable hip joint, what is the likelihood the infant will have hip dysplasia?
A: About 10% (1.5 children per 1000 live births).
Q: How effective is the Pavlik harness used within the first 4 months of life?
A: In patients with reducible hip dysplasia, results are excellent.

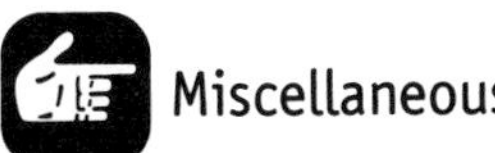

Miscellaneous

ICD-9 CODE

755.63

BIBLIOGRAPHY

Bennet GC. Screening for congenital dislocation of the hip. *J Bone Joint Surg Br* 1992;74:643–644.

Cotillo JA, Molano C, Albinana J. Correlative study between arthrograms and surgical findings in congenital dislocation of the hip. *J Pediatr Orthop B* 1998;7(1):62–65.

Darmonov AV, Zagora S. Clinical screening for congenital dislocation of the hip. *J Bone Joint Surg Am* 1996;78(3):383–388.

Author: Gregory F. Keenan

Eating Disorders

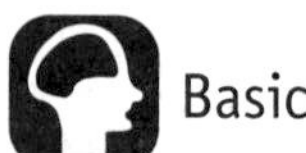

Basics

DEFINITION (DSM IV CRITERIA)

Anorexia Nervosa

- Weight less than 85% of normal for age and height
- Intense fear of gaining weight even though patient is underweight
- Body image disturbance and/or denial of current low weight status
- Secondary amenorrhea (defined as missing at least three consecutive menstrual cycles in a woman with established menses)
- Restricting type: mainly restricts intake to achieve weight loss
- Binge-eating/purging type: regularly uses binge-eating/purging to lose weight

Bulimia Nervosa

Recurrent episodes of binge eating with the following characteristics:

- Eating an abnormally large quantity of food within a 2-hour time period, and feeling unable to stop eating or control the amount of food eaten during this time
- Repeatedly uses inappropriate behaviors to compensate for the binge eating in order to prevent weight gain
- The above two behaviors occur at least twice a week for 3 months
- Body image disturbance
- The above characteristics do not occur only during episodes of anorexia nervosa
- Purging type: regularly uses self-induced vomiting, laxatives, diuretics, and/or enemas to control weight
- Nonpurging type: regularly uses fasting, excessive exercise, and/or other behaviors that do not include purging to control weight

Eating Disorder Not Otherwise Specified (NOS)

- Includes pathologic weight control disorders that do not meet the full criteria for anorexia nervosa or bulimia nervosa, yet may still have serious health implications

INCIDENCE/PREVALENCE

- Difficult to determine accurately due to secrecy surrounding these disorders
- In its 1998 guideline on eating disorders, NCAA reported at least one case of anorexia nervosa or bulimia in at least 40% of its member institutions.
- Anorexia occurs in 1% of general U.S. population.
- Bulimia occurs in 2% to 3% of general U.S. population.
- Eating disorder NOS and its subclinical variants occur in 5% to 10% of adolescents, and in 16% to 72% of female athletes

SIGNS AND SYMPTOMS

- Warning signs of anorexia: substantial weight loss; preoccupation or obsession about eating, food, or weight; loose or baggy fitting clothes; excessive exercise beyond the requirements for sport participation; mood swings; avoidance of food-related social activities
- Warning signs of bulimia: overly concerned about weight and/or body shape, frequent bathroom visits after meals, alternating episodes of strict dieting and binge eating, depressed mood

RISK FACTORS

- Genetic predisposition, environmental and social influences; family dynamics play a major role
- Certain sports have a higher predilection than others:
  - —Appearance sports such as ballet, figure skating, and gymnastics
  - —Sports that require weight classes such as wrestling, jockeying, martial arts
  - —Endurance sports such as long-distance running and swimming

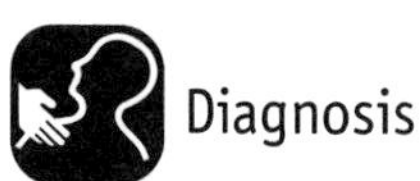

Diagnosis

DIFFERENTIAL DIAGNOSIS

- Gastrointestinal malabsorption syndromes
- Diabetes melitis
- Occult malignancies
- Psychiatric conditions (i.e., major depression or mood disorders)
- Female athlete triad: characterized by disordered eating, osteoporosis (often seen as stress fracture), and amenorrhea

HISTORY

- Amenorrhea
- Stress fractures
- Gastrointestinal problems
- Cardiac arrhythmias
- Orthostatic symptoms
- Cold intolerance
- Dental and gum disease

PHYSICAL EXAM

- Emaciation
- Lanugo hair
- Swollen parotid glands
- Hypercarotenemia
- Hypotension and bradycardia
- Electrolyte abnormalities
- Dehydration
- Poor dentition
- Russell's sign (callous on fingers due to self-induced vomiting)

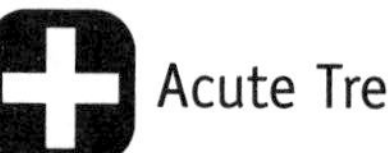

Acute Treatment

SPECIAL CONSIDERATIONS

- Explore the sports environment to determine situations that may foster or promote eating disorder behaviors.
- In athletes, look for the following performance effects of eating disorders: decreased muscle strength and endurance, diminished aerobic and anaerobic power, decreased coordination, impaired judgment and performance. On the other hand, many athletes with an eating disorder perform successfully.

MANAGEMENT STRATEGIES

- Return to play issues
- Athlete who refuses treatment: consider suspension from sport participation because the athlete's health should take precedence over sport.
- Athlete in treatment: multidisciplinary treatment team should address the key issues of assurance of medical stability before return to competition, involvement in intensive psychological therapy to address cognitive dysfunction, and maintenance of ongoing treatment with a dietitian to improve nutritional status.
- Whether to allow participation while the athlete is in treatment should be assessed on an individual basis according to problem severity and whether participation will put the athlete at risk or interfere with the treatment regimen.
- Allowing continued sport participation is advantageous in some athletes, but is detrimental in others.
- Health maintenance standards to return to full participation should be established between the athlete and multidisciplinary treatment team to include the following:
  - —Minimal weight for sports participation (90% of normal body weight as a guideline)
  - —Maintenance of caloric intake necessary to sustain the minimal weight
  - —Compliance with meal plan and nutritional requirements developed with dietitian
  - —Gynecologic evaluation if no menses for at least 6 months with consideration of hormone replacement therapy and evaluation of bone mineral density
  - —Maintenance of regular medical and psychological monitoring and treatment

Long-Term Treatment

REFERRAL/DISPOSITION

- Early referral to a mental health professional with experience with eating disorders
- Early referral to a dietitian with experience with eating disorders

MANAGEMENT STRATEGIES

- Prevention: be watchful of athletes who may be susceptible to eating disorders and those involved in high-risk sports.
- Weight loss programs in athletes should be agreed upon by the athlete, coach, and appropriate medical/nutritional personnel.
- Educate athletes, coaches, parents, administrators, and medical personnel about eating disorders.

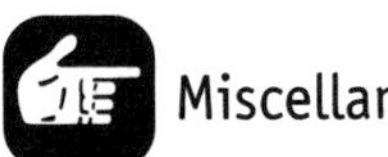

Miscellaneous

ICD-9 CODE

307.1 Anorexia nervosa
307.51 Bulimia
307.5 Eating disorder not otherwise specified

BIBLIOGRAPHY

Brownell KD, Steen SN, Wilmore JH. Weight regulation practices in athletes: analysis of metabolic and health effects. *Med Sci Sports Exerc* 1987;19:546–556.

Drummer GM, et al. Pathologic weight control behaviors of young competitors. *Phys Sports Med* 15:75–84.

Rosen LW, et al. Pathologic weight control behavior in female athletes. *Phys Sports Med* 14:79–86.

Thompson RA. *Helping athletes with eating disorders*. Champaign, IL: Human Kinetic Books, 1993.

Author: Lisa Barkley

Female Athlete Triad

Basics

DEFINITION

- A condition of the female athlete with the combined findings of disordered eating, amenorrhea, and osteoporosis

INCIDENCE/PREVALENCE

- Female athlete triad: unknown
- Disordered eating: 15% to 62% of female athletes, depending on defining criteria
- Amenorrhea: 3.4% to 66% of exercising females
- Osteoporosis: unknown in female athletes

SIGNS AND SYMPTOMS

- Amenorrhea
- Weight-control behaviors
- Stress fracture
- Cold intolerance
- Sore throat
- Constipation
- Light-headedness
- Fatigue
- Depression
- Decreasing athletic performance

RISK FACTORS

- Sports emphasizing leanness
- Sports requiring endurance
- Elite athletes
- Sports in which younger competitors excel
- Individual sports as opposed to team sports
- Unreasonable performance expectations by self or others
- Poor body self-image
- Social isolation
- Punitive measures imposed for weight gain
- Family history of eating disorder

Diagnosis

DIFFERENTIAL DIAGNOSIS

- Pregnancy
- Hyperthyroidism
- Pituitary disease
- Hypogonadism
- Polycystic ovary disease
- Adrenal dysfunction
- Anabolic steroid use/abuse
- Autoimmune disease
- Hyperparathyroidism
- Malabsorption syndromes
- Excess glucocorticoid administration
- Systemic infection
- Malignancy

HISTORY

- Absence of menses by age 16 in the presence of secondary sex characteristics
- Absence of secondary sex characteristics by age 14
- Secondary amenorrhea: the absence of three to six consecutive menstrual cycles or two or fewer cycles per year
- Pathogenic weight-control behavior involving food
- Stress fracture

PHYSICAL EXAM

- Vital signs for evidence of bradycardia and/or hypotension
- Height, weight, body composition measurement
- Dental examination for evidence of lingual enamel erosion secondary to vomiting
- Parotid gland palpation for hypertrophy secondary to vomiting
- Thyroid palpation
- Cardiac auscultation for evidence of dysrhythmia
- Abdominal examination for masses
- Skin examination for dryness and/or lanugo
- Evaluation for facial and/or extremity edema
- Neurologic examination for evidence of pituitary tumor
- Reflexes
- Tanner staging
- Pelvic examination

IMAGING

- Evaluation of bone mineral density using a standardized, recognized, reproducible method [World Health Organization criteria: 1–2.5 standard deviations (SD) below young adult mean = osteopenia; >2.5 SD below young adult mean = osteoporosis]
- Consider pituitary imaging
- Consider bone age imaging in delayed menarche

LABORATORY EVALUATION

- Pregnancy test
- Complete blood count
- Sedimentation rate (normal)
- Serum electrolytes, blood urea nitrogen, and creatinine
- Thyroid hormones
- Serum proteins
- Liver enzymes
- Luteinizing hormone and follicle-stimulating hormone levels (normal or low)
- Estradiol levels (low): progestin challenge test (10 mg Provera per day for 10 days) may be used in place of estradiol levels. If she bleeds, her estrogen level is satisfactory and her amenorrhea is probably not related to overzealous exercise. If she does not bleed, a cyclical estrogen-progesterone test can be conducted to assure she has a normal endometrium and vaginal outlet tract.
- Serum prolactin (normal)
- Serum testosterone and dehydroepiandrosterone sulfate (normal)
- Serum cortisol (normal or slightly elevated)

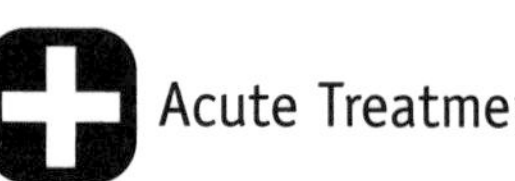

Acute Treatment

RECOGNITION

- High index of suspicion
- Condition-related questionnaire
- Open communication with athletes, teammates, coaches, trainers
- Specific education sessions with teams, trainers, and coaches

EMERGENT OR URGENT INTERVENTION

- Electrolyte disturbance
- Bradycardia or dysrhythmia
- Moderate to severe hypoproteinemia
- Dehydration
- Moderate to severe depression

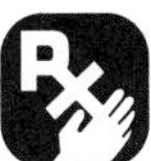

Long-Term Treatment

GENERAL MEASURES

- Multidisciplinary management optimal, with primary care physician coordinating care with other disciplines as necessary (consider nutritionist, behavioral medicine specialist)
- Outline treatment plan and contract in writing with patient.
- Educate athlete that incremental increases in caloric intake and decreases in exercise intensity may be all that is necessary to resolve symptoms.
- Monitor progress closely, as indicated by severity and response to treatment.
- Identify and modify specific behavior triggers or stressors.
- Treat associated depression when present.
- Communicate with support group (e.g., trainers, coaches, parents of adolescents).
- Prevention is best accomplished through education of athletes, coaches, trainers, and parents.

DISORDERED EATING

- Define specific nutritional goals.
- Specific education about nutrition and athletic performance
- Monitor weight gain.
- Nutritionist consult as necessary
- Behavioral medicine consult in severe or recalcitrant cases

ATHLETIC OR EXERCISE-ASSOCIATED AMENORRHEA

- Menstruation usually occurs with improved nutrition and decreased exercise intensity.
- Hormonal therapy with estrogen in conjugated oral contraceptives has been shown in a few studies to improve bone mineral density, but may mask an eating disorder.

OSTEOPOROSIS

- Return to normal estrogenic state
- Diet adequate in calories
- Total daily intake of 1,500 mg elemental calcium

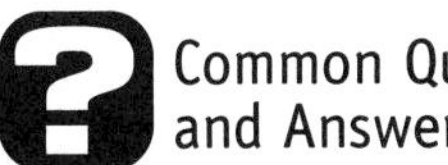

Common Questions and Answers

Physician responses to common patient questions:

Q: Why do I have to gain weight? My coach and I agree that less fat means better times and scores, or that I can compete more succcessfully in a lower weight class.

A: Although it is true that excess body weight and body fat percentage may adversely affect athletic performance, it is not true that improved athletic performance is inversely proportional in a linear fashion to weight loss. There is a range of acceptable weight for optimal performance, and excesses above and below that range can adversely affect performance.

Q: Why do I have to have a period? I like the convenience of not having to worry about having my period during competition. Besides, I don't want to get pregnant now.

A: The presence of amenorrhea is not a guarantee that pregnancy cannot occur. The hormonal corrections with effective treatment of the female athlete triad may permit ovulation prior to the next menses, and unprotected intercourse may result in pregnancy with that ovulation.

Q: Can't I wait until the season is over to start my periods again? Then my bones can regain their strength.

A: The resumption of menses (correction of the hypoestrogenic state) is no guarantee that lost deposition of bone mass density during amenorrhea will be fully corrected. In fact, there are studies indicating that bone losses during hypoestrogenic states cannot be fully recovered.

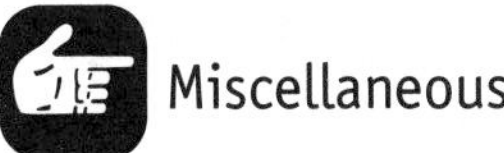

Miscellaneous

ICD-9 CODE

626.0 Amenorrhea
307.50 Eating disorder
733.0 Osteoporosis

BIBLIOGRAPHY

American College of Sports Medicine. Female athlete triad: position stand of ACSM. *Med Sci Sports Exerc* 1997;29:i–ix.

Agostini R. The athletic woman. *Clin Sports Med* 2000;19(2):199–213.

Agostini R, Titus S. *Medical and orthopedic issues of active and athletic women.* Philadelphia: Hanley & Belfus, 1994.

Joy E, Clark N, Ireland ML, et al. Team management of the female athlete triad: parts 1 & 2. *Physician Sportsmed* 1997;25 (3 & 4):94–110, 55–69.

Laughlin G, Yen S. Nutritional and endocrine-metabolic aberrations in amenorrheic athletes. *J Clin Endocrinol Metab* 1996;81:4301–4309.

Rencken M, Chestnut C, et al. Bone density at multiple skeletal sites in amenorrheic athletes. *JAMA* 1996;276:238–240.

Smith A. The female athlete triad: causes, diagnosis, and treatment. *Physician Sportsmed* 1996;24(7):67–76.

Author: Ross M. Patton

Greenstick Fracture

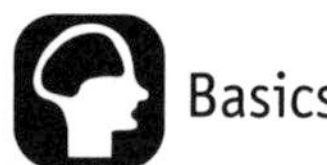

Basics

SIGNS AND SYMPTOMS

- Pain
- Inability to use or mobilize the affected extremity
- Localized tenderness
- Swelling
- Ecchymosis
- Palpation of bony deformities
- Crepitus
- Pseudoparalysis
- Ecchymosis

MECHANISM/DESCRIPTION

- An incomplete fracture of the diaphysis of a long bone
  —A break in the cortex and periosteum of one side
  —An intact periosteum on the other side of the fracture
- Compared with adults, children's bones are more
  —Porous
  —Compliant
  —Resilient
  —Soft
- Stresses and forces applied result often in incomplete fractures
  —These fractures are more stable
  —Somewhat less painful than complete fractures
  —May have some degree of angulation and rotation
- Most common type of pediatric fracture
  —50% of all fractures prior to the age of 12
  —May occur into the teenage years
- Complete healing is the most common outcome
- Complications
  —Plastic/bowing deformities
  —Reduction of limb mobility
  —Rarely growth plate disturbances

ETIOLOGY

N/A

PRE-HOSPITAL

- Cold packs to affected area
- Splint the injured extremity in the position found
  —Air cushions
  —Boards
  —Plain tape
  —Rolled towels

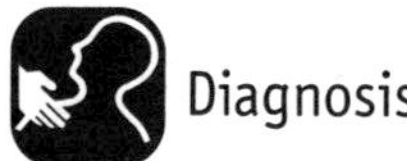

Diagnosis

ESSENTIAL WORKUP

- Assessment of the extremity distal to the injury
  —Circulation
  —Motor function
  —Sensation
- Assess for associated injuries
- Obtain appropriate radiographs

LABORATORY

N/A

IMAGING/SPECIAL TESTS

- AP and lateral radiograph of the involved limb
  —Cortical disruption
  —Periosteal tearing on the convex side of the bone
  —Intact periosteum on the concave side
  —Greenstick fractures are never compound
- Oblique views are sometimes helpful
- Repeat radiograph after reduction

DIFFERENTIAL DIAGNOSIS

- Contusions
- Sprains
- Bowing deformities
- Other fractures
- Infection
- Tumor

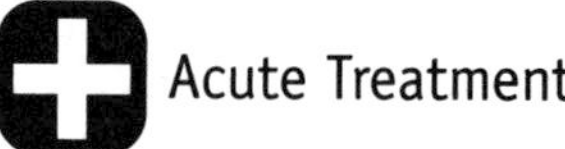

Acute Treatment

INITIAL STABILIZATION

- Immobilization of the injured extremity
- Pain control
- Reduction of angulation or rotation using conscious sedation

ED TREATMENT

- Splint or cast the injured limb
  —Immobilize the joints proximal and distal to the injury

MEDICATIONS

Conscious Sedation

- Fentanyl: 1–2 μg/kg IV
- Ketamine: 0.5–1 mg/kg IV
- Meperidine: 1–1.5 mg/kg IV
- Midazolam: 0.05–0.1 mg/kg (max 2.5 mg) IV
- Morphine sulfate: 0.1 mg/kg (max 15 mg) IV

Pain Control

- Acetaminophen with codeine: 0.5–1.0 mg/kg (max 60 mg) q 4 hrs po
- Ibuprofen: 4–10 mg/kg (max 3200 mg/24 hrs) po

HOSPITAL ADMISSION CRITERIA

- Suspicion of nonaccidental trauma

HOSPITAL DISCHARGE CRITERIA

- Pain is well controlled
- Immobilization does not severely impede the child
- Orthopedic referral within 1 week
- Splint or cast instructions
  —Ice/cold pack application
  —Elevation of the injured limb
  —Analgesic medication

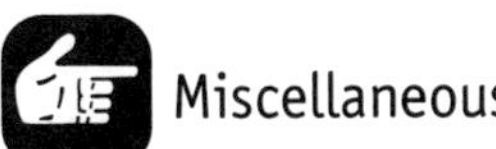

Miscellaneous

ICD-9-CM

N/A

CORE CONTENT CODE

N/A

BIBLIOGRAPHY

Davis D, Green D. Forearm fractures in children: Pitfalls and complications. *Clin Orthop* 1976;120:172.

England S, Sundberg S. Management of common pediatric fractures. *Pediatr Clin North Am* 1996;43:991.

Olney B. Musculoskeletal injuries. In: Buntain W, ed. *Management of pediatric trauma*. Philadelphia: WB Saunders, 1995.

Rang R. *Children's fractures*. Philadelphia: JB Lippincott, 1983.

Authors: William Sabina and Daniel L. Savitt

Kohler's Disease (Aseptic Necrosis of the Tarsal Navicular)

Basics

DEFINITION

- Idiopathic self-limiting ischemic necrosis of the tarsal navicular in young children

INCIDENCE/PREVALENCE

- Occurs in children 2 to 7 years of age (average age 5 years 10 months)
- Occurs more frequently in boys (4–6:1)
- Usually occurs unilaterally

SIGNS AND SYMPTOMS

- Insidious onset of foot pain and limp aggravated by activity
- Time to presentation varies from days to months after onset of pain.

RISK FACTORS

- May be caused by repetitive microtrauma to the maturing navicular ossification center
- Compression of the bony nucleus at a critical phase of growth may occlude the penetrating blood vessels and produce ischemia and aseptic necrosis of the bone.
- Delayed ossification leading to irregular ossification centers may predispose to this condition.
- Occurrence is not related to acute macrotrauma, age at first walking, foot type, or family history.

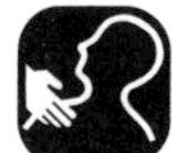

Diagnosis

DIFFERENTIAL DIAGNOSIS

- Normal variants: variations of size and shape of the navicular ossification center may be indistinguishable from Kohler's disease except for the absence of symptoms.
- Osteochondritis dissecans: localized involvement on the articular surface, well demarcated from the normal bone by a crescent-shaped area of radiolucency

HISTORY

- Location of pain? It is often difficult for young children to localize pain.
- Participation in sport activities? Repetitive microtrauma may be a risk factor.
- History of trauma? A history of macrotrauma should lead you to consider other causes of foot pain.

PHYSICAL EXAM

- Look for localized edema and warmth in the area of the tarsal navicular.
- Palpate the entire foot and ankle; tenderness should be localized to the medial mid-foot.
- Check the range of motion of the ankle and subtalar joints, which should be normal.
- Examine the knee and hip, which can be the source of referred pain and limp.

IMAGING

- Standard anteroposterior, lateral, and oblique radiographs of the foot: varying degrees of navicular sclerosis; diminished size or flattening of the navicular ("Alka-Seltzer-on-end" appearance); occasional loss of trabecular pattern and fragmentation
- Bone scintigraphy: decreased uptake in the navicular indicates decreased or interrupted blood supply.

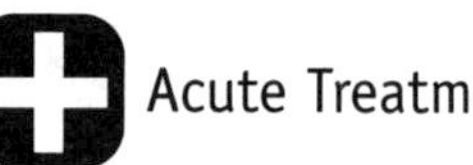

Acute Treatment

ANALGESIA

- Apply ice to mid-foot.
- Nonsteroidal antiinflammatory drugs
- Decrease activities that exacerbate foot pain.

IMMOBILIZATION

Short leg walking cast for 6 to 8 weeks decreases the duration of symptoms from approximately 15 to 3 months compared with treatment without casting.

SPECIAL CONSIDERATIONS

Orthoses have not been found to be effective.

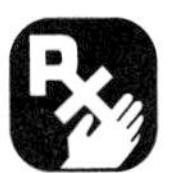

Long-Term Treatment

REHABILITATION
- Usually not indicated

SURGICAL TREATMENT
- Rarely required

REFERRAL/DISPOSITION
- Orthopedic referral indicated if symptoms do not resolve with conservative management

LONG-TERM OUTCOME
- Complete resolution of symptoms with reconstitution of the navicular can be expected in all patients.
- No evidence of cartilage degeneration in long-term follow-up studies

Common Questions and Answers

Physician responses to common patient questions:
Q: Is casting necessary?
A: Although all patients will eventually have complete resolution of symptoms, immobilization with a cast for 6 to 8 weeks shortens the duration of symptoms by approximately 1 year.
Q: When can I allow my child to return to sports?
A: Sports may be resumed once symptoms have resolved.
Q: Will my child develop arthritis when he is older?
A: Long-term follow-up studies have found no increase in the rate of arthritis or other chronic foot problems in adults who had Kohler's disease during childhood.

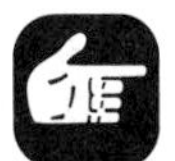

Miscellaneous

ICD-9 CODE
732.5 Juvenile osteochondroses of the foot

BIBLIOGRAPHY

Borges JP, Guille JT, Bowen JR. Kohler's bone disease of the tarsal navicular. *J Pediatr Orthop* 1995;15:596–598.

Ippolito E, Ricciardi Pollini PT, Falez PT. Kohler's disease of the tarsal navicular: long-term follow-up of 12 cases. *J Pediatr Orthop* 1984;4:416–417.

Kohler A. A frequent disease of individual bones in children. *Munch Med Wochenschr* 1908;55:1923–1925.

Manusov EG, Lillegard WA, Raspa RF, et al. Evaluation of pediatric foot problems: the forefoot. *Am Family Physician* 1996;54: 592–606.

Authors: Joyce Soprano and Lyle J. Micheli

Little Leaguer's Elbow (Medial Epicondylitis/Apophysitis)

Basics

DEFINITION

- Classic definition: valgus stress lesion of the medial epicondylar physis
- On a continuum with avulsion fracture of the medial epicondyle
- Now used as a catch-all phrase for elbow pain in a young athlete
- Medial epicondylar fragmentation and avulsion
- Delayed or accelerated apophyseal growth of the medial epicondyle
- Delayed closure of the medial epicondylar growth plate
- Osteochondrosis and osteochondritis of the capitellum (Panner's disease)
- Deformation and osteochondritis of the radial head
- Hypertrophy of the ulna
- Olecranon apophysitis

ANATOMY

- There are six distinct secondary centers of ossification in the elbow.
- The medial epicondyle may arise from more than one ossific nucleus and is commonly the last epiphyseal center to fuse with the humeral shaft in the normal child; it may fuse as late as 15 or 16 years of age.
- The medial epicondyle is the site of attachment for the flexor muscle origins and the ulnar collateral ligament.

SIGNS AND SYMPTOMS

- Pain in medial elbow
- Pain accentuated during early and late cocking of throwing motion
- Decrease in control of pitches or throwing distances

RISK FACTORS

- Position: shows magnitude of stress (pitcher > catcher > infielder > outfielder)
- Activity level: types of pitches, innings pitched, typical pitching rotation
- Handedness: occurs most commonly in the dominant arm, unless it is a traumatic event
- Family history of osteochondrosis

ASSOCIATED INJURIES AND COMPLICATIONS

If avulsion fragment is incarcerated in the joint, it can severely damage the articular surface.

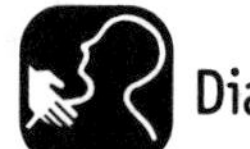

Diagnosis

DIFFERENTIAL DIAGNOSIS

- Medial epicondylitis
- Ulnar collateral ligament sprain/tear
- Ulnar nerve injury
- Neoplasms
- Referred pain: neck versus shoulder versus wrist

HISTORY

- Age: important because of the different ages at which each growth center appears and/or closes
- Location: most commonly, pain is located in the medial epicondyle; however, sometimes pain presents laterally or posteriorly.
- Duration (pain characteristics): the length of time that the athlete has had pain is usually an indirect measure of the severity of the problem. If the pain occurs during and after throwing as well as when the athlete is not throwing, it is an ominous sign.
- Radiation: if pain or numbness radiates into the last two fingers, consider ulnar nerve damage.
- Mechanism (acute vs. chronic): acute pain in young athlete in the medial elbow is more consistent with avulsion fracture of the medial epicondyle.

PHYSICAL EXAM

- Bilateral comparison of the elbows
- Inspection: note presence of swelling, muscle atrophy/hypertrophy, symmetry, carrying angle (normal = 5 to 10 degrees in males, 10 to 15 degrees in females); ecchymosis is indicative of an avulsion.
- Palpation: medial/lateral epicondyles (point tenderness along medial epicondyle consistent with avulsion fracture), olecranon process, radial head, collateral ligaments, ulnar nerve
- Range of motion: flexion/extension (flexion contracture >15 degrees consistent with avulsion fracture); supination/pronation usually normal; Assess for ulnar collateral ligament stability with valgus stress at 20 degrees of flexion
- Neurologic: check sensation along the ulnar nerve distribution; check Tinel's sign at the cubital tunnel; check interosseous muscle strength in the hand

IMAGING

- Radiography is indicated if there is decreased range of motion, or there is a suspicion of an avulsion fracture
- Anteroposterior/lateral views of the elbow
- Appearance of growth centers: CRITOC
  - —Capitellum: appears at 1 to 2 years of age
  - —Radial epiphysis (3–4 years)
  - —Inner epicondyle (medial epicondyle, 5–6 years)
  - —Trochlea (9–10 years)
  - —Outer epicondyle (lateral epicondyle >10 years)
  - —Common epiphysis (14–16 years)
- Obtain bilateral elbow views if needed for comparison.
- Assess for presence of anterior and posterior fat pads, which signify the presence of an effusion.
- Compare medial epicondylar ossification centers.
- Assess for displacement of epicondylar fragment.

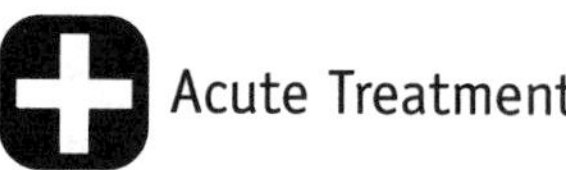

Acute Treatment

SPECIAL CONSIDERATIONS

- Treatment depends on the amount of displacement of the medial epicondylar physis.
- If fragment is minimally displaced (2–5 mm):
  - —Apply posterior splint until acute symptoms resolve (2–3 weeks)
  - —Gradual active motion
  - —Radiologic healing by 6 weeks; at this time start aggressive active motion
  - —When union is obvious, allow the patient to throw if pain free
  - —Allow return to competitive play when there is normal range of motion/strength/endurance while throwing
- If fragment is displaced more than 5 mm:
  - —Open reduction and internal fixation
  - —Two cancellous screws to prevent rotation
  - —Allow early gradual active motion
  - —After 6 weeks, aggressive rehabilitation program

Little Leaguer's Elbow (Medial Epicondylitis/Apophysitis)

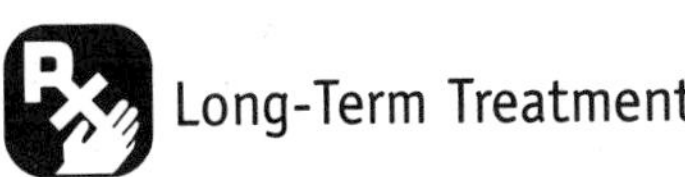

Long-Term Treatment

COMPLICATIONS

Closed reduction is associated with pseudoarthrosis, causing pain and instability, as well as formation of double epicondylar epiphyses.

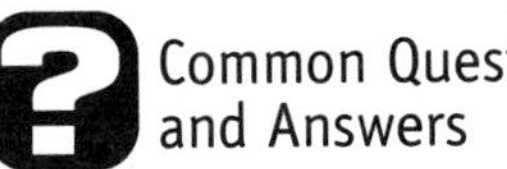

Common Questions and Answers

Physician responses to common patient questions:
Q: Does the type of pitch affect incidence?
A: In the adolescent, the type of pitch does matter because proper technique and muscle control have not yet been learned. Breaking pitches, such as the screwball, in the untrained adolescent pitcher will place more stress on the medial aspect of the elbow, increasing the likelihood of developing medial elbow pain.
Q: How many pitches should a little leaguer be allowed to throw?
A: There is no definitive answer, but at present, Little League rules that limit the number of innings per week and length of time between pitching has seemed to decrease the incidence of little league elbow.
Q: Are there any prevention strategies?
A: Follow the guidelines set by the Little League rules, and if pain does begin to occur, the player should rest and see a physician.

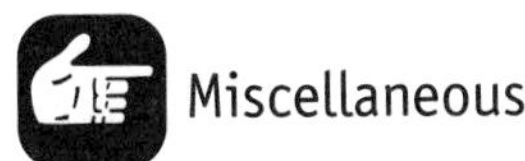

Miscellaneous

ICD-9 CODE

732.3 Juvenile
Osteochondrosis arm

BIBLIOGRAPHY

DaSilva M, et al. Pediatric throwing injuries about the elbow. *Am J Orthop* 1998;27: 90–96.

DeLee JC, Drez D Jr. *Orthopaedic sports medicine.* Philadelphia: WB Saunders, 1994.

Papavasiliou V. Fracture-separation of the medial epicondylar epiphysis. *Clin Orthop* 1982;171:172–174.

Authors: Sam Lin, Greg Crovetti, Robert G. Hosey, and Thomas D. Armsey

Menstrual Disorders in the Athlete

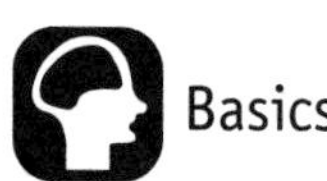

Basics

DEFINITION

- Female athlete triad is defined as disordered eating, amenorrhea, and osteoporosis.
- Disordered eating refers to a wide spectrum of harmful and ineffective eating behaviors used to lose weight or achieve a specific body appearance.
- Primary amenorrhea is the lack of spontaneous uterine bleeding (1) by the age of 14 years without development of secondary sexual characteristics, or (2) by the age of 16 years with otherwise normal development.
- Secondary amenorrhea is defined as a 6-month absence of menstrual bleeding in a woman with primary regular menses or a 12-month absence with previous oligomenorrhea.
- Osteoporosis is characterized by premature bone loss or inadequate bone formation, or both, resulting in microarchitectural deterioration, enhanced skeletal fragility, and increased risk of fracture.

INCIDENCE/PREVALENCE

- The exact incidence/prevalence is unknown due to a lack of a validated screening tool, disagreement on definitions, and the fact that the exact magnitude of all female athletes at risk is unknown.
- Based on limited data in the United States, the prevalence of disordered eating in athletes is 15% to 62% compared with 1% to 3% among the general population.
- Amenorrhea occurs in 3% to 66% of female college athletes compared with 2% to 5% of the general population.

SIGNS AND SYMPTOMS

- Amenorrhea
- Dry skin and hair
- Fat and muscle loss
- Cold, discolored hands and feet
- Lightheadedness
- Low body temperature
- Lanugo, especially on the trunk
- Bradycardia
- Impaired ability to concentrate
- Fatigue/depression
- Behavioral signs: preoccupation with food and weight, self-criticism, eating alone, excessive water/soda drinking, compulsive and excessive exercise, poor self-image, frequent bathroom trips during and after meals
- If anorexia nervosa is present, cachexia, hypotension, alopecia, pruritus, cold intolerance, and yellow skin (hypercarotenemia) also may be observed.
- If bulimia nervosa is present, abdominal pain, chest pain, parotid enlargement, scleral petechiae, tooth enamel erosion, pharyngitis/esophagitis, bloodshot eyes, knuckle scars, diarrhea/constipation, and face and extremity edema also may be observed.

RISK FACTORS

- Participation in sports in which low body weight, prepubertal body habitus, and subjective scoring is involved (gymnastics, ballet, figure skating, aerobics, dance, diving)
- Participation in sports that require endurance, body contour–revealing clothing, or weight categories (wrestling, cycling, track, swimming, cheerleading, cross-country running or skiing, rowing, martial arts, horse racing)
- Low self-esteem
- Family dysfunction
- Physical or sexual abuse
- Pressure from parents, coaches, peers, or the culture of the sport to lose weight, win at all costs, and be flawless during competition
- Traumatic events (e.g., loss of a coach or a mentor)
- Lack of self-identity outside of her sport

ASSOCIATED INJURIES AND COMPLICATIONS

- Stress fractures
- Osteoporosis
- Concomitant anxiety, depression, and/or obsessive-compulsive disorder

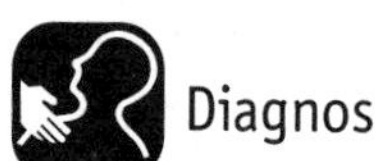

Diagnosis

DIFFERENTIAL DIAGNOSIS

- Pregnancy
- Hypothalamic dysfunction
  - —Gonadotropin-releasing hormone (GnRH) deficiency
  - —Hypogonadotropic hypogonadism (psychogenic, stress, weight loss, or exercise induced)
  - —Eating disorder
  - —Drugs (GnRH analogues, medroxyprogesterone acetate, danazol, or oral contraceptives) or systemic illness
  - —Kallmann's syndrome
  - —Idiopathic (e.g., head trauma)
  - —Space-occupying lesion or infection
- Pituitary dysfunction
  - —Pituitary neoplasm or prolactin-secreting tumor
  - —Sheehan's syndrome
  - —Empty-sella syndrome
  - —Granulomatous disease (e.g., sarcoidosis)
  - —Lawrence-Moon-Biedl syndrome
  - —Thalassemia major
  - —Mumps encephalitis
- Ovarian dysfunction
  - —Menopause or premature ovarian failure
  - —Polycystic ovary syndrome
  - —Ovarian neoplasm
  - —Turner's syndrome (45,X)
  - —Gonadal dysgenesis
  - —Autoimmune disease
- Uterine dysfunction
  - —Asherman's syndrome
  - —Absence of uterus or transverse vaginal septum
    - —Androgen insensitivity
    - —Imperforate hymen
    - —Mayer-Rokitansky-Kuster-Hauser syndrome (müllerian agenesis)
- Endocrine disease
  - —Hypothyroidism
  - —Cushing's syndrome
  - —Adrenal hyperplasia
  - —Adrenal tumors

HISTORY

- With amenorrhea, history is directed toward other causes besides hypothalamic amenorrhea: thyroid disease, androgen excess, anabolic steroids, and autoimmune and pituitary disorders.
- Menstrual history
  - —Age of menarche
  - —Last menstrual period
  - —Frequency and duration of menses
  - —Longest time between menses
  - —Physical signs of ovulation (cervical mucous change or menstrual cramps)
  - —Previous or current hormonal therapy
- Diet history
  - —Food list over the last 24 hours
  - —List of any forbidden foods
  - —Highest and lowest weight since menarche
  - —Patient's opinions of current weight and perception of ideal weight
  - —Disordered eating behaviors (binging and purging)
  - —Use of laxatives, diuretics, diet pills
- Exercise history
  - —Exercise patterns (intensity, hours/day, days/week)
  - —Additional exercise outside of required training
  - —History of previous fracture or overuse injuries

PHYSICAL EXAM

- Vital signs both supine and standing
- Weight and body fat composition by skinfold calipers
- Growth charts for pediatric patients
- A complete physical exam directed toward the physical signs listed above

IMAGING

- Consider dual-energy x-ray absorptiometry (DEXA) scan if osteoporosis is suspected or if amenorrhea is of more than 6 months' duration
- Normal bone mineral density is no more than 1 standard deviation below the mean for young adults.
- Triple-phase bone scan and MRI scan are useful for suspected stress fractures.

LABORATORY STUDIES

- Initial: pregnancy test, follicle-stimulating hormone, luteinizing hormone, thyroid-stimulating hormone, prolactin, complete blood count, chemistries
- If patient is hirsute, has acne, or if polycystic ovary syndrome is suspected, add free testosterone and dehydroepiandrosterone sulfate to the list of studies
- Electrocardiography

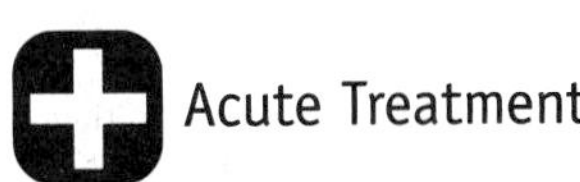

Acute Treatment

SPECIAL CONSIDERATIONS

- Treatment should involve a multidisciplinary team approach, involving the coach, primary care physician, dietitian, and psychiatrist or psychologist.
- Must identify issues that may have contributed to disordered eating and address those issues.
- Consider hospitalization under the following conditions: functional impairment, severe impairment of mental status, acute risk of bodily harm through reckless behavior or suicide, ineffective outpatient treatment.

PHARMACOLOGIC TREATMENT

- Hormone replacement therapy (HRT)
  —HRT is recommended because patients are typically estrogen deficient (including progestational therapy for all women with a uterus).
  —HRT induces regular menses and reduces the risk of stress fracture by leading to increase in bone mineral density.
  —Consider starting HRT in individuals who do not readily resume their menses with increased caloric intake and decreased exercise. Consider after 6 months of amenorrhea.
  —Patients who already have evidence of osteopenia on the basis of DEXA scanning should be strongly encouraged to start HRT.
  —Although HRT will treat amenorrhea, the ultimate goal is the return of regular menses through proper nutrition, revised training regimens, and maintenance of a reasonable body weight.
  —Avoid HRT in patients with endometrial cancer, breast cancer or a strong family history of breast cancer, recent deep venous thrombosis or recurrent thrombosis, and in adolescent patients within 3 years of menarche.
  —HRT option 1 is composed of one of the following, daily or cyclically (days 1–25): conjugated estrogen (0.625 mg), ethinyl estradiol (0.02 mg), transdermal estradiol (0.05 mg), or micronized estradiol (1 mg) plus oral progestin, daily (2.5–5 mg medroxyprogesterone) or cyclically (5–10 mg for 10–14 days each month).
  —HRT option 2 is composed of a combination of estrogen/progestin oral contraceptive with 25 to 35 μg of ethinyl estradiol.
- Vitamin D (400–800 IU/day)
- Calcium is recommended at a level of 1,200 to 1,500 mg/day. (Calcium carbonate contains the highest percentage of elemental calcium and is the least expensive.)
- Consider multivitamins
- Most will benefit from SSRIs for comorbid conditions such as anxiety, depression, and obsessive-compulsive disorder.
- Benzodiazepines have been advocated by some experts to control severe mealtime anxiety.

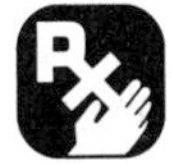

Long-Term Treatment

REHABILITATION

- A weight gain of 0.5 to 1.0 pound per week until goal weight is achieved.
- Exercise activity should be decreased by 10% to 20%, and weight should be monitored closely for 2 or 3 months.
- Family involvement is crucial to the success of treatment.
- Education about appropriate nutrition and exercise is crucial.

REFERRAL/DISPOSITION

Consider early referral to nutritionist and to a psychologist or psychiatrist.

Common Questions and Answers

Physician responses to common patient questions:

Q: If I'm amenorrheic just during my competitive years, won't I be OK as long as I resume my menses eventually?

A: You are at risk for irreversible bone loss after only 3 years of amenorrhea. This is especially important because your adolescence and early adulthood are times when you should be building bone for later life to prevent osteoporosis and its complications. Also, the amenorrhea may just be a symptom of more important issues that may prevail beyond your competitive years and should be addressed.

Q: If I gain too much weight, my coach or parent will be on my case.

A: There are certainly heavy societal and cultural expectations and misconceptions toward how certain athletes should behave and appear. But there is a fine line between being fit and being unhealthy. Physicians, trainers, and caretakers of athletes need to educate coaches, parents, and athletes on the potential dangers of the female athlete triad. They must also work on dispelling myths and changing accepted norms for certain sports.

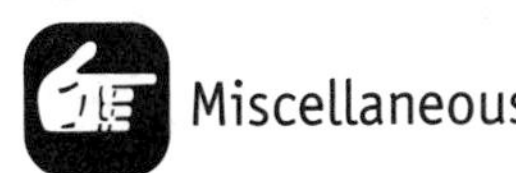

Miscellaneous

ICD-9 CODE

626.0 Amenorrhea
307.50 Eating disorder NEC
307.1 Anorexia nervosa
305.51 Bulimia nervosa
733.16 Stress fracture, tibia
733.14 Stress fracture, hip
733.0 Osteoporosis
733.9 Osteopenia

BIBLIOGRAPHY

Fagan KM. Pharmacologic management of athletic amenorrhea. *Clin Sports Med* 1998;17:327–341.

Hobart JA, Smucker DR. The female athlete triad. *Am Family Physician* 2000;61:3357–3364.

Otis CL, Drinkwater B, Johnson M, et al. American College of Sports Medicine position stand. The female athlete triad. *Med Sci Sports Exerc* 1997;29:i–ix.

Sanborn CF, et al. Disordered eating and the female athlete triad. *Clin Sports Med* 2000;19:199–213.

Authors: Thomas L. Pommering, Ken Taylor, and Timothy J. Linker

Nursemaid's Elbow

Basics

DEFINITION

- Results from a traumatic subluxation of the radial head, which is produced by sudden forcible traction on the pronated hand or wrist with the relaxed elbow extended
- Subluxation of the radial head only occurs in pronation, which is the position in which the diameter of the radial head is the most narrow in the anteroposterior plane.
- As the radial head subluxes, there is an interposition of the annular ligament in the radiocapitellar joint where it becomes entrapped.

INCIDENCE/PREVALENCE

- One of the most common musculoskeletal injuries in children under 4 years of age
- Rarely found in children over 5 years of age, probably because by this age the distal attachments of the orbicular ligament are sufficiently strong to prevent its proximal migration
- Peak incidence is between the ages of 1 and 3 years.
- Left side is more commonly affected than the right.

SIGNS AND SYMPTOMS

- Child cries in pain immediately at the time of injury.
- Child refuses to use the affected limb.
- An audible or palpable "click" may be heard by the person who pulled the child's arm.
- The forearm is always pronated and the elbow is partially flexed.
- The child typically holds the affected limb by his or her side, sometimes supporting the forearm with the other hand.

RISK FACTORS

- Frequently, the traction force occurs when the child suddenly attempts to pull away from a parent or drops to the ground.
- The necessary force also can occur while a child is being pulled by the hand or forearm such as in pulling a child as he or she stumbles, lifting him or her up by the hand, or swinging the child around.

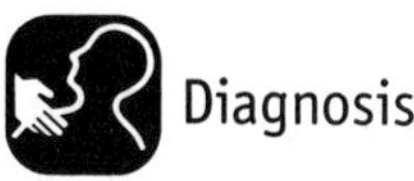

Diagnosis

DIFFERENTIAL DIAGNOSIS

- Posterior elbow dislocation
- Distal radial buckle fracture (torus) or other radial fracture
- Septic elbow
- Ulnar fracture
- Supracondylar fracture or other fracture of the humerus
- Avulsion of the medial or lateral epicondyle

HISTORY

- In more than 80% of cases, there is a history of sudden longitudinal traction to a pronated, extended forearm.
- May be a history of a "click" felt or heard by the person who pulled the child's arm.
- May be a history of an incidental fall in which the arm, elbow, and forearm were impacted between the ground and the child's trunk.
- Immediately following the injury, the child is usually tearful due to the pain and refuses to use the affected arm.
- Pain, if vocalized, may be referred toward the wrist.
- The child holds the forearm by his or her side, always in a pronated and partially flexed position (Nursemaid's position).
- Occasionally there is no history of trauma; the parents may simply notice the nonuse of the affected limb.

PHYSICAL EXAM

- The child may be tearful.
- The child also may appear content and playful, but declines to move the affected arm.
- Gentle palpation can reveal local tenderness over the anterolateral aspect of the radial head.
- By carefully avoiding movements involving the elbow and forearm, one can note painless range of motion of the wrist, hand, and shoulder.
- Typically no obvious swelling or deformity.
- There is minimal restriction to flexion and extension of the elbow, but supination of the forearm is markedly limited and resisted.

IMAGING

- Debate exists whether or not to obtain routine radiographs in straightforward clinical cases.
- Radiographs are not generally recommended if the mechanism of injury, body positioning, and examination are consistent with the diagnosis.
- Consider radiographic studies to rule out fracture or other abnormality. Radiographs should be obtained if the child exhibits point tenderness, soft tissue swelling, or ecchymosis of the elbow.
- Radiographs are typically normal. There is no distal displacement of the proximal radius from the capitellum.
- Reduction of the affected elbow may be performed by the x-ray technician who passively forces the forearm into full supination in an attempt to obtain a true anteroposterior view of the elbow.

POSTREDUCTION VIEWS

- Not usually indicated
- Postreduction views may be indicated if the child's arm does not return to normal function after reduction attempts are made.

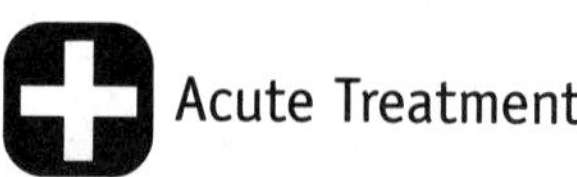

Acute Treatment

ANALGESIA

- Not typically necessary for reduction
- Consider acetaminophen (15 mg/kg) or ibuprofen (5–10 mg/kg) as needed.

REDUCTION TECHNIQUES

- The thumb is placed in the region of the radial head for palpation and the exertion of mild pressure (anterior to posterior).
- The child's forearm is gently but firmly rotated into full supination.
- The elbow is then flexed to 90 degrees by holding the child's forearm above the wrist and stabilizing the humerus and elbow with the other hand to prevent rotation of the shoulder. If any resistance is met, one should continue flexing the elbow to the point of maximal flexion.
- As reduction is achieved, a palpable and sometimes audible "click" can be felt in the region of the radial head.
- This maneuver will typically achieve instantaneous reduction of the radial head and sometimes instant relief of pain.

POSTREDUCTION EVALUATION

- The child should typically be observed for 15 minutes for a return of full function and use of the affected arm.
- If function has not normalized in 15 minutes, a repeated attempt at reduction is recommended.
- In some studies, the delay until normal use of the arm is achieved is longer when there has been a delay in treatment from the time of injury.
- If there is no evidence of recovery after several reduction attempts, the diagnosis must be reconsidered.

IMMOBILIZATION

- Immobilization is not usually necessary for the first occurrence of subluxation.
- If reduction is delayed for more than 12 hours following injury, an attempt is made to support the limb with a sling for 10 days with the elbow in 90 degrees of flexion and the forearm in full supination, but most toddlers discard the sling within minutes.
- Following reduction of recurrent cases, some clinicians recommend immobilization of the upper limb in an above-elbow cast for 2 to 3 weeks.

SPECIAL CONSIDERATIONS

- In a child under 6 months of age, consider abuse from a caretaker while evaluating the child. However, subluxation can occur while simply rolling over in this age group.
- Recurrence of subluxation as a result of subsequent pulls occurs in approximately 5% to 40% of cases.

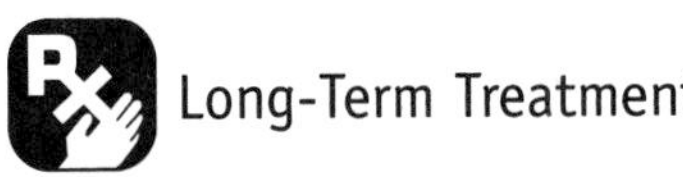

Long-Term Treatment

REHABILITATION

- Prevention is key. The parent should be advised to avoid longitudinal traction strains on the arm by not pulling on the hand or wrist, but rather pick the child up by the trunk.
- For the child who recovers fully after one or two reduction maneuvers, further therapy or intervention is unnecessary.

SURGICAL TREATMENT

- Very rarely, the subluxed radial head may be irreducible by manipulation, especially in recurrent cases, requiring surgical intervention.
- The need for open reduction is extremely rare.

REFERRAL/DISPOSITION

- Even when multiple attempts at closed reduction fail, spontaneous reduction almost always occurs.
- Usually no long-term sequelae
- Consider an occult fracture or cartilaginous injury if the response to treatment is not typical.

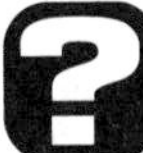

Common Questions and Answers

Physician responses to common patient questions:

Q: Now that my child has had one episode of nursemaid's elbow, is he at higher risk for having a second episode?

A: He is at slightly increased risk, but this can be minimized by avoidance of pulling on the child's hand or arm.

Q: Will my child have any long-term problems as a result of this episode?

A: There will most likely be no long-term sequelae.

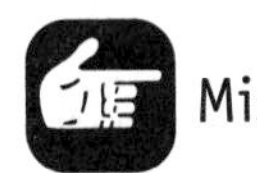

Miscellaneous

SYNONYMS

- Pulled elbow
- Radiocapitellar subluxation
- Subluxation of the head of the radius
- Subluxation of the radius by elongation
- Temper tantrum elbow
- Malgaigne's injury

ICD-9 CODE

832.0 Nursemaid's elbow
832.01 Closed dislocation, radius, proximal end

BIBLIOGRAPHY

Bachman D, Santora S. *Textbook of pediatric emergency medicine*. Baltimore: Williams & Wilkins, 1993.

Christoph RA. *Emergency medicine, a comprehensive study guide*. New York: McGraw-Hill, 1996.

Rand FF. *Emergency medicine*. Boston: Little, Brown, 1992.

Schunk JE. Radial head subluxation: epidemiology and treatment of 87 episodes. *Ann Emerg Med* 1990;19:1019–1023.

Tachdjian MO, ed. *Pediatric orthopedics*. Philadelphia: WB Saunders, 1990.

Authors: Timothy J. Linker and James E. Sturmi

Osgood-Schlatter Disease

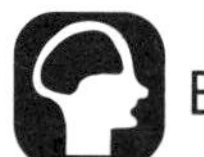

Basics

DEFINITION

- A disease process of late childhood and adolescence due to microfractures of the proximal tibial apophysis at the insertion point of the patellar tendon. This results in a reaction and an inflammation in the cartilage of this region.

INCIDENCE/PREVALENCE

- More prevalent in males in earlier studies
- Predominance in late childhood and adolescence

SIGNS AND SYMPTOMS

- Swelling and tenderness at tibial tubercle
- Increased prominence of tibial tubercle
- Unilateral or bilateral lower extremity pain
- Pain exacerbated by exercise, most notably running or jumping

RISK FACTORS

- Late childhood
- Male sex
- Athletic participation in sports that focus on repeated running or jumping

GENETICS

- Unknown genetic predisposition

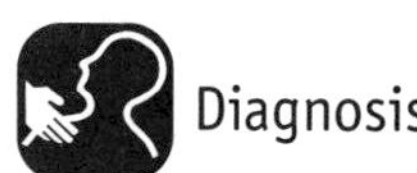

Diagnosis

DIFFERENTIAL DIAGNOSIS

- Pes anserinus bursitis
- Quadriceps tendon avulsion
- Patellofemoral stress syndrome
- Patellar tendonitis
- Osteomyelitis of proximal tibia
- Tibial plateau fracture
- Sindig-Larson-Johansson syndrome
- Patellar subluxation
- Proximal tibial neoplasm

HISTORY

- Worsening lower leg pain after exercise or increased activity
- Repetitive jumping or sprinting sports
- Unilateral or bilateral pain
- Typically pain is found in take-off leg.
- The patient may complain of mild swelling below the knee.
- History of suspicious trauma is usually absent.

PHYSICAL EXAM

Tenderness localized to the patellar tendon insertion is occasionally associated with mild swelling.

IMAGING

- Radiographs of the affected limb are only necessary to rule out other etiologies of leg pain.
- Radiographs demonstrate normal tibial apophysis in skeletally mature individuals.

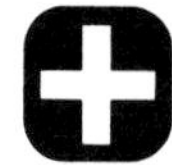

Acute Treatment

ANALGESIA

- Nonsteroidal antiinflammatory drugs are of minimal benefit.
- Ice application after exercise
- Treatment acutely consists of relative rest.

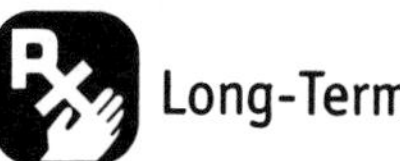

Long-Term Treatment

REHABILITATION

- Strengthening and stretching of quadriceps and hamstrings
- Few individuals will need long-term rest from athletic participation or knee immobilizers.

SURGICAL TREATMENT

- Surgical treatment has not been shown to improve outcome.
- Rarely, some individuals require intervention due to persistent discomfort after the physis fuses to remove remnants of bony ossicles.

REFERRAL/DISPOSITION

- Treatment may take up to several months to a year to completely resolve.
- When the physes close during late adolescence, the pain subsides.
- Overall a good prognosis is expected.

Common Questions and Answers

Physician responses to common patient questions:

Q: When can the patient return to activity?
A: Patients can return to activity when they can participate in activities without significant discomfort.
Q: Will the pain get better?
A: Complete resolution occurs when the physis closes.
Q: Will the patient need surgery?
A: Rarely, in some individuals who have persistent discomfort after the physis fuses, removal of any small bony ossicles that never fused with the tibia may be needed.
Q: Is the athlete at risk for complete avulsion of the apophysis when symptomatic with this condition?
A: No studies have demonstrated increased risk of avulsion with Osgood-Schlatter disease.
Q: What are alternate activities?
A: Biking, swimming, and isometric exercises.
Q: What are activities to avoid?
A: Running, sprinting, basketball, volleyball, and tennis.

Miscellaneous

SYNONYMS

- Osteochondritis of the tibial tubercle
- Jumper's knee or leg

ICD-9 CODE

732.4 Juvenile osteochondrosis of the lower extremity, excluding foot

BIBLIOGRAPHY

Bowers KD. Patellar tendon avulsion as a complication of Osgood-Schlatter disease. *Am J Sports Med* 1981;9:356–359.

King AG. A surgical procedure for the Osgood-Schlatter lesions. *Am J Sports Med* 1981;9:250–253.

Kujala UM. Osgood-Schlatter's disease in adolescent athletes. *Am J Sports Med* 1985;13:236–241.

Micheli L, Fehlandt AF. Overuse injuries to tendons and apophyses in children. *Clin J Sports Med* 1992;11:713–726.

Ryu RK. Adolescent and pediatric sports injuries. *Pediatr Clin North Am* 1998;45:1601–1635.

Stanitski CL. Pediatric and adolescent sports injuries. *Clin Sports Med* 1998;16:616–633.

Thomsen JEM. Operative treatment of osteochondritis of the tibia. *J Bone Joint Surg [Am]* 1956;38:142–148.

Authors: Harvey Leo and David T. Bernhardt

Osteoporosis

Basics

DEFINITION

- Systemic disorder characterized by decreased bone mass and microarchitectural deterioration of bone leading to bone fragility and increased susceptibility to fractures of the hip, spine, and wrist
- World Health Organization defines osteoporosis as bone mineral density (BMD) greater than 2.5 standard deviations below the mean for a particular age on dual-energy x-ray absorptiometry (DEXA) scan
- Osteoporosis is classified as either the primary, age-related type (postmenopausal estrogen deficiency, age-related vitamin D deficiency) or the secondary type (drug or concurrent medical condition etiology)

INCIDENCE/PREVALENCE

- In the United States, 1 in 4 women over age 50 have osteoporosis
- 1 in 8 men over age 50 have osteoporosis

SIGNS AND SYMPTOMS

- Usually late findings, such as an exaggerated kyphotic curvature (dowager's hump) indicating anterior wedge fractures of thoracic vertebrae

RISK FACTORS

- Female sex
- Non-Hispanic Caucasian race
- Asian race
- Family history
- Older age
- Diet low in calcium, low in vitamins C, D, and K, and decreased copper, manganese, and zinc mineral content
- Estrogen deficiency: postmenopausal or premenopausal secondary to overexercising and/or eating disorder
- Sedentary life-style, lack of weight-bearing exercise
- Female athlete triad: disordered eating, amenorrhea, and osteoporosis
- Medications: corticosteroids, anticonvulsants, cyclosporine, heparin, thyroid replacement drugs
- Excessive alcohol and tobacco intake
- Other diseases: diabetes, hyperparathyroidism, hyperthyroidism
- Impaired absorption of calcium, phosphate, and vitamin D from the gastrointestinal tract as in inflammed bowel disease, gastrectomy, celiac disease, jejunoileal bypass, or pancreatic insufficiency

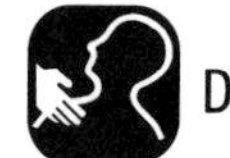

Diagnosis

HISTORY

- Atraumatic fracture/stress fracture
- Risk factor assessment

PHYSICAL EXAM

- Usually not evident on exam unless advanced stage and subsequent fracture

IMAGING

- DEXA measures bone mineral content of lumbar spine, femoral neck, and distal radius yielding BMD (g/cm^2).
- DEXA uses lower dose of radiation and costs less than quantitative computed tomography.
- Ultrasonography of the calcaneus may be useful as screening tool to identify patients at risk and those who would benefit from DEXA evaluation.

LABORATORY STUDIES

- Assessment of biochemical markers of bone turnover: osteocalcin, total and bone-specific alkaline phosphatase
- Serum type I collagen propeptide, pyridinoline levels in blood and urine, and plasma tartrate-resistant acid phosphatase levels are markers used in research settings.

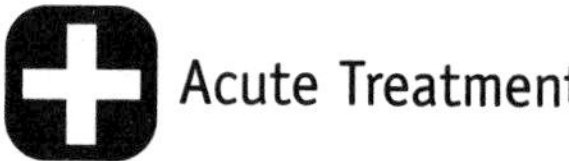

Acute Treatment

PHARMACOTHERAPY

- Pharmacologic interventions act by decreasing bone resorption, thus providing at most a 10% increase in BMD at any given site.
- Calcium carbonate and calcium citrate are essential adjuncts to other treatments: 1,500 mg for postmenopausal women, 1,000 mg for premenopausal women, 1,500 mg for female athletes.
- Vitamin D: particularly useful in vitamin D-deficient elderly (400–800 IU daily)
- Estrogen replacement: indicated for all women with premature or surgical menopause in the absence of contraindications, and for women immediately after menopause; conjugated estrogen 0.625 to 1.25 mg continuously in pill or patch form versus cyclic or continuous estrogen and progesterone administration for women with an intact uterus; combination estrogen-progesterone oral contraceptives in the estrogen-deficient amenorrheic female athlete
- Bisphosphonates: inhibit both osteoblast and, to a greater extent, osteoclast activity, thus decreasing bone turnover and increasing BMD; alendronate (Fosamax) 5 or 10 mg daily
- Selective estrogen receptor modulators: raloxifene (Evista); agonist activity in cardiovascular and bone tissue with antagonist activity in breast and uterine tissue; especially useful in women at high risk for breast cancer; short-term data only; long-term efficacy and safety limited; 60 mg daily with supplemental calcium
- Calcitonin: alternative treatment when estrogen contraindicated; 100 IU subcutaneously/intramuscularly daily or every other day; 200 IU intranasal spray daily with 1,000 mg calcium and 400 IU vitamin D

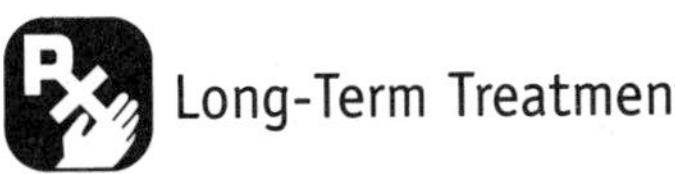

Long-Term Treatment

PREVENTIVE MEASURES

- Identification and treatment of risk factors/secondary causes of osteoporosis
- Weight-bearing exercise with additional resistance training can maintain bone mass and can help prevent falls when coupled with adequate calcium intake.
- When counseling young females, emphasize importance of achieving peak bone mass via calcium supplementation, good overall nutrition, and regular menstrual cycles.

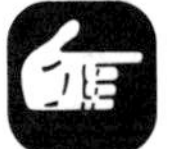

Miscellaneous

ICD-9 CODE

733.01 Osteoporosis, senile
782.81 Osteoporosis, screen

BIBLIOGRAPHY

Beck B, Shoemaker MR. Osteoporosis. Understanding key risk factors and therapeutic options. *Physician Sportsmed* 2000;28:69–84.

Iqbal MM. Osteoporosis: epidemiology, diagnosis, and treatment. *South Med J* 2000;93:2–18.

Keen AD, Drinkwater BL. Irreversible bone loss in former amenorrheic athletes. *Osteoporosis Int* 1997;7:311–315.

Otis CL, Drinkwater B, Johnson M, et al. American College of Sports Medicine position stand on the female athlete triad. *Med Sci Sports Exerc* 1997;29:i–ix.

Putukian M. Female athlete triad. *Sports Med Arthrosc Rev* 1995;3:295–307.

Rosen CJ, ed. *Osteoporosis. Diagnostic and therapeutic principles*. Totowa, NJ: Humana, 1996.

Voss LA, Fadale PD, Hulstyn MJ. Exercise-induced loss of bone density in athletes. *J Am Acad Orthop Surg* 1998;6:349–357.

West RV. The female athlete. The triad of disordered eating, amenorrhea, and osteoporosis. *Sports Med* 1998;26:63–71.

Author: Julie Kerr

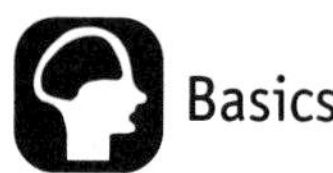

Basics

FOUR MAJOR AREAS OF THEORETICAL CONCERN

- Thermoregulation: Pregnancy increases a woman's metabolic rate and increases heat production. The increased heat production by exercising muscles may further increase maternal core temperature. Many clinicians quote a "teratogenic threshold" of 39.2°C. This temperature was set based on animal data. In addition, epidemiologic data suggest an increased incidence in neural tube defects in women using hot tubs in their first trimester of pregnancy.
- Cardiopulmonary changes: The primary theoretical concern is the redistribution of blood flow away from the uterus and other splanchnic organs toward muscles during exercise.
- Metabolic responses: The theoretical concern is substrate utilization and availability to the developing fetus. During exercise, substrates (such as glycogen and glucose) are mobilized to provide fuel for the musculature. With pregnancy, the converse is true: substrates are directed toward the developing fetus for storage and accretion. These two effects are apparently competitive.
- Endocrine changes: The body perceives exercise as an acute stress response. Serum epinephrine, norepinephrine, glucagon, and cortisol are increased; insulin and gonadotropin levels are decreased. During pregnancy, however, the body regulates uterine quiescence through decreased epinephrine, norepinephrine, glucagon, and cortisol levels. In addition, during pregnancy the levels of insulin and gonadotropins are increased. Again, these effects seem to contradict and potentially compete with each other.

1985 ACOG GUIDELINES

In 1985, because of these theoretical concerns coupled with available data (mostly animal and epidemiologic), the American College of Obstetricians and Gynecologists (ACOG) made recommendations for pregnant women who wished to exercise:

- Maintain maternal heart rate below 140 beats/min. This number was derived from the rationale that 140 beats/min reflects approximately 60% to 70% of age-predicted maximal heart rate.
- Maternal core temperature should not exceed 38°C, and women should not strenuously exert themselves for more than 15 minutes. The goal of this guideline was to avoid maternal core temperatures possibly injurious to the fetus.
- Avoid ballistic movements, supine activity and Valsalva maneuvers after the fourth month of pregnancy. Lying supine may compress the vasculature to the uterus and may reduce blood flow to the fetus during exercise.
- Avoid extremes of ranges of motion. During pregnancy, progesterone and relaxin cause changes to the musculoskeletal system that assist with carrying and delivery of the fetus. If extreme range of motion occurs, it may result in orthopedic injuries.
- Always perform an adequate warm-up and cool-down with exercise. In addition, provide enough hydration and nutrition to meet the extra needs associated with both pregnancy and exercise.

CURRENT LITERATURE: OUTCOMES

Since 1985, well more than 70 studies have been published evaluating these concerns and the effects of exercise on maternal and fetal outcomes.

- Thermoregulation: New data evaluating exercise-induced hyperthermia do not concur with animal and epidemiologic data. Proposed mechanisms include pregnancy-induced plasma volume expansion and decrease peripheral vascular resistance. These changes allow for more heat dissipation with pooling of blood in the lower extremities. The resultant heat transfer via the skin helps to regulate maternal core temperature. Hyperthermic stress is magnified by dehydration, improper clothing, exercise in hot/humid environment, and poor fitness levels. The magnitude of exercise-associated thermal stress for the developing fetus appears to be reduced by maternal physiologic adaptation to pregnancy and exercise.
- Cardiopulmonary changes: Although initial animal data suggested that uterine blood flow may, in fact, be reduced by 50%, this reduction in blood flow was limited to the myometrium. There was, however, no change in blood flow to the placental unit. This also may be related to pregnancy-associated plasma volume increase (resulting in a tenfold increase in uterine blood flow to begin with). Finally, an increase in oxygen extraction by the fetus rounds out a complex array of cardiopulmonary changes that protect the fetus during exercise.
- Metabolic responses: Current data suggest that blood glucose may decrease, but clinical hypoglycemia has never been demonstrated. In addition, there may be increased fat utilization for fuel (as demonstrated by the higher levels of serum triglycerides). Furthermore, the fetus appears to have an increased ability to extract glucose from the mother (similar to improved oxygen extraction above).
- Endocrine changes: Even with the theoretical concerns of increased epinephrine and norepinephrine levels associated with exercise, there has been no reported increase in the incidence of premature onset labor (POL), premature rupture of membranes (PROM), etc.
- Maternal outcomes: In general, current data demonstrate no clinically significant change in gestational length (up to 5 days) and gestational weight gain. There is no apparent increase in the incidence of spontaneous abortions, POL, or PROM. There are conflicting data on labor length. It does appear that exercisers exhibit a 50% reduction in medical interventions (Pitocin, forceps, cesarean section) during labor. In addition, there may be a slight decrease in the duration of the second stage of labor (pushing phase). Significant support for higher intensity and longer duration of exercise during pregnancy came from a meta-analysis evaluating 18 studies on pregnancy outcomes.
- Fetal outcomes: Current data do not demonstrate an increased incidence of birth defects, neural tube defects, etc. There has been no demonstrable difference in Apgar scores in exercising women. There are conflicting data on birth weight. Most studies indicate no adverse effect. Some studies demonstrate a reduction in birth weight by up to 400 g. Upon further examination, this weight decrement may have been secondary to a decrease in the size of the neonatal fat mass.

1994 ACOG GUIDELINES

Due to more substantial human studies supporting beneficial outcomes in the mother and fetus, the ACOG developed newer guidelines in 1994, which stand as the current guidelines today. The apparent rigidity of the 1985 guidelines and the increased use of those guidelines in legal terms led to more scientifically supported guidelines. The 1994 ACOG guidelines for exercise during pregnancy are much more vague, and less restrictive.

- Exercise of mild to moderate intensity at least 3 days a week. No mention of specific temperature or intensity duration. Recent data suggest that heart rate is less helpful in determining exercise intensity. More support is now given to rates of perceived exertion. The woman can exercise to a point where she can maintain relatively easy conversation.
- Modify exercise intensity/duration based on maternal symptoms.
- Avoid supine exercise after the fourth month of pregnancy; avoid exercise where loss of balance/blunt trauma may occur.

- Pregnancy requires an extra 300 calories per day of nutritional intake. Exercise further increases this requirement. Supplement nutritional intake to account for the added requirements.
- Provide adequate hydration and assist thermoregulation with proper clothing, fitness levels, etc.

CONTRAINDICATIONS TO EXERCISE DURING PREGNANCY

Most clinicians include the following list as contraindications to exercise in pregnancy:

- Pregnancy-induced hypertension
- POL
- PROM
- Incompetent cervix
- Persistent second- or third-trimester bleeding
- Intrauterine growth retardation
- Chronic/uncontrolled medical problems (such as cardiac, pulmonary, diabetic vascular and thyroid abnormalities)

THE TAKE HOME MESSAGE

Exercise has not been shown to increase the incidence of poor maternal and fetal outcomes. There is scientific support for exercise continued at prepregnancy levels without adverse effects. The clinician must individualize recommendations to each patient. Although theoretical concerns exist, the current literature demonstrates maternal and fetal adaptations that improve the efficiency of thermoregulation, cardiopulmonary systems, substrate use, and endocrine responses.

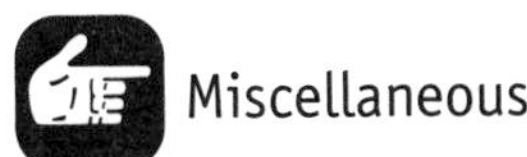

Miscellaneous

ORTHOPEDIC CONCERNS OF PREGNANT ATHLETES

- A number of changes occur with pregnancy that affect the musculoskeletal system of the exercising patient. Increases in serum progesterone and relaxin have been implicated in the occurrence of more musculoskeletal symptoms in the pregnant woman. The studies addressing this issue demonstrate conflicting results. In addition, biomechanical changes associated with the changing center of gravity (increased lordosis) have been implicated as a cause for orthopedic symptoms during pregnancy. Furthermore, increased plasma volume associated with pregnancy can exacerbate carpal tunnel symptoms.
- Low back pain has been reported in 50% to 70% of all pregnant women. Despite theories to the contrary, current data do not suggest an increased incidence of herniated nucleus pulposus. Some data support the theory that previously active women who continue their exercise/fitness level during pregnancy have less musculoskeletal symptomatology.
- Carpal tunnel syndrome is the second most common orthopedic symptom during pregnancy. It presents with night pain and paresthesias most prominent during the second and third trimesters. Most patients require nonoperative treatment, with swift spontaneous resolution of symptoms after delivery.
- Avoid nonsteroidal antiinflammatory drugs in treating musculoskeletal conditions during pregnancy (especially the first and second trimesters). Acetaminophen, supervised exercise routines, cryotherapy, and splinting may be helpful. Rarely, steroid injections may be useful for recalcitrant pain and dysfunction. Also consider alteration of activities as needed.

BIBLIOGRAPHY

Sternfeld B. Physical activity and pregnancy outcome—review and recommendations. *Sports Med* 1997;23:33–47.

Sternfeld B, Quesenberry CP, Eskenazi B, et al. Exercise during pregnancy and pregnancy outcome. *Med Sci Sports Exerc* 1995;27:634–640.

Wang TW, Apgar BS. Exercise during pregnancy. *Am Family Physician* 1998;57: 1846–1852.

Wolfe LA, Brenner IK, Mottola MF. Maternal exercise, fetal well-being and pregnancy. *Exerc Sport Sci Rev* 1994;22:145–194.

Authors: Guy Monteleone and Mark Bracker

Scoliosis and Kyphosis

Basics

DEFINITION

- Scoliosis is a fixed lateral curvature of the spine.
- Kyphosis is a fixed exaggerated anteroposterior (AP) curvature of the thoracic spine.
- Lordosis is a fixed exaggerated AP curvature of the lumbar spine.
- Kyphoscoliosis is a combination of lateral and AP curvature of the spine.

INCIDENCE/PREVALENCE

- Common occurrence in skeletally maturing patients; seen more often in adolescence as they transition through their secondary growth spurt
- More common in females than males
- Idiopathic scoliosis occurs in 2% to 4% of school-aged children.
- Categories:
  —Infantile scoliosis (<3 years old): less than 1% of all cases
  —Juvenile scoliosis (3–10 years old): 12% to 21% of all cases
  —Adolescent scoliosis (>10 years old): 75% to 85% of all cases

SIGNS AND SYMPTOMS

- Subtle findings, such as poorly fitting clothes, uneven shoulders, uneven waistlines, hip discomfort, leg length discrepancy
- Overt findings, such as a noticeable curve when seen from behind
- Pain is not a feature and should prompt a search for another cause.

RISK FACTORS

- Family history is the primary risk. Although the inheritance patterns have not been fully elaborated, current thinking favors an autosomal-dominant pattern involving many genes, resulting in variable expression within susceptible families.
- Adolescent patients with idiopathic scoliosis often demonstrate deficits in proprioception and vibratory sensation when compared with age-matched unaffected patients, which may suggest a causative factor in the development of this problem.

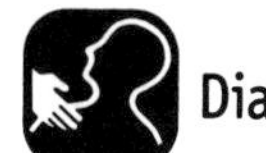

Diagnosis

DIFFERENTIAL DIAGNOSIS

- Congenital scoliosis: anomalies of vertebral segmentation and/or formation (Klippel-Feil syndrome, VACTERL syndrome).
- Spinal dysraphism (myelomeningocele).
- Neuromuscular scoliosis: upper motor neuron (Friedrich's ataxia, cerebral palsy, Charcot-Marie-Tooth syndrome, syringomyelia, muscular dystrophy) or lower motor neuron (poliomyelitis, spina bifida)
- Functional secondary scoliosis (leg-length inequality, unilateral muscle spasm)
- Scheuermann's: look for pathognomonic Schmorl's nodes
- Kyphosis secondary to bone demineralization (osteoporosis)
- Other causes: spondylolisthesis, herniated disk, discitis, osteoid osteoma

HISTORY

- Painless back curvature
- Often noticed by an observer, such as a parent
- Uneven shoulders, poorly fitting shirts, the prominence of one shoulder blade, or an overt curve may be evident.
- In many cases, it is discovered in school-based screenings or preparticipation examinations.

PHYSICAL EXAM

- Check posture, leg length discrepancy, abdominal reflexes.
- A complete neuroorthopedic exam (i.e., cavus feet seen in Charcot-Marie-Tooth syndrome)
- Marfanoid body habitus, hypermobile joints, or hyperflexible skin (i.e., Marfan's or Ehlers-Danlos syndrome)
- Café-au-lait spots (i.e., neurofibromatosis)
- Adams' forward bending test: Patient stands with legs locked, bends at the waist, arms toward feet. Examiner stands behind patient, lowers head and views across patient's back looking for elevated and rotated vertebral segments.
- A scoliometer may be used to measure the angle of trunk rotation (ATR). An ATR of 7 degrees or greater correlates (83% sensitive, 86% specific) to a clinically significant curve. The ATR multiplied by 3 estimates the curvature (Cobb angle).

IMAGING

- Scoliosis: a standing AP radiograph (36 inch) of the entire spine should be obtained for all patients with a scoliometer reading greater than 7 degrees (or predicted Cobb angle of 21 degrees).
- How to measure the Cobb angle to determines the severity of the curve:
  —Find the lowest transitional vertebra whose inferior surface tilts to the concavity of curve.
  —Erect a perpendicular from the inferior surface of the distal vertebrae. Repeat for the superior surface of the proximal transitional vertebra.
  —Measure the intersecting angle where the perpendicular lines cross.
- Types of scoliosis seen on films:
  —Thoracic (one curve)
  —Thoracolumbar (one curve)
  —Lumbar (one curve)
  —Double major (two curves: one lumbar, one thoracic)
  —Double thoracic (two curves in thorax)
- Kyphosis: a lateral standing 36-inch radiograph
- Make sure with radiographs to image the iliac crests, including the iliac epiphyses, so to help with the Risser scoring.

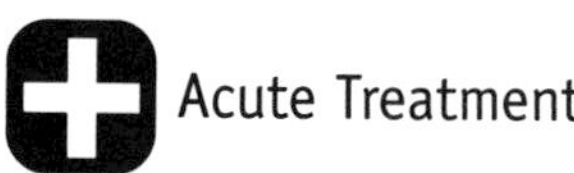

Acute Treatment

KYPHOSIS

- Rarely needs surgical intervention. Normal range for dorsal kyphosis falls between 20 and 40 degrees. Marginal kyphosis is between 40 and 50 degrees, and hyperkyphosis is above 50 degrees

SCOLIOSIS

- Depends on the severity of the curve, skeletal maturity, and the age of the patient
- Curvature and the probability it will progress:
  —Curvature of less than 19 degrees: 10 to 12 years = 25%; 13 to 15 years = 10%; 16+ years = 0%
  —Curvature of 20 to 29 degrees: 10 to 12 years = 60%; 13 to 15 years = 40%; 16+ years = 10%
  —Curvature of 30 to 59 degrees: 10 to 12 years = 90%; 13 to 15 years = 70%; 16+ years = 30%
  —Curvature of more than 60 degrees: 10 to 12 years = 100%; 13 to 15 years = 90%; 16+ years = 70%

RISSER SCORE

The Risser score can also be used to aid prediction of progression:

- 1 = completely open growth plates, immature skeleton.
- 2 = growth plates open, some vertical height to achieve.
- 3 = growth plates closing, near full height.
- 4 = growth plates closed, full height achieved.

PROGRESSION

Probability of progression (based on Risser grade and curve magnitude at detection):

- Risser grade 0 to 1: curve magnitude 5 to 19 degrees = 22%; curve magnitude 20 to 29 degrees = 68%
- Risser grade 2 to 4: curve magnitude 5 to 19 degrees = 1.6%; curve magnitude 20 to 29 degrees = 23%

MANAGEMENT

Scoliometer reading: multiply by 3. If greater than 20 degrees, then:

- 20 to 29 degrees = standing radiographs, measure Cobb angle, radiograph every 6 months.
- 30 to 39 degrees = bracing immediately, consider referral to an orthopedic/spine specialist.
- 40 degrees + = referral for consideration of internal fixation.
- Some clinicians advocate following juvenile patients with curves of 10 degrees at 4- to 6-month intervals. Curves of less than 10 degrees require little monitoring.

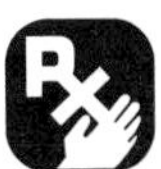

Long-Term Treatment

REHABILITATION

- Bracing should be continued as long as there is no progression of curvature and vertical growth is still occurring. In young women, this means a Risser stage of at least 3; in young men, a Risser stage of 4.

SURGICAL TREATMENT

- Surgical stabilization should be considered in skeletally mature patients with a Cobb angle of greater than 45 degrees.
- Surgical stabilization should be considered in skeletally immature patients with a Cobb angle of greater than 40 degrees.
- Surgery most commonly is the placement of one or two Harrington rods internally along the spine to correct the curvature. Anterior and posterior approaches are used.

REFERRAL/DISPOSITION

Refer to orthopedic/spine specialist when there is a:

- Nonbraceable curve of the thoracic spine (apex of curve higher than T6)
- Worsening curvature despite bracing
- Curvature in the newborn and infant; any children under 10 years old
- Curvature associated with severe trauma
- Curvature associated a high grade (3–4) spondylolisthesis

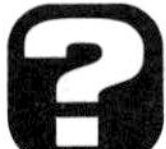

Common Questions and Answers

Physician responses to common patient questions:

Q: Can the athlete continue to play?
A: Athletes with curves of less than 30 degrees face little risk in sports. Athletes with curves of 30 to 39 degrees may participate in most sports as long as the brace can be tolerated. Athletes who have undergone surgical stabilization should strongly consider avoidance of contact/collision sports.
Q: Will bracing correct the curvature of the spine?
A: Braces have not been proven to permanently reduce curvatures, but can prevent progression in many cases. Compliance with bracing is critical to ensuring success of therapy.
Q: How long must the brace be worn daily to be effective?
A: Although it is ideal to wear the brace for 23 hours a day, studies have demonstrated good results when the brace is worn 18 hours a day.
Q: How long must the brace be worn until it can be discontinued?
A: Until the Risser score is 4 (closed growth plates).
Q: Does manipulation therapy help correct curvature of the spine?
A: As of this writing, there are few data to support the use of manipulative therapies to correct curvatures.

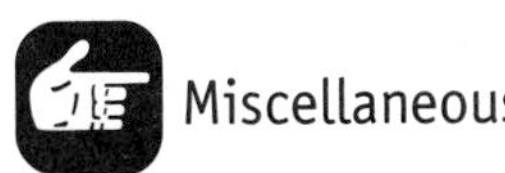

Miscellaneous

SYNONYMS

- Curvature of the spine
- Hunchback

ICD-9 CODE

737.30 Scoliosis, acquired, postural, idiopathic
754.2 Scoliosis, congenital
737.32 Scoliosis, infantile, progressive
737.31 Scoliosis, infantile, resolving
737.39 Scoliosis, paralysis
737.10 Kyphosis, acquired, postural
756.19 Kyphosis, congenital
737.30 Kyphoscoliosis, idiopathic

BIBLIOGRAPHY

Boachie-Adjei O, Lonner B. Spinal deformity. *Pediatr Clin North Am* 1996;43:883–896.

Dobbs MB, Weinstein SL. Infantile and juvenile scoliosis. *Orthop Clin North Am* 1999;30:331–340.

Ferrel MC. Scoliosis. *Clin Sport Med* 1999;18: 389–393.

Miller NH. Cause and natural history of adolescent idiopathic scoliosis. *Orthop Clin North Am* 1999;30:343–350.

Nelson W. *Nelson's textbook of pediatrics*, 14th ed. Philadelphia: WB Saunders, 1992.

Roach JW. Adolescent idiopathic scoliosis. *Orthop Clin North Am* 1999;30:353–364.

Staheli L, ed. *Fundamentals of pediatric orthopedics*, 2nd ed. Philadelphia: Lippincott-Raven, 1998.

Stanitsky CL. Scoliosis. *Clin Sport Med* 1997;18:613–633.

Authors: Mark Lavallee and Brian A. Jacobs

Slipped Capital Femoral Epiphysis

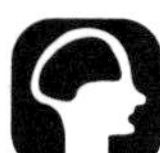

Basics

DEFINITION

- A disorder of unknown cause in which the proximal femoral epiphysis (head of the femur) begins to "fall off" the femoral neck. The slippage occurs at the epiphyseal plate, which begins to weaken as the plate matures.

INCIDENCE/PREVALENCE

- The disorder affects between 0.7 and 3.4 children per 100,000.
- The mean age at which it occurs is 11 years in girls, and 13 years in boys.
- It occurs during the rapid growth spurt.
- The disorder is bilateral in 20% to 40% of affected children.
- The disorder frequently occurs in two distinct body types: (1) slender, tall, rapidly growing boys, and (2) large, obese boys with or without undeveloped sexual characteristics. The second body type is more prevalent than the first.
- African-American boys are the group with the highest incidence.
- Endocrine disorders that weaken the physis are associated with slipped epiphyses and are particularly prevalent in preadolescent children.

SIGNS AND SYMPTOMS

- The most common presenting complaint is hip pain and a limp (antalgic gait).
- The pain is typically located in the groin area, but may be referred to the anterior thigh or medial knee area.
- Pain is usually gradual in onset, and symptoms occur even when a little displacement is present. Pain also may occur acutely with a dramatic onset of injury and sudden severe hip pain and inability to bear weight.

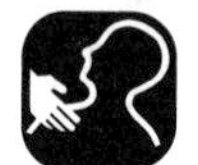

Diagnosis

DIFFERENTIAL DIAGNOSIS

- Femoral cutaneous nerve entrapment (more common in muscular girls)
- Growth hormone deficiency
- Hyperthyroidism
- Hypothyroidism
- Multiple endocrine neoplasia
- Panhypopituitarism
- Legg-Calve-Perthes disease (in younger age range)

PHYSICAL EXAM

- The physical exam reveals tenderness over the hip joint capsule, and an external rotation deformity of the lower extremity may be present.
- There is restricted hip motion, especially internal rotation, abduction, and forward flexion.
- The hip tends to rotate externally and abduct as it is flexed (Whitman's sign).
- In chronic cases, the affected leg may be 1 to 3 cm shorter than the normal leg, and the thigh muscles may be atrophied.

IMAGING

- Anteroposterior and frog-lateral views confirm the diagnosis. The affected side should be compared with the unaffected leg.
- The capital epiphysis is seen to displace posteriorly and downward, whereas the femoral neck displaces upward and anteriorly. In some patients, displacement is not obvious, but the physeal plate is widened (preslipping stage).
- Classification is based on the severity of the slip. Type 1 slips involve less than 33% of the width of the femoral epiphysis. Type 2 involves a 33% to 50% slip, and a type 3 involves more than 50% of the width of the femoral epiphysis.

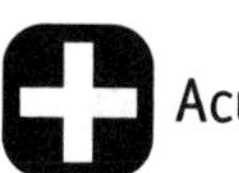

Acute Treatment

IMMEDIATE

- Acute treatment involves cessation of weight-bearing and surgical stabilization. A displaced epiphysis may require reduction before fixation. In the preslip phase, with widening of the physeal plate evident on radiographs, *in situ* operative fixation is recommended. Weight-bearing is begun at 6 weeks postsurgery.

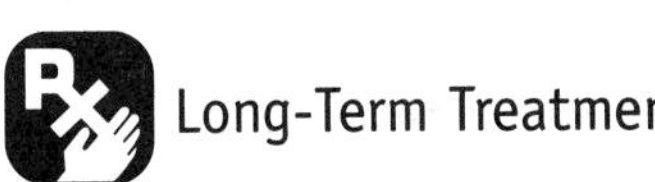

Long-Term Treatment

SURGICAL TREATMENT

Surgical stabilization is the mainstay of treatment for all types of slippages.

REFERRAL/DISPOSITION

Orthopedic referral should be done immediately upon diagnosis.

PROGNOSIS

Prognosis is usually good, except in those cases with acute traumatic separation. Slight shortening of the leg of less than 1.25 cm may result, along with a mild external rotation deformity. The internal fixation devices are removed after the physeal plate closes in 1 to 2 years.

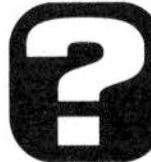

Common Questions and Answers

Physician responses to common patient questions:
Q: What are the complications of this condition?
A: In acute traumatic separations, avascular necrosis of the femoral head is a common complication, and this usually results in severe arthritis of the hip. Another complication is acute cartilage necrosis or lysis of the articular cartilage of the hip joint. A painful fibrous ankylosis of the hip joint is frequently the end result.

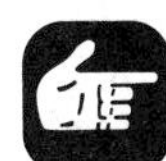

Miscellaneous

ICD-9 CODE

732.2 Nontraumatic
732.9 Traumatic
820.01 Fracture–separation

BIBLIOGRAPHY

Mercier L. *Practical orthopedics.* St. Louis: Mosby-Year Book, 1995.

Paletta GA Jr, Andrish JT. Injuries about the hip and pelvis in the young athlete. *Clin Sports Med* 1995;14:591–628.

Snider RK, Greene WB, Johnson TR, et al. *Essentials of musculoskeletal care.* Rosemont, IL: American Academy of Orthopedic Surgeons, 1998.

Stanitski CL, DeLee JC, Drez D Jr. *Pediatric and adolescent sports medicine.* Philadelphia: WB Saunders, 1994.

Authors: James Fambro and Ross M. Patton

Tillaux Fractures: Anterior Tibia-Fibula Ligament Avulsion

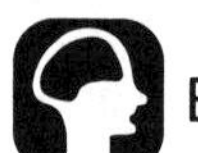

Basics

DEFINITION

- A Tillaux fracture is an avulsion of the lateral distal epiphysis of the tibia, which occurs in adolescents with partially closed physes, as a result of forced external rotation of the foot.
- This motion causes a significant stress to be applied to the anterior tibiofibular ligament, which inserts on the anterolateral aspect of the distal tibial epiphysis.
- When the distal tibial physis is undergoing physiologic closure (generally over a period of 18 months in adolescence), the stress applied to the ligament can result in a Salter-Harris type III physeal avulsion fracture.
- The Tillaux fracture is composed of a horizontal plane extending through the remainder of open physis and a vertical plane extending through the epiphysis, into the ankle joint.
- This fracture typically occurs in girls 13 to 15 years of age and boys 15 to 17 years of age, the ages that the distal tibia physes are undergoing physiologic closure.
- It is known as one of the transitional fractures, referring to the susceptibility of a partially closed physis.

INCIDENCE/PREVALENCE

- 2.9% (Speigel et al., 1978)

SIGNS AND SYMPTOMS

- Acute ankle pain, focal tenderness over anterolateral ankle, significant pain with weight bearing
- Swelling and ecchymosis may be seen, but are generally mild.
- Typically, little clinical deformity is noted, because the fibula prevents marked lateral displacement of the fragment.
- The patient may recall his or her foot being forced into external rotation, just prior to the onset of symptoms.

RISK FACTORS

- Girls 13 to 15 years of age
- Boys 15 to 17 years of age
- Rapid, forceful external rotation of the foot

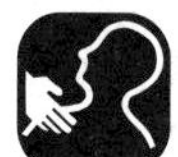

Diagnosis

DIFFERENTIAL DIAGNOSIS

- Ankle sprain, anterior tibiofibular ligament injury
- Triplanar fracture, likely a more severe version of Tillaux fracture; however, this injury has three fracture planes (the two planes described above for the Tillaux fracture and a vertical metaphyseal plane that exits the posterior cortex)
- Talar dome injury
- Distal fibular physeal injury

HISTORY

- Forceful external rotation of the foot, or internal rotation of the lower leg on a firmly planted foot
- Immediate pain in the anterolateral ankle joint region followed by pain with weight bearing, and mild to moderate swelling

PHYSICAL EXAM

Any of the following findings may be present: swelling, pain with palpation of anterolateral ankle, pain with passive ankle motion, inability to bear weight, or a significantly antalgic gait.

IMAGING

- Initial radiographs: anteroposterior (AP), lateral, and mortise views

POSTREDUCTION VIEWS

- AP, lateral, mortise
- Postreduction CT may be needed to accurately determine fracture pattern, amount of displacement, need for open reduction and fixation (ORIF)

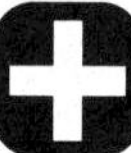

Acute Treatment

ANALGESIA

- Immobilization, ice, elevation, Tylenol
- For breakthrough pain, may require narcotics for first few days

REDUCTION TECHNIQUES

- Gently position the foot in internal rotation, prior to placement in a well-padded, bivalved, long leg cast.

POSTREDUCTION EVALUATION

- Neurovascular check of toes and foot
- Radiography: AP, lateral, mortise
- CT scan may be needed to determine the fracture pattern and amount of displacement, and to assess the need for ORIF

IMMOBILIZATION

- A long leg cast (due to the intraarticular component) with knee partially flexed
- Non-weight bearing for 4 weeks, weight bearing as tolerated for 2 to 4 weeks in a cam walker or rigid shell boot

SPECIAL CONSIDERATIONS

- Anatomic alignment of the articular surface is essential to minimize the risk of posttraumatic arthritis
- Physeal arrest is typically not a concern because the physis is, by definition, already in the process of closing. However, this should be evaluated periodically to monitor for the possibility of varus or valgus deformity long term.

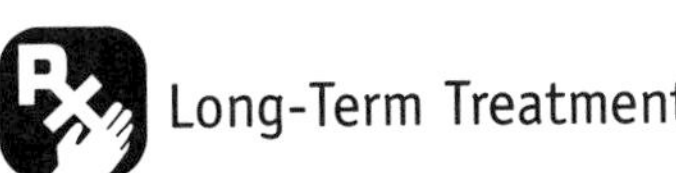

Long-Term Treatment

REHABILITATION

- Range of motion
- Strengthening
- Proprioception
- Endurance

SURGICAL TREATMENT

- Indicated if 2 mm of displacement or greater
- ORIF of fracture, typically using two cannulated screws.

REFERRAL/DISPOSITION

- After placement of the foot in internal rotation and application of a well-padded splint or cast, it is recommended that patients with this fracture be referred to an orthopedic surgeon experienced in treating pediatric fractures.
- If it is nondisplaced, referral within a week is appropriate.
- However, if there is displacement or if the treating physician is uncertain as to the amount of displacement, the patient should be referred to the orthopedist in 1 to 2 days. A CT scan is useful to determine displacement. Displacement of 2 mm or greater requires surgery (closed or open reduction and fixation).

Common Questions and Answers

Physician responses to common patient questions:

Q: What are possible complications?

A: Posttraumatic arthritis and asymmetric physeal growth.

Q: How long before weight bearing is allowed?

A: If the intraarticular fracture is treated nonoperatively, 4 weeks non-weight bearing, followed by 2 to 4 weeks in a walking cast or cam walker. If the intraarticular fracture is stabilized with internal fixation, 3 weeks non-weight bearing, followed by 3 weeks weight bearing in walking cast.

Q: How long before return to sports?

A: 12 weeks minimum. Must be healed on x-ray, be pain free with activity, and have full range of motion and strength.

Q: Precautions after this injury?

A: Peroneal strengthening and proprioception training is essential; proper mechanics in sport and proper shoe wear should be emphasized to prevent excessive stress to the anterior tibiofibular ligament. Consider use of an ankle support during early return-to-activity phase.

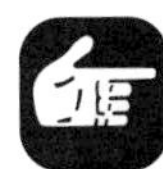

Miscellaneous

SYNONYMS

- Juvenile Tillaux fracture
- Transitional fracture of distal tibia

ICD-9 CODE

823.0

BIBLIOGRAPHY

Churchill JA, Mazur JM. Ankle pain in children: diagnostic evaluation and clinical decision making. *J Am Orthop Surg* 1995;3:183–193.

Morrisy RT, Weinstein SL. *Lovell and Winters' pediatric orthopaedics*. Philadelphia: Lippincott-Raven, 1996.

Rockwood C, Wilkins K, Beaty J. In: Rockwood CA, King RE (eds.). *Fractures in children* 4th ed. Philadelphia: Lippincott-Raven, 1996.

Speigel P, Cooperman D, Laros G. Epiphyseal fractures of the distal ends of the tibia and fibula. *J Bone Joint Surg [Am]* 1978;60:1046.

Authors: Aenor Sawyer and Lyle J. Micheli

SECTION III

General Medicine

Acne

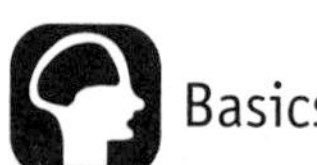

Basics

DEFINITION

- Acne is an inflammatory disorder of the pilosebaceous unit, resulting in comedones, apaules, and inflammatory pustules that may lead to scarring.

INCIDENCE/PREVALENCE

- Almost 100% of adolescents are affected.
- Intensity and duration can vary.
- Males are more commonly and severely affected than females.

SIGNS AND SYMPTOMS

- Open comedones (blackheads)
- Closed comedones (whiteheads)
- Papules (<5 mm in diameter)
- Pustules
- Nodules
- Scars

RISK FACTORS

- Adolescence
- Male sex
- Androgenic steroid use
- Some oral contraceptives (with more androgenic progesterone components)
- Rubbing or occluding skin surfaces: this occurs commonly with sports equipment (shoulder pads or helmets) or in wrestling when skin is frequently rubbed against the mat
- Occluding cosmetics (oil-based)
- Drugs: iodides or bromides, lithium, phenytoins
- Systemic corticosteroids
- Hot, humid climate

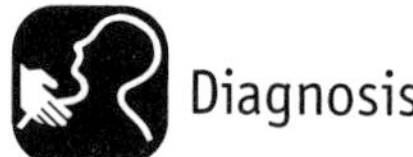

Diagnosis

DIFFERENTIAL DIAGNOSIS

- Contact dermatitis (tars, oils, grease)
- Folliculitis
- Acne rosacea
- Pseudofolliculitis barbae

HISTORY

- Onset typically at puberty as hormonal changes take place
- Females may have a flare-up just prior to menses.
- Athletes may have flare-ups when a new season or sport begins, correlating with activity or equipment used.

PHYSICAL EXAM

- Skin should be examined for which type of lesions are present and how many.
- Distribution of acne should be noted, especially if it seems to correlate with equipment used by the athlete.

PATHOGENESIS

- Hormonal changes stimulate increased production of sebum and increased keratin blocking follicular canals.
- *Proprionibacterium acnes*, a normal inhabitant of the follicular canal, may modify sebum, releasing potentially irritation-free fatty acids.
- *P. acnes* also produces chemotactic substances that contribute to inflammatory lesions.

GRADING

- Grade 1: comedonal (closed/open)
- Grade 2: papular (>25 lesions on face and trunk)
- Grade 3: pustular (>25 lesions, mild scarring)
- Grade 4: nodulocystic acne with extensive scarring

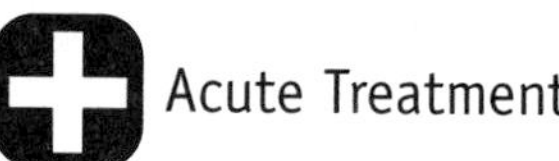

Acute Treatment

COMEDONAL ACNE

- Tretinoin (Retin-A): 0.025%, 0.05%, and 0.1% cream, 0.01% and 0.025% gel, 0.05% solution, apply at bedtime after washing
- Adapalene (Differin): 0.1% gel, apply at bedtime after washing
- Azelaic acid (Azelex): 20% cream twice daily
- Salicylic acid: 0.5% to 2.0% hydroalcoholic

MILD INFLAMMATORY ACNE

- Topical benzoyl peroxide 5% and 10% gel, apply at bedtime
- Topical antibiotic: erythromycin 2% gel or solution; clindamycin 1% gel, solution, or lotion twice daily; metronidazole gel (mostly for rosacea); azelaic acid 20% cream twice daily; benzoyl peroxide-erythromycin 5%/3% gel (very effective, must be refrigerated); tetracycline 0.22% solution twice daily (skin may flouresce under black light)

MODERATE INFLAMMATORY ACNE

- Topical tretinoin or adapalene, and
- Topical antibiotic/benzoyl peroxide, and/or
- Oral contraceptives (females): triphasic ethynyl estradiol/norgestimate (Ortho Tricyclen) has acne indication, or use 50-µg pill to increase sex hormone–binding globulin, which helps bind excess androgens
- Systemic (oral) antibiotic: tetracycline 500 to 1,000 mg daily; minocycline 50 to 200 mg daily; doxycycline 50 to 100 mg daily; erythromycin 500 to 1,000 mg daily

SEVERE INFLAMMATORY ACNE

- Isotretinoin (Accutane) 0.5 to 1.0 mg/kg twice daily, usually given for 12 to 20 weeks, total dose of 120 mg/kg; highly teratogenic
- Oral contraceptives (females >15 years of age)

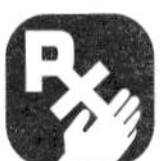

Long-Term Treatment

REFERRAL/DISPOSITION

- Dermatologist should be consulted if basic topical and systemic therapy fails.
- Dermatologic consultation is appropriate in cases of severe disfiguring lesions that may require intralesional injections.

EQUIPMENT MODIFICATIONS

- Equipment should be evaluated for potential alternative in acne that is clearly related to equipment (shoulder pads).
- Sometimes wearing a cotton undershirt beneath equipment can ameliorate the effects of equipment.

Common Questions and Answers

Physician responses to common patient questions:
Q: Is acne related to diet?
A: No.
Q: I started therapy, but my acne seemed to get worse. Is this normal?
A: Some therapies may cause an initial flare-up before improvement of acne. Ask your physician if you are on a medication that might cause this.
Q: How long will it take to see results?
A: Results are not obvious immediately. Typically a treatment needs to be continued for 6 to 8 weeks before a response is seen.

Miscellaneous

ICD-9 CODE

706.1 Acne NEC

BIBLIOGRAPHY

Dambro MR, Griffith JA. *Griffith's 5-minute clinical consult*. Philadelphia: Lippincott Williams & Wilkins, 1999.

Goroll AH, May LA, Mulley AG. *Primary care medicine*, 3rd ed. Philadelphia: Lippincott-Raven, 1995.

Habif TP. *Clinical dermatology*, 3rd ed. St. Louis: Mosby-Yearbook, 1996.

Author: Kimberly Harmon

AIDS and HIV

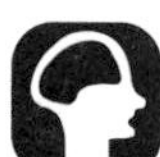

Basics

DEFINITION

- Human immunodeficiency virus (HIV) is the etiologic agent leading to the suppression of the immune system and to the development of the acquired immune deficiency syndrome (AIDS).

INCIDENCE/PREVALENCE

- With over 400,000 people in the United States living with HIV or AIDS, and over 100,000 HIV infection cases in 1999, the presence of HIV and AIDS in the United States is impossible to ignore.
- American football is the lone sport for which the risk of HIV transmission has been investigated. According to the frequency of bleeding injuries and player contact observed in one study, the risk of infection was estimated to be less than 1 per 85 million game contacts.
- There has been only one case of HIV transmission reported during sports contact. The report was of an Italian soccer player who allegedly seroconverted after a bloody head-to-head collision with an HIV-positive individual during a recreational soccer match. Health officials were unable to rule out other risk factors to verify the actual mode of transmission.

RISK FACTORS

- Modes of transmission include sexual contact, parenteral exposure to blood or blood components, contamination of infected blood on open wounds or mucous membranes, blood inoculation or needle sharing, and perinatal transmission from infected mother to fetus.
- There have been no definitive studies indicating transmission of the virus through bodily fluids such as sweat, tears, urine, sputum, vomitus, saliva, or respiratory droplets.

SIGNS AND SYMPTOMS

- The clinical spectrum of HIV infection ranges from a person being totally asymptomatic without any signs of infection, to specific clinical syndromes dependent on which opportunistic infections or neoplasms are present.
- Common opportunistic infections include oral thrush, pneumonia due to *Pneumocystis carinii* (PCP), diffuse lymphadenopathy due to mycobacteria or fungi, and characteristic neoplasms such as Kaposi's sarcoma or lymphoma.

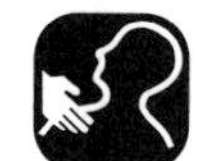

Diagnosis

DIFFERENTIAL DIAGNOSIS

The diagnosis of HIV infection is based on serologic studies (enzyme-linked immunosorbent assay with confirmatory Western blot), whereas the diagnosis of AIDS is based on the presence of certain opportunistic infections or neoplasms (such as Kaposi's sarcoma) and immunologic features (such as a depressed CD4+ count).

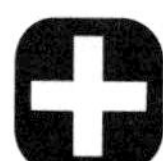

Acute Treatment

SPECIAL CONSIDERATIONS

Postexposure Prophylaxis

- Postexposure prophylaxis may be indicated after significant exposure of a patient to potentially infectious body fluids from an HIV-infected person (i.e., needlestick injury to health-care worker from a needle used on a patient with AIDS; sports participant with mucous membrane exposure to HIV-infected blood).
- Postexposure prophylaxis usually includes the administration of a multidrug antiretroviral regimen, preferably within 2 hours after injury/incident.

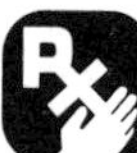

Long-Term Treatment

- Treatment of HIV infection includes specific antiretroviral therapy, and chemoprophylactic agents [depending on an individual's level of immunity (i.e., CD4+ count, viral load)].
- There are currently three classes of antiretroviral medications available: nucleoside reverse transcriptase inhibitors (zidovudine or AZT, ddI, d4T, and 3TC); non-nucleoside reverse transcriptase inhibitors (nevirapine and delavirdine); and protease inhibitors (indinavir, nelfinavir, saquinavir, and ritonavir).
- A combination of at least two drugs from different classes are commonly used to prevent the development of resistance and increase efficacy.
- Chemoprophylaxis for various opportunistic infections can be very effective; for example, trimethoprim/sulfamethoxazole for the prevention of PCP.

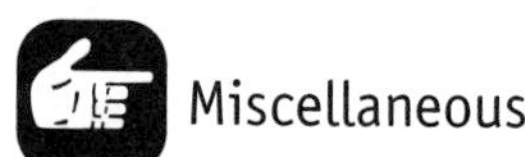

Miscellaneous

PREVENTION STRATEGIES

- Skin lesions should be immediately cleansed with suitable antiseptic and securely covered with occlusive dressing.
- If a bleeding wound occurs, the individual's participation should be interrupted until the bleeding has been stopped and the wound is both cleansed with antiseptics and securely covered or occluded.
- Any participant whose uniform is saturated with blood, regardless of the source, must have it changed before returning to competition.
- Coaches and athletic trainers should receive training in first aid and emergency care; they also should be provided with the necessary supplies to treat open wounds such as latex or vinyl gloves, disinfectant, bleach, antiseptic, designated receptacles for soiled equipment or uniforms, bandages and dressings, and a container for appropriate disposal of needles, syringes, or scalpels.
- Athletic equipment visibly contaminated with blood should be wiped clean and disinfected with a bleach solution before reusing.

- Gloves should be worn by persons attending to injuries when direct contact with blood or body fluids is anticipated.
- Gloves should be changed after treating individual participants and hands should be washed after every glove removal.
- Athletes should be encouraged to seek immunization against other blood-borne viral pathogens, such as the hepatitis B virus.
- The physician should respect the rights of patients to confidentiality.
- Athletes should not be restricted from participating in sports merely on the basis of their HIV status.
- Emergency care should never be delayed.
- Education of high-risk behaviors and their prevention (e.g., condoms and sexually transmitted HIV infection) is the primary preventative strategy to date, because no acceptable vaccine yet exists.

LEGAL CONSIDERATIONS

- Testing for the presence of HIV antibodies generally requires written consent from a patient, but specific regulations vary from state to state (in the United States).
- Disclosure of a patient's HIV status, without written consent, may be punishable by law in certain areas.
- AIDS is defined as a disability under U.S. Federal law.

ICD-9 CODE

042 HIV syndrome, AIDS, AIDS-related complex
V08 Asymptomatic HIV+

BIBLIOGRAPHY

American Academy of Pediatrics. In: Pickering LK, ed. *2000 Red book report of the Committee on Infectious Diseases,* 25th ed. Elk Grove Village, IL: American Academy of Pediatrics, 2000:124–127.

American Academy of Pediatrics Committee on Sports Medicine and Fitness. Human immunodeficiency virus and other blood-borne viral pathogens in the athletic setting. *Pediatrics* 1999;1400–1403.

American Medical Society for Sports Medicine (AMSSM) and the American Academy of Sports Medicine (AASM). Human immunodeficiency virus (HIV) and other blood-borne pathogens in sports. Joint position statement. *Am J Sports Med* 1995;23:510–514.

Brown LS Jr, Drotman DP, Chu A, et al. Bleeding injuries in professional football: estimating the risk of HIV transmission. *Ann Intern Med* 1995;122:271–274.

Brown LS Jr, Phillips RY, Brown CL Jr, et al. HIV-AIDS policies and sports: the National Football League. *Med Sci Sports Exerc* 1994;26:403–407.

Calabrese LH, Kelley D. AIDS and athletes. *Phys Sportsmed* 1989;17:126.

Centers for Disease Control and Prevention. HIV/AIDS Surveillance Report. June 13, 2000. September 21, 2000.

Goldsmith MF. When sports and HIV share the bill, smart money goes on common sense [news]. *JAMA* 1992;267:1311–1314.

Jones WK, Curran JW. Epidemiology of AIDS and HIV infection in industrialized countries. In: Pine JJ, ed. *Textbook of AIDS medicine*. Baltimore: Williams & Wilkins, 1994:91–108.

McGrew CA, Dick RW, Schniedwind K, et al. Survey of NCAA institutions concerning HIV/AIDS policies and universal precautions. *Med Sci Sports Exerc* 1993;25:917–921.

Minooee, Arezou, Rickman, et al. Transmission of infectious diseases during sports. In: Schlossberg D, ed. *Infections of leisure,* 2nd ed. Washington, DC: American Society for Microbiology, 1999.

Scott MJ, Scott MJ Jr. HIV infection associated with injections of anabolic steroids [Letter]. *JAMA* 1989;262:207–208.

Torre D, Sampietro C, Ferraro G, et al. Transmission of HIV-1 infection via sports injury [Letter]. *Lancet* 1990;335:1105.

World Health Organization consensus statement-consultation on AIDS and sports [News]. *JAMA* 1992;267:1312.

Wormser GP, Bittker S, Forseter G, et al. Absence of infectious human immunodeficiency virus type 1 in "natural" eccrine sweat. *J Infect Dis* 1992;165: 155–158.

Authors: Elizabeth Austin and Leland S. Rickman

Airway Obstruction, Partial and Complete

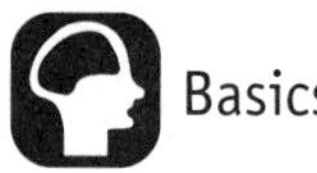

Basics

SIGNS AND SYMPTOMS

Clinical Conditions Requiring Airway Management

- Failure to maintain or protect the airway
  - —Stridor
  - —Oropharyngeal swelling
  - —Absence of a gag reflex
  - —Inability to handle secretions
- Hypoxia or ventilatory failure
  - —Shortness of breath
  - —Cyanosis
  - —Altered mental status
  - —Status epilepticus

Recognition of a Difficult Airway

- Congenital
  - —Pierre Robin syndrome
  - —Treacher Collins' syndrome
  - —Goldenhar's syndrome
  - —Down's syndrome
  - —Klippel-Feil syndrome
  - —Goiter
- Anatomic
  - —Mallampati criteria
    - —Faucial pillars, soft palate visible only (Class II)
    - —Only soft palate visible (Class III)
    - —Rule of 3, 3, and 2
    - —Mouth can not be opened more than 3 finger breadths
    - —Horizontal length of the mandible >3 finger breadths
    - —Thyromental distance <2 finger breadths
- Acquired
  - —Infections
    - —Supraglottitis
    - —Croup
    - —Abscess (intraoral, retropharyngeal)
    - —Ludwig's angina
  - —Arthritis
    - —Rheumatoid arthritis
    - —Ankylosing spondylitis
  - —Benign tumor
    - —Cystic hygroma
    - —Lipoma
    - —Adenoma
    - —Goiter
    - —Malignant tumors
    - —Facial injury
    - —Cervical spine injury
    - —Laryngeal-tracheal trauma
    - —Obesity
    - —Acromegaly
    - —Acute burns

MECHANISM/DESCRIPTION

- Oral and nasopharyngeal airways
  - —Lift the base of the tongue off the hypopharynx
  - —Facilitate bag-valve-mask ventilation
  - —Insert if a gag response is absent
- Oral rapid sequence intubation
  - —Induction of anesthesia and paralysis
  - —Minimize the risk of aspiration
  - —Method of choice for trauma patients with suspected head injury
  - —Contraindicated in patients who should not be paralyzed
- Oral awake intubation
  - —Oral intubation with sedation only
  - —Ketamine, a dissociative anesthetic, is ideal for this purpose
    - —Contraindicated in the head-injured patient due to intracranial pressure (ICP) elevation
  - —Indicated when paralysis is hazardous due to airway distortion (penetrating neck trauma)
- Blind nasotracheal intubation
  - —Indications
    - —Oral intubation is unsuccessful
    - —Neuromuscular blockade is dangerous
    - —Sitting or semi-reclined in patients who cannot tolerate the supine position: COPD; CHF; asthma
    - —Oral cavity is not accessible to allow oral intubation
    - —Limited cervical mobility: rheumatoid arthritis
  - —Contraindications
    - —Apnea
    - —Anticoagulation
    - —Massive facial trauma
    - —Nasal trauma
    - —Head trauma
    - —Upper airway abscess
    - —Acute epiglottitis
- Lighted stylet
  - —Light wand
  - —Transilluminate the neck
  - —Guide tube placement
  - —Alternative to laryngoscopic intubation
  - —Verifies ET tube placement
  - —Indications
    - —Blood in the oropharynx
    - —Failed airway
    - —Cricothyrotomy
  - —Surgical procedure
  - —Incision is made in the cricothyroid membrane
  - —Shiley tracheostomy tube is inserted in the airway
  - —Failed airway
  - —Massive facial trauma
  - —Total upper airway obstruction
  - —Contraindications
  - —Laryngeal crush injury
  - —Expanding zone II or III neck hematoma
- Percutaneous translaryngeal ventilation (PTV)
  - —A temporizing measure
  - —Percutaneous placement of a 12- or 14-gauge catheter through the cricothyroid membrane
  - —Intermittent ventilation via a high-pressure oxygen source
  - —Indications
    - —Failed oral or nasal intubation until cricothyrotomy is complete
  - —Contraindication
    - —Upper airway obstruction that prevents expiration
- Fiberoptic intubation
  - —ET tube placed over the bronchoscope
  - —Performed via the nasotracheal or orotracheal approach
  - —Indications
  - —Anatomic limitations to visualization of the glottis
  - —Limited movement of the mandible or cervical spine
  - —Contraindications
    - —Patients who need immediate airway management
    - —Significant airway hemorrhage
- Retrograde tracheal intubation
  - —Another technique available when others have failed
  - —Retrograde advancement of a guidewire through a translaryngeal catheter
- Laryngeal mask airway
  - —A device that is inserted blindly into the oropharynx
  - —The patient is ventilated through a tube connected to a small inflatable mask
    - —The mask forms a low pressure seal around the laryngeal inlet
  - —Used to ventilate the patient if other airway methods have failed, until a definitive airway can be established

ETIOLOGY

N/A

PEDIATRIC CONSIDERATIONS

- An estimation of ET tube size is 16 + age/4
- Uncuffed ET tubes should be used in patients <8 years old
- For children <3 years old, the straight Miller blade is preferred
- For children <12 years old the preferred surgical airway is PTV

CAUTIONS

- Indications for airway management and different methods are limited by available techniques
- Bag-mask ventilation only (COMMA) for basic life support providers
- Options for patients in cardiac and respiratory arrest for advanced life support providers

—Bag-mask ventilation and definitive airway management in the ED
—Oral intubation
—Pharyngotracheal lumen airway (PTLA)
  —A device with two tubes and two balloons
  —Blindly placed in either the trachea or the esophagus
  —Functions as an ET tube or an esophageal obturator
  —When endotracheal intubation is not available
—PTLA contraindications
  —Pediatric patients
  —Caustic ingestions
  —Esophageal disease
  —Presence of a gag reflex

CONTROVERSIES

- Rapid sequence intubation
  —Used in the field primarily by flight crews
  —Its use remains controversial for urban EMS systems in which transport times are short

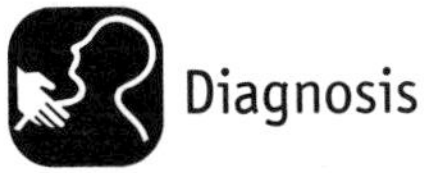

Diagnosis

ESSENTIAL WORKUP

- Verification of correct tube placement
  —Auscultation over both axillae, the anterior lung fields, and the stomach
  —Observation of chest wall movement
  —Condensation on the tube during ventilation

LABORATORY

- End-tidal CO_2 colorimetric devices
  —In cardiac arrest, low CO_2 production may prevent color change with a correctly placed endotracheal tube
- Rise in pulse oximetry after intubation

IMAGING/SPECIAL TESTS

- Syringe aspiration technique
  —Detects esophageal intubation
  —A catheter-tipped 60-cc syringe is inserted through the adapter at the proximal end of the ET tube
  —Resistance to aspiration indicates occlusion from esophageal collapse
- Chest radiography
  —Indicated to exclude a main stem bronchus intubation
  —Esophageal intubation may incorrectly appear to be in the trachea

DIFFERENTIAL DIAGNOSIS

- Esophageal intubation
- Right mainstem intubation
- Extratracheal placement through a tear in a pyriform sinus or the trachea
- Pneumothorax

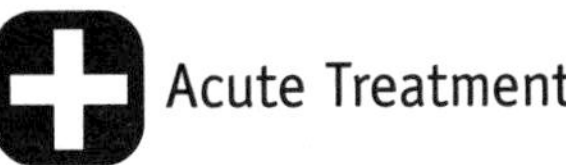

Acute Treatment

INITIAL STABILIZATION

- Maintain line cervical immobilization
- Check all intubation equipment
  —Suction
  —Bag-valve-mask
  —Various sizes of ET tubes
  —Laryngoscope blades
  —Stylets
  —Oxygen
  —Medications
  —Monitoring equipment

ED TREATMENT

- Rapid sequence intubation
- Preoxygenation
  —100% FIO_2 for 5 minutes
- Premedication
  —Performed 2–3 minutes prior to administration of SCh
  —Minimize the rise in ICP
    —Defasciculating dose of vecuronium or pancuronium
    —Fentanyl
    —Lidocaine
  —Reactive airway disease
    —Lidocaine
  —Attenuate the vagal effect in children
    —Atropine
- Paralysis/Induction
  —Administration of an induction agent followed immediately by SCh
  —Thiopental
    —Contraindicated in the hypovolemic or hypotensive patient
  —Relative contraindications
    —Anticipated difficult oral intubation
    —Open globe injury
    —Organophosphate poisoning
    —Burns >3 days old
- Apply Sellick's maneuver
  —Digital cricoid pressure to occlude the esophagus and prevent regurgitation
- Mask ventilation should be avoided because it will increase the aspiration risk
- Intubation
  —45–60 seconds after SCh administration when the patient has lost muscle tone
  —Use a stylet with the endotracheal tube
  —Inflate the cuff once the tube is placed before bagging
  —Confirm correct placement of endotracheal tube
- For continued paralysis after intubation use vecuronium and a sedative agent

PEDIATRIC CONSIDERATIONS

- Atropine should be given with ketamine to decrease secretions
- A defasciculating dose of neuromuscular blocking agent is not needed for children ≤5 years old

MEDICATIONS

- Atracurium: 0.4–0.5 mg/kg IV
- Atropine: 0.02 mg/kg IV
- Diazepam: 2–10 mg IV (peds: 0.2–0.3 mg/kg)
- Etomidate: 0.3 mg/kg IV
- Fentanyl: 3 μg/kg IV
- Ketamine: 1–2 mg/kg IV or 4–7 mg/kg IM
- Lidocaine: 1.5 mg/kg IV
- Midazolam: 1–5 mg (0.07–0.3 mg/kg for induction) IV
- Propofol: 2–2.5 mg/kg IV
- Pancuronium: 0.01 mg/kg (defasciculating dose) IV; 0.1 mg/kg (paralyzing dose) IV
- Succinylcholine: 1.5 mg/kg (peds: 2 mg/kg) IV; 2.5 mg/kg IM or subcutaneous; 0.15 mg/kg (defasciculating pretreatment dose)
- Thiopental: 3 mg/kg IV
- Vecuronium: 0.01 mg/kg (defasciculating dose) IV; 0.1 mg/kg (paralyzing dose) IV

HOSPITAL ADMISSION CRITERIA

- All intubated patients should be admitted to an ICU

HOSPITAL DISCHARGE CRITERIA

- Certain ED patients who have been intubated for airway protection or to facilitate diagnostic workup may be extubated in the ED after a period of observation, and then discharged

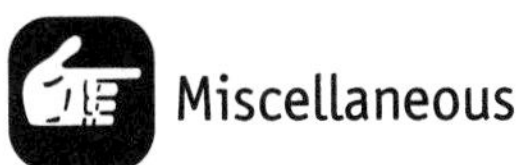

Miscellaneous

CORE CONTENT CODE

23.1

BIBLIOGRAPHY

Benumof JL, ed. *Airway management. Principles and practice*. St. Louis: CV Mosby, 1996.

Dailey RH, et al., eds. *The airway: Emergency management*. St. Louis: CV Mosby, 1992.

Walls RM. Airway management. In: Rosen P, et al., eds. *Emergency medicine: Concepts and clinical practice*. 3rd ed. St. Louis: CV Mosby, 1992:2–24.

Walls RM. Rapid sequence intubation in head trauma. *Ann Emerg Med* 1993;22:1008.

Author: Carlo Rosen

Allergic Rhinitis

 Basics

DEFINITION

- Allergic rhinitis is an immunoglobulin E-mediated immunologic response occurring after exposure to immunogenic proteins (allergens).

INCIDENCE/PREVALENCE

- Allergic rhinitis affects anywhere from 10% to 30% of American adults.
- Onset usually at 10 to 20 years of age
- Can occur in conjunction with atopic dermatitis, allergic conjunctivitis, or asthma

SIGNS AND SYMPTOMS

- Common symptoms include rhinorrhea (usually clear), postnasal drip, sneezing, itching of the nose and palate, and coughing.
- Nasal congestion also can be a prominent feature.
- Less common symptoms include headache and fatigue.

RISK FACTORS

- Positive family history, especially if both parents are affected
- Prior treatment for allergic rhinitis
- Prior treatment for atopic dermatitis
- Prior history of recurrent tonsillitis and/or tonsillectomy (or adenoidectomy), or recurrent otitis media and/or tympanostomy tubes
- Athletes and active people often have greater exposure to allergens due to the outside nature of many sports.

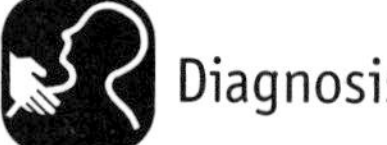

Diagnosis

DIFFERENTIAL DIAGNOSIS

- Upper respiratory infection (viral, bacterial, or fungal)
- Sinusitis
- Rhinitis medicamentosa from overuse of topical decongestants, certain blood pressure medications, or aspirin/nonsteroidal antiinflammatory drug sensitivity
- Chronic sniffing of cocaine
- Mechanical obstruction from nasal polyps, septal deviation, or foreign body
- Vasomotor rhinitis (etiology unclear); no identifiable allergen, often associated with dry atmosphere
- Rare causes: hypothyroidism, pregnancy, oral contraceptives

HISTORY

- Timing of symptoms during the year and with certain exposures or activities
- Typical allergens include pollens (spring), grasses (summer), ragweed (fall), animal dander, dust mites, soaps, and smoke.
- Possible exposures during practices and games ("away" events provide opportunities for allergen exposures)
- College athletes away from home and professional athletes who move to new cities are often exposed to new allergens.
- Response to previous treatments, both prescription and over the counter
- When evaluating allergic rhinitis, also screen for exercise-induced asthma or bronchospasm by history of coughing, wheezing, or shortness of breath during or after exercise. The incidence of exercise-induced bronchospasm can be as high as 40% in those with allergic rhinitis.

PHYSICAL EXAM

- Temperature: normal in allergic rhinitis but may be elevated in acute infections
- Clear rhinorrhea
- Edematous nasal mucosa and turbinates, often described as "pale" or "blue"
- Examine nares for nasal polyps or other mechanical obstruction.
- Examine posterior nasopharynx for postnasal drip and/or lymphoid hyperplasia.
- Congestion
- Check ears for acute or chronic otitis.
- Examine eyes for evidence of conjunctivitis.
- Auscultate for wheezing.

IMAGING

- Imaging usually is necessary only to rule out other causes of rhinitis.
- Plain sinus films or limited CT scan (CT often more cost effective)
- Nasal endoscopy

OTHER EVALUATION

- Further workup often unnecessary if history and physical exam provide adequate evidence for diagnosis.
- Examination of nasal smears for eosinophils
- Allergy testing

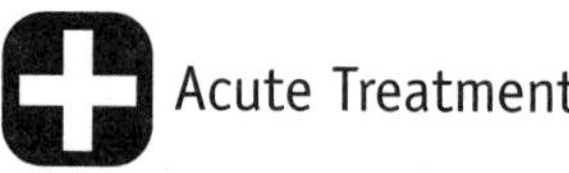

Acute Treatment

ENVIRONMENTAL CONTROL

- If possible, minimize exposure by limiting outdoor activity when pollen, dust, and mold counts are high.
- Athletes may need to train indoors or cross-train with swimming, stationary biking, or elliptical fitness machines.
- Allergen counts are usually lower after it rains, which provides an opportunity for outdoor activities.
- Physical barriers such as a filter mask can be effective but are usually not acceptable to athletes because they may affect performance.

PHARMACOLOGIC TREATMENT

- Selection depends on symptoms and side effects.
- Antihistamines (oral or topical): Oral antihistamines are the most commonly used drugs for allergic rhinitis. Second-generation antihistamines are less sedating. Topical antihistamines include nasal preparations such as Astelin.

- Decongestants (oral or topical). Limit use of topicals to 3 or 4 days to prevent rebound congestion.
- Nasal corticosteroids: Probably most effective therapy, especially long term, but usually takes 3 to 4 days to begin working
- A "burst" of oral corticosteroids may occasionally be used for severe symptoms.
- The best way to treat allergic rhinitis is to anticipate exposures in susceptible athletes and pretreat with the most appropriate medicine.

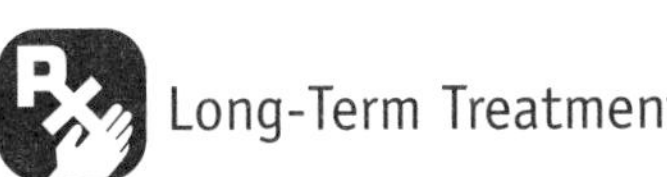

Long-Term Treatment

PHARMACOLOGIC TREATMENT

- Oral antihistamines, topical antihistamines, and nasal corticosteroids as noted above
- Cromolyn sodium: topical mast cell stabilizer; has no affect on acute symptoms but can be very effective for prophylaxis

OTHER

- Allergy testing is useful in those patients willing to commit to long-term immunotherapy treatment and in children with significant food allergies for avoidance purposes.

Common Questions and Answers

Physician responses to common patient questions:

Q: How long will treatment last?

A: For seasonal allergies, treatment may last a few weeks to a few months but could need to be repeated on a yearly basis if symptoms recur. For perennial rhinitis, treatment may need to be on a continuous basis.

Q: Will these drugs affect my performance?

A: It is certainly possible for drug side effects to limit performance. Some antihistamines can be sedating while decongestants may give a "pumped up" feeling. Oral corticosteroids may cause mild fluid retention.

Q: Are there any medicines for allergic rhinitis that athletes cannot take?

A: Certain drugs used for allergic rhinitis are banned or have restrictions at the competitive level. For example, decongestants are banned by the USOC due to their stimulant effects but are permitted by the NCAA in cough and cold preparations. Sedating antihistamines are not allowed in shooting sports. Oral corticosteroids are banned by the USOC but are generally not restricted by the NCAA. Nasal steroids are generally not restricted. Cromolyn is not restricted currently. The governing bodies of the individual sports should be contacted if there is any concern regarding use of a medication.

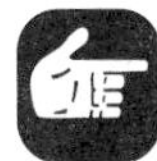

Miscellaneous

SYNONYMS

- Hayfever

ICD-9 CODE

477.9

BIBLIOGRAPHY

Barker LR, Burton JR, Zieve PD. *Principles of ambulatory medicine,* 4th ed. Baltimore: Williams and Wilkins, 1995.

O'Kane JW, Woodford GA. Allergen mediated disease. *Physician Sportsmed* 1999;27: 49–67.

Rosenberg JM. *Athletic drug reference '99.* Durham, NC: Clean Data, 1999.

Authors: Douglas Reeves Jr., Susan Glockner, and T. Jeff Emel

Altered Mental Status

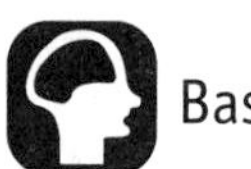

Basics

SIGNS AND SYMPTOMS

Confusion

- Difficulty in maintaining a coherent stream of thinking and mental performance
  —Remember to consider the level of education and language
- Inattention
- Memory deficit
  —Inability to recall any of the following
    —The date, inclusive of month, day, year, and day of week
    —The precise place
    —Items of generally acknowledged and universally known information
    —Why the patient is in the hospital
    —Address, zip code, telephone number, or social security number
- Impaired mental performance
  —Difficulty retaining seven digits forward and four backward
  —Serial calculations
    —Holding the result of one calculation in a working memory in order to pursue the next step
    —Serial 3-from-30 subtraction test
- Disorganized and rambling language
  —May be mistaken for aphasia

Findings that Suggest an Underlying Cause

- Fever
  —Infectious etiologies, drug toxicities, endocrine disorders, heat stroke
- Severe hypertension
  —Suggestive of an intracranial structural lesion
- Hypotension
  —Infectious and toxicological etiologies
- Eye resting position
  —Dysconjugate gaze in the horizontal plane occurs with drowsiness
  —Dysconjugate gaze in the vertical plane occurs with pontine or cerebellar lesions
  —Sustained conjugate downward eye deviation occurs with a variety of neurologic disorders
  —Sustained conjugate upward gaze occurs with hypoxic encephalopathy
  —Ocular bobbing
    —Cyclical brisk conjugate caudal jerks of the globes followed by a slow return to midposition
    —Bilateral pontine damage, metabolic derangement, and brainstem compression
  —Ocular dipping
    —Slow, cyclical, conjugate, downward movement of the eyes followed by a rapid return to midposition
    —Diffuse cortical anoxic damage
- Pupillary examination
  —Normal size, shape, and response to light indicates intact midbrain function
  —Nearly all toxic and metabolic causes of coma leave the pupillary reflexes sluggish but bilaterally intact
- Focal findings
  —Hemiparesis
  —Hemianopia
  —Aphasia
  —Myoclonus
  —Convulsions
- Asterixis
  —Arrhythmic flapping tremor
  —Caused by metabolic encephalopathy
    —Hepatic failure
    —Anticonvulsant drug ingestion
- Myoclonic jerking and tremor
  —Uremic encephalopathy
  —Antipsychotic drug ingestion

MECHANISM/DESCRIPTION

- Dysfunction in either the reticular activating system in the upper brainstem or a large area of one of the cerebral hemispheres
- Definitions
  —Clouding of consciousness
    —Confusion: a behavioral state of reduced mental clarity, coherence, comprehension, and reasoning
  —Diminished consciousness
    —Drowsiness: the patient cannot be easily aroused by touch or noise and cannot maintain alertness for some time
    —Stupor: the patient can be awakened only by vigorous stimuli, and an effort to avoid uncomfortable or aggravating stimulation is displayed
    —Coma: the patient cannot be aroused by stimulation and no purposeful attempt is made to avoid painful stimuli

ETIOLOGY

- Hypoxic
  —Severe pulmonary disease
  —Anemia
  —Shock
- Metabolic
  —Hypoglycemia
  —Diabetic ketoacidosis
  —Nonketotic hyperosmolar coma
  —Thiamine deficiency
  —Hyperammonemia
  —Uremia
  —CO_2 narcosis
  —Hyperglycemia
  —Hyponatremia; hypernatremia
  —Hypocalcemia; hypercalcemia
  —Hypomagnesemia; hypermagnesemia
  —Hypophosphatemia
  —Acidosis; alkalosis
- Toxicologic
  —Ethanol
  —Isopropyl alcohol
  —Methanol
  —Ethylene glycol
  —Salicylates
  —Sedatives and narcotics
  —Anticonvulsants
  —Psychotropics
  —Isoniazid
  —Heavy metals
  —Carbon monoxide
  —Cyanide
- Endocrine
  —Myxedema coma
  —Thyrotoxicosis
  —Addison's disease
  —Cushing's disease
  —Pheochromocytoma
- Environmental
  —Hypothermia
  —Heat stroke
  —Neuroleptic malignant syndrome
  —Malignant hyperthermia
- Intracranial hypertension
- Hypertensive encephalopathy
- Pseudotumor cerebri
- CNS inflammation
- Meningitis
- Encephalitis
- Encephalopathy
- Cerebral vasculitis
  —TTP
  —Subarachnoid hemorrhage
  —Carcinoid meningitis
  —Traumatic axonal shear injury
  —Primary neuronal or glial disorders
  —Creutzfeldt-Jakob disease
  —Marchiafava-Bignami disease
  —Adrenoleukodystrophy
  —Gliomatosis cerebri
  —Progressive multifocal leukoencephalopathy
  —Seizures and postictal state
  —Supratentorial lesions
  —Hemorrhage
  —Infarction
  —Tumors
  —Abscess
  —Subtentorial lesions
  —Cerebellar hemorrhage
  —Posterior fossa subdural or extradural hemorrhage
  —Cerebellar infarct
  —Cerebellar tumor
  —Cerebellar abscess
  —Basilar aneurysm
  —Pontine hemorrhage
  —Brainstem infarct
  —Basilar migraine
  —Brainstem demyelination

CAUTIONS

- Airway management if loss of airway patency
- Supplemental oxygen
- Bag-mask ventilation with cricoid pressure
- Endotracheal intubation if no response to coma cocktail
- Intravenous access
- Coma cocktail
  - —Dextrose
  - —Naloxone
  - —Thiamine
- Monitor patient
- Look for signs of an underlying cause
  - —Medications
  - —Medic alert bracelets
  - —Document a basic neurologic examination
  - —GCS
  - —Pupils
  - —Extremity movements

CONTROVERSIES

- Empirical dextrose should not be held or delayed if dextrostix is not available
  - —Glucose can be safely administered before thiamine
  - —Glucose does not worsen outcome in patients with stroke

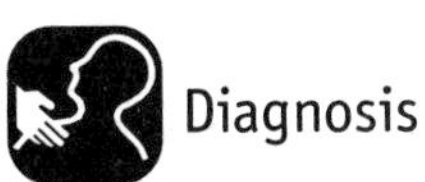

Diagnosis

LABORATORY

- Dextrostix and glucose
- CBC
- Electrolytes
- BUN, creatinine
- Calcium
- Arterial blood gases
- Toxicologic screen
- Alcohol screen if toxic alcohols are suspected and serum osmolarity

IMAGING/SPECIAL TESTS

- Caloric stimulation of the vestibular apparatus
- Indicated to assess unresponsive patients
- Tympanic membrane perforation and cerumen impaction should be excluded
- Irrigate the external auditory canal with 10 cc of ice-cold water after elevating the head to 30°
- Bilateral tonic deviation of the eyes toward the stimulus indicates an intact brainstem
- Nystagmuslike quick corrective phases indicates intact cerebral hemispheres
- A normal response in an unresponsive patient raises the suspicion of psychogenic coma
- CT scan
  - —Noncontrast only to rule out hemorrhage and mass effect
- Lumbar puncture
  - —Indicated when the etiology remains unclear after laboratory and CT scan
  - —Empiric antibiotics should be administered before the lumbar puncture to avoid any delay in therapy in patients with meningitis

DIFFERENTIAL DIAGNOSIS

- Locked in syndrome
  - —Rare disorder caused by damage to the corticospinal, corticopontine, and corticobulbar tracts resulting in quadriplegia and mutism with preservation of consciousness
  - —Communication may be established through eye movements
- Psychogenic unresponsiveness
  - —Conversion reactions
  - —Catatonia
- Malingering
- Akinetic mutism
- Dementia
  - —The mental status waxes and wanes
  - —Confusion due to poor recollection
  - —Attention is preserved in the early stages

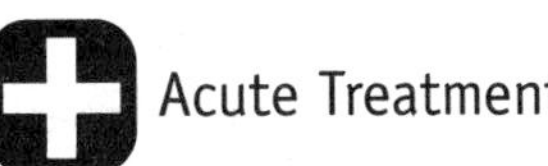

Acute Treatment

INITIAL STABILIZATION

- Intravenous D_{50}
  - —Empiric use when not administered in the field or dextrostix is unavailable
- Naloxone
- Thiamine

ED TREATMENT

- Consider empirical use of antibiotics for altered mental status of undetermined etiology
  - —Broad spectrum with good CSF penetration such as ceftriaxone
- Empiric treatment if a toxic ingestion is suspected
  - —Activated charcoal
  - —Alcohol drip if methanol or ethylene glycol is suspected
- Correct body temperature
  - —Warmed humidified O_2 if hypothermic
  - —Ice packs and forced air movement over exposed wetted skin if severe hyperthermia
- Specific therapy directed at underlying cause once identified

MEDICATIONS

- Ceftriaxone: 100 mg/kg IV
- Dextrose: 1–2 ml/kg of D_{50}W IV; neonate: 10 ml/kg D_{10}W IV; peds: 4 ml/kg D_{25} W IV
- Diazepam: 0.1–0.3 mg/kg slow IV (max 10 mg/dose) q 10–15 min × 3 doses
- Lorazepam: 0.05–0.1 mg/kg IV (max 4 mg/dose q 10–15 min)
- Naloxone: 0.01 mg/kg IV/IM/SC/ET
- Thiamine: 100 mg IM or 100 mg thiamine 1000 ml of intravenous fluid wide open

HOSPITAL ADMISSION CRITERIA

All patients with acute changes in mental status require admission

HOSPITAL DISCHARGE CRITERIA

Chronic altered mental status (e.g., dementia) without change from baseline

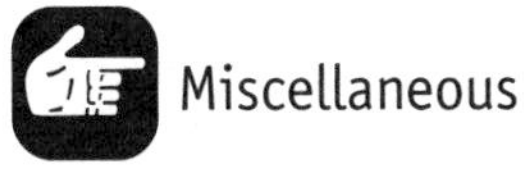

Miscellaneous

ICD-9 CODE

293.0
293.81
293.82
294.1
294.8

BIBLIOGRAPHY

Hoffman RS, Goldfrank LR. The poisoned patient with altered consciousness. Controversies in the use of a "coma cocktail." *JAMA* 1995;274:562–69.

Samuels MA. The evaluation of comatose patients. *Hosp Pract* 1993;28:165–82.

Authors: Richard Wolfe and David Brown

Anaphylaxis

Basics

SIGNS AND SYMPTOMS

- Symptoms begin within seconds to minutes after contact with an offending antigen
- Some patients may have an initial sensation of impending doom followed by more clearly definable symptomatology
- Respiratory: bronchospasm, laryngeal edema
- Cardiovascular: hypotension, dysrhythmias, myocardial ischemia
- Gastrointestinal: nausea, vomiting, diarrhea
- Cutaneous: urticaria, angioedema
- Hematological: activation of intrinsic coagulation pathway sometimes leading to DIC, thrombocytopenia
- Neurological: seizures
- Death can occur from airway obstruction or circulatory collapse

MECHANISM/DESCRIPTION

- An acute, widely distributed form of shock which occurs within minutes of exposure to antigen in a sensitized individual
- There are approximately 400–800 deaths annually in the United States attributed to anaphylaxis
- Release of bioactive molecules such as histamine, leukotrienes, and prostaglandins from inflammatory cells
  —Mediator release results in increased vascular permeability, vasodilation, smooth-muscle contractions, and increased epithelial secretion
  —Physiologically this is manifested in a decrease in total peripheral resistance, venous return and cardiac output, as well as intravascular volume depletion

ETIOLOGY

- IgE-mediated
  —Antibiotics (especially penicillin family)
  —Venom
  —Latex
  —Vaccines
  —Foodstuffs (shellfish, soybeans, nuts, wheat, milk, eggs, nitrates/nitrites)
- Non-IgE mediated
  —Iodine contrast media
  —Opiates
  —Vancomycin
  —Quaternary ammonium muscle relaxants

CAUTIONS

- Early intubation is paramount as laryngeal edema and spasm can progress rapidly
- Laryngeal edema can be managed with racemic epinephrine prior to intubation
- Subcutaneous epinephrine (0.5 mg of 1:1000 solution) can be administered en route even prior to establishment of an IV

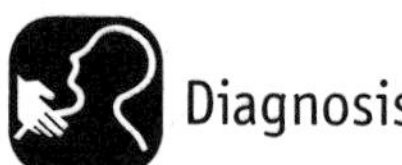

Diagnosis

ESSENTIAL WORKUP

- Diagnosis is made based on clinical symptoms
  —It is important not to underestimate the potential severity of an allergic reaction in its early stages
- EKG in patients with previous cardiac history or ischemic symptoms

LABORATORY

- While there are no specific tests necessary to make the diagnosis of anaphylaxis, an arterial blood gas may be helpful in evaluating ventilatory status
- These changes can be noted during anaphylaxis
  —Elevation of plasma histamine
  —Increase in hematocrit secondary to fluid extravasation

IMAGING/SPECIAL TESTS

- Hyperinflation on CXR
- EKG abnormalities including dysrhythmias, ischemic changes, infarction

DIFFERENTIAL DIAGNOSIS

- Pulmonary embolism
- Acute myocardial infarction
- Airway obstruction
- Asthma
- Tension pneumothorax
- NSAID reaction
- Vasovagal collapse
- Hereditary angioedema
- Serum sickness
- Systemic mastocytosis
- Pheochromocytoma
- Carcinoid syndrome

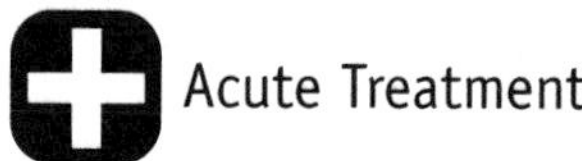

Acute Treatment

INITIAL STABILIZATION

- ABCs
  —Assure adequate ventilation
  —Endotracheal intubation may be required but difficult because of laryngeal edema or spasm
  —Transtracheal jet insufflation or cricothyrotomy may be necessary to control the airway
- Epinephrine IV/SQ or endotracheal administration
  —Direct injection into the venous plexus at the base of the tongue is an option
- Volume resuscitation with crystalloids or colloids
- A tourniquet can be used to decrease venous return from the site of antigen entry

ED TREATMENT

- Continuous cardiac and vital sign monitoring until stable
- Persistent bronchospasm can be treated with β_2-agonist bronchodilators
- Hypotension should be treated with volume repletion
  —Vasopressors, MAST garments and Trendelenburg positioning are useful adjuncts
- Antihistamines (both H_1 and H_2 blockers) have been shown to be helpful in preventing histamine interactions with target tissues
- Corticosteroids help prevent the progression or recurrence of anaphylaxis
- Glucagon is particularly useful in epinephrine-resistant anaphylaxis from ß-adrenergic blocking agents

MEDICATIONS

- Diphenhydramine: adult: 50 mg IV; peds: 1–2 mg/kg slow IVP
- Epinephrine: 0.3–0.5 mg (use 1:1000 dilution for SQ route, and 1:10000 for IV route); peds: epinephrine 0.01 mg/kg SC/IV
- Glucagon: adult: 1 mg IV
- Hydrocortisone: adults: 500 mg IV; peds: 4–8 mg/kg/dose IV
- Methylprednisolone: adult: 125 mg IV; peds: 1–2 mg/kg IV
- Prednisone: adult: 60 mg po; peds: 1 mg/kg po
- Ranitidine: adult: 50 mg IV or cimetidine 300 mg IV

HOSPITAL ADMISSION CRITERIA

- Intubated patients, or patients in respiratory distress should be admitted to an ICU setting
- A monitored bed may be necessary for the patient who has not had substantial response to initial therapy
- Patients with significant generalized reactions and persistent symptoms should be admitted for observation for 24 hours

HOSPITAL DISCHARGE CRITERIA

- Patients with complete resolution of symptoms may be discharged after several hours of ED observation
- Patients with allergic reactions should have follow-up within 48 hours of discharge to evaluate effectiveness of outpatient therapy
- A follow-up visit with an allergist is also recommended
- Patients should be advised to carry some type of treatment which can be self-administered in the event of future reactions such as the prefilled syringe *epi-pen*
- Patients with a known trigger should be counseled on strict avoidance of that trigger

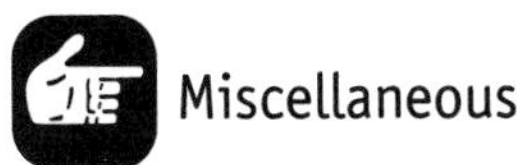

Miscellaneous

ICD-9 CODE

995.0

CORE CONTENT CODE

8.8.1

BIBLIOGRAPHY

Barach EM, et al. Epinephrine for the treatment of anaphylactic shock. *JAMA* 1984;251:2118.

Bochner BS, Lichtenstein LM. Anaphylaxis. *N Engl J Med* 1991;324:1785–1790.

Muelleman RL, et al. Allergy, hypersensitivity and anaphylaxis. In: Rosen P, Barkin R, eds. *Emergency medicine*. St. Louis: CV Mosby, 1998:2759–2776.

Author: Sean-Xavier Neath

Arrhythmias

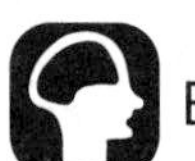

Basics

DEFINITION

- Arrhythmias are defined as any deviation from the normal (sinus) rhythm of the heart. Arrhythmias can be broadly categorized as tachyarrhythmias (fast) or bradyarrhythmias (slow).

INCIDENCE/PREVALENCE

Bradyarrhythmias

- Bradyarrhythmias are more common in aerobically trained athletes than the general population and are related to an elevated resting vagal tone.
- Sinus bradycardia (50%–65% of athletes vs. 23.7% in general population)
- Sinus arrhythmias (13.5%–69% of athletes vs. 2.4%–20% in the general population)
- Sinus pause of more than 2 seconds (37.1% of athletes vs. 5.7% in the general population)
- First-degree atrioventricular (AV) block (6%–33% of athletes vs. 0.65% in the general population)
- Second-degree AV block, Mobitz I (2.4%–10% of athletes vs. 0.003% in the general population)
- Third-degree AV block (0.017% of athletes vs. 0.00002% in the general population)
- Junctional rhythms (0.031%–7% of athletes vs. 0.06% in the general population)
- These changes are readily reversible with exercise when seen in the athlete's heart, because increased sympathetic drive overcomes baseline vagal tone. They may not be reversible in underlying cardiac disease.

Tachyarrhythmias

- Atrial fibrillation is found more commonly in competitive athletes (0%–0.063%) than the general population (0.004%).
- Other supraventricular atrial or AV nodal tachyarrhythmias are not more common in athletes than the general population.
- Wolff-Parkinson-White syndrome (characterized on electrocardiography (ECG) by a short PR interval and wide QRS complex with a slurred upstroke or delta wave) is no more frequent in athletes than the general population (average 0.15%).
- Premature ventricular contractions occur with a similar frequency in athletes and the general population.
- Complex ventricular arrhythmias are abnormal and should always prompt cardiologic examination in search of underlying cardiac disease.
- Increased QRS voltage, incomplete right bundle branch block, early repolarization, and peaked T waves are also common ECG findings found in well-conditioned athletes related to an increase in overall cardiac mass.

SIGNS AND SYMPTOMS

- Arrhythmias present with a broad scope of clinical scenarios, ranging from transient palpitations to the unconscious athlete on the playing field.
- Most tachyarrhythmias cause palpitations and may cause chest pain if cardiac ischemia is involved.
- Lightheadedness or syncope may occur, especially with unstable ventricular tachyarrhythmias.
- Syncope that occurs during exercise (rather than immediately after) is a more ominous sign of underlying cardiac abnormalities.

RISK FACTORS

- Structural heart disease (hypertrophic cardiomyopathy, anomalous coronary artery, arrhythmogenic right ventricular dysplasia, Marfan's syndrome, aortic stenosis, myocarditis, dilated cardiomyopathy)
- Atherosclerotic coronary artery disease (especially in the population >35 years of age)
- Drugs (amphetamines, cocaine, ephedrine)
- Long QT syndrome (congenital or iatrogenic from class IA antiarrhythmics, tricyclic antidepressants, antifungals, nonsedating antihistamines, antibiotics, and promotility agents) with QTc of more than 0.46 seconds
- Commotio cordis (direct nonpenetrating trauma to the chest wall)
- Metabolic abnormalities (hyperthyroidism and severe electrolyte disturbances)

SPECIAL CONSIDERATION

- The heart of a well-conditioned athlete undergoes normal physiologic and morphologic changes termed athlete's heart. These adaptations are related to an increase in resting parasympathetic (vagal) tone and an overall increase in cardiac mass and cause characteristic ECG changes that must be considered when interpreting ECGs in athletes.

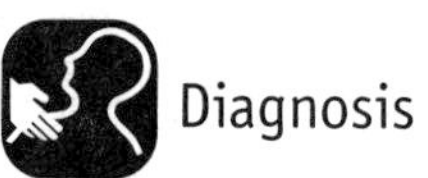

Diagnosis

DIFFERENTIAL DIAGNOSIS

- Anxiety disorder/panic attacks
- Angina
- Costochondritis
- Neurocardiogenic syncope
- Heat stroke
- Seizure

HISTORY

- Patients should be questioned as to the presence of palpitations, chest pain, lightheadedness, or syncope, and whether the symptoms occur at rest or with exertion.
- Family history of structural heart disease, sudden cardiac death, atherosclerotic heart disease, and long QT syndrome should be investigated.
- Prescription and over-the-counter medications (especially the use of cold or diet remedies) and the use of nutritional supplements, ergogenic aids, and recreational drugs should be noted.

PHYSICAL EXAM

- Vital signs (pulse, blood pressure, respiration rate, and temperature)
- Auscultation of the heart in both the sitting and supine positions
- Any cardiac murmur should be further evaluated during a Valsalva maneuver or while moving the patient from a squatting to standing position.
- The murmur in hypertrophic cardiomyopathy increases with maneuvers that decrease venous return (i.e., Valsalva or moving from the squatting to standing position), whereas the murmur in aortic stenosis decreases with these same maneuvers.
- Palpation of the femoral pulses (to rule out coarctation of the aorta)

FURTHER INVESTIGATIONS

- Workup of a suspected arrhythmia begins with an ECG.
- Home 24-hour cardiac monitoring or an event monitor can help establish the diagnosis when symptoms are intermittent.
- Exercise treadmill testing can identify exertional arrhythmias and ischemic heart disease; or (if normal) provide reassurance before return to play.
- Bradyarrhythmias seen in athlete's heart (due to increased vagal tone) usually resolve on exercise testing, whereas those from underlying cardiac disease may not.
- Echocardiography may identify structural heart disease.
- Rarely, cardiac catheterization, MRI, or electrophysiologic studies are needed.

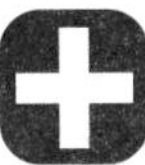

Acute Treatment

- Symptomatic athletes should be initially stabilized with the ABCs (airway, breathing, and circulation).
- Unstable athletes may require ACLS, immediate DC cardioversion, and transport to a medical facility.
- Suspected supraventricular tachycardias may respond to Valsalva maneuver, carotid massage, or facial ice water immersion.

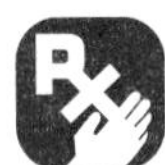

Long-Term Treatment

Long-term treatment may require antiarrhythmic medications, electrophysiologic cardiac ablation, or treatment of underlying coronary artery disease.

RETURN-TO-PLAY GUIDELINES

- Cardiac arrhythmias and underlying structural heart disease may place an individual at risk of sudden cardiac death with exercise.
- Recommendations for determining eligibility for competition presented jointly by the American College of Cardiology and the American College of Sports Medicine at the 26th Bethesda conference should be followed when cardiovascular abnormalities are found.

REFERRAL

Referral to a cardiovascular specialist should be considered for any tachyarrhythmia, any structural abnormality identified or suspected, any systolic murmur grade 3/6 intensity or greater, any diastolic murmur, or a family history of sudden cardiac death.

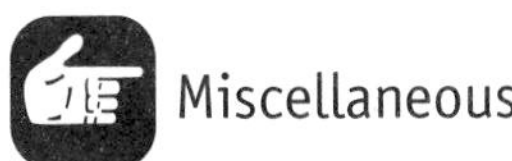

Miscellaneous

SYNONYMS

- Arrhythmias
- Conduction disorders

ICD-9 CODE

ICD-9 coding should be based on the specific diagnosis under the subheadings "Arrhythmias" or "Conduction Disorders," or coded based on symptoms (i.e., Palpitations 785.1).

BIBLIOGRAPHY

Huston TP, Puffer JC, Rodney WM. The athletic heart syndrome. *N Engl J Med* 1985;313:24–32.

Maron BJ, Mitchell JH. 26th Bethesda conference. *J Am Coll Cardiol* 1994;24: 845–899.

Zehender M, Meinertz T, Keul J, et al. ECG variants and cardiac arrhythmias in athletes: clinical relevance and prognostic importance. *Am Heart J* 1990;119: 1378–1391.

Authors: Jonathan Drezner and Michelle Look

Arteriosclerotic Heart Disease

Basics

DESCRIPTION

Arteriosclerosis is a group of diseases characterized by thickening and loss of elasticity of the arterial walls which progressively blocks the coronary arteries and their branches. Arteriosclerosis is the most common form of coronary arteriosclerosis. The process is chronic, occurring over many years, and is the most common cause of cardiovascular disability and death. Other forms of arteriosclerosis include arteriosclerosis and medialcalcific stenosis, both of which are uncommon in the coronary vasculature.
System(s) affected: Cardiovascular
Genetics: Tendency is inheritable
Incidence/Prevalence in USA: Common. Causes 35% of deaths in men age 35–50. Death rate age 55–64—1:100.
Predominant age: Men 50–60, women 60–70, for peak clinical manifestations
Predominant sex: Male > Female

SIGNS AND SYMPTOMS

- Variable. May remain clinically asymptomatic even in advanced disease states, e.g., silent ischemia.
- Clinical manifestations
  —Substernal chest pain
  —Exertional dyspnea
  —Orthopnea
  —Paroxysmal nocturnal dyspnea
  —Cardiac arrhythmias
  —Systolic murmur
  —Cardiomegaly
  —Pedal edema

CAUSES

- Atherosclerosis
- Narrowing of coronary arteries
- Embolism compromising coronary arteries at orifices
- Subintimal atheromas in large and medium vessels

RISK FACTORS

- Elevated low density lipoprotein (LDL)
- Decreased high density lipoprotein (HDL)
- Elevated triglycerides
- Smoking
- Family history of premature arteriosclerosis
- Obesity
- Hypertension
- Stress
- Sedentary life style
- Increasing age
- Male sex
- Postmenopausal female not on estrogen replacement therapy
- Diabetes mellitus

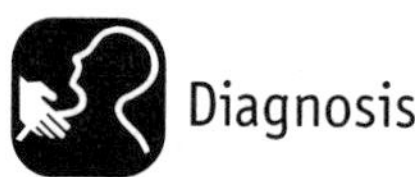

Diagnosis

DIFFERENTIAL DIAGNOSIS

N/A

LABORATORY

- Elevated triglycerides
- Elevated total cholesterol
- Elevated low density lipoproteins
- Decreased high density lipoproteins
- Elevated cholesterol/HDL ratio

Drugs that may alter lab results: N/A
Disorders that may alter lab results: N/A

PATHOLOGICAL FINDINGS

- Gross—narrowed coronary arteries
- Micro—cholesterol plaques on intima of coronary vessels
- Fibrotic subendothelial connective tissue of intima with plaque

SPECIAL TESTS

- ECG—variable. May be normal or may see ST segment elevation/depression and/or T wave inversion.
- Exercise stress test—positive

IMAGING

- Angiography—narrowed coronary arteries
- Echocardiography—wall motion abnormalities
- Pharmacologic stress tests (dobutamine, dipyridamole, adenosine)—positive
- Stress thallium test—positive

DIAGNOSTIC PROCEDURES

N/A

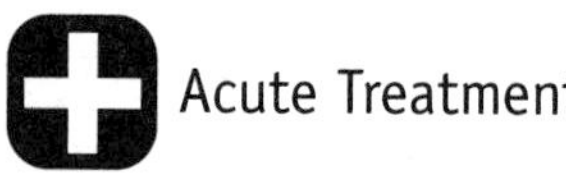

Acute Treatment

APPROPRIATE HEALTH CARE

- Outpatient for management of risk factors
- Inpatient for acute ischemic syndromes

GENERAL MEASURES

- Prevention of further progression of the disease
  —Smoking cessation
  —Treatment of hypercholesterolemia (diet, drugs)
  —Increase high density lipoprotein (diet, exercise)
  —Control of blood pressure
  —Diabetes mellitus treated early and adequately
  —Exercise
  —Prophylactic aspirin
  —Stress reduction
  —Diet changes
  —Weight loss
  —Estrogen replacement therapy in postmenopausal women is currently controversial
- Treatment of complications
  —Covered elsewhere under the individual topics (e.g., angina pectoris, myocardial infarction, heart failure, stroke, peripheral arterial occlusion, etc.)

SURGICAL MEASURES

N/A

ACTIVITY

Exercise may be helpful in preventing clinical coronary disease and useful for therapeutic measures.

DIET

- Low-fat (20–30 grams of fat/day total intake)
- Weight-loss diet, if obesity a problem
- Increase soluble fiber

PATIENT EDUCATION

For patient education materials favorably reviewed on this topic, contact: American Heart Association, 7272 Greenville Avenue, Dallas, TX 75231, (214)373-6300

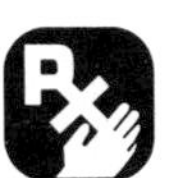

Long-Term Treatment

DRUG(S) OF CHOICE

- Aspirin, 160–325 mg/day, unless contraindicated
- Cholesterol-lowering agents
  —Cholestyramine or colestipol (bile acid sequestrants), 12–32 gm orally BID-QID
  —Niacin 2–6 gm daily in divided doses (highly efficacious, but side effects restrict use)
  —Gemfibrozil 600 mg bid
  —Probucol 500 mg bid
  —HMG-CoA reductase inhibitors (dose varies with product); atorvastatin (Lipitor), cerivastatin (Baycol), fluvastatin (Lescol), lovastatin (Mevacor), pravastatin (Pravachol), simvastatin (Zocor)

Contraindications: Refer to manufacturer's literature
Precautions: SR form of niacin may be linked to hepatotoxicity. Refer to manufacturer's literature.
Significant possible interactions: Refer to manufacturer's literature

ALTERNATIVE DRUGS

- Ticlopidine—antiplatelet activity

PATIENT MONITORING

Monitor cholesterol, triglyceride levels, other preventive programs (weight loss, smoking cessation)

PREVENTION/AVOIDANCE

See General measures

POSSIBLE COMPLICATIONS

- Myocardial infarction
- Ventricular fibrillation
- Congestive heart failure
- Angina pectoris
- Sudden cardiac death

EXPECTED COURSE/PROGNOSIS

Guardedly favorable. Many risk factors can be modified.

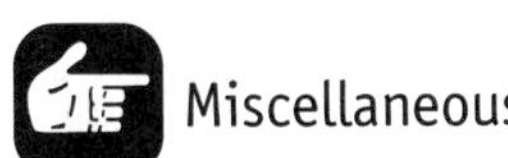

Miscellaneous

ASSOCIATED CONDITIONS

- Obesity
- Hypertension
- Diabetes
- Hypercholesterolemia

AGE-RELATED FACTORS

Pediatric: Preventive measures can begin early (proper nutrition, exercise, weight control, smoking deterrent programs, etc.)
Geriatric: Greatest incidence in this age group
Others: N/A

PREGNANCY

Rare in pregnant women
Miscellaneous

SYNONYMS

- Coronary artery disease (CAD)
- Coronary heart disease
- Coronary arteriosclerosis

ICD-9 CODE

414.0 arteriosclerotic heart disease

See also: Atherosclerotic Heart Disease

BIBLIOGRAPHY

Hurst JW, et al. *The heart*. 8th Ed. New York, McGraw-Hill, 1994.

Braunwald E. ed. *Heart disease: A textbook of cardiovascular medicine*. 4th Ed. Philadelphia, WB Saunders Co, 1992.

Goldman L, Braunwald E. *Primary cardiology*. 1st Ed. Philadelphia, WB Saunders Co, 1998.

Internet references: http://www.5mcc.com

Author: Peter Kozisek

Athletic Heart Syndrome

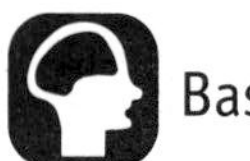 Basics

DEFINITION

- A benign condition consisting of physiologic adaptations to the increased cardiac workload of exercise. Its primary features are biventricular hypertrophy and bradycardia associated with normal systolic and diastolic function.

INCIDENCE/PREVALENCE

- These changes are almost universal in highly trained athletes.
- Often mistaken for pathologic conditions

SIGNS AND SYMPTOMS

- Vagally mediated arrhythmias such as sinus bradycardia, first- and second-degree atrioventricular block
- Laterally displaced left ventricular impulse
- Signs of left ventricular hypertrophy on electrocardiography
- Mid-systolic murmurs, third and fourth heart sounds are quite common

RISK FACTORS

- Chronic endurance exercise
- Genetic predisposition

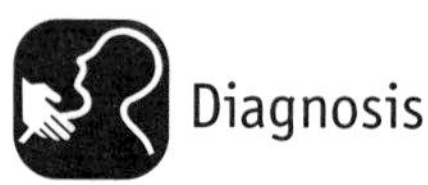 Diagnosis

DIFFERENTIAL DIAGNOSIS

- Hypertensive cardiac hypertrophy
- Hypertrophic cardiomyopathy
- Dilated cardiomyopathy

HISTORY

- Palpitations, presyncope or syncope? Search for a cause.
- Family history of sudden death or recurrent syncope? Clue for hypertrophic cardiomyopathy
- Prior rheumatic fever? Look for evidence of rheumatic heart disease.

PHYSICAL EXAM

- Decreased body fat and increased muscle mass (generally very physically fit)
- Pulse slow and often irregular (sinus bradycardia or bradycardia with first- and second-degree blocks)
- Grade I or II mid-systolic murmurs (benign functional ejection murmur resolves with Valsalva maneuver)
- Third and fourth heart sounds very common (benign filling sounds)
- Blood pressure typically remains normal

IMAGING

- Electrocardiogram rhythm
  —Sinus bradycardia of 40 to 55 beats/min while at rest
  —Sinus pauses of more than 2.0 seconds due to increased vagal tone
  —Wandering atrial pacemaker, found only in dynamic athletes
  —First-degree atrioventricular block present only at rest; P-R interval normalizes with exercise
  —Second-degree atrioventricular block present only at rest; Mobitz I (Wenckebach block) common in marathon runners; Mobitz II rare in athlete's heart
- Voltage
  —Left ventricular hypertrophy found in 85% of Olympic marathon runners
  —Right ventricular hypertrophy, common in dynamic athletes but rarely seen in sedentary controls and static athletes
- Repolarization
  —S-T segment elevation with peaked T waves, normalizes with exertion
  —S-T segment depression with depressed J points, rarely found in athletes
  —T-wave inversion in lateral leads associated with interventricular septal hypertrophy in static athletes (can be normal finding in dynamic athletes)
- Chest radiography
  —Heart is globular in appearance, particularly in endurance athletes.
  —Cardiomegaly (cardiothoracic ratio >0.50)
- Echocardiography
  —Dynamic athletes: left and right ventricular dilation with left, right ventricular and septal hypertrophy
  —Static (weight lifting) athletes: left ventricular and septal hypertrophy with either decrease or no change in left ventricle chamber size; similar changes occur with chronic hypertension
  —Female athletes: both dynamic and static athletes exhibit a lesser degree of left ventricular and septal hypertrophy than male athletes. Other changes are very similar between genders.
- Cardiac catheterization
  —May be necessary to determine the nature or extent of disease in individuals with known organic heart disease
  —Frequently this information can be obtained by noninvasive cardiac tests.

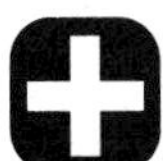

Acute Treatment

ANALGESIA

- Not indicated

REASSURANCE

- If pathologic evidence of heart disease is absent, then reassure the athlete that the observed changes are normal physiologic adaptations to exercise.
- Do not encourage the athlete to stop exercising.

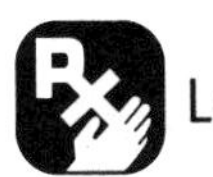

Long-Term Treatment

REFERRAL/DISPOSITION

- Many of the physiologic adaptations observed in athletic heart syndrome resolve when exercise is stopped.
- Because the adaptations that occur in the resistive or static athlete are similar to those caused by chronic hypertension, the long-term effects could be damaging. Therefore, these individuals should be encouraged to incorporate dynamic components to their weight-lifting routine.

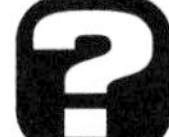

Common Questions and Answers

Physician responses to common patient questions:
Q: Is something wrong with my heart?
A: Far from being diseased, your heart is healthy and well equipped for strenuous exercise. These changes will not cause heart disease.

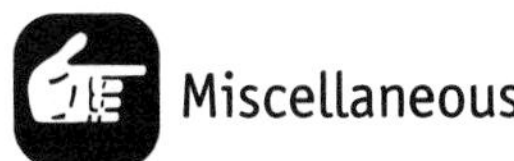

Miscellaneous

SYNONYMS

- Athlete's heart
- Physiologic cardiac hypertrophy

ICD-9 CODE

Athletic Heart Syndrome: none
427.89 Bradycardia

BIBLIOGRAPHY

Bryan G, Ward A, Rippe JM. Athletic heart syndrome. *Clin Sports Med* 1992;11: 259–272.

George KP, Wolfe LA, Burggraf GA, et al. Electrocardiographic and echocardiographic characteristics of female athletes. *Med Sci Sports Exerc* 1995;27:1362–1370.

George KP, Wolfe LA, Burggraf GW. The athletic heart syndrome: a critical review. *Sports Med* 1991;11:300–330.

Huston TP, Puffer JC, Rodney WM. The athletic heart syndrome. *N Engl J Med* 1985;313:24–32.

Author: John Hill

Barotitis Media

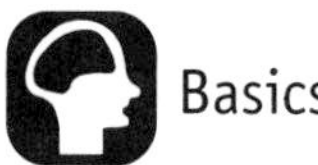

Basics

SIGNS AND SYMPTOMS

- Middle ear (barotitis media)
- Begins as a clogged sensation
- Increasingly painful as the pressure differential across the tympanic membrane (TM) increases
- Progresses to rupture of the TM
  —Tympanic membrane appearance: TM congestion→TM edema→gross hemorrhage→TM rupture
- External ear
  —Canal mucosa becomes edematous, then hemorrhagic, and ultimately tears
- Inner ear
  —Sudden, severe vertigo
  —Tinnitus
  —Sensineural hearing loss in the affected ear
- Paranasal sinuses
  —Sinus congestion
  —Pain
  —Epistaxis
- External objects
  —Mask: conjunctival hemorrhage, facial edema and swelling
  —Tight fitting dive suit: edema and erythema of the skin
- Teeth (barodontalgia)
  —Severe tooth pain
- Gastrointestinal (aerogastralgia)
  —Excessive belching
  —Flatulence
  —Abdominal distention
- Pulmonary
  —Dyspnea
  —Cough with a frothy red sputum
  —Subcutaneous emphysema
  —Delayed symptoms including a bull neck appearance, dysphagia, and changes in voice character

DESCRIPTION/MECHANISM

- Injury to the body as a result of the expansion and contraction of gas in an enclosed space
- Boyle's law states that at a constant temperature, pressure (P) is inversely related to volume (V)
  —PV = K (constant) or $P_1V_1 = P_2V_2$
  —Increase of pressure mandates a reduction of volume by same factor
- Gas-filled cavities in the body are subject to expansion/contraction
  —Lung
  —Middle ear
  —Sinus
- Solid and liquid-filled spaces distribute the pressure equally
- Volume changes experienced during ascent are greatest in the few feet nearest the surface

ETIOLOGY

- Middle ear
  —Barotrauma of descent
  —Most common type of barotrauma
  —Seen in 30% of inexperienced divers and 10% of experienced divers
  —Results from inadequate equalization of pressure between the middle ear and the external ear canal
  —Eustachian tube provides the sole route of pressure equalization for the middle ear
- External ear
  —Barotrauma of descent
  —Due to the presence of a tight fitting hood, ear plugs, or a cerumen plug
  —Pressure cannot equalize throughout the canal and a relative intracanal vacuum is created as the pressure differential across the obstruction increases
- Inner ear
  —Barotrauma of descent
  —Results from forceful attempts at equalizing middle ear pressure
  —Increased middle ear pressure can raise intracranial pressure and cause rupture of the round or labyrinth windows allowing perilymph to enter the middle ear
- Paranasal sinus
  —Barotrauma of descent
  —Nasal ostia act as a valve to regulate sinus pressure
  —If the ostia fail to allow pressure equalization, congestion, edema, and hemorrhage can occur
- External objects
  —Air pockets in dive suit/mask expand and contract
- Teeth
  —Air trapped inside a filling
- Gastrointestinal
  —Barotrauma of ascent
  —Swallowed air in the GI tract expands as external pressure decreases
- Pulmonary barotrauma (PBT or POPS—Pulmonary Over Pressurization Syndrome)
  —Occurs with ascent
  —Lungs expand against a closed glottis
  —Cause for arterial gas embolism (see Embolism Chapter)
  —Divers with decrease lung compliance/ increase lung volumes at increased risk (COPD, asthma)

CAUTION

- For barotrauma of descent, unless an air-filled cavity has ruptured, no progression of the disease upon return to normal atmospheric pressure expected
- If patient transport requires air evacuation, maintain air cabin pressure at 1 atmosphere or fly below 1000 feet to avoid aggravating barotrauma

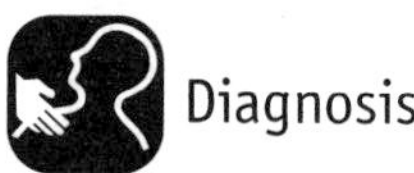

Diagnosis

ESSENTIAL WORKUP

- HEENT exam with particular attention paid to the TM to determine if rupture has occurred
- Pulmonary exam looking for signs of subcutaneous emphysema and pneumothorax
- Neurological exam looking for signs of inner ear pathology

LABORATORY

- ABG for pulmonary symptoms

IMAGING/SPECIAL TESTS

- Sinus imaging
  —CT
  —Plain films
- CXR for pneumothorax
- Abdominal series (upright, decubitus) for free air from a ruptured viscus

DIFFERENTIAL DIAGNOSIS

- Decompression sickness
- Otitis media
- Otitis externa
- Sinusitis

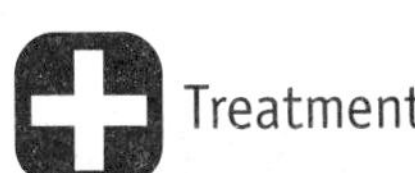

Treatment

INITIAL STABILIZATION

- ABCs
  —100% oxygen for ill-appearing patients
  —Intubation for in-patients with massive subcutaneous emphysema of the neck
  —Immediate needle thoracostomy for evidence of tension pneumothorax

ED TREATMENT

- Establish IV access for unstable patients
- Control bleeding from the ear or nose
- Oral decongestants for middle ear or sinus congestion
- Antibiotics with TM or sinus rupture
- Analgesics

MEDICATIONS

- Amoxicillin: 250–500 mg (peds: 40 mg/kg/24 hrs) po TID
- Bactrim DS 1 tablet (peds: 40/200 per 5 ml-5 ml/10 kg/dose) po BID
- Pseudoephedrine (Sudafed) 60 mg (peds: 6–12 yrs old, 30 mg; 2–5 yrs old, 15 mg/dose) po q4–6 hrs

HOSPITAL ADMISSION CRITERIA

- Pulmonary barotrauma

HOSPITAL DISCHARGE CRITERIA

- Discharge nonpulmonary barotrauma
- ENT follow-up for severe TM or sinus pathology

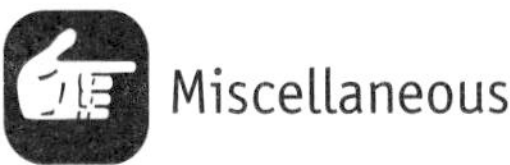

Miscellaneous

PATIENT CODE

993.2

CORE CONTENT CODE

5.1

BIBLIOGRAPHY

Bradley ME. Pulmonary barotrauma. In: Bove AA, Davis JC. *Diving medicine*. 2d ed. Philadelphia: WB Saunders, 1990:188–191.

Edmonds C, Lowry C, Pennefather J. *Diving and subaquatic medicine*. Oxford: Butterworth-Heinemann, 1992.

Jerrard DA. Diving medicine. *Emerg Med Clin North Am* 1992;10(2):329–338.

Raymond LW. Pulmonary barotrauma and related events in divers. *Chest* 1995;107: 1648–1652.

Author: Jeffrey Gordon

Bites and Stings

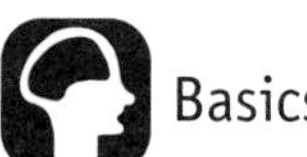

Basics

DESCRIPTION

Arthropods affect man by being pests, inoculating poison, invading tissue, or transmitting disease. Inoculation of poison may occur as either a bite or a sting. This discussion is limited to the irritative, poisonous, allergic effects of these pests.

- Harmful arthropods of the U.S. include:
  —Bees: Bumblebees, sweat bees, honeybees
  —Wasps: Hornets, wasps
  —Ants: Fire ants, harvester ants
  —Brown recluse spider
  —Black widow spider
  —Hobo spiders
  —Scorpions
  —Mosquitoes
  —Flies: Deer, horse, black, stable, and biting midges
  —Lice: Body, head, pubic
  —Bugs: Kissing, bed, wheel
  —Fleas: Human, cat, dog
  —Mites: Itch mite (scabies), red bugs (chiggers)
  —Ticks
  —Caterpillars: Puss, browntail, buck, moth saddleback
  —Centipedes
- Characteristic reactions include:
  —Local tissue imitation, inflammation and destruction
  —Systemic effects related to inoculated poisons
  —Allergic reactions: Immediate or delayed

System(s) affected: Skin/Exocrine
Genetics: N/A
Incidence/Prevalence in USA: Widespread (seasonal and regional variance)
Predominant age: All ages
Predominant sex: Male = Female

SIGNS AND SYMPTOMS

- Local reactions:
  —Erythema
  —Pain
  —Heat
  —Swelling
  —Itching
  —Blisters
  —Secondary infection—cellulitis, abscess
  —Necrosis
  —Ulceration
  —Drainage
- Toxic reactions: Non-antigenic
  —Nausea
  —Vomiting
  —Headache
  —Fever
  —Diarrhea
  —Lightheadedness
  —Syncope
  —Drowsiness
  —Muscles spasms
  —Edema
  —Convulsions
- Systemic reactions: Allergic
  —Itching eyes
  —Facial flushing
  —Generalized urticaria
  —Dry cough
  —Chest/throat constriction
  —Wheezing
  —Dyspnea
  —Cyanosis
  —Abdominal cramps
  —Diarrhea
  —Nausea
  —Vomiting
  —Vertigo
  —Chills/fever
  —Stridor
  —Shock
  —Loss of consciousness
  —Involuntary bowel/bladder action
  —Frothy sputum
  —Respiratory failure
  —Cardiovascular collapse
  —Death
- Delayed reaction:
  —Serum-sickness-like reactions
  —Fever
  —Malaise
  —Headache
  —Urticaria
  —Lymphadenopathy
  —Polyarthritis
- Unusual reactions:
  —Encephalopathy
  —Neuritis
  —Vasculitis
  —Nephrosis
  —Extreme fear/anxiety

CAUSES

- Local tissue inflammation and destruction from poison
- Allergic reaction from previous sensitization
- Toxic reaction from large inoculation of poison

RISK FACTORS

- Living environment
- Climate
- Season
- Clothing
- Lack of protective measures
- Perfumes, colognes
- Previous sensitization
- Young or elderly at more risk

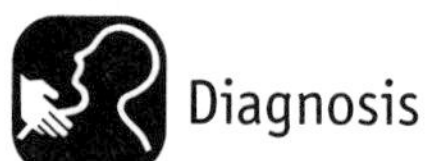

Diagnosis

DIFFERENTIAL DIAGNOSIS

- Local reaction: Infection, cellulitis, dermatoses, punctures, foreign bodies
- Toxic reaction: Chemical exposure/ ingestion, medications, IV drug abuse, environmental, plants
- Allergic reaction: Medications, illicit drugs, foods, topical products, environmental, plants, chemicals

LABORATORY

Leukocytosis, thrombocytopenia, hypofibrinogenemia, abnormal coagulation, DIC, proteinuria, hemoglobinemia, hemoglobinuria, myoglobinemia, myoglobinuria, and azotemia are uncommon but possible manifestations in severe reactions
Drugs that may alter lab results: N/A
Disorders that may alter lab results: N/A

PATHOLOGICAL FINDINGS

Inflammation, ulceration, vesiculation, pustulation, rupture, eschar, swelling

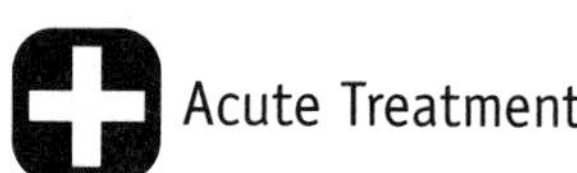

Acute Treatment

APPROPRIATE HEALTH CARE

- Outpatient or inpatient, depending on individual response to injury
- Hospitalize for severe systemic reactions with threatened airway obstruction, bronchospasm, hypotension, severe angiodermatitis or pain

GENERAL MEASURES

- First aid measures, local treatment, activate emergency services in severe reactions. If history of allergy or large envenomations, don't wait to seek emergency care.
- Use ANA kit and over-the-counter antihistamines, if available and required
- Local (depending on severity)
  —Remove stinger (scrape it out—don't squeeze with tweezer)
  —Cleanse wound
  —Ice packs to bite or sting site (alternate 10 minutes on/10 minutes off)
  —Elevation of affected part
  —Rest the affected area
  —Debride ulcers
  —Drain abscesses

- Systemic (depending on severity, and type of reaction); home use—Epi-Pen
  - —Adequate airway (intubation, tracheostomy)—if needed to bypass obstruction
  - —Oxygen (4-6 L/min)—if needed for respiratory distress
  - —Hospitalize and observe 24-48 hours

SURGICAL MEASURES

Optimal treatment of necrotic spider bites is not well defined. Surgical repair may be required of severe ulcerative lesions, but not until primary necrotizing process is complete.

ACTIVITY

Rest to limit spread of poison

DIET

No special diet; nothing by mouth if severe systemic reaction

PATIENT EDUCATION

- Protective measures, ANA kit use, risks
- Individuals with known sensitivity should wear medical identification (bracelet, tag) or carry a card

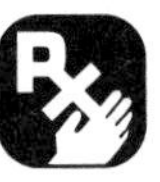

Long-Term Treatment

DRUG(S) OF CHOICE

- Local (depending on severity)
  - —Analgesics
  - —Antihistamines—diphenhydramine (Benadryl) 25-50 mg qid
  - —Steroids topical or oral—prednisone 20-40 mg/day
  - —Antibiotics
- Systemic (depending on severity and reaction type)
  - —Epinephrine [1:1000] subcutaneous: to combat urticaria, wheezing, angioedema—child 0.01 mL/kg, adult 0.3-0.5 mL
  - —Diphenhydramine: 25-50 mg IV or IM, to combat urticaria, wheezing, angioedema
  - —Aminophylline: adult 500 mg IV over 20-30 minutes, child 7.5 mg/kg, if needed for bronchospasm
  - —IV fluids (Ringer's lactate): if needed for hypotension, hypovolemia
  - —Dopamine: 200 mg in 250 mL at 5 mcg/kg/min—to correct vascular collapse.

  Titrate to maintain systemic blood pressure over 90 mm Hg.
  - —Hydrocortisone: 100-250 mg IV, if needed for severe urticaria or spider bite
  - —Tetanus prophylaxis and antibiotics: if indicated
  - —Diazepam (Valium): 5-10 mg, if needed for severe muscle spasms
  - —Morphine or meperidine (Demerol): if needed for pain
- Antivenins (e.g., Black Widow spider, scorpion) are available and appropriate in certain cases based on availability and identification of organism
- Topical insecticides
  - —Lice: 1% permethrin (Nix, Elimite) is drug of choice, but 1% lindane (Kwell) or pyrethrin (Rid) are effective.
  - —Scabies: 5% permethrin is drug of choice, but 10% crotamiton (Eurax) or lindane are effective

Contraindications: Refer to manufacturer's literature
Precautions:

- Dosing appropriate to age
- If severe reaction, don't delay treatment
- Severe vascular collapse may require central pressure monitor

Significant possible interactions: Refer to manufacturer's literature

ALTERNATIVE DRUGS

- Other antihistamines, e.g., loratadine (Claritin), fexofenadine (Allegra), etc.
- Oral ivermectin (Mectizan) appears effective for lice and scabies, but is not FDA approved for this purpose

PATIENT MONITORING

Followup wound care

PREVENTION/AVOIDANCE

- Avoid re-exposure in known hypersensitive individuals
- Prescribe anaphylactic (ANA kit) or Epi-Pen, if indicated
- Educate on risks of increasing anamnestic responses in future
- Consider desensitization with immunotherapy in severe cases
- DEET or other proven insect repellants
- Permethrin applied to clothes is better against ticks than DEET

POSSIBLE COMPLICATIONS

- Infection
  - —Bacterial
  - —Arthropod associated diseases with tick, fly, bug and mosquito bites, e.g., lyme borreliosis, rickettsial disease (Rocky Mountain spotted fever), arboviral encephalitis, malaria, leishmaniasis, trypanosomiasis, dengue
- Scarring
- Drug reactions
- Multisystem failure
- Death

EXPECTED COURSE/PROGNOSIS

- Minor reactions—excellent
- Severe reactions—excellent with early, appropriate treatment

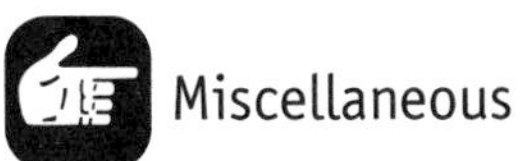

Miscellaneous

ASSOCIATED CONDITIONS

N/A

AGE-RELATED FACTORS

Pediatric: More at risk
Geriatric: More at risk
Others: N/A

PREGNANCY

Not a contraindication to appropriate management

ICD-9 CODE

989.5 insect sting (venomous)
910-919 (injury superficial by site, plus 4th digit 0-9 for subdivision)

See also: Pediculosis; Scabies

OTHER NOTES

- Imported fire ants and Africanized bees in endemic areas of the Southern United States pose increased risks to persons living in these areas

BIBLIOGRAPHY

- Tintinalli JE, Krome RL, eds: *Emergency medicine*. New York, McGraw-Hill, 1988.
- Schroeder SA, Krupp MA, Tieme LM, McPhee SJ, eds. *Current medical diagnosis and treatment*. Norwalk, CT: Appleton & Lange, 1989.
- MMWR: Necrotic arachnidism-Pacific Northwest, 1996;45(21).
- Isselbacher KJ, et al., eds: *Harrison's principles of internal medicine*. 13th ed. New York, McGraw-Hill, 1994.
- The Medical Letter. Vol 40 (issue 1017) Jan 2, 1998.
- Mosquitoes and mosquito repellants: A clinician's guide. *Annals of internal medicine* 1198;Jun 1:128(11):931-940.

Internet references: http://www.5mcc.com

Author: Robert L. Weston

Calluses and Corns

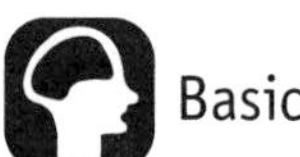

Basics

DEFINITION

- A callus is a plaque of hyperkeratosis of relatively even thickness caused by repeated friction, pressure, or trauma.
- A corn is a localized, tender, sharply defined area of hyperkeratosis over a bony prominence caused by trauma, found usually on the hand or foot. It has a central core that penetrates into the dermis, causing pain.

SIGNS AND SYMPTOMS

- The most common site for calluses is under the metatarsal heads, but they may occur anywhere on the skin as a result of friction.
- A callus may be asymptomatic or painful, often appearing as a yellowish plaque.
- Corns are tender when direct pressure is applied but not when squeezed.
- A hard corn is a dry horny mass found commonly over the interphalangeal joints (dorsally) or the fifth toe (dorsolaterally).
- Soft corns are extremely painful and occur interdigitally. The skin appears white and macerated, seen commonly between the fourth interdigital space (often mistaken for tinea).

RISK FACTORS

- Activity level: occupational (manual workers); athletes
- Ill-fitting footwear: tight, loose, irregularities in shoe
- Bony prominences
- Faulty foot mechanics
- Toe deformities

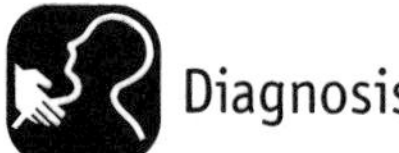

Diagnosis

DIFFERENTIAL DIAGNOSIS

- Verruca vulgaris or plantaris (differentiated by paring the skin: the corn becomes more normal in appearance and the wart displays the characteristic tiny red dots when pared)
- Tinea pedis (interdigital)
- Psoriatic plaque: hyperkeratosis with red base

HISTORY

- Location: is it consistent with a site of friction, pressure, repeat trauma, or bony prominence?
- Provoking factors: type of sport, occupation, or leisure activity causing repeated friction or pressure?
- Ask about footwear.
- Any previous treatments?
- Are there any coexisting illnesses (e.g., diabetes)?
- Inherited disposition? (autosomal-dominant inheritance)

PHYSICAL EXAM

- Observe gait and the alignment of the feet for any faulty mechanics.
- Note the location and appearance of the hyperkeratotic lesions.
- Palpate for any abnormal bony prominences.
- Assess for pain or tenderness.
- Common sites for corns and calluses: plantar surface (over the metatarsal heads, sides of the arch and the heel) and dorsum of the foot (over the interphalangeal joints)
- Common sites for calluses on hands: palmar surface and over metacarpophalangeal joints

IMAGING

- Usually not necessary
- Radiographs: weight-bearing views of the feet used to identify bony prominences or abnormalities

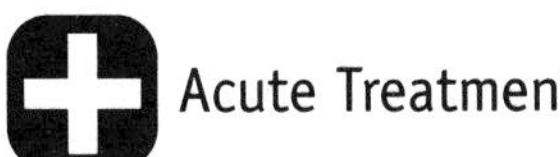

Acute Treatment

TREATMENT

- Salicylic acid (10%–20%): careful application or pads containing keratolytic agents
- Careful and regular paring
- Soft corn: toe separator or lamb's wool
- Doughnut-shaped corn pads
- Proper footwear with soft upper and a roomy toebox
- Orthotics can reduce pressure by redistributing forces.
- Surgery may be required to eliminate bony abnormalities or deformities, and is indicated only if all conservative measures fail.

PREVENTION

- Proper footwear
- Orthotics
- Toe separators
- Lamb's wool

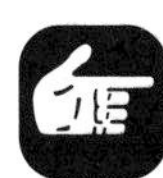

Miscellaneous

ICD-9 CODE

700 Corns and callosities
11055 Paring corn or callus: single lesion
11056 Paring corn or callus: two to four lesions
11057 Paring corn or callus: more than four lesions

BIBLIOGRAPHY

Champion RH, Burton JL, Burns DA, et al. In: Rook, Wilkinson, Ebling, eds. *Textbook of dermatology,* 6th ed. Oxford: Blackwell Science, 1998.

Sallis RE, Massimino F, eds. *Essentials of sports medicine.* St. Louis: CV Mosby, 1997.

Singh D, Bentley G, Trevino SG. Callosities, corns, and calluses. *BMJ* 1996;312: 1403–1406.

Author: Kathleen Weber

Cellulitis

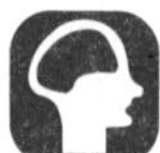

Basics

DEFINITION

- Cellulitis is a localized area of soft tissue inflammation. It involves the infiltration of an area of skin by white blood cells, as well as capillary dilation and a proliferation of bacteria.

MECHANISMS

- The bacteria responsible for most cases of cellulitis are *Staphylococcus aureus* and *Streptococcus pyogenes*.
- Cellulitis induced by other bacteria is possible, but uncommon.

RISK FACTORS

- The presence of an open wound permits *Staphylococcus aureus* or *Streptococcus pyogenes* to enter the epidermis and cause infection.
- Exposure of an open laceration to fresh water in a lake or similar environment may cause cellulitis due to *Aeromonas hydrophilia*.
- A laceration exposed to seawater may develop an infection related to *Vibrio vulnificus*.

ASSOCIATED INJURIES AND COMPLICATIONS

- Once an individual has developed cellulitis, the infection may spread away from the laceration. Cellulitis caused by *Streptococcus pyogenes* may spread particularly rapidly.
- Cellulitis may spread through the bloodstream and lymphatics.
- In older patients, cellulitis of the lower extremities may be complicated by thrombophlebitis.
- In patients with chronic dependent edema, cellulitis may spread very rapidly.

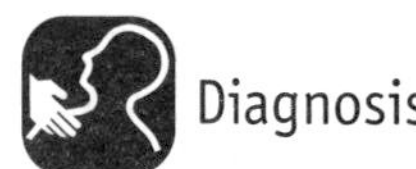

Diagnosis

DIFFERENTIAL DIAGNOSIS

- Within a few days of infection, local tenderness, pain, and erythema may develop.
- The lesion is hot and swollen, and the involved area often becomes extensive.
- Later symptoms may include malaise, fever, and chills.
- Positive swab culture or Gram stain

PHYSICAL EXAM

Check for elevated or sharply demarcated area borders. Cellulitis can be distinguished from erysipelas by the lack of elevated or clearly defined borders in the affected region.

LABORATORY TESTING

- Gram stain and culture from port of entry can often provide a definite diagnosis.
- Needle aspiration and punch biopsy of cellulitis only identify bacteria 20% of the time.

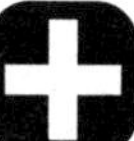

Acute Treatment

- Immobilize and elevate the affected limb.
- Apply a cool sterile saline dressing.

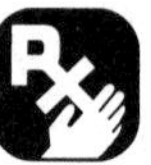

Long-Term Treatment

ANTIBIOTICS

- If cellulitis is mild, early, and of streptococcal origin, start with an initial dose of aqueous penicillin injection (600,000 units). Follow by intramuscular procaine penicillin (600,000 units every 8–12 hours).
- If infection is not severe, but suspected to be staphylococcal or of unknown etiology, consider a penicillinase-resistant penicillin (e.g., dicloxacillin 0.25–0.5 g orally every 6 hours).
- For more severe infections in which both staphylococcal and streptococcal etiologies are possible, parenteral administration of a penicillinase-resistant penicillin [e.g., nafcillin 1.0 g intravenously (IV) every 4 hours or oxacillin 1.0 g every 4 hours IV] or cefazolin 1.0 g every 8 hours IV is indicated; ceftriaxone 1 g intramuscularly or IV is an alternative

- For a freshwater injury with a rapidly progressive infection, consider gentamicin, along with a penicillinase-resistant penicillin.
- In patients with severe penicillin allergy, vancomycin (1.0–1.5 g/day IV) may be used.
- Alternatives to the above include erythromycin, azithromycin, clarithromycin, or parenteral or oral cephalosporins, amoxicillin/clavulanate, clindamycin; fluoroquinolones such as gatifloxacin, levofloxacin, or moxifloxacin also may be effective.

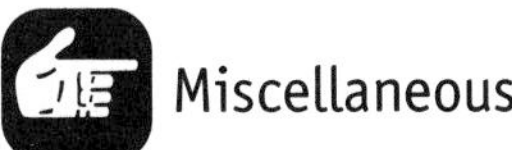

Miscellaneous

ICD-9 CODE

686 Other local infections of the skin and subcutaneous tissue

BIBLIOGRAPHY

Gilbert DN, Moellering RC Jr, Sande MA, eds. *The Sanford guide to antimicrobial therapy 2000,* 30th ed. Hyde Park, VT: Antimicrobial Therapy, 2000.

Minooee A, Arezou, Rickmans LS, et al. Transmission of infectious diseases during sports. In: Schlossberg D, ed. *Infections of leisure,* 2nd ed. Washington, DC. American Society for Microbiology, 1999.

Reese RE, Betts RF, eds. *A practical approach to infectious diseases,* 4th ed. Boston: Little Brown, 1996.

Stevens DL. Cellulitis, pyoderma, and other skin and subcutaneous infections. In: Armstrong D, Cohen J, eds. *Infectious diseases*. Vol. 1. Mosby/Harcourt Publishers, 1999:2.2.6–2.2.8.

Swartz NN. Cellulitis and subcutaneous tissue. In: Mandell GL, Bennet JE, Dolin R, eds. *Mandell, Douglas, and Bennett's principles and practice of infectious disease,* 5th ed. Vol. 1. Philadelphia: Churchill Livingstone, 2000.

Authors: Elizabeth Austin and Leland S. Rickman

Chest and Breast Lacerations and Contusions

Basics

DEFINITION

- Direct trauma from, for example, collision with an opposing player, a fall, contact with a ball, bat or stick to the chest or breast area may result in contusions, hematomas, abrasions, and lacerations, as well as pain.

INCIDENCE/PREVALENCE

- Chest and breast injuries are rarely reported in sports literature. This may be explained by decreased severity of injury, rare occurrence, or gender differences.
- There is a report of a horse bite in equestrian sports as a cause for breast injury.
- Accident-prone sports such as biking, road racing, mountain biking, skiing, and rodeo are thought to increase risk.
- Although most collision sports such as hockey, football, baseball, and field hockey provide some chest protection for at-risk players, trauma can occur.
- Sports with running and jumping components may contribute to breast pain, especially in large-breasted women.
- Nipple injuries such as jogger's nipples (i.e., irritated nipples due to chafing of clothing) and biker's nipples (i.e., irritated nipples due to thermal injury) have both been reported in the literature.

SIGNS AND SYMPTOMS

- Deformity of the chest or breast (hematoma)
- Pain of chest, breast, or nipples
- Blood on clothing

RISK FACTORS

- Large-breasted women (C and D cup)
- Lack of or poor fitting protective equipment
- Collision sports
- Sports with running, jumping or possibility of collision
- Bra parts such as straps, metal hooks, clips, and underwires
- Chafing, especially from cold, wet clothing over the nipples

ASSOCIATED INJURIES AND COMPLICATIONS

- Contact with a high-velocity missile can cause deep tissue and organ damage, such as cardiac contusion, lung contusion, great vessel rupture, or rib fracture.
- Rupture of breast implants has been known to rarely occur. Breast pain following trauma in athletes with implants is usually the result of rupture of scar tissue. However, any asymmetry of breasts should be followed closely.
- Rarely, hematomas in this area may become secondarily infected.
- Trauma of the chest and breast may lead to Mondor's disease (thrombophlebitis of superficial breast veins).
- Occasionally, breast trauma and pain lead to discovery of tumors and masses. There is no good evidence that trauma or exercise contributes to breast cancer. However, breast cancers may be identified in athletes with trauma because of closer surveillance.
- Complications following trauma include fat necrosis, induration, mastitis, scarring, and calcification.

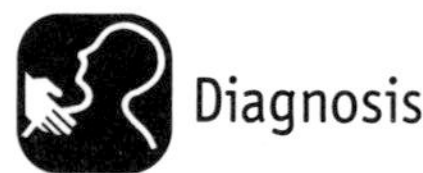

Diagnosis

DIFFERENTIAL DIAGNOSIS

- Pain (Mastodynia)
  —Achalasia
  —Cervical radiculopathy
  —Cholelithiasis
  —Coronary artery disease
  —Cervical rib
  —Cooper's ligament strain
  —Costochondritis (Tietze's syndrome)
  —Cyclic mastodynia
  —Fractured rib (stress fracture)
  —Fourth rib dysfunction
  —Hiatal hernia
  —Mondor's disease
  —Myalgia
  —Mastitis/infection
  —Neuralgia
  —Phantom pain
  —Pleurisy
  —Psychological disorder
  —Pregnancy
  —Trauma (contusion)
  —Tumor/neoplasia (rare)
  —Tuberculosis
- Mass
  —Adenocarcinoma
  —Angiosarcoma
  —Dermatofibromatosis
  —Ductal adenocarcinoma
  —Fat necrosis
  —Fibrocystic change
  —Fibroadenoma
  —Gynecomastia
  —Granular cell myoblastoma
  —Hematoma
  —Hemangioma
  —Intraductal papilloma
  —Interstitial fibrosis
  —Lipoma
  —Lymphangioma
  —Mammary duct ectasia
  —Mastitis
  —Metastatic disease
  —Mondor's disease
  —Nipple adenoma
  —Nipple keratoma
  —Neurofibromatosis
  —Papilloma sarcoidosis
  —Pregnancy
  —Sclerosing adenosis
  —Tuberous mastitis
  —Tumor/neoplasia

HISTORY

- Localized pain
- Trauma
- Skin changes
- Associated lumps
- Nipple complaints
- Cyclic versus noncyclic pain
- Assess for risk factors of breast cancer.
- Family history of breast cancer
- Personal history of breast cancer
- Hormone therapy
- Previous breast surgery
- Last mammogram
- Menstrual history
- Gynecomastia
- Age of athlete

PHYSICAL EXAM

- Observation/palpation
- Localization of dominant mass
- Axillary lymphadenopathy
- Consider need for pelvic exam to rule out ovarian tumor.

IMAGING

- Radiography: Usually normal, but may show healing stress fracture
- Mammography (if breast mass is suspected in male or older female)
- Ultrasonography (in younger female with discrete mass)
- Bone scan (if bony tenderness and stress fracture is suspected)

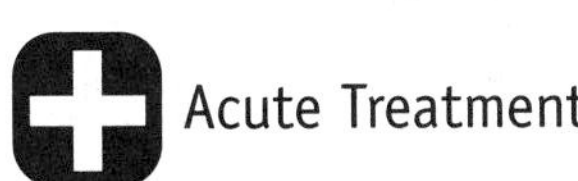

Acute Treatment

ANALGESIA

- Contusion and hematoma: ice, oral pain medications as needed
- Laceration: local anesthetic for cleaning, debriding and repair; ice, oral pain medications if needed; close either with suture or Steri-Strips; suture may be best option to close subcutaneous dead space
- Abrasion: direct pressure to control bleeding; clean, cover, and dress appropriately
- Jogger's nipple: treat as above if open wound present; otherwise, cover nipple with lubricating cream or ointment and replace irritating clothing.
- Biker's nipple: treat as above if open wound is present, otherwise, replace cold, wet, or irritating clothing; dry, rewarm, and lubricate nipple if necessary.
- Cyclic breast pain may be managed with evening primrose oil or contraceptive hormones.
- Cyclic breast pain may respond to other treatments such as diuretics, diet changes (e.g., elimination of methylxanthines and vitamins E, A, and B complex), thyroid hormones, tamoxifen, and gonadotropin-releasing hormone analogues.

IMMOBILIZATION

- Contusion and hematoma: supportive bra, especially in large-breasted women
- Laceration: firm dressing and support to control hematoma, wear bra at night

SPECIAL CONSIDERATIONS

- Laceration: check for signs of infection, check tetanus status
- Large breast hematomas should be aspirated given the risk of subcutaneous fat necrosis.
- In the case of the athlete with breast augmentation, consider the possibility of breast implant rupture, and early referral.
- Implant rupture in the augmented breast is associated with a gradual decrease in breast size and/or new localized masses.

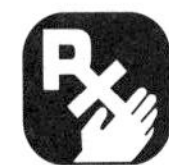

Long-Term Treatment

REHABILITATION

No specific rehabilitation required. In most cases, the athlete may return to activities to tolerance with adequate protection.

SURGICAL TREATMENT

- Although most hematomas resolve spontaneously, surgical aspiration may be indicated if the mass is growing, the mass appears infected, or calcifications are present.
- Masses thought to be cysts or hematomas may be aspirated under local anesthesia.

REFERRAL/DISPOSITION

Suspicious masses should be referred for biopsy and excision.

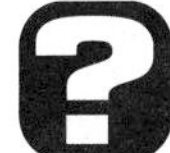

Common Questions and Answers

Physician responses to common patient questions:
Q: Do I have a higher risk of breast cancer because of this injury?
A: There is no evidence that trauma increases the risk of breast cancer.
Q: Is my breast pain a sign of cancer?
A: Although pain alone is a rare presentation of breast cancer, breast cancers may be identified by more diligent patient exam.

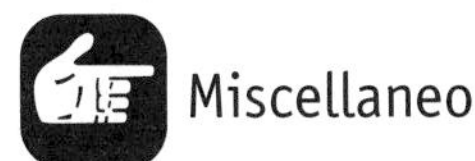

Miscellaneous

SYNONYMS

- Open wound of chest wall or breast
- Chest pain, musculoskeletal
- Mastalgia, mastodynia (breast pain)
- Breast hematoma
- Chest wall hematoma

ICD-9 CODE

875.0 Chest wall wound, open
875.1 Chest wall wound, open, complicated
786.59 Chest pain, musculoskeletal
786.52 Chest pain, wall
922.1 Chest wall contusion
879.0 Breast wound, open
879.1 Breast wound, open, complicated
611.71 Breast pain
307.89 Breast pain, psychogenic
922.0 Breast contusion

BIBLIOGRAPHY

BeLieu RM. Mastodynia. *Obstet Gynecol Clin North Am* 1994;21:461–477.

Dellon AL, Cowley RA, Hoopes JE. Blunt chest trauma. *J Trauma* 1980;20:982–985.

Greydanus DE, Patel DR, Baxter TL. The breast and sports: issues for the clinician. *Adolesc Med State Art Rev* 1998;9:533–550.

Steinbrunn BS, Zera RT, Rodriguez JL. Mastalgia: tailoring treatment to type of breast. *Postgrad Med* 1997;102:183–194.

Thune I, Lund E, Gaard M. Physical activity and the risk of breast cancer. *N Engl J Med* 1997;336:1269–1275.

Authors: Robert Baker

Chronic Lung Disease

Basics

DESCRIPTION

Chronic obstructive pulmonary disease encompasses several diffuse pulmonary diseases including chronic bronchitis, asthma, cystic fibrosis, bronchiectasis, and emphysema. The term usually refers to a mixture of chronic bronchitis and emphysema.

- Chronic bronchitis is defined clinically by increased mucus production and recurrent cough present on most days for at least three months during at least two consecutive years.
- Emphysema is the destruction of interalveolar septa. The disease occurs in the distal or terminal airways and involves both airways and lung parenchyma.

System(s) affected: Pulmonary
Genetics:

- Chronic bronchitis is not a genetic disorder although some studies have hinted at a predisposition for development of this condition.
- A rare form of emphysema, antiprotease deficiency (due to alpha 1-antitrypsin deficiency), is an inherited disorder that is an expression of two autosomal codominant alleles.

Incidence/Prevalence in USA:

- 10–20% of adults; more than 60,000 deaths/year
- 8 million people have chronic bronchitis; 2 million people have emphysema

Predominant age: Over 40 years
Predominant sex: Male > Female

SIGNS AND SYMPTOMS

- Chronic bronchitis
  - —Cough
  - —Sputum production
  - —Frequent infections
  - —Intermittent dyspnea
  - —Pedal edema
  - —Plethora
  - —Cyanosis
  - —Wheezing
  - —Weight gain
  - —Diminished breath sounds
- Emphysema
  - —Minimal cough
  - —Scant sputum
  - —Dyspnea
  - —Often significant weight loss
  - —Occasional infections
  - —Barrel chest
  - —Minimal wheezing
  - —Use of accessory muscles of respiration
  - —Pursed lip breathing
  - —Cyanosis is slight or absent
  - —Breath sounds very diminished

CAUSES

- Cigarette smoking
- Air pollution
- Antiprotease deficiency
- Occupational exposure (i.e., firefighters)
- Infection possibly (viral)

RISK FACTORS

- Passive smoking (especially adults whose parents smoked)
- Severe viral pneumonia early in life
- Aging
- Ethyl alcohol (EtOH) consumption
- Airway hyperactivity

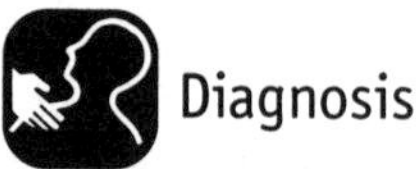

Diagnosis

DIFFERENTIAL DIAGNOSIS

Acute bronchitis, asthma, bronchiectasis, bronchogenic carcinoma, acute viral infection, normal aging of lungs, occupational asthma, chronic pulmonary embolism, sleep apnea, primary alveolar hypoventilation, chronic sinusitis

LABORATORY

- Chronic bronchitis
  - —Hypercapnia
  - —Polycythemia
  - —Hypoxia can be moderate to severe
- Emphysema
  - —Normal serum hemoglobin or polycythemia
  - —Normal $PaCO_2$; unless FEV1 < 1 L/sec, then can be elevated
  - —Mild hypoxia

Drugs that may alter lab results: Sedatives including alcohol
Disorders that may alter lab results: Obesity, concurrent restrictive lung dysfunction, primary pulmonary hypertension, acute infections, anemia, pulmonary embolism sleep apnea, congestive heart failure

PATHOLOGICAL FINDINGS

- Chronic bronchitis
  - —Bronchial mucous gland enlargement
  - —Increased number of secretory cells in surface epithelium
  - —Thickened small airways from edema and inflammation
  - —Smooth muscle hyperplasia
  - —Mucus plugging
  - —Bacterial colonization of airways
- Emphysema
  - —Entire lung affected
  - —Bronchi usually clear of secretions
  - —Anthracotic pigment
  - —Alveoli enlarged with loss of septa
  - —Cartilage atrophy
  - —Bullae

SPECIAL TESTS

- Pulmonary function testing
  - —Decreased FEV1 with concomitant reduction in FEV1/FVC ratio
  - —Poor or absent reversibility to bronchodilators
  - —FVC may be normal or reduced
  - —Normal or increased total lung capacity
  - —Increased residual volume
  - —Diffusing capacity is normal or reduced
- Nocturnal oximetry

IMAGING

- Chronic bronchitis chest x-ray shows increased bronchovascular markings and cardiomegaly
- Emphysema chest x-ray shows small heart, hyperinflation, flat diaphragms and possibly bullous changes
- CAT scan may show bullous changes

DIAGNOSTIC PROCEDURES

- Pulmonary function tests
- ABGs
- Chest x-ray

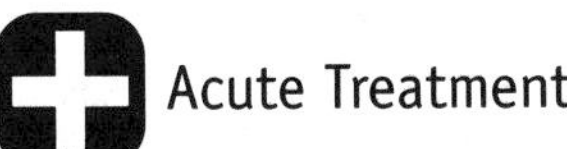

Acute Treatment

APPROPRIATE HEALTH CARE

- Outpatient treatment is usually adequate. However, hospitalization may be required for exacerbation, infection, or diagnostic procedures (i.e., transbronchial lung biopsy).
- Acute respiratory failure may require an intensive care unit and possibly a mechanical ventilator to support the patient

GENERAL MEASURES

- Smoking cessation
- Aggressive treatment of infections
- Treat any reversible bronchospasm
- Reduction of secretions through good pulmonary hygiene
- Cor pulmonale may necessitate use of home oxygen
- Pulmonary rehabilitation
- Appropriate vaccinations
- Adequate hydration

SURGICAL MEASURES

- Lung reduction surgery (selected cases)
- Lung transplantation (selected cases)

ACTIVITY

As tolerated. Full activity should be encouraged.

DIET

A well balanced, high protein diet is suggested. Low carbohydrates may benefit those with hypercarbia.

PATIENT EDUCATION

- Printed material is available from the National Jewish Hospital in Denver, Colorado. The local branch of the American Lung Association also has educational material.
- Coach patients in pulmonary rehabilitation

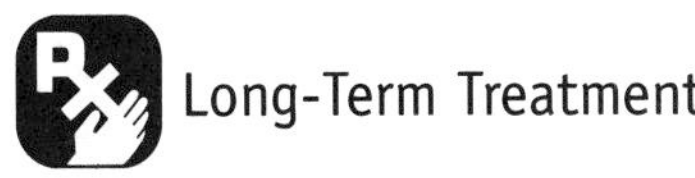

Long-Term Treatment

DRUG(S) OF CHOICE

- Theophylline (Theo-Dur, Slo-bid, Uni-Dur, Uniphyl) 400 mg/day. Increase by 100–200 mg in one to two weeks if necessary.
- Sympathomimetics—e.g., metaproterenol (Alupent), albuterol (Proventil, Ventolin), pirbuterol (Maxair), terbutaline (Brethaire). 1–2 puffs from the metered dose inhaler every 4–6 hrs. May be increased to every 3 hrs. Use of spacer device (AeroChamber, InspirEase) may be beneficial. (Up to 4 puffs recommended by some.) Long acting sympathomimetics—salmeterol (Serevent) to be considered.
- Anticholinergics—ipratropium (Atrovent). Two puffs (36 mg) 4 times daily. May take additional inhalations not to exceed 12 in 24 hrs.
- Corticosteroids—prednisone (Deltasone). Given orally 7.5–15 mg/day. Most useful in bronchitis with some reversibility.

Contraindications:

- Theophylline—hypersensitivity
- Sympathomimetics—cardiac arrhythmias associated with tachycardia; hypersensitivity
- Anticholinergics—hypersensitivity to atropine or its derivatives
- Corticosteroids—systemic fungal infections; hypersensitivity

Precautions:

- Theophylline—reduce dosage in patients with impaired renal or liver function; age over 55; CHF. Therapeutic drug level is 5–15 mg/mL (55.5–111 mmol).
- Rifampin—may cause a decrease in theophylline levels by increasing theophylline metabolism. Monitor serum theophylline level.
- Sympathomimetics—excessive use may be dangerous. May need to reduce dose in patients with cardiovascular disease, hypertension, hyperthyroidism, diabetes or convulsive disorders.
- Anticholinergics—narrow angle glaucoma, prostatic hypertrophy, bladder-neck obstruction
- Corticosteroids—may mask infection or predispose to infection, especially fungal; subcapsular cataracts; glaucoma; adrenocortical insufficiency, psychic derangements; gastrointestinal bleeding; diabetes mellitus, reactivation of tuberculosis

Significant possible interactions:

- Theophylline—lithium carbonate; propranolol; erythromycin; cimetidine; ranitidine; rifampin; ciprofloxacin
- Addition of cimetidine, ciprofloxacin, or erythromycin will decrease theophylline clearance causing theophylline levels to rise. Careful monitoring of serum theophylline levels is warranted. (Note: cimetidine is now an OTC drug.)
- Sympathomimetics—other sympathomimetics, monoamine oxidase inhibitors or tricyclic antidepressants
- Anticholinergics—refer to manufacturer's profile
- Corticosteroids—NSAIDs (indomethacin), aspirin, synthetic thyroid hormone

ALTERNATIVE DRUGS

- Theophylline may be given orally, intravenously or by rectal suppository
- Sympathomimetics may be given as aerosolized solution (albuterol, metaproterenol [Metaprel], levalbuterol, isoetharine) when mixed with saline; orally (Alupent, Proventil, Brethine, Ventolin) or subcutaneously (terbutaline)
- Anticholinergics—atropine sulfate, glycopyrrolate. Ipratropium (Atrovent) now available in aerosolized solution and may be mixed with albuterol.
- Corticosteroids may be given intravenously (hydrocortisone, methylprednisolone) or inhaled (beclomethasone, flunisolide, triamcinolone acetonide)
- Home oxygen

PATIENT MONITORING

- Severe or unstable patients should be seen monthly
- When stable, may be seen biannually
- Check theophylline level with each dose adjustment until the desired level (or result) is achieved, then check every 6–12 months
- With home oxygen, check arterial blood gasses yearly or with any change in condition. Monitor oxygen saturation (pulse oximetry) more frequently.
- Some patients only desaturate at night thereby only needing nocturnal oxygen.
- Avoid travel at high altitude. Air travel with oxygen requires pre-arrangement.
- Discuss advanced directive in severe cases.

PREVENTION/AVOIDANCE

Avoidance of smoking is the most important preventive measure. Passive smoke also has been shown to be harmful.

POSSIBLE COMPLICATIONS

- Infection is common
- Cor pulmonale, secondary polycythemia, bullous lung disease, acute or chronic respiratory failure, pulmonary hypertension, malnutrition, pneumothorax

EXPECTED COURSE/PROGNOSIS

- The patient's age and post-bronchodilator forced expiratory volume (FEV1) are the most important predictors of prognosis. Young age and FEV1 > 50% predicted have a good prognosis. Older patients with more severe lung disease do worse.
- Supplemental oxygen, when indicated, has been shown to increase survival
- Smoking cessation is also important for an improved prognosis
- Malnutrition, cor pulmonale, hypercapnia and pulse >100 indicate a poor prognosis

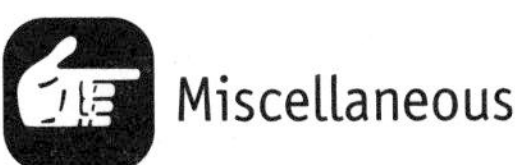

Miscellaneous

ASSOCIATED CONDITIONS

- Lung cancer
- Coronary artery disease
- Peptic ulcer disease
- Chronic sinusitis
- Malnutrition
- Laryngeal carcinoma

AGE-RELATED FACTORS

Pediatric: Repeated childhood respiratory illnesses make COPD a greater risk
Geriatric: Relative risk is 1.2 to 2.3 times greater than in younger person
Others: Unusual under age 25 unless antiprotease deficiency is present. Incidence increases as age approaches 60.

PREGNANCY

N/A

SYNONYMS

- Bronchitis
- COLD (Chronic obstructive lung disease)
- OAD (Obstructive airways disease)
- COPD

ICD-9 CODE

496 COPD
492.8 Emphysema

See also: Asthma; Bronchitis, acute

OTHER NOTES

- Albuterol is also known as salbutamol
- Other important considerations for treatment include adequate hydration, supplemental oxygen, antibiotics when indicated, mucolytic agents, pulmonary rehabilitation, good pulmonary hygiene

ABBREVIATIONS

FVC = forced vital capacity
FEV1 = forced expiratory volume at 1 second
COPD = chronic obstructive pulmonary disease
ABG = arterial blood gases

REFERENCES

Fishman A. *Pulmonary diseases and disorders*, 2nd Ed. New York, McGraw-Hill, 1988.

Chodosh S. Treatment of chronic bronchitis: state of the art. *Am J Med* 1991;91(6A):875.

Internet references: http://www.5mcc.com

Author: Alan J. Cropp

Claudication

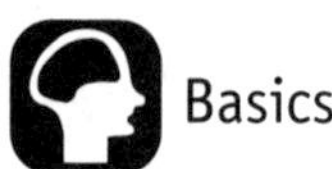

Basics

DESCRIPTION

The feeling of muscle fatigue after a period of minimal exercise of an extremity. The feeling may progress to a cramp-like pain, usually in the calf muscles. It is always relieved by resting the extremity. It can be reproduced by undergoing a similar exercise pattern. It may occur in the arms, but is more common in the legs, calf > thigh.

System(s) affected: Cardiovascular, Musculoskeletal
Genetics: N/A
Incidence/Prevalence in USA: Common
Predominant age: Common in males >55, females >60
Predominant sex: Male < Female (4:1)

SIGNS AND SYMPTOMS

- May start gradually or suddenly
- Unable to walk distances
- Pain varies from muscle tiredness to a frank cramp in muscle group involved
- May be a loss of hair on toes
- Foot may show rubor on dependency
- Pedal pulses absent
- Popliteal pulse absent
- With thigh claudication, femoral pulse absent
- Absent pulses in the distal extremity, secondary to more proximal arterial occlusion. The occlusion is usually from an arterial plaque.

CAUSES

- Lower extremity claudication—blockage of superficial femoral artery, secondary to arteriosclerosis in 95% of cases
- Other causes of arterial blocks—embolus, popliteal entrapment, adventitious cystic disease of popliteal artery, thromboangiitis obliterans
- Thigh and hip claudication—blockage of aortic and iliac vessels
- Upper extremity claudication—similar blocks of subclavian, axillary, and brachial artery

RISK FACTORS

- Smoking
- Diabetes
- Hypertension
- Hyperlipidemia
- Obesity
- Preexisting heart disease

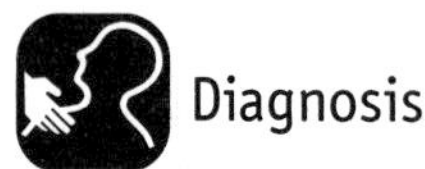

Diagnosis

DIFFERENTIAL DIAGNOSIS

- Pseudoclaudication, sometimes secondary to some form of spinal stenosis, usually impinging on the cauda equina portion of the spinal cord. The pain in the legs is characteristically relieved by squatting or sitting. The latter relieves tension on spinal nerve roots.
- Osteoarthritis of hips and knees sometimes can be confused with claudication, but pain starts immediately on weight bearing.

LABORATORY

N/A
Drugs that may alter lab results: None
Disorders that may alter lab results: Arterial calcinosis, often found in diabetics, will cause a falsely high ankle/arm index

PATHOLOGICAL FINDINGS

N/A

SPECIAL TESTS

- Noninvasive vascular tests—pulse volume recordings. Measurement of blood pressure in the arm compared to pedal arterial pressures before and after exercise establish the diagnosis as well as the severity of occlusion. The patient with one to two block claudication will have an ankle/arm index of 0.7–0.4 with 1.0 being normal. If below 0.4, there is a major threat of losing part of the leg if left untreated. Pseudoclaudication does not affect the pulses in the extremity.

IMAGING

- Duplex ultrasound
- Intra-arterial arteriography

DIAGNOSTIC PROCEDURES

- Arteriography—when surgical correction is anticipated
- Noninvasive vascular tests

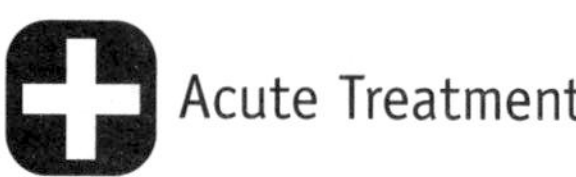

Acute Treatment

APPROPRIATE HEALTH CARE

Outpatient, except for severe cases or advanced disease

GENERAL MEASURES

- Conservative measures: stop smoking, initiate walking and exercise program, control of hyperlipidemia
- Reduce risk factors

SURGICAL MEASURES

- Surgical treatment with bypass of arterial obstruction may be appropriate in selected cases
- Angioplasty

ACTIVITY

Ambulatory

DIET

None

PATIENT EDUCATION

Prevention methods

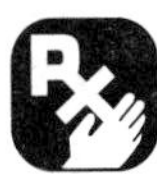

Long-Term Treatment

DRUG(S) OF CHOICE

- Aspirin—to reduce platelet aggregation: low dose 80 mg/day
- Pentoxifylline (Trental)—to decrease internal configuration of red cells—400 mg bid-tid.
- Administer for at least 6–8 weeks to determine if therapy is effective.
- Cilostazol (Pletal) 50–100 mg bid

Contraindications:

- Cilostazol is contraindicated in patient's with congestive heart failure
- Pantoxifylline is contraindicated in patient's with recent cerebral and/or retinal hemorrhage

Precautions:

- Headache occurs in up to 1/3 of patients taking cilostazol

Significant possible interactions:

- Cilostazol: Metabolized via the cytochrome P-450 isoenzymes. Use caution during coadministration of other inhibitors of CYP3A4 (e.g., grapefruit juice, ketoconazole, itraconazole, erythromycin and diltiazem), and during coadministration of inhibitors of CYP2C19 (e.g., omeprazole).
- Pentoxifylline: theophylline levels may rise

ALTERNATIVE DRUGS

- Ticlopidine
- Vasodilators
- Calcium channel blockers
- Anticoagulants

PATIENT MONITORING

Peripheral non-invasive vascular studies every 6 months

PREVENTION/AVOIDANCE

- Institute walking program of 4–5 miles
- Avoid smoking

POSSIBLE COMPLICATIONS

Only 10% of people without diabetes will progress to some amputation of the involved extremity

EXPECTED COURSE/PROGNOSIS

Gradual improvement in walking distance or progression of problem to gangrene, rest pain and/or tissue necrosis

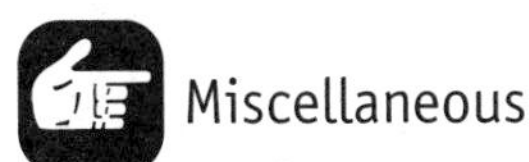

Miscellaneous

ASSOCIATED CONDITIONS

Other manifestations of arteriosclerotic vascular disease—history of myocardial infarction(s), carotid disease, renal vascular hypertension

AGE-RELATED FACTORS

Pediatric: N/A
Geriatric: More common with advancing age
Others: N/A

ICD-9 CODE

443.9 Peripheral vascular disease, unspecified (intermittent claudication)

See also: Thromboangiitis obliterans (Buerger's disease)

BIBLIOGRAPHY

Rutherford RB, ed: *Vascular surgery*. 4th Ed. Philadelphia, WB Saunders, 1995.

Internet references: http://www.5mcc.com

Author: Mark R. Dambro

Cluster Headache

Basics

SIGNS AND SYMPTOMS

- Unilateral, excruciating, nonthrobbing, incapacitating headache
- Pain is ocular or retro-ocular
- Rarely lasts longer than 2 hours
- Associated with nasal congestion, lacrimation, rhinorrhea, conjunctival injection, or facial flushing on the same side
- Horner's syndrome may be seen
- Headaches occur in clusters; several times per day for weeks or months at a time
- Occurs predominantly in middle-aged males
- Attacks are more likely after ingestion of alcohol, nitroglycerine, or histamine-containing compounds
- Episodes are often nocturnal, and are more common in spring and fall
- More likely in times of stress, prolonged strain, overwork, and upsetting emotional experiences
- No prodrome or aura

MECHANISM/DESCRIPTION

- Not clearly understood, but may be the result of vasoactive substances released from mast cells

ETIOLOGY

- Etiology is unclear at present
- Affects 0.1% of the population

CAUTIONS

- Recognize more severe life-threatening causes of headache
- Administration of oxygen by face mask may alleviate symptoms

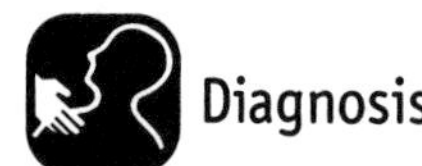

Diagnosis

ESSENTIAL WORKUP

- An accurate history and physical examination should confirm the diagnosis

LABORATORY

- Lumbar puncture (if meningitis or subarachnoid hemorrhage is suspected)
- ESR (if temporal arteritis is suspected)

IMAGING/SPECIAL TESTS

- CT scan/MRI (to rule out hemorrhage, tumor)

DIFFERENTIAL DIAGNOSIS

- Migraine headache
- Trigeminal neuralgia
- Meningitis
- Temporal arteritis
- Intracerebral mass lesion
- Herpes zoster
- Intracerebral bleed
- Hypertension
- Dental causes
- Orbital/ocular disease (acute glaucoma)
- Temporal mandibular joint syndrome

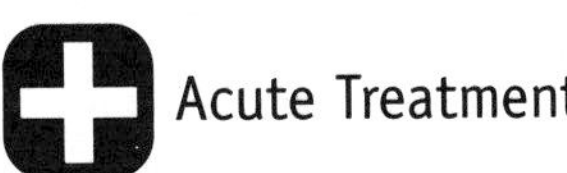

Acute Treatment

INITIAL STABILIZATION

- ABCs
- Rule out life-threatening causes of headache
- Administration of supplemental oxygen

ED TREATMENT

- Pain management

MEDICATIONS

- Ergots: DHE 1cc IM or IV; the repeat in 1 hour if necessary
- Fentanyl: 2–3 μg/kg IV
- NSAIDs: Ketorolac 15–30 mg IM or IV
- Meperidine: 50–75 mg IM or IV
- Morphine: 2–4 mg IV or IM, may repeat q 10 min
- Oxygen: 100% via face mask
- Prochlorperazine: 10 mg IM or IV
- Sumatriptan: 6 mg sq, may repeat in 1 hr (max of 2 doses in 24 hrs)

HOSPITAL ADMISSION CRITERIA

- Persistent headache unresponsive to usual measures
- Suicidal ideation associated with unremitting headache or severe depression

HOSPITAL DISCHARGE CRITERIA

- Patients with moderate to complete pain relief and with a confident diagnosis of cluster headache
- Follow-up with a neurologist should be arranged

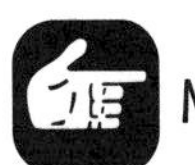

Miscellaneous

ICD-9 CODE

346.20

CORE CONTENT CODE

11.10

BIBLIOGRAPHY

Diamond S. The management of migraine and cluster headaches. *Compr Ther* 1995;21(9):492–498.

Kumar KL. Recent advances in the acute management of migraine and cluster headaches. *J Gen Intern Med* 1994;9(6): 339–348.

Mathews NT. Cluster headaches. *Neurology* 1992;42(3):22–31.

Authors: Gary D. Johnson and George Kondylis

Constipation

Basics

SIGNS AND SYMPTOMS

- Infrequent passage of dry, hard stools or straining at defecation
- Change of stool pattern
- Poorly localized abdominal pain, often spasmodic
- Abdominal distention/fullness
- Vomiting or decreased passage of flatus
- Firm hard stool on digital exam
  —May have empty rectum
- Tenesmus
- Encopresis in children
- Signs of peritonitis are not seen with constipation

MECHANISM/DESCRIPTION

- Perceived as a decrease in the frequency of bowel movements or as increased straining/pain with defecation
- 99% of normal population have a bowel frequency ranging from 3 bowel movements per day to 3 per week

ETIOLOGY

- Due to muscle disorders that affect the sphincter mechanism or may be secondary to delayed transit time in the colon
- Associated with
  —Immobility
  —Deficiency of dietary fiber
  —Dehydration
  —Depression
  —Degenerative neurologic diseases
- Decrease colonic motility due to medications (anticholinergics, opiates)
- Impaired colonic motor function (Hirschsprung's disease)
- Laxative abuse may damage the colonic myenteric plexus
- Pain produced by fissures or thrombosed hemorrhoids may cause avoidance of defecation
- Electrolyte abnormalities
  —Hypercalcemia
  —Hypokalemia
- Hormonal abnormalities
  —Hypothyroidism
  —Diabetes mellitus

PEDIATRIC CONSIDERATIONS

- Normal bowel habits different in children
  —First 2–3 months 1 bowel movement per feeding to 1 every other day is normal
  —2 months to 1 year: 2–3/day is normal
  —1–5 years: 1–2/day is normal
- In infancy consider
  —Effect of maternal drugs
  —Congenital gastrointestinal anomalies
  —Cystic fibrosis
  —Hirschsprung's disease
  —Poor intake
  —Anal fissures

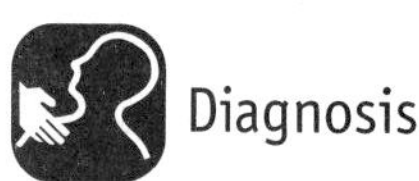

Diagnosis

ESSENTIAL WORKUP

- Thorough history and physical examination; note abdominal distention, presence of bowel sounds and masses
- Digital examination for
  —Rectal tone
  —Stool consistency
  —Masses
  —Occult blood

LABORATORY

- Only necessary when considering underlying disorders
- CBC may show
  —Leukocytosis with inflammatory processes
  —Anemia with colon neoplasm
- Electrolytes and calcium indicated if at risk for
  —Hypokalemia
  —Hypercalcemia
- Thyroid function tests indicated if patient appears to be hypothyroid

IMAGING/SPECIAL TESTS

- Rarely indicated unless suspect underlying process
- Abdominal radiograph—large amount of stool in the colon
- Barium enema examination for anatomical defects (tumor)

DIFFERENTIAL DIAGNOSIS

- Colonic disorders
  —Tumors
  —Intussusception
  —Inflammatory strictures
  —Diverticular disease
  —Irritable bowel syndrome
  —Bowel obstruction
- Metabolic/endocrine disorders
  —Hypothyroidism
  —Addison's disease
  —Cushing's syndrome
  —Diabetes mellitus
  —Hypercalcemia
- Anorectal disorders
  —Anal stenosis
  —Rectal prolapse
  —Anal fissure
  —Perianal abscess

- Drugs
  —Aluminum-containing antacids
  —Iron supplements
  —Opiates
  —Anticholinergics
  —Antiparkinson drugs
  —Antispasmodics

PEDIATRIC CONSIDERATIONS

- In differential diagnosis, consider breast feeding, effect of maternal drugs, meconium ileus/plug, GI anomalies, and sepsis
- Often occurs during period of toilet training

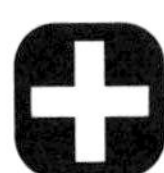

Acute Treatment

INITIAL STABILIZATION

N/A

ED TREATMENT

- Requires stepwise management
  —Initial clean out
  —Maintenance
  —Behavior modification
- Clean out can be "from above and below"
  —Enemas
  —Suppositories
  —Manual disimpaction
  —Laxatives
- Maintenance
  —Increase oral fluids and dietary fibers
  —Stool softeners
  —Bulk-forming agents
- Behavior modification
  —Dietary changes
  —Toilet training—place elderly and young on the toilet at regular intervals
- Change medications causing constipation

MEDICATIONS

Bulk Agents

- Bran/fiber
- Psyllium seeds (Metamucil): 30 g/day (peds: 0.5–1 tsp/day)

Enemas

- Fleet: 120 ml (peds: 60–120 ml) PR
- Tap water: 100–500 ml PR

Osmotic Agents

- Milk of magnesia: 15–30 ml (peds: 1 tsp–2 tbs) po
- Lactulose: 15–30 ml (peds: 1 tsp–2 tbs) po bid
- Polyethylene glycol (GoLYTELY): 2–6 L (peds: 150 ml/kg) po

Stool Softeners

- Docusate sodium (Colace): 60–360 mg/day (peds: 3–5 mg/kg/24 hrs tid) po
- Karo syrup (for infants): 1–2 tsp to each bottle
- Senna extract (Senokot): 1–2 tabs (peds: 0.5–1 tsp) po

HOSPITAL ADMISSION CRITERIA

- Severely constipated patients experiencing severe abdominal pain that cannot be relieved
- Neurologically impaired/elderly who cannot be cleaned out in the emergency department or at home
- Bowel obstruction or surgical emergencies

HOSPITAL DISCHARGE CRITERIA

- No comorbid illness requiring admission
- Pain-free
- Adequately cleaned out

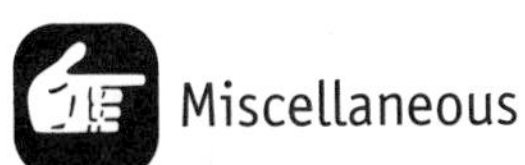

Miscellaneous

ICD-9 CODE

564.0

CORE CONTENT CODE

22.4.5

BIBLIOGRAPHY

Donatelle EP. Constipation: Pathophysiology and treatment. *Am Fam Physician* 1990; 1335–1342.

Orenstein JB. Constipation. In: Barkin R, et al., eds. *Pediatric emergency medicine: Concepts and clinical practice*. 2d ed. St. Louis: CV Mosby, 1997:804–807.

Read NW, Celik AF, Katsinelos P. Constipation and incontinence in the elderly. *J Clin Gastroenterol* 1995;20(1):61–70.

Author: Anthony Best

Contact Dermatitis

Basics

SIGNS AND SYMPTOMS

- *Acute lesions*: Skin erythema and pruritus. May see edema, papules, vesicles, bullae, serous discharge or crusting
- *Subacute*: Vesiculation less pronounced
- *Chronic lesions*: May see scaling, lichenification, pigmentation, or fissuring with little to no vesiculation. May have a characteristic distribution pattern

MECHANISM/DESCRIPTION

- An *eczematous eruption* (superficial inflammatory process primarily in the epidermis)
- Irritant
  - —Direct injury to the skin resulting in nonimmunologic inflammatory reaction
  - —Usually gradual onset with indistinct borders
- Allergic
  - —Delayed hypersensitivity reaction (requires prior sensitization)
  - —Usually rapid onset (12–48 hours), may correspond to exact distribution of contact (e.g., watchband)

ETIOLOGY

- Irritant
  - —Strong soaps, solvents, chemicals, certain foods, urine, feces, continuous exposure to moisture (diaper rash), etc.
- Allergic
  - —Common allergens include plants, cement (prolonged exposure may result in severe alkali burn), metals (especially nickel), solvents, epoxy, chemicals in rubber (e.g., elastic waistbands) or leather, lotions, cosmetics, topical medications (e.g., neomycin, benzocaine, parabens), some foods, etc.
  - —Poison ivy, oak, sumac (rhus dermatitis)
    - —Common form of allergic contact dermatitis
    - —Direct: Reaction to oleoresin from plant
    - —Indirect: Contact with pet or clothes with oleoresin on surface or fur, or in smoke from burning leaves
    - —Lesions may appear up to 3 days after exposure and may persist up to 3 weeks
    - —Fluid from vesicles is not contagious and does not produce new lesions
- Shoe dermatitis
  - —Common; identify by lesions limited to distal dorsal surface of foot usually sparing the interdigital spaces
- Photodermatitis
  - —Inflammatory reaction from exposure to an irritant (frequently plant sap) and sunlight

PEDIATRIC CONSIDERATIONS

- Allergic contact dermatitis is less frequent in children, especially infants, than adults
- Major sources of pediatric contact allergy
  - —Metals, shoes, preservatives or fragrances in cosmetics and topical medications, and plants
- Circumoral dermatitis: seen in infants and small children, may result from certain foods (irritant or allergic reaction)

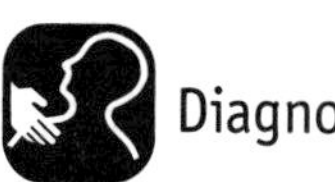

Diagnosis

ESSENTIAL WORKUP

- Medical history
  - —Include date of onset, time course, pattern of lesions, relationship to work, exposures (home and at work), new products (lotions, cosmetics, etc.), medications, and jewelry
- Physical examination
  - —Special attention to character and distribution of the rash

LABORATORY

- No specific tests in the ED are helpful

IMAGING/SPECIAL TESTS

- Patch testing
  - —Generally not done in the ED, refer to subspecialist
- When tinea is suspected consider evaluating for fluorescence with a Wood's lamp

DIFFERENTIAL DIAGNOSIS

- Atopic dermatitis: associated with family history of atopy
- Seborrheic dermatitis: scaly or crusting "greasy" lesions
- Nummular dermatitis: "coin-like" lesions
- Intertrigo: dermatitis where skin is in apposition
- Infectious eczematous dermatitis: dermatitis with secondary bacterial infection, usually *Staphylococcus aureus*
- Cellulitis: warm, blanching, painful lesion
- Impetigo: yellow crusting
- Scabies: intensely pruritic, frequently interdigital with "tracks."
- Psoriasis: silvery adherent, scaling, lesions well delineated, affecting extensor surfaces, scalp and genital region
- Herpes simplex: groups of vesicles, painful, burning
- Herpes zoster: painful, follows dermatomal pattern
- Bullous pemphigoid: diffuse bullous lesions
- Tinea: maximum involvement at margins, fluoresces under Wood's lamp
- Pityriasis alba: discrete, asymptomatic, hypopigmented lesions
- Urticaria: pruritic raised lesions (wheal) frequently with surrounding erythema (flare)
- Acrodermatitis enteropathica: vesiculobullous lesions of hands and feet, associated with failure to thrive, diarrhea, and alopecia
- Letterer-Siwe tumor (Langerhans cell histiocytosis)
  - —Associated with hepatosplenomegaly and adenopathy

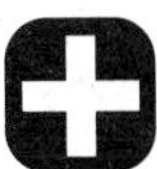

Acute Treatment

INITIAL STABILIZATION

- Rarely required in absence of concomitant pathology

ED TREATMENT

General

- Primarily symptomatic
- Wash area with mild soap and water
- Remove or avoid offending agent (including washing clothes)
- Cool, wet compresses, especially effective during acute blistering phase
- Antipruritic agents
  —Topical: calamine lotion, corticosteroids (does not penetrate blisters)
  —Systemic: Antihistamines, corticosteroids
- Aluminum acetate (Burrows) solution: weeping surfaces
- Avoid benzocaine-containing products—may further sensitize skin

Rhus Dermatitis

- Follow general measures plus
  —Aseptic aspiration of bullae may relieve discomfort
  —Severe reaction: systemic corticosteroids for 2–3 weeks with gradual taper.
- Premature termination of corticosteroid therapy may result in rapid rebound of symptoms

Shoe Dermatitis

- Follow general measures plus
  —Wear open toe, canvas, or vinyl shoes
  —Control perspiration—change socks, absorbent powder

MEDICATIONS

Systemic

- Antihistamine (H_1-receptor antagonist, 1st and 2nd generation)
- Diphenhydramine hydrochloride (Benadryl): Adult: 25–50 mg IV/IM/PO q 6 hr PRN; peds: 5 mg/kg/24 hrs divided q 6 hr PRN
- Hydroxyzine hydrochloride (Atarax): Adult: 25–50 mg po/IM up to qid PRN; peds: 2 mg/kg/24 hrs po divided qid or 0.5 mg/kg IM q 4–6 hr PRN
- Loratadine (Claritin): Adult: 10 mg po bid
- Corticosteroid
  —Prednisone: Adult: 40–60 mg po qd; peds: 1–2 mg/kg/24 hrs (max 80 mg/24 hrs) divided qd/bid

Topical

- Aluminum acetate (Burrows) solution: apply topically for 20 min tid until skin is dry
- Calamine lotion: qid PRN
- Corticosteroid
  —Hydrocortisone: cream 1%; ointment 0.5 or 1%; lotion 0.25, 0.5, or 1%; gel 0.5%; aerosol 0.5% tid qid
- Triamcinolone: ointment 0.025, 0.1%; cream 0.025, 0.1%; lotion 0.025, 0.1% tid qid

HOSPITAL ADMISSION CRITERIA

- Rarely indicated unless severe systemic reaction or significant secondary infection

HOSPITAL DISCHARGE CRITERIA

- Symptomatic relief
- Adequate follow-up with primary care physician or dermatologic specialist

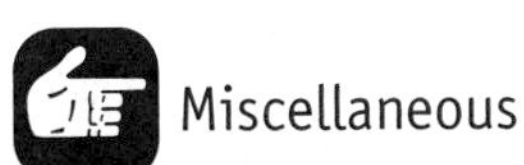

Miscellaneous

ICD-9 CODE

692.9

CORE CONTENT CODE

3.1.3

BIBLIOGRAPHY

Habif TP. *Clinical dermatology*. St Louis: CV Mosby, 1996:81–99.

Hurwitz S. *Clinical pediatric dermatology*. Philadelphia: WB Saunders, 1993:68–82.

Juckett G. Plant dermatitis. *Post Grad Med* 1996;100(3):159–171.

White IR. Occupational dermatitis. *BMJ* 1996;313:487–489.

Author: Jeffrey Horton

Corneal Abrasions

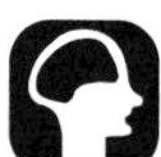

Basics

DEFINITION

- Removal or scraping away of the superficial layers of the cornea (stratified squamous epithelium). In the general population injury usually results from contact lens misuse, but can also be attributed to foreign bodies, tangential shearing injuries, and contusion to the globe. In sports the mechanism is more commonly direct trauma.

INCIDENCE/PREVALENCE

- More common in sports with projectiles/balls
- More common in collision sports than other contact sports

SIGNS AND SYMPTOMS

- Pain
- Redness
- Lacrimation
- Foreign body sensation
- Photophobia
- Blepharospasm

RISK FACTORS

- Collision/contact sports
- Contact lens use, especially soft lenses
- Failure to wear eye protection
- Sports with projectiles/balls

ASSOCIATED INJURIES AND COMPLICATIONS

- Hyphema (blood in the anterior chamber)
- Scleral rupture: look for vitreous leak
- Intraocular foreign body
- Perforation: look for vitreous leak
- Orbital fracture
- Iridodialysis: defect of the iris caused by its separation from the scleral spur
- Superinfection
- Recurrent erosion syndrome

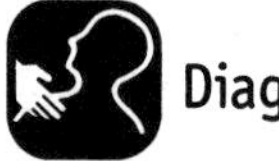

Diagnosis

DIFFERENTIAL DIAGNOSIS

- Foreign body
- Corneal laceration
- Perforation
- Viral keratitis (usually herpes)

HISTORY

- Mechanism of injury: guides physical exam for associated injuries and delineates the need for further studies
- History of previous injuries: possible viral keratitis or recurrent erosion syndrome
- Contact lens history

PHYSICAL EXAM

- General bony orbital exam
- Cranial nerve assessment
- Cardinal ocular movements
- Topical anesthetic and cycloplegic agents: may be needed to decrease pain and photophobia for optimal exam
- Visual acuity
- Loupe with good light or slit lamp (preferable)
- Fluorescein drops/strips: sharply demarcates defects in corneal epithelium and helps differentiate from herpes keratitis (dendritic pattern)
- Anterior chamber and corneal exam: slit lamp preferred to rule out associated injuries (hyphema, perforation)
- Eversion of upper and lower lids: identify any foreign bodies under tarsal plate
- Intraocular pressure: unless suspect perforation/scleral rupture

IMAGING

- Orbital series: only if history or physical exam suggests fracture
- Ultrasonography (B-scan)/CT/MRI: if occult intraocular foreign body is suspected

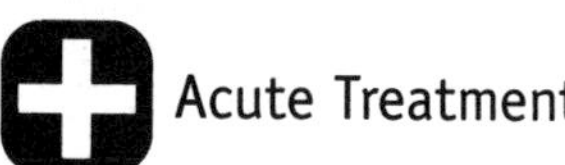

Acute Treatment

ANALGESIA

- Topical anesthesia: for exam only, see warnings
- Oral analgesia as needed

ANTIBIOTICS

- Broad-spectrum topical antibiotics: aid with lubrication and used for infection prophylaxis (sulfacetamide/quinolones)
- Contact lens associated: gram-negative coverage is essential (gentamicin/cefazolin)
- Water sport associated: pseudomonal coverage (gentamicin/quinolones)

SPECIAL CONSIDERATIONS

- Cycloplegic agent: for comfort, optional (initially given for first few days then discontinued)
- Pressure patch: patching is for patient comfort, and prevents retearing of healing epithelium. However, patching should not be used if the injury is contact lens induced because of the increased frequency of antibiotic dosing so frequent observation can be implemented.

WARNINGS

- No topical anesthetics: long-term use compromises epithelial healing

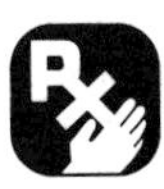

Long-Term Treatment

GENERAL

- Daily monitoring: until reepithelialization (48–72 hours) and no infection potential exists
- Topical antibiotics: continued for 1 week after reepithelialization
- Watch for recurrent erosion: sudden pain, redness, tearing, which may lead to recurrent erosion syndrome, requiring debridement and further specialized treatment.

REFERRAL/DISPOSITION

- Hyphema
- Intraocular foreign body
- Perforation
- Recurrent erosion syndrome

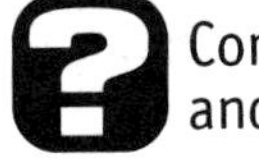

Common Questions and Answers

Physician responses to common patient questions:
Q: How long before I play?
A: It is based on your comfort. Once your pain is under control and you are not having any visual difficulties you may return to play.
Q: How long before I wear my contact lenses again?
A: The abrasion has to fully heal without complications (usually 3–5 days) before wearing your contact lenses again. Furthermore, if the abrasion is related to old, worn contact lenses, new lenses may be of great benefit.
Q: Should I wear protective eyewear?
A: There is no increased risk of another corneal abrasion after an initial injury, but anyone in a collision/contact sport or a sport with a projectile/ball should wear protective eyewear.
Q: What are the requirements for good protective eyewear?
A: The optimal protective eyewear is made of a sturdy frame that will not allow posterior dislocation of the lens of the eyewear. The lenses should have a 2- to 3-mm center thickness and be made of polycarbonate.

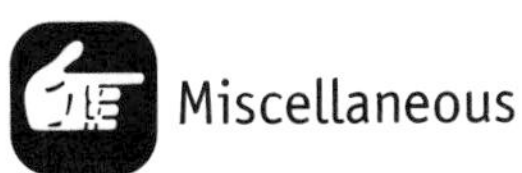

Miscellaneous

ICD-9 CODE

918.10 Corneal abrasion
918.11 Corneal abrasion with infection

BIBLIOGRAPHY

Vaughan D, Asbury T, Riordan-Eva P. *General ophthalmology*. Stamford, CT: Appleton & Lange, 1999.

Zagelbaum BM. Treating corneal abrasions and lacerations. *Physician Sports Med* 1997;25:38–44.

Authors: Nilesh Shah and James E. Sturmi

Dentoalveolar Trauma

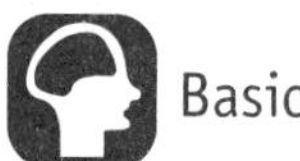

Basics

INCIDENCE/PREVALENCE

- 5% to 35% of the population; 75% under 15 years old
- 3:1 male:female; equal or higher rates sometimes reported for females than males when corrected for exposure rates

SIGNS AND SYMPTOMS

- Pain and tenderness to percussion or palpation
- Temperature sensitivity
- Color changes
- Tooth loosening

RISK FACTORS

- Protection: mouthguards are associated with a 7- to 10-fold reduction in risk.
- Sports: Baseball, basketball, cycling, hockey, soccer, skiing, rugby, and football, especially if proper protection is not used
- Anatomy: protruding maxillary incisors, lip incompetence, class II malocclusion
- Previous injury

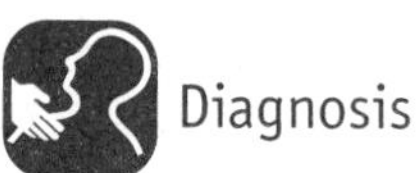

Diagnosis

DIFFERENTIAL DIAGNOSIS

- Associated trauma: ruled out by history, physical examination, and radiography
- Mandibular fractures and TMJ damage: check occlusion, limitation of jaw motion, mobility of multiple teeth or jaw fragments, maxillary/hard palate mobility, anesthesia/paresthesia of the cheek and lip, as well as radiography.
- Soft tissue injuries: include radiographs if not all tooth fragments are accounted for.

HISTORY

- Mechanism of injury and associated injuries
- Time since injury, time tooth was out of mouth, method of storage and transport
- Past dental history, past general medical and surgical history
- Medications and allergies
- Last tetanus shot

PHYSICAL EXAM

- Multiple types of injuries to each tooth must be suspected.
- Tenderness to percussion: nonspecific
- Bleeding from gingival sulcus: nonspecific
- Mobility: root and alveolar fractures; also with luxation injuries to a lesser degree; palpate tooth for nature and extent of fracture
- Alignment: may indicate luxation injury or fracture
- Electrical and thermal stimulation: lack of normal response is seen in pulpal injury (i.e., necrosis, root fracture, etc.).
- Modular movement of adjacent teeth: alveolar fractures

IMAGING

- Routine radiographs may not show root fractures; dental films (panoramic film with selected periapical views at multiple angles) are indicated with a low index of suspicion. Fractures may not be evident initially; negative films may be repeated 1 to 2 days after injury.

POSTREDUCTION VIEWS

Rule out root or alveolar fractures and confirm placement after reimplantation or splinting of an avulsed tooth.

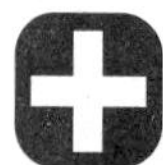

Acute Treatment

ANALGESIA

- Injection of 1 to 2 mL of lidocaine (0.5–1 mL for primary teeth) into the buccal gingival mucosa over the injured tooth's root apex, with epinephrine if not contraindicated; less effective with mandibular teeth
- Inferior alveolar nerve block may be required for pain relief of mandibular teeth, with 2 to 4 mL of lidocaine injected just superior to the lingula of the mandible
- Orthodontic wax may be applied to protect exposed dentin or pulp and sharp edges

SPECIAL CONSIDERATIONS

- Photographs and meticulous documentation are particularly important in cases of assault or motor vehicle accidents.
- Aspiration: if an avulsed tooth is not accounted for, a chest film may be indicated. Swallowed teeth rarely require treatment.
- Damage to primary teeth may result in damage to permanent teeth in 25% to 70% of injuries.

REFERRAL

- Patients should be advised to see their dentist as soon as possible.
- Urgent surgical referral may be necessary due to associated injuries.

TOOTH AVULSIONS

- Avulsed primary teeth should not be replaced due to risk of injury to permanent teeth.
- Replantation should be performed as soon as possible (good prognosis within 20 minutes but poor after 2 hours). Firmly (but not forcefully) reinsert into socket after local anesthesia and saline irrigation. Bite gently on gauze to seat tooth in socket.
- Handling: avoid touching root surface.
- Cleaning: may rinse in saline or tap water for up to 10 seconds, but not brushed off
- Storage: if reinsertion is not possible, tooth may be stored in milk for 3 to 6 hours or in saliva for up to 2 hours (pH, osmolarity, and bacteria make milk preferable). If low risk for aspiration and no other alternatives are available, store sublingually or in buccal vestibule to prevent drying. Water causes osmotic lysis of periodontal ligament cells. If available, Hanks' balanced salt solution is optimal
- 5 to 10 days of antibiotics (penicillin V or alternatives) reduce risks of root resorption

SPLINTING/IMMOBILIZATION

- Semirigid: acid-etch resin is used with wire along the labial surface to passively splint the injured tooth
- Duration of splinting varies with injury: semirigid splints should be applied for 7 to 10 days after avulsion and extrusion and for 2 to 3 weeks with lateral luxation. Rigid splinting is required for 4 to 6 weeks for alveolar fractures and 2 months after root fractures.

TOOTH FRACTURES

- Enamel only (Ellis class I): nonurgent referral to smooth rough edges, with cosmetic repair 4 to 8 weeks later if needed
- Enamel and dentin (Ellis class II): exposed dentin is sealed as soon as possible; delay may allow bacterial contamination of the pulp via dentinal tubules, especially in immature teeth. Acid-etch composite is used (possibly with tooth fragments) for definitive restoration (see Storage)
- Enamel, dentin, and pulp (Ellis class III): direct pulp capping may allow pulp vitality with small pulp exposures. Partial pulpotomy with calcium hydroxide treatment may be indicated in immature teeth to delay root canal treatment until after apex maturation (if pulp remains vital). Teeth with moderate pulp exposure and closed apices necessitate root canal treatment

- Crown-root fractures: fractures near the alveolar crest rarely heal without either root canal therapy and post/crown placement or extraction and prosthodontic treatment.
- Root fracture: coronal portion should be repositioned after local anesthesia with radiographic confirmation and rigid immobilization for 2 to 3 months (shorter for more apical fractures).

LUXATION

- Lateral luxation (subluxation of the dentoalveolar joint): local anesthesia, firm repositioning, and splinting with close follow-up
- Extrusion injuries: repositioning and splinting with anesthesia as needed
- Intrusion injuries: record the distance of intrusion, use local anesthesia, and luxate the tooth with gentle twisting if it is not already slightly mobile. Do not splint. Tooth may spontaneously reerupt over the next 2 to 3 months.

ALVEOLAR FRACTURES

- Immediate reduction with manual pressure after clinical diagnosis followed by radiographs and rigid splinting for 1 to 2 months reduces pulp necrosis.
- Empiric antibiotic therapy against oral flora is recommended to reduce contamination.

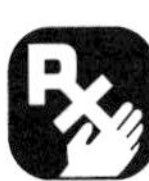

Long-Term Treatment

PREVENTION

- Mouth guards: reduce oral lacerations, and tooth fracture and displacement, and cushion impacts, which could result in condylar displacement and subsequent injury; reports of fewer jaw fractures, concussions, and neck injuries; dramatically reduced injury rates when mandated
- Behavior modification: highly variant among athletes and coaches due to difficulty speaking, breathing, drinking, and perception that they do not prevent injury
- Stock mouthguards: least expensive, often bulky; interfere with speech and breathing; held in place by biting
- Mouth-formed mouthguards: molded to mouth after placed in boiling water, then set in cold. May be reformed. Often too thin over biting surfaces
- Custom-fitted mouthguards: fit in two-stage process by dentist for maxillary (class I or II occlusion) or mandibular (class III occlusion) arches; increased comfort, compliance, and protection; last 1 to 2 years; may be impractical for children under 13 years of age due to rapid dental changes

TOOTH AVULSION

- Endodontic treatment is usually required at 1 to 2 weeks in teeth with a closed apex (after pulpal ischemic necrosis, before infection) to prevent periapical abscess formation and root resorption. Teeth with an open apex may reestablish blood supply; thermal sensitivity testing is performed every 3 to 4 weeks, with root canal treatment delayed until clinical or radiographic signs of disease. Calcium hydroxide treatment also may be considered to prevent inflammatory root resorption.
- Follow-up is essential at least every 6 months for several years; potential root resorption must be monitored and alveolar bone optimized for prosthetic implantation considerations.

TOOTH FRACTURES

- Crown fractures: definitive restoration should be performed as soon as possible, especially if the arch is crowded, because delay may allow encroachment of adjacent teeth and necessitate orthodontic treatment before restoration. Root canal treatment may be required in 1 to 2 weeks in cases of pulp exposure.
- Root fractures: monthly clinical and radiographic evaluation should be performed during splinting, then every 3 to 6 months for at least 2 years; 20% to 45% have pulpal necrosis and require pulpotomy, root canal treatment, or prosthesis. Hard tissue union is more likely with pulpal vitality, younger patients, closer fragment opposition, and increased root diameter.

TOOTH LUXATION

- Intrusion: radiographic monitoring for pulp necrosis or root resorption should occur every 3 weeks. Orthodontic extrusion is required if reeruption is not satisfactory after 3 months. Root canal treatment is required in 2 to 3 weeks for 95% of teeth with mature roots and 65% of teeth with immature roots due to pulp necrosis.
- Lateral luxation requires follow-up with radiographs every 3 months for 2 years to ensure that root resorption or loss of pulp vitality is not evident.

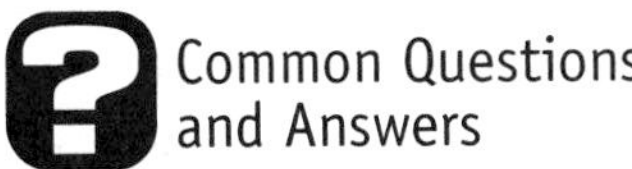

Common Questions and Answers

Physician responses to common patient questions:
Q: Will my tooth change color?
A: If the pulp becomes devitalized, the tooth will rapidly change color, along with associated symptoms. If root canal treatment is needed, a slight and gradual darkening may be noticed.

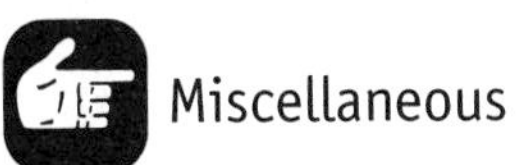

Miscellaneous

ICD-9 CODE

- Not commonly used

BIBLIOGRAPHY

Camp JH. Management of sports-related root fractures. *Dental Clin North Am* 2000;44:95–109.

Dewhurst SN, Mason C, Roberts GJ. Emergency treatment of orodental injuries: a review. *Br J Oral Maxillofac Surg* 1998;36:165–175.

Donly KJ. Management of sports-related crown fractures. *Dental Clin North Am* 2000;44:85–94.

Torg JS, Greenberg MS, Springer PS. *Diagnosis and management of oral injuries*. St. Louis: Mosby-Year Book, 1991.

Trope M. Clinical management of the avulsed tooth. *Dental Clin North Am* 1995;39: 93–112.

Authors: David Wallis, Donald H. Wallis, and Michelle Look

Diabetes Mellitus

Basics

DEFINITION

- Group of metabolic diseases characterized by hyperglycemia resulting from defects in insulin secretion, insulin action, or both

Type 1

- Autoimmune disease characterized by cellular antibodies against islet cells, insulin, and enzymes

Type 2

- Hepatic and peripheral insulin resistance with triad of
  —Impaired insulin secretion
  —Increased hepatic glucose production
  —Decreased muscle glucose uptake

INCIDENCE/PREVALENCE

- Most common endocrine disorder
- Increasing in incidence
- Estimated 16 million patients in the United States

Type 1

- 10%
- Diagnosis usually before age 30 years

Type 2

- 90%
- Diagnosis usually after age 40 years

SIGNS AND SYMPTOMS

Type 1

- Metabolically unstable with classic symptoms
  —3 P's: polyuria, polyphagia, polydipsia
  —Fatigue
  —Weight loss

Type 2

- Weight gain/loss
- Complications often present at time of diagnosis of
  —Serious infection
  —Pregnancy
  —Acute coronary syndrome
  —Sudden vision loss

RISK FACTORS

Type 1

- With/without family history
- Autoantibodies often present before clinical diagnosis
- Diagnosis or exacerbation of disease during adolescence or periods of stress

Type 2

- Genetic factors
  —Family history
  —Familial hyperlipidemia
- Environmental factors
  —Sedentary lifestyle
  —Inappropriate, calorie-laden diet
  —High association with insulin resistance and syndrome X

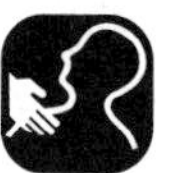

Diagnosis

- Fasting plasma glucose >125 mg/dL
- Casual plasma glucose >199 mg/dL together with classic symptoms of disease
- Two-hour oral glucose tolerance test glucose >199 mg/dL following 75-g glucose load
- Definitive diagnosis requires any two abnormal values preferably on 2 separate days.

DIFFERENTIAL DIAGNOSIS

- Nonketotic hyperosmolar coma
- Secondary causes (other pancreatic disease, drug-induced)

HISTORY

- Classic symptoms (3 P's)
- Unexplained weight loss and ketoacidosis (type 1)
- Family history
- Coexisting problem, e.g., serious infection, acute coronary syndrome

PHYSICAL EXAMINATION

- May be normal in mild or controlled cases
- Acute signs
  —Ketoacidosis
  —Weight loss
  —Volume depletion
  —Mental status changes
  —Hypotension
  —Abdominal pain
- Chronic signs
  —Obesity (type 2)
  —Diabetic retinopathy (microaneurysms, retinal hemorrhages)
  —Cardiac arrhythmia
  —Congestive heart failure
  —Chronic infections, fever
  —Neurologic sensation loss to monofilament testing
  —Foot ulcers/infections
  —Hypertension
  —Microalbuminuria
  —Renal failure
  —"Stiff man" syndrome, i.e., limited joint mobility

LABORATORY TESTS/UNDIAGNOSED/UNCONTROLLED CASES

- Elevated plasma glucose
- Elevated hemoglobin A_{Ic}
- Glycosuria, ketonuria
- Microalbuminuria/proteinuria (>30 μg albumin/mg creatinine in a.m. spot urine collection)
- Abnormal lipid profile
- Acidosis/decreased HCO_3^-
- Decreased K^+ and Mg^{2+}
- Elevated BUN and Na^+

MEDICAL RISKS OF EXERCISE

- Hypoglycemia
- Hyperglycemia/ketoacidosis in insulinopenic patients
- Asymptomatic coronary artery disease
- Peripheral vascular disease
- Exacerbation of retinopathy (weight-lifting, high-altitude sports)
- Foot injuries
- Autonomic dysfunction (abnormal sweating mechanisms, asymptomatic heart disease or hypoglycemia, lack of normal heart rate response to exercise)
- Specific activities (rock climbing, scuba diving)

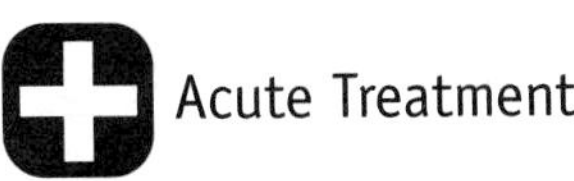

Acute Treatment

VENUE EVALUATION/TREATMENT

- Check for hypoglycemia, hyperglycemia, and dehydration
- Measure glucose; administer oral glucose, subcutaneous/intramuscular (i.m.) glucagon, intravenous (i.v.) glucose, and i.v. fluids as indicated

HOSPITAL EVALUATION/TREATMENT

- Dehydration: i.v. fluids (normal saline)
- Hypoglycemia
  —Immediate (occurs during or immediately after sporting event)
  —Treat with oral energy sources (fruit juices, sugar, Quick-surge, soft drinks)
  —Parenteral energy sources (i.m. or subcutaneous glucagon, i.v. glucose)
  —Delayed (occurs 6–28 hours after exercise)
  —Prevention/therapy: immediate repletion of glycogen in postexercise period Continued glucose monitoring during next 12–24 hours
- Hyperglycemia
  —Treat with i.v. fluids, insulin
  —Correct associated acidosis
  —Correct electrolyte abnormalities including potassium and magnesium

SPECIAL CONSIDERATIONS: DOZEN DIABETIC TIPS

- Have preexercise evaluation and exercise stress test, if indicated:
  —Age >35 years
  —Type 1 diabetes >15 years' duration
  —Type 2 diabetes >10 years' duration
  —Presence of any additional risk factor for coronary artery disease
  —Presence of microvascular disease
  —Presence of macrovascular disease
- *Always* exercise with a partner
- Wear identification (Med-Alert) and have strategy for treating hypoglycemia
- *Use,* do not simply possess, glucose-monitoring device with exercise
- Well-controlled type 1 athletes <10 years' duration usually have few complications
- Type 1 athletes >10 years' duration often have dysregulation
- Injection sites in type 1 athletes *may* affect absorption rate with exercise; certain medications in type 2 athletes may cause hypoglycemia.
- Meals should be ingested 3–4 hours before exercise.
- Avoid exercising during times of peak insulin activity (consider Humalog insulin)
- Check blood sugar before exercise.
  —Ideal range for type 1 athlete is 120–180 mg/dL.
  —If <100 mg/dL, snack before exercise (20 g of CHO)
  —If 100–250 mg/dL, exercise
  —If >250 mg/dL, delay exercise, check ketones, treat hyperglycemia and dehydration
  —Treat with glucose-containing fluids for each 30 minutes of strenuous exercise (ingest 30–75 g of CHO per hour of exercise)
  —Precompetition anxiety may mimic hypoglycemia: check glucose.
- Be aware of *delayed hypoglycemia.* Replenish glycogen stores after exercise based on duration/intensity of activity.
- Each diabetic athlete must be aware of personal pattern in blood glucose response to exercise.

Diabetes Mellitus

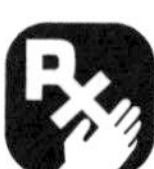

Long-Term Treatment

TREATMENT GOALS

- Control blood glucose
  - —Avoid blood glucose <60 mg/dL or >200 mg/dL
  - —Maintain hemoglobin A_{Ic} within 1% of the upper limits of normal for reference laboratory
- No severe hypoglycemia
- Treat associated problems
  - —Strive to normalize weight
  - —Avoid excessive alcohol use
  - —Cease smoking
- Treat associated diseases
  - —Hypertension
    - —Maintain blood pressure <130/85
    - —Select angiotensin-converting enzyme (ACE) inhibitors for treatment
    - —Avoid use of diuretics, beta blockers, verapamil, and calcium channel blockers in exercising persons
  - —Hyperlipidemia
    - —Maintain total cholesterol <200 mg/dL Strive for LDL cholesterol <100 mg/dL Strive for HDL cholesterol >45 mg/dl
- Monitor/prevent macrovascular complications
  - —Coronary artery disease
    - —Common but often asymptomatic
    - —Screen with exercise testing according to ADA/ACSM recommendations
    - —Use aspirin therapy in *primary prevention* for type 1 or type 2 patients with family history of coronary artery disease, cigarette smoking, hypertension, obesity, micro- or macroalbuminuria, hyperlipidemia, or age >30 years, or in *secondary prevention* for diabetics with macrovascular disease.
  - —Peripheral vascular disease
  - —Cerebrovascular disease
- Monitor/prevent microvascular complications
  - —Retinopathy
    - —Screen diabetic patients ≤29 years within 3–5 years of diagnosis and then yearly thereafter; diabetic patients ≥30 years at time of diagnosis and then yearly; pregnancy in preexisting diabetic patient before conception, during first trimester, and thereafter based on ophthalmologist's recommendation.
    - —Avoid activities in patients with moderate nonproliferative retinopathy (power-lifting, heavy Valsalva), severe nonproliferative retinopathy (boxing, heavy competitive sports), and proliferative retinopathy (weight-lifting, jogging, high-impact aerobics, racquet sports).
  - —Nephropathy
    - —Screen diabetic patients for microalbumin: type 1 at puberty, after 5 years' duration, then yearly thereafter; type 2 at diagnosis and yearly thereafter.
    - —Screening can be done as either a 24-hour urine collection, timed urine collection, or spot urine collection in a.m.
    - —Treat nephropathy with blood pressure control, good glycemic control, use of ACE inhibitors, and mild protein restriction.
  - —Neuropathy
- Treat special foot problems

Common Questions and Answers

Physician responses to common patient questions:

Q: Can diabetic athletes carbohydrate-load before competition?
A: Some diabetic athletes in good metabolic control can carbohydrate-load without ill effects.
Q: When is the ideal time to exercise?
A: Early a.m. or when in basal state (>3 hours since last meal).
Q: How should one adjust insulin regimens for exercise?
A: Short-acting insulin is decreased by 25% to 75%; intermediate-acting insulin is decreased by 50% before exercise. Further insulin adjustments are tailored to the individual athlete's response.
Q: How should one adjust agents for exercise in type 2 athletes?
A: As type 2 patients exercise, improve physical fitness, reduce body fat, and improve insulin resistance, the dosage of oral medications or insulin may be decreased.
Q: What is the best method to determine metabolic needs?
A: Careful testing during training to determine individual's metabolic response to exercise.
Q: Which diabetic agents cause hypoglycemia?
A: Insulin, sulfonylureas
Q: How is the insulin pump regulated during exercise?
A: Decrease basal infusion rate by 50% during exercise and for 1–2 hours afterward; reduce subsequent meal time bolus by 30% to 50%.
Q: What error is most common among diabetic athletes?
A: *Not* measuring glucose before, during, and after exercise.

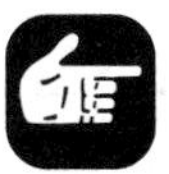

Miscellaneous

SYNONYMS

Type 1

- Juvenile-onset diabetes
- Insulin-dependent diabetes mellitus (IDDM)
- Childhood diabetes
- Ketosis-prone diabetes
- Autoimmune diabetes

Type 2

- Adult-onset diabetes
- Maturity-onset diabetes
- Noninsulin-dependent diabetes mellitus (NIDDM)
- Nonketosis-prone diabetes

ICD-9 CODE

250.0X Without complications
250.1X With ketoacidosis without coma
250.2X With hyperosmolarity
250.3X With other coma
250.4X With renal manifestations
250.5X With ophthalmic manifestations
250.6X With neurologic manifestations
250.7X With peripheral vascular disorders
250.8X With other specified manifestations (hypoglycemia)
250.9X With unspecified complications
Add fifth digit (X) to specify disease type: 0 = type 2 controlled; 1 = type 1 controlled; 2 = type 2 uncontrolled; 3 = type 1 uncontrolled

BIBLIOGRAPHY

Sherman WM, Ferrara C, Schneider B. Nutritional strategies to optimize athletic performance. In: Ruderman N, Devlin JT, eds. *The health professional's guide to diabetes and exercise.* Alexandria, VA: American Diabetes Association, Inc., 1995:9.

American College of Sports Medicine and American Diabetes Association. Joint position statement: diabetes mellitus and exercise. *Med Sci Sports Exerc* 1997;29:i–vi.

American Diabetes Association. Diabetes mellitus and exercise. *Diabetes Care* 2000;23[Suppl 1]:S50–S54.

Author: Russell D. White

Epistaxis

Basics

DEFINITION

- Bleeding from injured nasal mucosa overlying a blood vessel
- Typically from direct (blow, self) or indirect (sneeze) trauma; self-limited
- May be related to underlying pathologic condition

INCIDENCE/PREVALENCE

- Anterior bleed (Kiesselbach plexus at anterior inferior septum) accounts for 90%
- 10% incidence in general population
- Incidence increases with sports; in the young and elderly

SIGNS AND SYMPTOMS

- Bleeding may be brisk and profuse.
- Bleeding from nostrils suggests anterior bleed.
- Blood in pharynx (spitting and/or swallowing) suggests posterior bleed.
- Anxiety
- Nasal or facial deformity with fracture
- Orthostasis (may have significant blood loss)
- Exsanguination rare

RISK FACTORS

- Digital trauma most common cause
- Cold dry air: mucosal drying and nasal ciliary action decrease
- Substance abuse: alcohol, cocaine, inhalants
- Medication: abuse of nasal inhalers, nonsteroidal anti-inflammatory drugs, anticoagulants
- Infection: rhinitis, sinusitis
- Allergic rhinitis: creates two-fold risk epistaxis
- Coagulopathy: von Willebrand, hemophilia, liver disease
- Platelet abnormalities: thrombocytopenia
- Family history: Osler-Weber-Rendu (hereditary telangiectasias)
- Tumor: polyps, angiofibroma
- Anatomic abnormalities: deviated septum creates two-fold risk bleed; aneurysm
- Chemical irritants: cigarette smoke, ammonia
- Iatrogenic: instrumentation

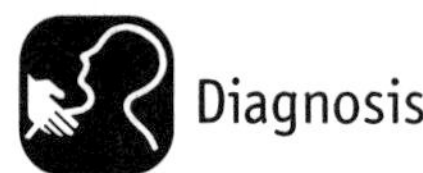

Diagnosis

DIFFERENTIAL DIAGNOSIS

- Fracture: nasal alae, ethmoid, Le Fort
- Foreign body
- Bleeding disorder: coagulopathy, platelet abnormality, angiofibroma, hereditary
- Upper gastrointestinal bleed
- Anatomic abnormality: septal perforation
- Tumor

HISTORY

- Ascertain nature of trauma: determine any associated or underlying injury, such as closed head injury or fracture
- Identify bleeding site: unilateral or bilateral, anterior or posterior; will guide treatment decisions
- Estimate extent of bleeding: hypovolemia suggests urgency of care/supportive care.
- Prior bleeding: number, frequency, duration, severity, treatments
- Identify any risk factors, including medication, substances, infection, allergy
- Family history of bleeding (hereditary coagulopathy, Osler-Weber-Rendu)

PHYSICAL EXAMINATION

- General: demeanor (anxious?), vitals (orthostatic)
- Inspect skin for signs of significant blood loss (pallor, turgor), signs of trauma, coagulopathy (bruising, petechiae), evidence of nasal/facial deformity or trauma
- Gently palpate nasal/facial structures
- Carefully examine nasal and oral cavities: identify bleeding source; requires good lighting and removal of clot

IMAGING

- Radiographs usually not helpful unless suspect nasal/facial fracture
- Waters view best single view
- Computed tomographic scan best for facial fractures and anatomic abnormalities
- Endoscopic evaluation may be necessary to identify bleeding site

LABORATORY

- For severe or recurrent bleeds
- Complete blood count, platelets, prothrombin and partial thromboplastin times, bleeding time

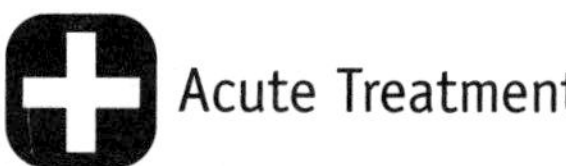

Acute Treatment

ANTERIOR BLEED

- Have athlete lean forward
- Apply pressure by pinching nasal alae and anterior septum for 5 minutes
- Apply pressure over upper lip for 5 minutes
- Apply ice to nasal bridge and back of neck
- Decongest using spray or pledget soaked with pseudoephedrine, phenylephrine, oxymetazoline, or epinephrine (1:10,000). Up to 65% success rate with this technique alone.

- Consider cautery (see Follow-Up/Recurrent Bleed)
- Pack if continued bleeding
  —Caution: can create complications, including pain, trauma, vagal response, infection, aspiration, and hypoxia
  —Consider anesthetizing with topical lidocaine or tetracaine
  —Materials: nasal tampons best, conformable sponge, petroleum jelly gauze in 0.5- or 1-inch strips with or without antibiotic, hemostatic agent (thrombin, cellulose, collagen) if available
  —Technique: use bayonet or small alligator forceps; good lighting; grasp packing 5 inches from end, insert so that loops are posterior; begin posterior—inferior; layer/fold in anterior superior direction
  —Tips: leave in no more than 72 hours; most would begin oral antibiotics (penicillin or first-generation cephalosporin) and analgesics (avoid NSAIDs and aspirin)
- Bleed continues: consider posterior pack or balloon; admission; and ear, nose, and throat (ENT) consult

FOLLOW-UP/RECURRENT BLEED

- Search for and address underlying causes and risk factors
- Cautery
  —Anesthetize with topical lidocaine or tetracaine
  —Remove clots
  —Decongest
  —Silver nitrate sticks work well. Be precise, work peripheral to central on bleeding area, hold 3–5 seconds, and remove any residual silver nitrate.
  —Do not use bilateral cauterization, which may disrupt blood supply.
  —Avoid excessive cautery due to risk of perforation
  —May use electrocautery but has increased risk of perforation
- Preventive measures
  —Facial protection
  —Limit/eliminate risk factors
  —Limit self-trauma
  —Humidification
  —Petroleum jelly to septum

POSTERIOR BLEED

- Follow initial management steps for anterior bleed
- Apply posterior packing: difficult due to anatomy, is painful, may require significant anesthesia, and may be ineffective
- Stabilize, transport, and refer for ENT consult/surgery

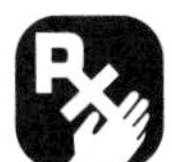

Long-Term Treatment

RECURRENT, NOT RESPONDING TO TREATMENT

- Endoscopic cauterization requires deep local or general anesthesia
- Angiographic embolization of external carotid branches (95% success, 6% neurologic sequelae)
- Surgery: remove anterior wall of maxillary sinus, ligate artery (Caldwell-Luc), and correct anatomic deformity

Common Questions and Answers

Physician responses to common patient questions:

Q: When can I play after an acute (anterior) bleed?
A: Assuming no significant facial trauma or underlying condition, may return to play upon cessation of bleeding.
Q: How about return to play after cautery?
A: It is possible to return to activity immediately, but most recommend 2–3 days.

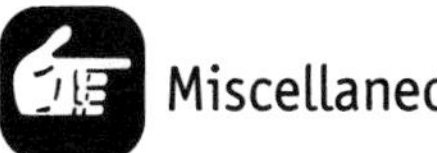

Miscellaneous

SYNONYMS

- Nosebleed

ICD-9 CODE

784.7

BIBLIOGRAPHY

Alvi A, Joyner-Triplett N. Acute epistaxis. *Postgrad Med* 1996;99;5:83–96.

Davidson TM, Davidson D. Immediate management of epistaxis. *Physician Sportsmed* 1996;24:74–83.

Josephson GD, Godley FA, Stiema P. Practical management of epistaxis. *Med Clin North Am* 1991;75:1311–1320.

Randall DA, Freeman S. Management of anterior and posterior epistaxis. *Am Fam Physician* 1991;43:2007–2014.

Rothenhaus T, James T. Epistaxis. *Emedicine.com*

Tan LK, Calhoun KH. Epistaxis. *Med Clin North Am* 1999;83:43–56.

Wurman LH, Sack JG, Flannery JV, et al. The management of epistaxis. *Am J Otolaryngol* 1992;13:193–209.

Author: William W. Dexter

Exercise-Induced Anaphylaxis

Basics

DEFINITION

- Distinct form of physical allergy characterized by a spectrum of exercise-induced symptoms, ranging from mild skin symptoms such as pruritus and urticaria to hypotension, syncope, and death

INCIDENCE/PREVALENCE

- Approximately 1,000 cases reported
- Only one death attributed to exercise-induced anaphylaxis (EIA) in the literature

SIGNS AND SYMPTOMS

- Generalized itching
- Gastrointestinal colic
- Headache
- Choking sensation
- Urticaria or angioedema with hypotension or respiratory obstruction is hallmark of classic EIA
- Patient may present in full anaphylactic shock.

RISK FACTORS

- Previous episodes
- Atopic individuals may be at slightly increased risk.

ASSOCIATED FACTORS

- Ingestion of certain foods or medications (particularly aspirin or nonsteroidal anti-inflammatories) before exercise may be a predisposing factor.
- Family variant may exist.

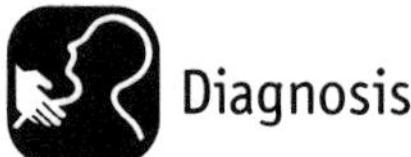

Diagnosis

DIFFERENTIAL DIAGNOSIS

- Cholinergic urticaria
- Exercise-induced asthma
- Environmental allergy

HISTORY

Q: What symptoms occur and when?
A: Transient exercise-induced itching, cutaneous erythema, with or without urticaria is suggestive of EIA. Progression of these symptoms to dyspnea, dizziness, gastrointestinal colic, or syncope is further suggestive of EIA.
Q: Does urticaria occur with warm shower or with anxiety?
A: Urticaria that occurs in these situations is consistent with cholinergic urticaria.
Q: In what environment does the patient exercise?
A: Identification of any provacative allergen aids in treatment. Patients may suffer from a different form of physical allergy, such as cold, solar, or aquagenic urticaria.
Q: Do symptoms occur during all episodes of physical activity?
A: Generally EIA does not occur with each bout of exercise, but may occur at any level of physical activity.

PHYSICAL EXAMINATION

- In acute setting, assess airway, breathing, and circulation (ABCs).
- Hypotension or respiratory difficulty may signify impending anaphylactic shock.
- Perform dermatologic examination
- Identifying urticarial size and presence of angioedema aids in diagnosis

DIAGNOSTIC TESTING

- Diagnosis generally is made by history.
- Abnormal laboratory tests include elevated serum histamine and serum tryptase levels. Serum tryptase levels should be drawn within 2 to 3 hours of the event.
- Passive warming test (warm shower or sauna) can be helpful in differentiating cholinergic urticaria and EIA.
- Exercise challenge test using a treadmill or stationary bike can be performed. Positive test (reproduction of symptoms and urticaria) is helpful in diagnosis, but negative test does not exclude a diagnosis of EIA, as reproducibility of symptoms is variable. Emergency equipment should be immediately available if exercise test is performed.

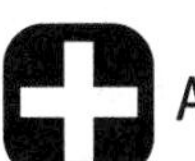

Acute Treatment

GENERAL CONSIDERATIONS

- Cessation of physical activity
- Subcutaneous administration of 0.3–0.5 mL epinephrine 1:1,000 if systemic symptoms of anaphylaxis are present
- Treat symptoms of anaphylactic shock as necessary in appropriate medical setting (fluid support for hypotension, assisted ventilation for respiratory obstruction)

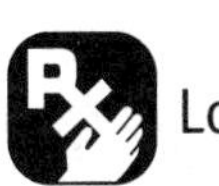

Long-Term Treatment

GENERAL CONSIDERATIONS

- Avoid exercise for 4–6 hours after eating
- Avoid anti-inflammatory drugs before exercise
- Always exercise with a partner and carry injectable epinephrine
- Possible role for desensitization to physical activity

MEDICATIONS

- Nonsedating antihistamines on a daily basis have been shown to be at least partially effective in prevention of symptoms (cetirizine 5–10 mg p.o. qday, loratidine 10 mg p.o. qday)
- Cromolyn sodium metered dox inhaler 2–4 puffs q.i.d.
- Possible role for use of leukotriene inhibitors (montelukast 10 mg p.o. q.p.m., zafirlukast 20 mg p.o. b.i.d.)

REFERRAL/DISPOSITION

- Referral to allergist for identification of possible associated triggers may be beneficial
- Follow-up to assess recurrence of symptoms and success of drug therapy

Common Questions and Answers

Physician responses to common patient questions:

Q: Can a patient with EIA continue to exercise?

A: Qualified "yes." Because symptoms may vary significantly from episode to episode and among patients, some patients may not feel comfortable returning to activity knowing that they could have repeat attacks. In addition, patients who have experienced anaphylactic response to exercise should be cautioned about returning to activity. For those whose symptoms are controlled with medication, it is recommended they continue to carry injectable epinephrine and exercise with a partner.

Q: Are there specific activities or foods that should be avoided?

A: EIA can occur with any level of activity and may be precipitated by the ingestion of many foods. Unless a specific trigger is identified, there are no restrictions placed on diet or type of activity. A general rule of thumb is to avoid eating for 4–6 hours before exercise.

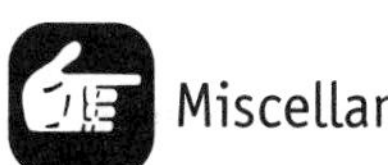

Miscellaneous

ICD-9 CODE

999.4 Anaphylactic shock
999.5

See also: Physical allergy

BIBLIOGRAPHY

Sheffer AL, Soter NA, McFadden ER, et al. Exercise induced anaphylaxis: a distinct form of physical allergy. *J Allergy Clin Immunol* 1983;71:311–316.

Briner WW. Physical allergies and exercise: clinical implications for those engaged in sports activities. *Sports Med* 1993;15: 365–373.

Nichols AW. Exercise induced anaphylaxis and urticaria. *Clin Sports Med* 1992;11:303–312.

Authors: Robert G. Hosey and Thomas D. Armsey

Exercise-Induced Asthma

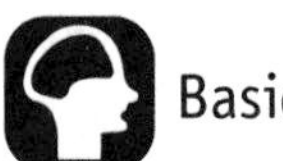

Basics

DEFINITION

- Airway bronchoconstriction characterized by wheezing, coughing, and/or chest tightness occurring during or after exercise

INCIDENCE/PREVALENCE

- 10% to 50% of recreational and elite athletes
- 70% to 80% of asthmatics
- 40% of patients with allergic rhinitis

SIGNS AND SYMPTOMS

- Coughing
- Wheezing
- Shortness of breath
- Chest tightness
- Stomachache
- Headache
- Fatigue
- Muscle cramps
- Feeling out of shape
- Chest pain and discomfort

RISK FACTORS

- High asthmogenic sports, such as long-distance running, cycling, soccer, basketball, rugby, ice hockey, ice skating, cross-country snow skiing
- Environmental factors, such as tobacco smoke, sulfur dioxide, nitrogen oxide, pollens and molds, cold weather, low humidity, duration of exercise, high-intensity exercise

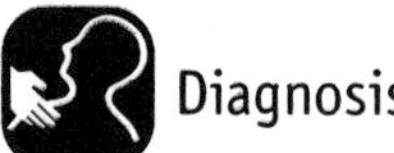

Diagnosis

DIFFERENTIAL DIAGNOSIS

- Asthma with exercise exacerbation
- Vocal cord dysfunction
- Gastroesophageal reflux
- Cardiac conditions (cardiomyopathy, congestive heart failure, arrhythmia) could mimic the exercise incapacibility of EIA
- General state of deconditioning

HISTORY

- Personal or family history of allergies or asthma
- Positive response to above signs and symptoms
- Symptoms occur during or after exercise, typically appearing after 6–8 minutes of exercise

PHYSICAL EXAMINATION

- Look for sinusitis or other underlying infection
- Lung examination typically normal; if wheezing, consider chronic asthma
- On the field or after exercise challenge, physical examination is more likely to be positive.

DIAGNOSTIC TESTS

- Pulmonary function tests before and after exercise
- Spirometry more accurate than peak expiratory flow rate
- FEV_1 at rest should be normal in patients with EIA, above normal in athletes, and below normal in those with chronic asthma.
- 10% to 15% reduction in FEV_1 or 15% to 20% reduction in peak expiratory flow rate from before to after exercise is diagnostic of EIA.
- Best to test athletes during sport-specific exercise.
- Exercise at a workload of 80% of predicted VO_2 max for 6–8 minutes during testing

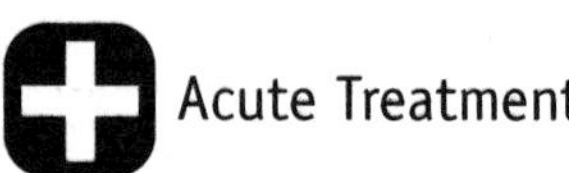

Acute Treatment

SPECIAL CONSIDERATIONS

For elite athletes, check the United States Olympic Committee or National Collegiate Athletic Association list of banned substances to be sure the medications used are in compliance with their rules.

MANAGEMENT STRATEGIES

Preexercise Medications

- Short-acting β agonist: 2–4 puffs 15–30 minutes before exercise; may repeat during exercise as needed
- Cromolyn: 4–10 puffs 10–20 minutes before exercise
- Nedocromil: 2–4 puffs 10–20 minutes before exercise
- For aerobic activities lasting >3–4 hours or for all-day tournaments, salmeterol 2 puffs 30–60 minutes to hours before exercise
- If needed, short-acting β agonists can be added to salmeterol.

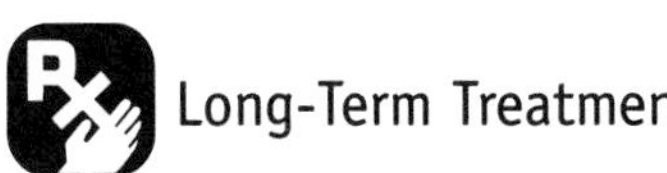

Long-Term Treatment

REFERRAL/DISPOSITION

- Consider another diagnosis if symptoms do not respond to more than one drug.
- Have patient return if use of short-acting β agonist increases

MANAGEMENT STRATEGIES

Daily Medication

- Cromolyn: 2 puffs q.i.d. or 4 puffs b.i.d.
- Nedocromil: 2 puffs q.i.d.
- Salmeterol: 2 puffs b.i.d.
- Inhaled corticosteroids: 2–16 puffs b.i.d. or t.i.d. depending on drug
- Ipratropium: use as additive treatment 2 puffs 30–60 minutes before exercise
- Oral theophylline: rarely used
- Leukotriene modifiers: Controlled studies show long-lasting benefits, but currently not approved by the United States Food and Drug Administration.
- Refractory period: Teach how to induce a refractory period by having athlete exercise to the point of inducing bronchospasm during warmup. This can result in less severe or no bronchospasm during full exercise and the effect can last 30–90 minutes.
- Educate on proper use of inhalers and spacers
- Maximize therapy of underlying asthma

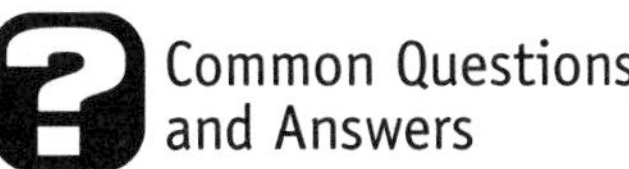

Common Questions and Answers

Physician responses to common patient questions:
Q: Do I have asthma?
A: Athletes with EIB only have symptoms around exercise and do not have chronic asthma; however, many people with baseline asthma have exercise-related symptoms.
Q: Can I play sports with EIB?
A: Yes, this is a highly manageable disorder that rarely limits participation in any sport.
Q: How should I use my inhaler around exercise?
A: Use short-acting β agonist, perform a 15-minute warmup, take a 15-minute rest period, then perform main form of exercise. If symptoms do not improve, see your doctor to reevaluate.

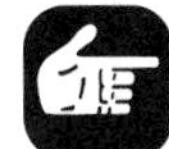

Miscellaneous

SYNONYMS

- Exercise-induced bronchospasm

BIBLIOGRAPHY

Beck K. Control of airway function during and after exercise. *Med Sci Sports Exerc* 31[Suppl]:S4–S11.

De Benedictis F, et al. Combination drug therapy for the prevention of exercise-induced asthma. *Ann Allergy Asthma Immunol* 1998;80:352–326.

Garcia de la Rubia S. Exercise induced asthma in children: a comparative study of the free and treadmill running. *Ann Allergy Asthma Immunol* 1998;80:232–236.

Guill M. Exercise induced bronchospasm in children: effects and therapies. *Pediatr Ann* 1996;25:146–153.

Kumar A, Busse W. Recognizing and controlling exercise induced asthma. *J Respir Dis* 16:1087–1096.

Mannix E, et al. Exercise induced asthma in figure skaters. *Chest* 1996;109:12–15.

Nelson J, et al. Effect of long term salmeterol treatment on exercise induced asthma. *N Engl J Med* 1998;339:141–146.

Pearlman D, et al. The leukotriene D4-receptor antagonist zafirlukast. *J Pediatr* 1999;134:273–279.

Rupp N. Diagnosis and management of exercise induced asthma. *Phys Sports Med* 24:77–87.

Schaanning J, et al. Efficacy and duration of salmeterol powder inhalation. *Ann Allergy Asthma Immunol* 1996;76:57–60.

Storms W. Exercise induced asthma: diagnosis and treatment for the recreational athlete. *Med Sci Sports Exerc* 1999;31[Suppl]: S33–S38.

Wright R, et al. Exercise induced asthma. Is gastroesophageal reflux a factor? *Dig Dis Sci* 1996;41:921–925.

Author: Lisa Barkley

Exercise-Induced Diarrhea

Basics

DEFINITION

- Increased stool frequency or volume often accompanied by lower abdominal cramping, urge to defecate, or rectal bleeding associated with strenuous physical activity

INCIDENCE/PREVALENCE

- Primarily associated with running sports
- Prevalence of diarrhea reported from 8% to 60%.
- Prevalence in control subjects reported up to 40%.

SIGNS AND SYMPTOMS

- Increased stool frequency
- Increased stool volume
- Loose or explosive stools
- Urge to defecate, often necessitating the athlete to cease exercise.
- Abdominal cramping
- Rectal bleeding

RISK FACTORS

- Underlying bowel pathology may worsen with strenuous exercise
- Worse with dehydration
- Occurs more frequently with increased exercise intensity
- Occurs more frequently in untrained participants
- Type of exercise (running > cycling, swimming, speed skating, cross-country skiing)
- Meals rich in fat, protein, and fiber taken shortly before exercise worsen symptoms.

DIFFICULTY WITH EXISTING RESEARCH

- Difficult to control all variables (diet, exercise intensity, underlying pathology such as irritable bowel syndrome)
- Studies often lack a denominator, making a true incidence of symptoms difficult to determine.
- Many studies are surveys with low response rates, which introduces a selection bias.
- Subject's dietary recall often is inaccurate.

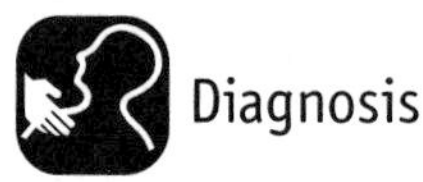

Diagnosis

DIFFERENTIAL DIAGNOSIS

- Irritable bowel disease
- Inflammatory bowel disease
- Infection
- Colon cancer
- Superior mesenteric or portal venous thrombosis

HISTORY

- Increased stool frequency or volume, or loose stools after exercise
- Often accompanied by abdominal cramping and urge to defecate
- May occur just with competition and not with training
- Normal bowel function at other times

PHYSICAL EXAMINATION

- Unremarkable physical examination

LABORATORY/IMAGING

- Exercise-induced diarrhea is a diagnosis of exclusion.
- Stool cultures are negative.
- Additional studies, such as barium enema, sigmoidoscopy, or colonoscopy, should be ordered as indicated.

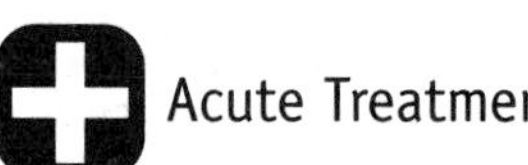

Acute Treatment

ACTIVITY MODIFICATION

- Acute symptoms usually rapidly resolve with cessation of activity.
- Hyoscyamine (Levsin) 0.125 mg sublingually sometimes is helpful in stopping abdominal cramping after exercise.

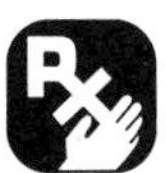

Long-Term Treatment

DIETARY CHANGES

- Stay well hydrated.
- Avoid caffeine, which is both a diuretic and a cathartic.
- Avoid foods that exacerbate symptoms (e.g., lactose in lactose-intolerant athlete).
- Eat small, low-fat, low-fiber meal several hours before competition; use low-osmolar sports drink between meal and competition or training.
- If athlete still has difficulty with diarrhea or urge to defecate, try complete nutritional liquid that is low in fiber during the day preceding competition.

MEDICATIONS

- Opiate/atropine combinations (diphenoxylate [Lomotil]) should be avoided.
- Opiates are habit forming, may be banned depending on governing body of the sport, and may adversely affect performance.
- Atropine may cause hyperthermia, tachycardia, and heat regulation problems.
- Antispasmodics dicyclomine (Bentyl) and hyoscyamine (Levsin) may be helpful, but have anticholinergic side effects and should be used with caution. The athlete should remain well hydrated; use in hot/humid conditions is not ideal.
- Loperamide (Imodium) decreases intestinal motility and affects water and electrolyte absorption. Take 30 minutes before exercise. Side effects are rare.
- All athletes should consult with the governing bodies of their sports regarding banned substances.

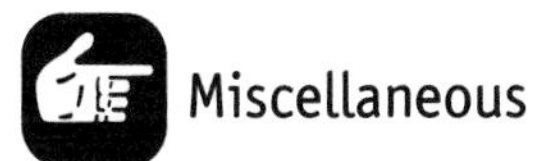

Miscellaneous

SYNONYMS

- Runner's diarrhea
- Runner's trots

ICD-9 CODE

787.91 Diarrhea
564.5 Functional diarrhea
306.4 Hyperperistalsis (nervous)

BIBLIOGRAPHY

Housner JA, Green GA. Gastrointestinal problems in athletes. In: Sallis SE, Massimino F, eds. *Essentials of sports medicine.* St. Louis: Mosby, 1996,80–92.

Swain RA. Gastrointestinal disorders in the athlete. *Clin Sports Med* 1992;11:453–471.

Swain RA. Exercise-induced diarrhea: when to wonder. *Med Sci Sports Exerc* 1993;26:523–526.

Author: Kimberly Harmon

Exercise-Induced Urticaria

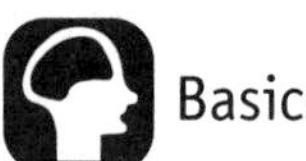

Basics

DEFINITION

- Spectrum of allergic response to exercise ranging from itching, flushing, and cutaneous warmth to development of well-circumscribed wheals (large papular lesions with pale centers and erythematous ring) and angioedema to severe anaphylactic shock
- Elevation of serum histamine levels with exercise
- Mast cell degranulation seen in skin biopsies suggesting immunoglobulin E-mediated sensitization
- Described with almost any type of physical exercise
- Distinguishable from cholinergic urticaria, which also has exercise as a possible trigger
- Certain foods, in combination with exercise, may cause symptoms in susceptible individuals.

INCIDENCE/PREVALENCE

- Incidence and prevalence unknown
- Gender distribution: males = females
- Seen more frequently in young adults, but has been described as early as 4 years of age

SIGNS AND SYMPTOMS

- Pruritus
- Urticaria
- Wheezing
- Hypotension
- Flushing
- Angioedema
- Headaches
- Nausea
- Choking
- Profuse sweating

RISK FACTORS

- Atopic history (eczema, asthma, allergic rhinitis)
- Other forms of physical allergy
- Food allergy

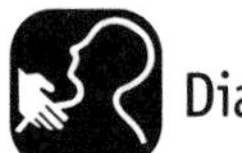

Diagnosis

DIFFERENTIAL DIAGNOSIS

- Physical urticaria (cold, dermographism, delayed pressure, solar, aquagenic, idiopathic)
- Exercise-induced asthma
- Cholinergic urticaria
- Vocal cord dysfunction
- Insect bites
- Drug eruption
- Urticaria pigmentosa
- Systemic lupus erythematosus
- Erythema multiforme

HISTORY

- Diagnosis usually made by history
- Initially patients describe generalized feeling of tingling, warmth, and itching.
- May start as early as 5 minutes after initiating exercise or can occur after exercise has been completed
- May have history of food ingestion within previous 6–8 hours before exercise
- Often (>50%) have atopic history (eczema, asthma, allergic rhinitis)
- Foods reported to be associated include eggs, lentils, shellfish, hazelnuts, wheat, peaches, apples, grapes, celery, and cheese sandwiches. Cases have been reported with many other foods.
- Usually resolves within 30 minutes to 4 hours after exercise
- Headaches may continue for up to 3–4 days after a severe reaction

PHYSICAL EXAMINATION

- Generally distinguished from cholinergic urticaria as larger (>10 mm) wheals are seen in exercise-induced urticaria while fine punctate (<5 mm) lesions are seen in cholinergic urticaria
- Wheals are not reproducible with generalized heat application or sweating, which is more characteristic of cholinergic urticaria.
- Respiratory examination may demonstrate stridor, wheezing, and retractions during acute attack.
- Angioedema seen in more severe acute attacks

LABORATORY TESTS

- Not necessary in acute attacks
- Skin testing for foods may be beneficial as an outpatient.
- Positive skin testing does not always mean a cause-and-effect relationship. Suspicious positive skin tests may need to be followed by an exercise challenge, as patients with positive food skin tests may not always develop urticaria with exercise and consumption of that food.

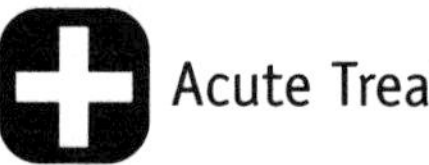

Acute Treatment

GENERAL MEASURES

- Acutely, care is targeted to ensure airway protection if severe anaphylaxis is present.
- Treatment with epinephrine, diphenhydramine, or hydroxyzine may improve symptoms.

MEDICATIONS

- Epinephrine (Epi-Pen) 0.3 mg i.m. for severe anaphylactic reaction
- Diphenhydramine (Benadryl) 25–50 mg p.o. every 4–6 hours (children 5 mg/kg/day divided every 6–8 hours, not exceeding 300 mg/day)
- Hydroxyzine (Atarax) 25–100 mg p.o. every 6 hours (children 2 mg/kg/day divided every 6–8 hours)

SPECIAL CONSIDERATIONS

- One reported death from severe anaphylactic reaction

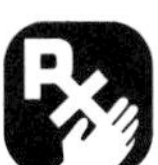

Long-Term Treatment

MEDICATIONS

- During exercise, patients should carry an epinephrine kit (Epi-Pen) with them at all times
- H1 antihistamines as prophylaxis have shown mixed results (fexofenadine 60 mg p.o. b.i.d., loratadine 10 mg p.o. daily, and cetirizine 10 mg p.o. daily).
- Cromolyn taken orally reported to be of some benefit.
- H2 antihistamines may be of help (cimetidine, ranitidine, famotidine).
- Doxepin, which has both H1- and H2-blocking abilities, may be of value.

PREVENTION/PRECAUTIONS

- Stop exercise with first onset of symptoms
- Avoid foods 6–8 hours before exercise. Exercising first thing in the morning after evening fast is preferable.
- Avoid known problematic food triggers at least 12 hours before exercise
- Preventive antihistamine therapy may be useful.
- Patients should always have an epinephrine kit with them while exercising; Benadryl also may be reasonable to have.
- Exercise with a companion knowledgeable in cardiopulmonary resuscitation (CPR) is recommended.

REFERRAL/DISPOSITION

Referral to allergist may be beneficial for skin testing and controlled exercise challenge testing.

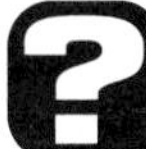

Common Questions and Answers

Physician responses to common patient questions:
Q: Do I need to stop exercising?
A: No, exercise may be continued as long as precautions are taken by avoiding all food 6–8 hours before exercise and 12 hours after eating food suspected of causing reactions. Epinephrine should be carried at all time with the patient when exercising, and a companion who knows CPR ideally would be exercising with the patient. Patients who had severe life-threatening reactions more likely need counseling to discuss curtailing exercise.
Q: Are these reactions preventable?
A: Not always. Despite premedication with various antihistamines, patients can still develop urticarial lesions and have anaphylaxis. Initiating antihistamine therapy on a daily basis for those who frequently exercise is a worthwhile start to hopefully reduce the number of occurrences of this phenomenon.
Q: What types of food should I avoid?
A: Each individual may react to different foods. Reported reactions occur more frequently with celery and shellfish, but also with hazelnuts, eggs, apples, peaches, grapes, wheat, and even cheese sandwiches. Some patients have been reported to react to any food they eat. If a food seems to be a trigger a reaction, it is best to avoid that food at least 12 hours before exercise. It is reasonable to see an allergist for skin testing and an exercise challenge with suspicious food items.

Miscellaneous

SYNONYMS

- Exercise-induced anaphylaxis
- Hives

ICD-9 CODE

708.8 Other specified urticaria

BIBLIOGRAPHY

Briner WW. Physical allergies and exercise: clinical implications for those engaged in sport activities. *Sports Med* 1993;15: 365–373.

Briner WW. Exercise-induced anaphylaxis. *Med Sci Sports Exerc* 1992;24:849–850.

Horan RF, Sheffer AL, Briner WW. Physical allergies. *Med Sci Sports Exerc* 1992;24: 845–848.

Kaplan AP. *Allergy: principles and practice,* 5th ed. St. Louis: Mosby-Year Book, 1998.

Nichols AW. Exercise-induced anaphylaxis and urticaria. *Clin Sports Med* 1992;11:303–312.

Tilles SA, Schocket AL. *Food allergy: adverse reactions to foods and food additives.* Cambridge: Blackwell Science, 1997.

Tilles S, Shocket A, Milgrum H. Exercise-induced anaphylaxis related to specific foods. *J Pediatrics* 1995;27: 587–589.

Authors: Mark Halstead and David T. Bernhardt

External Ear Chondritis/Abscess

Basics

SIGNS AND SYMPTOMS

- Initially a dull pain that increases in severity
- Pinna
  - —Painful
  - —Exquisite tenderness
  - —Erythematous
  - —Warmth
  - —Loss of contours caused by edema often with sparing of the lobule
- Increase of the auriculocephalic angle
- Fluctuant areas develop with eventual breakdown and suppuration
- Entire ear involvement if untreated
  - —Disfigurement can occur
- Fever
- Chills

MECHANISM/DESCRIPTION

- Inflammation and infection of the pinna
- Cartilage of the external ear is easily damaged due to
  - —Lack of overlying subcutaneous tissue
  - —Relative avascularity
  - —Exposed position
- Chondritis
  - —Most commonly a secondary complication of otic trauma and burns
  - —Onset often insidious and may be delayed until apparent healing has occurred

ETIOLOGY

- Common causes of chondritis include
  - —Chemical or thermal burns
  - —Frostbite
  - —Hematoma formation
  - —Mastoid surgery
  - —Human bites
  - —Deep abrasions
  - —External otitis
  - —High piercing of the ear lobe
- Bacteria involved
  - —*P. aeruginosa*
  - —Staphylococcus
  - —Proteus

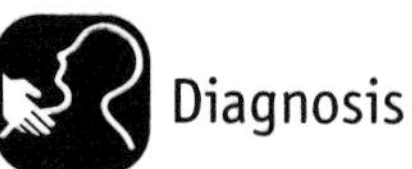

Diagnosis

ESSENTIAL WORKUP

- Clinical diagnosis
  - —Typical physical findings in combination with above causes

LABORATORY

- CBC for systemic symptoms
- Blood culture if systemic signs of infection

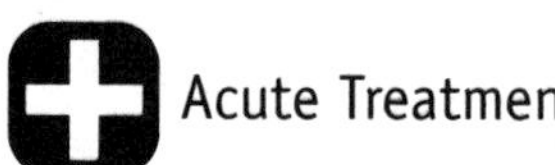

Acute Treatment

ED TREATMENT

Antibiotics

- Oral antibiotics for minor cases of early ear lobe inflammation
  - —Ciprofloxacin preferred (<18 years old)
  - —First-generation cephalosporin or dicloxacillin
  - —IV antibiotics for severe infection
  - —Apply topical antibiotics when break in skin barrier

ENT Consult

- For chondritis, abscess, and necrosis of the involved cartilage
- Early surgical drainage for chondritis
- Aggressive early management may prevent gross ear deformity

General Postinjury Preventive Measures

- Prevention of chondritis is of the utmost importance
  - —Difficult management and disfiguring potential
- Avoid pressure to the injured ear
- Minimize active débridement of eschars and crusts
- Gentle washing twice daily with antibacterial soap and water followed by complete drying and application of topical antibiotics
- Keep hair away from the ear

Complications

- Disfiguration of the pinna
  - —Occurs without proper treatment
  - —Ranging from being shriveled, cauliflower-like ear to complete loss of the external ear and possible stenosis of the auditory meatus

MEDICATIONS

- Ciprofloxacin: 500 mg po tid (adult)
- Cephalexin: 500 mg (peds: 50 mg/kg/24 hrs) po qid
- Dicloxacillin: 500 mg (peds: 25 mg/kg/24 hrs) po qid

HOSPITAL ADMISSION CRITERIA

- Parenteral antibiotics and early surgical drainage for patients with chondritis
- Edema, erythema, and significant ear tenderness
- Toxic patient with fever and chills
- Immunocompromised patient
- Unreliable patient or caretaker

HOSPITAL DISCHARGE CRITERIA

- Stable patient without systemic signs with close ENT followup

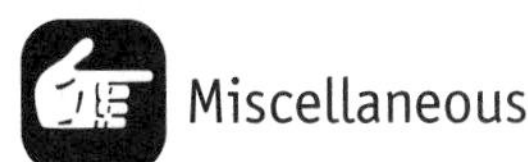

Miscellaneous

ICD-9 CODE

733.99

CORE CONTENT CODE

6.1.1

BIBLIOGRAPHY

Bentrem DJ, Bill TJ, Himel HN, et al. Chondritis of the ear: a late sequela of deep partial thickness burns of the face. *J Emerg Med* 1996;14:469–471.

Staley R, Fitzgibbon JJ, Anderson C. Auricular infections caused by high ear piercing in adolescents. *Pediatrics* 1997;99:610–611.

Author: Assaad J. Sayah

External Genital Trauma

Basics

SIGNS AND SYMPTOMS

- Prior history of trauma
- Pelvic pain, inability to void
- Blood at the meatus, high-riding prostate, perineal or genital swelling

MECHANISM/DESCRIPTION

- Females: injuries to the urethra are rare due to the short, unexposed, and mobile urethra
  - —Usually occur at the bladder neck
- Males: urethra is divided into sections
  - —Posterior urethra
    - —Prostatic
    - —Membranous
    - —Injuries more common
  - —Anterior urethra
    - —Bulbar
    - —Penile
    - —Rarely injured due to its mobility
- Posterior injuries are much more common and have the classification system detailed below
- *Classification of posterior urethral injuries*
  - —Type I: urethra stretched but not ruptured
  - —Type II: prostatic/membranous portions ruptured (either partially or completely); urogenital diaphragm intact
  - —Type III: both the prostatic/membranous urethra and urogenital diaphragm are ruptured, frequently with damage to the proximal bulbar urethra

ETIOLOGY

- Females
  - —Childbirth or vaginal surgery
  - —Straddle injuries
  - —Rare with pelvic fracture
- Males
  - —Trauma, especially straddle injuries
  - —Mutilation injuries
  - —Sexual activity
  - —Instrumentation
  - —Approximately 95% of posterior urethral injuries are caused by pelvic fractures
    - —As many as 25% of pelvic fractures have concomitant urethral injuries

POTENTIAL COMPLICATIONS

- Impotence
- Incontinence
- Strictures
- Infection

PEDIATRIC CONSIDERATIONS

- Urethral damage, frequently caused by traumatic mechanisms similar to adults
- Nonaccidental trauma or sexual abuse, especially females, may be contributory
- Majority of posterior urethral injuries are type I

PRE-HOSPITAL

- Similar considerations as for major trauma victims

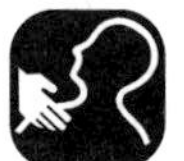

Diagnosis

ESSENTIAL WORKUP

- Female
  - —A meticulous vaginal examination to exclude vaginal laceration as the bleeding source
  - —Radiographic evaluation of the integrity of the urethra should be performed prior to urinary catheter placement if urethral injury is suspected
    - —If this is not possible, suprapubic aspiration, or cystostomy should be done
- Male
  - —Determine if the prostate is normally positioned (not high-riding) and examine for blood at the external meatus
  - —Radiographic evaluation of the integrity of the urethra should be performed prior to urinary catheter placement if urethral injury is suspected
    - —If this is not possible, suprapubic aspiration or cystostomy should be done

LABORATORY

- Urinalysis
- Hematocrit
- BUN and Cr

IMAGING/SPECIAL TESTS

- Retrograde urethrography (RUG)
- Water-soluble contrast is injected via a catheter-tipped syringe at the urethral meatus
- Extravasation of contrast and its relation to the prevesical space and urogenital diaphragm should be noted
- Proximity of the extravasation to the meatus and the bladder should be appreciated
- If the urethral tear is complete, there will be no contrast within the bladder and marked extravasation will occur
- A partial tear will demonstrate contrast material within the bladder
- Excretory urethrography to define proximal urethral tears
- Cystography
  - —40% of urethral injuries have concomitant bladder injuries

DIFFERENTIAL DIAGNOSIS

- Perineal and vaginal trauma
- Bladder trauma
- Ureter or kidney trauma

PEDIATRIC CONSIDERATIONS

- If an examination of the introitus and perineum cannot easily be performed, examination under anesthesia should occur
- An examination in the OR, in addition to being better tolerated by the patient, allows the physician to rule out sexual abuse and to confirm that the injury is consistent with the history
- The workup of male pediatric patients should also include an examination in the operating room if an adequate ED examination does not occur or if suspicion of abuse exists

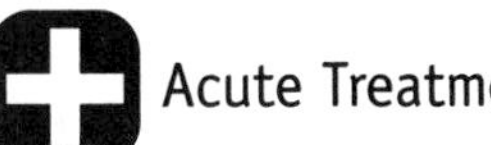

Acute Treatment

INITIAL STABILIZATION

- ABCs of trauma care take precedence

ED TREATMENT

- After RUG, the urologist should be contacted
- Urethral contusions, lacerations, and avulsions are best managed by an experienced urologist
- Catheter placement, if appropriate, or suprapubic aspiration/cystostomy followed by laboratory evaluation comprise the ED treatment

MEDICATIONS

- No specific medications for this injury

HOSPITAL ADMISSION CRITERIA

- Concurrent closed head injury, blunt abdominal trauma, or pelvic fracture
- Need for operative management of urethral, penile, or bladder injuries

HOSPITAL DISCHARGE CRITERIA

- Isolated urethral injuries frequently may be managed in the outpatient setting after appropriate urinary catheterization or suprapubic cystostomy with urologic follow-up

Miscellaneous

ICD-9 CODE

867.0

CORE CONTENT CODE

18.4.11.11

BIBLIOGRAPHY

Avanoglu A, Ulman I, Herek O, Ozok G, Gokdemir A. Posterior urethral injuries in children. *Br J Urol* 1996;77:598–600.

Carter CT, Schafer N. Incidence of urethral disruption in females with traumatic pelvic fractures. *Am J Emerg Med* 1993;11(3): 218–20.

Goldman SM, Sandler CM, Corriere JN Jr, McGuire EJ. Blunt urethral trauma: A unified, anatomical mechanical classification. *J Urol* 1997;157:85–89.

Lynch JM, Gardner MJ, Albanese CT. Blunt urogenital trauma in prepubescent female patients: More than meets the eye. *Pediatr Emerg Care* 1995;11(6):372–375.

Watnik NF, Coburn M, Goldberger M. Urologic injuries in pelvic ring disruptions. *Clin Orthop* 1996;329:37–45.

Authors: Kenneth Bramwell and Roscoe Nelson

Felon

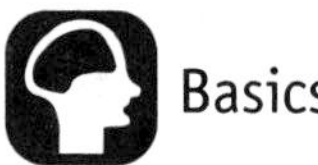

Basics

SIGNS AND SYMPTOMS

- Swelling and tension of distal finger tip
- Throbbing pain
- Patients often elevate the finger to avoid increased pain in the dependent position
- Kanavel's signs of pyogenic flexor tenosynovitis
  —Flexed resting position of involved digit
  —Tenderness over flexor sheath
  —Fusiform swelling
  —Severe pain in passive extension

MECHANISM/DESCRIPTION

- A felon is a palmer closed-space infection of the distal pulp of the finger
- Felons can develop into serious infections resulting in significant patient disability. Neglect or incomplete incision and drainage may result in soft tissue and bony tuft necrosis, osteomyelitis, septic arthritis, lymphangitis, and flexor tenosynovitis. Improper surgical interventions can also result in an insensate, unstable palmer pad

ETIOLOGY

- The distal finger is anatomically a closed compartment, separate from the rest of the finger
- Multiple fibrous septa connect the volar skin fat pad to the periosteum
- Septa form compartments causing infections to be closed-space
- Worsening infection increases compartmental pressure resulting in ischemia and necrosis
- Spread of the infection can result in osteomyelitis
- Inoculating site rarely identified; wooden or glass splinters, minor cuts, or repeated trauma from fingerstick blood testing are common etiologies
- *S. aureus* is the most common organism; Streptococcus and Gram-negatives are also reported

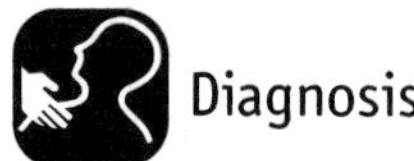

Diagnosis

ESSENTIAL WORKUP

- Thorough neurologic and vascular examination of finger pulp and digit function
- Cessation of pain indicates extensive tissue necrosis and nerve damage
  —Orthopedic consult should be obtained

LABORATORY

- Culture from I & D should be routinely performed because of the increased risk of osteomyelitis and prolonged infections

IMAGING/SPECIAL TESTS

- Finger radiographs should be obtained if there is suspicion of retained foreign body or osteomyelitis

DIFFERENTIAL DIAGNOSIS

- Herpetic whitlow—examine for vesicles
- Osteomyelitis
- Flexor tenosynovitis

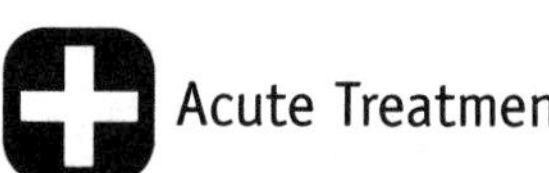

Acute Treatment

INITIAL STABILIZATION

No specific measures indicated

ED TREATMENT

- Digit block utilizing a long-acting agent (bupivacaine)
- Apply a tourniquet for the procedure to provide a bloodless field during incision
- Establish a sterile field
- Unilateral incision along side of the finger from 0.5 cm distal to the DIP crease to the free edge of the nail
  —Incision must be dorsal to neurovascular bundle of the fingertip
- Bluntly dissect subcutaneous tissue to break up loculations in the septa
- Débride necrotic tissue
- Frank pus may not be evident
- The incision and dissection must not cross the DIP flexor crease; increased risk of inoculating the flexor tendon sheath
- Pack wound with sterile gauze or packing strip
- Splint finger to immobilize both digit and wrist

- Previously advocated fishmouth and lateral through-and-through incisions are associated with severe iatrogenic complications (i.e., unstable finger pad, permanent anesthesia) and should not be part of initial management

MEDICATIONS

- Antibiotics for 5–7 days
  —Dicloxacillin: adult: 250–500 mg q 6 hrs po; peds: 25–100 mg/kg/d (qid) po
  —Nafcillin: adult: 1–2 g q 4–6 hrs IV; peds: 50 mg/kg q 6 hrs IV
  —Clindamycin: adult: 150–300 mg q 6 hrs po; peds: 10–25 mg/kg/d (qid) po
- Alternative antibiotics
  —Cephalexin: adult: 250–500 mg q 6 hrs po; peds: 25–50 mg/kg/d (qid) po
  —Cefazolin: adult: 1 g q 8 hrs IV; peds: 100 mg/kg/d (q 8 hrs) IV
  —Erythromycin: adult: 250–500 mg q 6 hrs po; peds: 20–50 mg/kg/d (qid) po
- While wound culture results are pending, coverage for *S. aureus* is mandatory

HOSPITAL ADMISSION CRITERIA

- Flexor tenosynovitis, frank necrosis or other reasons for debridement in the OR

HOSPITAL DISCHARGE CRITERIA

- Provided that reliable follow-up can be ensured and no indications of extension of infection from pulp, felons can be managed as an outpatient
- Wound check in 48 hours to include packing removal and wound irrigation
- Replace packing if continued drainage and follow up in 24 hours
- Otherwise, warm soaks and dressing changes
- Adjust antimicrobial coverage as indicated by cultures
- Symptoms usually resolve quickly; healing process can take up to 2 weeks
- Early consultation recommended for resistant infections

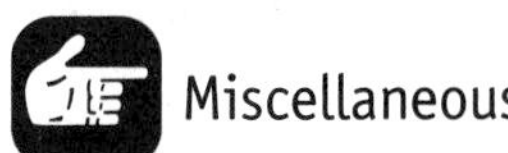

Miscellaneous

ICD-9 CODE

681.01

CORE CONTENT CODE

10.6.4

BIBLIOGRAPHY

Abrams RA, Botte MJ. Hand infections: Treatment recommendations for specific types. *J Am Acad Orthop Surg* 1996;4(4): 219–230.

Canales FL, Newmeyer WI, Kilgore ES. The treatment of felons and paronychias. *Hand Clin* 1989;5(4):515–523.

Lammers RL, Freemyer BC. Hand. In: Rosen P, et al. *Emergency medicine: Concepts and clinical practice*. 3rd ed. St. Louis: CV Mosby, 1992:580–581.

Warden TM, Fourré MW. Incision and drainage of cutaneous abscesses and soft tissue infections. In: Roberts H, ed. *Clinical procedures in emergency medicine*. 2d ed. Philadelphia: WB Saunders, 1991:605–608.

Author: Allen Marino

Folliculitis

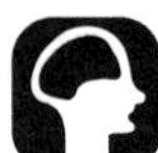

Basics

DEFINITION

- Infection of hair follicles usually caused by *Staphylococcus aureus*
- May be caused by gram-negative organisms, as in the case of "hot tub" folliculitis

INCIDENCE/PREVALENCE

- Lesions usually occur on areas of skin traumatized by maceration occurring under shoulder pads or sweaty garments
- May develop on the legs, arms, and trunk of wrestlers
- Infection does not spread in epidemic proportions, but may be transmitted through skin trauma.
- Hot tub folliculitis is associated with the use of hot tubs, whirlpools, Jacuzzis, and swimming pools.

RISK FACTORS

Furuncles occur in skin areas containing hair follicles subject to friction and perspiration.

ASSOCIATED INJURIES AND COMPLICATIONS

- Deep folliculitis lesions ultimately may produce furuncles or boils.
- Boils may combine to form a large, exquisitely painful group of furuncles called a carbuncle.
- Furunculosis, an infection pertaining to hair follicles, sebaceous glands, or skin compromised by abrasions, wounds, or burns, may arise from existing areas of folliculitis.

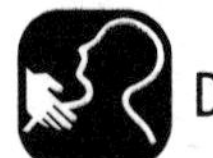

Diagnosis

DIFFERENTIAL DIAGNOSIS

- Folliculitis lesions consist of small (2–5 mm) erythematous, sometimes pruritic papules often topped by a central pustule.
- Cultures (if taken) will show the presence of *S. aureus* (or *Pseudomonas aeruginosa* for suspected hot tub folliculitis)
- Furuncles appear as deep, inflammatory nodules.
- Carbuncles extend into the subcutaneous fat; multiple abscesses are separated by connective tissue septa.

HISTORY

Q: Was equipment worn over the affected area?
A: Maceration caused by sports equipment is a common cause of folliculitis. This knowledge may lead to a definitive diagnosis.

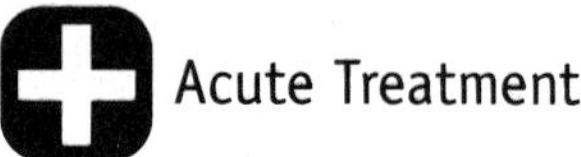

Acute Treatment

TREATMENT OF MILD FOLLICULITIS

- Most cases of mild folliculitis heal spontaneously within 5 days.
- To prevent furuncle formation, astringent lotions or drying agents that remove the tops of pustules can be used.
- Hot tub folliculitis is self-limiting and lasts only 7–10 days. It requires no specific treatment other than avoiding persistent hot tub use.

TREATMENT OF FURUNCLE OR CARBUNCLE FORMATION

- Aspiration or incision and drainage may be required for fluctuant lesions.
- Cleanse affected area with benzoyl peroxide.
- Oral antibiotics may be prescribed, but usually no more than 14 days are necessary to prevent recurrence. Agents effective against *S. aureus* include penicillinase-resistant penicillins such as oral dicloxacillin, cephalexin, and erythromycin (or other macrolides). Fluoroquinolones such as moxifloxacin, levofloxacin, and gatifloxacin may be effective.
- Warm compresses can be applied.

- Clothing and dressings that have come in contact with the affected area should be cleansed daily at high temperatures.
- Hand washing should be performed regularly by all who come into contact with affected area.

Common Questions and Answers

Physician responses to common patient questions:

Q: Is it contagious?

A: Personal contact rarely causes transmission of *S. aureus* from a patient with folliculitis, but cases of transmission through skin trauma have been documented. Infected areas should be kept clean and covered. To prevent spread of infection, athletes with furuncles or carbuncles should be strongly discouraged from participation in contact sports until lesions have resolved.

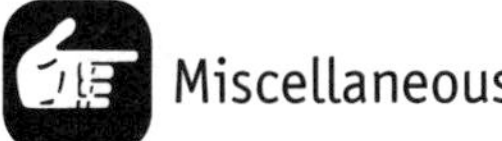

Miscellaneous

BIBLIOGRAPHY

Adler AI, Altman J. An outbreak of mud-wrestling-induced pustular dermatitis in college students. Dermatitis palaestrae limosae. *JAMA* 1993;269:502–504.

Bartlett PC, Martin RJ, Cahill BR. Furunculosis in a high school football team. *Am J Sports Med* 1982;10:371–374.

Chandrasekar PH, Rolston KV, Kannangara W, et al. Hot tub-associated dermatitis due to Pseudomonas aeruginosa. *Arch Dermatol* 1984;120:1337–1340.

Decker MD, Lybarger JA, Vaughn WK, et al. An outbreak of staphylococcal skin infections among river rafting guides. *Am J Epidemiol* 1986;124:969–976.

Heeb MA. Deep soft tissue abscesses secondary to nonpenetrating trauma. *Surgery* 1971;69:550–553.

Minooee A, Rickman LS. Transmission of infectious diseases during sports. In: Scholssberg D, ed. *Infections of leisure,* 2nd ed. Washington, DC: American Society for Microbiology, 1999.

Stevens DL. Cellulitis, pyoderma, and other skin and subcutaneous infections. In: Armstrong D, Cohen J, eds. *Infectious diseases, vol. 1.* St. Louis: Mosby/Harcourt Publishers, 1999:2.2.3–2.2.4.

Swartz NN. Cellulitis and subcutaneous tissue. In: Mandell GL, Bennett JE, Dolin R, eds. *Mandell, Douglas, and Bennett's principles and practice of infectious disease, vol. 1,* 5th ed. Philadelphia: Churchill Livingstone. 2000.

Sosin DM, Gunn RA, Ford WL, et al. An outbreak of furunculosis among high school athletes. *Am J Sports Med* 1989;1:828–832.

Authors: Elizabeth Austin and Leland S. Rickman

Gastroenteritis

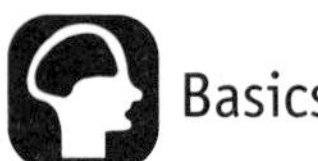

Basics

SIGNS AND SYMPTOMS

- Nausea, vomiting, diarrhea
- Bloody/mucous diarrhea
- Abdominal cramps or pain
- Fever
- Malaise, myalgias, headache, anorexia
- Tachycardia, hypotension, lethargy, and dehydration (severe cases)

ETIOLOGY

Infections

Viruses

- 50–70% of all cases

Invasive Bacteria

- Campylobacter: contaminated food/water, wilderness water, birds, and other animals
  - —Most common cause
  - —Gross or occult blood is found in 60–90%
- Salmonella: contaminated water, eggs, poultry or dairy products
  - —*Typhoid fever (S. typhi)* characterized by unremitting fever, abdominal pain, rose spots, splenomegaly, and bradycardia
  - —Immunocompromised susceptible
- Shigella: fecal-oral route
- Vibrio parahaemolyticus: raw and undercooked seafood
- Yersinia: contaminated food (pork), water, and milk
  - —May present as mesenteric adenitis or mimic appendicitis

Specific Food-Borne Disease (Food Poisoning)

- *Staphylococcal aureus*
  - —Most common toxin-related disease
  - —Symptoms 1–6 hours after ingesting food
- *Bacillus cereus*
  - —Classic source is fried rice left on steam tables
  - —Symptoms within 1–36 hours
- Cholera: profuse watery stools with mucous ("rice-water" stools)
- Ciguatera
  - —Fish intoxication
  - —Onset 5 minutes to 30 hours (average 6 hours) after ingestion
  - —Paresthesias, hypotension, peripheral muscle weakness
  - —Amitriptyline may be therapeutic
- Scombroid
  - —Caused by "blood fish": tuna, albacore, mackerel and mahi-mahi
  - —Flushing, headache, erythema, dizziness, blurred vision, and generalized burning sensation
  - —Symptoms last <6 hours
  - —Treatment includes antihistamines

Protozoa

- *Giardia lamblia*
  - —High-risk groups: travelers, day care children, homosexual men, and campers who drink untreated mountain water

Noninfectious Causes

- Toxins
  - —Zinc, copper, cadmium
  - —Organic chemicals: polyvinylchlorides
  - —Pesticides—organophosphates
  - —Radioactive substances
  - —Alkyl mercury
- Altered-host response to a food substance (tyramine, monosodium glutamate, tryptamine)

PEDIATRIC CONSIDERATIONS

- Focus evaluation on state of hydration
- Majority of viral origin and self-limited
- Rotavirus accounts for up to 50%
- *Shigella* infections associated with seizures

CAUTIONS

- Difficult IV access in severe dehydration
- Avoid exposure to contaminated clothes or body substances

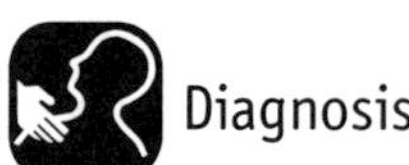

Diagnosis

ESSENTIAL WORKUP

- Digital rectal examination to determine the presence of gross or occult blood
- Fecal leukocyte determination
  - —Present with invasive bacteria
  - —Absent in protozoal infections, viral, toxin-induced food poisoning

LABORATORY

- CBC—indications
  - —Significant blood loss
  - —Systemic toxicity
- Electrolytes, glucose, BUN/Cr-indications
  - —Lethargy, significantly dehydration, toxicity, or altered mental status
  - —Diuretic use, persistent diarrhea, chronic liver or renal disease
- Stool culture—indications
  - —Presence of fecal leukocytes
  - —Historical markers (immunocompromised, travel, homosexual)
  - —Public health (food handler, day/health care worker)
- Blood cultures—indications
  - —Suspected bacteremia/systemic infections
  - —Ill patients requiring admission

IMAGING/SPECIAL TESTS

- Abdominal x-ray films have no value unless an obstruction or a toxic megacolon suspected

DIFFERENTIAL DIAGNOSIS

- Gastritis/peptic ulcer disease
- Milk and food allergies
- Appendicitis
- Irritable bowel syndrome
- Ulcerative colitis/Crohn's disease
- Malrotation with midget volvulus
- Meckel's diverticulum
- Drugs and toxins: mannitol, sorbitol, phenolphthalein, magnesium-containing anti-acids, quinidine, colchicine, mushrooms, mercury poisoning

PEDIATRIC CONSIDERATIONS

- Laboratory studies not required in most cases
- Rotazyme assay detects rotavirus
  - —Rarely indicated in managing outpatients
  - —Helpful to cohort and avoid cross-contamination among inpatients
- Stool cultures—indication
  - —Fecal leukocytes
  - —Toxic
  - —Infants
  - —Immunocompromised

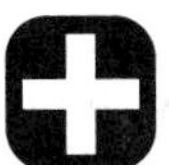

Acute Treatment

INITIAL STABILIZATION

- IV fluid with 0.9% NS resuscitation for severely dehydrated

ED TREATMENT

- Oral fluids for mild dehydration (Gatorade/Pedialyte)
- IV fluids for
  —Hypotension, nausea/vomiting, obtundation, metabolic acidosis, significant hypernatremia or hyponatremia
  —0.9% NS 500 ml-1 L bolus (peds: 20 ml/kg) for resuscitation then 0.9% NS or D5.45% NS (peds: D5.25% NS) to maintain an adequate urine output
- Bismuth subsalicylate (Pepto-Bismol)
  —Antisecretory agent
  —Effective clinical relief without adverse effects
- Kaolin-pectin (Kaopectate)
  —Reduces fluidity of stools
  —Does not influence the course of the disease
- Antimotility drugs (diphenoxylate (lomotil), loperamide (imodium), paregoric, and codeine)
  —Appropriate in noninfectious diarrhea
  —Initial use of sparse amounts to control symptoms in infectious diarrhea
  —Avoid prolonged use in infectious diarrhea—may increase the duration of fever, diarrhea, and bacteremia, and may precipitate a toxic megacolon
- Antiemetics: prochlorperazine (compazine) and promethazine (phenergan) for nausea/vomiting

Antibiotics for Infectious Pathogens

- Campylobacter: quinolone or erythromycin
- Salmonella: quinolone or trimethoprim/sulfamethoxazole (tmp/smx)
- Ceftriaxone for typhoid fever
- Shigella: quinolone, tmp/smx, or ampicillin
- *Vibrio parahaemolyticus*: tetracycline or doxycycline
- *Clostridium difficile*: vancomycin
- *Escherichia coli*: quinolone or tmp/smx
- *Giardia lamblia*: metronidazole or quinacrine

MEDICATIONS

- Ampicillin: 500 mg (peds: 20 mg/kg/24 hrs) PO/IV q 6 hrs
- Bactrim DS (trimethoprim/sulfamethoxazole): 1 tab (peds: 8–10 mg tmp/40–50 mg smx/kg/24 hrs) PO/IV bid
- Ciprofloxacin (quinolone): 500 mg PO/IV bid (>18 years old)
- Doxycycline: 100 mg PO/IV bid
- Erythromycin: 500 mg (peds: 40-50 mg/kg/24 hrs) po qid
- Metronidazole: 250 mg (peds: 35 mg/kg/24 hrs) po tid (>8 years old)
- Tetracycline: 500 mg PO/IV q 6 hrs
- Prochlorperazine (Compazine): 5–10 mg IVP q 3–4 hrs; 10 mg po q 8 hrs; 25 mg PR; q 12 hrs PRN (peds: >2 yrs: 0.06 mg/lb IM 1 dose only)
- Promethazine (Phenergan): 25 mg IM/IVP q 4 hrs, 25 mg PO/PR q 12 hrs PRN (peds: >2 yrs: 6.25–12.5 mg IM/IV q 4 hrs; 12.5–25 mg po PR q 12 hrs)
- Quinacrine: 100 mg (6 mg/kg/24 hrs) po tid

HOSPITAL ADMISSION CRITERIA

- Hypotension unresponsive to IV fluids
- Significant bleeding
- Signs of sepsis/toxicity
- Intractable vomiting or abdominal pain
- Severe electrolyte imbalance
- Metabolic acidosis
- Altered mental status
- Children with >10–15% dehydration

HOSPITAL DISCHARGE CRITERIA

- Mild cases requiring oral hydration
- Dehydration responsive to IV fluids

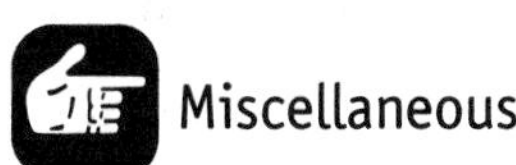

Miscellaneous

ICD-9 CODE

558.9

BIBLIOGRAPHY

Bitterman R. Acute gastroenteritis and constipation. In: Rosen P, Barkin RM, et al., eds. *Emergency medicine: Concepts and clinical practice*. 4th ed. St. Louis: Mosby-Year Book, 1998:1917–1958.

Blacklow NR, Greenberg HB. Viral gastroenteritis. *N Engl J Med* 1991;325:252.

DuPont H, Miranda A. Small intestine: Infections with common bacterial and viral pathogens. In: Yamada T, et al., eds. *Textbook of gastroenterology*. 2d ed. Philadelphia: JB Lippincott, 1995: 1605–1629.

Fleisher GR. Gastrointestinal infections. In: Fleisher G, Ludwig S, eds. *Pediatric emergency medicine*. 3rd ed. Baltimore: Williams & Wilkins, 1993:628–633.

Author: Isam Nasr

Gastroesophageal Reflux

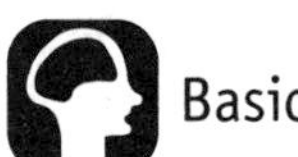

Basics

DEFINITION

- Reflux of gastroduodenal contents into the esophagus

INCIDENCE/PREVALENCE

- 65% of adults have suffered from heartburn.
- 24% have symptoms for >1 year.
- Can be induced or worsened by exercise

SIGNS AND SYMPTOMS

- Heartburn
- Regurgitation
- Dysphagia
- Angina-like chest pain
- Bronchospasm
- Cough

RISK FACTORS

- Endurance sports and high-intensity exercise.
- Preexisting gastroesophageal reflux without exercise
- Running/rowing > bicycling/weight-lifting

CAUSES

- Transient decrease in lower esophageal sphincter tone
- Delayed gastric emptying

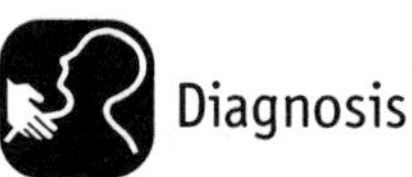

Diagnosis

DIFFERENTIAL DIAGNOSIS

- Esophagitis
- Gastritis
- Peptic ulcer disease
- Angina pectoris

HISTORY

Signs and symptoms may be present all the time or only with exercise.

PHYSICAL EXAMINATION

- Usually normal
- If patient experiences bronchospasm secondary to reflux, may hear wheezing with auscultation while symptomatic.

IMAGING

Barium swallow may show hiatal hernia, mucosal irregularity, or strictures.

SPECIAL TESTS

- Esophageal pH monitoring, especially with exercise, can establish diagnosis.
- Acid perfusion test can reproduce symptoms.
- Esophageal manometry
- Endoscopy can reveal mucosal changes consistent with reflux.

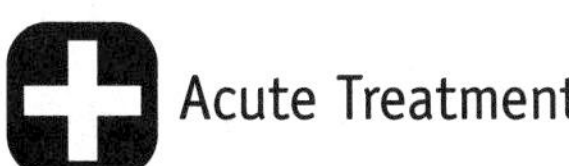

Acute Treatment

NONMEDICAL

- Reduce level of exertion initially, followed by gradual increase in intensity
- Athlete should have adequate fluid intake.
- Solid foods should be avoided during the last 3 hours before competition
- Avoid high-fat meals, caffeine, alcohol, chocolate, peppermint, onions, tobacco, and citrus juices

MEDICATION

- Typical history warrants initial empiric treatment
- H2 blockers: cimetidine (Tagamet), famotidine (Pepcid), ranitidine (Zantac), nizatidine (Axid)
- Proton pump inhibitors (reasonable as initial therapy): rabeprazole (Aciphex), lansoprazole (Prevacid), omeprazole (Prilosec). May need to use high doses.
- H2 blockers and proton pump inhibitors do not impair psychomotor or cardiovascular performance.

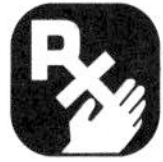

Long-Term Treatment

SURGERY

- Considered only after failed medication therapy and established diagnosis

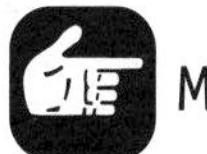

Miscellaneous

ICD-9 CODE

530.81

BIBLIOGRAPHY

Housner JA, Green GA. Gastrointestinal problems in athletes. In: Sallis RE, Massimino F, eds. *Essentials of sports medicine.* St. Louis: Mosby, 1997,80–88.

Lewis JH. Gastroesophageal reflux disease. In: Dambro MR, ed. *Griffith's 5-minute clinical consult 1999.* Philadelphia: Lippincott Williams & Wilkins, 1999,422–423.

Brouns F, Beckers E. Is the gut an athletic organ? *Sports Med* 1993;15:242–257.

Shawdon A. Gastro-oesophageal reflux and exercise. *Sports Med* 1995;20:109–116.

Author: Kimberly Harmon

Gonococcal Disease

Basics

SIGNS AND SYMPTOMS

Female

- Cervicitis
  - —Yellow or white thick mucopurulent endocervical discharge
  - —Cervical edema, congestion, and friability
  - —Abnormal vaginal bleeding
- Pelvic inflammatory disease
  - —Abdominal pain/tenderness
  - —Fever
  - —Cervical motion tenderness
  - —Bilateral adnexal tenderness
  - —Nausea/vomiting
  - —Fitz-Hugh-Curtis syndrome
    - —Right upper-quadrant pain/tenderness
- Vaginal itching
- Dysuria
- 30–40% asymptomatic carriers

Male

- Urethritis with yellow-white thick discharge
- Urinary tract infection symptoms
  - —Dysuria
- Prostatitis
- Epididymitis
- Proctitis

Disseminated

- Fever
- Chills
- Migratory tenosynovitis
  - —Involve flexor tendon sheaths of wrist/Achilles tendon
- Rash
- Two-thirds accompanies tenosynovitis
- Hemorrhagic, necrotic pustules on erythematous base
- Begin distally
- Resembles meningococcus
- Healing crust in 4 days
- Arthralgia
- Arthritis
  - —Especially of knees, ankle, and wrist
  - —Swollen, warm joint with effusion
- Endocarditis

Other

- Pharyngitis
- Conjunctivitis
  - —Severe purulent discharge
  - —Conjunctival injection/irritation

MECHANISM/DESCRIPTION

- Common sexually transmitted disease
- Often seen with Chlamydia
- Humans only known host for *Neisseria gonorrhea*
- 60–80% of females in contact with males with urethral gonorrhea develop infection
- 20–30% of males in contact with females with gonorrhea develop infection

ETIOLOGY

- *Neisseria gonorrhea*
  - —Gram-negative aerobic, diplococcus bacteria
  - —Die rapidly when outside normal environment

PEDIATRIC CONSIDERATIONS

- Ophthalmia neonatorum
  - —Bilateral conjunctivitis 2–5 days postbirth

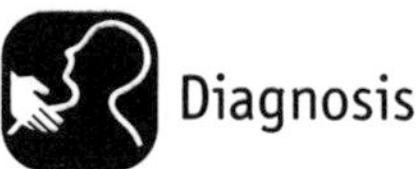

Diagnosis

ESSENTIAL WORKUP

- Clinical diagnosis in male gonorrhea
  - —Gram's stain of urethral exudate with 95% sensitivity and 97% specificity
- Cervical culture in female gonorrhea
  - —Gram's stain cervical discharge with 50% sensitivity and 90% specificity

LABORATORY

- Monoclonal antibodies and DNA probes
  - —From simple cervical or urethral swabs
  - —Accurate
- Blood cultures for disseminated GC
- Joint arthrocentesis/analysis
  - —Neutrophilic leukocytosis (usually 50,000 leukocytes/mm^3)
  - —Positive culture when 80,000 leukocytes/mm^3
- Pharyngeal/rectal cultures for local symptoms in high-risk individuals
- CBC for suspected PID
- Urinalysis for suspected PID/lower abdominal pain in females
- Pregnancy test for lower abdominal pain

DIFFERENTIAL DIAGNOSIS

- Urethritis
  - —Chlamydia
  - —Trichomonas
  - —Urinary tract infection
  - —Syphilis
- Disseminated GC
  - —Meningococcus (rash)
  - —Reiter's syndrome
  - —Rheumatic fever
  - —Systemic lupus
  - —Hepatitis

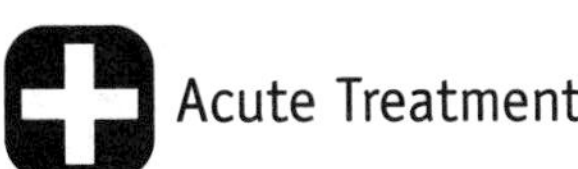

Acute Treatment

INITIAL STABILIZATION

- 0.9%NS 500 cc IV fluids bolus for dehydration due to nausea/vomiting

ED TREATMENT

Genital Infection

- Uncomplicated male genital or female/male pharyngeal/rectal infection
  - —1 dose of the following plus 7-day course of doxycycline or 1 dose of azithromycin
    - —Ceftriaxone 250 mg IM
    - —Cefixime 400 mg po
    - —Ofloxacin 400 mg po
    - —Ciprofloxin 500 mg po
- Salpingitis/pelvic inflammatory disease
  - —Outpatient options
    - —1 dose cefixime/ceftriaxone/spectinomycin plus 14-day course of doxycycline
    - —Ofloxacin 400 mg bid plus clindamycin 450 mg tid or metronidazole 500 mg bid for 14 days
  - —Inpatient options
    - —Cefoxitin IV plus doxycycline IV
- Gonorrhea in pregnancy
  - —1-dose ceftriaxone or spectinomycin plus 7-day course of erythromycin
- Treat sexual partners
- Recommend syphilis (RPR)/HIV testing

Nongenital Infections

- Disseminated GC
  - —Open drainage of septic joints rarely indicated
  - —Inpatient antibiotics for moderate to severe infection
    - —Oral outpatient antibiotics to conclude 7-day course once improvement
  - —Outpatient antibiotics for mild infection not involving weight-bearing joints
  - —Antibiotic options
    - —Ceftriaxone 1 g IM q 24 hrs
    - —Ceftizoxime 1 g IV q 8
    - —Cefotaxime 1 g IV q 8
    - —Spectinomycin 2 mg IM q 12 hrs
    - —Cefixime 400 mg po bid
    - —Ciprofloxacin 500 mg po bid
- Conjunctivitis
  - —Opthalmia neonatorum options
    - —Penicillin G 100,000 IU/kg/24 hrs q 6 hrs
    - —Ceftriaxone 25–50 mg/kg/24 hrs q day
    - —Ceftriaxone 125 mg IM/IV

MEDICATIONS

- Azithromycin: 1 g po
- Cefixime: 400 mg po
- Cefotaxime: 1 g IV 8 hrs
- Cefoxitin: 2 g IV q 6 hrs
- Ceftizoxime: 1 g IV q 8 hrs
- Ceftriaxone: 125–250 mg IM; 1 g (peds: 25–50 mg/kg/24 hrs) IV q 24 hrs
- Ciprofloxin: 500 mg po
- Clindamycin: 450 mg po tid
- Doxycycline: 100 mg IV/PO q 12 hrs
- Erythromycin: 500 mg po q 6 hrs
- Metronidazole: 500 mg po bid
- Ofloxacin: 400 mg po
- Penicillin G: 100,000 IU/kg/24 hrs q 6 hrs
- Spectinomycin: 2 g IM q 12 hrs

HOSPITAL ADMISSION CRITERIA

- Moderate to severe disseminated GC with arthritis involving weight-bearing joints
- PID with
  - —Peritoneal signs
  - —WBC $>15,000/mm^3$
  - —Vomiting
  - —Conjunctivitis requiring IV antibiotics

HOSPITAL DISCHARGE CRITERIA

- Uncomplicated genital, pharyngeal, or conjunctival infection
- Mild disseminated GC in nontoxic patient without arthritis in weight-bearing joints
- Encourage treatment of sexual partners

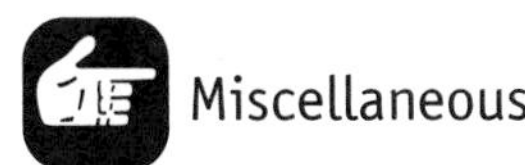

Miscellaneous

ICD-9 CODE

98.0

CORE CONTENT CODE

9.1.2

BIBLIOGRAPHY

Adimora AA, Hamilton H, Holmes KK, Sparling PF. *Sexually transmitted diseases—companion handbook*. New York: McGraw Hill, 1994.

Berger RE. Sexually transmitted diseases. *Adv Urol* 1997;2:97.

Centers for Disease Control and Prevention. 1993 Sexually transmitted disease treatment guidelines. *MMWR* 1993;42:1–102.

Author: David Levine

Gout/Pseudogout

Basics

SIGNS AND SYMPTOMS

- *Gout and pseudogout* both present abruptly as monoarticular arthritis
- Increased warmth, erythema, swelling of the joint
- Early attacks subside spontaneously within 3–10 days, even without treatment
- Later attacks may last longer, cluster, and be more severe
- Crystalline deposition presents as a subacute, acute, or chronic arthritis
  —Primarily affects articular cartilage, synovium, and nearby tendons or ligaments

Gout

- Symptoms present maximally within 12–24 hours
- Gout also affects bone and subcutaneous tissues (tophi and joint desquamation)
- In women, there is polyarticular predominance (up to 70%)
- Less dramatic presentations in the immunosuppressed and the elderly
- Most common: 1st metatarsophalangeal joint (75%) > ankle; tarsal area; knee > hand; wrist

Pseudogout

- Typically involves larger joints than gout
- Most common: knee > wrist > metacarpals; shoulder; elbow; ankle > hip; tarsal joints
- Monoarticular (25%)
- Asymptomatic (25%)
- Pseudo-osteoarthritis (45%): progressive degeneration, often symmetric
- Pseudorheumatoid arthritis (in the elderly): a polyarticular variant with fever and confusion

MECHANISM/DESCRIPTION

- Gout is the most common of the crystalline diseases
- Renal dysfunction due to urologic deposition of uric acid calculi
- It affects mainly middle-aged men and postmenopausal women
- Risk factors
  —Male:Female ratio = 9:1
  —Age: <40
  —Obesity; hypertension; diabetes; hyperlipidemia; vascular disease

Four Phases

- Asymptomatic hyperuricemia (up to 20 years)
- Acute gout
- Intercritical gout: initially no signs or symptoms
- Tophaceous gout (up to 45% of cases)
  —Attributed to inadequate treatment, and frequent or persistent attacks
  —Evident usually 10 years after first attack
  —A deforming arthritis
  —Associated with avascular necrosis
  —Tophi
    —Early in postmenopausal women
    —Most frequent in previously damaged joints; synovium; subchondral bone, bursae (olecranon; infrapatellar; prepatellar); Achilles tendon; extensor surface of the forearms; toes; fingers; ear; rarely CNS or cardiac (valves)
  —May coalesce later

Pseudogout (Chondrocalcinosis)

- The most common cause of acute monarthritis after age 60
- Risk factors
  —Hypercalcemia (e.g., hyperparathyroidism, familial); hemochromatosis; hemosiderosis;
  —Hypo- and hyperthyroidism, hypophosphatemia, hypomagnesemia, amyloidosis, or gout

ETIOLOGY

- Gout is caused by deposition of *monosodium urate crystals* in tissues from supersaturated extracellular fluid, due to
  —Underexcretion of uric acid
  —Any rapid change in uric acid levels (e.g., the initiation or cessation of diuretics, alcohol, salicylates, cyclosporine, lead acetate poisoning, and uricosurics or allopurinol)
- Pseudogout occurs secondary to excess synovial accumulation of *calcium pyrophosphate* crystals
- Precipitants for both gout and pseudogout include minor trauma and acute illnesses (e.g., surgery, ischemic heart disease)

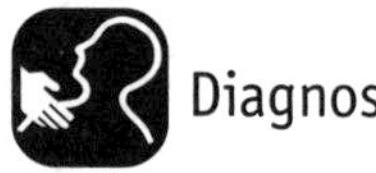

Diagnosis

ESSENTIAL WORKUP

- Arthrocentesis and aspiration pf tophi
  —Examine aspirant for crystals, Gram's stain, cultures, leukocyte count, and differential
  —Fluid is typically thick pasty white
  —*Gout:* 20,000–100,000 WBC/mm^3; poor string and mucin clot; no bacteria
  —*Pseudogout:* up to 50,000 WBC/mm^3; no bacteria
- Microscopic examination of crystals under polarized light
  —*Gout:* needle-shaped; strong birefringence; negative elongation
  —*Pseudogout:* rhomboid; weak birefringence; positive elongation

LABORATORY

- CBC often shows a leukocytosis that does not differentiate infectious from crystalline etiology
- Chemistry panel to assess for renal impairment
- Magnesium and calcium, TSH, and serum iron
- Uric acid level has limited value
  —It is normal in 30% of acute gouty attacks
  —In screening general populations, hyperuricemia is mostly asymptomatic (90% of cases)
- If infectious arthritis is suspected
  —Blood and urine cultures
  —Urethral, cervical, rectal, or pharyngeal gonococcal cultures

IMAGING/SPECIAL TESTS

- Plain radiographs to assess the presence of
  —Effusion
  —Joint space narrowing
  —The baseline status of the joint
  —Contiguous osteomyelitis

—Fractures or foreign body
—*Acute Gout:* soft tissue swelling; normal mineralization; joint space preservation
—*Chronic Gout:* calcified tophi; asymmetric bony erosions; overhanging edges; bony shaft tapering
—*Pseudogout:* chondrocalcinosis; subchondral sclerosis or cysts (wrist); radiopaque calcification of cartilage, tendons, and ligaments; radiopaque osteophytes
- 24-hour urine uric acid may detect uric acid underexcretion

DIFFERENTIAL DIAGNOSIS

- Infectious arthritis
- Trauma
- Osteoarthritis
- Reactive arthritis
- Miscellaneous crystalline arthritis
- Aseptic necrosis
- Rheumatoid arthritis
- Systemic lupus erythematosus
- Sickle cell
- Osteomyelitis

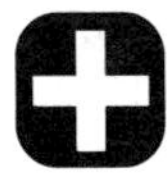

Acute Treatment

INITIAL STABILIZATION

- Relieve pain
- Rule out an infectious etiology

ED TREATMENT

- NSAIDs are the first line treatment
- If ineffective or contraindicated
  —Oral prednisone
  —Colchicine (limited by toxicity)
- Joint aspiration with or without intra-articular steroid injection
- Avoid aspirin
- The reduction of hyperuricemia and the long-term management of gout and pseudogout are not within the usual scope of ED care. Strategies include
  —The careful withdrawal of gout-producing agent
  —In gout, uricosurics or allopurinol can be used to reduce uric acid
  —Uricosurics (e.g., probenecid, sulfinpyrazone) increase uric acid excretion
  —Increased fluid intake and urine alkalization to prevent renal stones
  —Allopurinol is the most effective agent. It is recommended for overproducers, renal disease, those undergoing cytotoxic therapy, uricosuric failure, frequent attacks, and tophaceous disease
  —Long-term colchicine or NSAIDs may be effective prophylactically against pseudogout and gout

MEDICATIONS

- NSAIDs in maximal doses initially ×3 d, then taper over 4 d
  —Indomethacin: 50 mg po tid qid
  —Ketorolac: 15–30 mg IM/IV in ED, may × repeat 1 dose
  —Naproxen: 500 mg po tid
  —Sulindac: 200 mg po tid
- Corticosteroids
  —Prednisone: 40 mg po qd ×3–4 d; taper over 7–14 d
  —Methylprednisolone: 40 mg IM or IV qd ×3–4 d
  —Triamcinolone: 10–40 mg plus dexamethasone 2–10 mg intra-articular
- Colchicine: 0.5 mg/hr po up to pain relief, 8 mg total, or GI toxicity
- Probenecid: 250–500 mg po bid 1st dose
- Allopurinol: 100–300 mg po qd 1st dose

HOSPITAL ADMISSION CRITERIA

- Suspected infectious arthritis
- Acute renal failure
- Intractable pain

HOSPITAL DISCHARGE CRITERIA

- No evidence of infection
- Adequate pain relief

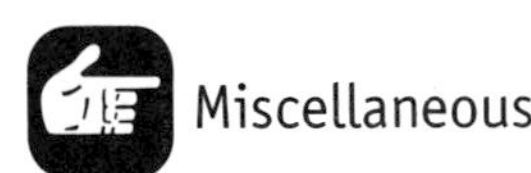

Miscellaneous

ICD-9 CODE

274.9
275.49

CORE CONTENT CODE

10.2.1.2

BIBLIOGRAPHY

Buckley TJ. Radiologic features of gout. *Am Fam Physician* 1996;54(4):1232–1238.

Joseph J, McGrath H. Gout or "pseudogout": How to differentiate crystal-induced arthropathies. *Geriatrics* 1995;50(4):33–39.

McGill NW. Gout and other crystal arthropathies. *Med J Aust* 1997;166:33–38.

Schumacher HR. Crystal-induced arthritis: An overview. *Am J Med* 1996;100(Suppl 2A):46S–51S.

Authors: Delaram Ghadishah and A. Antoine Kazzi

Hand Infection

Basics

SIGNS AND SYMPTOMS

Paronychia

- Localized edema, erythema, and pain in proximal portion of lateral nail fold
- Fluctuance may be present and may extend beneath the nail margin to the nail bed
- Systemic signs and symptoms are usually not present

Felon

- Erythema and tense swelling of the distal pulp space that does *not* extend proximal to the PIP
- Aching pain early, severe throbbing pain late
- Systemic signs and symptoms are usually not present

Herpetic Whitlow

- Distal pulp space is swollen, but remains soft
- Lateral nail folds may be affected
- Throbbing pain of the distal pulp space
- Vesicles containing nonpurulent fluid are present and may form bullae
- Systemic symptoms may be present, as fever, lymphadenopathy, and constitutional symptoms

Flexor Tenosynovitis

- Severe pain and symmetric edema of the digit, usually the thumb, index finger, or middle finger
- Severe tenderness over the course of the tendon sheath
- Flexed position of the finger at rest
- Pain on passive extension of the finger—may be the only finding in early infection

Clenched Fist Injury

- Laceration over the MCP from striking an object with a clenched fist
- Any laceration over the MCP must be assumed to be a human bite wound until proven otherwise

Web Space Abscess

- Pain and edema of the affected web space and adjacent palm
- Fingers are held abducted

Palmar Space Infections

- Thenar space infection
  - —Pain, tenderness, tense edema of thenar eminence
  - —Dorsal edema without tenderness
  - —Thumb is held abducted and flexed, and passive adduction is painful
- Midpalmar space infection
  - —Pain, edema, and tenderness of the midpalmar space
  - —Dorsal edema without tenderness
  - —Motion of middle and ring fingers is painful
- Hypothenar space infection
  - —Pain and fullness over hypothenar eminence
  - —No limitation of finger movement

ETIOLOGY

- Bacterial infection of the hand is associated with skin pathogens, *Staphylococcus* or *Streptococcus* species, and history of a puncture wound
- Anaerobes are identified in 75% of paronychia in children due to thumb sucking and nail biting
- Chronic paronychia may be caused by *Candida albicans*
- Herpetic whitlow is caused by type 1 or 2 herpes simplex virus
- Clenched fist injuries involve a variety of pathogens, including anaerobic *Streptococcus* and *Eikenella*

PRE-HOSPITAL

- No specific considerations

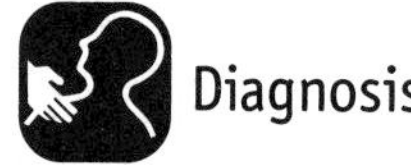

Diagnosis

ESSENTIAL WORKUP

- Most hand infections are diagnosed by history and physical examination with special attention to neurovascular status

LABORATORY

- Although usually not necessary, herpetic whitlow may be confirmed by Tzank test
- Gram stain and culture may guide antibiotic choice in felons
- Blood cultures are not routinely indicated

IMAGING/SPECIAL TESTS

- Radiographs are usually not helpful in paronychia unless there has been trauma or a suspected foreign body
- With felon, flexor tenosynovitis, and palmar space infection, radiograph may identify osteomyelitis or foreign body
- Radiographs in clenched fist injury may reveal a fracture

DIFFERENTIAL DIAGNOSIS

- Paronychia should be differentiated from herpetic whitlow and felon
- The differential for palmar space infection includes flexor tenosynovitis, cellulitis, and web space infection

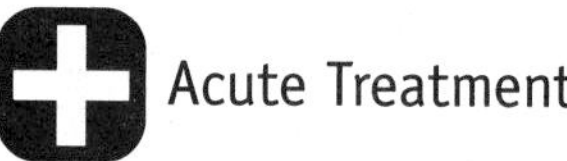

Acute Treatment

INITIAL STABILIZATION

- ABCs if patient is toxic or above conditions occur in the setting of sepsis or other injury

ED TREATMENT

Paronychia

- Early paronychia without purulence present may be managed with oral antibiotics and rest
  - —Cephalexin, dicloxacillin
  - —Clindamycin or erythromycin if associated with nail biting or oral contact
- Superficial infections are drained by inserting an 11-blade between nail and eponychium and lifting the eponychium from the nail
- If necessary, the lateral nail fold may be incised tangential to the curvature of the nail
- When pus is present under the adjacent nail, one-fourth of the nail should be removed
- When pus is present under the dorsal roof of the proximal nail, remove one-third of the proximal nail

Felon

- Felons are drained through a unilateral longitudinal incision which does not cross the DIP flexor crease
  —A lateral incision is preferred to drain distal pulp infection
  —Make sure the incision avoids the neurovascular bundle
- Disruption of fibrous septa is no longer recommended because it results in an unstable fingertip
- Give oral antibiotics to cover skin pathogens, place a drain, and recheck in 48 hours
  —Cephalexin, dicloxacillin

Herpetic Whitlow

- Usually self-limited; do not incise and drain
- Oral acyclovir may be given to patients with systemic infection

Flexor Tenosynovitis, Web Space Abscess, Palmar Space Infection

- Elevation, IV antibiotics, and pain control in the ED
  —Ampicillin/sulbactam, cefoxitin, ticarcillin/clavulanate
- All of these infections require consultation with a hand surgeon for admission and drainage

Clenched Fist Injury

- Elevation, IV antibiotics, tetanus prophylaxis, and pain control in the ED
  —Ampicillin/sulbactam, cefoxitin, ticarcillin/clavulanate
- All bite wounds with evidence of infection or joint involvement require emergent consultation with a hand surgeon
- If there are no signs of infection and no joint penetration, patients may be considered for outpatient treatment with oral antibiotics after appropriate irrigation and wound care
  —Ampicillin/clavulanate or penicillin V plus cephalexin or dicloxacillin
  —Do not primarily close lacerations associated with a human bite; delayed primary closure or healing by secondary intention is appropriate

MEDICATIONS

- Acyclovir: adult: 400 mg po tid for 10 d; peds: not recommended for herpetic whitlow
- Ampicillin/clavulanate: adult: 875/125 mg po bid; peds: 40 mg/kg/d po div q 6 hrs
- Ampicillin/sulbactam: adult: 2 g IV q 6 hrs; peds: safety not established
- Cefoxitin: adult: 2 g IV q 8 hrs; peds: 80–160 mg/kg/d IV or IM div q 6 hrs
- Cephalexin: adult: 500 g po qid for 7 d; peds: 40 mg/kg/d po div q 6 hrs
- Clindamycin: adult: 300 mg po qid for 7 d; peds: 20–40 mg/kg/d div q 6 hrs po, IV, IM
- Dicloxacillin: adult: 500 mg po qid for 7 d; peds: 12.5–50 mg/kg/d po div q 6 hrs
- Erythromycin: adult: 500 mg po qid for 7 d; peds: 40 mg/kg/d div q 6 hrs po
- Penicillin V: adult: 250 mg po qid; peds: 40 mg/kg/d po div q 6 hrs
- Ticarcillin/clavulanate: adult: 3.1 g IV q 6 hrs; peds: safety not established

HOSPITAL ADMISSION CRITERIA

- ***Flexor Tenosynovitis, Web Space Abscess, Palmar Space Infections***
  —All these infections require admission for IV antibiotics and drainage
- ***Clenched Fist Injury with Signs of Infection***
  —Requires admission for surgical debridement and IV antimicrobials

HOSPITAL DISCHARGE CRITERIA

- ***Paronychia and Felons***
  —Patients with uncomplicated paronychia or felon may be discharged from the ED with a recheck and drain removal in 48 hours
- ***Herpetic Whitlow***
  —Patients with herpetic whitlow may be discharged from the ED with appropriate follow-up
- ***Clenched Fist Injury Without Infection***
  —May be discharged on oral antibiotics with follow-up in 24 hours

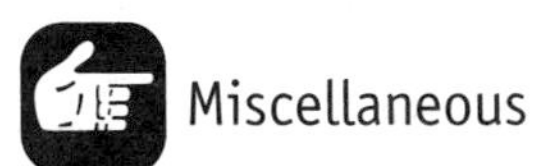

Miscellaneous

ICD-9-CM

136.9

CORE CONTENT CODE

3.2

BIBLIOGRAPHY

Brown DM, Young VL. Hand infections. *South Med J* 1993;86(1):56–66.

Hausman MR, Lisser SP. Hand infections. *Orthop Clin North Am* 1992;23(1):171–185.

Antosia RE, Lyn E. The hand. In: Rosen P, et al., eds. *Emergency medicine: Concepts and clinical practice*. 4th ed. St. Louis: CV Mosby, 1998:625–668.

Authors: Deborah Sanders and Robert Galli

Hematuria

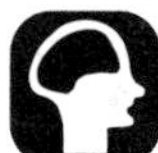

Basics

DEFINITION

- Presence of >2 red blood cells/high-power field (RBC/HPF) of sediment on a clean void specimen for males and nonmenstruating females, or >2 RBC/HPF on a catheter specimen for menstruating females.
- Note: 1 mL of blood per liter of urine can produce a visible color change.
- Microscopic or gross hematuria is a common occurrence in people who exercise strenuously; generally has benign prognosis if blood clears within 24–48 hours.
- Persistent, recurrent, symptomatic, or traumatic hematuria warrants further evaluation.

EXERCISE-INDUCED HEMATURIA

- Occurs with or without trauma in males and females; resolves with rest in 2–3 days.
- Although a benign condition, it is a diagnosis of exclusion.
- Directly correlated with intensity and duration of exertion
- Traumatic mechanisms
  —Direct kidney trauma
  —Contusion of the mobile bladder wall with the fixed wall in an empty bladder during running
- Atraumatic mechanisms
  —Physiologic decreased renal blood flow during exercise causing hypoxic damage to the nephron leading to increased permeability for RBCs and proteins
  —Relatively more marked constriction of the efferent arteriole leads to increased filtration pressure favoring excretion of RBCs and protein
- Hydration and a partially full bladder during exercise may help prevent or minimize this condition.

INCIDENCE

- Exercise-induced hematuria (EIH) = unknown
- All other causes
  —Age <40 usually infection
  —Age >40 increasing incidence of tumor
  —Males >60 usually prostatic obstruction, calculi, or tumor
  —Females >60 usually malignancy

SIGNS AND SYMPTOMS

- Fever
- Urethral discharge
- Flank ecchymosis
- Many patients will not have any signs.
- Painless red or brown urine
- Dysuria
- Frequency
- Hesitancy
- Flank pain
- Suprapubic pain
- Many are asymptomatic.

RISK FACTORS

- Chronic urinary tract infection
- Anticoagulation
- Strenuous exercise
- History of calculi, prostatitis, trauma, malignancy, coagulopathy, or sexually transmitted disease
- Family history of renal failure
- Travel to Africa, India, or the Middle East

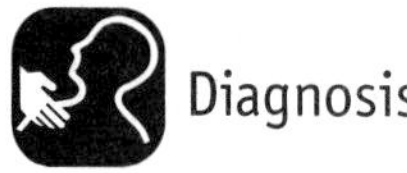

Diagnosis

DIFFERENTIAL DIAGNOSIS

Painful

- Pyelonephritis
- Prostatitis
- Cystitis
- Urethritis
- Calculi
- Trauma
- Bladder tumor
- Renal tumor
- Renal artery aneurysm
- Renal vein thrombosis

Painless

- Malignancies
- Glomerulonephropathy, especially in children
- Polycystic kidney disease
- Sickle cell trait or disease
- Coagulation defect (clotting factor deficiency, thrombocytopenia, polycythemia)
- Vasculitis (lupus, Goodpasture syndrome)
- Infection (endocarditis, tuberculosis [TB], syphilis)
- Iatrogenic: anticoagulation; catheterization; nonsteroidal anti-inflammatory drug (NSAID) nephritis: decrease in vasodilating prostaglandin causes decreased renal blood flow leading to nephron damage and hyperfiltration
- Early calculi formation (cause of microscopic damage): hypercalciuria (>4 mg Ca/kg/day in a 24-hour urine specimen); hyperuricosuria (>750 mg uric acid/day); hypocitruria (<450mg citrate/day for men, <650 mg/day for women; citrate helps prevent stone formation)
- EIH

Pseudohematuria

- Myoglobinuria due to rhabdomyolysis (no RBCs in HPF)
- Hemolysis and/or "march hematuria" (no RBCs in HPF; red cells are hemolyzed in foot capillaries during marching)
- Medication: phenothiazine, phenolphthalein laxatives, rifampin, phenazopyridine (Pyridium), phenytoin, quinine
- Porphyria
- Vegetable dyes (beets, rhubarb)
- Vaginal blood contamination

HISTORY

- Age (if age >40, warrants full workup for genitourinary malignancy)
- Trauma
- Onset with relation to recent exercise; EIH can occur any time between 0 and 12 hours after exercise.
- Recent upper respiratory infection suggests poststreptococcal glomerulonephritis or immunoglobulin A nephropathy.
- Unilateral flank pain suggests calculi or pyelonephritis.
- Family history of sickle cell trait or disease (papillary necrosis caused by sickling in the renal medulla)
- Hesitancy and dribbling (signs of prostatic obstruction)
- Family history of polycystic kidney disease or hereditary nephritis, primarily in males
- Dysuria or frequency suggest infection
- Fever, night sweats, or weight loss suggest TB or malignancy
- Bleeding disorder; anticoagulant or NSAID use
- Travel to Africa, India, the Middle East, or Indian Ocean Islands (possible *Schistosomiasis haematobium* infestation)

PHYSICAL EXAMINATION

- Vitals (fever, hypertension, tachycardia)
- Inspection of urethral meatus, flank, and abdomen for signs of trauma
- Auscultation for renal artery bruits, pericarditis, and endocarditis
- Prostate examination in males to evaluate for tenderness, mass, and size
- Pelvic examination in females to evaluate for tenderness and mass
- Stepwise approach to the patient
  —Step 1. History and physical examination (HPE) as above
    —If HPE reveals only a history of exercise in a patient <40 years, observe and repeat urinalysis after 48–72 hours.
    —If urinalysis is normal, no further studies are warranted. Observe the patient for recurrence.
    —If hematuria persists or HPE suggests cause other than EIH, proceed to step 2.

—Step 2. Obtain the following laboratory tests:
  —Urine culture and serum creatinine, blood urea nitrogen (BUN), complete blood count (CBC), prothrombin time (PT), partial thromboplastin time (PTT), sickle cell preparation
  —Consider serum creatine kinase to rule out rhabdomyolysis.
  —If serum creatinine normal, obtain intravenous pyelogram (IVP) to evaluate for obstruction, mass, and kidney function.
  —If results of these tests are normal, proceed to step 3.
—Step 3. Cystoscopy
  —If normal, proceed to step 4.
—Step 4. Ultrasound or computed tomographic (CT) scan
  —Include bladder, especially if patient >40
  —CT can detect early bladder tumors missed on cystoscopy.
  —If normal, proceed to step 5.
—Step 5. Consider renal arteriogram
  —Evaluate for vasculitis, atrioventricular malformation, and renal infarction/thrombosis
  —If normal, proceed to step 6.
—Step 6. Consider renal biopsy
  —Evaluate for interstitial kidney disease
  —If at any time concurrent proteinuria, dysmorphic RBCs, or casts are present
  —Obtain 24-hour urine for protein, creatinine, calcium, citrate, and uric acid
  —Consider serum Antistreptolysin Otiter, Venereal Disease Research Lab, antineutrophil cytoplasmic antibody complement levels, antiglomerular basement membrane antibody levels, Hepatitis B serology.
  —Consider renal biopsy if results of all above tests are negative.

IMAGING

- Plain x-ray views kidney shape, size, number, and radiopaque calculi.
- Ultrasound views size, shape, mass, obstruction, scarring due to pyelonephritis, and radiolucent stones.
- CT same as ultrasound plus detects early bladder tumors missed on cystoscopy
- IVP views size, shape, calyceal anatomy, obstruction, and function.
- Voiding cystourethrogram (VCUG) detects vesicoureteral reflux.
- Retrograde pyelogram determines site of obstruction.
- Arteriography detects renovascular hypertension, polyarteritis nodosa, thromboemboli, mass, and aneurysm.
- Cystoscopy provides direct visualization of bladder and urethra.

LABORATORY TESTS

- Urinalysis
  —Analyze within 30 minutes or refrigerate immediately to prevent change in bacterial count and hemolysis
  —Must include cell count to rule out pseudohematuria
  —RBC alone suggests prostatic disease, pelvic or ureteral calculi, trauma, heavy exercise, or malignancy.
  —White blood cells + RBC suggests infection.
  —RBC + protein/casts/dysmorphic RBCs/or absence of clots suggests glomerular disease.
  —RBC casts are virtually diagnostic of glomerulonephritis or vasculitis.
  —RBC clots usually indicate extraglomerular bleeding (urokinase in the glomeruli prevents clotting).
- Urine culture (consider acid-fast bacilli culture if suspect tuberculosis)
- 24-hour urine for protein (consider electrophoresis for Bence-Jones protein/multiple myeloma), creatinine, calcium, uric acid, and citrate
- CBC, PT, PTT to evaluate for coagulopathy
- Serum creatinine/BUN/electrolytes to evaluate renal function
- Three-tube test may help isolate the specific origin of bleeding in isolated hematuria.
  —Collection and comparative evaluation of the number of RBCs in three urine specimens of roughly equal volume
  —First few milliliters (indicates a urethral lesion), a midstream sample, and the last few milliliters (possible lesion at the trigone region of the bladder if this sample alone has most RBCs).
  —If all three samples have similar levels of RBCs, the lesion more likely is renal, ureteric, or diffuse bladder disease.

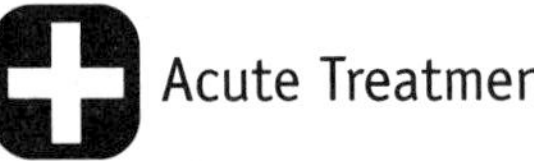

Acute Treatment

ANALGESIA

- Pyridium can be given for cystitis.
- Avoid NSAIDS until diagnosis is clear and renal insufficiency and nephritis have been ruled out.

SPECIAL CONSIDERATIONS

- Signs of shock (tachycardia, hypotension), expanding flank mass, or oliguria require emergent urologic referral.
- Prescribe rest until hematuria resolves if EIH suspected.
- Emphasize hydration during exercise and avoidance of urination within 15–20 minutes of onset of exercise.

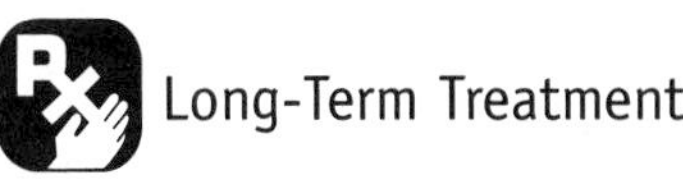

Long-Term Treatment

REFERRAL/DISPOSITION

- Referral to urologist or nephrologist where appropriate

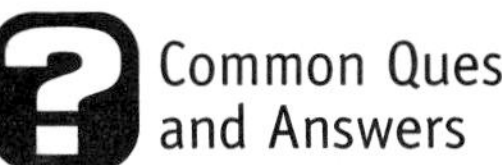

Common Questions and Answers

Physician responses to common patient questions:
Q: When can I return to play?
A: Acceptable if hematuria resolves after 48–72 hours of rest; otherwise counsel on an individual basis depending on the diagnosis.

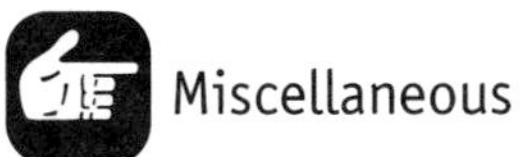

Miscellaneous

PEARLS

- Persistent hematuria must always be worked up.
- Transient hematuria can be normal in young people, but must be worked up in all patients >40 years.

ICD-9 CODE

None known for EIH, use 599.70
599.7 Hematuria, benign
595.0 Cystitis (acute = .01, chronic = .02)
120.0 Schistosomiasis due to *Schistosoma haematobium*

BIBLIOGRAPHY

Goldszer R, Siegel A. *Renal abnormalities during exercise, sports medicine.* Philadelphia: WB Saunders, 1991.

Healy P, Jacobsen E. *Proteinuria, common medical diagnosis, an algorithmic approach,* 2nd ed. Philadelphia: WB Saunders, 1994: 79.

Roy S, Noe N. Renal disease in childhood. In: Walsh PC, ed. *Campbell's urology.* Philadelphia: WB Saunders, 1998:1673.

Cianflocco AJ. Renal complications of exercise. *Clin Sports Med* 1992;11:437–451.

Abarbanel J, et al. Sports hematuria. *J Urol* 1990;143:887–890.

Authors: W. Mark Peluso and Michael J. Henehan

Hepatitis, Viral

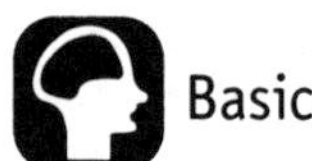

Basics

DESCRIPTION

A group of systemic infections involving the liver with common clinical manifestations; caused by different viruses with typically distinctive epidemiological patterns
System(s) affected: Gastrointestinal
Genetics: Some predisposition to immunologic manifestations; DR4 - positive increase with concurrent immunologic disease
Incidence/Prevalence in USA:

- HAV—33% of Americans have antibodies; 125,000–200,000 infections/yr; 70% symptomatic
- HBV—140,000–320,000 infections/year; 1–1.25 million chronically infected; >500,000 carriers (10% of infected). Post-transfusion HBV <1% of blood recipients.
- HCV—16% of sporadic hepatitis: 35,000–180,000 new infections year; 3.9 million chronically infected (85% of infected)
- HDV—present in 1% of HBV—co-infection or superinfection
- HEV—unknown

Predominant age: HAV rare in infants; susceptibility increases with age. HBV, HCV, HEV occur in all ages.
Predominant sex: Fulminant HBV: Male > Female (2:1)

SIGNS AND SYMPTOMS

- Fever (60%); unusual with HBV and HCV
- Malaise (67%)
- Nausea (80%)
- Anorexia (54%)
- Jaundice (in adults, 62%); 66% of HCV anicteric
- Dark urine (84%)
- Abdominal pain (56%)
- Fatigue (major complaint in HCV)
- Headache
- Meningismus (occasional)
- Vomiting

CAUSES

- Multiple viruses possible
- HAV and HEV transmitted enterically (fecal-oral); parenteral route rare
- Maximum infectivity 2 weeks before jaundice
- May be endemic in institutions
- HBV transmitted sexually or by blood products including infection acquired perinatally; also enterically. HDV coinfection increases HBV severity.
- HCV transmitted through blood or its products; in 40%, mode unknown
- HDV identified only with HBV infection
- HGV has similar patterns to HCV, not pathogenic
- Chronicity
  —HAV, HEV—no chronicity
  —HBV 2–5%
  —HDV—almost all
  —HCV—50–80%
- Primary liver cancer risk
  —HCV associated cirrhosis—1–3% per year, lifetime risk 20%
  —HBV—cancer may occur with or without preexisting cirrhosis
  —HBV positively increases cancer risk, needs therapy

RISK FACTORS

- Health care workers/other occupational risks
- Hemodialysis
- Recipients of blood and/or blood products
- IV drug users (53% of new infections); individuals with tattoos
- Sexually active homosexual males
- Household exposure
- Intimate exposure
- Positive needlestick
- Transplanted organs

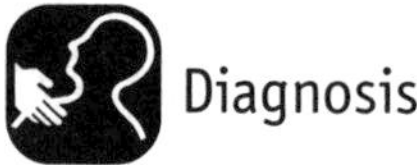

Diagnosis

DIFFERENTIAL DIAGNOSIS

Infectious mononucleosis, primary or secondary hepatic malignancy, ischemic hepatitis, drug-induced hepatitis, alcoholic hepatitis, autoimmune hepatitis, Wilson's disease

LABORATORY

- Marked elevation of AST/ALT (acute hepatitis, particularly ALT, 400-several thousand U/L); HCV may have normal ALT; AST/ALT ratio ⇒ 1 associated with cirrhosis in chronic HCV
- Mild elevation of alkaline phosphatase
- Bilirubin from normal to markedly elevated; with elevation, conjugated and unconjugated fractions usually increased
- Serological markers to identify viruses

Diagnosis Biochemical markers

HAV:	
A, R	Anti-HAV IgM
P	Anti-HAV IgG
HBV:	
A, E	HBsAg
A	Anti-HBc IgM, HBsAg, HBeAg
C	HBsAg, ± HBeAg
HCV:	
A, C, Rcv	Anti-HCV (ELISA)
HDV:	
A	HDAg, Anti-HDV IgM
P	Anti-HDV IgG
HEV:	Test not available
HGV:	Unnecessary

A = acute infection, R = recent infection, C = chronic infection, P = previous infection, E = early/carrier state, Rcv = Recovered

- For severe hepatitis, measure PT and PTT, albumin, electrolytes, glucose and CBC
- If HBV chronic, confirm by HBV-DNA titer
- Patients with severe HBV infection should be tested for coinfection or superinfection with HDV
- HBeAg indicates high infectivity (horizontal and vertical transmission)
- Persistence >10 weeks indicates probable: chronic liver disease
- Acute, ongoing HCV, confirm by other markers, RIBA, HCV-RNA (for chronic HCV); viral titers in genotypes 1a, 1b >2, 3e
- In early acute HCV infection, anti-HCV may be negative; may need retest in 3–6 months
- HCV-RNA becomes positive early in acute cases
- HCV genotypes may be useful. Genotypes with favorable prognosis—2a, 2b, 3a; less favorable 1a, 1b

Drugs that may alter lab results: N/A
Disorders that may alter lab results: N/A

PATHOLOGICAL FINDINGS

Liver biopsy in persistent or chronic disease shows wide range of histologic changes (variable inflammation and/or necrosis, cholestasis, lymphoid aggregate, steatosis, fibrosis, cirrhosis or chronic active hepatitis). Clinical course does not predict severity of histopathologic changes.

SPECIAL TESTS

Liver biopsy usually needed for determining type and extent of liver injury in persistent disease and to exclude other diseases. Also, usually necessary prior to start of interferon alfa treatment.

IMAGING

Usually helpful. Ultrasound may demonstrate ascites or exclude obstruction. Helpful when cancer is suspected.

DIAGNOSTIC PROCEDURES

- History; exposure source; exclude drugs
- Tenderness on list percussion over the liver; may be hepatomegaly
- Jaundice may not be present in most
- Serum "liver function tests" often elevated before bilirubin increases; measure aminotransferases in acute illnesses when there is no evident cause
- Serum biochemical markers for each virus, diagnosis in 90% of patients

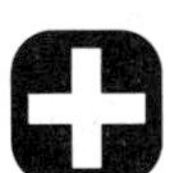

Acute Treatment

APPROPRIATE HEALTH CARE

- Outpatient care usual
- Segregation helpful for food handlers with HAV, or health care workers with HBV or HCV

GENERAL MEASURES

- Correct: coagulation defects, fluid and electrolytes, acid-base imbalance, hypoglycemia, impairment of renal function
- Report acute cases to public health dept

SURGICAL MEASURES

Consider liver transplantation in fulminant acute hepatitis/end-stage liver disease (HCV) and in early stages of primary liver cancer

ACTIVITY

As tolerated

DIET

Adequate calories; balanced nutrition

PATIENT EDUCATION

- Proper use and disposal of needles
- Proper hygiene, particularly food handlers
- HBV sexually transmitted; HCV sexual transmission low, but does occur
- HBV present in saliva also

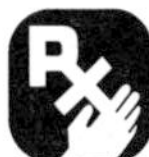

Long-Term Treatment

DRUG(S) OF CHOICE

- Interferon alfa-2b (IFN, Intron A) or Interferon alfa-2a (Roferon-A) (HCV), or with ribavirin (Virazole) 1 g/day. Induces remission (25–50% in HBV; 40% in HCV); decreases abnormal aminotransferase concentrations in chronic HBV/HCV. May be used safely post-transplant.
- Lamivudine 100 mg qid po is as effective as interferon
- Corticosteroids: in cholestatic HAV, a short course may shorten illness, but may be most effective in milder disease

Contraindications: Interferon: platelet count <50,000. Mouse immunoglobulin, egg protein or neomycin allergy. Corticosteroids may add to morbidity/increased mortality.
Precautions:

- Other disorders of coagulation, myelosuppression, seizures, depression (esp. suicide ideation), pregnancy, fertile age group, lactation.
- Increased serum triglycerides may occur during IFN therapy; may cause abnormal ALT. Measure HCV-RNA to assess response in such patients.
- Psychiatric evaluation may be prudent prior to IFN treatment in chronic HCV

Significant possible interactions: Refer to manufacturer's profile of each drug

ALTERNATIVE DRUGS

Famciclovir (Famvir) 500 mg tid for chronic hepatitis B

Hepatitis, Viral

PATIENT MONITORING

- Serial measurement of serum AST/ALT
- Appropriate serum viral markers useful for evaluation of recovery or progression
- Liver biopsies in chronic disease
- Monitor for metabolic complications
- WBC, platelets with interferon alpha therapy
- Chronic HBV, HBV-DNA valuable for prediction of favorable response to IFN. High pretreatment ALT and low pretreatment HBV-DNA associated with favorable response.
- With HCV, quantitative serum HCV-RNA levels monitor response and post-treatment relapse (if negative after 3 months, sustained response likely)

PREVENTION/AVOIDANCE

- General
  —Screen blood products
  —Proper disposal of needles
  —Good sanitation, hygiene
- HAV
  —Immune globulin (passive immunization): 0.02 mL/kg IM (given 1–2 weeks after exposure prevents illness in 80–90%). With prolonged exposure give q 5 months. Also use for close contacts, day care staff/children (if case occurs), institutions with multiple cases, travelers to areas of high prevalence (with 3 week lead time, use vaccine).
  —Hepatitis A vaccine (Havrix, Vaqta): 0.5 mL dose IM in children >2 yrs; 1 mL in adults IM; 2nd dose 6–12 mo later for >8 yrs. Separate syringe site from immune globulin. Use for travelers, day-care staff/children, custodial facility employees, sewage workers, military, homosexual men, food handlers, Native Americans/Alaskan natives.
- HBV
  —Hepatitis B vaccine: 3 doses at 0, 1, and 6 months. Dose dependent on manufacturer. Merck Recombivax: 0.5 ml (5 mcg)/dose age ≤19 and 1 mL (10 mcg)/dose age >19. SKB Engerix: 0.5 mL (10 mcg)/dose age ≤19 & 1 mL (20 mcg)/dose age >19.
  —High risk groups: hepatitis B human immune globulin within 24 hr of exposure (0.06 mL/kg IM)
  —HBV screening in pregnant women; vaccinate all infants at birth. Schedule: 3 injections—birth, 2 mo, 6–18 mo. Children/adolescents may start series anytime, but complete by age 11–12 yrs.
- HCV: No specifics on prevention/avoidance
- HDV: Preventing HBV will prevent HDV
- HEV: No specifics on prevention/avoidance

POSSIBLE COMPLICATIONS

Acute or subacute necrosis, chronic active or chronic hepatitis, cirrhosis, hepatic failure; hepatocellular carcinoma (HBV, HCV)

EXPECTED COURSE/PROGNOSIS

- Varies with causative virus
- Severity of hepatic encephalopathy best predictor of poor survival in hepatic failure
- HAV may cause mild disease at times, often no jaundice; no chronic liver disease; mortality <1%; lifetime immunity usual with recovery. 3 rare variants: relapsing, cholestatic, fulminant.
- HBV (mortality 1%) and HDV (with icterus, mortality 2–20%) more severe symptoms; often leads to persistent/chronic liver disease, cirrhosis, liver failure, hepatocellular carcinoma (HCC); more severe problems if impaired immune function. Follow treatment with HBV-DNA levels.
- In HCV, regardless of severity, >80% progress to chronic hepatitis, 20–50% to cirrhosis, and some, liver failure. Typically slow progression 10–30 years. May progress to HCC, but IFN may decrease HCC risk. Association with type II AI. Chronic HCV unlikely to clear HCV-RNA spontaneously. HCV after needlestick, usually sustained IFN response. Final phase HCV rare cause of fulminant hepatic failure.

- Alcohol may be factor for HCC in chronic HCV
- Chronic HDV, 70% develop cirrhosis; low incidence of HCC
- HEV does not result in chronic disease

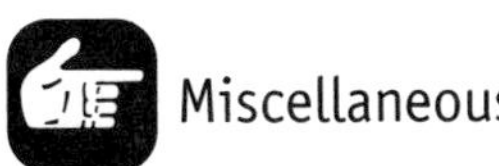

Miscellaneous

ASSOCIATED CONDITIONS

- Arthritis, urticaria, immune complex nephritis (particularly membranous glomerulopathy), anemias (including aplastic anemia), dermatitis and cardiomyopathy (usually with HBV, rare with HCV). HCV implicated in sporadic form of idiopathic mixed cryoglobulinemia, porphyria cutanea tarda, polyarteritis nodosa.
- HIV-HCV: more severe course

AGE-RELATED FACTORS

Pediatric: HAV milder; usually anicteric; may be unrecognized. HBV more acute, less prolonged, less complications, but may become chronic.
Geriatric: N/A
Others: Alcohol abuse a major factor for chronic liver disease from HBV and HCV. Measure viral biochemical markers in patients with alcoholic liver disease (esp. anti-HCV).

PREGNANCY

- Test, in later gestation, for HBsAg
- HBV transmitted vertically (<10%) as well as perinatally and produces carrier state in 30%. Give infant HBIg 0.5 mL and HBV vaccine (Recombivax HB; separate sites) within 12 hrs of birth followed by HBV vaccine, 0.5 mL IM at ages 1 and 6 months. Check HBsAg and HBsAb at age 1
- HCV vertical transmission increased in HIV

ICD-9 CODE

070 Viral hepatitis

ABBREVIATIONS

PCR = polymerase chain reaction; HCC = hepatocellular carcinoma; AI = autoimmune hepatitis

BIBLIOGRAPHY

Alter MJ, Mast EE. The epidemiology of viral hepatitis in the U.S. *Gastroenterol Clin North Am* 1994;23:437–455.

Seeff LP. Emerging and reemerging issues, infectious diseases: Hepatitis C: A meeting ground for the generalist and the specialist. *Amer J Med* 1999;107(6B):1s–100s.

Internet references: http://www.5mcc.com

Author: Rajiv R. Varma

Herpes Gladiatorum

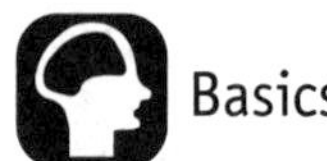

Basics

DEFINITION

- Variant of cutaneous herpes disease caused by herpes simplex virus type 1 (HSV-1) or type 2 (HSV-2) occurring among wrestlers and transmitted by direct skin-to-skin contact

INCIDENCE/PREVALENCE

- Affects 2.6% of high school wrestlers and 7.6% of collegiate wrestlers

SIGNS AND SYMPTOMS

- Incubation period for primary infection is 2–14 days.
- Prodrome of burning, stinging pain, or itching at the infected site, followed by clusters of vesicles on an erythematous base
- Common locations include head, neck, and upper body
- Symptoms of fever, localized lymphadenopathy, malaise, myalgia, or pharyngitis may accompany infection.
- Repeated outbreaks usually are less severe and involve a smaller area.
- Infections around the eye increase the risk of corneal or retinal involvement, such as keratoconjunctivitis or retinal necrosis.

RISK FACTORS

- Abrasions increase the likelihood of acquiring infection.
- Stresses of weight loss, competition, and school responsibilities can lead to recurrence.

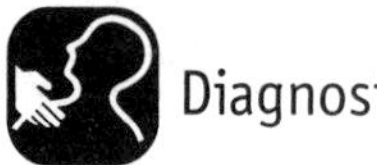

Diagnosis

DIFFERENTIAL DIAGNOSIS

- Impetigo
- Herpes zoster
- Folliculitis
- Allergic or contact dermatitis
- Cellulitis
- Think herpes if infection fails to improve after 3–4 days of oral antibiotic therapy and if lesions cross the midline and involve the face and scalp
- Definitive diagnosis can be made by viral culture or Tzanck smear of vesicle fluid.

HISTORY

- Initial versus recurrent eruption
- Similar location as previous infection
- Previous treatment and length of infection

PHYSICAL EXAMINATION

- Erythema and grouped vesicles, ulcers, or crusts on head, face, neck, or upper extremities most common, but may occur anywhere on the body

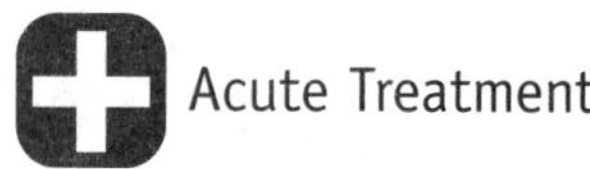

Acute Treatment

INITIAL INFECTION

- Started early in the clinical course, during vesicle formation, oral antiviral medications can arrest viral replication and shorten the duration of infection.
- Acyclovir 200 mg five times a day or 400 mg three times a day for 10 days
- Valacyclovir 1 g twice a day for 10 days
- During the ulcer stage, benzoyl peroxide and use of a hair dryer can help dry crusts more rapidly and minimize secondary bacterial infections.

RECURRENT INFECTION

- Antiviral medications begun during the prodromal phase can effectively shorten the duration of recurrent infections.
- Acyclovir 200 mg five times a day for 5 days
- Valacyclovir 500 mg twice a day for 5 days
- Famciclovir 125 mg twice a day for 5 days

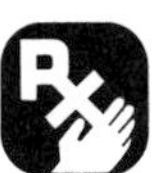

Long-Term Treatment

PROPHYLAXIS

- Isolate infected wrestler to prevent skin contact with other wrestlers
- Used to control outbreaks among previously infected wrestlers
- Acyclovir 200 mg twice a day
- Valacyclovir 500 mg daily
- Famciclovir 250 mg twice a day
- Consider using prophylactic antiviral medications during the wrestling season or before important tournaments
- Teach skin hygiene and protect other skin abrasions from secondary contact with HSV

Common Questions and Answers

Physician responses to common patient questions:
Q: When can I wrestle?
A: Wrestlers are disqualified if vesicles or ulcers are present. Participation is allowed only when the affected area is scabbed and dry. NCAA guidelines allow competition if no new lesions for 3 days; no active lesions; lesions crusted; taking medication at time of competition; and lesions covered with a gas-permeable membrane.

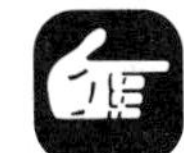

Miscellaneous

ICD-9 CODE

054.9

BIBLIOGRAPHY

Anderson BJ. The effectiveness of valacyclovir in preventing reactivation of herpes gladiatorum in wrestlers. *Clin J Sports Med* 1999;9:86–90.

Annunziato PW, Gershon A. Herpes simplex virus infections. *Pediatr Rev* 1996;17:415–423.

Becker TM, Kodsi R, Bailey P, et al. Grappling with herpes: herpes gladiatorum. *Am J Sports Med* 1988;16:665–669.

Belongia EA, Goodman JL, Holland EJ, et al. An outbreak of herpes gladiatorum at a high-school wrestling camp. *N Engl J Med* 1991;325:906–910.

Dienst WL Jr, Dightman L, Dworkin MS, et al. Pinning down skin infections: diagnosis, treatment, and prevention in wrestlers. *Physician Sportsmed* 1997;25:45–50.

Author: Julie Kerr

High-Altitude Illness

Basics

DEFINITION

- Clinical spectrum of signs and symptoms resulting from ascent to high altitude
- Hypobaric hypoxia is the physiologic basis for acute mountain sickness (AMS), high-altitude pulmonary edema (HAPE), and high-altitude cerebral edema (HACE).
- These high-altitude syndromes frequently overlap in presentation and can be considered as a continuum from mild AMS to severe AMS, HAPE, and HACE.
- Each syndrome can present independently and progress rapidly without the initial warning of milder symptoms.

INCIDENCE/PREVALENCE

- In general, 12% to 25% of unacclimatized individuals experience symptoms of AMS beginning at a threshold altitude of 8,000 ft (2,440 m).
- Incidence and severity increase with higher altitude.

SIGNS AND SYMPTOMS

AMS

- Headache
- Insomnia
- Nausea
- Anorexia
- Lassitude
- Fatigue
- Weakness
- Malaise
- Dizziness
- Light-headedness
- Memory impairment
- Concentration difficulties

HAPE

- 50% of HAPE victims experience symptoms of AMS, in addition to
- Severe dyspnea on exertion progressing to dyspnea at rest
- Nonproductive and persistent cough
- Chest tightness
- Fatigue
- Weakness

HACE

- Headache
- Lethargy
- Incoordination
- Vomiting
- Disorientation
- Irrational behavior
- Visual or auditory hallucinations
- Semicoma
- Unconsciousness

RISK FACTORS

- Rapid ascent to or at high altitude >8,000 ft (2,440 m)
- Sleeping altitude increase >3,000 ft/night (>1,000 m/night)
- Inadequate acclimatization
- Strenuous exertion upon arrival to high altitude
- Previous history and/or individual susceptibility to altitude illness
- Younger age
- Obesity
- Chronic illness

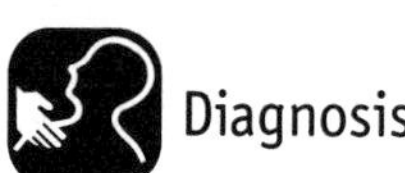

Diagnosis

DIFFERENTIAL DIAGNOSIS

- Dehydration
- Exhaustion
- Viral syndrome and viral upper respiratory tract
- Gastroenteritis
- Hangover
- Hypothermia
- Carbon monoxide intoxication

HAPE

- Can mimic pneumonia
- Uncomplicated HAPE usually does not present with high fever >101°F, chills, or mucopurulent sputum.

HACE

- Can mimic signs of a cerebrovascular accident
- Generally presents with other signs/symptoms (i.e., mental status changes) in addition to neurologically based motor deficits

HISTORY

Altitude Syndromes (AMS, HAPE, HACE)

- All associated with increased prevalence and more severe progression with rapid ascent to high altitude without proper acclimatization

AMS

- Ascent to high altitude with onset of symptoms in 12–24 hours

HAPE

- Symptoms usually begin 24–72 hours after arrival to high altitude and classically the second night sleeping at high altitude
- Characterized by insidious onset, with decreased exercise performance, cough, and progressive worsening of symptoms, especially at night.

HACE

- Previous symptoms of AMS, with progressive worsening of neurologic symptoms, including

—Ataxia
—Extreme lassitude
—Mental status changes
—Coma

- Commonly associated with APE
- Onset usually about 5 days after ascent to high altitude
- Uncomplicated HACE occurs at a mean altitude of 15,500 ft, which is generally higher than for AMS or HAPE.

PHYSICAL EXAMINATION

AMS

- Tachycardia possible
- Blood pressure normal
- Crackles in right middle lobe
- Peripheral edema

HAPE

- Cyanosis common
- Crackles in right middle lobe
- Tachycardia with resting heart rate >90/min
- Tachypnea >20/min in adults
- Low-grade fever
- Orthopnea
- Pink frothy sputum is a late finding

HACE

- Truncal ataxia demonstrated by poor heel-toe walking, mental status changes, occasionally focal neurologic deficits
- Abnormal extensor plantar reflex
- Funduscopic examination can demonstrate papilledema and retinal hemorrhages.

IMAGING

HAPE

Chest x-ray demonstrates homogenous or patchy confluent infiltrate in right middle lobe with normal heart size.

HACE

- Brain magnetic resonance imaging not necessary for diagnosis but shows characteristic white matter edema and cortical atrophy

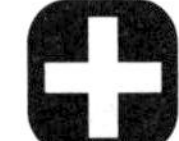

Acute Treatment

SPECIAL CONSIDERATIONS

Altitude Syndromes in General

- Descent to a lower altitude is mainstay of treatment

Severe AMS, HAPE, and HACE

- Require immediate descent and usually not reascending to high altitude

AMS

Mild

- No further ascent until symptoms resolve; consider descent of at least 1,500 ft
- Limit physical exertion and maximize hydration.
- Symptomatic medications: nonsteroidal anti-inflammatory drugs, aspirin, acetaminophen for headache, antiemetics for nausea/vomiting, acetazolamide (Diamox) 125–250 mg every 8–12 hours to speed acclimatization and provide symptomatic relief (usually within 24–48 hours).

Moderate-to-Severe AMS or Continued Mild Symptoms

- In addition to treatment of mild AMS, descend at least 1,500 ft or until symptoms improve
- Consider low-flow oxygen at 2–4 L/min
- Consider dexamethasone 4 mg p.o., i.m., or i.v. every 6 hours until symptoms resolve
- After stopping dexamethasone, ensure the patient remains symptom-free for 24–48 hours before reascending, as rebound symptoms of AMS can occur after discontinuing steroid use.
- Consider use of Gamow bag if O_2 not available and symptoms are severe

HAPE

Descent

- Assisted descent of at least 3,000–4,000 ft should occur as soon the diagnosis of HAPE is suggested.
- Early recognition of HAPE symptoms is essential to initiate immediate descent oxygen.
- Concomitant use of high-flow oxygen at 4–6 L/min is essential, if available.
- Keep pulse oximetry >90%
- High flow necessary to oxygenate the alveoli
- Nifedipine: if descent impossible or symptoms are severe or worsening, consider nifedipine 10 mg sublinguinal every 4 hours until symptoms improve or 10 mg sl once and then 30 mg extended release every 12–24 hours.
- Acetazolamide 250 mg every 6–8 hours may improve ventilation in mild cases.
- Gamov bag: hyperbaric therapy for 4–6 hours can be used if immediate descent is impossible and oxygen is unavailable; symptomatic medications as for AMS can be used.

HACE

Descent

- Early recognition of HACE is essential to initiate descent and avoid progression.
- Immediate descent is mandatory.
- Oxygen at 2–10 L/min

- Dexamethasone 4 mg every 6 hours p.o. or i.v.
- Acetazolamide 250 mg every 6–12 hours
- Gamov bag before descent; encourage hyperventilation if conscious; periodically record heart rate, blood pressure, respiration rate, and urine output.
- Observe for codevelopment of HAPE.
- After descent, hospitalization is recommended for appropriate workup, including computed tomography (CT) of head to rule out other cerebral pathology, if indicated.
- Continue oxygen, dexamethasone, acetazolamide, and possibly Lasix in intensive care unit setting and taper appropriately

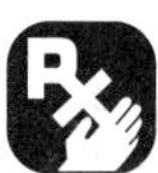

Long-Term Treatment

GENERAL PREVENTATIVE MEASURES

- Avoid heavy exertion for 2–3 days upon arrival to high altitude
- Maintain adequate hydration
- Eat frequent, small, high-carbohydrate meals
- Avoid alcohol
- Avoid sedative/hypnotics
- Avoid smoking
- Avoid daytime sleeping

ACCLIMATIZATION

- Planned acclimatization is the physiologic method of progressively increasing sleeping altitude.
- Proper acclimatization can prevent serious altitude illness.
- "Climb high and sleep low."
- Start by sleeping 1–3 nights at an intermediate altitude before ascending to higher altitudes. Plan on limiting sleeping altitude gain to no more than 1,000 ft/night.

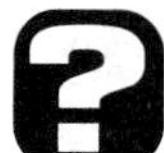

Common Questions and Answers

Physician responses to common patient questions:

Q: Does physical fitness and training prevent altitude illness?

A: No. Physically fit individuals have shown a predilection toward altitude illness because of a tendency to exert themselves more upon arrival at altitude and climb at a faster ascent rate. Physical fitness can be advantageous in performing at altitude when altitude illness is not present.

Q: Which type of athletes benefit the most from altitude training?

A: Athletes who have reached a performance plateau at sea level with a scheduled training regime (elite or pre-elite athletes) and compete in events requiring a high Vo_2 max are the most likely to benefit from altitude training. Recreational or occasional athletes will benefit most from a scheduled training program at their native altitude or sea level.

Q: How long do the effects of acclimatization last for the prevention of altitude illness?

A: The physiologic adaptations occurring as a result of acclimatization to prevent altitude illness depend on the elevation and time spent acclimatizing at high altitude. Generally most of the acclimatization process is complete by 1–2 weeks (near-total completion takes up to 80 days) and the effects last up to 2–6 weeks upon descent and return to sea level. Children tend to lose the acclimatization effect quicker and can develop HACE after spending 5 days at sea level and reascending to altitude.

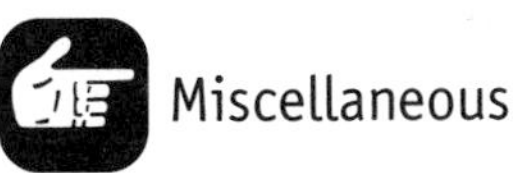

Miscellaneous

TRAINING AT ALTITUDE

Benefit

- Improved performance at sea-level competition is based on the physiologic acclimatization process to living at high altitude.
- Acclimatization process causes an increase in red cell mass and accordingly increases in oxygen-carrying capacity of blood, resulting in increases in aerobic power and exercise performance at sea level.
- There is a further increase in capillary density, mitochondrial number, and tissue myoglobin concentration and increase in 2,3-diphosphoglyceric acid, which results in increased oxygen uptake of exercising muscle.

Training Methods

- Train low and sleep high: lower-altitude training (optimally below 1,500 m) at high-intensity intervals will allow achievement of high VO_2 max, absolute workload, heart rate, and blood lactate concentration.
- Living and sleeping at high altitude will maximize the acclimatization response.
- High-altitude living optimally should occur at an altitude of 2,500–3,000 m. Higher altitude increases risk of altitude illness and should be avoided with preventative measures.

COMPETITION AT ALTITUDE

- VO_2 max will decrease at altitude.
- Acclimatizing at altitude adequately for 1–2 weeks can maximize the decreased performance occurring at altitude.
- Anecdotally, low-lander athletes report better performance at altitude by minimizing stay at altitude before the event and timing travel to compete as soon as possible upon arrival at high altitude.

BIBLIOGRAPHY

Hackett PH, Roach RC. High altitude medicine. In: Auerbach PS, ed. *Management of wilderness and environmental emergencies.* St. Louis: Mosby, 1995.

Hultgreen H. *High altitude medicine.* Stanford: Hultgreen Publications, 1998.

Levine BD, Stray-Gunderson J. "Living high–training low": the effect of moderate-altitude acclimatization with low-altitude performance. *J Appl Physiol* 1997;83:102–112.

Levine BD, Stray-Gunderson J. A practical approach to altitude training: where to live and train for optimal performance. *Int J Sports Med* 1992;13:s209–s212.

Stray-Gunderson J, Chapman RF, Levine BD. Hi lo altitude training improves performance in elite runners. *Med Sci Sports Exerc* 1998;30:s35.

Authors: R. Thole and Aaron L. Rubin

Hypertension

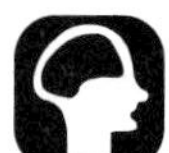

Basics

DEFINITION

- Persistent elevation in systemic blood pressure, currently defined as >140/90 mm Hg

INCIDENCE/PREVALENCE

- Most common cardiovascular disease worldwide
- Most common cardiovascular condition seen in athletes
- Prevalence may be as high as 25% of the population
- Higher incidence in males, older patients, African-Americans, and certain Asian populations

SIGNS AND SYMPTOMS

- Presence of hypertension generally is silent.
- Most patients are asymptomatic.
- With more significant blood pressure elevations, symptoms may include
  —Chest pain
  —Dyspnea
  —Orthopnea
  —Poor exercise tolerance
  —Headache
- In addition to persistently elevated blood pressure readings, signs may include development of S4 gallop or evidence of pulmonary edema.

RISK FACTORS

- Genetic predisposition
- Diet and salt consumption
- Alcohol intake
- Illicit drug use
- Associated with a number of comorbid conditions and cardiovascular risk factors, including
  —Hyperinsulinemia and glucose intolerance
  —Obesity
  —Hyperlipidemia

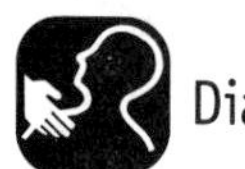

Diagnosis

DIFFERENTIAL DIAGNOSIS

- Once the presence of hypertension is established, must differentiate essential hypertension (comprising about 95% of cases) and hypertension due to a secondary cause.
- Essential hypertension has no identifiable cause and results from a complex process of hormonal, neurologic, and vascular changes.
- Secondary causes of hypertension include
  —Primary hyperaldosteronism
  —Cushing disease/syndrome
  —Hyperthyroidism
  —Renal parenchymal disease
  —Renal insufficiency
  —Renal artery stenosis
  —Coarctation of the aorta
  —Pheochromocytoma
  —Androgen or growth hormone use
  —Alcohol
  —Illicit vasoconstrictive drug use

HISTORY

- Often noncontributory, as most patients are asymptomatic and hypertension is found incidentally.
- Family history of hypertension may be helpful for surveillance.
- Historic data on diet, alcohol and tobacco use, recent weight changes, caffeine intake, sympathomimetic agents (nasal decongestants, ephedrine, ma huang), illicit drugs (cocaine, amphetamines, anabolic/androgenic steroids)

PHYSICAL EXAMINATION

- Important to accurately document the true presence of hypertension
- Blood pressure elevations should be recorded on three separate occasions using appropriately sized cuff (blood pressure will be artificially elevated if cuff size is too small)
- Measurement after at least 5 minutes of rest
- Hypertension classification
  —Stage I: >140/90
  —Stage II: >160/100
  —Stage III: >180/110
- Assess for presence of S4 gallop, arterial bruits (particularly renal), and tachycardia

LABORATORY EVALUATION

- At initial diagnosis, all patients require
  —Complete blood count
  —Electrolytes
  —Glucose
  —Renal function
  —Thyroid evaluation
  —Fasting lipids
  —Urinalysis for proteinuria/hematuria
- Baseline electrocardiogram to rule out evidence of structural/hypertensive heart disease

IMAGING

Ultrasonographic or angiographic evaluation for renal artery stenosis should be considered, particularly in older patients or those with accelerated hypertension.

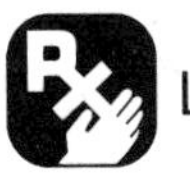

Long-Term Treatment

NONPHARMACOLOGIC

- Regular exercise
- Avoidance of excessive salt intake
- Limited alcohol consumption

PHARMACOLOGIC

Antihypertensive Agents Considered Safe in Athletes and Having no Significant Effect on Aerobic Capacity

- Angiotensin-converting enzyme inhibitors and angiotensin-receptor blockers
- Calcium channel blockers
- α_1-Receptor blockers
- Central α-receptor antagonists
- Cardioselective β blockers (metoprolol, atenolol)

Antihypertensive Agents to Be Avoided in Athletes

- Noncardioselective beta blockers (propranolol, nadolol), which impair aerobic capacity
- Diuretics (thiazides), which may cause electrolyte imbalances, dehydration, and potentiate the risk for heat illness in athletes

Common Questions and Answers

Physician responses to common patient questions:
Q: What level of hypertension is "acceptable" for athletic participation?
A: Stages I and II: full participation if no evidence of end-organ (i.e., cardiac, renal) disease is present. Stage III: discontinue activity until better blood pressure control is obtained, especially in high-static sports (boxing, cycling, rowing, weight-lifting, wrestling).

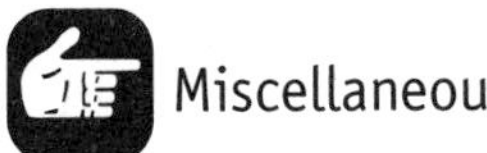

Miscellaneous

SYNONYMS

- High blood pressure

ICD-9 CODE

401.1 Benign hypertension
401.9 Unspecified hypertension

BIBLIOGRAPHY

Kaplan NM, Devereaux RB, Miller HS Jr. 26th Bethesda Conference: recommendations for determining eligibility for competition in athletes with cardiovascular abnormalities. Task Force 4: systemic hypertension. *Med Sci Sports Exerc* 1994;26:S268–S270.

American College of Sports Medicine Position Stand. Physical activity, physical fitness, and hypertension. *Med Sci Sports Exerc* 1993;25:i–x.

MacKnight JM. Hypertension in athletes and active patients. *Physician Sportsmed* 1999;27:35–44.

Author: John MacKnight

Hyperthermia: Heat Stroke, Exhaustion, and Cramps

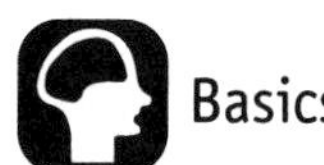

Basics

DEFINITION

- Body's inability to balance heat gain with heat loss
  —Heat gain: metabolic and environmental
  —Heat loss: radiation, conduction, convection, evaporation

INCIDENCE/PREVALENCE

- Common

SIGNS AND SYMPTOMS

Heat Cramps

- Severe involuntary cramping of skeletal muscles used most heavily during exercise

Heat Exhaustion

- Fatigue
- Shortness of breath
- Dizziness
- Emesis
- Syncope
- Cold/clammy or hot dry skin
- Elevated core (rectal) temperature (39°C, 102.2°F) common but not the rule

Heat Stroke

- Core temp >40°C (104°F)
- Rapid pulse
- Rapid respirations
- Hypertension (HTN)
- Central nervous system (CNS) signs (confusion, impaired consciousness)
- May have minimal perspiration or hot dry skin

RISK FACTORS

- Hot, humid weather
- Poorly trained and/or heavy athletes
- Improper attire (plastic suits)
- Equipment (football pads/helmet)
- Lack of acclimatization
- Medications/concurrent illness

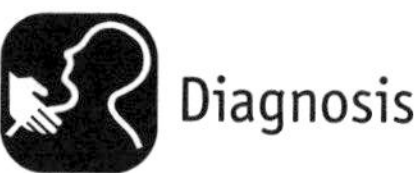

Diagnosis

DIFFERENTIAL DIAGNOSIS

- Dehydration
- Cardiovascular disease
- CNS lesion
- Electrolyte abnormality

HISTORY

- Cramps: sudden onset of cramping muscles, often in the gastrocnemius
- Exhaustion: fatigue, dyspnea, presyncope, emesis
- Stroke: confusion, impaired consciousness

PHYSICAL EXAMINATION

- Cramps: tense, tender, involuntary contraction of muscle belly
- Exhaustion: elevated core (rectal) temperature (39°C, 102.2°F) common; orthostatic; skin may be cold or hot, wet, or dry
- Stroke: core temp >40°C (104°F); rapid pulse and respirations; HTN; lack of sweating; hot dry skin

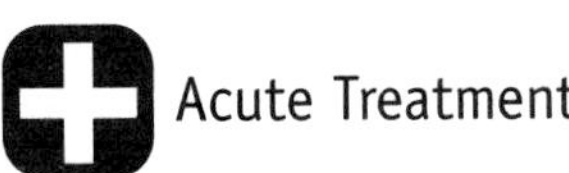

Acute Treatment

ENVIRONMENT

- Cramps: cool environment, fluid replacement, passive stretching
- Exhaustion: cool environment, rest, elevate lower extremity, oral or intravenous fluids; transfer to emergency room (ER) if unstable
- Stroke: support airway, breathing, and circulation; rapid cooling of body with cold water, ice, fanning, wet towels; transfer to ER if unstable.

TRIAGE

Use basic or advanced cardiac life support for all unstable patients and transfer them to the nearest medical facility.

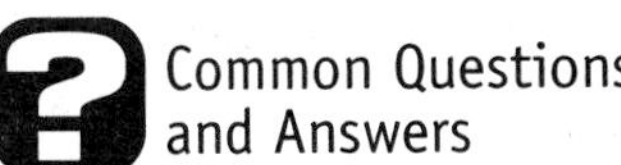

Common Questions and Answers

Physician responses to common patient questions:
Q: How can I avoid heat injury?
A: Prevention is the best medicine: acclimatization, proper breathable clothing, hydration, and early race times.

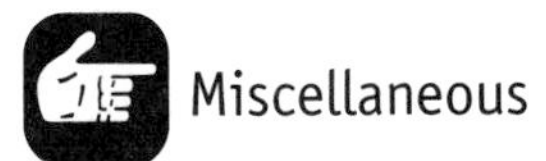

Miscellaneous

ICD-9 CODE

9932.1 Heat syncope
992.2 Heat cramps
992.3 Heat exhaustion (water depletion)
992.4 Heat exhaustion (salt depletion)
992.0 Heat stroke

BIBLIOGRAPHY

Wilmore JH, Costill D. *Physiology of sport and exercise*. Muncie: Human Kinetics, 1994.

Author: Dan Ostlie

Hypertrophic Cardiomyopathy

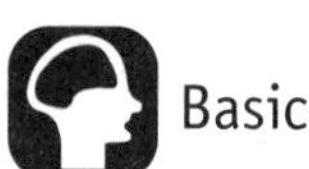

Basics

DEFINITION

- Genetically heterogeneous disease marked by left ventricular hypertrophy (LVH) without outflow obstruction
- Primary cause (35%) of sudden atraumatic death in athletes <35 years.
- Death results from ventricular tachycardia either due to or in the absence of LV outflow obstruction (some patients have arrhythmogenic foci).

INCIDENCE/PREVALENCE

- Incidence of hypertrophic cardiomyopathy (HCM) is 1–2 cases per 1,000 persons.
- Incidence of sudden cardiac death in athletes <35, mostly due to HCM, is 1:250,000.

SIGNS AND SYMPTOMS

- Most common initial presentation is syncope or sudden cardiac death (SCD) with exertion.
- Exertional chest discomfort secondary to diastolic dysfunction

RISK FACTORS

- Family history of unexplained or early (<40 years) cardiac death
- Severity of hypertrophy is related to risk of SCD.

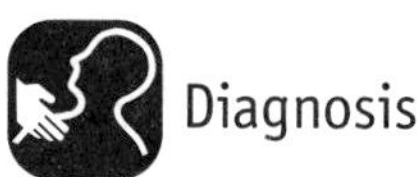

Diagnosis

DIFFERENTIAL DIAGNOSIS

- Athletic heart syndrome (AHS)
- Myocarditis/pericarditis
- Coronary artery anomalies
- Aortic stenosis
- Prolonged QT syndrome
- Rhabdomyolysis with sickle cell trait
- Marfan syndrome
- Wolff-Parkinson-White syndrome
- Arrhythmogenic right ventricular dysplasia

HISTORY

- History is negative for most patients.
- Exertional syncope is the only reliable warning sign when present in history.

PHYSICAL EXAMINATION

- Most patients with HCM have a completely normal physical examination.
- Murmur
  - —In rare cases where murmur is detected, it usually is midsystolic and heard at the mid left sternal border.
  - —Murmur is ominous if it increases with maneuvers to decrease LV end-diastolic (LVED) filling. These maneuvers cause dynamic obstruction in the LV outflow tract.
  - —Maneuvers include rising from squatting to standing and performing the Valsalva maneuver.
  - —Murmur decreases when LVED filling increases, while moving from standing to squatting (LV free wall moves away from the septum with increased filling).
  - —Benign murmurs usually become louder while squatting and decrease on rising.
  - —Such murmurs are common with improved fitness from training, as described with the AHS.
  - —Athletes with significant outflow obstruction eventually may have pansystolic blowing murmur of mitral regurgitation radiating to the axilla.
- As the HCM athlete ages, more signs of LVH are present, particularly lateral displacement of the apex beat.
- Any diastolic murmur indicates other cardiac pathology requiring workup.

IMAGING

- Echocardiogram shows LV wall thickening measured on the free wall as >13 mm.
- Concentric LVH may be present or the septum may be asymmetrically hypertrophied, producing LV outflow obstruction.
- Mitral regurgitation and left atrial dilation are seen.
- Unlike patients with HCM, athletes with AHS (fit young adults who also have murmurs) have right ventricular hypertrophy and increased LV volumes or total LV diameter. These findings represent physiologic adaptations to increased plasma volume.

ELECTROCARDIOGRAM

- LVH findings
- Increased voltage
- Repolarization abnormalities
- Prominent Q waves in inferior and anterolateral leads and giant negative T waves

HOLTER

- Not commonly used for screening but may reveal paroxysmal atrial fibrillation and ventricular tachycardia, which frequently are symptomatic.

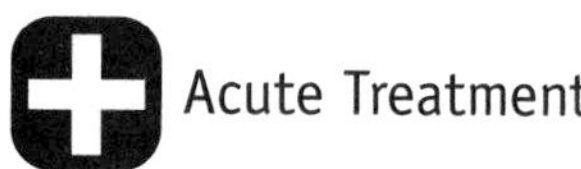

Acute Treatment

- Airway, breathing, and circulation for syncope or arrest

SPECIAL CONSIDERATIONS

- Exercise treadmill and adenosine thallium testing, with target accelerated heart rates, are relatively contraindicated due to higher risk for arrhythmia due to obstruction during induced tachycardia.
- Most important point of treating youthful survivors of exertional syncope is to ensure HCM is not present.

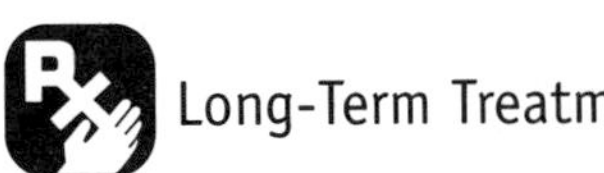

Long-Term Treatment

26TH BETHESDA CONFERENCE RECOMMENDATIONS FOR ACTIVITY FOR INDIVIDUALS WITH HCM

- Athletes with unequivocal HCM should not participate in most competitive sports, except possibly low-intensity sports. This recommendation includes athletes with and without symptoms or LV outflow obstruction.
- Given that the risk of SCD may be reduced in older individuals (>40 years) with HCM, an alternative of individual judgment may be used in selected older athletes only when each of the following clinical features is absent:
  —Ventricular tachycardia (sustained or nonsustained) on ambulatory electrocardiogram
  —Family history of SCD due to HCM, particularly if <40 years old.
  —History of syncope or other clinically relevant episodes of impaired consciousness
  —Severe hemodynamic abnormalities, including dynamic LV outflow tract gradient >50 mm Hg
  —Exercise-induced hypotension
  —Moderate-to-severe mitral regurgitation, enlarged left atrium (>50 mm), or paroxysmal atrial fibrillation
  —Presence of abnormal myocardial perfusion
  —These recommendations are not altered if medical or surgical treatment is undertaken in a given athlete.
- Small number of youthful members of families with HCM, who are free of typical morphologic features of the disease, will be identified in the future using DNA testing. The clinical significance of such findings is uncertain. Presently there is no available evidence to preclude such individuals from competitive athletics, in the absence of cardiac symptoms or a family history of sudden cardiac death.

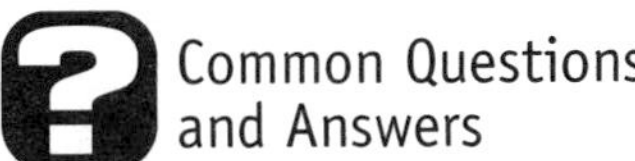

Common Questions and Answers

Physician responses to common patient questions:
Q: Since it takes a while to be sure about the diagnosis while getting an echocardiogram, what can I do while I wait for the results?
A: It is not safe to exert at all when HCM is suspected. Please be patient while we wait a few days for the reading.
Q: What does my child have?
A: A rare genetic disease that can cause abnormal beating of the heart, especially with exercise. This disease is difficult to control, and even those who are treated probably should avoid all strenuous exercise unless HCM is proven to not be the diagnosis.
Q: How dangerous is this?
A: There is a significant risk of death in people who have true HCM. Exercise increases this risk in some athletes. Certain exercises may be permitted after the true diagnosis and extent of the problem are clear.
Q: I want to stay fit. What activities are OK for people with HCM?
A: Currently only very low-intensity exercises are considered possibly acceptable, including golf, billiards, bowling, cricket, and curling.

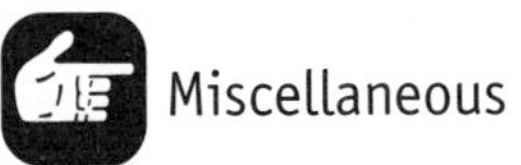

Miscellaneous

SYNONYMS

- Idiopathic subaortic stenosis
- Asymmetric septal hypertrophy

ICD-9 CODE

425.14 Nonobstructive
425.1 Obstructive
746.84 Congenital obstructive

BIBLIOGRAPHY

Marian AJ. *Conn's current therapy*. Philadelphia: WB Saunders, 1999.

Maron BJ, Isner JM, McKenna WI. Task Force 3: hypertrophic cardiomyopathy myocarditis, and other myopericardial diseases and mitral valve prolapse. 26th Bethesda Conference: recommendations for determining eligibility for competition in athletes with cardiovascular abnormalities. *Med Sci Sports Exerc* 1994;26:5223–5283.

O'Connor FG. Sudden death in young athletes, screening for a needle in a haystack. *Am Fam Physician* 1998;57:2763–2770.

Richman PB. The etiology of cardiac arrest in children and young adults: special considerations for ED management. *Am J Emerg Med* 1999;17:264–270.

Van Camp SP. Non-traumatic sports deaths in high school and college athletes. *Med Sci Sports Exerc* 1995;27:641–647.

Author: John Shelton

Hyponatremia

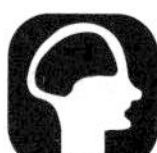

Basics

DEFINITION

- Decrease in serum sodium concentration to <136 mmol/L.
- Serum sodium concentration and serum osmolarity normally are maintained under precise control by homeostatic mechanisms involving thirst, antidiuretic hormone (ADH), and renal handling of filtered sodium.
- Increased serum osmolarity above normal (280–300 mosmol/kg) stimulates hypothalamic osmoreceptors, which then cause increased thirst and circulating levels of ADH.
- Can be associated with low, normal, or high tonicity.
- Effective osmolality or tonicity refers to the contribution to osmolality of solutes, such as sodium and glucose, that cannot move freely across cell membranes, thereby inducing transcellular shifts in water.
- Most common form is hypotonic (dilutional) hyponatremia.
  —Excess of water in relation to existing sodium stores, which can be decreased, normal, or increased.
  —Retention of water most commonly reflects presence of conditions that impair renal excretion of water.
  —Less commonly caused by excessive water intake, with normal or near-normal excretory capacity.
- Hypertonic hyponatremia results from a shift of water from cells to the extracellular fluid that is driven by solutes confined in the extracellular compartments (as occurs with hyperglycemia or retention of hypertonic mannitol).
- Pseudohyponatremia is a form of iso-osmolar and isotonic hyponatremia identified when severe hypertriglyceridemia or paraproteinemia is present, which affects accurate laboratory measurement of sodium concentration.

INCIDENCE/PREVALENCE

- Occurs in 10% to 40% of ultraendurance athletes after a race.
- 7% of healthy elderly persons
- Male = female
- More common in the very young and very old, who are less able to experience and express thirst and less able to autonomously regulate fluid intake.

SIGNS AND SYMPTOMS

- Varying range depending on the chronicity, cause, and the individual.
- Overhydration in athletes characterized by edema of the hands with swelling of the fingers
- Anorexia
- Headache
- Muscle cramps
- Nausea and vomiting
- Difficulty concentrating
- Confusion
- Lethargy
- Agitation
- Obtundation
- Coma
- Status epilepticus

RISK FACTORS

- Elite endurance athletes who consume excessive fluids
- In marathoners, more common in women, slower runners, and finishers who maintain or increase their body weight.
- Excess fluid losses (e.g., excessive sweating, vomiting, diarrhea, gastrointestinal fistulas or drainage tubes, pancreatitis, burns) that have been replaced primarily by hypotonic fluids
- Infants given inappropriate amounts of free water
- Thiazide diuretics, chlorpropamide, cyclophosphamide, clofibrate, carbamazepine, opiates, oxytocin, desmopressin, vincristine, selective serotonin reuptake inhibitor, or tolbutamide
- Those with history of hepatic cirrhosis, congestive heart failure, or nephrotic syndrome, who are subject to increases in total body sodium and free water stores
- Acute or chronic renal insufficiency in patients who may be unable to excrete adequate amounts of free water or those with salt wasting nephropathy
- Syndrome of inappropriate ADH secretion (SIADH)
- Uncorrected hypothyroidism or cortisol deficiency
- Consumption of large amounts of beer or use of the recreational drug methylenedioxy-methamphetamine (ecstasy)
- Nonsteroidal anti-inflammatory drug use

ASSOCIATED INJURIES AND COMPLICATIONS

- Hyponatremic encephalopathy associated with noncardiogenic pulmonary edema in healthy marathon runners
- Cerebral edema leading to brainstem herniation and death
- Permanent central nervous system dysfunction
- Central pontine myelinolysis characterized by weakness, muscle spasms, diplopia, confusion, delirium, or dysphagia
- Seizures
- Rhabdomyolysis

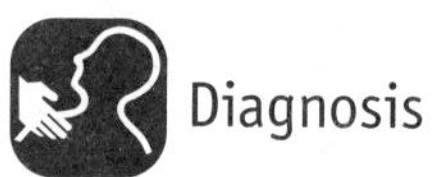

Diagnosis

DIFFERENTIAL DIAGNOSIS

- Adrenal insufficiency and adrenal crisis
- Congestive heart failure and pulmonary edema
- Gastroenteritis
- Hypothyroidism and myxedema coma
- Renal failure, acute
- Renal failure, chronic
- SIADH
- Cirrhosis
- Nephrotic syndrome
- Psychogenic polydipsia
- Pseudohyponatremia
- Iatrogenic
- Medication related

HISTORY

- Thorough past medical, past surgical, medication, and social history, with special attention to signs, symptoms, and differential diagnosis as listed above.

PHYSICAL EXAMINATION

- Most abnormalities are neurologic in origin.
- Assess level of alertness
- Assess degree of cognitive impairment
- Depressed deep tendon reflexes, ataxia, asterixis, pathologic reflexes, or pseudobulbar palsy (bilateral hemiplegia, dysarthria, dysphagia)
- Look for signs of focal or generalized seizure activity
- In patients with acute severe hyponatremia, signs of brainstem herniation may be apparent, including coma; fixed, unilateral, dilated pupil; decorticate or decerebrate posturing; and respiratory arrest.

IMAGING/LABORATORY STUDIES

- Measure serum sodium level and always consider possibility of laboratory error or improper sampling technique
- Measure blood urea nitrogen, creatinine, uric acid, urinary osmolality, and urinary Na
- Measure serum osmolality (low <280 mosmol)
  —If normal (280–285), measure blood sugar, lipid, and protein levels
  —If elevated (>280), measure blood sugar
- If serum hyperglycemia is present, then serum sodium must be corrected by a factor of 1.6 mEq/L for each 100 mg/dL increase in serum glucose.
- Consider chest x-ray, electrocardiogram, head computed tomographic scan, or other laboratory work based on history and physical examination.

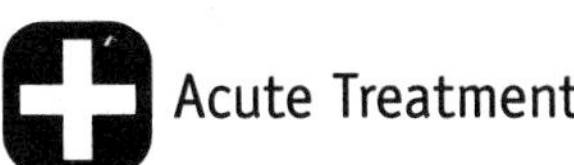

Acute Treatment

GENERAL

- Airway, breathing, and circulation
- Establish intravenous (i.v.) access
- Determine cause by history, physical examination, and laboratory data and direct treatment accordingly
- There is no consensus about the optimal treatment of symptomatic hyponatremia. Increase serum sodium rapidly by 1–2 mEq/L/hour over the first 1–2 hours for levels <120 mEq/L
- Patients with seizures or impending brainstem herniation should receive 3% saline (see Calculations) to accomplish rapid correction, but only enough to arrest progression of symptoms; usually 4–6 mEq/L is sufficient. Be aware of cardiac status with aggressive i.v. therapy.
- Patients with mild symptoms and serum sodium ≤125 mEq/L often have chronic hyponatremia and must be managed cautiously.
- Rapid increase in serum sodium can lead to central pontine myelinolysis, but risk appears minimal if correction is at rate <0.5 mEq/L/hour or 12 mEq/L/day. Isolated cases of osmotic demyelination after correction at 9–10 mEq/L/day have been reported; therefore, maximum correction of 8 mEq/L/day is a more conservative approach.
- Hypovolemic hyponatremia with mild-to-moderate symptoms is treated with normal saline (see Calculations), and frequent monitoring of serum sodium levels is important to assess rate of correction.
- Hypervolemic hyponatremia treatment consists of sodium and water restriction and attention to the underlying cause.
- Euvolemic hyponatremia treatment consists of free water restriction and correction of the underlying condition.

TRIATHLETE CONSIDERATIONS

- Unconscious athlete should have bladder catheterized and should be promptly moved to a hospital for definitive management.
- For severe hyponatremia (<126), patient should not receive fluids either orally or intravenously, except perhaps 3% saline solution (these athletes usually are volume overloaded).
- For less severe hyponatremia (>130), watchful waiting is the cornerstone of therapy, as most will self-correct.

CALCULATIONS

- Change in serum Na = (infusate Na − serum Na)/total body water + 1. Estimates effect of 1 L of any infusate on serum Na
- Total body water (in liters) is calculated as a fraction of body weight.
- Fraction = 0.6 in children; 0.6 and 0.5 in nonelderly men and women, respectively; and 0.5 and 0.45 in elderly men and women, respectively.
- Normally, extracellular and intracellular fluids account for 40% and 60% of total body water, respectively.

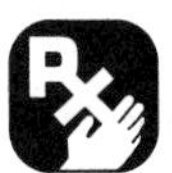

Long-Term Treatment

GENERAL

- Patients with severe, symptomatic hyponatremia should be admitted to an intensive care unit, with close monitoring of serum sodium levels.
- Proper management of underlying cause with close clinical follow-up
- Discontinue medications known to be associated with hyponatremia
- Clozapine appears to be effective in long-term treatment of schizophrenic patients with compulsive water drinking.

MANAGEMENT PEARLS AND PREVENTION STRATEGIES

- Although uncertainty about the diagnosis occasionally may justify a limited trial of isotonic saline, attentive follow-up is needed to confirm the diagnosis before substantial deterioration occurs.
- Isotonic saline is unsuitable for correcting the hyponatremia of SIADH.
- Great vigilance is required to recognize and diagnose hypothyroidism and adrenal insufficiency, which tend to masquerade as SIADH.
- Presence of hyperkalemia should always alert the physician to the possibility of adrenal insufficiency.
- Patients with persistent asymptomatic hyponatremia require slow paced management, but those with symptomatic hyponatremia must receive rapid but controlled correction.
- Education on fluid intake and appropriate placement of support stations was associated with a decreased incidence of symptomatic hyponatremia at ultraendurance sporting events.
- Hypotonic fluids and excessive isotonic fluids should be avoided after surgery.

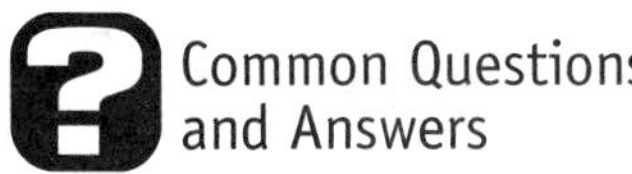

Common Questions and Answers

Physician responses to common patient questions:

Q: Use i.v. in ultraendurance athletes?

A: No, unless there are signs of dehydration, including cardiovascular instability.

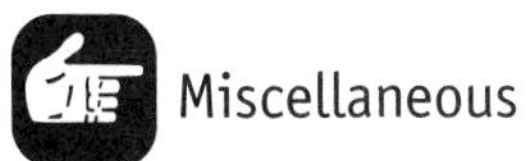

Miscellaneous

ICD-9 CODE

276.1

BIBLIOGRAPHY

Adrogue HJ, Madias N. Hyponatremia. *N Engl J Med* 2000;342:1581–1589.

Ayus JC, Varon J, Arieff AI. Hyponatremia, cerebral edema, and noncardiogenic pulmonary edema in marathon runners. *Ann Intern Med* 2000;132:711–714.

Craig S. http://www.emedicine.com/emerg/topic275.htm (hyponatremia). http://dynamicmedical.com Hyponatremia (hypotonic)

Kugler JP, Hustead T. Hyponatremia and hypernatremia in the elderly. *Am Fam Physician* 2000;61(12):3623–3630.

Noakes TD, Mayers LB. A guide to treating ironman triathletes at the finish line. *Physician Sportsmed* 2000;28.

Speedy DB, Rogers IR, Noakes TD, et al. Diagnosis and prevention of hyponatremia at an ultradistance triathlon. *Clin J Sports Med* 2000;10:52–58.

Authors: Tod Sweeney and William W. Dexter

Hypothermia and Frostbite

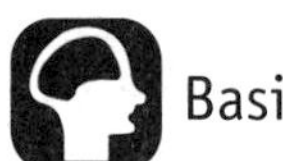

Basics

DEFINITION

Frostbite

- Severe local cold-related injury resulting in freezing of soft tissue

Hypothermia

- Systemic cold injury, classified as
  —Mild: core body temperature 32–35°C (90–95°F)
  —Moderate: 29–32°C (85–90°F)
  —Severe: <29°C (85°F)

INCIDENCE/PREVALENCE

- True incidence unknown
- Estimated 700 deaths per year in United States due to hypothermia

SIGNS AND SYMPTOMS

Frostbite

- Skin appears waxy, white, yellow, or blue-purple.
- Skin feels hard and cold to touch.
- Patient complains affected area is numb.

Hypothermia

- Mild: Patient displays shivering and mild mental status changes, including confusion, amnesia, dysarthria, and ataxia.
- Moderate: As core temperature declines, patient may develop severely impaired judgment or stupor, loss of deep tendon reflexes, loss of shivering with muscle rigidity, and cardiac arrhythmias.
- Severe: Patient may have dilated pupils and appear comatose, with nearly undetectable blood pressure and respiration.

RISK FACTORS

- Environmental factors: cold temperature, wind chill, prolonged exposure
- Wet clothing (increases heat loss 2–5 times) or immersion (increases heat loss 10–25 times)
- Dehydration
- Alcohol use (inhibits shivering, enhances heat loss through peripheral vasodilation, and may lead to false sense of warmth)
- Smoking
- Extremes of age (very young or elderly)
- Underlying medical disease (e.g., sickle cell anemia, peripheral vascular disease, diabetes, seizure disorder)

ASSOCIATED INJURIES AND COMPLICATIONS

Frostbite

- Limb and digit loss
- Premature closure of the epiphysis (younger athletes)
- Autonomic dysfunction of affected extremity

Hypothermia

- Cardiac arrhythmias
- Electrolyte and acid-base disorders
- Inefficient clotting leading to disseminated intravascular coagulation

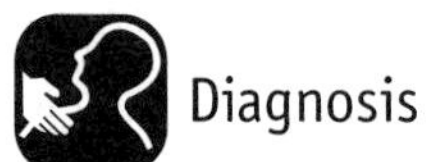

Diagnosis

DIFFERENTIAL DIAGNOSIS

Frostbite

- Frostnip: freezing injury to superficial skin layers
- Trenchfoot: swelling, cyanosis, and erythema of extremity without freezing of tissue
- Chilblains: local cold-related erythematous skin lesions

Hypothermia

- Altered mental status from metabolic abnormalities, alcohol/toxic ingestion, or closed head injury

HISTORY

Q: Duration and severity of cold exposure?
A: Prolonged exposure to very cold temperatures increases risk of severe frostbite or hypothermia.
Q: Recent alcohol or drug use?
A: Impairs judgment and increases susceptibility to cold injury.
Q: History of cold-water immersion?
A: Wet clothing and skin significantly increase continued heat loss.

PHYSICAL EXAMINATION

Measure Core Body Temperature

- For greatest accuracy, should be taken rectally with a thermometer capable of measuring hypothermic temperatures

Assess Pulse and Cardiac Rhythm

- Tachycardia may be seen with mild hypothermia.
- May progress to bradycardia, atrial fibrillation, or ventricular fibrillation with more severe hypothermia
- In severe hypothermia, may be difficult to manually palpate pulse

Assess Mental Status

- Degree of mental status alteration correlates with severity of hypothermia

Perform Complete Neurologic Examination

- Intact sensation to pinprick indicates a better prognosis for patients with frostbite.
- Decreased muscle coordination, delayed deep tendon reflexes, and slowed pupillary reflexes suggest more severe hypothermia.
- Focal neurologic deficit suggests etiology of mental status changes other than hypothermia.

Inspect Appearance of Skin

Cold, firm, yellow-white, or purple skin suggests frostbite.

TESTS

- Electrocardiogram: may see J wave (positive deflection occurring at junction of QRS complex and ST segment)
- Electrolytes and basic chemistries: hypothermic patients are at high risk for acid–base disturbances.

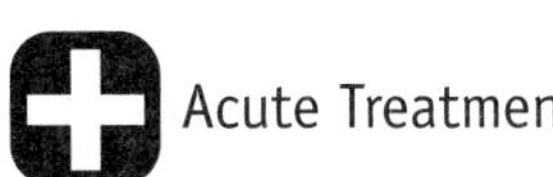

Acute Treatment

FROSTBITE

- Avoid thawing until no further risk of refreezing, then immerse affected part in 40°C (104°F) water for 15–30 minutes.
- Remove wet clothing and protect from further cold injury
- Arrange transport to emergency facility
- Monitor and treat for hypothermia
- After rewarming, debride white blisters and apply topical aloe vera. For hemorrhagic blisters, apply aloe vera without debridement.
- Administer tetanus prophylaxis, analgesics, and penicillin G (500,000 U every 6 hours for 48–72 hours)

HYPOTHERMIA

Field Treatment

- Passive external rewarming: prevent further heat loss with blankets, dry clothing, shared body heat, and moving patient to shelter. Avoid rubbing or massaging skin, which may compound tissue damage.
- Attempts at field rewarming should not delay transport to emergency facility for patients with moderate or severe hypothermia.
- Active external rewarming: direct application of heat sources (heating pad, hot water bottle, warm-water immersion, electric blanket) applied to trunk and used cautiously. Application of heat sources to extremities can result in rapid reversal of cold-induced peripheral vasoconstriction, leading to hypotension (rewarming shock) and further decreases in core temperature("afterdrop").
- Hot drinks for patients with normal gag reflex
- Avoid agitation or jarring because patient is at high risk for arrhythmia

Hospital Treatment for Moderate or Severe Hypothermia

- Continuous cardiac monitoring
- Active internal rewarming with heated [40°C (104°F)] intravenous fluid or heated humidified air or oxygen
- Peritoneal dialysis and extracorporeal blood rewarming may be used for severe hypothermia or in cases of cardiac arrest.
- Monitor electrolytes; rewarming usually corrects electrolyte and acid–base disturbances

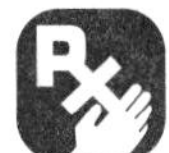

Long-Term Treatment

REHABILITATION

Range of motion and strengthening exercises may benefit frostbite-affected limbs.

SURGERY

Surgical debridement or amputation may be indicated for late treatment of necrotic or gangrenous tissue due to frostbite.

PREVENTION

- Best treatment for hypothermia and frostbite is prevention.
- Patients should be advised to wear proper clothing, including hats and multiple layers as necessary, maintain adequate hydration, and avoid alcohol during cold-weather exposure.

Common Questions and Answers

Physician responses to common patient questions:

Q: Can I get hypothermia if the temperature is not below "freezing" [32°F (0°C)]?

A: Yes. Hypothermia can occur even at moderate temperatures [50–65°F (10–18°C)] if wind, rain, sweat, or wet clothing lead to heat loss that is greater than metabolic heat production.

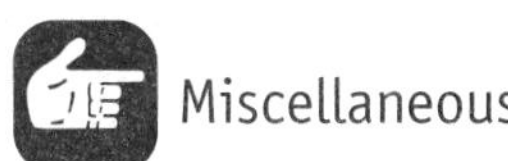

Miscellaneous

ICD-9 CODE

991.6 Hypothermia
991.3 Frostbite

BIBLIOGRAPHY

American College of Sports Medicine. Position Stand. Heat and cold illnesses during distance running. *Med Sci Sports Exerc* 1996;28:i–x.

Bracker MD. Environmental and thermal injury. *Clin Sports Med* 1992;11:419–436.

Sallis R, Chassay CM. Recognizing and treating common cold-induced injury in outdoor sports. *Med Sci Sports Exerc* 1999; 31:1367–1373.

Authors: Rania L. Dempsey and Craig C. Young

Impetigo

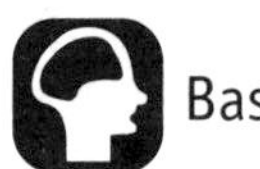

Basics

DEFINITION

- Superficial skin infection of the corneum stratum produced by group A β-hemolytic streptococci, *Staphylococcus aureus,* or a mixture of both.
- Two forms of impetigo are bullous and nonbullous.
- Nonbullous impetigo usually begins as an erythematous base with small vesicles filled with clear to amber-colored serous fluid that forms the characteristic honey-colored crust over the lesion.
- Removal of the crust shows an amber, serous fluid exuding from the erythematous base.
- Bullous form is less common and usually begins with superficial bullae 0.5–3.0 cm in diameter appearing on normal-looking skin. The bulla has a variable-colored fluid with a thin erythematous rim at the lesion's base.
- The bulla ruptures and a thin varnish-like coating forms over the denuded area. Regional lymphadenopathy is rare.
- Impetigo of Bockhart is a superficial staphylococcal folliculitis consisting of clusters of small pustules surrounding hair follicles.
- Ecthyma is a more advanced form of impetigo with lesions more deeply involved in the skin.
- Epidermis is eroded, which creates ulcerative, crusted lesions. Crusts form over the erosion and scarring occurs as the lesion heals.
- Children are more susceptible than adults.
- Legs are most commonly involved.

INCIDENCE/PREVALENCE

- Unreported, but most common in children and young adults
- Occurs most often in summer and fall seasons
- Incidence higher in tropical and semitropical climates
- Commonly seen in wrestlers, swimmers, gymnasts, football players, and soccer players

SIGNS AND SYMPTOMS

- Vesicles progressing to pustules
- Erythematous base
- Honey-colored serosanguineous crusts
- Insidious or rapid spread of lesions
- Thin-roofed vesicles with clear to cloudy fluid
- Weeping thin ulcer
- Satellite lesions

RISK FACTORS

- Hot, humid environment
- Tropical climates
- Summer and fall sports seasons
- Tight nonbreathable clothing
- Insect bites
- Contact sports
- Poor hygiene
- Epidemics
- Malnutrition
- Atopic dermatitis
- Diabetes mellitus
- Human immunodeficiency virus infection

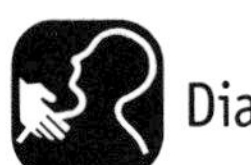

Diagnosis

DIFFERENTIAL DIAGNOSIS

- Folliculitis
- Insect bites
- Scabies
- Tinea corporis
- Varicella-zoster
- Herpes gladiatorum
- Scalded skin syndrome
- Contact dermatitis
- Burns
- Erythema multiforme
- Eczema
- Necrotizing fasciitis
- Stevens-Johnson syndrome

HISTORY

- 70% of impetigo cases account for nonbullous form
- *S. aureus* is the most common organism, followed by group A *Streptococcus*
- Lesions usually appear on the face and exposed skin.
- Occurs primarily in children and can spread to family members by close physical contact
- Bullous impetigo is caused exclusively by *S. aureus,* which is isolated from fluid cultures of the aspirates. Phage type 71 is most often reported, and the epidermolytic toxin produced by the bacteria forms the bullae.

PHYSICAL EXAMINATION

- Usually small vesicles appear on intact or compromised skin.
- Vesicles can progress to pustules filled with clear to amber fluid, which rupture and exude the serous fluid.
- Honey-colored crusts form over the thinly ulcerated lesion with an erythematous base.
- Diagnosis usually is made by clinical appearance.
- Cultures may be necessary if the lesion does not respond to appropriate therapy.
- Regional lymphadenopathy is common with the nonbullous form, and lymphadenitis is seldom seen on the physical examination.
- Poststreptococcal glomerulonephritis is more likely to follow impetigo than streptococcal pharyngitis.

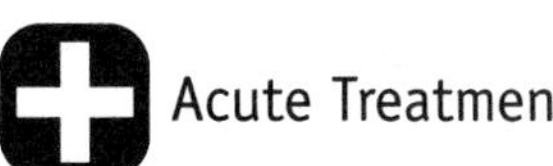

Acute Treatment

DRUGS OF CHOICE

- Topical antibiotic mupirocin (Bactroban) is applied t.i.d. for 7–10 days. Not as effective around the scalp and should not be applied to lesions around the mouth.
- If widespread lesions, consider oral antibiotics. Treat minor lesions for 7 days. If impetigo is widespread, treat for 10 days
- β-Lactamase–resistant antibiotics are used due to increasing incidence of penicillin-resistant staphylococci
- Dicloxacillin 250 mg q.i.d.; pediatric 12–25 mg/kg/day q6h.
- Cloxacillin 250 mg q.i.d. or 500 mg b.i.d.
- Intramuscular benzathine penicillin can be used as a single dose.
- Cephalexin 250 mg q.i.d. or 500 mg b.i.d.; pediatric 25–50 mg/kg/day q6h
- Other first-generation cephalosporins are effective.
- Erythromycin 250 mg q.i.d. or 500 mg b.i.d. for 7–10 days; pediatric 30–40 mg/kg/day q6h, but be aware that increasing erythromycin resistance may render this antibiotic ineffective.

COMPLICATIONS

- Septic arthritis
- Pneumonia
- Osteomyelitis
- Septicemia
- Cellulitis
- Suppurative lymphadenitis
- Erysipelas
- Ecthyma
- Poststreptococcal acute glomerulonephritis

MANAGEMENT

- Local cleansing and debridement with hydrogen peroxide
- Prevent spread of infection. Do not share athletic equipment and towels.
- Infected athletes should be discouraged from participating until lesion is dry and medically treated.
- NCAA guidelines state no new lesions for 48 hours and/or completion of 3 days of antibiotic treatment.

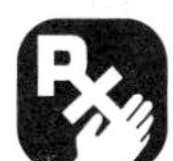

Long-Term Treatment

REFERRAL/DISPOSITION

- If no response to initial therapy, consider culture of the lesion and/or dermatologic referral.
- No increase of redeveloping infection if treated completely and patient is immune competent.

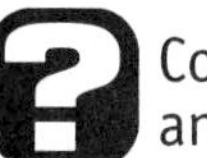

Common Questions and Answers

Physician responses to common patient questions:
Q: How did I get impetigo?
A: Impetigo is contracted by skin-to-skin contact with an infected person during athletic practice or competition.
Q: Can I participate while I have impetigo?
A: The crusty lesion of impetigo should not be weeping serous fluid and the athlete needs to be medically treated with the appropriate medication before return to sport.

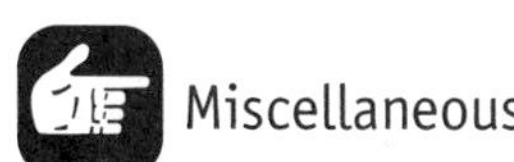

Miscellaneous

SYNONYMS

- Impetigo vulgaris
- Impetigo contagiosa

ICD-9 CODE

684 Impetigo

BIBLIOGRAPHY

Habif T. *Clinical dermatology.* St. Louis: Mosby, 1996.

Rosen P, ed. *Emergency medicine: concepts and clinical practice.* St. Louis: Mosby, 1998.

Sadick N. Current aspects of bacterial infections of the skin. *Dermatol Clin* 1997; 15:341–350.

Author: Paul Johnson

Inner Ear Injuries (Tympanic Membrane Perforation)

Basics

SIGNS AND SYMPTOMS

- Ear pain (mild)
- Decreased hearing (partial)
- Severe pain or complete hearing loss in the affected ear suggests additional injuries
- Purulent or bloody discharge from ear canal
- Tinnitus
- Vertigo
- Otorrhea

MECHANISM/DESCRIPTION

- Blunt trauma (slap to the ear)
- Penetrating trauma (Q-tip)
- Rapid pressure change (diving, flying)
- Extreme noise (blast)
- Lightning
- Spontaneous perforation of acute otitis media
- Acute necrotic myringitis

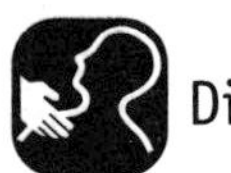

Diagnosis

ESSENTIAL WORKUP

- Clinical examination
  - —Direct visualization of tympanic membrane with otoscope
  - —Test hearing in both ears
  - —Note any nystagmus with changes of position or pressure on the tragus occluding the canal (fistula sign)

IMAGING/SPECIAL TESTS

- Insufflation via pneumatic otoscope
  - —Will not cause the perforated tympanic membrane to move normally
  - —Holding pressure for 15 seconds (the fistula test) may cause nystagmus or vertigo if the pressure is transmitted through the middle ear and into a labyrinthine fistula
- Weber test (tuning fork on midline bone)
  - —Sound should be equal or louder in the injured ear, consistent with decreased conduction
  - —Sound localizing to the opposite side of injury indicates possible otic nerve injury
- Rinne test
  - —Usually normal (air conduction detected after bone conduction fades) or shows a small conductive loss

DIFFERENTIAL DIAGNOSIS

- Temporal bone fracture
- Serous otitis media
- Infectious otitis media
- Otitis externa
- Cerumen impaction
- Barotrauma
- Acoustic trauma
- Foreign body
- Child abuse

Acute Treatment

INITIAL STABILIZATION

- ABCs of trauma care
  - —Immobilize C-spine and investigate for intracranial injury when indicated

ED TREATMENT

- Clean debris from the ear canal
- Prescribe antibiotics if there is evidence of infection
  - —Antibiotic choices (7–10 days administration)
    - —Amoxicillin
    - —Trimethoprim-sulfamethoxazole
    - —Cefixime
    - —Augmentin
  - —Prophylactic antibiotics not indicated
- Analgesics if needed for pain
- Do not prescribe topical steroids
- Arrange ENT follow up
  - —After detailed examination and formal audiometric tests, most otolaryngologists follow the perforation with monthly examinations
  - —Operative repair reserved for the 10–20% that do not heal spontaneously
- Provide detailed discharge instructions
  - —Occlude the ear canal with cotton coated in petroleum jelly or antibiotic ointment when showering to prevent entry of water into the middle ear, which can be painful
  - —Swim only with fitted earplugs
  - —Avoid forceful blowing of the nose

- Expected outcome
  - —Most perforations heal spontaneously over a few months
  - —A few require operative repair such as a collagen foam splint or a flap from the canal wall
  - —Perforations caused by molten metal or electrical burns are less likely to heal spontaneously
  - —Forceful entry of water, as in a water skiing accident, is more likely to lead to infection
  - —Complications include infection, dislocation of ossicles, perilymph leak, and cholesteatoma

MEDICATIONS

- Amoxicillin: 250–500 mg (peds: 20–40 mg/kg/24 hrs) po tid
- Trimethoprim-sulfamethoxazole (Bactrim DS): 1 tablet (peds: 6–12 mg/kg/24 hrs TMP) po bid
- Cefixime: 400 mg (peds: 8 mg/kg/24 hrs) q d
- Augmentin: 250–500 mg (peds: 20–40 mg/kg/24 hrs) po tid

HOSPITAL ADMISSION CRITERIA

- Associated injuries requiring admission
- Severe vertigo impairing ambulation

HOSPITAL DISCHARGE CRITERIA

- Almost all patients will be discharged

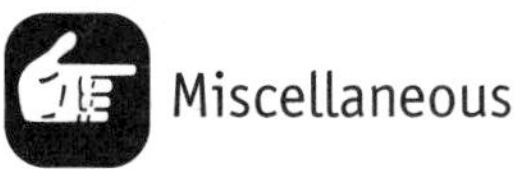

Miscellaneous

ICD-9 CODE

384.20

CORE CONTENT CODE

6.1.9

BIBLIOGRAPHY

Gladstone HB, Jackler RK, Varav K. Tympanic membrane wound healing: an overview. *Otolaryngol Clin North Am* 1995;28:913–933.

Kristensen S. Spontaneous healing of traumatic tympanic membrane perforations in man: a century of experience. *J Laryngol Otol* 1992;106:1037–1050.

Kristensen S, Juul A, Gamelgaard NP, et al. Traumatic tympanic membrane perforations: complications and management. *Ear Nose Throat J* 1989;68:503–516.

Turbiak T. Ear trauma. *Emerg Med Clin North Am* 1987;5:243–251.

Author: Thomas Osborne Stair

Intraocular Foreign Bodies

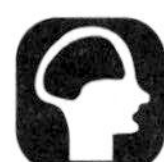

Basics

INCIDENCE/PREVALENCE

- Adults: often in industrial accidents, especially with hammering and machine tools
- Children: often with explosives, weapons
- 92% to 98% male
- Mostly work-related injuries, although increasingly related to leisure activity accidents

SIGNS AND SYMPTOMS

- Pain: ranges from asymptomatic or slight discomfort to severe pain
- Vision: ranges from asymptomatic or slight blurring to complete loss of vision
- Foreign body (FB) sensation: may be transient or persistent

RISK FACTORS

- Eye protection was worn by only 0% to 6% of patients at the time of injury.
- Nonsafety glasses may provide inadequate protection.

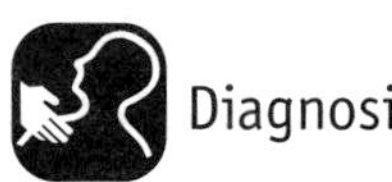

Diagnosis

DIFFERENTIAL DIAGNOSIS

- Corneal abrasion
- Conjunctival and corneal FBs
- Extraocular FB
- Ruptured globe
- Other trauma without retained intraocular foreign body (IOFB)

HISTORY

- Detailed history and high index of suspicion are very important with any periorbital soft tissue trauma or history suggestive of IOFB.
- Ophthalmologic history: prior vision with and without correction, prior surgeries, medications
- Vision correction: Does the patient usually wear glasses or contacts? Were they worn at the time of injury? When and how were they removed?
- Eye protection: Was the patient wearing eye protection? What type? Is it still intact?
- Mechanism: approximate the trajectory and velocity of the IOFB
- Composition:
  —Organic: injuries involving wood, soil, plants.
  —Glass or plastic: injuries with broken windshields, other shattered glass or plastic
  —Metal: injuries involving explosions, motor vehicle accidents
- Thorough medical history, including medications, allergies, date of last tetanus immunization, and last meal

PHYSICAL EXAMINATION

- Document findings as soon as possible, as hemorrhage or traumatic lens opacification may develop quickly.
- Minimize manipulation of the globe and exercise caution during examination to prevent prolapse of ocular contents.
- Document baseline visual acuity; visual fields; pupillary size, shape, and reactivity; corneal irregularities; wound location and size; depth of anterior chamber; iris and lens condition; blood in the anterior chamber or vitreous; gaze restriction; and external examination. Slit-lamp and funduscopic examinations should be performed as soon as possible.
- History, physical, and imaging studies should be used to assess number, size, shape, location, composition, visibility, trajectory, and accessibility of the IOFB.

IMAGING

- Computed tomographic (CT) scan: replaces many prior techniques due to superior localization and identification of IOFB and associated injuries
- Radiography: adjunctive test with low sensitivity, especially for small and nonmetallic objects
- Ultrasound: allows detailed evaluation of IOFB and associated ocular trauma; used adjunctively and intraoperatively. Caution due to risk of ocular prolapse.
- Magnetic resonance imaging: initially contraindicated due to risk of magnetic properties, but may be used to localize small nonmetallic IOFBs after metallic IOFBs ruled out by CT scan

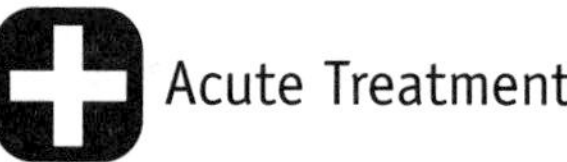

Acute Treatment

ANALGESIA

- No topical medications or ointments if globe perforation is suspected
- Ice may be applied (avoiding pressure on the globe) to minimize pain and reduce edema of periorbital soft tissues.
- Minimize nausea and vomiting to prevent resultant increases in intraocular pressure

IMMOBILIZATION

- Shield should be placed over involved eye, avoiding any pressure on the globe.
- Both eyes should be shielded if immobilization of the eye is desirable due to associated injury.

SPECIAL CONSIDERATIONS

- Retinal tears may be repaired by photocoagulation or cryotherapy (controversial).
- Retinal detachment is repaired by vitrectomy, retinopexy, gas tamponade, and scleral buckling.
- Lens capsule disruption may lead to infection, glaucoma, and sterile lens-induced endophthalmitis.
- Intraocular lens placement may be delayed if patient is at high risk for infection.

INFECTION

- Endophthalmitis reported in up to 13% of patients, with potential complete loss of vision. Signs suggestive of infection (hypopyon, severe eyelid edema, vitreous inflammation) only present initially in 60% to 90% of patients, as they may be subclinical or masked by trauma.
- Risk factors for endophthalmitis include age >50 years, particularly if IOFB removal is delayed >24 hours. Steel and organic IOFBs may confer higher risk.
- Causative pathogens include *Bacillus* (especially poor outcomes), *Staphylococcus* sp, and *Streptococcus* sp. Fungal infections must be considered with organic IOFBs.
- A 1- to 3-day course of broad-spectrum intravenous antibiotics is started as soon as possible. Short delays may be considered to increase culture sensitivity if IOFB removal is imminent. Recommended antibiotics include vancomycin, ceftazidime, cefazolin, and ciprofloxacin, alone or in combination, depending on the clinical suspicion of infection.

- Prophylactic intravitreal antibiotics may include vancomycin and either amikacin (synergistic against *Bacillus*) or ceftazidime (less retinotoxic), particularly with a "dirty" IOFB or delayed removal (>24 hours).
- Steroids (dexamethasone) may be administered topically, subconjunctivally, or intravitreously (controversial).
- Tetanus booster, if indicated

SURGERY

- Nothing by mouth (after acute injury) in preparation for surgery
- Early removal is preferable, even for inert "clean" IOFBs due to risk of infection or fibrous tissue enmeshment.
- Magnetic FBs may be removed by permanent magnets (force is coaxial with tip) or electromagnets (bulkier, wider, and stronger field of pull: requires adequate visibility and localization).
- Cornea: cut down directly over FB, using a magnet if possible
- Anterior or posterior chambers: removal through the limbus with a constricted pupil
- Intralenticular: removal of biologic lens; may consider sealing capsule with fibrin clot in young patients with nonmetallic IOFB
- Vitreous: vitrectomy often preferred, especially with endophthalmitis or if anterior segment material is displaced into posterior segment
- Intraretinal: removal with minimal retinal traction, often through scleral flap

REFERRAL

- Urgent ophthalmologic referral required for all cases of suspected IOFB.
- Delayed surgical removal (24 hours) is associated with significantly worse outcomes.
- Urgent neurosurgical or otolaryngologic referral may be indicated due to concomitant injuries.

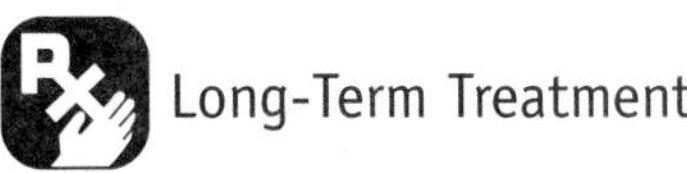

Long-Term Treatment

REHABILITATION

- Protect associated soft tissue wounds from the sun for 6 months
- Massage and vitamin E after 1 month may help reduce scarring.

SURGERY

Cosmetic surgery may be required for associated injuries, but should be delayed at least 6 months for resolution of inflammation and scar tissue maturation.

SPECIAL CONSIDERATIONS

Metallosis

- Usually with iron and copper alloys
- Lead, zinc, and nickel usually well tolerated, but may cause chronic nongranulomatous inflammatory reactions
- Testing may include electroretinography or x-ray spectrometry.

Chalcosis (from Retained Copper Alloy IOFB)

- May resemble Wilson disease, including (rarely) Kayser-Fleischer rings and sunflower cataracts due to extracellular, reversible copper deposition
- Pure copper IOFBs may cause acute sterile panophthalmitis.

Siderosis Bulbi (from Retained Iron IOFB)

- May resemble changes seen after intraocular hemorrhage due to uptake and intracellular, largely irreversible deposition in various epithelial tissues
- Signs include heterochromia, chronic open angle glaucoma, subcapsular cataracts, and various rusty-appearing corneal iron lines
- Consider retinal epithelial uptake leading to constricted visual fields, night blindness, and poor dark adaptation, clinically resembling retinitis pigmentosa

Proliferative Retinopathy

- Frequent cause of vision loss and retinal detachment, especially with intraretinal IOFBs
- Complete vitrectomy often performed prophylactically

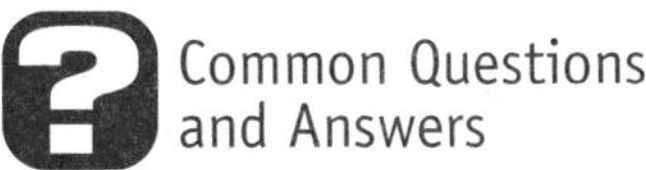

Common Questions and Answers

Physician responses to common patient questions:
Q: What is the prognosis?
A: Usually good prognosis. May be unpredictable, with some acute deteriorations seen years after IOFB removal.

- 80% to 85% recover vision to 20/200; 60% to 70% recover to 20/40
- Favorable prognostic indicators are initial visual acuity >20/200, anterior wound site, wound <10 mm, and sharp, metallic, nonmagnetic IOFBs.
- Poor prognostic indicators are initial visual acuity <5/200, posterior wound site, wound >10 mm, high blunt force, nonmetallic, organic, or magnetic FBs, afferent pupillary defect, disruption of lenticular capsule, vitreous hemorrhage, and intraretinal IOFBs.

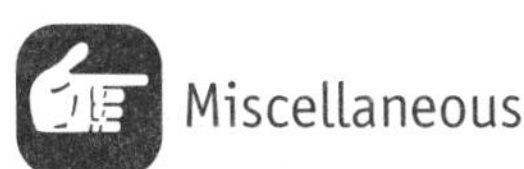

Miscellaneous

ICD-9 CODE

871.5 Current penetrating injury with magnetic foreign body
871.6 Current penetrating injury with nonmagnetic foreign body
871.7 Current penetrating injury with unspecified foreign body
360.5 Retained IOFB, magnetic
360.6 Retained IOFB, nonmagnetic
871.9 Unspecified open wound of eyeball

PREVENTION

- Use eye protection at home and at work when hammering, grinding, etc.
- Use particular caution with explosives

BIBLIOGRAPHY

Albert DM, Jakobiec FA, eds. *Principles and practice of ophthalmology*. Philadelphia: WB Saunders, 2000.

Behrens-Baumann W, Praetorius G. Intraocular foreign bodies: 297 consecutive cases. *Ophthalmologica* 1989;198:84–88.

Greven CM, Engelbrecht NE, Slusher MM, et al. Intraocular foreign bodies: management, prognostic factors and visual outcomes. *Ophthalmology* 2000;107:608–612.

Pavan-Langston D, ed. *Manual of ocular diagnosis and therapy*, 4th ed. Boston: Little, Brown and Company, 1996.

Williams DF, Mieler WF, Abrams GW, et al. Results and prognostic factors in penetrating ocular injuries with retained intraocular foreign bodies. *Ophthalmology* 1988;95:911–916.

Author: David Wallis

Lacerations and Soft Tissue Injuries

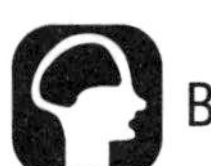

Basics

SIGNS AND SYMPTOMS

- Lacerations may be accompanied by
  - —Bleeding
  - —Tissue foreign bodies
  - —Hematoma
  - —Pain or numbness
  - —Loss of motor function
  - —Diminished pulses, delayed capillary refill

MECHANISM/DESCRIPTION

- A laceration is a disruption in skin integrity most often resulting from trauma
- May be single or multiple layered

CAUTIONS

- Obtain hemostasis, or control of bleeding with direct pressure
- Unkink any flaps of skin whose blood supply may be strangulated
- Universal precautions

PEDIATRIC CONSIDERATIONS

- Assess for possible nonaccidental trauma

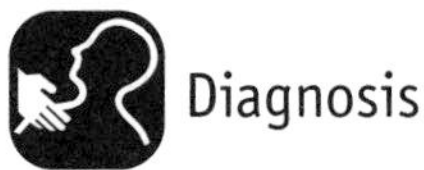

Diagnosis

ESSENTIAL WORKUP

- Mechanism and circumstances of injury
- Time of injury
- History of foreign body (glass, splinter, teeth)
  - —Avoid digital exploration if the object is believed to be sharp
- Tetanus immunization
- Comorbid condition that may impede wound healing
- Evaluate nerve and motor function
- Document associated neurovascular injury
- Assess presence of devitalized tissue, debris from foreign materials, bone or joint violation

LABORATORY

N/A

IMAGING/SPECIAL TESTS

Evaluation for Possible Foreign Bodies

- Plain radiography
  - —Soft tissue views may aid in visualization
  - —Objects with the same density as soft tissue may not be seen (wood, plants)
- Ultrasonography

DIFFERENTIAL DIAGNOSIS

- Skin avulsion
- Contusion
- Abrasion

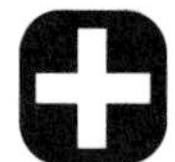

Acute Treatment

INITIAL STABILIZATION

- ABCs
- Control of hemostasis

ED TREATMENT

Time of Onset

- Lacerations may be closed primarily up to 8 hours old in areas of poorer circulation
- Lacerations may be closed up to 12 hours old in areas of normal circulation
- On face, lacerations may be closed up to 24 hours if clean and well irrigated
- If not closed, wound may heal by secondary intention, or delayed primary closure (DPC) in 3–5 days

Analgesia and Conscious Sedation

- Adequate analgesia is crucial for good wound management
- Conscious sedation may be required

Local Anesthetics

- Topical
  - —TAC (tetracaine, adrenaline, cocaine)
  - —EMLA ("eutectic mixture," lidocaine, prilocaine)
- Local/regional
  - —Lidocaine, bupivacaine
  - —Epinephrine will cause vasoconstriction and improve duration of action
  - —Avoid in the penis, digits, toes, ears, eyelids, skin flaps (necrosis), and severely contaminated wounds (impairs defense)
  - —For patient comfort, inject slowly with small gauge needle; buffer every 9 cc of 1% lidocaine with 1 cc 8.4% sodium bicarbonate

Exploration and Removal of Foreign Body

- Indications for removal of a foreign body include
  - —Potential or actual injury to tendons, nerves, vasculature
  - —Toxic substance, or reactive agent
  - —Continued pain

Irrigation and Debridement

- Clean surrounding skin with an antiseptic solution (betadine)
  - —Do not use antiseptic solution within the wound itself as it may impair healing
- Scrub with a fine-pore sponge only if significant contamination, or particulate matter
- Irrigation with 200 cc or more of NS
  - —Optimal pressure (5–8 psi) generated with 30 cc syringe through 18–20-gauge needle
  - —Debride devitalized tissue

Wound Repair

- Universal precautions
- Wounds that cannot be cleaned adequately should heal by secondary intention, or DPC
- Reapproximate all anatomic borders carefully (skin-vermilion border of lip, etc.)

Simple Layered Closure

- Simple interrupted sutures
  - —Avoid in lacerations under tension
- Horizontal mattress sutures (running or interrupted)
  - —Edematous finger and hand wounds
  - —Ideal in skin flaps where edges at risk for necrosis
- Vertical mattress
  - —For wounds under greater tension

Multiple Layered Closure

- Closes deep tissue dead space
- Lessens tension at the epidermal level, improves cosmetic result
- Buried interrupted absorbable suture, simple or running nonabsorbable sutures for epidermis

Dressing

- Dress wound with antibiotic ointment and nonadherent semiporous dressing
- Inform patient about scarring and risk of infection, use of sunscreen

Antimicrobial Agents

- Uncomplicated lacerations do not need antibiotic prophylaxis
- Lacerations with high likelihood of infection
  - —Human bite to hand
  - —Contaminated with dirt, bodily fluids, feces
    - —Polymicrobial, enteric prophylaxis
- Tetanus immunization

MEDICATIONS

- Tetanus (Td adults, DT peds): 0.5 cc IM

Local Anesthetics

- Topical, applied directly to wound with cotton, gauze
  - —TAC (0.5% tetracaine, (1:2000) adrenaline, (11.8% cocaine)): apply for 20 min
  - —EMLA ("eutectic mixture," 5% lidocaine and prilocaine): apply for 60 min
- Injected

Local/Regional	Maximum Dose (mg/kg)	Duration (Hours)
Lidocaine	4.5	1.5–3.5
Bupivacaine	2	3–10

MATERIALS

Suture Materials

Absorbable

- For use in mucous membranes and buried muscle/fascial layer closures
  - —Natural—dissolve <1 week, poor tensile strength, local inflammation
    - —Plain catgut
    - —Chromic
    - —Fast absorbing gut for certain facial lacerations where cosmesis is important
  - —Synthetic braided—tensile strength diminishing over 1 month, mild inflammation
    - —Polyglycolic acid (dexon)
    - —Polyglactin 910 (vicryl)
  - —Synthetic monofilament-tensile strength 70% at 1 month, inflammation degree unknown
    - —Polydioxanone (PDS)
    - —Polyglyconate (maxon)

Nonabsorbable

- Greatest tensile strength
  - —Monofilament
    - —Nylon (ethilon, dermalon)
    - —Polypropylene (prolene)
    - —Polybutester (novofil): can stretch with wound edema
  - —Polyethylene, stainless steel
  - —Multifilament
    - —Cotton
    - —Silk (local inflammation)

Needle Types

- Cutting (cuticular and plastic) are most often used in outpatient wound repair

Staples

- For linear lacerations of scalp, torso, extremities
- Avoid in hands, face, and areas requiring CT or MRI

Adhesive Tapes (Steri-Strips)

- For lacerations that are clean, small, and under minimal tension
- Avoid in wounds that have potential to become very swollen
- Pretreat wound edges with tincture of benzoin to improve adhesion

Tissue Adhesives

- Good cosmetic results have been achieved in simple lacerations with low skin tension
- An alternative to sutures/staples especially in children, if adhesive is available

HOSPITAL ADMISSION CRITERIA

- Few lacerations by themselves necessitate admission unless they require significant debridement, ongoing intravenous antibiotics, or are complicated by extensive wound care issues or comorbid processes (head injury, abdominal trauma)

HOSPITAL DISCHARGE CRITERIA

- Wounds at risk for infection or poor healing requiring a wound check within 48 hours
- Time of suture removal dependent upon location and peripheral perfusion
  - —Scalp: 7–10 days
  - —Face: 3–5 days
  - —Oral: 7 days
  - —Neck: 4–6 days
  - —Abdomen, back, chest, hands, feet: 7–10 days
  - —Upper extremity: 7–10 days
  - —Lower extremity: 10–14 days

PEDIATRIC CONSIDERATIONS

- If it is unsafe for a child to return home if nonaccidental trauma is suspected

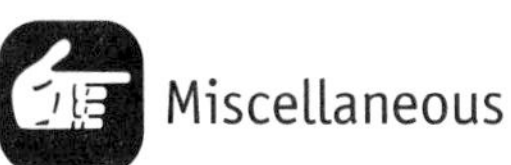

Miscellaneous

ICD-9 CODE

998.2

CORE CONTENT CODE

18.4.17.2

BIBLIOGRAPHY

Chisolm C, Howell JM. Soft tissue emergencies. *Emerg Med Clin North Am* 1992;10(4):665–705.

Roberts PA, Lamacraft G. Techniques to reduce the discomfort of pediatric laceration repair. *MJA* 1996;164(1):32–35.

Edich RF, Rodeheover GT, Thacker JG. Wound preparation. In: Tintinalli JE, Ruiz E, Krome RL, eds. *Emergency medicine: a comprehensive study guide*. 4th ed. New York: McGraw Hill, 1996:279–283.

Author: Gordon Chew

Lightning Injuries

Basics

SIGNS AND SYMPTOMS

Cardiorespiratory

- Cardiac asystole
  - —Due to direct current injury
  - —May resolve spontaneously as the heart's intrinsic automaticity resumes
- Respiratory arrest
  - —Due to paralysis of medullary respiratory center
  - —May persist longer than cardiac asystole and lead to hypoxic induced VFib
- Acute myocardial infarction rare
- Shock
  - —Neurogenic (spinal injury)
  - —Hypovolemic (trauma)
- Mottled or cold extremities
  - —Due to autonomic vasomotor instability
  - —Usually resolves spontaneously in a few hours

Neurological Injuries

- Confusion
- Memory defects
- Alteration of level of consciousness (>70% of cases)
- Flaccid motor paralysis
- Seizures
- Fixed dilated pupils due either to serious head injury or autonomic dysfunction

Traumatic Injuries

- Blunt trauma
  - —To the head or spine
  - —Fractures, dislocations, muscle tears, and compartment syndromes
- Ruptured tympanic membrane with ossicular disruption (up to 50%)
- Burns
  - —Discrete entrance and exit wounds uncommon
  - —Thermal burns due to evaporation of water on skin, ignited clothing, heated metal objects (buckles/jewelry)
- Feathering (fernlike pattern) "burns"
  - —Cutaneous imprints from electron showers that track over skin
  - —Pathognomonic of lightning injury
  - —Resolve within 24 hours

Ophthalmologic Injuries

- Cataracts occur days to years postinjury
- Corneal lesions
- Intraocular hemorrhages
- Retinal detachment

MECHANISM/DESCRIPTION

- Due to the brief duration (1–100 msec) of lightning
  - —Current passes over the skin rather than through the body (flashover)
  - —Deep tissue injuries are rare
- Mechanisms of injury
  - —Direct strike—strikes victim directly
  - —Splash injury—moves from object to victim of lesser resistance to current flow
  - —Ground strike—current moves through ground and may injure multiple victims
  - —Blunt injury due to direct explosive effect
  - —Thermal burning

CONTROVERSIES

- Field triage should rapidly focus on providing ventilatory support to unconscious victim(s) or those in cardiopulmonary arrest
  - —Prevents reversible asystolic cardiac arrest from degenerating into hypoxic induced VFib
- Conscious victims are at lower risk of imminent demise

CAUTIONS

- Spine immobilization for
  - —Cardiopulmonary arrest (suspected trauma)
  - —Significant mechanical trauma
  - —Suspected loss of consciousness at any time
- Cover superficial burns with sterile saline dressings
- Immobilize injured extremities
- Rapid extrication prevents exposure to repeat lightning strikes

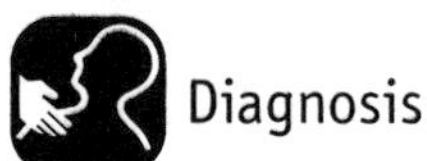

Diagnosis

ESSENTIAL WORKUP

- Confirmatory history from bystanders or rescuers of the circumstances of the injury

LABORATORY

- CBC for baseline Hct
- Urinalysis for myoglobin
- Electrolytes for acidosis
- BUN, Cr for baseline renal function
- CK and CKMb fraction for muscle/cardiac damage

IMAGING/SPECIAL TESTS

- CXR
- C-spine radiograph
- CT head for altered mental status or significant head trauma
- ECG should be performed in all cases
  - —Nonspecific ST changes common
  - —Acute myocardial infarction rare

DIFFERENTIAL DIAGNOSIS

- Consider lightning strike in unwitnessed falls, cardiac arrests, or unexplained coma in an outdoor setting

- Other causes of coma, cardiac dysrhythmia, or trauma
  —Hypoglycemia
  —Intoxication
  —Drug overdose
  —Cardiovascular disease
  —CVA

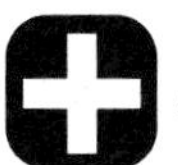

Acute Treatment

INITIAL STABILIZATION

- ABCs
- Standard ACLS measures for cardiac arrest
- Diligent primary and secondary survey for traumatic injuries
  —Maintain cervical spine precautions until cleared
- Treat altered mental status with glucose, naloxone, or thiamine as indicated
- Hypotension requires volume expansion and pressor agents

ED TREATMENT

- IV access for medication administration
- Volume expansion
  —Do not follow burn treatment formulas as flashover burns are rarely the cause of fluid loss
  —Occult deep burn injury is rare when compared to other types of electrical current injury
  —Titrate volume administration to urine output—fluid-loading may be dangerous with head injuries
- Clean and dress burns
- Tetanus prophylaxis
- Treat myoglobinuria with
  —Diuretics, such as furosemide or mannitol,
  —Alkalinization of urine to a pH $\geq$7.45
  —Maintain urine output with IV fluid administration
- Compartment syndrome
  —Must be distinguished from vasospasm, autonomic dysfunction, and paralysis which are usually self-limited phenomena
  —Delay fasciotomy if possible because it will rarely be necessary

MEDICATIONS

- Furosemide: 1 mg/kg IV slow bolus q 6 hrs
- Mannitol: 0.5 mg/kg IV, repeat PRN
- Sodium bicarbonate: 1 amp IVP (peds: 1 mEq/kg) followed by 2–3 amps/L of D5W IV fluid

HOSPITAL ADMISSION CRITERIA

- Seriously injured and postcardiac arrest victims
- History of change in mental status/altered level of consciousness
- Myoglobinuria
- Acidosis
- History dysrhythmias or ECG changes
  —May not resolve spontaneously
  —24–48-hour observation period to identify potentially unstable cases

HOSPITAL DISCHARGE CRITERIA

- Asymptomatic patients with no injuries
- Close follow-up due to the risk of delayed sequelae

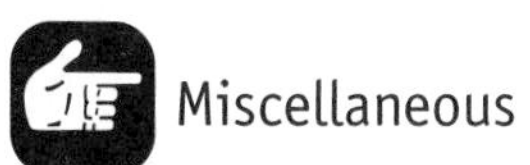

Miscellaneous

ICD-9 CODE

994.0

CORE CONTENT CODE

5.4

BIBLIOGRAPHY

Browne BJ, Gaasch WR. Lightning. *Emerg Med Clin North Am* 1992;10:2:211–230.

Cooper MA. Lightning injuries. In: Rosen P, Barkin R, Danzl D, et al., eds. *Emergency medicine: Concepts and clinical practice*. 4th ed. St. Louis: CV Mosby, 1998: 1010–1022.

Cooper MA, Andrew CJ. Lightning injuries. In: Auerbach P, ed. *Wilderness medicine*. St. Louis: CV Mosby, 1995:261–290.

Lichtenberg R, et al. Cardiovascular effects of lightning strikes. *J Am Coll Cardiol* 1993;21(2):531–536.

Author: Paul Arnold

Marfan's Syndrome

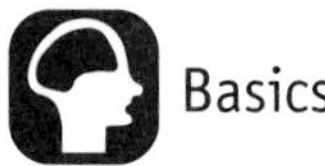

Basics

DESCRIPTION

A dominantly inherited disorder of connective tissue affecting primarily the musculoskeletal system, the cardiovascular system and the eye
System(s) affected: Musculoskeletal, Endocrine/Metabolic
Genetics: Autosomal dominant with high penetrance; 15% spontaneous mutation
Incidence/Prevalence in USA: 1 in 10,000–20,000 (estimated 1 in 15,000)
Predominant age: Congenital, so disorder is present from birth. However clinical manifestations do not usually become apparent until adolescence or young adulthood.
Predominant sex: No gender, ethnic or racial predilection

SIGNS AND SYMPTOMS

- Musculoskeletal
  —Tall stature
  —Thin, gangly body habitus (limb length out of proportion to trunk)
  —Arachnodactyly, i.e., long, thin fingers
  —Pectus deformity
  —High arched palate
  —Hyperextensible joints
  —Kyphoscoliosis
  —Joint laxity
- Cardiovascular
  —Aortic root dilatation
  —Aortic regurgitation
  —Aortic dissection
  —Mitral valve prolapse
  —Mitral regurgitation
- Ocular
  —Subluxation of lens, usually upward
  —Myopia
  —Retinal detachment (uncommon)
- Other
  —Easy bruising (uncommon)
  —Excessive bleeding (uncommon)

CAUSES

Genetic; at least 5% are obviously familial, the remainder arise from apparent spontaneous mutations

RISK FACTORS

Advanced paternal age gives rise to a slightly increased risk only in those cases which are not clearly familial

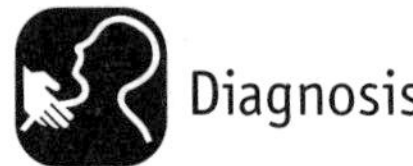

Diagnosis

DIFFERENTIAL DIAGNOSIS

Homocystinuria, contractural arachnodactyly, Ehlers-Danlos syndrome, trisomy, all of which are rare conditions and all of which have clear cut distinguishing clinical features from the Marfan's syndrome

LABORATORY

- There are no specific laboratory abnormalities in the Marfan syndrome
- It is recommended that suspected patients have urinary homocystine measured to rule out homocystinuria

Drugs that may alter lab results: N/A
Disorders that may alter lab results: N/A

PATHOLOGICAL FINDINGS

- Cystic medial necrosis of the aorta
- Myxomatous degeneration of the cardiac valves
- FBN1 gene on chromosome 15 codes for fibrillin, a large glycoprotein constituent of microfibrils. Mutations in this gene have been found in over 90% of patients with the Marfan's syndrome, when tested.

SPECIAL TESTS

Slit lamp examination is necessary to detect lens subluxation

IMAGING

- Plain x-rays of spine are necessary during growth years to detect and quantify scoliosis
- Annual screening echocardiograms are recommended beginning in adolescence in order to detect presymptomatic aortic root dilatation or valvular degeneration

DIAGNOSTIC PROCEDURES

N/A

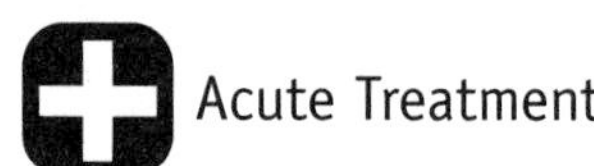

Acute Treatment

APPROPRIATE HEALTH CARE

Outpatient

GENERAL MEASURES

Multidisciplinary approach including primary care physician, cardiologist, ophthalmologist and possibly orthopedic surgeon. A clinical geneticist available, would be ideal as primary care physician.

SURGICAL MEASURES

Many, if not most, of these patients will ultimately require reconstructive cardiovascular surgery

ACTIVITY

- Fully active unless limited by symptoms
- Several highly-trained athletes with the Marfan syndrome have suffered sudden death during competition leading to some concern that people with the Marfan syndrome should be discouraged from participating in aerobically demanding sports

DIET

No special diet

PATIENT EDUCATION

Information available from the National Marfan Foundation, 382 Main St., Port Washington, NY 11959; 800-8MARFAN

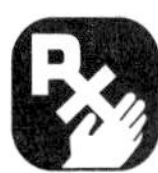

Long-Term Treatment

DRUG(S) OF CHOICE

- No specific medical therapy is available, however drugs are used to try to prevent certain complications
- Propranolol or other beta-adrenergic blocking drugs are used to decrease the force of cardiac contraction, in the hope of delaying the development or progression of aortic root dilatation. The dosage of these drugs are adjusted to target heart rate, i.e., resting rate of 60 per minute, with a rise to no more than 80 per minute after moderate exertion.
- Estrogen combined with progestogen has been used to induce puberty in pre-adolescent girls in an attempt to shorten the growth spurt thereby ameliorating scoliosis and preventing excessively tall stature. Do this only under the supervision of an endocrinologist.

Contraindications:

- Congestive heart failure, asthma, diabetes for the beta-adrenergic blocking drugs
- Thromboembolic disease for the estrogen/progestogen

Precautions: Refer to manufacturer's profile of each drug.

Significant possible interactions: Amphetamines, antihistamines, antidiabetics, oral contraceptives

ALTERNATIVE DRUGS

N/A

PATIENT MONITORING

- Frequent examinations (at least twice a year) while growing, with particular attention to cardiovascular system and scoliosis
- When cardiac symptoms develop or aortic root diameter becomes >50 mm, surgical intervention must be considered
- When lens subluxation is detected, surgical correction is possible. However a high incidence of glaucoma results, so surgery should be offered only to those who cannot be treated with corrective lenses.

PREVENTION/AVOIDANCE

- No prenatal diagnosis yet available, but presymptomatic diagnosis may be possible at research centers using linkage analysis techniques
- Each child has a 50% chance of inheriting the disorder from an affected parent. Clinical manifestations are variable, however, so children may be more or less severely affected.
- Antibiotic prophylaxis for endocarditis should be prescribed for all Marfan's syndrome patients with either a heart murmur or echocardiographic evidence of valvular or aortic root abnormalities

POSSIBLE COMPLICATIONS

- Bacterial endocarditis
- Aortic dissection
- Aortic or mitral valve insufficiency
- Dilated cardiomyopathy
- Retinal detachment

EXPECTED COURSE/PROGNOSIS

- Life-threatening complications are cardiovascular. Before routine corrective surgery was available most Marfan's syndrome patients died before reaching the age of 35.
- With appropriate surgical intervention most patients can live a normal life span

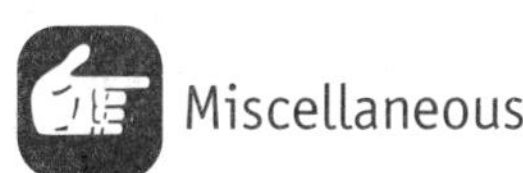

Miscellaneous

AGE-RELATED FACTORS

Pediatric: Early medical or surgical intervention may reduce the degree of scoliosis
Geriatric: N/A
Others: N/A

PREGNANCY

Pregnant women with the Marfan syndrome need to be managed as high-risk patients, preferably with involvement of a cardiologist. The outcome is usually excellent.

ICD-9 CODE

759.82 Marfan syndrome

BIBLIOGRAPHY

Pyeritz RE, McKusick VA. The Marfan syndrome: diagnosis and management. *New Engl J Med* 1979;300:772–777.

Scriver RC, et al., eds. *The metabolic basis of inherited disease*. 7th Ed. New York, McGraw Hill, 1995.

Internet references: http://www.5mcc.com

Author: Mark R. Dambro

Migraine Headache

 Basics

SIGNS AND SYMPTOMS

- *Common migraine*
  - —Unheralded onset of headache that is recurrent, throbbing, and frequently unilateral
  - —Usually associated with photophobia, phonophobia, nausea, anorexia, and vomiting
- *Classic migraine:* common migraine, which is preceded by a prodrome; usually visual symptoms such as bright lights or jagged lines
- *Complicated migraine:* migraine headache with associated neurologic symptoms such as numbness, weakness, paralysis, or aphasia

MECHANISM/DESCRIPTION

- The prevailing theory is that a migraine begins with intracranial artery vasoconstriction, which results in reduced cerebral blood flow. This produces the *aura*, the type of which is dependent on the area of reduced flow
  - —This is followed by a rebound vasodilation of the arteries during which the headache occurs
  - —The arterial dilation gives rise to pain

ETIOLOGY

- Idiopathic
- May be precipitated by chocolate, cheese, nuts, alcohol, sulfites, MSG, stress, tension, or puberty
- There is a family history of migraines in 60%
- Affects 5–15% of the population (women 3 times more than men)

PEDIATRIC CONSIDERATIONS

- Migraines do present in the pediatric age group, but are less common
- The typical pediatric patient is a prepubertal female with a strong family history of migraine

CAUTIONS

- It is important to recognize life-threatening causes of headache and transport rapidly
  - —Sudden onset of symptoms, altered mental status, neck stiffness, fever, or neurologic deficits are useful signs that suggest a more serious cause of headache
  - —Prior history of similar headache, absence of above symptoms, or strong family history is more suggestive of migraine
- Allow patients with migraine headache to be in a calm, dark environment

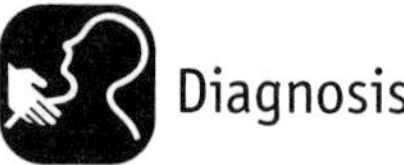

Diagnosis

ESSENTIAL WORKUP

- An accurate history and physical exam should confirm the diagnosis
- Patients with new onset of headache syndrome need an objective evaluation to rule out more serious causes of severe headaches
  - —Complete neurologic examination
  - —CT or MRI of the head
  - —Lumbar puncture
  - —If the patient can be assured of close follow-up, imaging studies and LP can be done as an outpatient if the clinical presentation does not suggest a life-threatening cause of headache

LABORATORY

- Not needed for classic migraine or established migraines with typical symptoms
- Lumbar puncture if suspect meningitis, intracranial hemorrhage, or pseudotumor cerebri
- ESR if suspect temporal arteritis
- Carbon monoxide (CO) level if there is history or suspicion of CO exposure

IMAGING/SPECIAL TESTS

- CT scan or MRI to rule out intracranial hemorrhage or tumor

DIFFERENTIAL DIAGNOSIS

- Meningitis
- Subarachnoid/intracranial hemorrhage
- Cerebral ischemia
- Hypertension
- Brain tumor
- Arteriovenous malformation
- Dental cause
- Temporal mandibular joint (TMJ) syndrome
- Pseudotumor cerebri
- Temporal arteritis

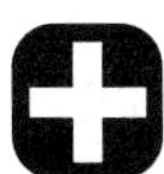

Acute Treatment

INITIAL STABILIZATION

- ABCs
- Patients with evidence of increased intracranial pressure may need rapid sequence intubation and therapeutic hyperventilation

ED TREATMENT

- Abortive therapy and pain management are the primary issues for patients in which life-threatening causes of headache have been ruled out
- Generally, abortive therapy options such as sumatriptan should be attempted first
- Narcotic pain medications may be administered as rescue therapy
- Intravenous saline hydration is often a helpful adjunct for migraine headaches

MEDICATIONS

- Abortive therapy in ED
  —Ergot alkaloids: DHE 1 mg IM or IV, then repeat in 1 hr if necessary
  —Metoclopramide: 10 mg IV
  —NSAIDs: ketorolac 15–30 mg IM/IV
  —Prochlorperazine: 10 mg IV
  —Sumatriptan: 6 mg SQ, may repeat in 1 hr (max of 2 doses per 24 hrs)
- Rescue pain medication
  —Meperidine: 25–100 mg IM/IV per dose
  —Morphine: 2–10 mg I/IV per dose
- Prophylactic therapy
  —β-blockers: propranolol 40 mg po bid
  —Ca^{++} channel blockers: verapamil 40 mg po tid
  —Cyclic antidepressants: amitriptyline 25 mg po tid

HOSPITAL ADMISSION CRITERIA

- Severe intractable headache pain
- Intractable vomiting, electrolyte imbalance, or inability to take oral food or fluid
- Suicidal ideation secondary to unremitting headache

HOSPITAL DISCHARGE CRITERIA

- Patients with moderate to complete pain relief and a confident diagnosis of migraine

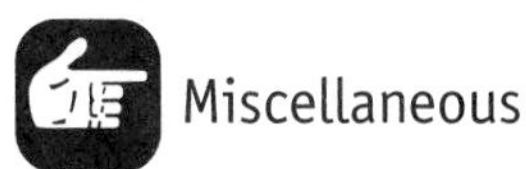

Miscellaneous

ICD-9 CODE

346.90

CORE CONTENT CODE

11.10

BIBLIOGRAPHY

Goadsby PJ, Olesen J. Diagnosis and management of migraine. *Br Med J* 1996;312(7041):1279–1283.

Noack H, Rothrock JF. Migraine: Definitions, mechanisms, and treatment. *So Med J* 1996;89(8):762–769.

Silberstein SD, Lipton RB. Overview of diagnosis and treatment of migraine. *Neurology* 1994;44(Suppl 7):S6–16.

Singer HS. Migraine headaches in children. *Pediatr Rev* 1994;15(3):94–101; quiz 101.

Spierings EL. Symptomatology and pathogenesis of migraine. *J Pediatr Gastroenterol Nutr* 1995;21(Suppl 1): S37–S41.

Authors: George Kondylis and Gary Johnson

Molluscum Contagiosum

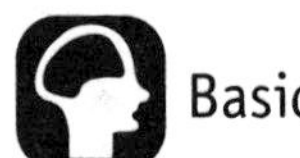

Basics

DEFINITION

- Superficial pox virus skin infection

SIGNS AND SYMPTOMS

- Nonpruritic rash
- Located at the axilla/arm, chest wall, perineum, and upper thigh
- Approximately 1.5-mm, smooth, pearly, flesh-colored papules with umbilication
- No associated prodrome, fever, or illness

RISK FACTORS

- Close physical contact/sports (i.e., wrestling)
- Sexual contact
- Autoinoculation

ASSOCIATED COMPLICATIONS

- Sexually transmitted diseases possible

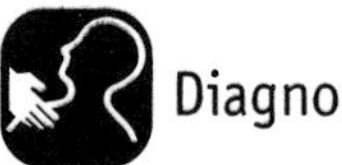

Diagnosis

DIFFERENTIAL DIAGNOSIS

- Acne/ectopic sebaceous glands
- Warts
- Ingrown hairs
- Molluscum contagiosum
- Basal cell epithelioma

HISTORY

- How long has it been there?
- Does it itch?
- Any blisters? (usually more associated with herpetic lesions)
- Do new lesions keep appearing?
- Sexually active or previous sexually transmitted disease (STD)?
- Contact sports participation?

PHYSICAL EXAMINATION

- Small, raised, 1- to 2-mm, flesh-colored umbilicated lesions containing white core substance

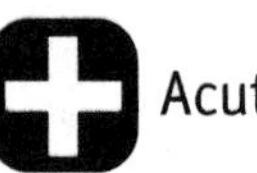

Acute Treatment

- Gentle destruction. Options include
  —Deroofing the lesion individually, which hastens resolution
  —Cryotherapy with liquid nitrogen
  —Chemical therapy, using retinoic acid or salicylic acid

Other
- —Refrain from contact activities until lesions are healed
- —Cover lesions
- —If untreated, usually last 6–9 months but can persist for years

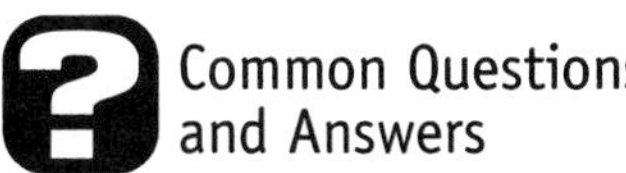

Common Questions and Answers

Physician responses to common patient questions:
Q: Does this mean I have an STD?
A: Not if it was contracted from another athlete via close contact, such as football or wrestling.

Q: Is it contagious to others?
A: Yes, it is spread by physical or sexual contact. Should keep them covered when participating; ideally, athletes should wait to resume contact sports for 48 hours after lesions are gone.

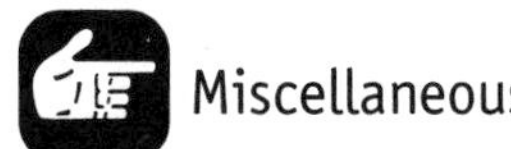

Miscellaneous

ICD-9 CODE

078.0

BIBLIOGRAPHY

Levandowski R, Keogh G, Mullane J. Sports dermatology. In: Mellion MB, ed. *Sports medicine secrets.* Philadelphia: Hanley & Belfus, 1994:189–193.

Mellman MF, Podesta L. Common medical problems in sports. *Clin Sports Med* 1997;16:635–662.

Author: Paul Stricker

Motion Sickness

Basics

DESCRIPTION

Not a true sickness but a normal response to an abnormal situation in which there is a sensory conflict about body motion between the visual receptors, vestibular receptors and body proprioceptors. It can also be induced when patterns of motion differ from those previously experienced.

System(s) affected: Nervous
Genetics: N/A
Incidence/Prevalence in USA: N/A
Predominant age: N/A
Predominant sex: N/A

SIGNS AND SYMPTOMS

- Nausea
- Vomiting
- Diaphoresis
- Pallor
- Hypersalivation
- Yawning
- Hyperventilation
- Anxiety
- Panic
- Malaise
- Fatigue
- Weakness
- Confusion

CAUSES

Motion (auto, plane, boat, amusement rides)

RISK FACTORS

- Travel
- Visual stimuli (i.e., moving horizon)
- Poor ventilation (fumes, smoke, carbon monoxide)
- Emotions (fear, anxiety)
- Zero gravity
- Other illness or poor health

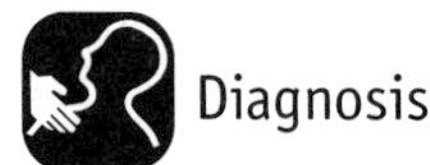

Diagnosis

DIFFERENTIAL DIAGNOSIS

- Mountain sickness
- Vestibular disease
- Gastroenteritis
- Metabolic disorders
- Toxin exposure

LABORATORY

N/A

Drugs that may alter lab results: N/A

Disorders that may alter lab results: N/A

PATHOLOGICAL FINDINGS

N/A

SPECIAL TESTS

N/A

IMAGING

N/A

DIAGNOSTIC PROCEDURES

N/A

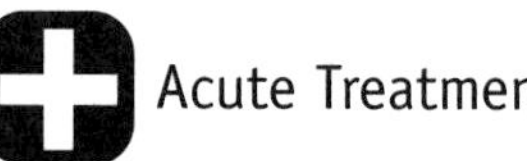

Acute Treatment

APPROPRIATE HEALTH CARE

Remove triggers or noxious stimuli

GENERAL MEASURES

- Minimize exposure (seat in middle of plane or boat)
- Improve ventilation

SURGICAL MEASURES

N/A

ACTIVITY

- Semi-recumbent seating
- Fix vision at 45 degree angle above horizon
- Avoid fixation of vision on moving objects (i.e., waves)
- Avoid reading

DIET

- Decrease oral intake or take frequent small feedings
- Avoid alcohol

PATIENT EDUCATION

N/A

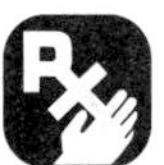

Long-Term Treatment

DRUG(S) OF CHOICE

- Scopolamine transdermal where available; apply patch 6 hours before travel and replace every 3 days
  or
- Dimenhydrinate (Dramamine) adults and adolescents 50–100 mg q4h, maximum 400 mg/day; children 6–12 years 25–50 mg q4h, maximum 150 mg/day
- Meclizine (Antivert) 25 mg qid

Contraindications: Glaucoma

Precautions:

- Young children
- Elderly
- Pregnancy
- Urinary obstruction
- Pyloric obstruction

Significant possible interactions:

- Sedatives (antihistamines, alcohol, antidepressants)
- Anticholinergics (belladonna alkaloids)

ALTERNATIVE DRUGS

- Antihistamines
  —Meclizine (Antivert)

PATIENT MONITORING

N/A

PREVENTION/AVOIDANCE

- Minimize exposure (seat in middle of plane or boat)
- Improve ventilation
- Semi-recumbent seating
- Fix vision at 45 degree angle above horizon
- Avoid fixation of vision on moving objects (i.e., waves)
- Avoid reading
- Minimize food intake prior to travel

POSSIBLE COMPLICATIONS

- Hypotension
- Dehydration
- Depression
- Panic

EXPECTED COURSE/PROGNOSIS

- Symptoms should resolve when motion exposure ends
- Resistance to motion sickness seems to increase with age

Miscellaneous

AGE-RELATED FACTORS

Pediatric: Children more susceptible to motion sickness

Geriatric: Age confers some resistance to motion sickness

Others: N/A

SYNONYMS

- Car sickness
- Sea sickness
- Air sickness
- Space sickness

ICD-9 CODE

994.6 Motion sickness

BIBLIOGRAPHY

Dundee JW, McMillan C. Positive evidence for P6 acupuncture antiemesis. *Postgrad Med* 1991;67:417–422.

Bennett JC, Plum F, eds. *Cecil textbook of medicine*. 20th Ed. Philadelphia, W.B. Saunders Co., 1996.

Kohl RL, Calkins DS. Control of nausea & autonomic dysfunction with terfenadine, a peripherally acting antihistamine. *Aviation, Space and Environmental Medicine* 1991; 62(5):392–396.

Internet references: http://www.5mcc.com

Author: Marshall Godwin

Mononucleosis

Basics

DEFINITION

- Acute viral syndrome classically resulting from infection with the Epstein-Barr virus (EBV)
- EBV is a lymphotrophic γ-herpesvirus that replicates in epithelial cells and B lymphocytes; may establish latent infection with possibility of reactivation
- Characterized by classic triad of fever, pharyngitis, and lymphadenopathy

INCIDENCE/PREVALENCE

- Peak incidence in the United States (U.S.) is between ages 15 and 19 years
- Estimated prevalence 1% to 3% of adolescent/young adult population. U.S. incidence 45:100,000.
- Evidence of infection via EBV antibody seroconversion occurs earlier in lower socioeconomic groups.
- In all populations, >90% seroconversion by the end of the third decade of life

SIGNS AND SYMPTOMS

- Classic triad: fever, pharyngitis, and cervical lymphadenopathy (anterior and posterior)
- Many patients manifest a prodrome of disabling fatigue/malaise.
- Pharyngitis characterized by yellow-gray tonsillar exudate and palatal edema
- Fevers of 39–40°C with evening peaks, typically for 10–14 days
- Splenomegaly present in at least 50% of patients, peaking in the second and third weeks
- Notable decline in exercise tolerance

RISK FACTORS

- Transmission via passage of infected secretions, most commonly saliva ("the kissing disease"); incubation period typically 30–50 days
- EBV also felt to be passed via respiratory tract secretions, blood, rectal and potentially genital secretions, raising the possibility of sexual transmission. No aerosol transmission has been found.
- Lack of mononucleosis epidemics supports concept of low-level contagiousness.
- Relative risk of contracting EBV increased by factors negatively affecting the overall status of the immune system: baseline fatigue, overtraining, poor nutritional status.

COMPLICATIONS

- Edema of Waldeyer's ring, resulting in airway compromise
- Splenomegaly and risk of splenic rupture
- Guillain-Barré syndrome
- Cranial nerve palsies
- Aseptic meningitis
- Meningoencephalitis

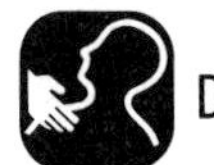

Diagnosis

DIFFERENTIAL DIAGNOSIS

- Primarily must be differentiated from nonspecific viral syndromes, lymphoma, leukemia, and *Streptococcus* pharyngitis
- Many infectious agents may cause mononucleosis-like syndromes: cytomegalovirus, adenovirus, hepatitis A, human herpesvirus 6, human immunodeficiency virus, rubella, toxoplasmosis
- Medications causing mononucleosis-like syndromes: phenytoin, sulfa drugs

HISTORY

- Prodrome of malaise/fatigue followed by development of the classic triad of fever, pharyngitis, and lymphadenopathy
- Patient often does not have known history of EBV exposure.
- Athlete may complain of poor exercise performance.
- Fatigue is often disabling, even for activities of daily living.

PHYSICAL EXAMINATION

General/Vital Signs

- Fever often demonstrable
- Patient may appear fatigued and mildly to moderately ill but generally nontoxic

Head, Eyes, Ears, Nose, Throat, and Neck

- Exudative pharyngitis (intense swelling of Waldeyer ring may create respiratory compromise and dysphagia)
- Palatal petechiae
- Periorbital edema
- Prominent anterior and posterior cervical lymphadenopathy

Abdomen

- May display right and left upper quadrant tenderness, with or without evidence of hepatosplenomegaly.
- Should be no evidence of an acute abdomen
- With splenic rupture, may develop Kehr sign (patient supine, raise left leg, intra-abdominal blood tracks up to diaphragm, creates referred pain to left shoulder)

Derm

- Viral exanthem skin
- Maculopapular rash may often develop with administration of ampicillin or amoxicillin.

IMAGING

- No routine imaging used for diagnosis or management of mononucleosis.
- Questions regarding splenic size should be evaluated with ultrasonography; contrasted abdominal computed tomography for concerns about splenic rupture (incidence of 1–2 per 1,000 cases of mononucleosis, often spontaneous).

LABORATORY EVALUATION

- Primary means of laboratory testing via nonspecific heterophile antibody studies (i.e., monospot qualitative agglutination slide test)
- Heterophile antibody (+) 60% to 70% at 1 week, 80% to 90% by 3–4 weeks
- Definitive diagnosis: EBV viral capsid antigen (VCA) immunoglobulin M (+) for acute infections, (−) for recent or past infections
- EBV VCA immunoglobulin G confirms past infection and generation of protective antibody
- May use more specific EBV-associated antigens if necessary to determine exact phase of illness
- Classic hematologic findings include >10% atypical lymphocytes [Downey cell-activated cytotoxic suppressor (CD8) T lymphocytes], relative leukocytosis (up to 20,000), followed by mild neutropenia during week 2 of illness, mild hemolytic anemia, and mild thrombocytopenia (100,000–140,000/mm^3)
- Mild hepatitis (two- to three-fold increase in liver function tests) may be seen in week 2–3 of illness

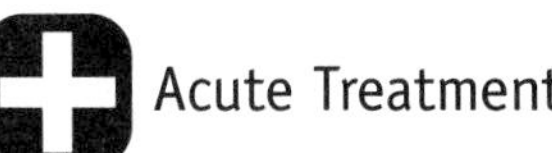

Acute Treatment

GENERAL CONSIDERATIONS

- Care is primarily supportive/symptomatic.
- No effective treatment presently is available.
- Care should be taken to avoid splenic trauma; avoid exercise and activities with jarring movements; use stool softeners to avoid increasing intra-abdominal pressure.
- Avoid alcohol

SPECIAL CONSIDERATIONS

- Acyclovir has been shown to decrease viral shedding but has no effect on the natural course of the illness.
- Pulse dose steroids (e.g., prednisone 40 mg q.d. for 5 days) may be used for pharyngeal edema and airway compromise as well as for painful prominent splenomegaly.

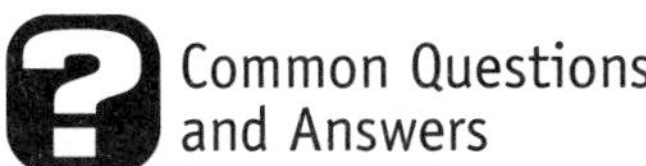

Common Questions and Answers

Physician responses to common patient questions:

Q: When can the athlete safely return to full participation?

A: As the risk for splenic rupture (most feared complication of mononucleosis in athletes) is greatest during days 4–21 of clinical illness, all athletes should be disqualified for a minimum of 3 weeks from onset of illness. Athletes may resume low-level conditioning at 3 weeks if fatigue is resolving, no airway compromise is present, there is no hepatosplenomegaly, and there are no persisting hematologic or hepatic laboratory abnormalities. In an uncomplicated case, the athlete should be able to resume full participation, even in contact sports, at 4 weeks from onset of illness.

Q: Can mononucleosis in the athlete population be prevented?

A: Fortunately, because of the nature of transmission, epidemics of mononucleosis are uncommon. Care should be taken to avoid shared water bottles, utensils, etc. Teams that travel extensively together have greater potential contacts for transmission. As the incubation period is lengthy, identifying index cases is difficult. It is not practical or necessary to exclude infected teammates if appropriate measures are taken to avoid spread of the virus.

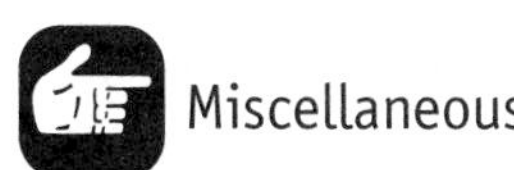

Miscellaneous

SYNONYMS

- "Mono"
- Glandular fever

ICD-9 CODE

075 Infectious mononucleosis

BIBLIOGRAPHY

Haines JD. When to resume sports after infectious mononucleosis. *Postgrad Med* 1987;81:331–333.

Hickey SM, Strasburger VC. What every pediatrician should know about infectious mononucleosis in adolescents. *Pediatr Clin North Am* 1997;44:1541–1556.

Peter J, Ray CG. Infectious mononucleosis. *Pediatr Rev* 1998;19:276–279.

Author: John MacKnight

Nasal Septal Hematomas

Basics

DEFINITION

- Bleeding between cartilaginous and mucosal layers of nasal septum resulting from trauma to the nose that collects to form a hematoma
- Septal hematomas can occur bilaterally or unilaterally.

SIGNS AND SYMPTOMS

- Epistaxis, nasal deformity and swelling, ecchymosis, pain, and crepitant to palpation, usually from associated nasal fracture
- Difficulty breathing through one or both sides of the nose

IMPORTANCE

- Hematoma contained in the tight submucosal space can lead to pressure necrosis or abscess. This results in cartilage destruction and collapse of the nasal dorsum or a "saddle nose" deformity.
- Dorsal nose deformity causes significant cosmetic and functional morbidity that usually is permanent. Although rare, monitor for presence of septal hematoma in every case of nasal trauma and treat promptly when it is diagnosed.

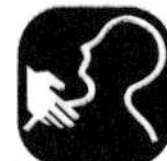

Diagnosis

HISTORY

- Trauma to the nose, most often an inferior blow, as the supportive structure of the lower two thirds of the nose is composed entirely of cartilage

PHYSICAL EXAMINATION

- Control bleeding with direct pressure, topical decongestants, or cautery, as indicated.
- Visualize the anterior septum, preferably using a nasal speculum or otoscope with the tip inserted past the nasal vestibule, if necessary. Sufficient lighting and suction are helpful.
- Septal hematoma will appear as a bluish-red bulge from the septum into the nasal vestibule. Palpation with a cotton swab can help differentiate between a firm deviated septum and a boggy hematoma.

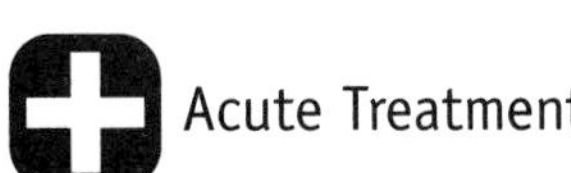

Acute Treatment

PROMPT INTERVENTION

- Needle aspiration or sharp incision and drainage under local or general anesthesia followed by suction of the clot, if needed, irrigation, and wick placement
- Anterior nasal packing to hold mucosa in place and prevent recurrence of the hematoma
- Systemic antibiotic coverage of *Staphylococcus aureus* and sinus pathogens for sinusitis prophylaxis and to help treat or prevent infection of the septum itself

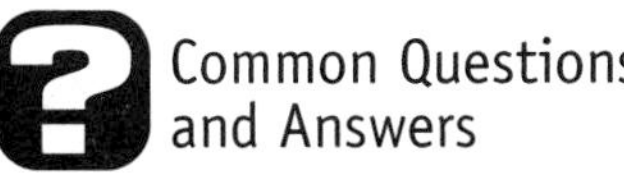

Common Questions and Answers

Physician responses to common patient questions:
Q: How long will I need to leave the nose packing in?
A: Usually about 2–4 days so that the mucosa can heal and fill in the space where the hematoma formed.
Q: When can I return to play?
A: Not advised until the packing is removed due to impaired breathing and the need to protect the septal mucosa while it heals. After removal of packing, return to play is based on consideration of the associated nasal fracture and whether or not an infection is present.

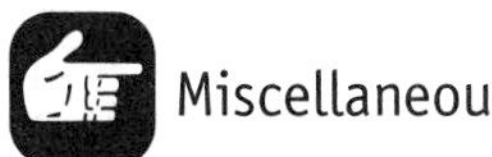

Miscellaneous

ICD-9 CODE

920 Septal hematoma

CPT CODE

30020 Incision and drainage of a septal hematoma or abscess

BIBLIOGRAPHY

Ehrlich A. Nasal septal abscess: an unusual complication of nasal trauma. *Am J Emerg Med* 1993;11:149–150.

Kaufman BR, Heckler FR. Sports-related facial injuries. *Clin Sports Med* 1997;16:543–562.

Stackhouse T. On-site management of nasal injuries. *Physician Sportsmed* 1998;26: 69–74.

Authors: Douglas Browning and Daryl A. Rosenbaum

Near-Drowning

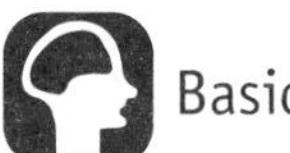

Basics

DEFINITION

- Drowning: to die from suffocation in water
- Near-drowning: to survive, at least temporarily, after suffocation by submersion in water
- Secondary drowning: delayed death (>24 hours after submersion) due to rapid deterioration of respiratory status (respiratory insufficiency); occurs in about 5% of near-drowning patients
- Immersion syndrome: sudden death following contact with icy-cold water
- Major pathophysiologic event in near-drowning is hypoxemia, with or without aspiration, secondary to immersion in any fluid medium.
- Period of hypoxemia generally is only as long as the immersion incident itself. If ventilation can be reestablished before development of injury secondary to hypoxemia, recovery generally is rapid and uneventful (if aspiration does not occur).
- When aspiration occurs, the pathophysiologic processes are markedly different. The victim who aspirates remains hypoxemic, even after ventilation is reestablished. Secondary damage caused by prolonged hypoxemia is more likely to occur.
- With both salt- and fresh-water aspiration, it is believed that the surfactant is washed out with collapse of alveoli, and there may be transudation of fluid into the alveoli.
- Aspiration of sand, algae, and other particles can result in a reactive exudate.
- In both circumstances above, there is resulting low ventilation/perfusion (V/Q) ratios and areas of shunt, resulting in hypoxemia.

INCIDENCE/PREVALENCE

- In some states, drowning is the second most common cause of death in children 4–14 years of age (after motor vehicle accidents). In other states, drowning is the leading cause of death.
- Drowning is responsible for more than 7,000 deaths each year in the United States. Near-drowning incidents approach 90,000 per year.
- Approximately 80% of drownings occur in places other than those designated for swimming.
- Majority of drowning incidents in the toddler group occur in residential pools.
- Male-to-female ratio in drowning is 5:1. Black-to-white drowning ratio is 2:1.
- Major factor responsible for drowning in adults is alcohol.
- Hypothermia and hyperventilation before breath-hold diving are associated with drowning and near-drowning episodes.

SIGNS AND SYMPTOMS

- Victims of near-drowning frequently suffer from cardiac asystole, tachycardia, bradycardia, or ventricular/atrial fibrillation.
- It is not uncommon for these patients to respond to, but require prolonged, cardiopulmonary resuscitation (CPR).
- Patients who respond to CPR or never develop cardiac arrest frequently suffer from sinus tachycardia due to hypoxemia and acidosis.
- Patients with water aspiration may present with either minimal symptoms or severe pulmonary edema (labored breathing; pink froth from mouth and nose; wet, gurgling sounds; or frank cardiopulmonary arrest).
- Neurologic status can be documented using the following classification scheme:
  —A: Awake
  —B: Blunted
  —C: Comatose; further subdivided according to best motor response
  —C1: Decorticate response
  —C2: Decerebrate response
  —C3: No motor response
- Ischemic injury to the kidney may result in acute renal insufficiency; the patient may become anuric, oliguric, or polyuric. Renal failure may develop in severe cases.
- Life-threatening electrolyte abnormalities occur when the amount of aspirated fluid is >22 mL/kg of body weight. This amount of water is only aspirated in about 15% of the cases.
- Vomiting is common.
- Hypothermia may be present.

RISK FACTORS

- With scuba-related drowning, the most common factor is the diver's running out of air at depth from reasons such as entanglement or becoming lost in a cave or wreck.
- Intentional hyperventilation before breath-hold diving
- Cold-water immersion or hypothermia
- Contamination of scuba air supply with toxic gases (most commonly carbon monoxide).
- Oxygen-induced seizures have been described in divers using oxygen-enriched air mixtures.
- Idiopathic seizure disorders
- Diabetes (hyperglycemia- or hypoglycemia-induced unconsciousness)
- Any traumatic event in the water
- Inability to swim
- Panic/anxiety
- Cardiac arrhythmias/myocardial infarction
- Cerebrovascular accident
- Alcohol
- Improper fencing of pools
- Inadequate adult supervision of children

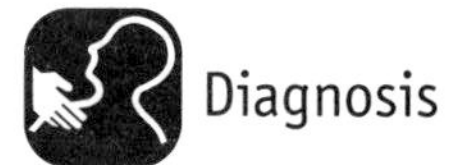

Diagnosis

DIFFERENTIAL DIAGNOSIS

- Consider a potential underlying cause of near-drowning, such as alcohol or drug intoxication, myocardial infarction, or hypoglycemia
- Pulmonary edema
- Sudden acute illness (e.g., epilepsy, myocardial infarction, stroke)
- Head or spinal cord injury/trauma
- Venomous stings by aquatic animals
- Decompression sickness or arterial gas embolism from scuba diving
- Nitrogen narcosis from scuba diving

HISTORY

- See Risk Factors

PHYSICAL EXAMINATION

- Depends on severity; ranging from sinus tachycardia to cardiac arrest and apnea

IMAGING

- Chest x-rays may be normal or show infiltrates ranging from a patchy distribution to global pulmonary edema
- Pulmonary edema is a form of adult respiratory distress syndrome.
- Computed tomographic scan of head may be needed to rule out acute or chronic intracranial process in unconscious patients.
- Obtain cervical spine (C-spine) films if you suspect head/neck trauma.

SPECIAL TESTS

- Electrocardiogram
- Electroencephalogram

LABORATORY TESTS

- Arterial blood gases may reveal hypoxemia (low PO_2), hypercarbia (high PCO^2), and a mixed acidosis picture (both respiratory and metabolic), with increased A-a gradient.
- Chemistry panels may show hypokalemia, hypernatremia or hyponatremia, or signs of renal failure.
- Urinalysis rarely shows albuminuria and/or hemoglobinuria.

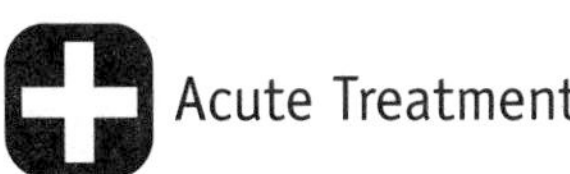

Acute Treatment

CARDIOPULMONARY RESUSCITATION

- Establish an adequate airway and supply 100% oxygen immediately. Follow C-spine precautions, if needed.
- In the comatose patient, there is always the threat of aspiration of stomach contents. Endotracheal intubation is preferred in these patients. Concomitant unstable neck injury is possible.
- The near-drowning patient who presents in cardiac arrest should be resuscitated vigorously. Although unusual, recovery with normal neurologic function has been reported even after prolonged cardiac arrest.
- Check for hemodynamic instability. If the patient is hypotensive, it is better to insert a Swan-Ganz catheter to check pulmonary artery wedge pressure and cardiac output (insert catheter when patient is normothermic to avoid inducing arrhythmias). Giving fluids to a near-drowning victim with pulmonary edema may not be appropriate.
- Positive end-expiratory pressure (PEEP) can be effective in reversing the abnormal V/Q relationships leading to hypoxemia. Only small amounts of PEEP usually are required to achieve adequate oxygenation. PEEP also allows for lower levels of inspired oxygen that is not toxic to the lung.
- In patients who are alert, nasal continuous positive airway pressure may be needed for ventilatory support. Risk for aspiration is still present.
- If bronchospasm present or suspected, give nebulized β_2-agonist treatments.
- Near-drowning victims with cardiac arrest usually have profound metabolic acidosis, and large doses of bicarbonate may be needed to correct it after vigorous CPR efforts. Arterial blood gas (ABG) determinations are needed to calculate the exact dose of bicarbonate. Give bicarbonate only if the other measures of resuscitation (ventilation and perfusion) do not correct the acidosis.
- There are insufficient data to warrant the use of the Heimlich maneuver (subdiaphragmatic thrust) or postural drainage in near-drowning patients. Avoid these maneuvers unless airway obstruction from a foreign body is present. Insert a nasogastric tube to decompress the stomach.
- Insert Foley catheter, if needed.
- Check body temperature to assess for hypothermia. A hypothermic patient should be aggressively resuscitated for prolonged periods.
- Check and correct severe electrolyte abnormalities and monitor acid–base balance.
- Antibiotics needed only in those patients who become febrile, develop new pulmonary infiltrates, or have purulent secretions. Prophylactic antibiotics do not improve morbidity or mortality. Corticosteroids to treat the lung injured by near-drowning is unwarranted at this point.

CEREBRAL RESUSCITATION

- Management of patients with suspected hypoxic brain injury includes
  —Hyperventilation (maintain P_aCO_2 at 25–30 mm Hg)
  —Head elevation (if no C-spine injury is present)
  —Diuretics
  —Muscle relaxants

LABORATORY TESTS

- Obtain ABG, complete blood count, electrolytes, urinalysis, and prothrombin time

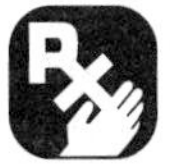

Long-Term Treatment

REFERRAL/DISPOSITION

- Asymptomatic patients with normal ABG and chest radiography may be discharged after a 6-hour observation period.
- All other patients should be admitted to the hospital.

PROGNOSIS

- Prognosis of near-drowning patients is related to degree of damage secondary to the anoxic episode and the duration of immersion.
- Estimated immersion time $\geq$5 minutes is associated with poor prognosis.
- Victims of near-drowning who had prolonged hypoxemia should remain under close hospital observation for 2–3 days after all supportive measures have been discontinued and clinical and laboratory findings are stable.
- Patients who are alert or mildly obtunded at the time of presentation have an excellent prognosis.
- Residual complications of near-drowning may include intellectual impairment, convulsive disorders, and pulmonary or cardiac complications.
- No prediction of eventual outcome can be made in the presence of severe hypothermia.

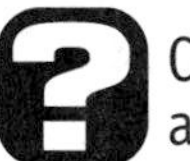

Common Questions and Answers

Physician responses to common patient questions:
Q: What is the difference between salt-water and fresh-water drowning?
A: None! Again, the focus should be on the resulting hypoxemia.

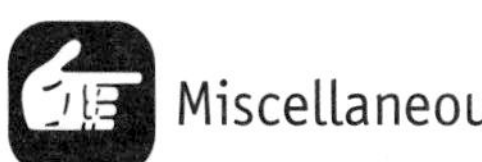

Miscellaneous

ICD-9 CODE

994.1 Drowning and nonfatal submersion
518.5 Pulmonary insufficiency due to trauma and surgery

BIBLIOGRAPHY

Bove AA. *Diving medicine.* Philadelphia: WB Saunders, 1997.

Modell JH. Drowning. *N Engl J Med* 1993; 328:253–256.

Strange GR, Ahrens WR, Lelyveld S, et al. *Pediatric emergency medicine.* New York: McGraw-Hill, 1996.

McPhee SJ, Papadakis MA. In: Tierney LM Jr, ed. *Current medical diagnosis and treatment 2000.* New York: Lange Medical Books/ McGraw-Hill, 2000.

Author: James Fambro

Neck Lacerations and Penetrating Injuries

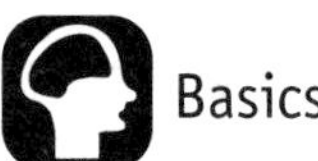

Basics

SIGNS AND SYMPTOMS

- Signs and symptoms vary depending on the specific structures injured
- Vascular injury
  - —Active hemorrhage or hematoma
  - —Tracheal deviation, loss of normal anatomic landmarks
  - —Pulse deficits in upper extremities
  - —Thrills or bruits in neck
- Laryngotracheal injury
  - —Respiratory distress
  - —Hoarseness, voice changes
  - —Hemoptysis
  - —Neck pain or tenderness
  - —Crepitance
- Pharyngoesophageal injury
  - —Dysphagia
  - —Odynophagia
  - —Hematemesis
- Neurologic injury
  - —Central or peripheral nervous system deficits

MECHANISM/DESCRIPTION

- Penetrating neck trauma is defined as a wound that penetrates the platysma muscle
- The neck is divided into *three zone*s based on superficial landmarks
  - —Zone I extends from the top of the sternum to the sternal notch or cricoid cartilage
    - —Penetrating trauma in this zone carries the highest mortality due to injury to thoracic structures
  - —Zone II extends from the sternal notch or cricoid cartilage to the angle of the mandible
    - —The majority of penetrating neck wounds occur in this zone
    - —Zone II wounds have a lower mortality because hemorrhage can be controlled with direct pressure and structures are easily accessible for surgical exploration
    - —Zone III extends from the cephalad to the angle of the mandible

ETIOLOGY

- Gunshot wounds
- Stab wounds
- Miscellaneous (glass shards, metal fragments)

PEDIATRIC CONSIDERATIONS

- In the pediatric patient, the larynx is located higher in the neck and receives better protection from the mandible and hyoid bone

PRE-HOSPITAL

- Frequent suctioning to clear airway of blood, secretions, or vomitus
- Lateral decubitus or prone positioning may be required to prevent aspiration
- The airway must be vigilantly monitored as edema or expanding hematoma can progress to airway compromise
- Early oral intubation is indicated for clinical signs of respiratory distress, such as stridor, air hunger, or labored breathing, or if an expanding neck hematoma is present

CAUTIONS

- Nasotracheal intubation should be avoided because of potential rupture of an expanding hematoma and is difficult to perform because of distortion of anatomy
- Occlusive dressings should be applied to lacerations over major veins to prevent air embolism

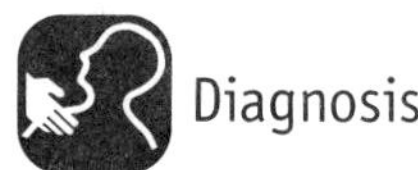

Diagnosis

ESSENTIAL WORKUP

- Careful examination of the wound determine the extent of injury and if it penetrates the platysma
  - —Wounds should never be blindly probed as this may result in uncontrolled hemorrhage
- Lateral neck radiograph to evaluate soft tissue injury and detect foreign bodies
- Chest radiograph to detect hemopneumothorax, mediastinal air, or bleeding that extends into the upper mediastinum

LABORATORY

- Type and crossmatch
- Baseline CBC and chemistry panel

IMAGING/SPECIAL TESTS

- Angiography
  - —Considered the Gold Standard to evaluate arterial injury
  - —Indicated for penetrating wounds in Zone I or Zone III
- Color duplex ultrasound is a noninvasive, rapid screening test for arterial injury
- Bronchoscopy can be helpful to evaluate tracheal injury but it may increase airway edema and is difficult in patients with respiratory distress
- Esophagram with Gastrografin or dilute barium
  - —Low sensitivity
  - —Combine with esophagoscopy to include injury
  - —Indications
    - —wound approaches/crosser midline
    - —subcutaneous air
- Esophagoscopy to evaluate for esophageal injury

DIFFERENTIAL DIAGNOSIS

- Vascular injury
- Pharyngoesophageal injury
- Laryngotracheal injury
- Peripheral or central nervous system injury
- Cervical spine injury
- Associated head or thoracic trauma

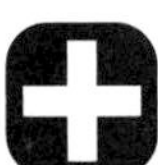

Acute Treatment

INITIAL STABILIZATION

Airway Management with C-spine Control

- Patients who are comatose or in respiratory distress require immediate intubation
- Stable patients without evidence of respiratory distress may be aggressively managed with prophylactic intubation or closely observed with airway equipment at the bedside
- Orotracheal intubation with rapid sequence induction or sedation is the method of choice for securing
- The airway in penetrating neck trauma
- Nasotracheal intubation is contraindicated with apnea, severe facial injury, or airway distortion because of the risk of puncturing an expanding hematoma
- Endoscopic intubation is contraindicated with active bleeding that may obscure the scope
- Percutaneous transtracheal ventilation may be useful when oral or nasotracheal intubation fails
  —Leaves the airway unprotected and is contraindicated in cases of upper airway obstruction as it may cause barotrauma
  —Cricothyroidotomy, tracheostomy, or intubation via a penetrating wound may be required in cases of severe facial injury, laryngotracheal injury, or uncontrolled upper airway hemorrhage

Breathing

- Zone I injury can cause pneumothorax or subclavian vein injury and hemothorax, requiring needle decompression and tube thoracostomy

Circulation

- External hemorrhage should be controlled with direct pressure. Blind clamping of vessels is contraindicated due to the risk of further neurovascular injury
- Patients with uncontrollable bleeding or hemodynamic instability must go directly to the operating room
- Following intubation, the throat can be packed with heavy gauze to tamponade the bleeding
- Tube thoracostomy for bleeding into the chest

ED TREATMENT

- Nasogastric tube should not be placed due to risk of rupturing a pharyngeal hematoma
- Prophylactic antibiotics are recommended (cefoxitin, clindamycin, penicillin G plus metronidazole)
- Surgical consult for all wounds that penetrate the platysma muscle
- There is controversy in mandatory versus selective surgical exploration in stable patients
  —Mandatory approach
  —Surgical exploration is indicated in all cases of penetrating neck trauma because significant injury may not manifest outward signs or symptoms
  —Selective approach
    —Surgical exploration for specific indications including expanding or pulsatile hematoma, active bleeding, absence of peripheral pulses, hemoptysis, Horner's syndrome, bruit, subcutaneous emphysema, respiratory distress, or air bubbling through a wound
- Tetanus prophylaxis

MEDICATIONS

- Cefoxitin: adult: 2 g IV q 8 hrs; peds: 80–160 mg/kg/day IM/IV div q 6 hrs *or*
- Clindamycin: adult: 600–900 mg IV q 8 hrs; peds: 25–40 mg/kg/day IV div q 6–8 hrs *or*
- Penicillin G: adult: 24 million IU/day div q 4–6 hrs; peds: 150,000–250,000 IU/kg/day div q 4–6 hrs *plus*
- Metronidazole: adult: 1 g load then 500 mg IV q 6 hrs; peds: 30 mg/kg/day IV div q 12 hrs

HOSPITAL ADMISSION CRITERIA

- All patients with penetrating neck trauma should be admitted and observed for at least 24 hours
- Observation must take place in a facility capable of providing definitive surgical care
- Patients with suspicion of airway or vascular injury must be admitted to the ICU

HOSPITAL DISCHARGE CRITERIA

- Asymptomatic patients who have negative studies may be discharged after at least 24 hours of observation

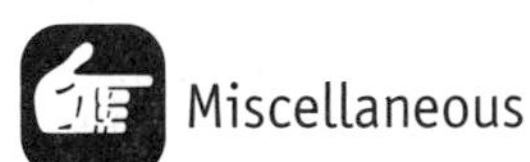

Miscellaneous

ICD-9-CM

959.09

CORE CONTENT CODE

18.4.8.2

BIBLIOGRAPHY

Carducci B, Lowe RA, Dalsey W. Penetrating neck trauma: Consensus and controversies. *Ann Emerg Med* 1986;15:208.

Jorden RC. Neck trauma. In: Rosen P, et al., eds. *Emergency medicine: Concepts and clinical practice*. 4th ed. St. Louis: CV Mosby, 1998:505–513.

Roon AJ, Christensen N. Evaluation and treatment of penetrating cervical injuries. *J Trauma* 1979;19:391.

Author: Tamaki Kimbro

Nonsteroidal Anti-Inflammatory Drug Poisoning

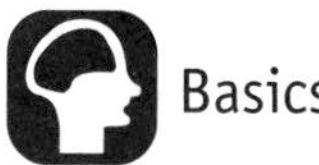

Basics

DEFINITION

- Indicated as antipyretic, analgesic, and anti-inflammatory agents
- Main action is to reversibly inhibit the enzyme cyclooxygenase responsible for production of prostaglandins from arachidonic acid
- This ultimately results in reduction of pain, inflammation, fever, and gastrointestinal (GI) cytoprotection.
- Prostacyclin and thromboxane production is inhibited, resulting in platelet aggregation and vasodilation, respectively.
- Classification
  —Carboxylic acids
    —Salicylic acids: aspirin, diflunisal (Dolobid)
    —Phenylacetic acids: diclofenac (Voltaren)
  —Carbocyclic and heterocyclic acetic acids: indomethacin (Indocin), sulindac (Clinoril), tolmetin (Tolectin), ketorolac (Toradol)
    —Propionic acids: ibuprofen (Motrin, Advil, Nuprin), naproxen (Naprosyn, Anaprox), flurbiprofen (Ansaid), fenoprofen (Nalfon), ketoprofen (Orudis), oxaprozin (Daypro), suprofen
    —Fenamic acids: mefenamic acid (Ponstel), meclofenamate (Meclomen)
    —Enolic acids
    —Pyrazolones: phenylbutazone (Butazolidin), oxyphenbutazone
    —Oxicams: piroxicam (Feldene)
- Over-the-counter nonsteroidal anti-inflammatory drugs (NSAIDs) include ibuprofen and naproxen.

INCIDENCE/PREVALENCE

- >30 billion NSAIDs consumed annually in the United States
- >70 million prescriptions written each year
- 6-billion dollar per year industry
- NSAID poisoning is relatively rare despite their extensive use.
- Less toxic than salicylate and acetaminophen
- American Association of Poison Control Centers reported >50,000 exposures to ibuprofen in 1998; >13,000 required treatment; and four deaths were reported.

RISK FACTORS

- Overzealous use for treatment of pain and inflammation
- Suicide attempt/gesture

TOXICITY

- Acute overdoses of ibuprofen in adults resulted in 60% remaining asymptomatic, 30% to 40% developing mild-to-moderate symptoms, and <3% suffering severe symptoms.
- Phenylbutazones (pyrazolones) and fenamic acids (mefenamic acid, meclofenamate) cause the most serious and life-threatening poisoning.

Gastrointestinal

- Most common adverse effects are GI, including nausea, vomiting, dyspepsia, diarrhea, and constipation.
- Gastric, duodenal, and large intestinal ulceration may occur.
- Relative risk of serious hemorrhage is increased three- to ten-fold.
- Other factors increasing the risk of GI bleeding include elderly population; chronic high dosing; previous ulcer, alcohol, and steroid use; and use of more than one agent.

Renal

- Second most common class of adverse effects
- Inhibition of prostaglandins interferes with renal blood flow and glomerular filtration rate.
- Acute and chronic intersitial nephritis, nephrotic syndrome, and acute renal failure may result.
- Retention of sodium, potassium, and water may lead to congestive heart failure exacerbation.

Central Nervous System

- Central nervous system (CNS) depression is very common with NSAID overdose.
- The elderly are at particular risk.
- Manifestations include headache, confusion, delirium, psychosis, hallucinations, tremor, and seizures.
- One series reports 30% of ibuprofen poisonings result in altered mental status ranging from drowsiness to coma.
- Other effects include tinnitus, transient hearing loss, and aseptic meningitis.

Pulmonary

- Respiratory depression/arrest is rare.
- Adult respiratory distress syndrome has been reported with multiorgan failure.
- Asthmatics are at particular risk for bronchospasm, as leukotriene production is increased with blockade of cyclooxygenase.

Hepatic

- Rarely seen in acute overdose
- Elevation of transaminase levels, hepatitis, and fulminant hepatic failure

Hematologic

- Aplastic anemia, agranulocytosis, hemolytic anemia, and thrombocytopenia have been associated.
- Decreased platelet aggregation may exacerbate GI bleeding.

Metabolic

Increased anion gap metabolic acidosis has been reported in both adults and children.

Drug Interactions

- Concurrent use with anticoagulants increases risk of GI bleeding.
- Levels of digoxin, lithium, oral hypoglycemics, and aminoglycosides increase when combined with NSAIDs.
- NSAIDs reduce the antihypertensive effects of diuretics, β blockers, and angiotensin-converting enzyme inhibitors.

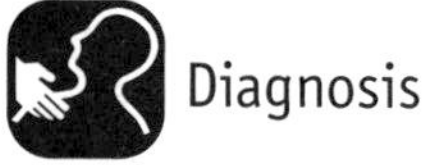

Diagnosis

HISTORY

- Agent ingested may help dictate the severity of poisoning (more serious if phenylbutazone or mefenamic acid).
- Other NSAIDs tend to be less toxic.
- Amount ingested is important information, even though there is a poor correlation between quantity ingested and toxic poisonings. Significant symptoms may occur after ingestion of >5–10 times the usual therapeutic dose.
- Time of ingestion may help with acute management strategies. Use of nomograms correlating drug levels with time are not reliable in management or predicting outcome. Most authorities believe patients with acute ingestions show symptoms within 4 hours.
- Why the agent was ingested will help determine final disposition. Also inquire about the patient's past medical history (peptic ulcer disease renal insufficiency, etc.) and concurrent medications.

PHYSICAL EXAMINATION

- Airway protection, breathing, and circulatory status are essential in any overdose patient.
- Vital signs, with close attention to blood pressure and respiratory rate
- Thorough neurologic examination assessing mental status changes and level of arousal
- Mandatory rectal examination, including Hemoccult test, to assess for GI bleeding

IMAGING

- Abdominal x-ray series necessary only if physical examination suggests a perforated viscus

LABORATORY TESTS

- Complete blood count, electrolytes, glucose, blood urea nitrogen, creatinine, urinalysis liver transaminases, coagulation profile (PT/PTT)
- Electrocardiogram, especially if potassium level is abnormal
- Plasma levels of NSAIDs are not useful. Patients without coingestion who are asymptomatic need no serum or urine toxicity screens. Consider acetaminophen and salicylate levels in all patients.
- Consider arterial blood gas if anion gap is elevated.

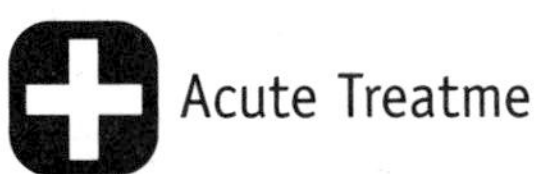

Acute Treatment

SUPPORTIVE MEASURES

- There is no antidote.
- Supportive care usually is all that is necessary.
- Maintain a patent airway, ventilatory assistance, if necessary, and fluid replacement for hypotension.
- Intravenous benzodiazepines for seizures

DECONTAMINATION

- Consider gastric lavage only if presentation is within 1 hour of ingestion and/or massive overdose
- Activated charcoal: 1 g/kg for adults; 0.5–1 g/kg in children. In adults, add a cathartic (70% sorbitol).
- No role for dialysis or charcoal hemoperfusion

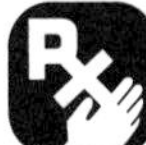

Long-Term Treatment

DISPOSITION

- Admission criteria include presentation with signs and symptoms of toxicity (abnormal vital signs, altered mental status, electrolyte abnormalities, acute renal failure).
- Mild gastrointestinal or CNS symptoms may warrant observation in the emergency department as an alternative to admission.
- Asymptomatic patients should be observed for 4–6 hours in the emergency department before discharge, especially those with possible coingestants.
- Psychiatric consultation for all suicide attempts/gestures.

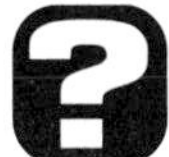

Common Questions and Answers

Physician responses to common patient questions:
Q: Is syrup of ipecac useful in NSAID poisoning?
A: Only useful if administered at the scene within minutes of the exposure.
Q: How much is too much ibuprofen?
A: In children, doses <100 mg/kg are very unlikely to induce symptoms. Adults present with CNS symptoms after ingesting >3 g and with renal effects after >6 g. Life-threatening complications have occurred in overdoses of 6.8 g in a child and 24 g in an adult.
Q: When should I really worry and not hesitate presenting to the emergency department?
A: After ingestion of fenamic acids or pyrazolones, which are the most toxic NSAIDs and warrant aggressive management.

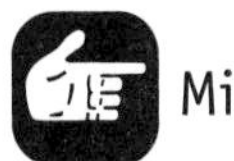

Miscellaneous

ICD-9 CODE

977.9 Drug overdosage
965.1 Poisoning, salicylates
965.4 Poisoning, aromatic analgesics
965.61 Poisoning, propionic acid derivative (ibuprofen, naproxen, fenoprofen, ketoprofen, flurbiprofen)
965.69 Poisoning, indomethacin, diclofenac, tolmetin
965.7 Poisoning, other nonnarcotic analgesics
965.9 Poisoning, unspecified analgesic and antipyretic
See also: Specific E-Codes

BIBLIOGRAPHY

Carson JL, Willet LR. Toxicity of nonsteroidal anti-inflammatory drugs. *Drugs* 1993;46[Suppl 1]:243–248.

Palmer ME, Howland MA. In: Goldfrank LR, ed. *Goldfrank's toxicologic emergencies.* Stamford: Appleton & Lange, 1998.

Donovan JW. In: Haddad LM, ed. *Clinical management of poisoning and drug overdose.* Philadelphia: WB Saunders, 1998.

Hall AH, Smolinske SC, Conrad FL, et al. Ibuprofen overdose: 126 cases. *Ann Emerg Med* 1986;15:1308–1313.

Hall AH, Smolinske SC, Stover B, et al. Ibuprofen overdose in adults. *J Clin Toxicol* 1992;30:23–37.

Keller KH. In: Olson KR, ed. *Poisoning and drug overdose.* Stamford: Appleton & Lange, 1999.

Polisson R. Nonsteroidal anti-inflammatory drugs: practical and theoretical considerations in their selection. *Am J Med* 1996;100[Suppl 2A]:31S–36S.

Seger DL, Murray L. In: Rosen P, ed. *Emergency medicine: concepts and clinical practice.* St. Louis: Mosby, 1998.

Bruno GR, Carter WA. In: Tintinalli JE, ed. *Emergency medicine: a comprehensive study guide.* New York: McGraw-Hill, 2000.

Authors: Sean Bryant and Timothy J. Linker

Oral Lacerations

Basics

DEFINITION

- Soft tissue injury in the orofacial area
- Typically results from a direct blow to the mouth resulting from a fall or impact by an opponent or object
- Lacerations may be an indirect result of an individual biting the cheek or lip.

INCIDENCE/PREVALENCE

- Most common in contact sports (football, hockey, lacrosse, soccer, wrestling)
- 50% of all injuries sustained in sports occur around the oral cavity; 58% to 75% of these injuries are soft tissue lacerations

SIGNS AND SYMPTOMS

- Significant hemorrhage due to the abundant blood supply in the face and maxillofacial areas
- Visible defects with "through and through" lacerations (lacerations involving all layers mucosa, muscular, subcutaneous, and skin)
- Patient distress

RISK FACTORS

- Participation in collision or contact sports
- *Not* using a mouth guard (use of a mouth guard is estimated to prevent 150,000 oral injuries yearly in football)

ASSOCIATED INJURIES

- Fracture of the mandible, dental arch, palate
- Dental luxation or avulsion
- Tooth fracture
- Temporomandibular (TMJ) trauma
- Vessel injury
- Nerve transection
- Salivary gland duct injury

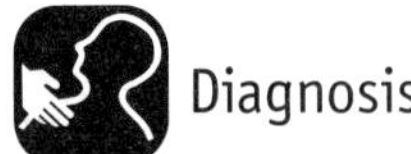

Diagnosis

DIFFERENTIAL DIAGNOSIS

- Contusion
- Abrasion
- Dental trauma (luxation, avulsion, fracture)

HISTORY

- Determine where and how injury was sustained. Common in sports, but also seen as result of fighting, assault, and abuse.
- Determine areas of numbness or loss of muscle control to evaluate for nerve injury.
- Determine last tetanus immunization, as wounds often are contaminated from the environment as well as from the oral cavity.
- Need for prophylactic antibiotics when under going dental procedures
- Sensitivity of teeth (assess for occult dental trauma)

PHYSICAL EXAMINATION

- Head and neck examination for signs of neural injury
- Palpate over TMJ to evaluate for subcondylar mandibular fracture
- Test mobility of jaw
- Evaluate laceration for length and depth as well as for affected structures, including nerves and vessels (transected nerves need to be referred for surgical repair)
- Buccal lacerations need to be evaluated for parotid salivary flow from Stenson duct. Orifice is located opposite the maxillary first molar. Saliva should flow from opening when parotid gland is palpated (disruptions of the duct should be referred to an oral and maxillofacial surgeon for repair).
- Evaluate for normal occlusion of the teeth. Basic dental examination to check for fractured, loose, or avulsed teeth.

IMAGING

- If there is a clinical suspicion of a fracture, appropriate studies should be ordered.
- Bone fixation/repair, if needed, should be performed before soft tissue closure.

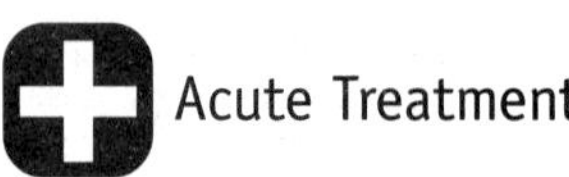

Acute Treatment

LACERATION CLOSURE POINTS

- Copious irrigation of the wound to remove foreign debris and wound contaminants
- Clean with antiseptic scrub

SIMPLE LACERATIONS OF THE ORAL MUCOSA

- Simple interrupted stitches using 3-0 chromic or similar absorbable suture material

"THROUGH AND THROUGH" LACERATIONS

- Inside-out and bottom-up technique; eliminating dead spaces helps prevent hematoma and subsequent infection
- Oral mucosa: 3-0 or 4-0 chromic or other absorbable suture material on a cutting needle
- Oral mucosa should be closed to seal off oral cavity and reduce risk of contamination from oral flora.
- Muscular layer: 4-0 slow-absorbing suture; polyglactic suture breaks down more slowly than chromic suture, maintaining wound strength for approximately 30 days.
- Subcutaneous layer: 3-0 or 4-0 plain gut on a cutting needle
- Skin: 4-0 to 6-0 nylon

LIP LACERATIONS

- Suture orbicularis oris first; see above suture suggestions
- Loosely approximate the vermilion border (very important for cosmetic appearance) with a suture at the junction with the skin
- Proceed in layers as above

TONGUE LACERATIONS

- Superficial lacerations <1 cm do not require sutures.
- Lacerations involving the muscular layer or labial margin require sutures.
- Repair in layers: 4-0 slow-resorbing polyglactic suture for the muscle and chromic suture for the mucosa

FRENULUM LACERATIONS

- Typically "V" shaped
- Small lacerations can be allowed to close by secondary intention.
- Hemorrhage typically from disruption of the muscular layer may require a stitch to obtain hemostasis.
- Large gapping lacerations can be repaired with one or two vertical sutures.

SPECIAL CONSIDERATIONS

- Tetanus immunization status
- Prophylactic antibiotics for severe or grossly contaminated laceration (coverage for the oral flora amoxicillin, penicillin, clindamycin, erythromycin)
- If fracture is present, leave wound open until fixation is completed.

INITIAL MANAGEMENT

- Evaluate airway, breathing, and circulation
- Control hemorrhage

ANALGESIA

- Regional anesthesia via nerve block is preferred over local injection to minimize tissue distortion, making approximation easier (especially for the vermilion border).
- Infraorbital nerve block numbs the upper lip.
- Mental nerve block numbs the lower lip and teeth.
- Maxillary nerve second division numbs the entire maxilla on the blocked side.

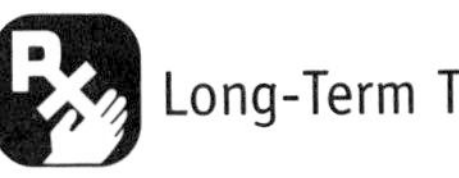

Long-Term Treatment

REFERRAL/DISPOSITION

- Laceration associated with fracture or involving nerves or salivary ducts should be referred for management as soon as possible.
- Refer dental trauma to a dentist.

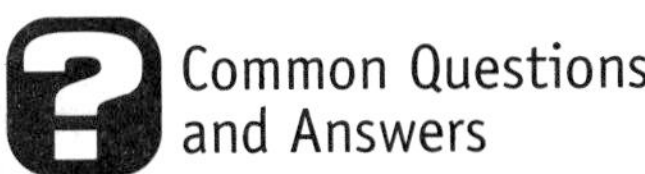

Common Questions and Answers

Physician responses to common patient questions:
Q: How long will the stitches be in?
A: Those placed inside the mouth will come out on their own. Sutures in the skin should be removed in 4–5 days to prevent significant scarring.
Q: When can I return to play?
A: Return to play depends on the severity of the injury, chance of reinjury, and availability/feasibility of protection for the wound.

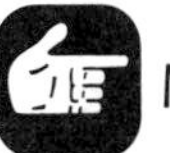

Miscellaneous

ICD-9 CODE

873.60 Mouth unspecified wound, simple
873.70 Mouth unspecified wound, complex
873.61 Buccal mucosa laceration, simple
873.71 Buccal mucosa laceration, complex
873.64 Tongue or floor of mouth laceration, simple
873.74 Tongue or floor of mouth laceration, complex
873.43 Lip laceration, simple
873.53 Lip laceration, complex
873.74 Tooth broken

BIBLIOGRAPHY

Balkland LK, Boyne PJ. Trauma to the oral cavity. *Clin Sports Med* 1989;8:25–41.

Banks K, Merlino PG. Minor oral injuries in children. *Mt Sinai J Med* 1998;65–66: 333–342.

Bringhurst C, Herr RD, Aldous JA. Oral trauma in the emergency department. *Am J Emerg Med* 1993;11:486–490.

Lephart SM, Fu FH. Emergency treatment of athletic injuries. *Dent Clin North Am* 1991;35:707–717.

Grant FC. In: Pfenniger JL, ed. *Procedures for primary care physicians.* St. Louis: Mosby, 1994.

Author: Bradley Kocian

Osteoarthritis

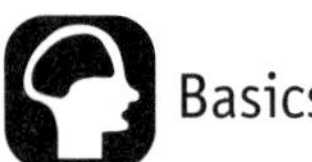

Basics

DEFINITION

- Slowly progressive degeneration of the articular cartilage of a joint
- Hypertrophy of the underlying bone (via Wolfe's law) may contribute to irregularities such as subchondral sclerosis and osteophytes.
- The term osteoarthritis (OA) implies an inflammatory process, but the arthropathy typically does not involve inflammation (<15% to 20% of cases exhibit adjacent synovitis).
- The term degenerative joint disease implies that the symptoms are due to a destructive process.
- Reparative process (osteophytes, etc.) may cause the pain.

INCIDENCE/PREVALENCE

- Radiographic evidence for OA can be seen in up to 40 million Americans, although only 25 million will actually experience symptoms.
- Reports demonstrate that 65% to 85% of patients >65 years will be affected by OA.

SIGNS AND SYMPTOMS

Joint Predilection

- Most commonly affected joints include the distal interphalangeal (DIP) and proximal interphalangeal (PIP) joints of the hands, metacarpophalangeal joints of the thumb, and the hallux, hips, knees, cervical and lumbar spine.
- Articular changes can progress to nodule formation in the DIP and PIP joints, termed Heberden and Bouchard nodes, respectively.

History

- Most common symptoms are pain and joint swelling.
- There is typically stiffness with immobilization (i.e., upon awakening).
- Early morning stiffness and pain typically lasts ~30 minutes, but improves with mobilization.
- Crepitus and grinding are characteristic of OA.
- Some patients experience muscular weakness in the surrounding soft tissue.
- There may be a history of antecedent trauma (ligament tears, fractures, meniscal tears).

PHYSICAL EXAMINATION

- May yield biomechanical changes (such as genu varum), effusions, disuse atrophy of surrounding musculature (especially the knees), crepitus, and decreased range of motion
- In the knees, joint line tenderness is common.
- In the hips, decreased internal rotation may be the first harbinger.

RISK FACTORS

- Multiple risk factors have been proposed.
- Lack of well-controlled human studies make definitive assessment of risk difficult.
- Proposed risk factors include
  —Age
  —Previous injury/internal derangement
  —Obesity
  —Genetics
  —Exercise
    —Question of whether exercise (such as jogging, etc.) causes OA has not been fully answered.
    —Available prospective, controlled human trials do not support a cause-and-effect relationship.
    —There appears to be increased risk of OA in joints with prior injury and internal derangement.

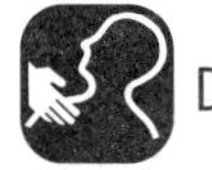

Diagnosis

DIFFERENTIAL DIAGNOSIS

- With the dearth of systemic signs and symptoms, as well as the classic joint involvement, diagnosis of OA in a joint is fairly straightforward.
- Differential should include
  —Trauma
  —Rheumatoid arthritis
  —Collagen vascular diseases
  —Crystal deposition disease
  —Gout
  —Calcium pyrophosphate deposition disease

IMAGING

X-rays

- Plain films are the standard imaging technique.
- Radiographic severity does *not* correlate with symptom severity.
- X-ray characteristics include osteophytes, joint space narrowing, subchondral sclerosis (eburnation), and cyst formation.

Computed Tomography and Magnetic Resonance Imaging

- Do not play a large role in diagnosis of OA
- Their sensitivity, specificity, and predictive values are not sufficient as they relate to subtle changes and disease progression.

LABORATORY ASSESSMENT

- Diagnosis generally is made through thorough history and physical examination and confirmed by plain films.
- Laboratory assessment is more helpful to rule out other disorders.
- Complete blood count, chemistry profile, and urinalysis are normal.
- Markers of inflammation (erythrocyte sedimentation rate [ESR], C-reactive protein) usually are normal, but may be slightly elevated during the acute phase of erosive OA.
- ESR increases with age.
- Rheumatoid factor and antinuclear antibody titers are negative.
- Arthrocentesis not routinely necessary. Unless the diagnosis is in question, there is a possibility of septic arthritis/crystal deposition disease, or for treatment of tense effusion.

CLASSIFICATION

- Primary (idiopathic): accounts for most of cases
- Secondary: causes include previous trauma/internal derangement, metabolic disorder, and deposition diseases

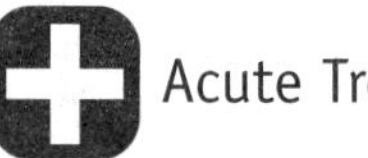

Acute Treatment

NONPHARMACOLOGIC

- Nonpharmacologic treatment issues are the keystone of therapy for a patient with OA. Because of the chronicity and risks from comorbid conditions in this age group, non-pharmacologic measures in some ways may be more important than pharmacologic measures.
- Weight reduction is paramount to treatment of OA. Obesity is considered a risk factor, and reduction of weight decreases contact pressure through all weight-bearing joints.
- Aerobic conditioning
- Joint specific rehabilitation (see below)
- Thermal and cryotherapy: Use of heat may desensitize nociceptive fibers, decrease muscle spasm and stiffness, and increase joint range of motion. It increases vascular congestion and may be less well tolerated in patients with acute inflammation. Cryotherapy is useful in both the acute inflammatory and rehabilitation phases. It provides analgesia, decreases inflammation and edema, and reduces local metabolism.
- Social and emotional support
- Physical support: Appropriate use of braces, canes, and walkers is essential to overall treatment.

PHARMACOLOGIC TREATMENT

- A number of different categories of medications are used for treatment. Most have significant potential side effects that need to be considered within each patient's clinical profile. These medicines are for symptomatic improvements. No medication or therapy has been shown to be "chondroprotective."

- Acetaminophen: as effective as aspirin and salicylates for analgesic and antipyretic properties. No anti-inflammatory properties. There is support for use of acetaminophen as a first-line agent for treatment, with a good side-effect profile.
- Nonacetylated salicylates
- Nonsteroidal anti-inflammatory drugs (NSAIDs): one of the most commonly prescribed drugs in the United States (U.S.). Onset of anti-inflammatory effect of most NSAIDs is ~7 days. Allow for an adequate trial. When one class of NSAIDs does not work, consider switching to a different class. Greatest drawback of traditional NSAIDs is their risk for GI toxicity (perforation, ulceration, and bleeding). The newer COX-2 inhibitors, celecoxib and rofecoxib, are NSAIDs with equal efficacy to naproxen and diclofenac, but with a significantly lower rate of GI toxicity. Rate of dyspepsia is high at 10%.
- Opiates: may be helpful for short-term analgesia. May be sedating and increase the risk for falls/fractures.
- Antidepressants: This category of drugs has an analgesic effect distinct from their antidepressant effect. Typical analgesic dose is less than the antidepressant effect. May potentiate the analgesic effects of other medications.
- Tramadol (Ultram): centrally acting analgesic with two main mechanisms of action: weak agonist of opiate receptors and interference with neurotransmitter reuptake (norepinephrine and serotonin).
- Glucosamine/chondroitin sulfate: Most research demonstrates modest reductions in pain and improvements in function, but most studies are small and poorly controlled.
- Topical therapies (e.g., capsaicin)
- Intra-articular injections (see below)

SPECIAL CONSIDERATIONS

Intra-articular Therapies

- Includes corticosteroids and hyaluronic acid derivatives

Corticosteroids

- Intra-articular steroids have been used for years.
- Taking into account experimental design flaws, they may offer modest benefit.
- Optimal type, dosing, and frequency are not known, but most authors suggest no more than 2–3 injections per weight-bearing joint per year.

Hyaluronic Acid Derivatives

- Two current hyaluronic acid derivatives exist in the U.S.: sodium hyaluronate (Hyalgan) and hylan G-F 20 (Synvisc).
- They require a series of injections (five for sodium hyaluronate; three for hylan G-F 20), each spaced 1 week apart.
- Most of the studies are from Europe and Asia, and are small, not well controlled, and unblinded.
- Large placebo response rates up to 55% reported.
- Results are conflicting, but there appear to be modest improvements in pain and function for 5–26 weeks in the hyaluronate and hylan G-F studies.
- Adverse reactions are limited to local transient pain and swelling.

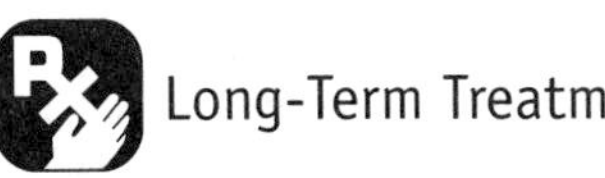

Long-Term Treatment

REHABILITATION

- Primary goals are to decrease pain and improve range of motion, strength to facilitate joint stability, gait, and aerobic capacity.
- Exercise: aerobic, weight-training or resistance exercise, flexibility, postural training, and gait training. All must be incorporated into a long-term lifestyle modification.
- Joint-specific exercises should concentrate on balance of training and strengthening muscular groups of opposing action. For example, strength training in knee OA should concentrate on quadriceps and hamstring musculature.

SURGERY

- Indicated in patients with recalcitrant pain despite maximizing medical management (nonpharmacologic and pharmacologic).
- Indicated when pain and dysfunction interfere with activities of daily living
- Options include arthroscopic debridement, high tibial osteotomy (for OA of the knee), and total joint replacement.
- Autogenous transplantation attempts to transplant the patient's own normal articular cartilage (typically from nonweight-bearing areas of the index joint) into the degenerative articular cartilage. Seems to be more promising for localized defects. Further research is pending.

PROGNOSIS AND NATURAL HISTORY

- OA is considered a progressive arthropathy.
- Rapidity of progression is highly variable.
- Progression is not guaranteed, with radiographic regression reported in some patients.

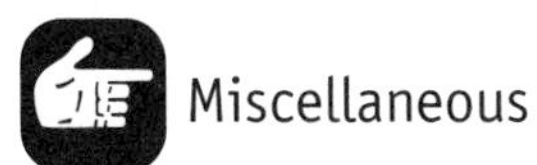

Miscellaneous

SYNONYMS

- Osteoarthritis
- Arthritis
- Degenerative joint disease

ICD-9 CODE

715.1X OA localized (X refers to specific site)
721.0 OA spine
719.4X Joint pain
729.4 Pain in limb

BIBLIOGRAPHY

Balint G, Szebenyi B. Non-pharmacological therapies in osteoarthritis. *Baillieres Clin Rheumatol* 1997;11:795–815.

Brandt KD. Nonsurgical management of osteoarthritis, with an emphasis on nonpharmacologic measures. *Arch Fam Med* 1995;4:1057–1064.

Creamer P, Hochberg MC. Osteoarthritis. *Lancet* 1997;350:503–509.

Felson DT, Zhang Y, Hannan MT, et al. Risk factors for incident radiographic knee osteoarthritis in the elderly: the Framingham Study. *Arthritis Rheum* 1997;40:728–733.

Felson DT, McAlindon TE, Anderson JJ, et al. Defining radiographic osteoarthritis for the whole knee. *Osteoarthritis Cartilage* 1997;5:241–250.

Griffin MR, Brandt KD, Liang MH, et al. Practical management of osteoarthritis. *Arch Fam Med* 1995;4:1049–1055.

Katz WA. Pharmacology and clinical experience with tramadol. *Drugs* 1996;52[Suppl 3]:39–47.

Lane NE, Thompson JM. Management of osteoarthritis in the primary-care setting. *Am J Med* 1997;103:25S–30S.

LaPrade RF, Swiontkowski MF. New horizons in the treatment of osteoarthritis of the knee. *JAMA* 1999;281:876–878.

McAlindon TE, LaValley MP, Gulin JP, et al. Glucosamine and chondroitin for the treatment of osteoarthritis: a systematic quality assessment and meta-analysis. *JAMA* 2000;283:1469–1475.

Oddis CV. New perspectives on osteoarthritis. *Am J Med* 1996;100[Suppl]:10S–15S.

Puett DW, Griffen MR. Published trials of nonmedicinal and noninvasive therapies for hip and knee osteoarthritis. *Ann Intern Med* 1994;121:133–140.

Wollheim FA. Current pharmacologic treatment of osteoarthritis. *Drugs* 1996;52[Suppl 3]:2738.

Author: Guy Monteleone

Osteomyelitis

Basics

DEFINITION

- Acute, subacute, or chronic infection of the bone or bone marrow

Acute Osteomyelitis

- Usually a disorder of childhood; less common in adults
- Usual cause is hematogenous dissemination, but may be caused by direct contamination (open fracture, nail puncture wound).
- Presents within 2 weeks of disease onset

Subacute Osteomyelitis

- More balanced response between host and organism resulting in a quasi-contained lesion in the bone
- Children with subacute osteomyelitis typically present after 1 to several months.
- Two categories of subacute osteomyelitis
  —Cavitary osteomyelitis occurs in the epiphysis or metaphysis and is characterized by small, localized lucency surrounded by reactive, dense-appearing bone (Brodie abscess).
  —Second category simulates a neoplastic process and, therefore, mandates a biopsy with or without debridement. Lesions typically are diaphyseal but also may be metaphyseal.

Chronic Osteomyelitis

- Presents after 1 to several months
- Characterized by sequestrum of necrotic bone harboring bacteria
- Occasionally can be the end result of an acute hematogenous osteomyelitis; more commonly is caused by an open fracture or wound; rarely caused by a surgical procedure

INCIDENCE/PREVALENCE

- Metaphysis of long bones is the most common location of osteomyelitis in children.
- Primary hematogenous osteomyelitis occurs mainly in infants and children, due to the sluggish circulation at the metaphyseal-physeal barrier. Metaphyseal arteries lack phagocytic lining cells, and sinusoidal veins (in growth plate) contain functionally inactive phagocytic cells.
- Primary hematogenous osteomyelitis also seen in adults. Usually begins in the diaphysis, but may spread to involve the entire medullary canal.
- Secondary hematogenous infections in adults are more common and represent reactivation of a quiescent focus of hematogenous osteomyelitis initially developed in infancy or childhood.
- In patients >50 years, the spine becomes the most common site of infection. Patients often have a history of genitourinary disease or manipulation. Onset is insidious.

SIGNS AND SYMPTOMS

- Children with acute hematogenous osteomyelitis may present with abrupt fever, irritability, lethargy, and local signs of inflammation ≤3 weeks in duration.
- 50% of children present with vague complaints, including pain of the involved limb 1–3 months in duration and minimal if any temperature elevation.
- Adults usually present with vague complaints of nonspecific pain and few constitutional symptoms. Pain, swelling, erythema, fever, chills, nausea, and generalized malaise are seen occasionally.
- In a young child, a limp or refusal to walk may be observed if the spine, pelvis, or lower extremity is involved.
- Pseudoparalysis (failure to use a limb despite normal neuromuscular structures) is observed in the upper extremity, especially in young children.
- Limitation of joint motion usually is present, especially if the infection involves the spine or if primary lesions are particularly close to joint spaces where sympathetic effusions may occur.
- In chronic osteomyelitis, local bone loss, persistent drainage through fistulas or sinus tracts, chronic pain, low-grade fever (if present), and mild systemic symptoms usually are present.
- External physical findings in chronic osteomyelitis may be minimal, but soft tissue inflammation and tenderness usually develop.

RISK FACTORS

- Open or compound fractures
- Intravenous drug use (predominantly spondylitis or intervertebral disc infection)
- Immunocompromised
- Infections of the genitourinary or biliary tracts
- Any surgical manipulation (particularly colorectal surgery, discectomy, joint replacement, and genitourinary procedures)
- Sickle cell anemia (*Salmonella* osteomyelitis)
- Low socioeconomic status
- History of tuberculosis (Pott disease)
- Infancy
- Elderly

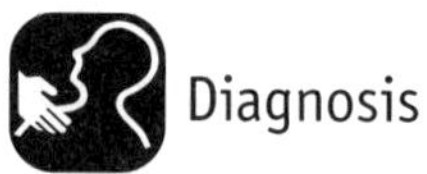

Diagnosis

DIFFERENTIAL DIAGNOSIS

- Acute leukemia
- Acute rheumatic fever
- Acute rheumatoid arthritis, adult or juvenile
- Acute gout
- Cellulitis
- Malignant bone tumors (Ewing sarcoma, osteosarcoma)
- Septic arthritis
- Multiple myeloma (older patients)
- Sepsis (in early osteomyelitis)

PHYSICAL EXAMINATION

- Fever with temperature >100.4°F (not always present)
- Tenderness, swelling, and erythema over the involved area
- Limited movement of adjacent joint
- Look for other foci of infection

IMAGING

- Obtain anteroposterior and lateral radiographs of the suspected area
- In early disease, x-rays may be normal or show only soft tissue swelling.
- Osseous changes usually appear 7–10 days after symptom onset and include periosteal elevation and/or destruction of bone with radiolucency, fading cortical margins, and no surrounding reactive bone.
- In acute osteomyelitis in children, classic findings include deep, circumferential soft tissue swelling with obliteration of muscular planes.
- In adults, plain radiographs are of less value because at least 50% to 75% of the bone matrix must be destroyed before radiographs show lytic changes.
- Radioisotope bone scans are the test of choice for early diagnosis of osteomyelitis or if x-ray studies are ambiguous.

- Consider magnetic resonance imaging (MRI) if bone scan is negative or when very minor destructive changes are present. The spatial resolution of MRI makes it useful in differentiating between bone and soft tissue infection (which is often a problem with bone scans).
- Computed tomographic scanning may play a role in diagnosis of osteomyelitis and assist the surgeon in planning an approach for debridement.
- Ultrasound may show periosteal thickening and elevation. It can provide direction for aspiration that will confirm infection with gram stain and cultures.

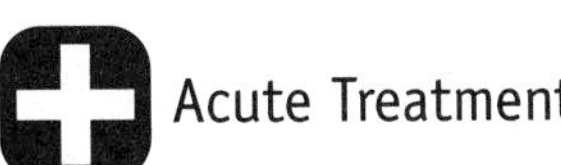

Acute Treatment

MEDICAL

- Immobilization of the affected part, hydration, fever control, and intravenous antibiotics directed by culture and sensitivity results (when available).
- Empiric treatment is guided by the age of the patient, severity of disease, and suspected organisms.
- For children >4 years old, nafcillin or oxacillin is recommended. If allergic to penicillin, use vancomycin or clindamycin. Add a third-generation cephalosporin if gram-negative bacteria are seen on gram stain.
- In adults >21 years, infection usually is vertebral. Recommended empiric antibiotics are nafcillin, oxacillin, or cephazolin. If allergic to penicillin, use vancomycin. If gram stain shows gram-negative bacilli, add a third-generation cephalosporin or ciprofloxacin (Cipro) plus rifampin.
- Osteomyelitis secondary to a nail puncture wound through a tennis shoe strongly suggests contamination with *Pseudomonas aeruginosa*. Administer ceftazidime or cefepime; alternatively use ciprofloxacin, except in children.
- Duration of treatment is usually 4–6 weeks, but may be longer, depending on the clinical response and laboratory values.

SURGICAL

- Surgical drainage and debridement is needed for tissue culture identification of the offending organism, evacuation of abscesses, and removal of necrotic bone.
- Reconstruction of large bony defects may be required.

HYPERBARIC OXYGEN THERAPY

- Has shown some promising results in treating chronic osteomyelitis
- Provides oxygen to promote collagen production, angiogenesis, and ultimately wound healing

SICKLE CELL ANEMIA PATIENTS

- Most common culprit is *Salmonella* sp. inoculation, followed by *Staphylococcus aureus*.
- Use a fluoroquinolone (not in children); alternatively use a third-generation cephalosporin

SKELETAL TUBERCULOSIS

- Any bone can be involved
- In children and adolescents, it usually involves the metaphysis of long bones.
- In adults, the axial skeleton most often is involved, followed by the proximal femur, knee, and small bones of the hands and feet.
- Tissue for histologic and microscopic examination almost always is required for diagnosis.

FUNGAL OSTEOMYELITIS

- Bone infections may be caused by coccidioidomycoses, blastomycosis, cryptococcosis, candidiasis, or sporotrichosis.
- Most common presentation is a cold abscess overlying an osteolytic lesion.
- Treatment involves surgical debridement and antifungal chemotherapy.

VERTEBRAL OSTEOMYELITIS

- Biopsy and debridement cultures dictate choice of antibiotic(s).
- Percutaneous transpedicular debridement and discectomy by removing infected necrotic bone accelerates healing and prevents progression of bone destruction and deformity in the early stages of vertebral osteomyelitis and spondylodiscitis.

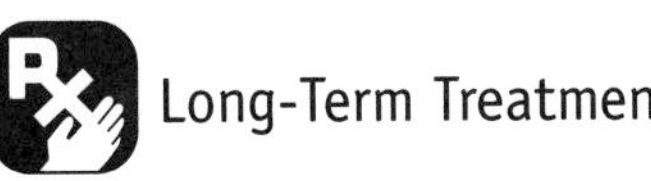

Long-Term Treatment

CHRONIC OSTEOMYELITIS

- Treatment is similar to that of the acute form, but some experts say that empiric treatment is not indicated. Base treatment on results of cultures and sensitivities.
- May be treated with surgical incision and drainage, sequestrectomy, and appropriate antibiotic coverage for 4–6 weeks.

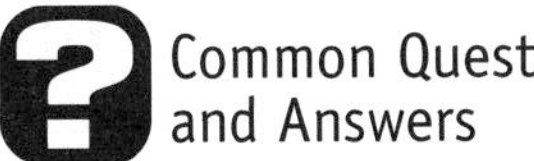

Common Questions and Answers

Physician responses to common patient questions:

Q: What are the adverse outcomes of the disease?

A: Adverse outcomes include growth disturbance and leg length discrepancy, destruction of adjacent joints, pathologic fractures, and bone defects leading to limb dysfunction. Chronic draining of sinuses that persist into adulthood may result in squamous cell carcinoma.

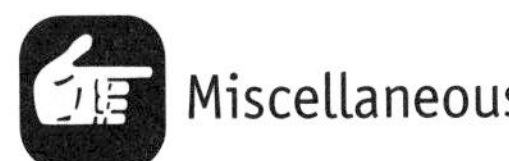

Miscellaneous

ICD-9 CODE

730.2 General/infective/localized/neonatal/purulent/pyogenic/septic/staphylococcal/streptococcal/suppurative/with periostitis
730.3 Acute/subacute
730.1 Chronic/old
731.8 Due to or associated with diabetes mellitus
Use fifth digit subclassification with category 730: 0 = site unspecified; 1 = shoulder region; 2 = upper arm; 3 = forearm; 4 = hand; 5 = pelvic region and thigh; 6 = lower leg; 7 = ankle and foot; 8 = other unspecified sites; 9 = multiple sites

BIBLIOGRAPHY

Gilbert DN, Moellering RC Jr, Sande MA. *The Sanford guide to antimicrobial therapy, 1999*. Hyde Park, VT: Antimicrobial Therapy, 1999.

Mandell GL, Bennet JE, Dolin R. *Principles and practice of infectious diseases,* 5th ed. Philadelphia: Churchill Livingstone, 2000, 1182–1184.

Pettid FJ, Tamisea DF, Heieck JJ. In: Mercier LR, ed. *Practical orthopedics,* 4th ed. St. Louis: Mosby, 1995.

Greene WB, Lieberman JR, Johnson TR, et al. In: Snider RK, ed. *Essentials of musculoskeletal care.* Rosemont, IL: American Academy of Orthopedic Surgeons, 1997.

Author: James Fambro

Otitis Media

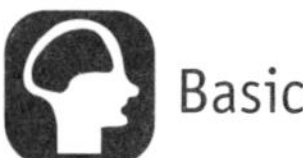

Basics

DEFINITION

Acute Otitis Media

- Fluid in the middle ear accompanied by signs or symptoms of ear infection

Recurrent Otitis Media

- ≥3 episodes of acute otitis media in 6 months

Otitis Media with Effusion

- Fluid in the middle ear without signs or symptoms of ear infection

INCIDENCE/PREVALENCE

- Almost all (93%) children experience ≥1 episode of otitis media by age 6 years.
- Most frequent primary diagnosis at U.S. office visits in children <15 years
- Peak incidence in children age 6–18 months

SIGNS AND SYMPTOMS

Acute Otitis Media

- Cough or rhinitis
- Irritability, fever, earache
- Most reliable is tympanic membrane (TM) appearance: bulging, full, red, and immobile under positive pressure using pneumatic otoscopy
- Cloudy appearance with decreased mobility also reliable
- Redness alone not reliable

Otitis Media with Effusion

- Absence of signs and symptoms of acute infection
- Reduced hearing may be present
- TM neutral or retracted in appearance; fluid in middle ear space

RISK FACTORS

- Bottle feeding
- Passive smoking
- Group child-care facility attendance
- Previous episodes of acute otitis media, especially if first when <1 year old
- Sibling history of recent infection

ETIOLOGY

- Usually eustachian tube dysfunction after viral upper respiratory infection (URI), which results in fluid in the middle ear that acts a culture medium for bacterial superinfection
- *Streptococcus pneumoniae* (increased incidence of drug resistance 30% to 60% in some communities)
- *Haemophilus influenzae*
- *Moraxella catarrhalis*
- *Streptococcus pyogenes*
- *Mycoplasma pneumoniae*
- Otitis media with effusion may have underlying bacterial component. Can follow treatment for acute otitis media.

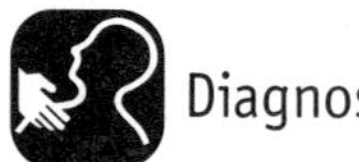

Diagnosis

DIFFERENTIAL DIAGNOSIS

- Redness: crying, fever, cerumen removal with irritation of external canal
- Earache: referred pain from throat, jaw, teeth, other nearby structures
- Tympanosclerosis
- Mastoiditis: tenderness in mastoid area may be due to otitis media.

HISTORY

- Patient with or without recent URI symptoms complains of otalgia, fever, decreased hearing, or occasional vertigo
- May have history of otitis media
- TM may spontaneously rupture, leading to resolution of pain.

PHYSICAL EXAMINATION

Acute Otitis Media

- TM bulging, full, red, and immobile; may be cloudy.
- TM rupture may lead to signs of otorrhea on examination.
- May have tenderness in mastoid area

Otitis Media with Effusion

- TM neutral or retracted
- Fluid behind TM may be present.
- May need tympanometry or acoustic reflectometry to confirm diagnosis

TESTS

Tympanocentesis may be helpful in selected refractory or recurrent cases to make microbiologic diagnosis.

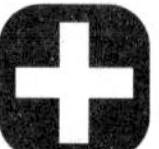

Acute Treatment

GENERAL

- Outpatient management except in cases requiring surgical intervention.
- Modification of environmental risk factors (see Risk Factors)

Acute Otitis Media

- Usually treated empirically with antibiotics (see Etiology)
- Amoxicillin: 500 mg three times a day is first-line drug. High dose may be needed to treat resistant pneumococcus. Peds: 40–80 mg/kg/day. Not effective against *H. influenzae* or *M. catarrhalis* (B-lactamase producers).
- Penicillin allergy: erythromycin 250 mg four times a day or trimethoprim-sulfamethoxazole (Bactrim or Septra) two tablets twice a day
- Decongestants, acetaminophen, or ibuprofen
- Cortisporin otic suspension: four drops three times a day may be added if TM is ruptured.

Acute Otitis Media Treatment Failures

- Center for Disease Control (CDC) recommendations
- Switch in empiric therapy recommended on day 3 or days 10 to 28 after initial diagnosis if clinically defined treatment failure
- Agents selected should be effective against *S. pneumoniae,* including drug-resistant strains, and *H. influenzae* and *M. catarrhalis*.
- Drugs of choice: amoxicillin-clavulanate (Augmentin), cefuroxime axetil (Ceftin), and intramuscular ceftriaxone (Rocephin)

Otitis Media with Effusion

- Initial diagnosis may be confirmed with tympanometry; usually observe or treat with oral antibiotic.
- Decongestants, antihistamines, and oral steroids not indicated
- May need grommet placement after 3 months following complete ear, nose, and throat (ENT) evaluation.

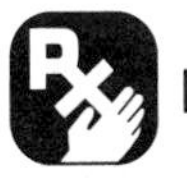

Long-Term Treatment

SURGERY

- Consider tympanocentesis for treatment failures, especially if several recent courses of antibiotics; allows for pathogen-directed treatment

REFERRAL/DISPOSITION

Age 1–3 years

- If effusion present for >6 weeks, consider hearing evaluation
- If effusion present for >3 months, need hearing evaluation and possible ENT referral for tympanostomy tube (grommet) placement

Older Individuals

- May need grommet placement after 3 months following complete ENT evaluation to exclude other causes of effusion

Common Questions and Answers

Physician responses to common patient questions:
Q: What about acute otitis media and diving?
A: Avoid diving until normal TM mobility because of increasing risk of rupture at depths >4.3 feet.
Q: Which decongestants and/or antihistamines are banned by sports governing bodies?
A: Be careful with over-the-counter decongestants. Drugs containing ephedrine or pseudoephedrine are banned by International Olympic Committee (IOC). Sedating antihistamines banned by IOC for shooting sports. If in doubt, call the United States Anti-Doping Agency Drug Reference Line at 1-800-233-0393.
Q: What about water sports in athletes with grommets?
A: No evidence of increased development of otorrhea; possibly decreased incidence in swimmers versus nonswimmers. Decreased incidence of infection with use of polymyxin B-Neosporin-hydrocortisone (two drops at night after swimming).
Q: What about water sports and ear plugs?
A: No evidence of decreased infection rate with ear plug use. Surface swimming only; increased pressure in diving may increase infection rate.

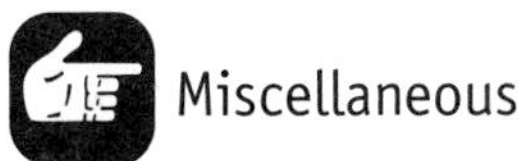

Miscellaneous

SYNONYMS

- Serous otitis media
- Suppurative otitis media
- Secretory otitis media

ICD-9 CODE

382.9 Acute otitis media
382.00 Acute suppurative otitis media
381.01 Acute or subacute serous otitis media

BIBLIOGRAPHY

American Academy of Pediatrics practice guideline: managing otitis media with effusion in young children. *Pediatrics* 1994;94.

Karl KB, Fricker PA. *Medical problems in athletes.* Malden, MA: Blackwell Science, 1997.

Lister PD, Pong A, Chartrand SA, et al. Rationale behind high-dose amoxicillin therapy for acute otitis media due to penicillin-nonsusceptible pneumococci: support from in vitro pharmacodynamic studies. *Antimicrob Agents Chemother* 1997;41:1926–1932.

Nelson W. *Nelson textbook of pediatrics,* 15th ed. Philadelphia: WB Saunders, 1996.

Pichichero ME. Acute otitis media, part I: improving diagnostic accuracy. *Am Fam Physician* 2000;61:2051–2056.

Pichichero ME. Acute otitis media, part II: treatment in an era of increasing antibiotic resistance. *Am Fam Physician* 2000;62: 2410–2416.

Roger G, Carles P, Pangon B, et al. Management of acute otitis media caused by resistant pneumococci in infants. *Pediatr Infect Dis J* 1998;17:631–638.

Authors: Darin Rutherford and Craig C. Young

Overtraining

Basics

DEFINITION

- Process of training at a level beyond which an athlete can adapt with adequate recovery, both physiologically and psychologically
- Overtraining syndrome (OTS) refers to the final stage in a proposed continuum of overtraining characterized by a variety of symptoms and physiologic abnormalities that always include performance decrements refractory to normal regeneration cycles.

INCIDENCE/PREVALENCE

- Career prevalence in elite distance runners up to 60%
- May be more common in high school and collegiate athletes who are subjected to rigid overload stimuli without benefit of individualized training

SIGNS AND SYMPTOMS

- Because OTS is a spectrum of disease, the clinical presentation varies among individual athletes.
- Increased resting heart rate, poor sleep, and later time to bed may be the most sensitive markers, but few athletes complain until athletic performance declines.

Psychological

- Generalized fatigue
- Loss of motivation
- Poor sleep
- Poor appetite
- Loss of confidence
- Decreased mood as measured by the Profile of Mood States

Physiologic

- Increased resting heart rate
- Increased resting blood pressure
- Weight loss
- Postural hypotension
- Chronic muscle soreness
- Frequent illness/injuries

Performance

- Performance decrements
- Decreased maximum work output
- Prolonged reaction time
- Increased perceived exertion at given workload
- Decreased coordination

RISK FACTORS

- Highly motivated athletes who respond to poor athletic performance by increasing training loads
- Athletes subjected to generic overload stimuli, without individualized training
- Increased psychological stressors (i.e., finances, scholastics, relationships)

PATHOPHYSIOLOGY

- Previously thought to occur in two clinical forms: parasympathetic and sympathetic
- Currently, hypothesized that both types reflect different stages in OTS
- Early overtraining associated with heightened sympathetic tone
- Advanced overtraining produces an inhibition in sympathetic tone resulting in a predominance of the parasympathetic nervous system.

ASSOCIATED FACTORS

- Frequent overuse injuries (i.e., soft tissue injuries, stress fractures)
- Frequent illness (i.e., recurrent upper respiratory infection)

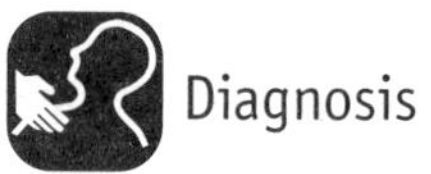

Diagnosis

DIFFERENTIAL DIAGNOSIS

- Major depression
- Organic disease (mononucleosis, hypothyroidism, anemia)
- Drug abuse

HISTORY

- Any recent changes in intensity, frequency, duration, and/or mode of training?
- Any changes in social stressors? Financial problems, family illness, relationship problems, scholastic concerns?
- Any changes in sleep pattern?
- Recent exposure to infection?
- Changes in menstruation?

PHYSICAL EXAMINATION

- Oral temperature to rule out systemic infection
- Evaluate resting heart rate and blood pressure
- Chest auscultation to rule out pneumonia, bronchitis, and asthma
- Abdominal examination to evaluate spleen and liver
- Neurologic examination to rule out central nervous system disease

DIAGNOSTIC TESTING

- Profile of Mood States may document decreased mood.
- Serologic testing if clinically indicated to rule out organic disease

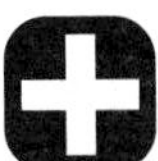

Acute Treatment

GENERAL CONSIDERATIONS

- OTS can only be treated with rest.
- Severity of overtraining will dictate the recovery period
  - —Severest cases need weeks to months of absolute rest
  - —Mild cases needing alteration in intensity, frequency, duration, and/or mode of training sessions

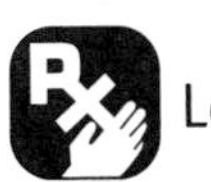

Long-Term Treatment

PREVENTION AND EARLY DETECTION

Daily Training Logs

- Helpful in determining the cumulative strain involved with training
- To be useful in early detection of OTS, systematic documentation of subjective and objective factors must be completed at baseline (when the athlete has no signs or symptoms) and reevaluated periodically.
- Although small daily variations occur in athletes, training logs can identify an individual athletes' abnormal response to training at an early stage.
- Once identified, interventions can be made to prevent further deterioration of performance and normalization of subjective and objective criteria.
- Training logs should include
  - —Resting heart rate
  - —Daily workout schedule (including intensity, duration, and mode of training)
  - —Borg perceived exertion scale (BPE), which correlates physiologic responses with training but also accounts for outside stressors that are difficult to quantify objectively

Proper Coaching and Training Techniques

- Recognize overtraining early and intervene
- Avoid monotony in training
- Avoid punishing poor training performance with higher levels of training
- Training goals should be formulated on a week-to-week basis during times of increased training
- Training loads should display day-to-day variability
- Alternate hard day/easy day and include 1 rest day per week (hard day = BPE >5; easy day = BPE <5)
- If athlete begins to show strain (performance decrements, increasing BPE at low-level training, elevated resting heart rate), reduce training to a lower level.

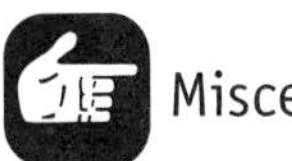

Miscellaneous

ICD-9 CODE

780.79 Fatigue

BIBLIOGRAPHY

Mellion M, ed. *The team physician handbook,* 2nd ed. Philadelphia: Hanley & Belfus, 1997:243–247.

Foster C. Monitoring training in athletes with reference to overtraining syndrome. *Med Sci Sports Exerc* 1998;30:1164–1168.

Kuipers H. Training and overtraining: an introduction. *Med Sci Sports Exerc* 1998;30:1137–1139.

Authors: Thomas D. Armsey and Robert G. Hosey

Paronychia

 Basics

DESCRIPTION

Infectious inflammation of the folds of skin surrounding the fingernail or toenail. May be acute or chronic.
System(s) affected: Skin/Exocrine
Genetics: No known genetic pattern
Incidence/Prevalence in USA: Common
Predominant age: All ages
Predominant sex: Female > Male (3:1)

SIGNS AND SYMPTOMS

- Separation of nail fold from nail plate
- Red, painful swelling of skin around nail plate
- Purulent
- Secondary changes of nail plate
- Green changes in nail (pseudomonas)

CAUSES

- Acute—Staphylococcus aureus. Less frequently by Streptococci and Pseudomonas
- Chronic—Candida albicans. Less frequently by fungi—dermatophytes and occasionally, by molds (Scytalidium Fusarium)

RISK FACTORS

- Acute—trauma to skin surrounding nail, ingrown nails
- Chronic—frequent immersion of hands in water, diabetes mellitus

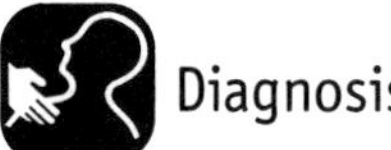 Diagnosis

DIFFERENTIAL DIAGNOSIS

- Herpetic whitlow
- Felon
- Reiter's disease
- Psoriasis

LABORATORY

- Gram stain
- Culture and sensitivity
- KOH preparation plus fungal culture

Drugs that may alter lab results: Use of over-the-counter antimicrobials or antifungals
Disorders that may alter lab results: N/A

PATHOLOGICAL FINDINGS

N/A

SPECIAL TESTS

None

IMAGING

N/A

DIAGNOSTIC PROCEDURES

N/A

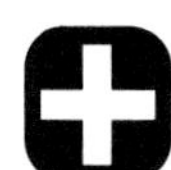 Acute Treatment

APPROPRIATE HEALTH CARE

Outpatient

GENERAL MEASURES

- Acute—warm compresses or vinegar soak's, elevation
- Chronic—keep fingers dry

SURGICAL MEASURES

Incision and drainage (I&D) of abscess, if present. If there is a subungual abscess or ingrown nail present, will need partial or complete removal of nail.

ACTIVITY

Full activity

DIET

No special diet

PATIENT EDUCATION

Chronic—keep fingers dry

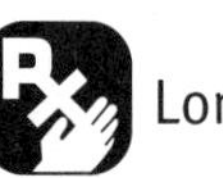 Long-Term Treatment

DRUG(S) OF CHOICE

- Acute (if diabetic, suppurative or more severe cases):
  - —Dicloxacillin 125–500 mg q6h
  - —Cloxacillin 250–500 mg q6h
  - —Erythromycin 500 mg q6h
  - —Cephalexin (Keflex) 250 mg q6h
- Chronic:
  - —Bacterial—mupirocin (Bactroban)
  - —Yeast or dermatophyte—topical imidazoles (econazole, ketoconazole, terbinafine)
- Systemic:
  - —Itraconazole (Sporanox) 200 mg/day for 90 days (may have longer action because incorporated in nail plate). Pulse therapy may be useful: 200 mg BID for 7 days, repeated monthly for 2 months
  - —Terbinafine (Lamisil) 250 mg q/d for 90 days
  - —Fluconazole (Diflucan) 150 mg/week for 4–6 months

Contraindications: Allergy to antibiotic

Precautions: Erythromycin may cause significant gastrointestinal upset

Significant possible interactions:

- Erythromycin affects levels of theophylline and effects of carbamazepine, digoxin and corticosteroids. Cardiac toxicity with terfenadine or astemizole.
- Ketoconazole, astemizole, itraconazole, fluconazole—terfenadine,

ALTERNATIVE DRUGS

Antipseudomonal drugs, e.g., third generation cephalosporin, aminoglycosides

PATIENT MONITORING

Routine follow-up until healed

PREVENTION/AVOIDANCE

- Chronic—avoid frequent wetting of hands, wear rubber gloves with cloth liner
- Good diabetic control

POSSIBLE COMPLICATIONS

- Acute—subungual abscess
- Chronic—secondary ridging, thickening and discoloration of nail, nail loss

EXPECTED COURSE/PROGNOSIS

With adequate treatment and prevention, healing can be expected

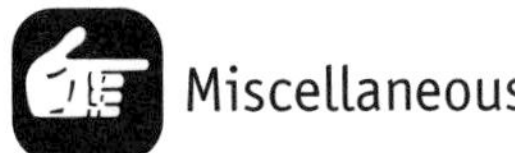

Miscellaneous

ASSOCIATED CONDITIONS

Diabetes mellitus

AGE-RELATED FACTORS

Pediatric: Anaerobes may be involved in cases with thumb/finger sucking
Geriatric: N/A
Others: N/A

SYNONYMS

- Eponychia
- Perionychia

ICD-9 CODE

681.02 Onychia and paronychia of finger
112.3 Candidiasis of skin and nails

See also: Onychomycosis

OTHER NOTES

May be considered work-related in bartenders, waitresses, nurses and others who often wet their hands

BIBLIOGRAPHY

Fitzpatrick TB, et al., eds. *Dermatology in general medicine*. 3rd Ed. New York, McGraw-Hill, 1987.

Moschella SC, Hurley HJ, eds. *Dermatology*. 3rd Ed. Philadelphia, W.B. Saunders Co., 1992.

Baran R, Dawber RPR, eds. *Diseases of the nail and their management*. 2nd Ed. Boston, Blackwell Scientific, 1994.

Internet references: http://www.5mcc.com

Author: Larry Milikan

Pericarditis

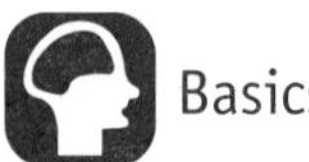

Basics

SIGNS AND SYMPTOMS

- Chest pain
  - —Retrosternal or precordial
  - —Usually sharp
  - —Pleuritic
  - —Radiating to the shoulder or the trapezial ridge
  - —Worsened with cough or inspiration
  - —Increased with recumbency
  - —Improved with leaning forward
- Fever
- Mild dyspnea
- Cough
- Hoarseness
- Nausea
- Anorexia
- Tachypnea
- Tachycardia
- Odynophagia
- Friction rub
  - —Heard best at lower left sternal border
  - —Any of three components
    - —Presystolic
    - —Systolic
    - —Early diastolic
  - —Intermittent and exacerbated by leaning forward
- Beck's triad with the accumulation of pericardial fluid
- Muffled heart sounds
- Increased venous pressure (distended neck veins)
- Decreased systemic arterial pressure (hypotension)
- Worsened dyspnea
- Ewart's sign
- Dullness and bronchial breathing between the tip of the left scapula and the vertebral column
- Pulsus paradoxus
- Exaggerated decrease (>10 mm Hg) in systolic pressure with inspiration
- Constrictive pericarditis
- Signs of both right- and left-sided heart failure
- Pulmonary and peripheral edema
- Ascites
- Hepatic congestion

MECHANISM/DESCRIPTION

- Inflammation, infection, or infiltration of the pericardial sac which surrounds the heart
  - —Pericardial effusion may or may not be present
- Acute pericarditis
  - —Rapid in onset
  - —Potentially complicated by accumulation of pericardial fluid leading to cardiac tamponade
- Constrictive pericarditis
  - —Results from chronic inflammation causing thickening and adherence of the pericardium to the heart

ETIOLOGY

- Idiopathic (most common)
- Viral
  - —Echovirus
  - —Coxsackie
  - —Adenovirus
  - —Varicella
  - —Epstein-Barr
  - —Cytomegalovirus
  - —Hepatitis B
  - —AIDS
- Bacterial
  - —Staphylococcus
  - —Streptococcus
  - —Haemophilus
  - —Salmonella
  - —Legionella
  - —Tuberculosis
- Fungal
  - —Candida
  - —Aspergillus
  - —Histoplasmosis
  - —Coccidioidomycosis
  - —Blastomycosis
  - —Nocardia
- Parasitic
  - —Amebiasis
  - —Toxoplasmosis
  - —Echinococcosis
- Neoplastic
  - —Lung
  - —Breast
  - —Lymphoma
  - —Leukemia
  - —Melanoma
- Uremia
- Myxedema
- Myocardial infarction, Dressler's syndrome
- Connective tissue disease
  - —Systemic lupus erythematosus
  - —Rheumatoid arthritis
  - —Scleroderma
- Radiation
- Chest trauma
- Postpericardiotomy
- Aortic dissection
- Pancreatitis
- Inflammatory bowel disease
- Drugs
  - —Procainamide
  - —Cromolyn sodium
  - —Hydralazine
  - —Dantrolene
  - —Methysergide
  - —Mesalamine
- Amyloidosis

CAUTIONS

- Differentiation between acute pericarditis and myocardial infarction necessitates rapid transport to the ED for evaluation with a 12-lead ECG
- Treat the hypotensive patient in cardiac tamponade with aggressive prehospital fluid resuscitation and rapid transport to point of definitive care

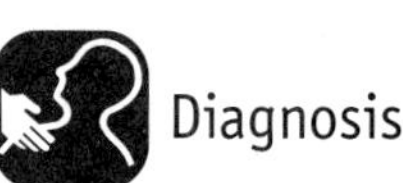

Diagnosis

ESSENTIAL WORKUP

- ECG
  - —Stage 1
    - —ST segment elevation diffusely except AVR and V1
    - —ST segments concave up
    - —No reciprocal ST segment depression in other leads (in contradistinction to the changes seen in acute myocardial infarction)
  - —Stage 2
    - —ST segments return to normal
    - —T waves flatten
    - —PR segments may become depressed
  - —Stage 3
    - —T-wave inversion

—Stage 4
 —Eventual resolution of all changes
 —Differentiation from myocardial infarction
 —No Q waves formed
 —T-wave inversion occurs after the resolution of the ST segment changes

LABORATORY

- CBC
- Leukocytosis
- ESR may be elevated
- Cardiac enzymes
  —Helpful in distinguishing pericarditis from myocardial infarction
  —Reported elevated with the inflammation of pericarditis

IMAGING/SPECIAL TESTS

- CXR
  —Can be normal
  —May show enlargement of the cardiac silhouette
  —No change in heart size until >250 ml of fluid have accumulated in the pericardial sac
- Echocardiography
  —Diagnostic method of choice for the detection of pericardial fluid
  —Can detect as little as 15 ml of fluid in the pericardial sac
- Chest CT
  —Useful for the detection of calcifications or thickening of the pericardium
- Pericardiocentesis
  —Used to obtain fluid for protein, glucose, culture, cytology, Gram and acid-fast stains, and fungal smears

DIFFERENTIAL DIAGNOSIS

- Acute myocardial infarction
- Pulmonary embolism
- Pneumothorax
- Aortic dissection
- Pneumonia
- Empyema
- Cholecystitis
- Pancreatitis

Acute Treatment

INITIAL STABILIZATION

- ABCs
- Pericardiocentesis for hemodynamic compromise secondary to cardiac tamponade
  —Removal of even a small amount of fluid can lead to a dramatic improvement
- Guided ultrasound is safest

ED TREATMENT

- Treatment dependent on the underlying etiology
- Idiopathic, viral, rheumatologic, and posttraumatic
  —Nonsteroidal antiinflammatory drug regimens effective
  —Corticosteroids reserved for refractory cases
- Bacterial
  —Aggressive treatment with intravenous antibiotics along with drainage of the pericardial space
  —Search for primary focus of infection
  —Therapy guided by determination of pathogen from pericardial fluid tests
- Neoplastic
  —Treat underlying malignancy
- Uremia
  —Intensive 2-6-week course of dialysis
  —Caution should be used if using nonsteroidal medications
- Expected course/prognosis
  —Majority of patients will respond to treatment within 2 weeks
  —Most have complete resolution of symptoms
  —Small number progress to recurrent bouts with eventual development of constrictive pericarditis or cardiac tamponade

MEDICATIONS

- Aspirin: 350–500 mg po q 3–4 hrs
- Ibuprofen: 400–600 mg po q6–8 hrs
- Indomethacin: 25–50 mg po q 6 hrs

HOSPITAL ADMISSION CRITERIA

- ICU
  —Hemodynamic instability
  —Cardiac tamponade
  —Associated malignant arrhythmia
  —Any suspicion of myocardial infarction
  —Severe pain unresponsive to oral medications
  —Suspicion of bacterial etiology
  —Patients having undergone pericardiocentesis due to the relatively high incidence of complications

HOSPITAL DISCHARGE CRITERIA

- Mild symptoms in patients without any hemodynamic compromise
- Close follow up
- Able to tolerate a regimen of oral medication

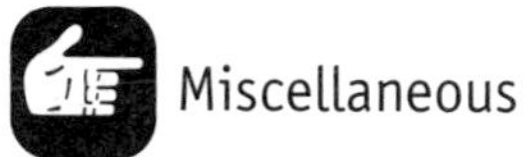

Miscellaneous

ICD-9 CODE

423.9

CORE CONTENT CODE

2.3.1

BIBLIOGRAPHY

Jourilles NJ. Pericardial and myocardial disease. In: Rosen P, et al., eds. *Emergency medicine: concepts and clinical practice*. 4th ed. St. Louis: CV Mosby, 1998; 1716–1726.

Maisch B. Myocarditis and pericarditis—old questions and new answers. *Herz* 1992; 17(2):65–70.

Maisch B. Pericardial diseases, with a focus on etiology, pathogenesis, pathophysiology, new diagnostic imaging methods, and treatment. *Curr Opin Cardiol* 1994;9:379–88.

Sternbach GL. Pericarditis. *Ann Emerg Med* 1988;17(3):214–20.

Author: Andrew T. McAfee

Periorbital Cellulitis

Basics

SIGNS AND SYMPTOMS

- Erythema
- Warmth
- Tenderness
- Swelling
- Unilateral location

Bacteremic Periorbital Cellulitis

- Children <2 years old
- Preceding upper respiratory infection
- Fever (>39°C)
- Erythematous or violaceous swelling of the eyelid
  —Obscured eye from swelling within 12 hours

Complication of Sinusitis

- URI
- Low grade fever
- Gradual swelling over days
  —Inflammatory edema in the periorbital tissue does not contain actual infection
  —Secondary to vascular and lymphatic congestion

Orbital Cellulitis

- Proptosis
- Limitation of eye movement
- Eye pain
- Abnormal pupillary reaction
- Decreased visual acuity
- Diplopia
- Toxicity
- Fever
- Leukocytosis
- Chemosis
  —Associated with both periorbital and orbital cellulitis

MECHANISM/DESCRIPTION

- Periorbital (preseptal) cellulitis
  —Inflammatory process of the tissues anterior to the orbital septum
- Orbital septum
  —Connective tissue extension of the orbital periosteum that is reflected into the upper and lower eyelids
  —Represents a nearly impervious barrier to the spread of infection into the orbit
- Orbital cellulitis
  —Inflammatory process in the structures posterior to the orbital septum

Three Mechanisms

- Localized infection of the eyelid or adjacent structures
  —Blepharitis
  —Hordeolum
  —Chalazion
  —Dacryoadenitis
  —Dacryocystitis
  —Impetigo
  —Abscess
  —Surrounding skin disruptions (minor trauma, insect bites, dermatologic disorders)
  —Organisms include
    —*S. aureus*
    —*S. pyogenes*
    —Less commonly *S. epidermidis*, anaerobes
- Hematogenous dissemination
  —Pathogens migrate to the periorbital tissues
  —Organisms include
    —*S. pneumoniae*
    —*S. pyogenes*
    —*Haemophilus influenzae* type b (Hib)
- Inflammation and edema from an underlying sinusitis
  —Organisms include
    —*S. pneumoniae*
    —Nontypeable *H. influenzae*
    —*M. catarrhalis*

ETIOLOGY

- Prior to *H. influenzae* type b (Hib) immunization *H. influenzae* accounted for 80% of bacteremic periorbital cellulitis cases
- Currently *Streptococcal* infections (group A and pneumococcus) are the primary causative organisms
- Consider nonbacteremic causes

PEDIATRIC CONSIDERATIONS

- Child who has had at least the second Hib vaccination a week prior to the onset of the cellulitis is unlikely to have *H. influenzae* b infection

CAUTIONS

- Establish IV access and administer oxygen if associated serious complications
  —Sepsis
  —Meningitis

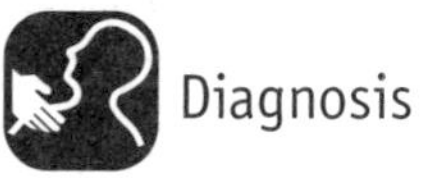

Diagnosis

ESSENTIAL WORKUP

- Clinical diagnosis
  —Typical signs/symptoms
  —Perform thorough neurologic exam
  —Assess for orbital involvement

LABORATORY

- CBC
  —WBC >15,000 is usually associated with bacteremic periorbital cellulitis
- Blood culture
- Gram stain and culture of either a tissue aspirate or swab of draining purulent material
- Lumbar puncture/CSF evaluation
  —If ill-appearing
  —Signs of meningeal irritation
  —Without adequate Hib vaccinations

IMAGING/SPECIAL TESTS

- Sinus x-rays
- CT scan
  - —Indicated if
    - —Concern for orbital cellulitis or traumatic penetration of the orbital septum
    - —Failure to respond to parenteral antimicrobial therapy
  - —Demonstrates
    - —Sinusitis
    - —Subperiosteal abscess
    - —Presence of a foreign body
    - —Proptosis

DIFFERENTIAL DIAGNOSIS

- Lack of fever and leukocytosis suggest noninfectious causes
  - —Trauma
  - —Insect bite
  - —Allergy
  - —Tumor
  - —Local eye/eyelid infection
- Early orbital cellulitis
  - —May have the same appearance as periorbital cellulitis

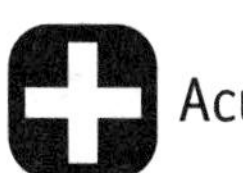

Acute Treatment

INITIAL STABILIZATION

- 0.9%NS IV bolus (500 cc or 20 cc/kg) for dehydration, sepsis, hypotension

ED TREATMENT

- Administer IV antibiotics for toxic/ill appearing bacteremic periorbital cellulitis
  - —Consider vancomycin in geographic areas with prevalent penicillin-resistant pneumococci
- Children with signs of orbital cellulitis require
  - —Parenteral antibiotics
  - —CT scan
  - —Ophthalmologic consultation
  - —Prompt surgery may be necessary

MEDICATIONS

- Augmentin: 500 mg (peds: 45 mg/kg/24 hrs) po bid
- Cefazolin: 1 g (peds: 100 mg/kg/24 hrs) IV q 6–8 hrs
- Cefotaxime: 1–2 g (peds: 150 mg/kg/24 hrs) q 6–8 hrs
- Ceftriaxone: 1 g (peds: 50–100 mg/kg/24 hrs) IV q 24 hrs or q 12 hrs
- Cephalexin: 500 mg (peds: 100 mg/kg/24 hrs) po qid
- Clindamycin: 600 mg (peds: 40 mg/kg/24 hrs) IV q 6 hrs; 300 mg (peds: 20 mg/kg/24 hrs) po qid
- Dicloxacillin: 500 mg (peds: 100 mg/kg/24 hrs) po qid
- Nafcillin: 1–2 g (peds: 150 mg/kg/24 hrs) IV q 6 hrs
- Oxacillin: 1–2 g (peds: 150 mg/kg/24 hrs) IV q 6 hrs
- Vancomycin: 500 mg (peds: 40 mg/kg/24 hrs) q 6 hrs

HOSPITAL ADMISSION CRITERIA

- Toxicity
- Signs of orbital cellulitis
- Progression of infection on oral antibiotics

HOSPITAL DISCHARGE CRITERIA

- Oral antibiotics for modest swelling, nontoxic appearance, and reliable parents
- Monitor for progressive swelling, irritability, increased fever, or vision changes

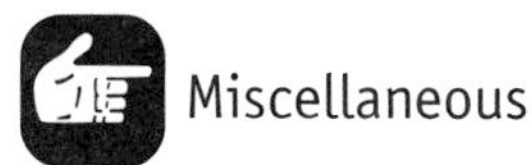

Miscellaneous

ICD-9 CODE

376.01

CORE CONTENT CODE

6.4.4.2

BIBLIOGRAPHY

Powell KR. Orbital and periorbital cellulitis. *Pediatr Rev* 1995;16:1163–1167.

Schwartz GR, Wright SW. Changing bacteriology of periorbital cellulitis. *Ann Emerg Med* 1996;28:6:617–620.

Author: Joseph Wathen

Pharyngitis

Basics

SIGNS AND SYMPTOMS

- Sore throat
- Odynophagia
- Dysphagia
- Fever
- Cervical adenopathy
- Rash
- Diminished oral intake
- Fatigue
- Pharynx
  —Erythematous
  —Exudates
- Cervical adenopathy
- Fever
- Scarlatiniform rash
- Diphtheria
  —Exuberant gray, airway-threatening pharyngeal membrane
- Mononucleosis
  —Hepatosplenomegaly
- Gonococcal pharyngitis
  —In children with signs of sexual abuse
  —In adults with sexually transmitted disease

MECHANISM/DESCRIPTION

- Inflammation/infection of the pharynx
- Third most common complaint of patients seeking medical attention

ETIOLOGY

- Viral
  —Most common cause of infectious pharyngitis
  —Influenza
  —Adenovirus
  —Epstein Barr virus (mononucleosis)
- Bacterial
  —Many bacterial pathogens cause pharyngitis
  —Direct attention toward organisms with potentially serious sequelae
- *Group A β-hemolytic streptococcus*
  —Strep throat
  —Causes <10% of adult pharyngitis and <30% of childhood pharyngitis
- *Corynebacterium diphtheriae* (diphtheria)
- *Neisseria gonorrhoeae* (gonococcal pharyngitis)
- Noninfectious
  —Chemical burns
  —Foreign bodies
  —Inhalants
  —Postnasal drip

CAUTIONS

- Direct attention to airway control for difficulty with respirations
- Initiate 0.9%NS IV fluid for hypotension or significant signs of dehydration

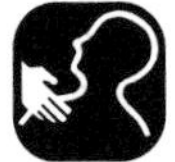

Diagnosis

ESSENTIAL WORKUP

- Physical exam
  —Does not allow physician to differentiate between various etiologies of pharyngitis
  —Ability to differentiate *Group A β-hemolytic streptococcus* from nonstreptococcal etiologies
    —50% false-negative rate
    —75% false-positive rate when attempting to differentiate *Group A β-hemolytic streptococcus* based solely on clinical grounds

LABORATORY

- Throat culture
  —Gold standard
  —Cumbersome due to 48-hour delay and difficulties with ER followup
  —False-negative rate = 10%
  —False-positive rate = 20%
- Rapid strep tests (RST)
  —Convenient
  —Results within 30 minutes
  —Sensitivity = 85–95%
  —Specificity = 96–99%
  —Few false-positives and many false-negatives
  —Treat all positive-RST
  —Confirm all negative-RST by throat culture and treated empirically
- Monospot for suspected mononucleosis

DIFFERENTIAL DIAGNOSIS

- Epiglottitis
- Peritonsillar/retropharyngeal abscess
- Diphtheria
- Acute leukemia
- Oropharyngeal cancer
- Foreign body
- Postnasal drip

IMAGING/SPECIAL TESTS

- Lateral neck x-ray for suspected epiglottitis or foreign body

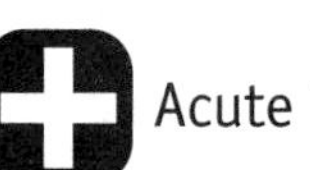

Acute Treatment

INITIAL STABILIZATION

- ABCs
- Administer 1-L (peds: 20 cc/kg) 0.9%NS fluid bolus for signs of volume depletion or if patient is unable to tolerate oral solutions

ED TREATMENT

- Administer antipyretics
  - —Acetaminophen
  - —Ibuprofen

Group A β-Hemolytic Streptococcus

- Administer antibiotics for confirmed or highly suspicious
  - —Objectives of treatment
    - —Prevent rheumatic fever
    - —Diminish symptoms
    - —Prevent the suppurative complications
  - —Options
    - —Penicillin
    - —Erythromycin
- Corticosteroids
  - —Dexamethasone 10 mg IM × 1
  - —Provides symptomatic relief in patients with severe streptococcal pharyngitis
- Children should not return to school until they have had at least 24 hours of antibiotics
- Complications
  - —Acute rheumatic fever
    - —Usually occurs 2.5 weeks following infection
    - —Attack rate 0.5–3.0% in untreated patients
    - —Preventable if patients are treated within 9 days of infection
  - —Poststreptococcal glomerulonephritis
    - —Rarely causes permanent renal failure
    - —Antibiotics do not prevent occurrence
  - —Peritonsillar/retropharyngeal abscess
    - —<1% of those treated
    - —Retropharyngeal abscess occurs primarily in children <3 years old
    - —Retropharyngeal nodes regress after age 3

Diphtheria

- Goals of therapy
  - —Protect patient against the local dangers of the airway-compromising membrane
  - —To treat the infection
  - —Counteract the exotoxin which, unabated, causes myocarditis and neuritis
- Horse antitoxin
  - —Dose dictated by illness severity
- Penicillin or erythromycin
- Complications
  - —Myocarditis
    - —Occurs in two-thirds
    - —Clinically significant in 10%
  - —Peripheral neuritis usually involves the cranial nerves

Gonococcal Pharyngitis

- Treat as per usual sexually transmitted disease protocol
  - —third-generation cephalosporin/azithromycin

MEDICATIONS

- Penicillin
  - —Intramuscular
    - —<27 kg: Pen G benzathine (LA) 0.6 million units × 1
    - —>27 kg: Pen G benzathine (LA) 1.2 million units × 1
  - —Oral
    - —<12 years: 250 mg bid × 10 d
    - —>12 years: 500 mg bid × 10 d
- Erythromycin
  - —Erythromycin base 500 mg po qid × 10 d (peds: erythroethylsuccinate 40 mg/kg/d po + tid × 10 d)

HOSPITAL ADMISSION CRITERIA

- Airway compromise
- Severe dehydration
- Child sexual abuse

HOSPITAL DISCHARGE CRITERIA

- Able to tolerate oral intake

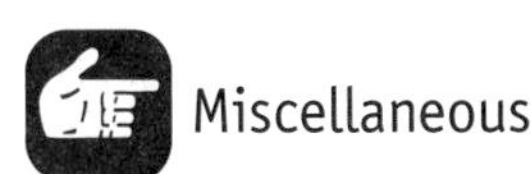

Miscellaneous

ICD-9 CODE

462

CORE CONTENT CODE

6.3.9

BIBLIOGRAPHY

Kline J. Streptococcal pharyngitis: a review of pathophysiology, diagnosis and management. *J Emerg Med* 1994;12: 665–680.

Quayle K. Otitis and pharyngitis in children. In: Tintinalli J, et al., eds. *Emergency medicine: a comprehensive study guide*. 4th ed. 1996:604–610.

Shulman S. Evaluation of penicillins, cephalosporins, and macrolides for therapy of streptococcal pharyngitis. *Pediatr Infect Dis J* 1994;13(Suppl 1):955–959.

Slay R. Upper respiratory tract infection. In: Rosen P, et al., eds. *Emergency medicine: concepts and clinical practice*. 3rd ed. St. Louis: CV Mosby, 1997.

Authors: Annie Jewel Sadosty and Brian I. Browne

Photodermatitis

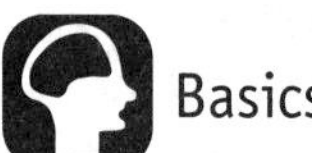

Basics

DESCRIPTION

Light-induced eruptions seen in a pattern of photo-distribution

- Phototoxic reactions—result of the acute toxic effect on skin of ultraviolet light alone (sunburn) or together with a photosensitizing substance (non-allergic)
- Photoallergic eruptions—a form of allergic dermatitis resulting from combined effects of a photosensitizing substance (drugs or chemical) plus ultraviolet light (immunologic/delayed hypersensitivity)
- Polymorphous light eruption (PLE)—chronic, intermittent light-induced eruption with erythematous papules, urticaria, or vesicles on areas exposed to sunlight

System(s) affected: Skin/Exocrine
Genetics: Predisposition occurs in inbred populations (e.g., Pima Indians)
Incidence/Prevalence in USA: Unknown
Predominant age: All ages
Predominant sex: Male = Female

SIGNS AND SYMPTOMS

- Phototoxic
- Erythema
- With increasing severity—vesicles and bullae
- Classic example—sunburn
- Nails may exhibit onycholysis
- Chronic—epidermal thickening, elastosis, telangiectasia and pigmentary changes
- Sharp lines of demarcation between involved and uninvolved skin (sunlight exposure)
- Phototoxic eruption due to topicals—area of application
- Usually develops shortly after sun exposure
- Hyperpigmentation may follow resolution
- Pain
- Photoallergic
  —Papules with erythema and occasionally vesicles
  —Area exposed to light with less distinct borders
  —Usually delayed—24 hours or more after exposure
  —May spread to unexposed areas
  —Pruritus
- Polymorphous light eruption (PLE)
  —Erythematous papules
  —Occasionally urticaria or vesicles
  —Scattered over sun exposed areas with normal skin in between
  —Can spread to non-exposed areas
  —Often flares in spring or early summer
  —Desensitization affect (less over the course of the summer)
  —Burning or pruritus may precede lesions

CAUSES

- Sunlight
- Phenothiazines
- Diuretics
- Tetracyclines
- Sulfonamides
- Oral contraceptives
- Topicals—psoralens, coal tars, photo-active dyes (eosin, acridine orange)

RISK FACTORS

N/A

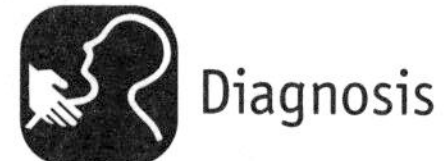

Diagnosis

DIFFERENTIAL DIAGNOSIS

Systemic lupus erythematosus

LABORATORY

Antinuclear antibody (ANA) to rule out systemic lupus erythematosus
Drugs that may alter lab results: N/A
Disorders that may alter lab results: N/A

PATHOLOGICAL FINDINGS

Nonspecific

SPECIAL TESTS

- Photo-testing
- Photopatch testing
- Skin biopsy—to rule out other disorders

IMAGING

N/A

DIAGNOSTIC PROCEDURES

Physical examination and medical history

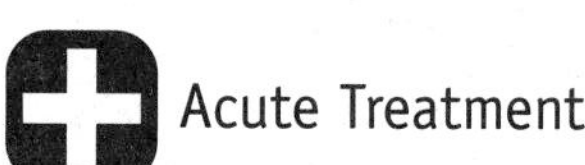

Acute Treatment

APPROPRIATE HEALTH CARE

Outpatient

GENERAL MEASURES

- Avoid sunlight/limit exposure
- Protective clothing/sunscreens
- Ice packs/cold water compresses

SURGICAL MEASURES
N/A

ACTIVITY
Avoid sunlight

DIET
No special diet

PATIENT EDUCATION
- Avoidance of sunlight
- Avoidance of photosensitizing drugs
- Protective clothing
- Sunscreens

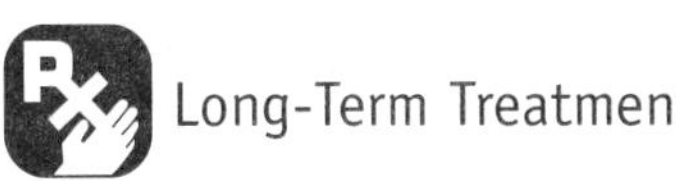

Long-Term Treatment

DRUG(S) OF CHOICE
- Topical corticosteroids (betamethasone valerate 0.1% cream)
- NSAIDs (indomethacin 25 mg tid; aspirin; others)
- Prednisone for severe reactions (0.5–1 mg/kg/d) for 3–10 days
- Antihistamines for pruritus (hydroxyzine 25–50 mg qid)
- Sunscreens for prevention. Use broad-spectrum sunscreen to block both UVA and UVB. PABA may aggravate photodermatitis in sensitized patients (due to the sulfa moiety).

Contraindications: Refer to manufacturer's profile of each drug
Precautions: Refer to manufacturer's profile of each drug
Significant possible interactions: Refer to manufacturer's profile of each drug

ALTERNATIVE DRUGS
N/A

PATIENT MONITORING
As necessary for persistence or recurrence

PREVENTION/AVOIDANCE
- Sunlight avoidance/protective clothing
- Identification and avoidance of causative drugs (see under Causes)
- Sunscreens—apply before exposure
  - —Zinc oxide—opaque, cosmetically less acceptable
  - —Chemical—use sun-protective factor >15 for maximum protection; substantively resistant to sweat and swimming; cosmetically more acceptable

POSSIBLE COMPLICATIONS
N/A

EXPECTED COURSE/PROGNOSIS
Good with avoidance/protection measures

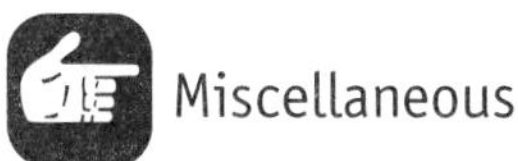

Miscellaneous

ASSOCIATED CONDITIONS
- Sunlight aggravation of systemic lupus
- Persistent light reactivity
- Actinic reticuloid

AGE-RELATED FACTORS
Pediatric: N/A
Geriatric: More likely to experience adverse reactions to causative drugs
Others: N/A

SYNONYMS
- Sun poisoning

ICD-9 CODE
692.79 Due to solar radiation, other
692.89 Due to other specified agents, other

ABBREVIATIONS
NSAID = nonsteroidal anti-inflammatory drugs

REFERENCES
Bondi J, Jegasothy B, Lazarus G. *Dermatology, Diagnosis and Therapy*. Norwalk, CT: Appleton & Lange, 1991.

Internet references: http://www.5mcc.com
Author: Jeffrey A. Stearns

Pneumothorax and Hemothorax

Basics

DEFINITION

- Air (pneumothorax), blood (hemothorax), or both (hemopneumothorax) in the pleural space between the lung and chest wall
- If mediastinal shift toward the uninvolved lung is present on x-ray, then "tension pneumothorax" is present.

INCIDENCE/PREVALENCE

- Rare, but potentially serious
- <4% of all sports injuries involve chest or abdomen
- Usually due to rib fracture with subsequent lung puncture
- Can be "spontaneous"; generally secondary to ruptured apical blebs

SIGNS AND SYMPTOMS

- Pain in chest, especially on deep inspiration
- Dyspnea
- Tachycardia

RISK FACTORS

- Congenital apical lung blebs

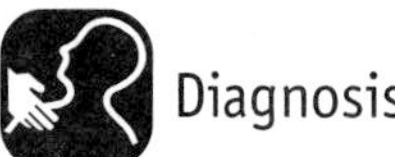

Diagnosis

DIFFERENTIAL DIAGNOSIS

- Chest wall contusion
- Lung contusion

HISTORY

- Trauma to thoracic wall?
- Persistent pain at injury site?
- Shortness of breath?

PHYSICAL EXAMINATION

- Decreased breath sounds on affected side
- Possible pallor/tachycardia

IMAGING

- Posteroanterior and lateral chest films; expiration film may help detect small pneumothorax
- Rib x-rays on affected side

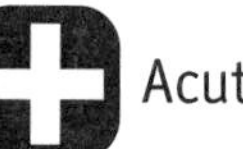

Acute Treatment

VENUE EVALUATION

- Determine diagnostic possibilities; transfer to hospital (x-ray) facility if suspicious for pneumothorax
- Semi-Fowler position
- Oxygen if available and if patient is dyspneic

HOSPITAL EVALUATION

- Small (<20%) tension-free pneumothorax (no mediastinal shift) can be treated expectantly with follow-up films and no chest tube
- All others (>20% pneumothorax) should be treated with closed thoracostomy-chest tube insertion with Heimlich valve or, preferably, underwater seal
- Analgesia: Tylenol #3 by mouth; lidocaine (Xylocaine) 1% for chest tube insertion

SPECIAL CONSIDERATIONS

- Hemothorax with even a small pneumothorax requires a chest tube to preclude development of "trapped lung," which eventually may require decortication.

- Avoid chest binders, taping, etc., which tend to compromise deep inspiration and may contribute to development of atelectasis.
- Chest tube can be removed when air leak has stopped and x-ray confirms lung expansion.

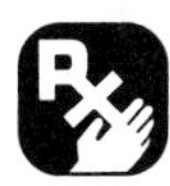

Long-Term Treatment

SURGERY

- Rarely necessary unless congenital blebs contributed to development of pneumothorax
- Persistent air leak may require thoracoscopy or, very occasionally, thoracotomy.
- Pleurodesis (creation of adherence between parietal and visceral pleurae) required in some cases

REHABILITATION

- Advise patient that pain likely will be present at least 6 weeks, especially if rib fracture produced the pneumothorax
- Encourage resumption of noncontact exercises
- Recheck chest x-ray in 6 weeks

Common Questions and Answers

Physician responses to common patient questions:
Q: How long before I can play ball again?
A: 3–6 weeks
Q: How long before I can fly?
A: 4–6 weeks after chest tube removal (if repeat x-ray is OK)
Q: When can I scuba dive?
A: Find a different sport to enjoy.

Miscellaneous

SYNONYMS

- Collapsed lung

ICD-9 CODE

512.8 Spontaneous pneumothorax
860 Traumatic pneumothorax
860.4 Traumatic pneumothorax with hemothorax

BIBLIOGRAPHY

Culpepper MI. High school football injuries in Birmingham, Alabama. *South Med J* 1983;76:873–875.

Amaral JF. Thoracoabdominal injuries in the athlete. *Clin Sports Med* 1997;16:739.

Cohen RG, DeMeester TR, Lafontain E. Pneumothorax. In: *Sabiston and Spencer's surgery of the chest,* 6th ed. Philadelphia: WB Saunders, 1995:524.

Authors: Richard Norenberg and Russell D. White

Proteinuria

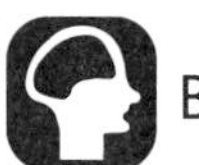

Basics

DEFINITION

- Excretion >150 mg/day of urinary protein (adults normally excrete 45–150 mg urinary protein daily)

Exercise-Induced Proteinuria

- Relatively common, benign finding
- Occurs in 70% to 80% athletes after exercise
- Incidence highest with strenuous, rather than prolonged, exercises
- 2+ to 3+ dipstick immediately after exercise; resolves over the first 24–48 hours <100–300 mg protein/24 hours
- Due to increased glomerular permeability and decreased tubular resorption of protein as a result of reversible physiologic changes in the kidney
- No known long-term sequelae

INCIDENCE/PREVALENCE

- Variable; highest in children, adolescents, and athletes
- 4% to 7% of asymptomatic adults have proteinuria that resolves on further examination

SIGNS AND SYMPTOMS

- Peripheral edema; indicates hypoalbuminemia and possibly nephrotic syndrome
- No symptoms directly attributable or specific for proteinuria

RISK FACTORS

- Pregnancy
- Diabetes
- Fever
- Exposure to cold
- Emotional stress
- Exercise

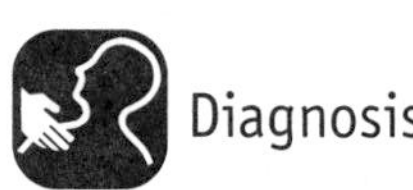

Diagnosis

DIFFERENTIAL DIAGNOSIS

<3 g Protein/24 Hours

- Exercise-induced proteinuria (range 100–300 mg protein/24 hours)
- Orthostatic proteinuria (thought to be due to increased pressure on the renal vein while standing)
- Multiple myeloma (monoclonal light chain proteins)
- Light chain nephropathy (polyclonal light chain, as can occur with hepatic cirrhosis)
- Minimal change disease/glomerulonephritis
- β-Microglobulinuria/tubular proteinuria
- —Hereditary: Wilson disease, cystinosis, oxalosis, medullary cystic disease
  —Congenital: Fanconi syndrome, renal tubular acidosis
  —Acquired: pyelonephritis, interstitial nephritis, obstructive uropathy, radiation nephritis, vitamin D intoxication

>3 g Protein/24 Hours: Glomerulonephritis/Nephrotic Syndrome

- Loss of negative charge on capillary wall and increased permeability allow large negatively charged proteins to pass through glomerulus.
- Patients exhibit edema, hypoalbuminemia, hyperlipidemia, and possibly hyponatremia, hypocalcemia, coagulation abnormalities.
- Minimal change disease
- Focal sclerosis
- Membranous glomerulonephritis
- Membranoproliferative glomerulonephritis
- Congenital nephrotic syndrome (first 3 months of life)
- Unclassified glomerulonephritis

>3 g Protein/24 Hours: Multisystem Disease

- Caused by direct renal trauma or by deposition of antigen–antibody complexes on the glomerulus
- Diabetes mellitus
- Hypertension
- Lupus
- Henoch-Schönlein purpura
- Sarcoidosis
- Amyloidosis
- Goodpasture syndrome
- Takayasu syndrome
- Polyarteritis
- Myxedema

>3 g Protein/24 Hours: Infectious Related

- Poststreptococcal glomerulonephritis
- Immunoglobulin A (IgA) nephropathy
- Bacterial endocarditis
- Syphilis

>3 g Protein/24 Hours: Iatrogenic

- Nonsteroidal anti-inflammatory drugs (NSAIDs)
- Probenecid
- Penicillamine
- Mephenytoin

>3 g Protein/24 Hours: Neoplasm

- Carcinomas of the breast, lung, and colon
- Lymphoma
- Leukemia
- Wilms tumor

>3 g Protein/24 Hours: Familial Disorders

- Fabry disease
- Sickle cell disease
- Alport syndrome

HISTORY

- Onset with relation to exercise; exposure to cold, stress, fever
- Recent upper respiratory infection suggests poststreptococcal glomerulonephritis or IgA nephropathy
- Unilateral flank pain suggests calculi or pyelonephritis
- Family history of sickle cell trait or disease, polycystic kidney disease, or renal failure
- Hesitancy and dribbling (signs of prostatic obstruction)
- Dysuria and frequency suggest infection
- Fever, night sweats, and weight loss suggest tuberculosis or malignancy
- NSAID use

PHYSICAL EXAMINATION

- Vitals (fever, hypertension)
- Palpation of flank and abdomen for tenderness
- Auscultation for renal artery bruits, pericarditis, endocarditis, congestive heart failure
- Prostate examination in males to evaluate for tenderness, mass, and size
- Pelvic examination in females to evaluate for tenderness and mass

APPROACH TO PATIENT

General

- Rule out benign causes before referral to nephrologist

Step 1

- Repeat urinalysis on two occasions after 24–48 hours of rest
- If proteinuria resolves on subsequent specimens, further testing is not required (exercise-induced proteinuria likely).
- If persists, continue to step 2.

Step 2

- Rule out orthostatic proteinuria (see Test Protocol).
- If proteinuria persists in supine position, proceed to step 3.

Step 3

- 24-hour urine collection for protein, creatinine, and creatinine clearance
- Serum creatinine, blood urea nitrogen (BUN), complete blood count, electrolytes, albumin, lipids, fasting blood glucose
- Intravenous pyelogram (IVP) to view kidney number, size, and function
- Based on 24-hour total protein:
  —<150 g/day: normal; generally no follow-up required
  —>150 g/day: follow annually with blood pressure (BP) and urinalysis
  —1–2 g/day: follow closely every 6–12 months for BP, urinalysis, BUN, creatinine
  —3 g/day: refer to nephrologist; consider renal biopsy
  —Tubular protein: refer to nephrologist

Step 4

- Consider urine protein electrophoresis to qualitatively and quantitatively determine type of protein

IMAGING

- IVP is first choice in atraumatic setting; shows structure and function.
- Consider ultrasound or computed tomographic scan in setting of trauma or if low creatinine clearance prohibits IVP

LABORATORY TESTS

Urinalysis/Dipstick

- Excellent screening test, but mainly screens for albumin
- False-positive results caused by highly concentrated urine (specific gravity >1.025), alkaline urine (pH >8.0), hematuria, or use of phenazopyridine (Pyridium); these factors less important with readings ≥3+.
- Dipstick test is primarily sensitive for albumin and may underestimate degree of proteinuria if large amounts of undetectable globulins or light chains are present (as in amyloidosis or multiple myeloma).

Sulfosalicylic Acid Test

- Detects all proteins
- Trace urine dipstick test and ≥3+ sulfosalicylic acid test indicate large amounts of nonalbumin proteins in the urine.

Microscopy

Casts, dysmorphic red blood cells, and absence of clot suggest glomerulonephritis.

24-Hour Urine Collection

- Quantitative assessment of renal function, loss of protein, creatinine, and creatinine clearance

Urine Protein Electrophoresis

- Quantitative and qualitative assessment of various forms of urinary proteins to help differentiate Bence-Jones from tubular proteins

Test for Orthostatic Proteinuria

- Void before bedtime; collect, label, and refrigerate urine for dipstick.
- Void, collect, and label; have partner refrigerate urine while patient remains supine on three separate occasions: midnight, 5 a.m., and 7 a.m. Patient must remain supine during this entire phase of the test.
- Void mid morning (approximately 2–3 hours after rising); collect, label, and refrigerate urine for dipstick.
  —Positive test: positive for protein only while standing; no proteinuria while supine.
  —Negative test: constant proteinuria

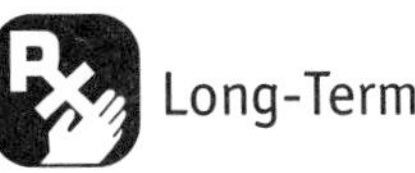

Long-Term Treatment

REFERRAL/DISPOSITION

- Treat underlying issue
- Only general medical care is indicated for transient, orthostatic, and exercise-induced proteinuria.
- Nephrology referral where appropriate

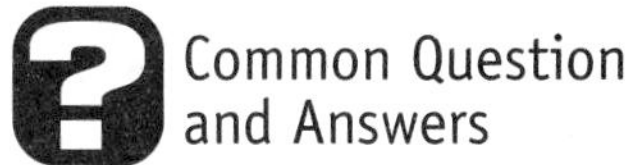

Common Questions and Answers

Physician responses to common patient questions:

Q: When can I return to play?

A: There are no absolute contraindications for athletes with exercise-induced proteinuria or for children with transient or orthostatic proteinuria. Return to play once a diagnosis is made. All other cases warrant review of the inherent risks of participation before return and should be made on a case-by-case basis.

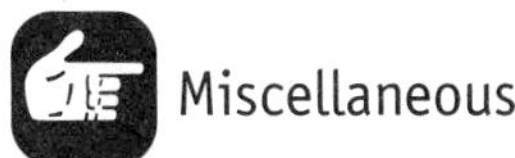

Miscellaneous

ICD-9 CODE

None known for Exercise-induced proteinuria; use 791.0

791.0 Proteinuria, NOS

791.0 Proteinuria, Bence-Jones

593.6 Proteinuria, orthostatic

646.2 Proteinuria, gestational

BIBLIOGRAPHY

Healy P, Jacobsen E. *Proteinuria, common medical diagnosis, an algorithmic approach,* 2nd ed. Philadelphia: WB Saunders, 1994: 80–81.

Cianflocco AJ. Renal complications of exercise. *Clin Sports Med* 1992;11:438–443.

Roy S, Noe N. Renal disease in childhood. In: Walsh PC, Retik AB, Vaughan ED Jr, Weln AJ. *Campbell's urology.* Philadelphia: WB Saunders, 1998:1677–1679.

Brendler C. Evaluation of the urologic patient. In: Walsh PC, Retik AB, Vaughan ED Jr, Weln AJ. *Campbell's urology.* Philadelphia: WB Saunders, 1998:149–152.

Goldszer R, Siegel A. Renal abnormalities during exercise. In: *Sports medicine.* Philadelphia: WB Saunders, 1991.

Authors: W. Mark Peluso and Michael J. Henehan

Pseudoanemia

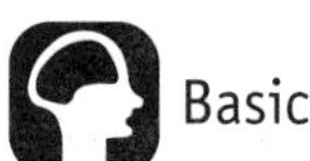

Basics

DEFINITION

- Dilutional phenomenon in endurance athletes causing decreased hemoglobin and hematocrit
- Plasma volume expansion with little change in red cell numbers (i.e., oxygen-carrying capacity)
- Contributing factors include
  - —Exercise-induced release of aldosterone, renin, and vasopressin
  - —Increased size of vascular bed due to muscle hypertrophy
  - —Retention of crystalloids and colloids governed by hormones
- Hemodilution occurs over the 48 hours after every episode of endurance exercise and may persist for as long as 1 week.
- Theoretically, this increased blood volume decreases viscosity, thereby maximizing stroke volume, cardiac output, and subsequent oxygen delivery.

INCIDENCE/PREVALENCE

- Elite athletes involved in endurance training
- Previously sedentary individuals starting an exercise program
- Athletes increasing intensity of training

SIGNS AND SYMPTOMS

- Hemoglobin levels 13–14 g/100 mL in men and 11–12 g/100 mL in women
  Dose–response relationship between amount/intensity of exercise and hemoglobin drop.
- Elite endurance athletes have a greater degree of dilutional pseudoanemia than more moderate endurance athletes.

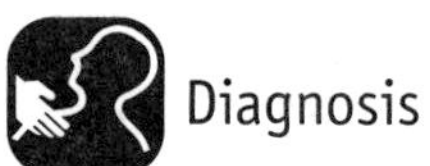

Diagnosis

DIFFERENTIAL DIAGNOSIS

- Iron deficiency anemia
- Gastrointestinal bleeding
- Hematuria
- Foot strike hemolysis

HISTORY

- Check exercise schedule, type of training activity, and occurrence of any symptoms

PHYSICAL EXAMINATION

- No particular symptoms or physical findings

LABORATORY STUDIES

- Performed if etiology unclear or symptoms present
- Normal mean corpuscular volume
- No hematuria or hemoglobinuria on urinalysis
- Normal bilirubin and haptoglobin
- Ferritin may be lower in endurance athletes due to the same relative dilutional effect. Values often <60 μg/L, occasionally <30, but <15 = iron deficiency.

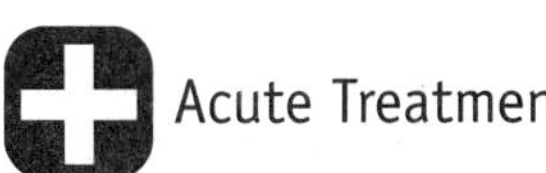

Acute Treatment

SPECIAL CONSIDERATIONS

- Rule out iron deficiency anemia
- Self-limited condition; indexes return to pretraining levels after training discontinued
- Normal physiologic response; no treatment required

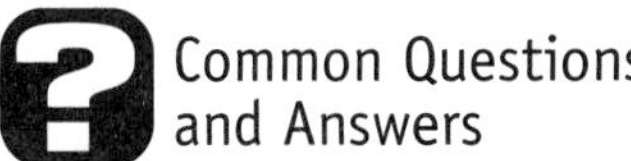

Common Questions and Answers

Physician responses to common patient questions:
Q: Should I start taking iron supplements?
A: Iron supplementation does not affect occurrence.

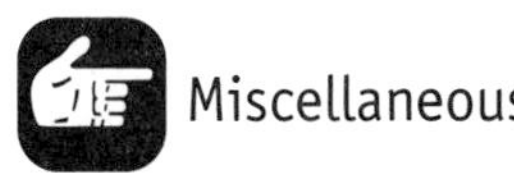

Miscellaneous

ICD-9 CODE

285.9 Anemia

SYNONYMS

- Sports anemia
- Athletes' pseudoanemia

BIBLIOGRAPHY

Balaban EP. Sports anemia. *Clin Sports Med* 1992;11:313–325.

Carlson DL, Mawdsley RH. Sports anemia: a review of the literature. *Am J Sports Med* 1986;14:109–112.

Chatard JC, Mujika I, Guy C, et al. Anaemia and iron deficiency in athletes. Practical recommendations for treatment. *Sports Med* 1997;27:229–240.

Raunikar RA, Sabio H. Anemia in the adolescent athlete. *Am J Dis Child* 1992;146: 1201–1205.

Watts E. Athletes' anaemia. A review of possible causes and guidelines on investigation. *Br J Sports Med* 1989;23: 81–83.

Weight LM, Darge BL, Jacobs P. Athletes' pseudoanemia. *Eur J Appl Physiol* 1991;62: 358–362.

Author: Julie Kerr

Pulmonary Contusion

Basics

DEFINITION

- Blunt trauma to the chest causing disruption of alveolar capillary interface, resulting in collection of blood, edema, and protein in the interstitium and alveoli

INCIDENCE/PREVALENCE

- Incidence of pulmonary contusion is low compared to chest wall contusion.
- 26% of rib fractures are associated with pulmonary contusion.
- 32% are associated with hemothorax/pneumothorax in one study.

SIGNS AND SYMPTOMS

- Dyspnea or tachypnea must be present for diagnosis.
- Airway and vascular spasm lead to pulmonary vascular bed shunting away from the affected lung.
- Hemoptysis may occur but is not invariably present.
- Palpable and pleuritic chest wall pain invariably are present due to the force required to produce a pulmonary contusion.
- Arm or trunk movement may worsen chest pain.

RISK FACTORS

- High-speed contact sports, football, cycling, equestrian, "extreme" sports

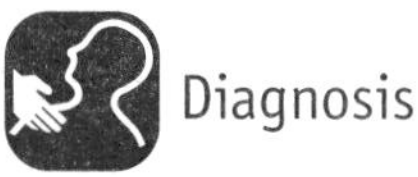

Diagnosis

DIFFERENTIAL DIAGNOSIS

- Rib fracture or contusion: pain predominates, minimal dyspnea, no hemoptysis
- Naso-oropharyngeal trauma when hemoptysis is primary sign
- Tracheobronchial mucosal avulsion: hemoptysis with normal chest x-ray (CXR) and without dyspnea. Most often from acceleration/deceleration of the blow to the chest. Observed on bronchoscopy.
- Traumatic pneumothorax hemothorax
- Diaphragmatic, splenic, or hepatic injury suggested by shoulder or scapular angle pain
- When trauma history is vague or unwitnessed, consider viral syndrome, spontaneous pneumothorax, and pericarditis.
- Pulmonary emboli when risk factors are present with dyspnea and hemoptysis or if there is no other cause such as trauma

HISTORY

- Blunt nonpenetrating trauma is required, usually reported by athlete or witnessed.
- Hemoptysis may be present only 12% of the time.
- Pain in the shoulder or scapular angle suggests abdominal or diaphragmatic injury. If fever is present, consider other infectious differential.
- Chest wall contusion is the usual initial diagnosis.
- Consider pulmonary parenchymal contusion when dyspnea is progressive over hours or days or if hemoptysis occurs.

PHYSICAL EXAMINATION

- Dyspnea persists after rest.
- Chest wall region is tender.
- Ecchymosis usually will not be present initially, but crepitus or more severe point tenderness often is present when ribs are fractured.
- Auscultation should be normal in absence of asthma history. Consider hemo pneumothorax if abnormal lung sounds are present.
- Inspect and record naso-oropharyngeal findings, as onset of hemoptysis may be delayed. Note any evidence of bleeding in the nose or mouth. Nasal trauma or bites of cheeks or tongue are far more common than pulmonary contusion as etiologies of "hemoptysis."
- Inspect range of motion of neck and palpate to rule out other injury in the presence of significant blunt trauma to chest.
- Record vital signs serially if athlete is unable to return to play to observe for deterioration. Pulse oximetry <91% suggests contusion with A/V shunting.
- Penetrating injury occurring anteriorly at rib interspace 5 or below may penetrate the abdomen. Abdominal examination for tenderness or guarding is critical.

IMAGING

- Posterior, anterior, and lateral CXR is not indicated for chest pain in absence of dyspnea or hemoptysis. Rib films do not contribute to management in absence of pulmonary symptoms or clinical flail fracture.
- PAL CXR reveals peripheral infiltrate in area of trauma when significant contusion occurs.
- Hemopneumothorax is ruled out by CXR. If hemoptysis is recurrent over >48 hours, bronchoscopy may be indicated.
- Ventilation perfusion scan shows matched ventilation perfusion defect.

FOLLOW-UP IMAGING

- Daily when hospitalized, consider every other day when managing outpatient, depending on respiratory effort

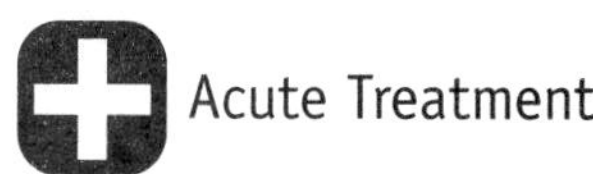

Acute Treatment

ANALGESIA

- Acetominophen, nonsteroidal anti-inflammatory drugs, or narcotics for comfort and to allow sleep. In cases of severe pain, particularly rib fracture, careful infiltration of local at the rib may help in the short term.
- Anyone requiring narcotics or local should not return to play until able to function at preinjury levels.

IMMOBILIZATION

- Rib taping and other attempts at immobilization are not effective and may be harmful by predisposing to atelectasis and pneumonia.

SPECIAL CONSIDERATIONS

- Complications: Rib fractures are associated with severe blunt trauma.
- Flail chest is a rare but serious complication requiring hospitalization to observe for pulmonary deterioration and need for intubation with respiratory support.
- Pneumothorax due to rib fracture-induced pulmonary laceration is rare.
- Pulmonary laceration: with transfer of energy from the chest wall, shear forces often are generated that can tear the lung. Most lacerations heal without complications, but elastic recoil of the lung may extend the laceration to form a pulmonary pseudocyst, which may result in infection, abscess, hemoptysis, air leak, adult respiratory distress syndrome, and death.

- Airway avulsion or rupture: Hemoptysis is more likely due to tracheobronchial epithelial disruption than pulmonary contusion. Most common site is within 2.5 cm of the carina between tracheal rings. Findings include subcutaneous emphysema and hemoptysis.
- Pneumothorax is uncommon with blunt trauma due to dense fibroconnective tissue surrounding carina and mainstem bronchi.

PRIMARY ON-FIELD CONCERNS

- Primary concerns with severe trauma are airway, breathing, and circulation.
- Expose by removing equipment, if needed
- Place in a comfortable position until adequate assessment is completed
- Observe for need to transport
- Report any increase in dyspnea; may need support, oxygen, and ventilation.

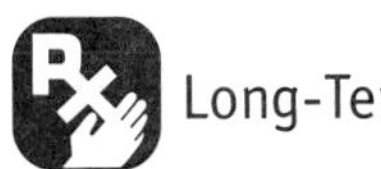

Long-Term Treatment

REHABILITATION

- Rest from strenuous exercise at least 7 days to allow pulmonary healing. A/A shunt limits exertion.
- Light exercise or walking promotes deep breathing and retards atelectasis.

SURGERY

Chest tube may be required emergently if hemopneumothorax is present.

REFERRAL/DISPOSITION

- Pulmonary consultation for bronchoscopy if hemoptysis persists

EXPECTED COURSE

- Most mild pulmonary contusions probably go undiagnosed and heal without incident.
- Dyspnea and tachypnea are the most important signs of deterioration.
- Serial films are not needed as long as the athlete is improving.
- Recheck PAL CXR for any dyspnea, fever, and increase in pain.
- After 4–6 weeks, consider follow-up film for clearing, especially if symptoms recur.
- Chest wall pain usually persists for 6 weeks but may not interfere with function.

RETURN TO PLAY

Simple Chest Wall Contusions

- Same day
- Athlete must be nondyspneic, able to perform usual movements as required for the sport, and able to tolerate pain without narcotics or local.
- On return to play, rib pads, flak jacket, or equestrian chest protector may decrease discomfort and reinjury during contact.
- Remove from activity for recurrent dyspnea; consider CXR.
- Athlete makes this decision, not the coach.
- Player must not be apprehensive.

Contusions Hemoptysis by CXR or Hemoptysis

- Field-side diagnosis with hemoptysis or persistent pain precludes return to that contest.
- Athlete should avoid strenuous activity for 1 week after the last episode.
- Lung heals in 7–10 days.
- After 7 days, if not dyspneic at rest, resume conditioning to maximum effort.
- After strenuous exercise is tolerated for 48 hours and athlete is able to perform at a level appropriate for contact sports, return to play in contact may be allowed.

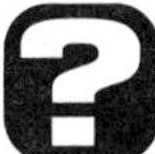

Common Questions and Answers

Physician responses to common patient questions:
Q: Could this injury get worse?
A: Yes. Pulmonary dysfunction of contusion may take 24–48 hours to develop as fluid accumulates in the air spaces. Serial reevaluations daily may be needed to detect worsening tachypnea and tachycardia. Get emergency follow-up evaluation if delayed deterioration occurs rapidly.

Q: Will this affect my future ability to play?
A: Lung healing is complete in 1–3 weeks without residual effects on pulmonary function. Return to peak conditioning depends on ability to reach maximum exertion effort. Involuntary guarding of pleuritic pain during healing may delay recovery to peak form by 6 weeks.

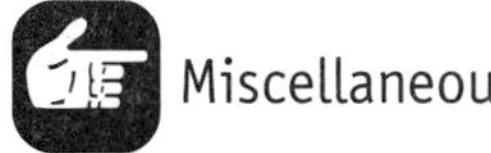

Miscellaneous

SYNONYMS

- Bruised lung

ICD-9 CODE

861.21 Pulmonary contusion without open wound, NS
860.0 Pneumothorax, traumatic without open wound, NS
807.0 Fractured ribs, closed injury, NS

BIBLIOGRAPHY

Dorshimer G. News briefs, lung injuries in contact sports. *Physician Sportsmed* 1999;27(6):10.

Dubinsky I, Low A. Non-life-threatening blunt chest trauma: appropriate investigation and treatment. *Am J Emerg Med* 1997;15: 240–243.

Fishman A, ed. *Fishman's pulmonary diseases and disorders,* 3rd ed. New York: McGraw Hill, 1997.

Rosen P, ed. *Emergency medicine: concepts and clinical practice,* 3rd ed. St. Louis: Mosby-Yearbook, 1998.

Ziegler DW, Agarwal NN. The morbidity and mortality of rib fractures. *J Trauma* 1994; 37:975–979.

Author: John Shelton

Red Eye

Basics

SIGNS AND SYMPTOMS

- Discharge
- Pruritus
- Pain
  - —Foreign body sensation
- Ectropion
- Entropion
  - —Eyelash against globe (trichiasis)
  - —Conjunctival injection
  - —Corneal abrasion, ulcer or opacity
  - —Anterior chamber cells or flare
  - —Photophobia (from movement of an inflamed iris)
  - —Proptosis
  - —Preauricular or submandibular lymphadenopathy
  - —Rosacea (may cause blepharitis)
  - —Facial skin lesions (herpes)
- Associated
  - —Sinusitis
  - —Otitis
  - —Pharyngitis

MECHANISM/DESCRIPTION

- Red eye
  - —May be caused by almost any eye disorder
  - —Often benign
  - —May represent systemic disease
- Pathophysiology—conjunctival vascular engorgement (common to all nontraumatic red eyes) which may be associated with
  - —Inflammatory diseases
    - —Uveitis (anterior and posterior)
    - —Episcleritis (70% idiopathic)
    - —Scleritis (50% associated with systemic disease)
  - —Inflammation/allergy
    - —Histamine release and increased vascular permeability, which results in swelling of the conjunctiva (chemosis), sometimes with watery discharge and pruritus
  - —Infection
    - —Bacterial—purulent mucous discharge
    - —Viral—watery or no discharge, pruritus
  - —Trauma
    - —Corneal abrasion
    - —Conjunctival hemorrhage
    - —Foreign bodies

ETIOLOGY

- Categorize by location of conjunctival injection
  - —Perilimbal
    - —Anterior uveitis (iritis)
    - —Sectorial
    - —Pinguecula
    - —Pterygium
    - —Hemorrhage
    - —Episcleritis
    - —Scleritis
      - * Occult perforation
    - —Diffuse
    - —Bacterial or viral conjunctivitis
    - —Blepharitis
    - —Dry eye syndrome
    - —Acute angle closure glaucoma
    - —Endophthalmitis
- Categorize red eyes by the presence of discharge or pain
  - —With discharge
    - —More common
      - * Conjunctivitis
      - * Ophthalmia neonatorum
      - * Blepharitis
  - —Less common
    - * Allergic reaction
    - * Dacryocystitis
    - * Caniculitis
  - —Without discharge
    - —No pain
      - * Subconjunctival hemorrhage
      - * Conjunctival tumor
    - —Mild to moderate pain
      - * Inflamed pinguecula/pterygium
      - * Blepharitis
      - * Dry eye syndrome conjunctivitis
      - * Foreign body
      - * Corneal disorder
      - * Episcleritis
      - * Posterior uveitis
      - * Orbital cellulitis
    - —Moderate to severe pain
      - * Corneal ulcer/abrasion/erosion
      - * Anterior uveitis
      - * Scleritis
      - * Acute angle-closure glaucoma
      - * Endophthalmitis

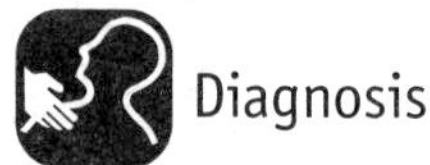

Diagnosis

ESSENTIAL WORKUP

- Visual acuity
  - —Pupil exam
  - —Confrontational visual field exam
  - —Extraocular muscle function
  - —Slit-lamp examination with fluorescein
  - —Lid eversion
- Funduscopy and tonometry when applicable

IMAGING/SPECIAL TESTS

- Direct towards the suspected etiology of the red eye
  - —Dacryocystitis: culture discharge
  - —Corneal ulcers: ophthalmologist should scrape the cornea for cultures
  - —Bacterial conjunctivitis: obtain conjunctival swab
  - —Moderate discharge: routine culture and sensitivity (usually *S. aureus*, *Streptococcus*, and *H. influenzae* [children])
  - —Severe discharge: Neisseria gonorrhea and Chlamydia
    - —Treat systemic infection and sexual partners
  - —Foreign body or orbital disease: Plain films or CT scan of the orbits
  - —Uveitis
    - —If unilateral, nongranulomatous, and history and physical are unremarkable: no systemic workup is necessary
    - —If bilateral, recurrent, or granulomatous: CBC, ESR, ANA, VDRL, FTA Ab. PPD, ACE level, CXR (sarcoidosis and TB), Lyme titer and HLA B-27, Toxoplasma and CMV titers

DIFFERENTIAL DIAGNOSIS

- Trauma
- Uveitis
- Arthritic disease
- Ankylosing spondylosis
- Ulcerative colitis
- Reiter's syndrome
- TB
- Herpes

- Syphilis
- Sarcoidosis
- Toxoplasma
- CMV
- Lyme

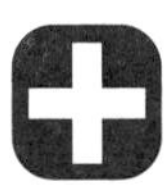

Acute Treatment

INITIAL STABILIZATION

N/A

ED TREATMENT

- Direct therapy toward specific etiology
  - —Differentiate between a corneal abrasion and a corneal ulcer
    - —Most abrasions will heal with or without patching
    - —Ulcers will get worse and may perforate if patched
  - —Never patch an eye with significant infection risk
    - —Contact lens wearers
    - —Abrasions from tree branch
    - —Fingernails
  - —Do not spread infection from the affected eye to the unaffected eye
- Trauma or uveitis
  - —Rule out intraocular foreign body
- Antibiotic drops
  - —Polytrim
  - —Gentamycin 0.3%
  - —Ciprofloxacin 0.35%
  - —Sulfacetamide 10%
  - —Trifluridine 1%
- Antibiotic ointments
  - —Bacitracin
  - —Erythromycin
  - —Gentamycin
  - —Neosporin
  - —Polysporin
  - —Sulfacetamide
  - —Vidarabine
- Mydriatics and Cycloplegics
  - —Atropine
  - —Cyclopentolate
  - —Homatropine
  - —Phenylephrine
  - —Tropicamide
- Corticosteroid drops (always with ophthalmology consultation)
  - —Cortisporin
  - —Maxitrol
  - —Metimyd
  - —Neo-decadron
  - —Prednisolone
  - —TobraDex
- Glaucoma agents (always with ophthalmology consultation)
  - —Acetazolamide
  - —Betaxolol
  - —Carteolol
  - —Dipivefrin
  - —Pilocarpine
  - —Timolol
  - —Mannitol
  - —Pilocarpine (only if mechanical closure is ruled out)
- Consult ophthalmologist for
  - —Dacryocystitis
  - —Corneal ulcer
  - —Scleritis
  - —Angle-closure glaucoma
  - —Uveitis
  - —Proptosis
  - —Orbital cellulitis
  - —Vision loss
  - —Uncertain diagnosis

HOSPITAL ADMISSION CRITERIA

- Endophthalmitis
- Perforated corneal ulcers
- Orbital cellulitis

HOSPITAL DISCHARGE CRITERIA

- Depends on the diagnosis
  - —If the diagnosis is certain and visual loss will not result, the patient may be discharged without consultation

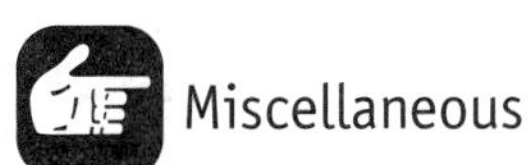

Miscellaneous

ICD-9 CODE

N/A

CORE CONTENT CODE

22.2.18

BIBLIOGRAPHY

Bertolini J, Pelicio M. The red eye. *Emerg Med Clin North Am* 1995;13(3):561–579.

Cullom R, Chang B. *The Wills eye manual: office and emergency room diagnosis and treatment of eye disease*. 2nd ed. Philadelphia: JB Lippincott, 1994.

Juang P, Ahn D, Rosen P. Ocular examination techniques for the emergency department. *J Emerg Med* 1997;15:793–810.

Author: Pascal S.C. Juang

Renal Trauma

Basics

DEFINITION

- Back or abdominal trauma due to collision with other players or equipment may result in injury to the kidney and its collecting system. Because signs and symptoms may initially be subtle, a high level of suspicion is warranted, especially if other commonly associated injuries such as splenic trauma, rib fractures, or vertebra fractures are present.

INCIDENCE/PREVALENCE

- 5% to 10% of renal trauma occurs in sports.
- About 8% to 10% of all blunt and penetrating injuries to the abdomen involve the kidney. The kidney is the most commonly injured organ in the urogenital system. Blunt trauma accounts for 80% to 90% of kidney injuries.
- The most common blunt trauma mechanism is rapid deceleration, especially to the upper abdominal area.
- Vascular injury of renal vessels has been reported in 1% to 3% of patients with blunt trauma. Venous injuries following blunt or penetrating trauma to the kidney can result in rapid and massive blood loss with relatively few symptoms.
- Injuries to the renal pedicle can lead to life-threatening blood loss. Fortunately, these injuries account for only 1% to 2% of all renal injuries.
- Among children, 16% to 25% of renal trauma is sports related. The majority of injuries involve boys 11 to 17 years of age. Of children with renal trauma, 8% to 22% have congenital anomalies.

SIGNS AND SYMPTOMS

- Diffuse abdominal tenderness with or without hematuria is the most common sign and symptom of kidney trauma.
- Associated injuries such as lower rib fractures, vertebral body fractures, and flank trauma with or without other internal injuries is common.
- Major injury to the renal vasculature may occur in the absence of hematuria. Hematuria, when present, is usually an early indicator of renal injury. The degree of hematuria, however, does not correlate with the severity of the injury.
- Significant renal trauma may result in hypovolemic shock.

RISK FACTORS

- Multiple fractures and injuries to abdominal organs, the vascular system, chest, and head make kidney trauma more likely.
- Ectopic placement of kidneys elsewhere in the abdomen may predispose to injury due to lack of protection usually afforded by the ribs.
- Preexisting renal anomalies have been shown to be associated with injury in 0.1% to 23% of adult cases and in 0.4% to 23% of pediatric cases.

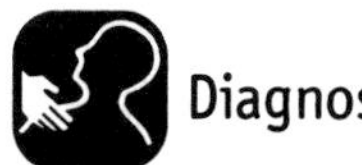

Diagnosis

DIFFERENTIAL DIAGNOSIS

- Hematuria
  —Renal: congenital anomalies, polycystic kidney, tumor, pyelonephritis, glomerulonephritis, Alport's syndrome, nephrolithiasis
  —Collecting system: bladder rupture, exercise induced, tumor, ureteral laceration, urethral laceration, blood dyscrasias
- Organ injury: splenic fracture, ruptured viscera, pulmonary contusion, liver fracture.
- Musculoskeletal injury: fractured rib(s), fractured vertebral body, fractured posterior spinal elements, contusion, muscle strain

HISTORY

- Flank pain and tenderness is usually present.
- The athlete may complain of gross hematuria.
- History of a collision or fall is described.

PHYSICAL EXAM

- The athlete may initially present as pale, perspiring, tachycardic, and nauseated.
- Tenderness to palpation of the flank and back is usually present.
- Muscle guarding may be present.
- Reflex ileus may occur with a loss of bowel sounds.
- A mass may be palpable representing either a hematoma or other renal abnormality.
- Hypotension and shock may be present if there is significant blood loss.
- Assess for associated injuries to the abdomen, chest, and back.

IMAGING AND LABORATORY TESTS

- Blood counts may show slight leukocytosis with a left shift. Hematocrit may be normal or decreased depending on fluid status. Serum blood urea nitrogen and creatine, as a baseline, help evaluate for preexisting renal abnormalities.
- Gross or microscopic hematuria has been reported in over 95% of patients with kidney injuries.
- Athletes with hematuria, gross or microscopic, following blunt trauma, should undergo radiologic assessment.
- Microscopic hematuria without shock does not necessarily require radiographic evaluation, but can be managed conservatively.
- Renal imaging is required in all pediatric patients.
- Renal imaging is required in all adult patients with penetrating trauma and hematuria, gross or microscopic.
- If physical exam or associated injuries suggest renal injury, renal imaging should be performed for staging.
- High resolution CT scan with contrast is the preferred method of renal evaluation following trauma.
- CT scan is noninvasive, sensitive to hematoma, and sensitive to urine extravasation, and provides additional information regarding other possible organ damage.
- CT scan is not reliable in evaluating possible renal vein injuries. If venous injury is suspected, venography should be performed.
- Arteriography is the definitive study to identify parenchymal and vascular injuries.
- Sonography provides less information compared with CT scan and does not accurately detect vascular injuries.
- Radionuclide scanning gives limited information and is not especially helpful in staging renal injuries.
- Although retrograde pyelography is useful in evaluating ureteral injuries, it is not helpful in evaluating renal injuries.

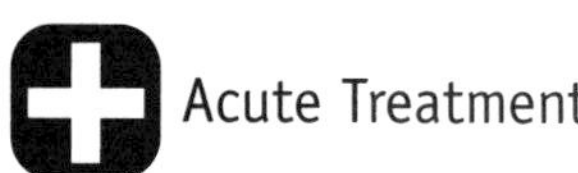

Acute Treatment

- Aggressive fluid resuscitation in athletes with hypotension or shock
- Often conservative management if renal contusion is present

- If staging evaluation of the kidneys show evidence of vascular involvement, surgical intervention may be required.
- Evidence of renal venous compromise necessitates emergent intervention.
- Athletes should be followed until hematuria resolves. Some recommend IVP at 3 months.
- Athletes with serious renal trauma should be followed at 3-month intervals with urinalysis and IVP for at least 1 year.

SPECIAL CONSIDERATIONS

Renal injuries are classified according to five grades:

- Grade I: renal contusion
- Grade II: minor lacerations
- Grade III: lacerations greater than 1.0 cm without collecting system rupture
- Grade IV: parenchymal laceration through renal cortex, medulla, and collecting system
- Grade V: complete kidney fracture with vascular compromise

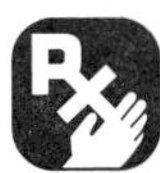

Long-Term Treatment

REHABILITATION

- Generalized return to conditioning may be required following prolonged convalescence.
- Specific rehabilitation of chest, abdomen, and back muscles for associated injuries

SURGICAL TREATMENT

- Contusions represent 85% to 90% of blunt renal injuries. These can be managed nonoperatively.
- Surgical management of minor and major renal lacerations is controversial. Most clinicians avoid operating unless bleeding is life threatening.
- In those cases when surgery is performed, a nephrectomy is usually required.
- Indications for surgical intervention of complications include expanding uncontained hematoma, pulsatile hematoma, urinary extravasation, vascular injury, nonviable parenchyma, and incomplete staging.
- Renal exploration is required in about 2.5% of cases of blunt trauma.
- Of those requiring renal exploration, the salvage rate is about 87%.

REFERRAL/DISPOSITION

Vascular injuries to the main renal artery carry a poor chance of reconstruction if diagnosis is delayed or the patient is older.

RETURN TO PLAY

- Athletes with renal contusions should refrain from participating in contact sports for 6 weeks after hematuria resolves.
- Athletes with extensive renal trauma should be withheld from contact or collision sports for 6 to 12 months.
- Although athletes with a solitary kidney may participate in sports, the decision to participate in contact and collision sports should be weighed on an individual basis.
- Athletes with solitary kidneys or previous kidney trauma should seriously consider special protective equipment use when they return.

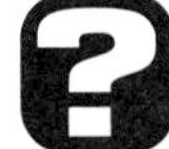

Common Questions and Answers

Physician responses to common patient questions:

Q: Will I be able to return to sports?
A: Depending on the seriousness of your injury, your time to return may be longer. If surgery (particularly nephrectomy) was required, you may want to consider not returning to contact or collision sports.
Q: Why did this happen to me?
A: Often abnormal anatomy can contribute to renal trauma. However, sometimes it's just bad luck or being in the wrong place at the right time.
Q: How long do I need to be followed for this injury?
A: Your doctor will want to see you on a regular basis until all symptoms clear. After that, depending on how serious your injury was, he or she may want to continue monitoring your kidney function periodically.

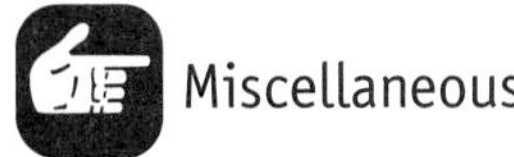

Miscellaneous

SYNONYMS

- Nephroptosis: floating kidney, mobile kidney
- Renal trauma: kidney trauma, nephric trauma

ICD-9 CODE

593.0 Nephroptosis
593.81 Vascular disorders of the kidney (renal artery embolism, hemorrhage, thrombosis, or renal infarction)
866.00 Injury, internal, kidney (subcapsular)
866.03 Injury, internal, kidney (subcapsular) with disruption of parenchyma (complete)
866.13 Injury, internal, kidney (subcapsular) with open wound into cavity
866.01 Injury, internal, kidney with hematoma (without rupture of capsule)
866.11 Injury, internal, kidney with hematoma with open wound into cavity
866.02 Injury, internal, kidney with laceration
866.12 Injury, internal, kidney with laceration with open wound into cavity
866.10 Injury, internal, kidney with open wound into cavity
868.04 Injury, internal, multiple, retroperitoneum
868.14 Injury, internal, multiple, retroperitoneum with open wound into cavity

BIBLIOGRAPHY

Armstrong PA, Litsher LJ, Key DW, et al. Management strategies for genitourinary trauma. *Hosp Physician* 1998;34:19–25.

Cianflocco AJ. Renal complications of exercise. *Clin Sports Med* 1992;11:437–451.

Danzl DF, Rosen P, Barkin R. *Emergency medicine: concepts and clinical practice*. St. Louis: CV Mosby, 1998.

Feliciano DV, Moore EE, Mattox KL. *Trauma*. Stamford, CT: Appleton & Lange, 1996.

Gillenwater JY, Grayhack JT, Howards SS, et al. *Adult and pediatric urology*. St Louis: CV Mosby, 1998.

Mandell J, Cromie WJ, Caldamone AA, et al. Sports-related genitourinary injuries in children. *Clin Sports Med* 1982;1:483–493.

Moeller JL. Contraindications to athletic participation. *Physician Sportsmed* 1996; 24:57–75.

Author: Nick Carter

Retinal Detachments and Tears

Basics

SIGNS AND SYMPTOMS

- Flashes of light
- Floaters
- "Curtain" or shadow over visual field
- Peripheral or central vision loss
- Visual field defects
- May be asymptomatic, especially in tractional retinal detachments

MECHANISM/DESCRIPTION

- Three distinct classifications of retinal detachments—treatments for each are different and exclusive
  - —Rhegmatogenous retinal detachments (RRD)
  - —Tractional retinal detachments (TRD)
  - —Exudative retinal detachments (ERD)
- RRD
  - —Most common
  - —Occur when a break in the sensory retina allows fluid from the vitreous to separate the rods and cones from the villi of the pigment epithelium
  - —Occur as an acute event, with symptoms of flashes due to the separation of the nerve fibers, and spots due to bleeding from the rupturing of retinal blood vessels
- TRD
  - —Occur because of contraction of fibrous vitreous bands pulling the sensory retina off of the pigment epithelium
  - —Chronic progressive disorder
  - —May remain without symptoms unless hemorrhage or retinal tear occurs
- ERD
  - —Abnormal collections of fluid are produced, separating the layer of the retina
  - —Usually asymptomatic until involvement of the macula occurs, with impairment of the central vision
  - —Occasionally, the retina can become so elevated and anteriorly displaced by underlying fluid as to be visible with a penlight just behind the lens

ETIOLOGY

- RRD occurs as a result of either structural/developmental abnormalities of the eye
  - —High myopia
  - —Marfan's syndrome
  - —Structural degeneration of the underlying anatomy of the eye (including the pigment epithelium, the sensory retina, and the vitreous body, or occasionally as a result of trauma)
- TRD occur in association with
  - —Diabetes
  - —Vasculopathy
  - —Perforating injury
  - —Severe chorioretinitis
  - —Retinopathy of prematurity, sickle cell retinopathy, or toxocariasis
- ERD arise from
  - —Tumors of the choroid (e.g., melanoma) or retina (e.g., retinoblastoma)
  - —Inflammatory disorders as Coats' or Harada's diseases

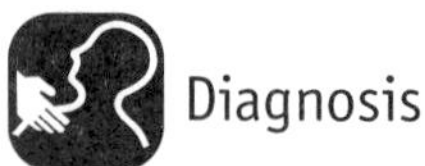

Diagnosis

ESSENTIAL WORKUP

- History, especially
  - —Age
  - —Speed of onset of symptoms
  - —Associated symptoms
  - —Previous episodes
- Complete ophthalmologic examination, especially
  - —Assessment of pupillary function
  - —Evaluation of the vitreous for cells
  - —Dilated retinal exam

LABORATORY

- As indicated for underlying disease

IMAGING/SPECIAL TESTS

- Visual field testing

DIFFERENTIAL DIAGNOSIS

- Senile retinoschisis (retinoschisis—a splitting of the retina)
- Juvenile retinoschisis
- Choroidal detachment

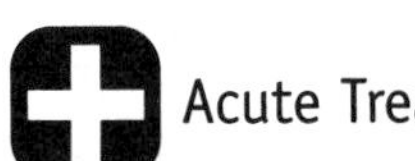

Acute Treatment

INITIAL STABILIZATION

N/A

ED TREATMENT

- Bedrest
- Urgent ophthalmologic consultation

HOSPITAL ADMISSION CRITERIA

- Admit acute RRDs that threaten the macula for bedrest pending urgent repair of the detachment
- Admit TRDs involving the macula for bedrest and urgent repair

HOSPITAL DISCHARGE CRITERIA

- RRDs that do not threaten the macula may be repaired at the earliest convenience, ideally within 1–2 days
- Chronic retinal detachments may be repaired or treated within 1 week
- Exudative retinal detachments will generally resolve with successful treatment of the underlying condition

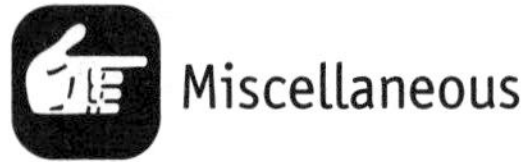

Miscellaneous

ICD-9 CODE

361.9

CORE CONTENT CODE

6.4.3.4

BIBLIOGRAPHY

LaVene D, Halpern J, Jagoda A. Loss of vision. Emergency treatment of the eye. *Emerg Med Clin North Am* 1995;13(3):539–560.

Lincoff H, Kreissig I. Retinal detachment. In: Fraunfelder, FT. *Current Ocular Therapy*. 4th ed. Philadelphia: WB Saunders, 1995: 474–476.

Author: Evan Liu

Rhabdomyolysis

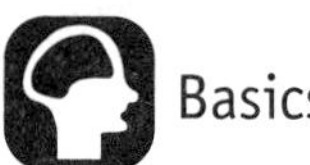

Basics

SIGNS AND SYMPTOMS

- Can vary dramatically, reflect underlying disease process
- Obvious crushing injury
- Hypothermia/hyperthermia
- Alert/obtunded
- Muscle pain (only 50%), tenderness, swelling
- Hypovolemic state, dry mucous membrane, poor skin turgor, tachycardia, hypotension
- Decreased urine output
- Change in urine color

MECHANISM/DESCRIPTION

- Syndrome associated with muscle injury and systemic release of its content (CPK)
- Combination of myoglobinuria, hypovolemia, and aciduria lead to acute renal failure
- Direct release of potassium from damaged muscle tissue may lead to dysrhythmias and sudden death

ETIOLOGY

- Muscle injury due to trauma, exercise, seizure, burn, electrical shock
- Hypothermia, hyperthermia
- Prolonged immobile state
- Drugs/toxins (alcohols, cocaine, amphetamines, opiates, antihistamines, barbiturates, PCP, caffeine, carbon monoxide, cholesterol lowering agents, succinylcholine, snake venom, bee/hornet venom, etc.)
- Neuroleptic malignant syndrome
- Metabolic disorder (hypokalemia, hypophosphatemia, hyperthyroid state, DKA, hyperosmolar state, hypoxia)
- Infections (viral, bacterial, parasitic, protozoan, rickettsial)
- Genetic disorders (McArdle's disease, Tarui's disease)
- Immunological disorders (dermatomyositis, polymyositis)
- Idiopathic

PRE-HOSPITAL

- Need for rapid extrication in case of crush injury
- *Early IV fluids* to prevent complications of restored blood flow to injured limb (hypovolemia, acute renal failure (ARF), hyperkalemia, etc.)

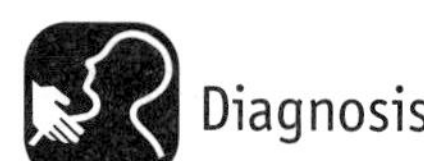

Diagnosis

ESSENTIAL WORKUP

- History and physical are insensitive in making the diagnosis
- *Serum CPK level is criterion standard and must be sent if any clinical suspicion exists*
- Urine dipstick which is positive for heme but absent for RBCs suggests rhabdomyolysis
  - —Because of rapid urinary excretion of myoglobin, up to 26% of patients with rhabdomyolysis have negative urine dipstick
  - —Serum electrolytes (potassium, calcium, magnesium, phosphorus, bun, creatinine, uric acid)

LABORATORY

- Arterial blood gas
- Urine/serum myoglobin is too transient to be useful
- Serum glucose, LDH, SGOT, albumin, toxicology screen in absence of physical injury
- PT/PTT, platelet count, fibrinogen, fibrin-split products if DIC is suspected

IMAGING/SPECIAL TESTS

- MRI is 90–95% sensitive in visualizing muscle injury, but does not change initial ED treatment

DIFFERENTIAL DIAGNOSIS

- The following conditions may present with elevated serum CPK but may not lead to complications of rhabdomyolysis
  - —Nontraumatic myopathies
  - —Renal failure
  - —Intramuscular injections
  - —Myocardial injury
  - —Hypothyroidism
  - —Hyperthyroidism
  - —Stroke
  - —Surgery

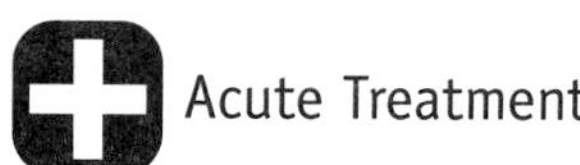

Acute Treatment

INITIAL STABILIZATION

- ABCs
- Immobilization of trauma/crush injuries
- IV fluids for hypotension and hypovolemia

ED TREATMENT

- Directed toward treating or reversing the cause of rhabdomyolysis
- *Prevent ARF*: IV fluid, mannitol, furosemide (keep urine output >30 cc/hr)
- *Hyperkalemia*: IV fluid, dextrose, insulin, kayexalate, calcium gluconate, monitor/EKG
- *Acidocis*: bicarbonate IV (keep urine PH >6.5)
- *Overdose*: activated charcoal, lavage, antidote
- *Infection*: broad spectrum antibiotics
- *Compartment syndrome*: fasciotomy (compartment pressure >35 mmHg)
- *Neuroleptic malignant syndrome*: dantrolene, bromocriptine
- *Need for hemodialysis*: refractory to treatment, hyperkalemia, hyperphosphatemia, hyperuricemia, volume overload, overdose

MEDICATIONS

- Bicarbonate: 50–100 cc of 8.4% solution IV; peds: 1 mEq/kg up to 50–100 mEq
- Furosemide: 20 mg IV bolus; peds: 1 mg/kg/dose IV

HOSPITAL ADMISSION CRITERIA

- *Because it is impossible to predict which patients will develop complications all patients with significant elevated CPK or suspicion for rhabdomyolysis must be admitted*
- Admit to monitored bed for patients with electrolyte abnormalities
- Admit to ICU bed for patients who might require hemodialysis or closer fluid and electrolyte monitoring

HOSPITAL DISCHARGE CRITERIA

- No patients suspected of having rhabdomyolysis should be discharged from the ED

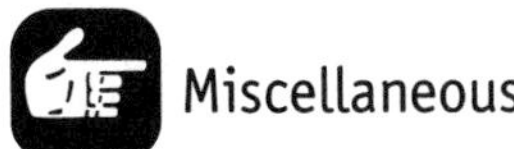

Miscellaneous

ICD-9 CODE

728.89

CORE CONTENT CODE

10.5.2

BIBLIOGRAPHY

Cheney P. Early management and physiologic changes in crush syndrome. *Crit Care Nurs Q* 1994;17(2):62–73.

Pina EM, Mehlman CT. Rhabdomyolysis—primer for the orthopaedist. *Orthop Rev* 1994;23(1):28–32.

Prendergast BD, George CF. Drug-induced rhabdomyolysis—Mechanisms and management. *Postgrad Med J* 1993; 69(811):333–336.

Sinert R, Kohl L, Rainone T, Scalea T. Exercise-induced rhabdomyolysis. *Ann Emerg Med* 1994;23(6):1301–1306.

Zager RA. Rhabdomyolysis and myohemoglobinuric acute renal failure [Editorial Review]. *Kidney Int* 1996; 49(2):314–326.

Authors: Marcelo Sandoval and Nicholas K. Han

Rheumatoid Arthritis

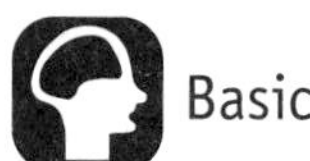

Basics

DEFINITION

Rheumatoid arthritis (RA) is a chronic, systemic, inflammatory disorder, classically presenting as a symmetric polyarthritis affecting the small joints of the hands and feet.

INCIDENCE/PREVALENCE

- Prevalence approximately 1%
- Female:male ratio 3:1
- 80% present at 35 to 50 years of age

SIGNS AND SYMPTOMS

- For two thirds of patients, onset of RA is insidious (over weeks or months), with inflammation of the small joints of the hands [metacarpophalangeal (MCP), proximal interphalangeal (PIP)], wrists, knees, and feet, as well as morning stiffness (an hour or more), swelling, pain, and warmth.
- About 10% to 15% of patients have fulminant onset of polyarticular arthritis.
- Constitutional symptoms of fatigue, anorexia, and low-grade fever are common.
- Extraarticular manifestations: rheumatoid nodules, digital vasculitis, Sjogren's syndrome (dry eyes and mouth), pericarditis, pleural effusion, peripheral entrapment neuropathies, Felty's syndrome (RA splenomegaly, neutropenia)
- Later in disease course, damage to joints and periarticular structures may result in deformities (swan neck, boutonniere, Z deformity thumb, ulnar drift of fingers).

RISK FACTORS

- Female sex (improves during pregnancy and with oral contraceptive use)
- HLA DR4 allele
- Positive family history

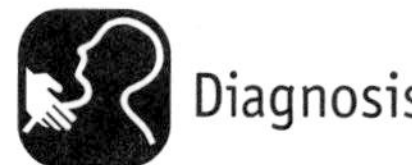

Diagnosis

DIFFERENTIAL DIAGNOSIS

- Acute: reactive arthritis, viral arthritis (parvovirus B19, EBV), systemic lupus erythematosus (SLE), Lyme disease
- Chronic: polyarticular spondyloarthropathies, SLE, polyarticular gout or pseudogout, erosive osteoarthritis, rheumatic fever

HISTORY

- Morning stiffness (>1 hour), swelling, warmth (inflammatory vs. mechanical joint pain)
- Pattern of joint involvement is MCPs, wrists, PIPs, knees, metatarsal phylangeal joints, and ankles. RA is a clinical diagnosis. The pattern of joints involved is central to making an accurate diagnosis.
- Extraarticular manifestations (dry eyes/mouth, skin changes, chest pain, breathlessness)

PHYSICAL EXAM

- Locomotor exam: joint swelling, warmth, erythema, tenderness (inflammatory vs. mechanical joint pain)
- General physical exam: nail fold infarcts, splinter hemorrhages (vasculitis), RA nodules, splenomegaly, pericardial rub, pleural effusion (accurate diagnosis and severity)

LABORATORY INVESTIGATIONS

- Rheumatoid factor (RhF) positive in 75% to 85% of patients with RA (5% of the general population is RhF positive). High titer RhF associated with aggressive disease (erosions, extraarticular involvement). RhF is associated with other conditions, such as Sjogren's syndrome (90%), SLE (25%–50%), and pulmonary diseases (e.g., tuberculosis; 10%–25%).
- Complete blood count: normochromic normocytic anemia (of chronic disease), neutropenia (Felty's syndrome)
- Erythrocyte sedimentation rate (ESR) and C-reactive protein (CRP): help estimate prognosis and gauge response to therapy

IMAGING

- Radiography
  - —Early: soft tissue swelling, joint effusions, periarticular osteopenia
  - —Later: joint space narrowing, erosions (70% of patients develop erosions in first 2 years)
- MRI may detect erosions before plain radiographs.

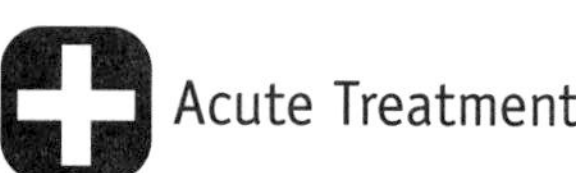

Acute Treatment

ANALGESIA

- Goals of treatment for RA patients are relief of pain, reduction of inflammation, and preservation of function
- Analgesia, nonsteroidal antiinflammatory drugs, corticosteroids (oral, intraarticular, intramuscular, intravenous), and joint or systemic bed rest often helps in acute flare-ups.

SPECIAL CONSIDERATIONS

- Patients with prognostic factors of poor outcome (high titer RhF, high ESR/CRP, erosions, nodules, HLA DR4 alleles) should also be treated with one (or more) second-line drug (disease modifying antirheumatic drugs) (e.g., methotrexate, sulphasalazine, gold, hydroxychloroquine, cyclosporine, azathioprine)
- The choice of drugs often depends on the severity and comorbidity of the patient
- Side effects are common and may be severe. Monitoring is often required, and many patients fail to remain on a given DMARD long term due to adverse effects or lack of efficacy.

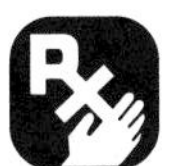

Long-Term Treatment

REHABILITATION

- Although pain and inflammation may be controlled, joint destruction and functional decline may progress.
- Physical and occupational therapy, splints, orthotics, periods of rest, exercise, education, and walking assistive devices may all help.

SURGICAL TREATMENT

- Synovectomy may be considered for uncontrolled synovitis, which may be tendon threatening.
- Tendon repair
- Arthrodesis and arthroplasty may be required for severely damaged joints. The main indication for surgery is for pain relief.

Common Questions and Answers

Physician responses to common patient questions:
Q: Are there any new drugs available for the treatment of RA?
A: Several new drugs have recently been licensed for the treatment of RA, including the pyrimidine synthesis inhibitor leflunomide and the two tumor necrosis factor–blocking agents etanercept and infliximab. These drugs represent an improvement over existing therapies but are more expensive.

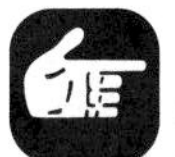

Miscellaneous

ICD-9 CODE

714.0 Rheumatoid arthritis

BIBLIOGRAPHY

Breedveld FC. Future trends in the treatment of rheumatoid arthritis: cytokine targets. *Rheumatology* 1999;38(suppl 2):11–13.

Brooks PM. Clinical management of rheumatoid arthritis. *Lancet* 1993;341: 286–290.

D'Cruz D, Hughes G. Rheumatoid arthritis: the clinical features. *J Musculoskel Med* 1993; 10:85–95.

Smolen J, Kalden J, Scott D, et al. Efficacy and safety of leflunomide compared with placebo and sulphasalazine in active rheumatoid arthritis: a double blind, randomized, muticentre trial. *Lancet* 1999; 353:259–266.

Author: Nick Carter

SCUBA Diving Injuries: DCS and AGE

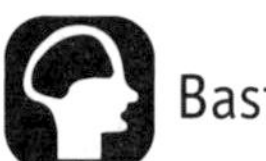

Basics

DEFINITION

- Decompression sickness (DCS): The formation of gas bubbles in anatomic spaces unsuited to the presence of gas. The term *DCS* is used in a general sense to denote all forms of injury due to bubble formation occurring as a consequence of a sudden reduction in ambient pressure. Type I DCS is characterized by musculoskeletal pain (vague, intense pain), dermal complications (pruritis, rash, blebs), and constitutional symptoms (fatigue, malaise, anorexia, fatigue). Extreme fatigue may be a sign or forerunner of a more severe decompression illness. Type II DCS is characterized by neurologic, cardiorespiratory, and vestibular symptoms.
- Arterial gas embolism (AGE): A central nervous system injury (usually cerebral) or systemic injury (usually cardiac) as a consequence of pulmonary barotrauma. Barotrauma refers to injury produced by mechanical forces caused by a change of pressure in a gas-filled space (the lungs). Air released from an overpressurized alveolus enters the pulmonary circulation and causes occlusion of the organ's blood supply. AGE can be confused with type II DCS.
- It is sometimes difficult to tell the difference between the two, because both can cause similar symptoms. The time of onset of symptoms may be more informative. The time course of air embolism symptoms from lung overexpansion is usually short (immediately or within minutes after surfacing). Decompression sickness usually develops later after a dive, sometimes up to several hours later.
- Some clinicians advocate grouping the two into one clinical entity called decompression illness (DCI). The two are treated the same (recompression).

INCIDENCE/PREVALENCE

- DCI is estimated to occur in approximately 4 in 100,000 sport divers per year (Divers Alert Network statistics).
- Predominant age is young adulthood (20–29 years).
- Predominant sex is male (95%), but there is no evidence to suggest that men are more susceptible.

SIGNS AND SYMPTOMS

- Gas deposition in joints and soft tissues may manifest as a "pain only" syndrome (limb bends), or simple pruritus (cutis marmorata), blebs (or skin bends), fatigue, or vague soreness.
- Gas deposition in the cerebral circulation causes strokelike symptoms (cerebral bends).
- Gas deposition in the spinal cord (or autochthonous bubbles) can cause transverse paresis (spinal cord bends or spinal decompression sickness).
- Development of bubbles in the inner ear can cause deafness or equilibrium dysfunction, nausea, vomiting, and nystagmus (inner ear bends or "staggers").
- Excessive venous bubbles develop and release vasoactive substances causing pulmonary irritation and bronchoconstriction. Symptoms may include chest pain, dyspnea, and cough (lung bends or "chokes").
- Other symptoms include headache, ataxia, delirium, coma, convulsions, confusion, patchy numbness, coughing paroxysms (Behnken's sign), arrhythmias, cardiac arrest, tachy- or bradycardia, vertigo, aphasia, blindness, and rapidly ascending paraplegia.

RISK FACTORS

- Rapid ascent from SCUBA diving
- Flying too high too soon after SCUBA diving
- Tunnel work (caisson disease)
- Inadequate pressurization/denitrogenation when flying
- Prolonged dive at depth of greater than 33 feet
- Obesity
- Multiple/repetitive dives
- Diving in cold water
- Strenuous physical activity while diving
- Poor physical conditioning
- Dehydration
- Panicking while diving
- Holding breath while diving
- Intracardiac septal defects
- Patent foramen ovale
- Chronic obstructive pulmonary disease (increases risk for pulmonary barotrauma)

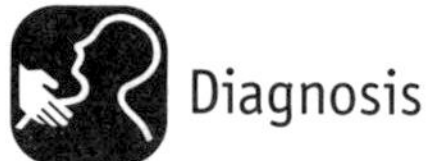

Diagnosis

DIFFERENTIAL DIAGNOSIS

- Traumatic injury to extremity
- Cerebrovascular accident
- Acute myocardial infarction
- Musculoskeletal strains
- Urticaria/anaphylaxis
- Malingering
- Contaminated breathing gas (carbon monoxide)
- Near drowning and hypoxic brain injury
- Seafood toxin poisoning (ciguatera, puffer fish, paralytic shellfish, sea snake, cone shell)
- Migraine
- Guillain-Barré syndrome
- Porphyria
- Multiple sclerosis
- Transverse myelitis
- Spinal cord compression (from disk protrusion, hematoma, or tumor)
- Middle ear or sinus barotrauma with cranial nerve compression
- Inner ear barotrauma
- Unrelated seizure (hypoglycemia, epilepsy), and postictal state from unrelated seizure
- Cold water immersion pulmonary edema

HISTORY

- The history should include the dive profile, rate of ascent, time of onset of symptoms, and changes in the type or intensity of symptoms.
- An independent account from a dive buddy or dive instructor is often useful, especially if the patient's consciousness is impaired.
- Obtaining information from a dive computer (if the patient was wearing one) is also very useful.
- Note any history of previous dives in the past few days, any exposure to altitude (which can precipitate decompression sickness), and any previous health problems.

PHYSICAL EXAM

- Skin lesions: painful, pruritic, red rash on torso, burning blebs on skin, lymphedema. Also palpate skin for subcutaneous emphysema.
- Joints: erythema and edema on periarticular surfaces. There is usually pain with movement.

- Neurologic: various manifestations of a cerebrovascular accident, including numbness, weakness, aphasia, paralysis, paraplegia, confusion, personality changes, etc.
- Cardiac: arrhythmias, tachy- or bradycardia, findings of congestive heart failure
- Pulmonary: decreased breath sounds if pneumothorax present

IMAGING

- Chest radiography (to look for pneumothorax, mediastinal emphysema, heart enlargement)
- CT scan (of the brain to look for cerebral abnormalities)
- Ultrasonography (to look for gas bubbles in joints, tendons, bursae, muscles)

SPECIAL TESTS

- Electroencephalography (irregular slowing in cerebral bends)
- Audiography and electronystagmography are extremely helpful in tracking the course of inner ear bends.

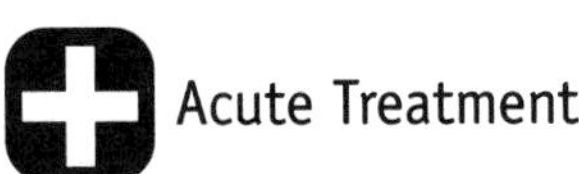

Acute Treatment

SPECIAL CONSIDERATIONS

- Call the Diver's Alert Network [DAN; (919) 684-8111] for referral to nearest hyperbaric facility for recompression.
- Patients may be sent home if cutaneous manifestations only are present, and the appropriate response to therapy is observed in the emergency department.

GENERAL MEASURES

- Administer 100% oxygen by nonrebreather mask
- Give intravenous (IV) fluids (avoid glucose-containing solutions unless treating hypoglycemia). Glucose solutions may worsen neurologic outcome in patients with central nervous system (CNS) conditions. Isotonic solutions (normal saline, lactated Ringer's) are preferred.
- Give diazepam 5 to15 mg IV for inner ear bends (symptomatic relief from vertigo, nausea, and vomiting).
- Place the patient in a recumbent or Trendelenburg position if cerebral symptoms are present.
- Transport (via ground preferably) to nearest hyperbaric facility. Aircraft that can be pressurized to sea level also can be used for transport.
- Intravenous lidocaine administration to achieve standard plasma drug levels has been shown to improve short-term neurologic outcomes in dogs and cats. Studies in humans are not yet complete, but are promising.
- Deep venous thrombosis and pulmonary embolism prophylaxis is recommended for patients with severe CNS bends with leg weakness.
- Do not give nonsteroidal antiinflammatory drugs to patients with pain-only symptoms of DCS, until hyperbaric treatment has been instituted.
- The cause of a fever in a patient with DCS should be determined and vigorously treated (outcome is significantly worsened by hyperthermia).

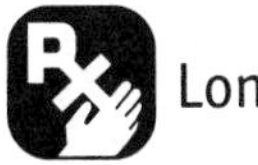

Long-Term Treatment

REHABILITATION

Rehabilitation of the injured diver is more successful than that of the patient with a traumatic spinal cord injury. The patient may continue to improve slowly after recompression treatments for up to 2 years.

REFERRAL/DISPOSITION

- Referral to the nearest hyperbaric chamber facility should be done as soon as possible.
- Follow-up should be made with a physician knowledgeable in dive medicine.

PROGNOSIS

- The prognosis is excellent for early symptomatic presentation, referral, and treatment.
- The duration and severity of symptoms prior to presentation and treatment negatively affects outcome.

COMPLICATIONS

- Oxygen toxicity (rare)
- Residual neurologic deficits in CNS bends (46%–75%)
- Long-term risk for aseptic necrosis of bone

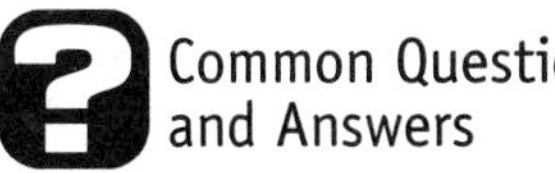

Common Questions and Answers

Physician responses to common patient questions:

Q: When can I return to diving?

A: The conditions for a safe return to diving include (a) no significantly increased risk of recurrence and (b) no risk of augmenting tissue damage. With both DCS and AGE, the diver should be evaluated for risk factors.

Q: When can I fly again?

A: After treatment of DCS and AGE, exposure to altitude can precipitate symptoms. After reaching a clinical plateau with treatment, an additional period of 3 to 4 days at sea level pressure is usually sufficient, but occasionally exposure to altitude can precipitate symptoms. In-flight oxygen supplementation may provide additional safety.

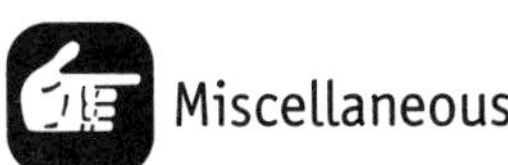

Miscellaneous

SYNONYMS

- The bends
- Air embolism
- Caisson disease

ICD-9 CODE

993.3 Decompression sickness
958.0 Arterial gas embolism

BIBLIOGRAPHY

Bookspan J. *Diving physiology in plain English*. Kensington, MD: Undersea and Hyperbaric Medical Society, 1995.

Bove AA. *Diving medicine*, 3rd ed. Philadelphia: WB Saunders, 1997.

Shilling CW. *The physician's guide to diving medicine*. New York: Plenum, 1984.

Author: James Fambro

Seizures and Epilepsy

Basics

DEFINITION

A seizure is an abnormal paroxysmal electrical discharge in the brain, usually with mental status changes. Individuals who have, two or more seizures are deemed to have epilepsy.

INCIDENCE/PREVALENCE

- Over 10% of the population will have at least one seizure during their lifetime
- Approximately 3% will have epilepsy by age 70

SIGNS AND SYMPTOMS

- Fever: suggests infectious etiology
- Focal neurologic deficit: possible localized trauma or tumor
- Meningismus: may be present in meningitis
- Papilledema: secondary to increased intracranial pressure

RISK FACTORS

- Previous head injury
- Low seizure threshold is impossible to quantify. It may represent a genetic or acquired brain disorder.

ASSOCIATED INJURIES

- Abrasions, lacerations, contusions: occur from uncontrolled contact with objects during seizure
- Tongue lacerations: tongue is often bitten during a seizure.

COMPLICATIONS

- Status epilepticus: recurrent generalized seizures without return to consciousness

SEIZURE TYPES

- Generalized: sudden onset involving an altered level of consciousness, usually bilateral and symmetrical
- Partial: either simple (no alteration of consciousness) or complex (alteration/loss of consciousness often with semipurposeful inappropriate movements)

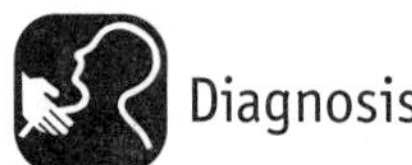

Diagnosis

DIFFERENTIAL DIAGNOSIS

- Alcohol withdrawal
- Arteriovenous malformation
- Electrolyte abnormalities
- Hepatic failure
- Hypoglycemia
- Hyponatremia
- Illicit drug use/abuse/withdrawal
- Intracranial swelling /second impact syndrome
- Primary/secondary brain tumor
- Syncope
- Uremia
- Vascular disease

HISTORY

- Actual account by first-hand observer is extremely helpful.
- Previous history of seizure
- Previous history of head trauma
- Medications
- Social/family history

PHYSICAL EXAM

- Look for injuries that may have occurred during the seizure.
- Look for evidence of acutely increased intracranial pressure, such as pupillary dilation or posturing, indicating an emergency.
- Expect postictal confusion that gradually clears after a seizure.
- Thorough neurological exam to document focal deficits.

LABORATORY

- Electrolytes, including glucose, calcium, magnesium, and phosphorus
- Liver function tests, including ammonia level
- Blood toxicology
- Urine toxicology
- Anticonvulsant level: inadequate levels are a significant cause of recurrent seizures

IMAGING

- CT scan: rule out acute bleeding or intracranial masses
- MRI: may better define posterior fossa tumors, vascular abnormalities, and temporal lobes
- Electroencephalography (EEG) may define true seizure activity and focus, although a negative EEG result does not rule out seizure disorder. Sometimes a sleep-deprived patient EEG may be required.

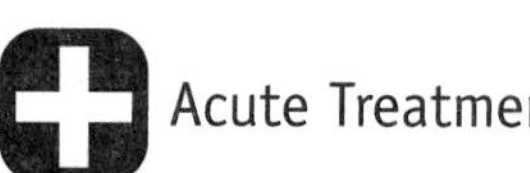

Acute Treatment

IMMEDIATE ACTIONS

- Supportive: Airway, breathing, and circulation
- Keep area clear: ensure the patient does not injure self or others
- Once stable, workup begins as above

SPECIAL CONSIDERATIONS

Transfer to emergency department if the patient has no known seizure disorder.

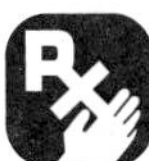

Long-Term Treatment

GENERAL

- If no reversible cause is found, place patient on antiepileptic drugs (AEDs).
- Monitor levels of AEDs, especially in first couple months of training.
- Follow up with neurologist.

REFERRAL/DISPOSITION

If no reversible cause is found, the patient should be referred to a neurologist for an initial visit and EEG.

Common Questions and Answers

Physician responses to common patient questions:

Q: What sports can I play or not play?
A: There is no definitive evidence of any relationship between repetitive minor head injury and deterioration of the epileptic patient; therefore, most collision/contact sports are acceptable (but no boxing). Swimming is acceptable only with a certified lifeguard who should be made aware of the situation. Motor sports should be undertaken only by individuals with well-controlled seizures. Sports in which falling is a potential (gymnastics, rock climbing, hang gliding) should be judged on an individual basis, based on the type and frequency of seizure.

Q: Should my child with a seizure disorder play sports?
A: Your child will obtain all of the physiologic benefits of exercise, including increased cardiovascular fitness, stronger muscles, and weight control. Improving overall health may actually reduce the number of seizures experienced by your child. He or she may also benefit from the increased self-esteem and social integration, so important to all youngsters, available with participation in sports.

Q: Will AEDs impair my performance?
A: Many of the medications have side effects that may impair concentration or coordination. Most are approved by the NCAA and IOC.

Q: How do you decide if sport/exercise is OK?
A: The following questions need to be asked: Are there any other impairments to modify the athlete's participation (i.e., ventricular shunts or vascular malformations)? What type of seizures occur? How often do seizures occur? Do AEDs significantly impair the athlete's perception and alertness? Overall the decision is individualized, but the physiologic and psychological benefits of sport and exercise usually far outweigh the risk to athletes or their competitors.

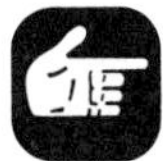

Miscellaneous

SYNONYMS

- Convulsions
- Epilepsy
- Fits
- Spells

ICD-9 CODE

780.3 Seizure
345.9 Epilepsy (idiopathic)

BIBLIOGRAPHY

Cantu RC. Epilepsy and athletics. *Clin Sports Med* 1998;17:61–69.

Sirven JI, Varrato J. Physical activity and epilepsy—what are the rules? *Physician Sports Med* 1999;27:63,64,67–70.

Authors: Nilesh Shah and James E. Sturmi

Septic Arthritis and Bursitis

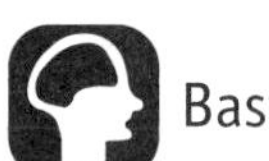

Basics

DEFINITION

- Infection of articular joints or bursae with a bacterial, mycobacterial, spirochetal, fungal, or viral source
- May be an indication of systemic infection

INCIDENCE/PREVALENCE

- Usually a monoarticular or oligoarticular pattern for acute bacterial infection, chronic mycobacterial infection, or fungal infection
- Acute polyarticular involvement usually signifies disseminated neisserial infection or acute hepatitis B.
- Neisserial involvement is responsible for approximately 50% of infectious arthritis.

SIGNS AND SYMPTOMS

- Various degrees of pain in region of joint or bursa
- Swelling
- Decreased range of joint motion
- Erythema overlying joint or bursa
- Localized or systemic fever
- Possible associated skin lesions (petechial or pustular rash, Kaposi's sarcoma)
- Concomitant urethral discharge

RISK FACTORS

- Sexually active person at risk for sexually transmitted disease
- Joint penetration or recent surgery
- Trauma
- Immunocompromised patient
- History of arthritis in affected joint (greatest incidence in patients with rheumatoid arthritis)
- Intravenous drug abuse
- Significant comorbid diseases (diabetes, malignancy, hepatic failure, sickle cell disease, immunocompromised states)

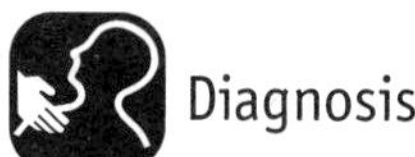

Diagnosis

DIFFERENTIAL DIAGNOSIS

- Cellulitis
- Osteomyelitis
- Gout
- Pseudogout (calcium pyrophosphate deposition disease)
- Rheumatoid arthritis
- Juvenile rheumatoid arthritis
- Rheumatic fever
- Lyme disease
- Spondyloarthropathy (Reiter's syndrome, psoriatic arthritis, ankylosing spondylitis, IBD)
- Sarcoidosis
- Synovitis
- Synovial papilloma
- AIDS

HISTORY

- Rapid or insidious onset (patient may describe crescendo-like throbbing pain)
- Single joint involvement in more than 90% of patients
- Most commonly involves knee > hip > shoulder, wrist, or elbow joints

PHYSICAL EXAM

- Erythema and tenderness to palpation of affected joint or bursa
- Joint effusion
- Decreased range of motion (usually secondary to pain or effusion/swelling)
- Local warmth or generalized fever
- Cutaneous lesions (Lyme disease, meningococcal infection, gonorrhea)

IMAGING

- Plain radiographs may show soft tissue swelling, joint space widening, or displacement, radiolucent areas indicating presence of gas, erosions, or joint space loss.
- Ultrasonography is useful for identifying hip effusions.
- CT and MRI are useful for evaluation of sacroiliac joint and vertebral joints.
- Bone scan is indicated for identification of region affected by inflammatory process.

LABORATORY EVALUATION

- Laboratory evaluation of joint or bursal aspirate is essential for diagnosis.
- Laboratory specimens should be collected prior to antibiotic administration.
- Complete blood count and blood cultures
- Prompt collection of joint or bursal aspirate if clinical suspicion of infectious process
- Contaminated overlying tissue (i.e., cellulitis) should be avoided during arthrocentesis or bursal aspiration.
- Synovial or bursal fluid aspirate should be sent for Gram stain and examination for crystals, chemistry (LDH, protein, and glucose), and culture.

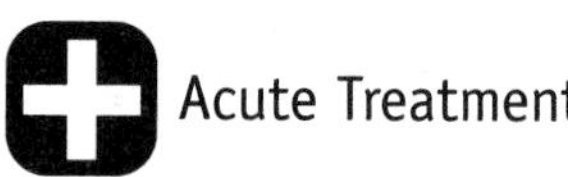

Acute Treatment

SEPTIC BURSITIS

- Most common organisms include *Staphylococcus aureus*, beta-hemolytic *Streptococcus*, and *Staphylococcus epidermidis*. Rarely mycobacterial infection is identified.
- Potential exists for overwhelming sepsis or extension of infection into the adjacent joint.
- Primary therapy includes penicillinase-resistant penicillins (nafcillin or dicloxacillin) or first-generation cephalosporins.
- Therapy should be continued for a minimum of 2 to 3 weeks.
- Hospitalization for parenteral therapy is required when signs of systemic or bony extension of infection are observed.

SEPTIC ARTHRITIS

- Usually requires hospitalization for parenteral antibiotics
- Treatment based on Gram stain results if positive
- If Gram stain is negative, cover with full dose penicillin or cephalosporin plus gentamicin.
- Infection eradication complicated by presence of joint prosthesis, and removal of prosthesis may be necessary
- No indication for intraarticular antibiotics
- Antibiotics are to be continued for 1 to 2 weeks after resolution of symptoms.
- Longer treatment is required for joints affected by arthritis.
- Surgical intervention via arthrotomy indicated only if needle drainage ineffective (fluid loculation or inaccessible joint)

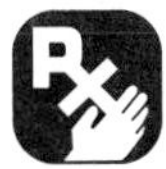

Long-Term Treatment

FOLLOW-UP

- Recurrent arthrocentesis is recommended as joint fluid reaccumulates to rule out persistent/recurrent infection.
- Regular office visits are recommended after hospital discharge for reevaluation and early recognition of persistent or new problems.
- Prosthesis replacement possible in future after clearance of infection

OUTCOMES

- Complete resolution and restoration of joint function is the goal.
- Possible adverse outcomes include death, impaired joint function (decreased motion, fusion, dislocation), septic necrosis, sinus formation, ankylosis, osteomyelitis, synovitis, and limb length changes.

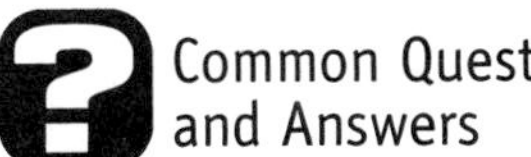

Common Questions and Answers

- Complete restoration of joint function is expected if early diagnosis and treatment before articular damage occur.
- Prophylaxis may be indicated in certain conditions.
- Protection from sexually transmitted diseases should be discussed with all high-risk patients.

Miscellaneous

SYNONYMS

- Infectious arthritis
- Infectious bursitis

ICD-9 CODE

711.0 Septic arthritis

BIBLIOGRAPHY

Dambro MR, Rothschild BM. *Griffith's 5-minute clinical consult*. Philadelphia: Lippincott Williams & Wilkins, 1999.

Gilbert DN, Moellering RC Jr, Sande MA. *The Sanford guide to antimicrobial therapy*. Hyde Park, NY: Antimicrobial Therapy, Inc., 2000.

Pioro MH. Septic arthritis. *Rheum Dis Clin North Am* 1997;23:239–258.

Stell IM, Gransden WR. Simple tests for septic bursitis. *BMJ* 1998;316:187–189.

Thaler SJ, Maguire JH. *Harrison's principles of internal medicine*. 14th ed. New York: McGraw-Hill, 1998.

Authors: Douglas McKeag and Kevin B. Gebke

Sinusitis

Basics

SIGNS AND SYMPTOMS

- Facial pain
- Headache
- Cough
- Purulent nasal discharge
- Fever
- Edema of the nasal mucous membranes
- Pus in the nares or posterior pharynx
- Warmth, tenderness and possibly cellulitis over the affected sinus
- Frontal sinusitis
  —Pain of the lower forehead
- Maxillary sinusitis
  —Malar facial pain
  —Maxillary dental pain
  —Referred ear pain
- Ethmoid sinusitis
  —Retro-orbital pain
- Sphenoid sinusitis (very uncommon)
  —Pain over the occiput or mastoid
- Recent history of nasotracheal intubation suggests nosocomial sinusitis
  —Involves atypical pathogens such as Pseudomonas and gram negative organisms
- Rhinocerebral mucomycosis
  —Rare but rapidly progressive fungal infection
  —Occurs in diabetic and other immunocompromised patients
  —Orbital and facial pain out of proportion to physical signs
  —Lethargy, headache in a systematically ill appearing patient
  —Black eschar or pale area on the palate or nasal mucosa

MECHANISM/DESCRIPTION

- Sinusitis is inflammation of the mucous membranes lining the paranasal sinuses
- Acute bacterial sinusitis is diagnosed when signs and symptoms last less than 3 weeks
- Chronic sinusitis occurs when signs and symptoms last longer than three weeks
- Nosocomial sinusitis is associated with nasogastric and nasotracheal tubes

ETIOLOGY

- Complication of simple viral upper respiratory tract infection or allergic rhinitis
- As mucous membranes become inflamed, sinus ostia narrow and block drainage
- Air is absorbed and negative pressure develops, resulting in transudate formation
- Bacteria are trapped and multiply resulting in suppuration
- Foreign bodies, nasal polyps, tumors, or traumatic fractures can lead to obstruction of ostia
- Immunocompromised patients and patients with impaired mucociliary movement are also predisposed to sinusitis
- Pathogens
  —Acute sinusitis: *H. influenza, Strep pneumoniae, Moraxella catarrhalis, S. aureus*
  —Chronic sinusitis: *Peptostreptococcus, Fusobacterium, Bacteroides, Aspergillus*
  —Nosocomial sinusitis: *S. aureus, Pseudomonas, klebsiella*

COMPLICATIONS

- Osteomyelitis
- Extension into the CNS
  —Seizures
  —Focal neurologic signs
  —Cranial nerve palsies
  —Altered level of consciousness
  —Meningitis, subdural empyema, epidural abscess
  —Cavernous sinus thrombosis
  —Brain abscess
- Periorbital cellulitis
- Orbital cellulitis
  —Periorbital swelling, fever, ptosis, proptosis, and painful or decreased extraocular movements
  —Most frequently a complication or ethmoid sinusitis in children
- Pott's puffy tumor
  —A focal, doughy mass localized to the forehead
  —Indicative of osteomyelitis of the frontal bone

SPECIAL PEDIATRIC CONSIDERATIONS

- Ethmoid and maxillary sinuses are present at birth
- Frontal and sphenoid sinuses do not emerge until age 6–7
- Periorbital/orbital cellulitis is a common complication of ethmoid sinusitis in children
  —Periorbital swelling, fever, ptosis, proptosis, and painful or decreased extraocular movements

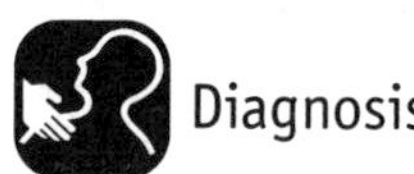

Diagnosis

ESSENTIAL WORKUP

- Clinical diagnosis based on history and physical exam
- Transillumination is not a reliable indicator of sinus disease
- Imaging is unnecessary in uncomplicated cases (see below)

LABORATORY

- White blood cell count if the patient appears toxic

IMAGING/SPECIAL TESTS

- Plain film radiography
  —Normal plain films do not rule out bacterial involvement
  —A water's view may help in the diagnosis of maxillary sinusitis
  —Opacification or air fluid level in involved sinus
- Computed tomography
  —Preferred to plain films if imaging is necessary
  —May assist in diagnosing complications of sinusitis

DIFFERENTIAL DIAGNOSIS

- Migraine and cluster headache
- Dental pain
- Trigeminal neuralgia
- TMJ disorders
- Temporal arteritis
- Uncomplicated viral or allergic rhinitis
- Nasal polyp, tumor, or foreign body
- CNS infection

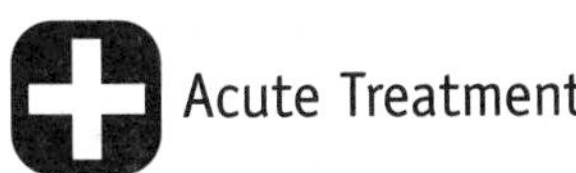

Acute Treatment

INITIAL STABILIZATION

- Toxic-appearing patients may require airway intervention and fluid resuscitation
  - —First dose of antibiotics in ED

ED TREATMENT

- Cost-effective approach favors appropriate antibiotic therapy and no testing
- Establishing good drainage with topical or oral decongestants and mucoevacuants
- Reducing edema with topical corticosteroids in chronic sinusitis
- Humidification and saline spray are beneficial adjunct to pharmacologic therapy

MEDICATIONS

Antibiotics

- Antibiotics listed are considered first-line drugs, except for amoxicillin where there is known drug resistance
  - —Acute sinusitis
    - —Amoxicillin: adults: 500 mg po tid; peds: 40 mg/kg/day po divided tid for 10–14 days
    - —Amoxicillin-clavulanate: adults: 500 mg po tid; peds: 40 mg/kg/day po divided tid for 10–14 days
    - —Azithromycin: adults: 500 mg po day 1, 250 mg po days 2–5; peds: 10 mg/kg po day 1, 5 mg/kg po qd days 2–5
    - —Trimethoprim-sulfa DS: adults: 1 tab po bid; peds: 5 cc/10 kg (40/200 per 5 cc) po bid 10–14 days
    - —Cefuroxime: adults: 500 mg po bid; peds: 20–30 mg/kg/day po divided bid for 10–14 days
  - —Chronic
    - —Amoxicillin-clavulanate: adults: 500 mg po bid; peds: 40 mg/kg/day po divided tid for 21 days
    - —Cefaclor: adults: 500 mg po tid; peds: 20–40 mg/kg/day po divided tid for 21 days

Decongestants

- Topical: not to be used for more than 3 days
- Oxymetazoline hydrochloride 0.05%: 2–3 drops/sprays per nostril bid
- Phenylephrine hydrochloride 0.5%: 2–3 sprays per nostril q 3–4 hrs; oral: if longer than 3 days of treatment
- Phenylpropanolamine: 25 mg po q 4 hrs
- Pseudoephedrine: 60 mg po q 4–6 hrs

Mucoevacuants

- Guaifenesin: adults: 5–20 ml po q 4 hrs; peds: 5–10 ml/dose if 6–12 years old, 2.5–5 ml if 2–6 years old

Corticosteroids for Chronic Sinusitis

- Beclomethasone dipropionate: 1 spray/nostril bid/tid
- Dexamethasone sodium phosphate: 2 sprays/nostril bid/tid

HOSPITAL ADMISSION CRITERIA

- Evidence of spread of infection beyond the sinus cavity
- Toxic-appearing patients
- Immunocompromised/diabetic patients with extensive infection
- ENT evaluation and aspiration if patient is severely ill, immunocompromised, or pansinusitis and ill-appearing

HOSPITAL DISCHARGE CRITERIA

- Most cases of uncomplicated sinusitis may be managed as outpatients
- Followup with primary care physician or ENT if symptoms persist greater than 7 days despite antibiotic therapy

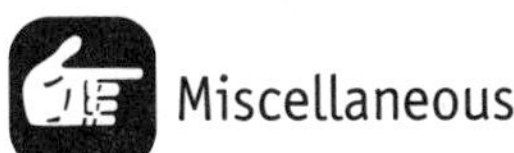

Miscellaneous

ICD-9 CODE

473.9

CORE CONTENT CODE

6.2.5.1

BIBLIOGRAPHY

Brook I. Microbiology and management of sinusitis. *J Otolaryngol* 1996:25(4):249–56.

Gershwin ME, Incaudo GA, eds. *Diseases of the sinuses*. Totowa, NJ: Humana Press, 1996. pp. 215–233.

Reuter JB, Lucas LM, Kumar KL. Sinusitis: a review for generalists. *West J Med* 1995; 163(1):40–48.

Authors: Cara Deckelman and Michael Rolnick

Splenic Contusion and Rupture

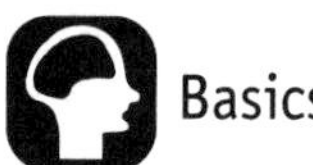

Basics

DEFINITION

Injury to the spleen typically occurs due to blunt trauma. This may be seen in high-velocity sports such as skiing, biking, and motor sports, or more commonly in contact sports. Injuries to the spleen range from contusions and lacerations to complete avulsion of the vascular supply.

INCIDENCE/PREVALENCE

- Most commonly injured organ in blunt abdominal trauma
- Up to 50% of all organ injuries

SIGNS AND SYMPTOMS

- Left upper quadrant pain
- Left shoulder pain (referred pain, Kerr's sign)

RISK FACTORS

- Overlying rib injury, especially if displaced
- Splenomegaly (mononucleosis, etc.)

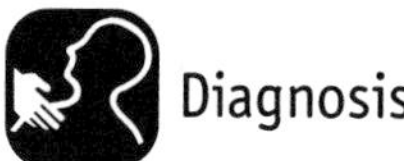

Diagnosis

DIFFERENTIAL DIAGNOSIS

- Rib fracture
- Abdominal wall injury (rectus, obliques)
- Renal contusion or laceration

HISTORY

- Obtain mechanism of injury
- Any lightheadedness or weakness? Signs of hypotension suggest vascular involvement and emergent transport.
- Any recent illnesses? Helps to determine if patient is at risk for splenic rupture (i.e., infectious mononucleosis, etc.).

PHYSICAL EXAM

- Check pulse and respirations. Assess hemodynamic status. Patient is at risk for hypovolemic shock if bleeding is significant.
- Observe for superficial lacerations, ecchymosis, and swelling.
- Auscultate for bowel sounds and breath sounds. Hypoactive bowel sounds indicate peritoneal irritation. Decreased breath sounds indicate possible pneumothorax.
- Palpate abdomen: note tenderness, rebound tenderness, and presence of guarding. Evaluate size of spleen. Exquisite tenderness, rebound tenderness, and guarding are all suggestive of peritoneal irritation and possible organ injury.
- Palpate ribs, checking for possible rib fracture and resulting displacement.

IMAGING

Abdominal CT scan, if spleen is injured, will require serial studies.

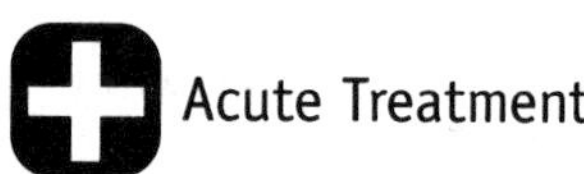

Acute Treatment

ANALGESIA

- Acetaminophen and oral/intravenous (IV) narcotics as needed.
- Avoid nonsteroidal antiinflammatory drug use due to risk of bleeding.

SPECIAL CONSIDERATIONS

- Any question of a splenic injury necessitates emergent transport to a hospital for further evaluation.
- If unstable (hypotension, tachycardic), attempt IV placement and bolus with isotonic IV fluid if available. Use two large-bore IVs.
- Splenic salvage (conservative treatment) is now more common. Decision is based on hemodynamic stability.

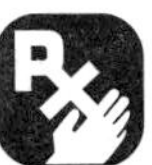

Long-Term Treatment

SURGERY

- Emergent if patient is hemodynamically unstable
- Failure of nonoperative treatment typically occurs in first 48 to 72 hours, but may occur 2 or more weeks later.
- Will need immunization prophylaxis against *Streptococcus pneumoniae* and *Neisseria meningitidis*.
- Rest for 6 to 8 weeks postsurgery; return to play in 3 months

CONSERVATIVE TREATMENT

- Frequent hemodynamic monitoring and hemograms
- Serial abdominal exams
- Strict bed rest
- Repeat CT scan in 5 to 7 days; if improved, patient may be discharged
- Continued rest and avoidance of contact sport until complete resolution seen on CT scan
- Nonoperative management successful in 90% of children and around 70% of adults

Common Questions and Answers

Physician responses to common patient questions:

Q: How long before I can play again?

A: Typically 3 to 4 months either if managed conservatively or surgically. Training may be started earlier and will depend on the severity of the initial injury and the treatment course.

Q: Do I need my spleen?

A: The spleen is an organ involved with the immune system. You'll need to be vaccinated against certain types of bacteria. However, there is no evidence that you will have any long-term problems with your health after your splenectomy.

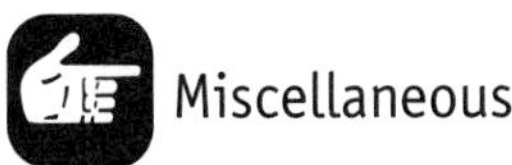

Miscellaneous

ICD-9 CODE

865.00

BIBLIOGRAPHY

Amaral JF. Thoracoabdominal injuries in the athlete. *Clin Sports Med* 1997;16:739–746.

Ryan JM. Abdominal injuries and sport. *Br J Sports Med* 1999;33:155–160.

Author: William W. Dexter

Spondyloarthropathies

Basics

DEFINITION

Spondyloarthropathy (SpA) is a generic term applied to the clinical, radiologic, and immunogenetic features shared by a group of diseases that include ankylosing spondylitis (AS), reactive arthritis (ReA), psoriatic arthritis (PsA), and enteropathic arthritis (EnA). These conditions are variably associated with the HLA B27 antigen. Individuals with these conditions frequently exhibit overlapping clinical and radiologic features

INCIDENCE/PREVALENCE

- AS prevalence: 0.5 to 5 in 1,000
- PsA develops in 5% of patients with psoriasis
- ReA incidence: 3.5 in 100,000 men
- SpA is seen in all age groups, but most present at 20 to 50 years of age

SIGNS AND SYMPTOMS

- Low back pain at night with prominent early morning stiffness (sacroiliitis, spondylitis)
- Peripheral joint pain and swelling (often lower limb and asymmetric)
- Pain and inflammation at the insertion of tendons or ligaments (enthesitis), sausage digits (dactylitis)
- Ocular: conjunctivitis, iritis
- Gastrointestinal: oral ulcerations, gut inflammation
- Skin and nails: psoriasis, keratoderma blennorrhagica, psoriatic nail dystrophy
- Genitourinary: urethritis, cervicitis, circinate balanitis

RISK FACTORS

- HLA B27 positivity: AS 90%, ReA 70% to 80%, spondylitic EnA and PsA 50%. No association between peripheral EnA and PsA. Note: 8% of the general population is HLA B27 positive.
- Family history: AS develops in 1% to 2% of HLA B27-positive individuals and 12% of HLA B27 positive siblings of AS patients.

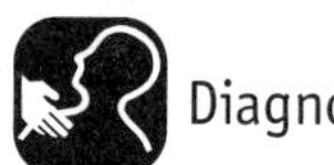

Diagnosis

DIFFERENTIAL DIAGNOSIS

- AS: other SpA, osteitis condensans ilii, diffuse ideopathic skeletal hyperostosis
- PsA: other SpA erosive osteoarthritis, gout, rheumatoid arthritis (RA)
- ReA: other SpA, septic (gonococcal) arthritis, gout, sarcoidosis, seronegative RA
- EnA: other SpA, seronegative RA, Behçet's syndrome

HISTORY

- Insidious onset of low back pain, often worse at night, with morning stiffness (>30 minutes), eased by exercise and nonsteroidal antiinflammatory drugs (NSAIDs) (inflammatory vs. mechanical back pain)
- Other joint or enthesis involvement, eye, bowel, skin, mucous membrane, gut, genitourinary symptoms (diagnosis SpA is clinical)

PHYSICAL EXAM

- Lumbar spine: restricted range of motion
- Peripheral joints: involvement in 30% (hip and shoulder most common)
- Skin and nails: psoriatic nail changes and plaques (scalp, umbilicus, natal cleft may be subtle)

IMAGING

- Radiographic changes of sacroiliitis (AS, axial PsA, EnA, ReA; erosions, sclerosis, ankylosis) may take years to develop. Sacroiliitis may be asymmetrical (PsA, ReA).
- MRI may detect up to 75% of early sacroiliitis not seen on plain radiography.
- Lumbar squaring and bridging syndesmophytes in axial disease
- Peripheral arthritis with soft tissue swelling, juxtaarticular osteopenia, joint space narrowing, and erosions.
- Areas of periostitis or osteitis are not uncommon (PsA, ReA).

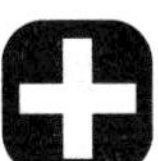

Acute Treatment

ANALGESIA

Acute flare-ups of SpA are treated with NSAIDs, intraarticular/topical steroids, joint rest, or splinting.

SPECIAL CONSIDERATIONS

- Antibiotic therapy may be indicated for proven *Yersinia-* or *Chlamydia*-induced ReA for up to 3 months.
- ReA due to *Salmonella* and *Shigella* do not benefit from antibiotics.
- Eye, genitourinary, and bowel involvement should be treated accordingly.
- Disease-modifying antirheumatic drugs (DMARDs; e.g., sulfasalazine and methotrexate) maybe used for chronic, progressive, or refractory peripheral arthritis/enthesitis. They have little effect on axial disease.

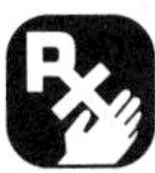

Long-Term Treatment

REHABILITATION

- The goal of treatment is to reduce pain and stiffness and maintain posture and function.
- Appropriate exercise with physical therapy are central to this.
- Patients with spondylitis should engage in a lifelong program of exercise to preserve posture and mobility.

SURGICAL TREATMENT

Joint arthroplasty may be required for those with severe peripheral joint disease (hip, knee).

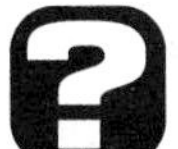

Common Questions and Answers

Physician responses to common patient questions:
Q: After the initial acute episode (of reactive arthritis), will I develop a chronic arthritis?
A: In most patients the initial episode is short lived and settles within weeks to months. Some may go on to experience recurrent attacks, and these occur more frequently in HLA B27–positive individuals. Less than 30%, however, develop a chronic arthritis.

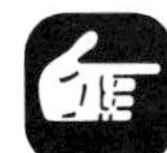

Miscellaneous

SYNONYMS

- Seronegative spondyloarthropathies
- HLA B27-related spondyloarthropathy

ICD-9 CODE

720.0 Ankylosing spondylitis
099.3 Reactive arthritis
696.1 Psoriatic arthritis

BIBLIOGRAPHY

Carter N, Williamson L, Kennedy LG, et al. Susceptibility to ankylosing spondylitis. *Rheumatology* (Oxford) 2000 39(4):445.

Khan MA, van der Linden SM. A wider spectrum of spondyloarthropathies. *Semin Arthritis Rheum* 1990;20:107–113.

Lauhio A, Leirisalo-Repo M, Lahdevirta J, et al. Double blind placebo-controlled study of three-month treatment with lymecycline in reactive arthritis with special reference to *Chlamydia* arthritis. *Arthritis Rheum* 1991; 34:6–14.

Mau W, Zeidler H, Mau R, et al. Clinical features and prognosis of patients with possible ankylosing spondylitis. Results of a 10-year follow-up. *J Rheumatol* 1988;15: 1109–1114.

Oosteveen J, Prevo R, den Boer J, et al. Early detection of sacroiliitis on magnetic resonance imaging and subsequent development of sacroiliitis on plain radiography. A prospective, longitudinal study. *J Rheumatol* 1999;26:1953–1958.

Author: Nick Carter

Sports Hernias

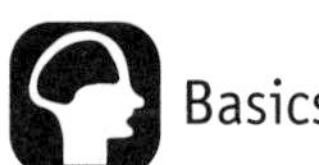

Basics

DEFINITION

The sports hernia is a syndrome of chronic pain due to weakness or injury to the posterior inguinal canal and conjoined tendon. It is considered to be an early direct inguinal hernia.

INCIDENCE/PREVALENCE

- Unknown; far more common in soccer players

SIGNS AND SYMPTOMS

- Groin pain with exercise
- Exacerbated by sudden movements
- Usually unilateral
- Often insidious in onset, but may occur after sudden tearing sensation
- Chronic in nature; may progress to affect daily activities, even getting out of bed
- In soccer players, pain worse with long kicks and hard shots

RISK FACTORS

- Activities with high speed twisting and turning, such as soccer and rugby

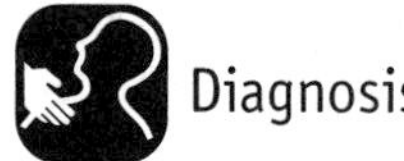

Diagnosis

DIFFERENTIAL DIAGNOSIS

- Inguinal hernia
- Chronic adductor strain
- Chronic rectus abdominis strain
- Bursitis: especially iliopectineal bursa
- Ilioinguinal nerve entrapment
- Femoral hernia
- Femoral neck stress fracture
- Pubic ramus fracture
- Osteitis pubis
- Intraarticular hip pathology
- Testicular/ovarian pathology
- Referred pain from herniated disk or spondyloarthropathy
- Chronic groin pain is often multifactorial. Sports hernia often coexists with one or more of these diagnoses.

HISTORY

- See Signs and Symptoms.
- Early in course, groin pain is felt after activity, or toward end of activity.
- As condition progresses, pain is more severe and occurs earlier in activity. Decreased ability to twist, turn, or stride out is observed. Later in course, pain occurs with running and may progress to affect daily activities.
- Pain may radiate to uninvolved side or scrotum.
- Painful intercourse
- Pain with coughing/Valsalva maneuver
- Often more intense and felt more "internally" than groin strains
- Resolves with prolonged abstinence from training, but recurs with return to activity

PHYSICAL EXAM

- Inversion of scrotal skin, and palpation along inguinal canal
- Most tender posteriorly in mid-inguinal canal
- May also have tenderness of external inguinal ring, conjoined tendon, or pubic tubercle
- Pain worse with cough or sit-ups, with possible bulge palpable
- Lack of palpable hernia
- Careful hip/genitourinary exam

IMAGING

- Plain films to rule out fracture and pubic symphysis asymmetry
- Herniography used in Europe

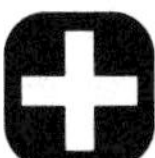

Acute Treatment

SPECIAL CONSIDERATIONS

Conservative measures are generally ineffective, but a rest period of several weeks followed by a rehabilitation program and slow return to activities are usually attempted.

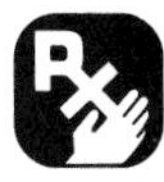

Long-Term Treatment

REHABILITATION

- Mainly postsurgical
- Pelvic strength/flexibility exercises
- Non-weight-bearing exercises as tolerated
- Return to running at 4 to 5 weeks, avoiding twisting and cutting movements
- Return to prior level of activity at 6 to 8 weeks, possibly sooner with close attention to functional rehabilitation

SURGICAL TREATMENT

Herniorrhaphy is the definitive treatment. Anatomic repair of all layers of tissue must be undertaken. Anchoring sutures to the pubic symphysis are usually necessary.

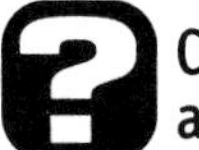

Common Questions and Answers

Physician responses to common patient questions:

Q: What's the difference between a sports hernia and a regular hernia?

A: In a true hernia, there is protrusion of bowel into the inguinal canal. A sports hernia is a weakness or injury of the posterior inguinal canal, with no protrusion of bowel into the canal. It is generally considered to be an early form of a hernia.

Q: What are my treatment options other than surgery?

A: Your symptoms are likely to resolve with prolonged rest. However, they usually recur with resumption of activity. Therefore, surgery with herniorrhaphy is the treatment of choice.

Q: What are my chances for success with surgery?

A: The answer is somewhat debated, but studies seem to indicate at least an 80% to 90% rate of return to prior level of activity. Although groin pain is often multifactorial, if sports hernia is the only source of pain, surgery is curative. Although there is no definitive diagnostic test readily available in the United States, surgery is often both diagnostic and therapeutic. If there are other components to the pain, they also need to be addressed, ideally prior to surgery.

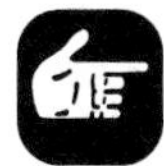

Miscellaneous

SYNONYMS

- Sportsman's hernia
- Inguinal ligament sprain
- Gilmore's groin
- Footballer's groin/hernia
- Pubalgia

ICD-9 CODE

550.9 Direct inguinal hernia

BIBLIOGRAPHY

Hackney RG. The sports hernia: a cause of chronic groin pain. *Br J Sports Med* 1993; 27:58–62.

Lacroix VJ. A complete approach to groin pain. *Physician Sports Med* 2000;28:66–86.

Lynch SA, Renstrom PA. Groin injuries in sport: treatment strategies. *Sports Med* 1999;28:137–144.

Authors : William W. Briner Jr. and Jason D. Johnson

Subconjunctival Hemorrhage

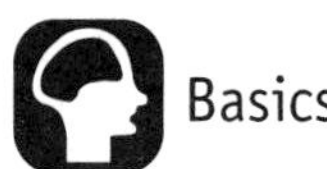

Basics

DEFINITION

Rupture of vessels leading to an accumulation of blood in the potential space between the episclera and conjunctiva

INCIDENCE/PREVALENCE

- One of the most frequently encountered eye problems in primary care offices; accounted for 2.9% of visits to outpatient eye clinics in one study

SIGNS AND SYMPTOMS

- Extreme redness of eye without change in vision
- Extensive subconjunctival hemorrhage may cause a protruding sac of blood, possibly beyond the lid margin
- May be present with pain, blurred vision, and systemic symptoms in cases of acute hemorrhagic conjunctivitis

RISK FACTORS

- Local trauma to the eye, including blunt trauma, eye rubbing, etc.
- Hypertension
- Acute conjunctivitis
- Aspirin or anticoagulant use (or overdose thereof)
- Vigorous coughing, sneezing, straining, or vomiting
- Underlying hematologic or systemic disorders

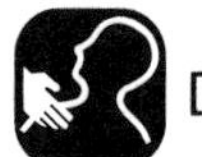

Diagnosis

DIFFERENTIAL DIAGNOSIS

- Acute hemorrhagic conjunctivitis: a highly contagious disease caused by enterovirus 70 and coxsackievirus A24. Pain, photophobia, blurred vision, and epiphora develop acutely, with 80% developing bilateral disease within 24 hours. Ocular signs may include subconjunctival hemorrhage as well as discharge, punctate corneal epithelial keratitis, and lid edema. Patients also may complain of fever, headache, upper respiratory infection symptoms, and myalgia, and may have tender preauricular lymphadenopathy. Symptoms usually resolve without treatment over 5 to 7 days, with persistent subconjunctival hemorrhages resolving over an additional 1 to 2 weeks.
- Scleral rupture should be suspected in a posttraumatic patient with a bullous subconjunctival hemorrhage, especially in the presence of blood in the vitreous, decreased intraocular pressure, or a shallow anterior chamber.
- Orbital hemorrhage may present with massive subconjunctival hemorrhage as well as proptosis and limitation of extraocular movements, usually after trauma.
- Infrequently, adenoviral conjunctivitis, bacterial conjunctivitis, and even allergic conjunctivitis may present with an associated subconjunctival hemorrhage.

HISTORY

- Vision: unchanged
- Eye trauma, including rubbing
- Medications, especially aspirin or other anticoagulants
- Medical conditions leading to high blood pressure or straining, including uncontrolled hypertension, constipation, prostatic hypertrophy, cough, sneezing, and vomiting
- Predisposing exercise or activities involving exertional straining (i.e., weight lifting, etc.)
- Diagnosis of or symptoms suggestive of bleeding disorders, such as easy bruising, menorrhagia, etc.

PHYSICAL EXAM

- Bright red area of blood, either focally or diffusely in potential space under conjunctiva
- Blood pressure
- Stigmata of bleeding or other hematologic disorders (petechiae, bruising, etc.)
- Associated signs suggestive of acute hemorrhagic conjunctivitis

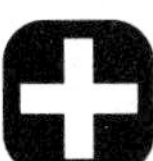

Acute Treatment

ANALGESIA

- Compresses (cool initially, warm later) may reduce discomfort
- Ophthalmic ointment or artificial tears for lubrication and discomfort
- Topical steroids are contraindicated, especially with suspicion of acute hemorrhagic conjunctivitis, due to risk of clinical deterioration and permanent side effects

GENERAL

- Reassurance: hemorrhages usually resolve spontaneously in 1 to 3 weeks.
- Further treatment should be directed at reduction of risk factors (above) and treatment of any identified underlying etiology (bleeding problems, hypertension).
- With suspicion of acute hemorrhagic conjunctivitis, education on prevention of transmission should be provided; the patient may be contagious for 2 weeks from symptom onset.
- Treat secondary bacterial conjunctivitis and allergic conjunctivitis as indicated.

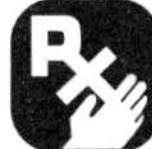

Long-Term Treatment

REFERRAL/DISPOSITION

- Consider ophthalmology consultation if history of significant ocular trauma is present or in the presence of associated ocular injury.
- Consider hematology consultation if hemorrhages are idiopathic and recurrent.

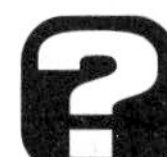

Common Questions and Answers

Physician responses to common patient questions:

Q: How long until I can expect this to go away?

A: Most cases resolve completely over the course of 5 days to 3 weeks.

Miscellaneous

SYNONYMS

- Conjunctival hemorrhage

ICD-9 CODE

372.72

BIBLIOGRAPHY

Fukuyama J, Hayasaka S, Yamada K, et al. Causes of subconjunctival hemorrhage. *Ophthalmologica* 1990;200:63–67.

Goroll AH, May LA, Mulley AG Jr, eds. *Primary care medicine*. Philadelphia: JB Lippincott, 1995.

Pavan-Langston D, ed. *Manual of ocular diagnosis and therapy*, 4th ed. Boston: Little, Brown, 1996.

Wright PW, Strauss GH, Langford MP. Acute hemorrhagic conjunctivitis. *Am Fam Physician* 1992;45:173–178.

Author: David Wallis

Syncope

Basics

DEFINITION

Sudden, transient loss of consciousness characterized by unresponsiveness and loss of muscular tone with rapid spontaneous recovery

INCIDENCE/PREVALENCE

- A common condition, accounting for 3% of emergency room visits and 6% of hospital admissions
- Recurrence rate of 30%
- Incidence rises with age
- Estimated that 15% of children experience syncope prior to adulthood

SIGNS AND SYMPTOMS

- Patients may develop prodromal symptoms such as "graying" of vision, nausea, diaphoresis, pallor, and lightheadedness/dizziness prior to the syncopal episode.
- Some patients have abrupt onset of syncope without any prodrome or warning.

ETIOLOGIES

- Primary mechanism is decreased cerebral perfusion or impaired glucose or oxygen delivery.
- Often multifactorial; specific etiology is not found in 38% to 47% of cases.
- Etiologies divided into cardiac (with and without structural heart disease) and noncardiac
- Cardiac etiologies without structural heart disease: vasovagal reaction (increased vagal tone leading to hypotension and bradycardia), vasodepressor syncope (enhanced sympathetic tone leading, paradoxically, to decreased cardiac function), situational (cough, defecation, micturition, postprandial, sneeze, swallow), carotid sinus syncope (via stimulation of carotid baroreceptors), orthostatic hypotension, heat syncope (in association with heat illness), drug induced (antihypertensives, diuretics, antidepressants, phenothiazines, antiarrhythmics, insulin, drugs of abuse)
- Cardiac etiologies with structural heart disease: aortic dissection, aortic stenosis, cardiac tamponade, hypertrophic cardiomyopathy, left ventricular dysfunction, myocardial infarction, atrial myxoma, pulmonary embolism, pulmonary hypertension, pulmonary stenosis, arrhythmias (Wolff-Parkinson-White syndrome, atrial fibrillation/flutter, ventricular tachycardia, ventricular fibrillation)
- Noncardiac etiologies: metabolic (hyperventilation, hypoglycemia, volume depletion, hypoxia), neurologic (cerebrovascular insufficiency, diabetic neuropathy, normal pressure hydrocephalus, seizure, subclavian steal syndrome, increased intracranial pressure), psychiatric (hysteria, panic attacks, major depression)

Diagnosis

DIFFERENTIAL DIAGNOSIS

True syncope must be differentiated primarily from sleep and seizure disorders in order to identify the presence of potentially life-threatening etiologies.

HISTORY

- Patients may report prodromal symptoms or a definitive "trigger" to the event.
- Patients may have recently suffered from one of the etiologies noted above.
- Prodromal symptoms are most commonly associated with vasovagal syncope.
- Abrupt onset of syncope without prodrome raises concern for a significant cardiac etiology.
- Exercise-associated syncope should raise suspicion for aortic stenosis, hypertrophic cardiomyopathy, left ventricular dysfunction, or arrhythmia.
- Syncope with bending or stretching of the neck suggests a carotid sinus etiology.

PHYSICAL EXAM

- Comprehensive examination should be performed on every syncopal patient; however, the physical exam may be completely normal.
- Attention to vital signs for evidence of altered cardiorespiratory status
- Careful cardiovascular examination to evaluate for the cardiac etiologies noted above [harsh systolic crescendo/decrescendo murmur (aortic stenosis, apical systolic murmur increased by Valsalva maneuver), hypertrophic cardiomyopathy, S3 gallop (impaired left ventricular function, ectopy), and arrhythmia]
- Thorough neurologic exam to assess for predisposing factors or residual dysfunction (carotid bruits, focal deficits, hypertension)
- Relative hypotension and bradycardia consistent with vasovagal response
- Carotid sinus sensitivity may result in sinus pauses of more than 3 seconds or a 30 to 50 mm Hg decrease in systolic blood pressure with unilateral carotid massage.

ANCILLARY STUDIES

- If history and physical exam fail to reveal a definitive diagnosis, the initial focus of additional testing centers on ruling out a significant cardiac etiology. An electrocardiogram (ECG) and echocardiogram are considered standard initial studies
- When the initial evaluation is negative, continued symptoms suggesting a cardiac etiology may then warrant use of 24-hour Holter monitoring, continuous cardiac loop event recording, signal-averaged ECG, formal electrophysiology testing (to assess for arrhythmogenic etiologies), or head-upright tilt table testing (to evaluate for vagal/vasodepressor syncope).

- Hematologic and metabolic testing is not routinely indicated but should be explored if no diagnosis is made by other means.
- Unless significant neurologic findings are present by history or physical exam, or loss of consciousness is prolonged, neurologic imaging (head CT/MRI) or functional testing (electroencephalography) is not routinely recommended.

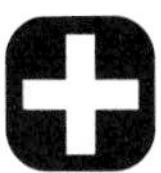

Acute Treatment

GENERAL

- Initial care is generally supportive.
- Supine positioning for maintenance of blood pressure and cerebral perfusion
- Other measures as dictated by specific etiologies: correction/management of acute cardiac or neurologic conditions

SPECIAL CONSIDERATIONS

- If complete resolution of symptoms does not occur immediately after the syncopal episode, other diagnoses must be entertained and the patient should be transported to a medical facility for further evaluation.

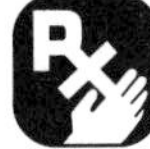

Long-Term Treatment

REFERRAL/DISPOSITION

- Long-term management of recurrent syncope is based on the specific etiology.
- Correction/management of underlying cardiac or neurologic conditions
- Volume expansion and consideration of salt tablet use or Florinef (fludrocortisone) for vasovagal syncope
- Beta blockade for vasodepressor syncope

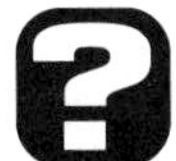

Common Questions and Answers

Physician responses to common patient questions:

Q: Can the athlete with syncope continue to participate?

A: Athletes with a definitive diagnosis of a benign cause of syncope may resume sports activity when appropriately managed. Those athletes who have been thoroughly evaluated and have had no diagnosis made may resume sports activities with the understanding that additional events may occur and may require additional testing or may warrant disqualification. Those athletes who neither carry a firm diagnosis nor have completed a thorough but reasonable diagnostic evaluation should be restricted from participation.

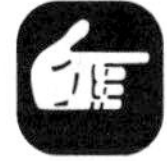

Miscellaneous

SYNONYMS

- Drop attacks

ICD-9 CODE

780.2 Syncope (cardiac)
780.2 Vasovagal/vasodepressor syncope
337.0 Carotid sinus syncope
992.1 Heat syncope

BIBLIOGRAPHY

Benditt DG, Lurie KG, Fabian WH. Clinical approach to diagnosis of syncope. *Cardiol Clin* 1997;15:165–176.

Kapoor WN. Evaluation and management of the patient with syncope. *JAMA* 1992;268: 2553–2560.

Maron BJ, Mitchell JH. 26th Bethesda Conference: recommendations for determining eligibility for competition in athletes with cardiovascular abnormalities. *J Am Coll Cardiol* 1994;24:846–899.

Author: John MacKnight

Tension Headache

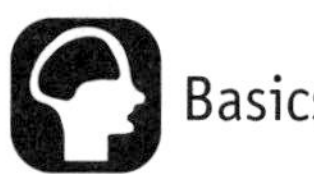

Basics

SIGNS AND SYMPTOMS

- Migraine
  —Aura (usually visual)
  —Recurring
  —Unilateral
  —Pulsating
  —Moderate to severe intensity
  —4–72-hr duration
  —Nausea and vomiting
  —Photophobia
  —Phonophobia
- Tension
  —Recurring
  —Bilateral
  —Nonpulsatile
  —Bandlike
  —Mild to moderate intensity
  —30 min to 7 days duration
  —Anorexia
  —Photophobia
  —Phonophobia
- Cluster
  —Recurring
  —Unilateral
  —Penetrating
  —Severe intensity
  —Sudden onset
  —45–60-min duration
  —Lacrimation
  —Conjunctival injection
  —Rhinorrhea
  —Ptosis
  —No aura
- Potentially life-threatening headaches
- Less common
- New onset severe headache or "worst headache of my life"
  —New onset in elderly
  —Abnormal vital signs, particularly diastolic BP >130 mm Hg or fever
  —Altered level of consciousness
  —Altered mental status
  —Abnormal neurologic findings or meningismus

MECHANISM/DESCRIPTION

- Vascular
  —Severe, throbbing headache
  —Divided into migraine (the majority) and vascular nonmigrainous
  —Triggered by stress, hormone fluctuations, lack of sleep, certain foods
- Tension (muscle contraction headache)
  —Most common type of chronic recurring headache
  —Secondary to sustained contraction of head and neck muscles
  —Triggered by poor posture, stress, anxiety, depression, cervical osteoarthritis
- Cluster headaches
  —Triggered by alcohol, certain foods, altered sleep habits, strong emotions
- Intracranial (traction)
  —Mass lesions inside the calvarium stretching arteries and other pain sensitive structures
- Extracranial (nontension)
  —Pathology from an extracranial site causing pain in a peripheral nerve of the head and neck

ETIOLOGY

- Vascular
  —Intra/extracranial vasodilatation and constriction of pain-sensitive blood vessels
- Tension
  —Unknown (possibly serotonin imbalance, decreased endorphins)
- Other headaches
  —Multiple etiologies depending on cause (see differential diagnosis)
  —Generally through traction, tension or inflammation of the pain-sensitive structures; the vasculature, meninges, and cranial nerves V, IX, and X

PEDIATRIC CONSIDERATIONS

- Migraine
  —Most common headache in children
  —70–90% have positive family history
  —May only manifest as cyclic vomiting or vertigo

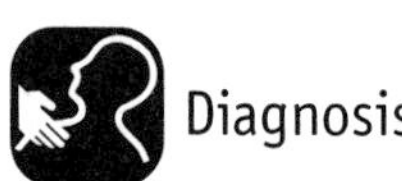

Diagnosis

ESSENTIAL WORKUP

- Detailed history and CNS examination
- Workup is strongly dependent on the clinical differential diagnosis

LABORATORY

- ESR
  —If temporal arteritis or other inflammatory disorders suspected
- Tests appropriate for patient's underlying medical condition (e.g., ABG, glucose)
- Tests appropriate for physical examination abnormalities

IMAGING/SPECIAL TESTS

- Head CT scan
  —Indications
    —Unclear diagnosis based on H&P
    —Signs of increased ICP
    —Worst or first headache
    —Acute onset
    —Focal neurologic abnormalities
    —Papilledema
    —Recurrent morning headache
    —Persistent vomiting
    —Headache associated with fever, rash, and nausea without systemic illness
    —Head trauma with LOC, focal neurologic findings, or lethargy
    —Altered mental status, meningismus
  —90% Sensitive for subarachnoid hemorrhage (SAH)
    —Must do LP if SAH suspected and CT is negative
- Lumbar puncture indications
  —Intracranial infections
  —Detect blood not evident on CT scan
- Sinus imaging
  —Suspect sinusitis
- Vascular assessment with angiogram or MR angiography
  —May be indicated if nonmigrainous vascular cause suspected
- MRI
  —Suspected posterior fossa lesion

DIFFERENTIAL DIAGNOSIS

- Vascular
  —Migraine: classic (with aura), common (without aura), cluster, ophthalmoplegic, hemiplegic, migraine equivalents
  —Hypertensive headache: throbbing, occipital, SBP >130 mm Hg
  —Anoxic: carbon monoxide toxicity, sleep apnea, anemia
- Tension
  —Muscular contraction
  —Conversion reaction
  —Chronic anxiety states
- Intracranial (traction)
  —Subarachnoid hemorrhage: "first or worst," sudden onset, vomiting, meningismus

—Aneurysm/AVM: sudden onset, unilateral, severe, decreased vision
—Meningitis/encephalitis: fever, nonfocal, meningismus
—Acute subdural hematoma: mental status, depression, or focal findings
—Chronic subdural hematoma: hemiparesis, focal seizures
—Epidural hematoma: trauma, brief LOC, rapid progression of neurologic symptoms
—Brain tumor: pain on awakening, progressively worsens, worse with Valsalva, ataxia
—Brain abscess: fever, nausea/vomiting, seizures
—Pseudotumor cerebri: young obese female, irregular menses, papilledema
- Extracranial
  —Trigeminal neuralgia: transient, shocklike facial pain
  —Temporal arteritis: elderly, severe, scalp artery tenderness/swelling
  —Sinusitis: stabbing/aching, worse with bending or coughing
  —Metabolic: fever, hypoglycemia, high altitude, acute anemia
  —Acute glaucoma: nausea/vomiting, eye pain, conjunctival injection, increased IOP
  —Cervical: spondylosis, trauma, arthritis
  —Temporomandibular joint syndrome

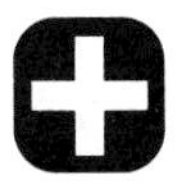

Acute Treatment

INITIAL STABILIZATION

- ABCs
- IV fluids, oxygen, and monitoring if necessary

ED TREATMENT

- Migraine
  —Abortive therapy
    —Ergotamine
    —Phenothiazine
    —Serotonin agonists
    —NSAID
  —Analgesia/comfort
    —Narcotics (most common but suboptimal)
    —Dark quiet room
  —Prophylactic measures
    —Not recommended for ED use
- Tension
  —Aspirin
  —Acetaminophen
  —NSAID
- Cluster
  —Oxygen
  —Intranasal lidocaine
  —Migraine medications excluding β-blockers
- Temporal arteritis
  —Steroids
- Intracranial infection: see meningitis chapter
- Intracranial hemorrhage: see subarachnoid hemorrhage chapter

MEDICATIONS

- Chlorpromazine: 25–50 mg IM/IV (peds: 0.5–1 mg/kg/dose IM/IV/PO) q 4–6 hrs
- Dihydroergotamine: 0.5–1.5 mg IM/IV, repeat hourly; max dose 3 mg
- Ergotamine: 2 mg PO/SL at onset, then 1 mg po q 30 min; max dose 10 mg/wk
- Ketorolac: 30–60 mg IM; 15–30 mg IV once, then 15–30 mg q 6 hrs
- Lidocaine 4%: 1 ml intranasal on same side as symptoms
- Meperidine: 50–150 mg (peds: 1–1.5 mg/kg/dose) PO/IV/IM/SC q 3–4 hrs
- Metoclopramide: 1–2 mg/kg IV q 2–4 hrs
- Morphine: 2.5–20 mg (peds: 0.1–0.2 mg/kg/dose) IM/IV/SC q 2–6 hrs
- Prochlorperazine (compazine): 10 mg IV
- Sumatriptan: 6 mg SQ, repeat in 1 hr, up to 12 mg/24 hrs

HOSPITAL ADMISSION CRITERIA

- Headache secondary to suspected organic disease
- Chronic daily headache, pain refractory to outpatient management
- Persistent migraine with intractable vomiting and dehydration
- Headache complicated by significant surgical or medical history
- Intracranial infection
- Intracranial hemorrhage
- Consider ICU admission
  —Suspected aneurysm
  —Acute subdural hematoma
  —Subarachnoid hemorrhage
  —Stroke
  —Increased ICP
  —Severe headache following trauma
  —Intracranial infection

HOSPITAL DISCHARGE CRITERIA

- Most migraine, cluster, and tension headaches after pain relief
- Local or minor systemic infections

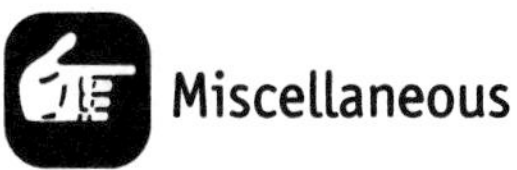

Miscellaneous

ICD-9 CODE

784.0

CORE CONTENT CODE

22.2.12

BIBLIOGRAPHY

Goadsby PJ, Olesen J. Diagnosis and treatment of migraine. *Br Med J* 1996; 312:1279–1283.

Henry GL. Headache. In: Rosen P, et al., eds. *Emergency medicine: concepts and clinical practice*. 4th ed. St. Louis: CV Mosby, 1997; 2119–2130.

Perkins AT, Ondo W. When to worry about headache: head pain as a clue to intracranial disease. *Postgrad Med* 1995;98(2):197–208.

Thomas SH, Stone CK. Emergency department treatment of migraine, tension, and mixed-type headache. *J Emerg Med* 1994; 12(5):657–664.

Authors: Matthew R. Harmody and Robert J. Vissers

Testicular Torsion

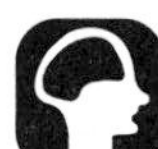

Basics

SIGNS AND SYMPTOMS

- Sudden onset of unilateral testicular pain and tenderness followed by scrotal swelling and erythema
- Less commonly, torsion may present with pain in the inguinal or lower abdominal area
- Up to 40% of patients may describe previous similar episodes of testicular pain that remitted spontaneously, representing spontaneous torsion and detorsion
- The affected testicle may be found to lie transversely as opposed to the normal vertical lie
- Nausea and vomiting occur in 50% of cases, and low-grade fever occurs in 25%
- There is a bimodal distribution with peak incidences in infancy and adolescence
  —Torsion is rare after age 30
- Symptoms of urinary infection (dysuria, frequency, and urgency) are absent
- In distinguishing torsion from epididymitis, localization of tenderness is helpful early in the course. However, once significant scrotal swelling occurs the anatomy becomes indistinct and some form of testicular flow study or surgical exploration is required
- The cremasteric reflex is frequently absent with testicular torsion
- The classic Prehn's sign, which consists of relief of pain on elevation of the testicle in epididymitis and worsening or no change in the pain with torsion, is considered unreliable

ETIOLOGY

- Most patients have a congenital abnormality of the genitalia with a high insertion of the tunica vaginalis on the spermatic cord and a redundant mesorchium that permit increased mobility and twisting of the testicle on its vascular pedicle
- The anatomic abnormality is generally bilateral, so that both testicles are susceptible to torsion

MECHANISM/DESCRIPTION

- Rotation generally occurs medially and ranges from incomplete (e.g., 90–180°) to complete (540–720°) torsion
- Depending on the degree of torsion, vascular occlusion occurs and the result is infarction of the testicle after 6 hours
- Testicular infarction leads to atrophy and may ultimately decrease fertility

PEDIATRIC CONSIDERATIONS

- Testicular torsion has been described in utero and in virtually every pediatric age group
- The peak incidence occurs in late childhood and adolescence (mode: 13-years old) with a smaller peak in infancy

CAUTIONS

- There is no definitive treatment that can be rendered in the field. However, pre-hospital personnel need to recognize the urgency of acute testicular pain in young patients
- These patients should be transported to the ED immediately as the outcome is time-dependent

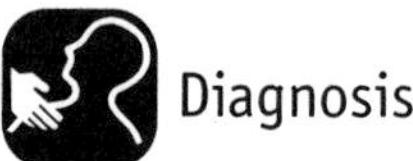

Diagnosis

ESSENTIAL WORKUP

- The presentation of an "acute scrotum" in a child or adolescent requires rapid assessment and immediate consultation with an urologist
- These patients will require noninvasive flow studies or surgical exploration to detect torsion
- 25–30% of these patients will ultimately prove to have testicular torsion

LABORATORY

- Urinalysis is usually normal, but up to 20% of cases of torsion have pyuria
- Elevated WBC count with a left shift is present in 50% of cases
- There are no laboratory tests specific for testicular torsion

IMAGING/SPECIAL TESTS

- The criterion standard imaging modality has traditionally been ^{99m}TC-pertechnetate radionuclide scans which shows decreased flow in the torsed testicle compared to the unaffected side
  —Epididymitis will reveal increased flow due to inflammation
  —This technique has an overall sensitivity and specificity of 98% and 100% respectively
- Because of the frequent time delays in obtaining nuclear scans, use of Doppler ultrasound to assess testicular blood flow has increasingly replaced nuclear scanning as a less invasive, more readily available test with comparable accuracy

- —Several modalities are available including color flow Doppler, power Doppler, and pulsed Doppler with mechanical sector scanning, although none of these modalities has demonstrated superiority
- —Color-flow Doppler is the most commonly available
- —Use of Doppler contrast material may soon become available and should enhance the accuracy of this modality
- —Overall sensitivity and specificity for color flow Doppler ranges from 86–100% and 97–100% respectively, although the accuracy tends to be lower in infants

- There are limitations of all flow studies in that they reflect only the current state of perfusion. Consequently, a spontaneously detorsed testicle may show normal or even increased flow and yet still be at high risk recurrent torsion

DIFFERENTIAL DIAGNOSIS

- Epididymitis/orchitis
- Torsion of the appendix testis
- Testicular trauma or rupture of the testicle
- Incarcerated inguinal hernia
- Testicular tumor
- Acute hydrocele
- Henoch-Schönlein purpura
- Other intra-abdominal conditions (appendicitis, pancreatitis, renal colic may rarely present with testicular pain)

PEDIATRIC CONSIDERATIONS

- All imaging techniques designed to evaluate testicular blood flow have technical limitations when applied to infants because the testicular vessels are very small and the amount of blood flow to the testicle under normal conditions is minimal
- Scrotal exploration may be required

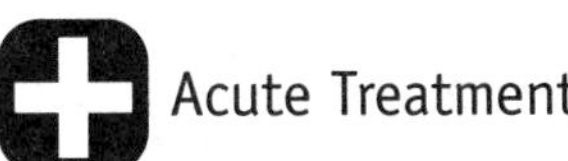

Acute Treatment

INITIAL STABILIZATION

- Intravenous fluid, analgesics as appropriate

ED TREATMENT

- Establish the diagnosis and mobilize appropriate urologic care
- In situations in which definitive care is likely to be delayed beyond 4-5 hours since the onset of torsion, manual detorsion may be attempted
  - —This is accomplished by externally rotating the affected testicle (opposite the usual medial direction of torsion) until pain is relieved or normal anatomy is restored. All patients who undergo manual detorsion must be surgically explored

HOSPITAL ADMISSION CRITERIA

- Any patient with confirmed testicular torsion must be admitted for scrotal exploration and bilateral orchiopexy
- Flow studies that are inconclusive or technical failures mandate further investigation by surgical exploration of the scrotum
- Admission for urgent surgical exploration of an acute scrotum is mandatory if there will be any potential delay in obtaining a flow study

HOSPITAL DISCHARGE CRITERIA

- Patients with negative scrotal exploration, or normal flow studies can be discharged with appropriate urologic follow-up
- Appropriate parameters for return to ED must be discussed because of the possibility of intermittent torsion
- Patients with an obvious diagnosis other than testicular torsion (e.g., a nonincarcerated inguinal hernia) can be referred for elective care

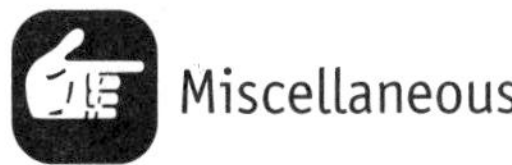

Miscellaneous

ICD-9 CODE

608.2

CORE CONTENT CODE

19.2.2.4
13.13.3.1

BIBLIOGRAPHY

Al Mufti RA, Ogedegbe AK, Laferty K. The use of Doppler ultrasound in the clinical management of acute testicular pain. *Br J Urol* 1995;76:625–627.

Coley BD, Frush DP, Babcock DS, et al. Acute testicular torsion: Comparison of unenhanced and contrast enhanced power Doppler US, color Doppler US, and radionuclide imaging. *Radiol* 1996;199: 441–446.

Patriquin HB, Yazbeck S, Trinh B, et al. Testicular torsion in infants and children: Diagnosis with Doppler sonography. *Radiol* 1993;188:781–785.

Rabinowitz R, Hulbert WC Jr. Acute scrotal swelling. *Urol Clin North Am* 1995;22: 101–105.

Schul MW, Keating MA. The acute pediatric scrotum. *J Emerg Med* 1993;11:565–577.

Author: Ed Newton

Thrombophlebitis, Superficial

Basics

DESCRIPTION

Superficial thrombophlebitis is an inflammatory condition of the veins with secondary thrombosis.

- Septic (suppurative) thrombophlebitis types:
  —Iatrogenic
  —Infectious, mainly syphilis and psittacosis
- Aseptic thrombophlebitis types:
  —Primary hypercoagulable states—disorders with measurable defects in the proteins of the coagulation and/or fibrinolytic systems
  —Secondary hypercoagulable states—clinical conditions with a risk of thrombosis

System(s) affected: Cardiovascular

Genetics

- Septic—no known genetic pattern
- Antithrombin III deficiencies—autosomal dominant
- Proteins C and S deficiency—autosomal dominant with variable penetrance
- Disorders of fibrinolytic system—congenital defects inheritance variable
- Dysfibrinogenemia—autosomal dominant
- Factor XII deficiency—autosomal recessive

Incidence/Prevalence in USA

- Septic
  —Up to 10% of all nosocomial infections
  —Incidence of catheter-related thrombophlebitis is 88/100,000
  —Develops in 4–8% if cut down is performed
- Aseptic primary hypercoagulable state
  —Antithrombin III and heparin cofactor II deficiency incidence is 50/100,000
- Aseptic secondary hypercoagulable state
  —Trousseau incidence in malignancy 5–15%
  —Trousseau in pancreatic carcinoma 50%
  —In pregnancy 49-fold increased incidence of phlebitis
  —Superficial migratory thrombophlebitis in 27% of patients with thromboangiitis obliterans

Predominant Age

- Septic
  —More common in childhood
- Aseptic primary hypercoagulable state
  —Antithrombin III and heparin cofactor II deficiency—neonatal period, but first episode usually at age 20–30 years
  —Proteins C and S—before age 30
- Aseptic secondary hypercoagulable state
  —Mondor's disease: women, ages 21–55 years
  —Thromboangiitis obliterans onset: 20–50 years

Predominant Sex

- Suppurative:
  —Male = Female
- Aseptic
  —Mondor's—Female > Male (2:1)
  —Thromboangiitis obliterans—Female > Male (1–19% of clinical cases)

SIGNS AND SYMPTOMS

- Swelling, tenderness, redness along the course of the veins
- May look like cellulitis or erythema nodosa
- Fever in 70% of patients
- Warmth, erythema, tenderness, or lymphangitis in 32%
- Sign of systemic sepsis in 84% in suppurative
- Red, tender cord
- Pain

CAUSES

- Septic
  —Staphylococcus aureus in 65–78%
  —Enterobacteriaceae, especially Klebsiella
  —Multiple organisms in 14%
  —Anaerobic isolate rare
  —Candida spp.
  —Cytomegalovirus in AIDS patients
- Aseptic primary hypercoagulable state
  —Antithrombin III and heparin II deficiency
  —Protein C and protein S deficiency
  —Disorder of tissue plasminogen activator
  —Abnormal plasminogen and co-plasminogen
  —Dysfibrinogenemia
  —Factor XII deficiency
  —Lupus anticoagulant and anticardiolipin antibody syndrome
- Aseptic secondary hypercoagulable states
  —Malignancy (Trousseau syndrome: Recurrent migratory thrombophlebitis). Most commonly seen in metastatic mucin or adenocarcinomas of the GI tract (pancreas, stomach, colon and gall bladder); lung, prostate, ovary.
  —Pregnancy
  —Oral contraceptive
  —Infusion of prothrombin complex concentrates
  —Behçet's disease
  —Buerger's disease
  —Mondor's disease

RISK FACTORS

- Nonspecific
  —Immobilization
  —Obesity
  —Advanced age
  —Postoperative states
- Septic
  —Intravenous catheter
  —Duration of intravenous catheterization (68% of cannulae have been left in place for 2 days)

—Cutdowns
—Cancer, debilitating diseases
—Steroid
—Incidence is 40 times higher with plastic cannula (8%) than with steel or scalp cannulas (0.2%)
—Thrombosis
—Dermal infection
—Burned patients
—Lower extremities intravenous catheter
—Intravenous antibiotics
—AIDS
—Varicose veins

- Antithrombin II and heparin cofactor II deficiency
  —Pregnancy
  —Oral contraceptives
  —Surgery; trauma; infection
  In pregnancy
  —Increased age
  —Hypertension
  —Eclampsia
  —Increased parity
- Thromboangiitis obliterans
  —Persistent smoking
- Mondor's disease
  —Breast abscess
  —Antecedent breast surgery
  —Breast augmentation
  —Reduction mammoplasty

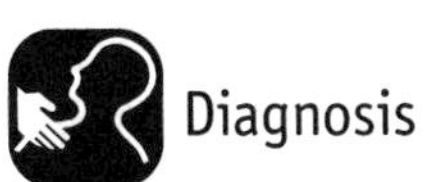

Diagnosis

DIFFERENTIAL DIAGNOSIS

- Cellulitis
- Erythema nodosa
- Cutaneous polyarteritis nodosa
- Sarcoid
- Kaposi's sarcoma
- Hyperalgesic pseudothrombophlebitis

LABORATORY

- Septic
  —Bacteremia in 80–90%
  —Culture of IV fluid bag
  —Leukocytosis
- Aseptic
  —Acute phase reactant
  —Factor levels
  —Thrombin activity
  —Platelet function test

Drugs that may alter lab results: In septic, broad spectrum antibiotics

Disorders that may alter lab results: N/A

PATHOLOGICAL FINDINGS

- The affected vein is enlarged, tortuous, and thickened
- Associated perivascular suppuration and/or hemorrhage
- Vein lumen may contain pus and thrombus
- Endothelial damage, fibrinoid necrosis and thickening of the vein wall

SPECIAL TESTS

Leukocyte imaging

IMAGING

- Septic and aseptic
  —Ultrasound of veins reveal an increase in the diameter of the lumen
  —Chest x-ray—multiple peripheral densities or a pleural effusion consistent with pulmonary embolism, abscess, or empyema
  —Bone and gallium scan—for associated subperiosteal abscess in septic thrombophlebitis
  —Evaluation of complications (deep vein thrombosis and others)

DIAGNOSTIC PROCEDURES

Skin biopsy

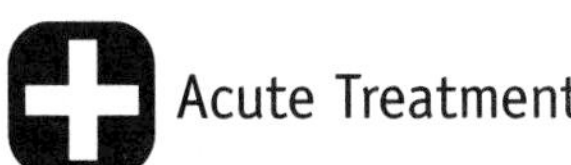

Acute Treatment

APPROPRIATE HEALTH CARE

Septic—inpatient
Aseptic—outpatient

GENERAL MEASURES

- Heat application
- Extremity elevation

SURGICAL MEASURES

- Septic
  —Excision of the involved vein segment and all involved tributaries
  —Excision from ankle to groin may be required in some burn patients
  —If systemic symptoms persist after vein excision, re-exploration is necessary with removal of all involved veins
  —Drainage of contiguous abscesses
  —Remove all cannulae
- Aseptic
  —Mondor's disease, consider surgical transection of the phlebitic cord
  —Management of underlying conditions

ACTIVITY

Bedrest

DIET

No restrictions

PATIENT EDUCATION

- Avoid trauma
- Be alert to change in skin color
- Be alert to tenderness over extremities

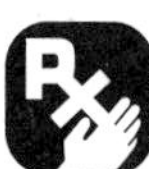

Long-Term Treatment

DRUG(S) OF CHOICE

- Septic
  —Initially: semisynthetic penicillin (e.g., nafcillin 2 g IV q6h) plus an aminoglycoside (e.g., gentamicin, 1.0–1.7 mg/kg IV)
  —Duration of therapy is empiric
  —If due to Candida albicans, consider a short course of amphotericin B, approximately 200 mg cumulative dose
  —If osteomyelitis documented, antibiotic therapy for at least 6 weeks
- Aseptic general
  —Nonsteroidal anti-inflammatories
  —Oral anticoagulant warfarin
  —Systemic anticoagulant heparin
- Antithrombin III and heparin cofactor II deficiency
  —IV heparin
  —Antithrombin III concentrate
  —Prophylaxis: warfarin, oxymetholone
- Proteins C and S
  —Long-term warfarin, lower dose, no loading
- Disorder of tissue plasminogen activator
  —Phenformin and ethylestrenol
  —Stanozolol and phenformin
  —Stanozolol alone
  —Ethylestrenol alone

PATIENT MONITORING

- Septic
  —Routine WBC and differential and culture
  —Repeat culture from the phlebitic vein
- Aseptic
  —Clinical followup to rule out secondary complications
  —Repeat of blood studies for fibrinolytic system, platelets and factors

PREVENTION/AVOIDANCE

- Use of scalp vein cannulae
- Avoidance of lower extremity cannulations
- Insertion under aseptic conditions
- Secure anchoring of the cannulae
- Replacement of cannulae, connecting tubing, and IV fluid every 48–72 hrs
- Neomycin-polymyxin B-bacitracin ointment in cutdown

POSSIBLE COMPLICATIONS

- Septic: Systemic sepsis, bacteremia (84%); septic pulmonary emboli (44%); metastatic abscess formation; pneumonia (44%); subperiosteal abscess of adjacent long bones in children
- Aseptic: Deep vein thrombosis; thromboembolic phenomena
- Dysfibrinogenemia
  —Acute attack—anticoagulation
  —Prophylaxis—stanozolol
- Abnormal plasminogen and plasminogenemia
  —Acute attack—anticoagulation
  —Prophylaxis—warfarin
- Factor XII deficiency
  —Standard therapy
- Lupus anticardiolipin
  —Prophylaxis—warfarin
- Trousseau's syndrome
  —Heparin
- For pregnancy
  —Heparin
- Behçet's disease
  —Phenformin
  —Ethylestrenol
  —Stanozolol
- Thromboangiitis obliterans
  —Stop smoking
  —Pentoxifylline

Contraindications: Refer to manufacturer's literature
Precautions: Refer to manufacturer's literature
Significant possible interactions: Refer to manufacturer's literature

ALTERNATIVE DRUGS

- Factor XII deficiency—streptokinase or alteplase [tissue plasminogen activator (tPA)]
- Behcet's—oral anticoagulants plus cyclosporine
- Thromboangiitis obliterans—corticosteroid, antiplatelets and vasodilating drugs

EXPECTED COURSE/PROGNOSIS

- Septic-high mortality (50%), if untreated
- Aseptic
  —Usually benign course; recovery 7–10 days

—Antithrombin III and heparin cofactor deficiency; recurrence rate is 60%
—Proteins C and S, recurrence rate 70%
—Prognosis depends on development of DVT and early detections of complications
—Aseptic thrombophlebitis can be isolated, recurrent or migratory

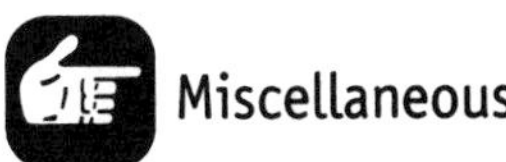

Miscellaneous

ASSOCIATED CONDITIONS

Varicose veins, manifestation of systemic disease, hypercoagulable states, surgery, trauma, burns, obesity, pregnancy

AGE-RELATED FACTORS

Pediatric: Subperiosteal abscesses of adjacent long bone may complicate
Geriatric: Septic thrombophlebitis is more common, prognosis poorer
Others: N/A

PREGNANCY

- Associated with increased risk of aseptic superficial thrombophlebitis
- Warfarin and NSAIDs are contraindicated

SYNONYMS

- Phlebitis
- Phlebothrombosis

ICD-9 CODE

451 Phlebitis and thrombophlebitis
451.0 Phlebitis and thrombophlebitis of superficial vessels of lower extremities
451.1 Phlebitis and thrombophlebitis of deep vessels of lower extremities

See also: Thrombosis, deep vein (DVT); Cellulitis

ABBREVIATIONS

DVT = deep vein thrombosis

REFERENCES

Samlaskie CP, James WD. Superficial thrombophlebitis II. Secondary hypercoagulable states. *J Am Acad Dermato* 1990;23(1)1–18.
Samlaskie CP, James WD. Superficial thrombophlebitis I. Primary hypercoagulable states. *J Am Acad Dermatol* 1990;22:975–989.
Mandell GL, ed. *Principles and practice of infectious diseases*. 4th Ed. New York: Churchill Livingstone, 1995.

Internet references: http://www.5mcc.com

Author: Abdulrazak Abyad

Thrombosis, Deep Vein (DVT)

Basics

SIGNS AND SYMPTOMS

- Extremity pain, swelling and fullness
  - —Greater than a 1–2-cm circumferential difference in legs
  - —Tenderness on compression of the calf
  - —Warmth
  - —Palpation of a venous "cord."

MECHANISM/DESCRIPTION

- Roughly 2 million cases of thrombophlebitis occur in the U.S. annually
- Part of a systemic process better known as venous thromboembolism
  - —Most significant complication is pulmonary embolism (PE) from which an estimated 60,000 Americans die annually
- Lower extremity deep venous thrombosis (DVT) is divided into distal (to the popliteal vein) or proximal
- DVT also occurs in pelvic and upper extremity veins

ETIOLOGY

- Risk factors
  - —Hypercoagulable states
    - —Cancer
    - —Nephrotic syndrome
    - —Sepsis
    - —Inflammatory conditions such as ulcerative colitis
    - —Increased estrogen (pregnancy, oral contraceptives)
    - —Various protein (S, C, and antithrombin 3) deficiencies
  - —Stasis
    - —Prolonged bed rest
    - —Immobility from a cast, long travel rides
    - —Neurologic disorders with paralysis
    - —Congestive heart failure
    - —Obesity
  - —Vascular damage
    - —Trauma
    - —Surgery
    - —Central lines
  - —Advancing age
  - —Prior thromboembolism
  - —Family history of DVT

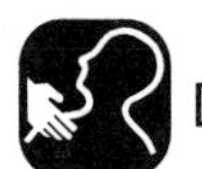

Diagnosis

ESSENTIAL WORKUP

- Doppler ultrasound (duplex scanning) of extremity

LABORATORY

- No blood test diagnoses or excludes DVT with certainty
  - —The absence of D-dimer (ELISA technique) suggests DVT is not present.
  - —CBC, PT/PTT baseline measurements

IMAGING/SPECIAL TESTS

- Duplex scanning (combination of color Doppler and B-mode ultrasound)
  - —Rapid, inexpensive, and highly accurate in detecting proximal DVT
- Impedance plethysmography (IPG)
  - —Nearly as accurate as duplex scanning
  - —Not as routinely available as US
- Venography is the historic gold standard
  - —Accurate but invasive
  - —Associated with dye reactions
  - —Can precipitate phlebitis

DIFFERENTIAL DIAGNOSIS

- Superficial thrombophlebitis
- Cellulitis
- Torn muscles and ligaments
- Ruptured Baker's cyst
- Bilateral edema (seen with heart, kidney, or liver disease) is rarely caused by DVT
- Prior DVT and postphlebitic syndrome

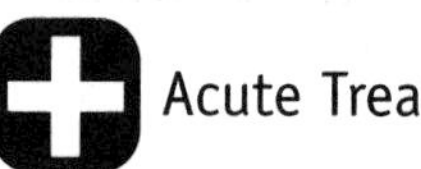

Acute Treatment

INITIAL STABILIZATION

- Patients with DVT rarely require immediate stabilization
  - —Phlegmasia alba dolens (painful white leg) or phlegmasia cerulea dolens (painful blue leg)
  - —Hypoperfusion with blanching and cyanosis
  - —May require fluid resuscitation, immediate anticoagulation, and thrombolysis or thrombectomy

ED TREATMENT

- Anticoagulation
  —Contraindications
    —Active internal bleeding
    —Uncontrolled hypertension
    —Significant recent trauma or surgery
    —CNS tumor
    —Initiate in the ED
- Recurrent thromboembolism despite documented adequate anticoagulation (defined as a aPTT of <1.5 times control for heparinized patients and an INR of <2 for warfarinized patients) requires vena caval interruption
- Low molecular-weight heparin (LMWH) is treatment of choice if cost is less important or outpatient management is considered
  —Enoxaparin
  —Does not require laboratory monitoring
  —May be administered as an outpatient
  —Initiate oral warfarin therapy same day

MEDICATIONS

- Enoxaparin: 1 mg/kg SQ bid
- Heparin: 80 IU/kg bolus followed by a drip of 18 IU/kg/hr (aPTT should be checked in 6 hours and tile infusion rate adjusted accordingly)
- Warfarin: 10 mg po, then 5 mg po q day, monitor PT

HOSPITAL ADMISSION CRITERIA

- Severely ill patients
- Patients with significant comorbid conditions
- Patients without the means for appropriate home administration of LMWH

HOSPITAL DISCHARGE CRITERIA

- Isolated DVT
- No significant comorbid conditions
- Resources available for home administration of LMWH
- Appropriate followup assured

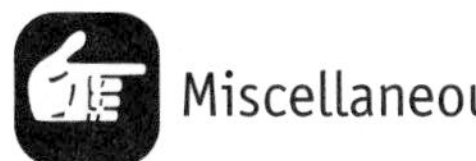

Miscellaneous

ICD-9 CODE

451.9

CORE CONTENT CODE

2.5.2.3

BIBLIOGRAPHY

Hirsh J, Hoak J. Management of DVT and PE. *Circulation* 1996;93:2212–245.

Levine M, et al. A comparison of LMWH administered primarily at home with unfractionated heparin administered in the hospital for proximal DVT. *N Engl J Med* 1996;334:677–81.

Pearson SP, et al. A critical pathway to evaluate suspected DVT. *Arch Int Med* 1995;155:1773–778.

Author: Jonathan Edlow

Thyroid Disease

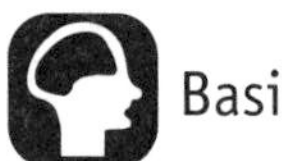

Basics

DESCRIPTION

A variety of inflammatory thyroid disorders that can cause thyroid enlargement and thyroid atrophy. May lead to hypothyroidism or hyperthyroidism. Complete resolution can occur.

- Hashimoto's disease—the most common form, an autoimmune disease, often presenting as an asymptomatic diffuse goiter. Often first detected after thyroid atrophy and hypothyroidism have occurred and occasionally as hyperthyroidism ("Hashitoxicosis").
- Granulomatous thyroiditis ("subacute")—probably related to viral infection and usually presenting with thyroid pain (which may be severe), involving one or both thyroid lobes, accompanied by hyperthyroidism, going through a phase of mild hypothyroidism and then to permanent resolution to normal
- "Silent" thyroiditis—one form is characterized by spontaneously resolving hypothyroidism and/or hyperthyroidism often associated with pregnancy. Another form has the characteristics of granulomatous thyroiditis without the pain.
- Rare forms of thyroiditis—suppurative, due to bacterial infection and radiation due to ingested radionuclides or external irradiation
- One form is postpartum onset of goiter and/or hypothyroidism that may resolve spontaneously. Another is painless granulomatous thyroiditis.
- Riedel's thyroiditis—dense infiltration of thyroid and surrounding tissues of unknown cause

System(s) affected: Endocrine/Metabolic
Genetics: N/A
Incidence/Prevalence in USA:

- Not known definitively
- Lymphocytic thyroiditis increases with age, probably up to 10% over age 65
- Granulomatous thyroiditis much less common, has an epidemic pattern

Predominant age: All ages, postpuberty
Predominant sex: Female > Male

SIGNS AND SYMPTOMS

- Lymphocytic thyroiditis
  - —Insidious onset of goiter, often detected incidentally
  - —Slow onset of hypothyroidism
  - —Association with other autoimmune diseases
- Granulomatous thyroiditis
  - —Pain, tenderness and enlargement of one or both thyroid lobes
  - —Malaise, fever
  - —Mild to moderate symptoms of hyperthyroidism
  - —History of recent respiratory infection

CAUSES

- Lymphocytic thyroiditis
  - —Autoimmune response of thyroid tissue
  - —Genetic susceptibility
- Granulomatous thyroiditis
  - —Chronic inflammatory response of thyroid tissue
  - —Preceding infection with any of a variety of viruses

RISK FACTORS

- Lymphocytic thyroiditis
  - —Positive family history of thyroid disease
  - —Preceding autoimmune diseases including type I diabetes, primary adrenal insufficiency, rheumatoid arthritis, pregnancy/delivery
- Granulomatous thyroiditis
  - —Recent viral respiratory infection
  - —Other known cases in the community

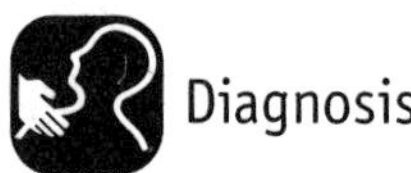

Diagnosis

DIFFERENTIAL DIAGNOSIS

- Lymphocytic thyroiditis
  - —Simple goiter
  - —Iodine-deficient goiter (especially in endemic areas)
  - —Early Graves' disease
  - —Lithium induced goiter
- Granulomatous thyroiditis
  - —Infections of oropharynx and trachea
  - —Hemorrhage into a thyroid cyst
  - —Subacute systemic illness
  - —Suppurative thyroiditis

LABORATORY

- Lymphocytic thyroiditis
  - —Elevated anti-thyroid antibodies (especially high titers of anti-TPO antibodies)
  - —Free thyroxine index (FTI, normal 4.5–12) less than 5 with TSH greater than 5 mcg/dl (normal 0.5–5 mcg/dl)
  - —Thyroid radioactive iodine uptake (RAIU) variable with scintiscan showing patchy distribution of radioiodine
  - —Positive cytopathology of fine needle aspirate or positive formal biopsy
- Granulomatous thyroiditis
  - —Elevated erythrocyte sedimentation rate
  - —Normal or moderately elevated WBC without a granulocyte shift to band forms
  - —FTI greater than 12, TSH undetectable, RAIU less than 5% in 24 hours (often nil) early in course. FTI less than 4.5 with RAIU above normal (greater than 35% in 24 hours in USA) late in course

Drugs that may alter lab results:

- Thyroid
- Corticosteroids
- Iodine containing drugs and contrast media
- Lithium

Disorders that may alter lab results:

- Iodine-deficiency
- Non-thyroidal illness

PATHOLOGICAL FINDINGS

- Lymphocytic thyroiditis
  - —Lymphocytic infiltration
  - —Oxyphilic changes in follicular cells
  - —Fibrosis
  - —Atrophy
- Granulomatous thyroiditis
  - —Giant cells
  - —Mononuclear cell infiltrate

SPECIAL TESTS

- Immunometric assays
- Anti-thyroid antibody titers
- Complete blood count with differential count
- Erythrocyte sedimentation rate

IMAGING

- Thyroid radioiodine uptake and scan in granulomatous thyroiditis
- Ultrasonography if hemorrhage into thyroid cyst suspected

DIAGNOSTIC PROCEDURES

Needle biopsy in confusing cases

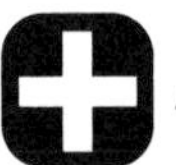

Acute Treatment

APPROPRIATE HEALTH CARE

Outpatient

GENERAL MEASURES

- Analgesics for pain
- Corticosteroids for severe granulomatous thyroiditis

SURGICAL MEASURES

N/A

ACTIVITY

Fully active

DIET

No special diet

PATIENT EDUCATION

N/A

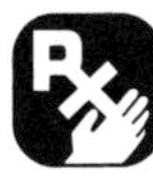

Long-Term Treatment

DRUG(S) OF CHOICE

- Lymphocytic thyroiditis:
  - —Levothyroxine if hypothyroid or goitrous. Generic levothyroxine may not be bioavailable. Carafate, iron preparations may decrease levothyroxine availability. Begin with 25 or 50 g/day and titrate to TSH suppression to lower limit of assay normal range.
  - —Propylthiouracil and propranolol if thyrotoxic and symptomatic
- Granulomatous thyroiditis:
  - —Analgesics, e.g., codeine for pain
  - —Propranolol 40 mg q6h for symptomatic hyperthyroidism
  - —Levothyroxine 80 g per 100 lbs (45.5 kg) body wt/day if hypothyroid phase is symptomatic
  - —Prednisone once daily in lowest effective dose, for severe symptoms
- Maintenance:
  - —Optimal dose can be established by measuring TSH at 6–8 week intervals until dosage level causes TSH to be at the lower level of normal for the assay used

Contraindications:

- Propylthiouracil—allergy or hypersensitivity to analgesics/narcotics
- Propranolol—insulin therapy, asthma
- Prednisone—adverse reactions
- Levothyroxine—none

Precautions: Reduce doses of corticosteroids, propranolol and narcotics as soon as feasible
Significant possible interactions: Sucralfate (Carafate) and iron preparations may decrease levothyroxine availability

ALTERNATIVE DRUGS

Methimazole for propylthiouracil

PATIENT MONITORING

- Repeat thyroid function tests every 3–12 months in lymphocytic thyroiditis
- Repeat thyroid function tests every 3–6 weeks in granulomatous thyroiditis until permanently euthyroid

PREVENTION/AVOIDANCE

N/A

POSSIBLE COMPLICATIONS

Treatment induced hypothyroidism or hyperthyroidism

EXPECTED COURSE/PROGNOSIS

- Lymphocytic thyroiditis—persistent goiter, eventual thyroid failure
- Granulomatous thyroiditis—eventual return to normal over weeks or months

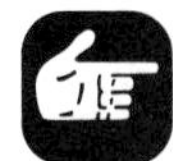

Miscellaneous

ASSOCIATED CONDITIONS

Other autoimmune diseases with lymphocytic thyroiditis including type I diabetes, primary adrenal insufficiency, premature ovarian failure

AGE-RELATED FACTORS

Pediatric: N/A
Geriatric: Remission of granulomatous thyroiditis may be slower in the elderly
Others: N/A

PREGNANCY

- Avoid radioisotope scanning
- Avoid hypothyroidism
- Minimize use of antithyroid drugs

SYNONYMS

- Lymphocytic thyroiditis
- Granulomatous thyroiditis
- Silent thyroiditis
- Hashimoto's disease

ICD-9 CODE

245.0 Acute thyroiditis

See also: Hypothyroidism, Adult; Hyperthyroidism

ABBREVIATIONS

RAIU = radioactive iodine uptake
FTI = free thyroxine index
TSH = thyroid stimulating hormone

BIBLIOGRAPHY

Wilson JD, Foster DW, Konenberg HK, Larson PR (eds). *Williams textbook of endocrinology*. 9th ed. Philadelphia: WB Saunders Co, 1998:454–457;476–478.
Greenspan FS, Strewler GJ, 1997. *Basic and clinical endocrinology*. 5th ed. Stamford, CT: Appleton & Lange, pp 233–247.
DeGroot LW, Larsen PR, Hennemann G. *The thyroid and its diseases*. 6th Ed. Churchill, Livingstone, 1996.
Jacobson DL, et al. Epidemiology and estimated population burden of selected autoimmune diseases in the United States. *Clin Immunol Immunopathol* 1997;84(3): 223–243.
Baker JR Jr: Autoimmune endocrine disease. *JAMA* 1997;10:278(22):1931–1937.

Internet references: http:/www.5mcc.com

Author: Richard P. Levy

Tinea Gladiatorum (Capitis, Corporis, Cruris, Pedis)

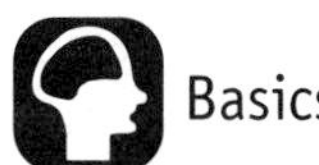

Basics

DEFINITION

This group of topical fungal infections commonly affect athletes, particularly wrestlers. They are classified by site of infection: tinea capitis involves the scalp and hairline; tinea corporis involves the trunk, face, or extremities; tinea cruris involves inguinal folds; tinea pedis involves the feet. Infection is caused by a dermatophyte, most commonly from the *Trichophyton, Epidermophyton,* and *Microsporum* species.

INCIDENCE/PREVALENCE

- Varies from 25% to 35% of all wrestlers during any given season
- 10% to 20% lifetime risk for nonathletes

SIGNS AND SYMPTOMS

Lesions present with erythema, pruritus, and scaling.

RISK FACTORS

- Spread by direct contact with a pet or human carrier
- Fomite transmission occurs from wrestling mat, piece of athletic equipment, shower floor, etc.

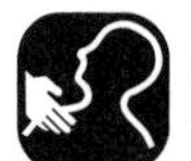

Diagnosis

DIFFERENTIAL DIAGNOSIS

- Tinea capitis: alopecia areata, impetigo, psoriasis, seborrhea, trichotillomania
- Tinea corporis: eczema, psoriasis, contact or atopic dermatitis, drug eruption, cutaneous herpes, lupus, pityriasis rosea
- Tinea cruris: contact dermatitis, candidal intertrigo, erythrasma, psoriasis, seborrhea
- Tinea pedis: eczema, contact or atopic dermatitis, dyshidrosis, pitted keratolysis, psoriasis

HISTORY

- Determine when and where lesions appeared and exposure history.
- Other wrestlers on the team are infected.

PHYSICAL EXAM

- Tinea capitis: erythematous, scaly lesions on scalp or hairline; may be associated with hair loss
- Tinea corporis: circular, erythematous, scaling plaques with central clearing on trunk, face, and extremities
- Tinea cruris: pruritic, scaling, erythematous patches in inguinal folds. If lesions present on penis or scrotum, consider candidal infection rather than tinea.
- Tinea pedis: pruritic, erythematous scaly skin along the sole of foot. Cracking and maceration of the web spaces also may be present.

DIAGNOSTIC TESTS

Scraping of skin lesion in KOH can be examined under the microscope. This will reveal hyphae and pseudohyphae, which are diagnostic of tinea infection. Fungal culture also can be used, but in athletes use is limited by time and expense involved. Tinea infections do not fluoresce under Wood's light examination.

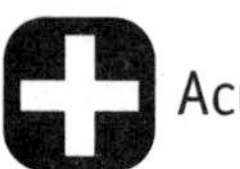

Acute Treatment

SPECIAL CONSIDERATIONS

- Return to play guidelines: length of time to keep out of competition is ill defined because cultures continue to be positive 4 to 6 weeks after treatment with both oral and topical antifungal agents.
- Areas that can be well covered, such as feet and inguinal folds, need not be withheld from competition.
- Tinea corporis should be under treatment for 48 to 72 hours, and the lesion should be well covered before return to contact sports.
- A 1-week pulsed dose of an oral antifungal agent at the beginning and middle of the season could be used to reduce the risk of an athlete acquiring the infection in season.
- Some physicians recommend fluconazole 100 mg once per week during the season. Further studies are needed prior to recommending this as a primary prevention strategy.

MANAGEMENT STRATEGIES

- Primary treatment is with topical antifungal agents.
- Imidazole class: clotrimazole 1% applied twice daily; miconazole 2% applied twice daily; econazole 1% applied once daily; ketoconazole 2% applied once daily; oxiconazole 1% applied once daily; sulconazole 1% applied once or twice daily.
- Benzylamine class: butenafine 1% applied once daily. Length of treatment varies from 2 to 6 weeks with no definitive research at this time to clarify optimal time course. Generally, continue treatment for several days after lesions disappear.
- Initial treatment also may include a topical corticosteroid to help reduce the associated pruritus and erythema.
- Tinea capitis and diffuse, multiple lesions in other areas, should be treated with oral antifungal agents.
- When using oral agents, give consideration to drug interactions, potential for toxicity, and cost of medication.

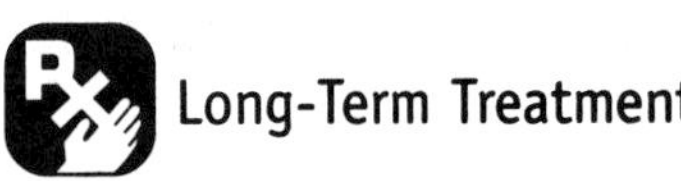

Long-Term Treatment

REFERRAL/DISPOSITION

Most infections are easily treated with topical or oral antifungal agents; therefore, referral is rare. However, for cases that do not respond as expected, further evaluation to rule out an immunocompromised state or other systemic illness should be considered.

MANAGEMENT STRATEGIES

- Prevention is key: emphasize proper personal hygiene, use dry, cotton clothing, and keep athletic equipment disinfected properly.

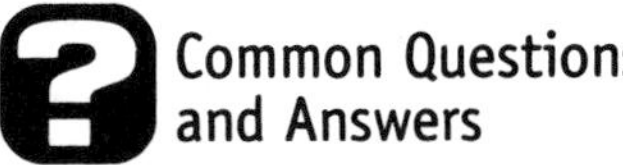

Common Questions and Answers

Physician responses to common patient questions:
Q: Is this infection contagious?
A: Tinea infections are spread from human or pet contact or from fomites. Good hygiene helps prevent these infections.

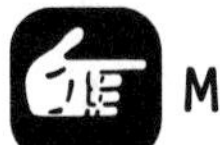

Miscellaneous

SYNONYMS

- Ring worm (tinea corporis)
- Jock itch (tinea cruris)
- Athlete's foot (tinea pedis)

ICD-9 CODE

110.0 Tinea capitis
110.5 Tinea corporis
110.3 Tinea cruris
110.4 Tinea pedis

BIBLIOGRAPHY

DeDoncker P, Gupta AK, Marynissen G, et al. Heremans: itraconazole pulse therapy for onychomycosis and dermatophytosis. *J Am Acad Dermatol* 1997;37:969–974.

Dienst WL, Dightman L, Dworkin MS, et al. Pinning down skin infections. *Phys Sportsmed* 25:45–56.

Hazen PG, Weil ML. Itraconazole in the prevention and management of dermatophytosis in competitive wrestlers. *J Am Acad Dermatol* 1997;36:481–482.

Kohl TD, Martin DC, Berger MS. Comparison of topical and oral treatments for tinea gladiatorum. *Clin J Sport Med* 1999;9: 161–166.

Lesher JL. Oral therapy of common superficial fungal infection. *J Am Acad Dermatol* 1999; 40(suppl):31–34.

Noble SL, Forbes RC. Diagnosis and management of common tinea infection. *Am Fam Physician* 1998;58:163–174.

Sallis RE, Knopp WD. *ACSM's essentials of sports medicine*. St. Louis: CV Mosby, 1997.

Authors: Lisa Barkley and Andrew Reisman

Tinea Versicolor

Basics

DEFINITION

A chronic, asymptomatic, superficial infection of the trunk, neck, and arms caused by the lipophilic yeast Pityrosporum orbiculare or Pityrosporum ovale (some believe that both are different forms of the same organism). Both were previously called Malassezia furfur. This organism is a normal inhabitant of the hair follicles and sebaceous glands.

INCIDENCE/PREVALENCE

Disease may occur at any age, but is much more common during the years of higher sebaceous activity (adolescence and young adulthood).

SIGNS AND SYMPTOMS

- Multiple small circular macules of various colors that enlarge radially
- Lesions may be hyper- or hypopigmented; the color is uniform in each individual.
- The upper trunk is most commonly involved, but it is not unusual for lesions to spread to the upper arms, neck, face, and abdomen.
- The lesions are usually asymptomatic, but they may be pruritic.

RISK FACTORS

- Excess heat and humidity
- Adrenalectomy
- Cushing's disease
- Pregnancy
- Malnutrition
- Burns
- Corticosteroid therapy
- Immunosuppression
- Oral contraceptives
- Individuals with oily skin

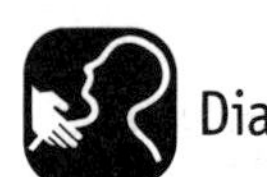

Diagnosis

DIFFERENTIAL DIAGNOSIS

- Vitiligo
- Pityriasis alba
- Seborrheic dermatitis
- Secondary syphilis
- Pityriasis rosea

HISTORY

- Usually asymptomatic, but patients may say that the rash "suddenly appeared," or that the rash appeared gradually.
- Older patients will sometimes have a history of treating this since early adolescence.

PHYSICAL EXAM

- A powdery scale can be easily demonstrated with a no. 15 surgical blade. Wood's light examination shows irregular yellow to white fluorescence; some lesions may not fluoresce.
- A microscopic exam with KOH preparation shows the typical "spaghetti and meatballs" appearance of fungal hyphae and spores.

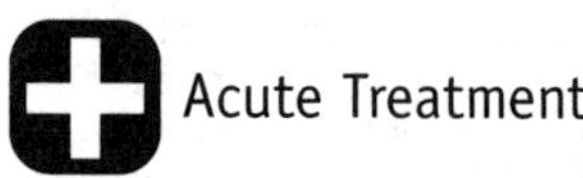

Acute Treatment

TOPICAL THERAPY

- Selenium sulfide shampoo 2.5% applied to the skin for 10 minutes a day for 7 days (87% cure rate). Another schedule is to apply the lotion and wash it off after 24 hours, repeated once a week for a total of 4 weeks.
- Miconazole, clotrimazole, econazole, or ciclopirox is applied to entire affected area twice daily for 2 to 4 weeks.
- Ketoconazole cream is applied once daily for 2 weeks.

SYSTEMIC THERAPY

- Itraconazole is also effective: give 200 mg a day for 5 days (>90% cure rate).

- Systemic treatments may be given to patients who fail topical therapies. Ketoconazole may be given as a single 400-mg dose, or 200 mg a day for 5 days (90% cure rate). The patient should be instructed to work out for an hour or more to facilitate drug excretion in the sweat. Refraining from bathing for an hour after workouts or "sleeping sweaty" allows the drug to accumulate in the skin.
- Fluconazole may be given as a single 400-mg dose (74% cure rate).
- The inability to produce a powdery scale with a no. 15 surgical blade indicates that the fungus has been eliminated. Recurrence rates are high (40% to 60%).

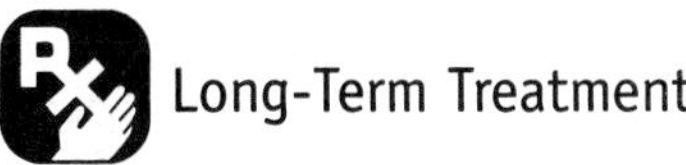

Long-Term Treatment

TOPICAL OR SYSTEMIC THERAPIES

Repeat above treatments as necessary. If patient has multiple recurrences and requires systemic treatments each time, check baseline liver function tests (especially with ketoconazole).

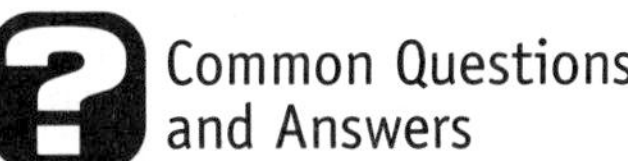

Common Questions and Answers

Physician responses to common patient questions

Q: Will the spots go away?
A: The spots will remain until the skin is exposed to sunlight (tanning accelerates repigmentation).
Q: What can I do to keep it from coming back?
A: Unfortunately, some individuals are predisposed to recurrences. Repeat a treatment program just before the summer months to avoid uneven tanning. Fungal elements may be retained in clothes that are frequently worn; discarding or boiling such clothing might decrease recurrences. Removing sweat-drenched or other wet clothing quickly can make a less favorable environment for fungal growth.
Q: Is it contagious?
A: This is unknown.

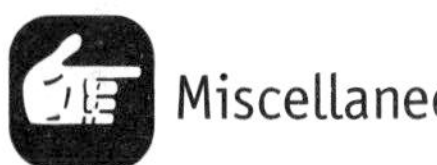

Miscellaneous

SYNONYMS

- Sun spots
- Pityriasis versicolor

ICD-9 CODE

111.0

BIBLIOGRAPHY

Fitzpatrick TB, Johnson RA, Wolff K, et al. *Color atlas and synopsis of clinical dermatology*. New York: McGraw-Hill, 1992.

Habif T. *Clinical dermatology*. St. Louis: Mosby-Year Book, 1996.

Scheinburg R. Stopping skin assailants: fungi, yeasts, and virus. *Physician Sportsmed* 1994;22:35–36.

Authors: Ross M. Patton and James Fambro

Tracheal and Laryngeal Injuries

Basics

DEFINITION

- Trauma to the middle airway involving the region from the hyoid bone superiorly to the trachea
- Injuries rare due to anatomic protection from superior mandible, lateral sternocleidomastoids, inferior clavicle and manubrium, and posterior cervical spine
- Even less common in children because the larynx at the level of C2 is well protected by the mandible (larynx at C6 in adults)
- Injury typically results from crush injury with anterior force compressing airway against rigid cervical spine posteriorly.

INCIDENCE/PREVALENCE

- 0.03% to 1.5% of all trauma patients experience airway injury
- Significant decrease noted with increased use of seat belts
- Hyoid bone and paramedian thyroid cartilage most common laryngeal fracture

SIGNS AND SYMPTOMS

- Subcutaneous emphysema, dysphonia, tachypnea, diaphragmatic breathing with decreased anteroposterior thoracic diameter with inspiration, paradoxic motion of the abdomen, cervical ecchymosis, loss of thyroid prominence
- Stridor and hemoptysis indicative of more significant injury in some studies
- Hoarseness, anterior neck pain, dyspnea, dysphagia, anxiety, foreign body sensation

MORBIDITY/MORTALITY

- Airway injuries second most common cause of death in head and neck trauma; 21% die in first 2 hours, overall mortality 24%
- Laryngeal dislocations, cricoid injuries, 44% mortality
- Isolated tracheal injuries 25%
- Isolated laryngeal injuries 8%
- Long-term morbidity, dysphonia

RISK FACTORS

- Motor vehicle accidents
- Hanging injuries, clothesline injuries
- Contact sports, especially with high-velocity projectiles (i.e., hockey, baseball)
- Weight lifting

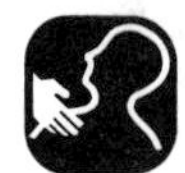

Diagnosis

DIFFERENTIAL DIAGNOSIS

- Soft tissue contusion
- Foreign body
- Asthma
- Upper airway injury (mandibular fracture)
- Lower airway injury (pneumothorax)
- Hyoid bone fracture
- Cricoid fracture
- Cricothyroid joint dislocations
- Laryngotracheal dislocations
- Cricoarytenoid dislocations
- Andolaryngeal hematoma
- Laryngeal cartilage fracture
- Tracheal laceration
- Vocalis muscle tear (especially with dysphonia)

HISTORY

- Mechanism, symptoms, high index of suspicion as often missed in multitrauma patients of injury

PHYSICAL EXAM

- Primary survey crucial: airway, breathing, circulation (ABCs)
- Observe: typically minimal external derangement, even in severe injuries. Examine for deformity, posture, expression, drooling/hemoptysis, respiratory rate, effort, accessory muscles (particularly diaphragm), and associated facial/chest injuries.
- Auscultate: chest (breath sounds, rales), neck (turbulent airflow, stridor)
- Palpate: point tenderness, deformity, subcutaneous emphysema

IMAGING

- Diagnosis is typically made by examination; acute treatment decisions often cannot await imaging studies.
- In less severe injuries, however, diagnostic testing may properly stratify surgical versus nonsurgical management.
- Plain films: obtained once the patient is clinically stabilized.
- Soft tissue lateral neck: often nonspecific, prevertebral/mediastinal air, prevertebral soft tissue swelling, foreign body, narrowed air column, laryngeal cartilage fracture
- Cervical spine films: rule out cervical spine injury before manipulating neck.
- Chest radiograph: rule out associated chest injuries.
- Computed tomography: more specific information, considered by some clinicians as test of choice. Cartilaginous injuries are visualized very well, are hematoma and deep focal paratracheal air. Most recommend CT if there is any suspicion of injury. Thin 2-mm cuts are made through hyoid to the lower edge of the cricoid. Very sensitive for cartilage fracture as well as degree of internal edema.
- Endoscopy: gold standard. Invaluable for assessing mucosal injury, immobile vocal cords, exposed cartilage, displaced fracture, arytenoid displacement, or disruption of anterior commissure, indicating need for operative intervention. Fiberoptic transnasal laryngoscopy is used in the emergency room for mild cases. In moderate/severe cases, it is best to proceed to the operating room (once the airway has been established with tracheotomy) for direct laryngoscopy.
- Barium swallow: may help rule out associated esophageal injury

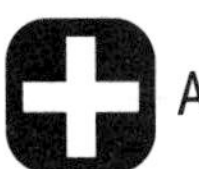

Acute Treatment

ANALGESIA

- Often not warranted in emergent setting
- Topicals avoided even in stable patients due to risk of aspiration
- Tracheotomy achieved with local anesthesia

EMERGENCY MANAGEMENT

- ABCs; stabilize and transport to emergency department
- Ensure adequate airway, most definitively with tracheostomy
- Emergent cricothyrotomy is rarely, but occasionally, necessary. A 14-gauge angiocatheter is inserted through the cricothyroid membrane; ventilate through catheter. The patient must have some patency of airway above for exhalation, and conversion to tracheostomy should be undertaken as soon as feasible. Avoid endotracheal intubation.
- Emergency ENT consultation
- Mild injuries (group I–II) without respiratory compromise: Transnasal fiberoptic laryngoscopy is performed in the emergency room. If there are mild/moderate hematoma/edema, no mucosa tears or displaced arytenoids, and patient remains stable, perform CT scan. If CT scan reveals no fracture, or a nondisplaced fracture, prescribe bed rest, absolute voice rest, head elevation, humidified air, steroids, antibiotics, and histamine blockers. Observation for 24 hours is advised because an initially stable airway may deteriorate rapidly.
- Moderate/severe injuries (group II–V): Ensure adequate airway, tracheostomy. Proceed directly to operating room for direct laryngoscopy. CT can help delineate pathology and help guide surgery. Some surgeons will go straight to open reduction and internal fixation (ORIF) without imaging if direct exam gives clear indications for it.

CLASSIFICATION

- Group I: minor endolaryngeal hematoma without detectable fracture
- Group II: edema, hematoma, minor mucosal disruption without exposed cartilage, nondisplaced fractures noted on CT scan
- Group III: massive edema, mucosal tears, exposed cartilage, cord immobility
- Group IV: more than two fracture lines, or massive trauma to laryngeal mucosa
- Group V: Complete laryngotracheal separation

SPECIAL CONSIDERATIONS

- Associated injuries to esophagus 21%, cervical spine 9% to 50%
- Airway injuries are dynamic, must be followed closely for first 24 to 48 hours

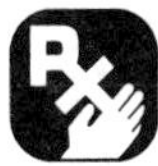

Long-Term Treatment

- Maintain adequate airway, prevent aspiration.
- Antireflux therapy until healed
- Refrain from activity until edema resolved, throat guard until appropriate callus formed
- Absolute voice rest for 2 to 3 days (no talking), relative rest 7 to 10 days (limited use)
- Restore phonation to preinjury quality; patients often require speech phonation therapy secondary to loss of control of true vocal cords due to recurrent laryngeal nerve injury.

SURGICAL TREATMENT

- Controversial, but typically recommended within first 24 hours
- Major indications: tracheotomy for definitive airway management; ORIF for displaced fracture of laryngeal skeleton, exposed cartilage, large mucosal lacerations, expanding subcutaneous emphysema, vocal cord paresis, cricoid cartilage fracture, cricoarytenoid joint disruption, anterior commissure laceration, laceration of free margin of vocal fold, persistent internal bleeding, defining extent of injury if still unclear after direct laryngoscopy and CT

BIBLIOGRAPHY

Bent JP, Silver JR. Acute laryngeal trauma: a review of 77 patients. *J Otolaryngol Head Neck Surg* 1993;109:441–449.

Cherian TA, Rupa V, Raman R. External laryngeal trauma: analysis of thirty cases. *J Laryngol Otol* 1993;107:920–930.

Fuhrman GM, Steig FH, Buerk CA. Blunt laryngeal trauma: classification and management protocol. *J Trauma* 1990;30:87–92.

Ganzel TM, Mumford LA. Diagnosis and management of acute laryngeal trauma. *Am Surgeon* 1989;55:303–306.

Hanft K, Posternack C. Diagnosis and management of laryngeal trauma in sports. *South Med J* 1996;89:631–633.

LeBlang SD, Nunez DB. Advances in emergency radiology. I. Helical CT of the cervical spine and soft tissue injuries of the neck. *Radiol Clin North Am* 1999;37:515–532.

Myers EM, Benny OI. The management of acute laryngeal trauma. *J Trauma* 1987;27:448–452.

Schaefer SD. The treatment of acute external laryngeal injuries: state of the art review series. *Arch Otolaryngol Head Neck Surg* 1991;117:35–39.

Schaefer SD. The acute management of external laryngeal trauma: a 27 year experience. *Arch Otolaryngol Head Neck Surg* 1992;118:598–604.

Sullivan CA, Gotta AW. Problems in the recognition and management of the traumatized airway. *Anesthesiol Clin North Am* 1996;14:13–28.

Yen PT, Lee HY. Clinical analysis of external laryngeal trauma. *J Laryngol Otol* 1994;108:221–225.

Authors: John Lombardo and Aarick Forest

Ultraviolet Keratitis

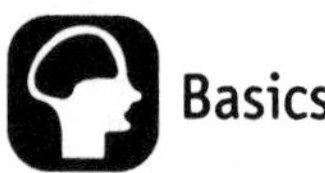

Basics

SIGNS AND SYMPTOMS

- Foreign body sensation
- Increased lacrimation
- Photophobia
- Severe pain
- Blepharospasm
- Decreased visual acuity
- 6–10-hour latent period between exposure and the onset of symptoms
- Worse symptoms associated with increased exposure time and more intense exposure

Ocular Findings

- Conjunctival injection
- Corneal edema
- Iritis (cell and flare in the anterior chamber or spasm of the pupillary sphincter)
- Punctate uptake of fluorescein in an interpalpebral pattern—pathognomonic
- Sloughing of large portions of the cornea may obliterate this finding later in severe cases

MECHANISM/DESCRIPTION

- Prolonged exposure to ultraviolet radiation leads to corneal edema and sloughing, followed by secondary inflammation of the iris
- Sources of ultraviolet radiation
  - —Sun lamps
  - —Welder's arcs
  - —Reflected sunlight (water or snow—worse at high altitude)

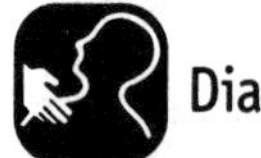

Diagnosis

ESSENTIAL WORKUP

- Accurate history including
  - —Type of exposure
  - —Timing and duration of exposure
- Visual acuity
- Complete ocular exam including
  - —Extraocular movements
  - —Conjunctiva/sclera/corneas with fluorescein
  - —Anterior chambers (checking for cell and flare)
  - —Lenses
  - —Eversion of the lids to check for foreign bodies

LABORATORY

N/A

IMAGING/SPECIAL TESTS

- Orbit radiographs/ultrasound/CT/MRI for suspected intraocular foreign body

DIFFERENTIAL DIAGNOSIS

- Foreign body of the cornea or eyelids
- Intraocular foreign body
- Corneal abrasion
- Chemical exposures
- Thermal burns

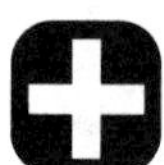

Acute Treatment

INITIAL STABILIZATION

- Topical anesthesia helps to obtain
  - —More accurate documentation of visual acuity
  - —More thorough eye exam and fluorescein staining
  - —Do not prescribe on outpatient basis—interferes with healing and worsens keratitis

ED TREATMENT

- Initiate short-acting cycloplegic for iritis, which usually develops
- Apply topical broad-spectrum antibiotic ointment or drops (less desirable)
- Apply eyepatch in severe cases
  - —Soft double-patching with mild pressure for patient comfort
  - —If both eyes involved, either patch both eyes or the eye that is more severely affected
- Analgesics (acetaminophen/NSAID/codeine/oxycodone)
- Tetanus prophylaxis if needed

MEDICATIONS

- Topical anesthetics
  - —Proparacaine (ophthaine) 0.5% (onset 20–30 seconds; duration 15 minutes)
  - —Tetracaine (pontocaine) 0.5% (onset 30–60 seconds; duration up to 20 minutes)
- Topical antibiotics
  - —Gentamicin, tobramycin
  - —Sulfacetamide
  - —Fluoroquinolones
- Topical cycloplegics
  - —Cyclopentolate 0.5% (onset 30–60 minutes; duration up to 24 hours)
  - —Homatropine 2% (onset 40 minutes to 3–4 hours; duration 24–48 hours)

HOSPITAL ADMISSION CRITERIA

- Patients requiring bilateral patching with severely decreased visual acuity and whose social circumstances make it impossible for the patient to take care of his or her own needs

HOSPITAL DISCHARGE CRITERIA

- Nearly all patients may be discharged from the ED following treatment with cycloplegics, topical antibiotics, and patching
  - —Lesions usually heal completely within 24 hours
- Ophthalmologist referral for patients who have other eye disorders, or for those who fail to improve significantly after 24 hours

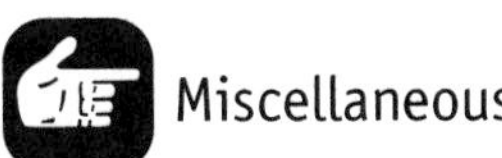

Miscellaneous

ICD-9 CODE

370.20

CORE CONTENT CODE

6.4.2.5

BIBLIOGRAPHY

Lerman S. Direct and photosensitized ultraviolet radiation. In: Fraunfelder FT, Roy FH, eds. *Current ocular therapy*. Sec. 16. 3rd ed. Philadelphia: WB Saunders, 1990:315–320.

Lubeck D, Greene JS. Corneal injuries. *Emerg Med Clin North Am* 1988;6(1):73.

Newell FW. Injuries caused by radiant energy. In: Newell FW, ed. *Ophthalmology: Principles and concepts*. Chap. 8. 7th ed. St. Louis: CV Mosby, 1992:184–185.

Author: Jeffrey Ellis

Ureteral, Bladder, and Urethral Trauma

Basics

DEFINITION

- Sports-related trauma to the trunk and/or perineum can result in contusion, laceration or complete transection of the ureter, bladder, or urethra.
- Ureteral, bladder, and urethral injuries may be associated with pelvic fractures.

INCIDENCE/PREVALENCE

- Fractures of the pelvis can result in injuries to the urethra, bladder, and ureters.
- Ureteral injuries rarely occur as isolated injuries following blunt abdominal trauma.
- Bladder contusion or rupture may occur as a result of lower abdominal blunt trauma and pelvic fractures.
- Although males are susceptible to blunt injury of the urethra, this type of injury is uncommon in females.
- Urethral injuries in children may result from a straddle mechanism (i.e., direct trauma to the perineum commonly due to contact with the cross-bar of a bicycle).
- Impingement of the bulbous urethra against the pubic symphysis results in urethral injuries from the straddle mechanism.
- Straddle injuries in females may result in labial hematoma and urinary retention.
- Most posterior urethral injuries occur by a shearing mechanism.

SIGNS AND SYMPTOMS

- Ureter: flank pain, flank mass (urine or hematoma), hematuria, fever, chills, rarely shock
- Bladder: hematuria, urethrorrhagia, or inability to void
- Urethral: urethrorrhagia and inability to void, especially if pelvic fracture is present or suspected

RISK FACTORS

- Especially in children with multiple injuries, genitourinary injuries are common.
- Although rare, avulsion of the ureter secondary to blunt trauma is known to occur in children.
- Rupture of the bladder may occur following blunt or penetrating trauma. The bladder is especially at risk for injury when full.
- The abdominal position of the bladder in childhood places it at great risk for traumatic injury.

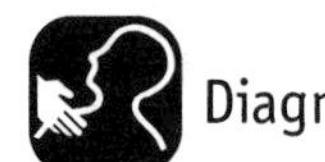

Diagnosis

DIFFERENTIAL DIAGNOSIS

- Hematuria: kidney contusion, kidney laceration, sports induced hematuria, kidney failure, renal calculi
- Inability to void: kidney failure, renal calculi, kidney laceration

HISTORY

- Ureter: trauma to the back or flank, hematuria, expanding flank mass
- Bladder: hematuria, urethrorrhagia, or inability to void following a traumatic injury to the abdomen
- Urethra: trauma to the pelvis possibly resulting in fracture, urethrorrhagia, hematuria, inability to void, lower abdominal or perineum pain.

PHYSICAL EXAM

- Localized tenderness: ureter, flank pain; bladder, abdominal pain; urethra, perineum pain
- Extravasation, especially of the bladder, may result in peritoneal signs.
- Ecchymosis in the pubic area or perineum
- Findings consistent with pelvic fracture
- Ureter: flank mass; lower abdominal pain, chills, fever, urgency, frequency, and pyuria
- Urethra: blood at the meatus; rectal exam reveals a floating or absent prostrate; ecchymosis and swelling of the external genitalia

IMAGING

- Ureter: intravenous pyelography (IVP) is diagnostic.
- Bladder: cystography can establish presence of bladder rupture.
- Urethra: retrograde urethrography is diagnostic.

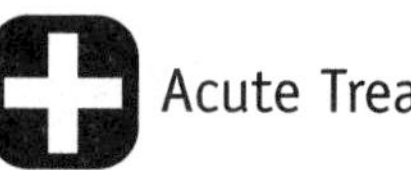

Acute Treatment

ANALGESIA

Oral analgesia may be adequate; however, pain from associated trauma may require intramuscular or intravenous administration of strong narcotics.

SPECIAL CONSIDERATIONS

- Ureteral fistulas and strictures can occur as a result of missed injuries or from entrapment associated with fibrosis from healed dislocation of sacroiliac joints.
- IVP should be performed prior to the cystogram.
- Retrograde urethrography should be performed prior to catheterization in the male athlete who has sustained a pelvic fracture and is unable to void following trauma.

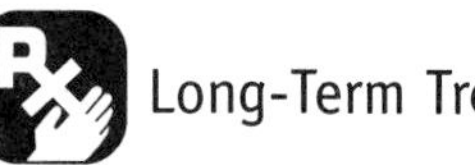

Long-Term Treatment

REHABILITATION

- No specific rehabilitation, but general reconditioning is usually required following the period of convalescence.
- Following surgical procedures, rehabilitation exercises directed at the back or pelvic musculature may be necessary.

SURGICAL TREATMENT

- Transection of the ureter requires prompt repair, ureteropyelostomy.
- Any bladder rupture associated with pelvic fracture where penetration of the bladder by a bony spicule is possible is best managed with surgical debridement.

- Intraperitoneal rupture of the bladder is appropriately treated with transperitoneal exploration, debridement, and repair.
- Initial management of urethral injuries remains controversial. Although early exploration and realignment has been successful, lower complication rates have been found with conservative treatment and delayed realignment.

REFERRAL/DISPOSITION

- Delayed diagnosis of ureteral injury can result in nephrectomy
- Small, uncomplicated, extraperitoneal rupture of the bladder may be managed nonoperatively with a urethral catheter for 7 to 14 days.

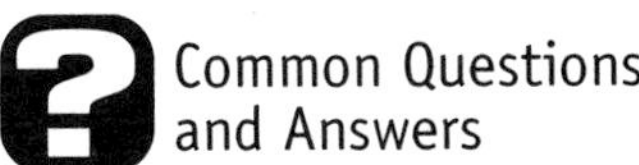

Common Questions and Answers

Physician responses to common patient questions:

Q: Can these types of injuries be prevented?
A: Using sport-specific protective equipment, along with appropriate coaching and officiating, will decrease the likelihood of these rare sports injuries.

Q: Are there any limitations to sports participation following such injuries?
A: Usually these injuries occur after significant trauma. Avoiding high-risk behaviors may decrease the occurrence. However, there is no specific limitation to participation.

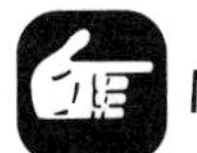

Miscellaneous

ICD-9 CODE

593.3 Stricture or kinking of the ureter
593.4 Other ureteric obstruction
593.82 Ureteral fistula
593.9 Unspecified disorder of kidney and ureter
867.2 Injury to ureter, without open wound into cavity
867.3 Injury to ureter, with open wound into cavity
595 Cystitis
595.9 Cystitis, unspecified
596.0 Bladder neck obstruction
596.6 Rupture of the bladder, nontraumatic
596.7 Hemorrhage into the bladder wall
867.0 Injury to bladder and urethra, without open wound into cavity
867.1 Injury to bladder and urethra, with open wound into cavity
597.8 Urethritis
598 Urethral stricture
598.1 Traumatic urethral stricture
599.1 Urethral fistula
599.7 Hematuria

BIBLIOGRAPHY

Gillenwater JY, Grayshack JT, Howards SS, et al. *Adult and pediatric urology*. St. Louis: CV Mosby, 1998.

Livine PM, Gonzales ET. Genitourinary trauma in children. *Urol Clin North Am* 1985;12: 53–65.

Mandell J, Cromie WJ, Caldamone AA, et al. Sports-related genitourinary injuries in children. *Clin Sports Med* 1982;1:483–493.

Rosen P, Barkin R, Danzl DF. *Emergency medicine: concepts and clinical practice*. St. Louis: CV Mosby, 1998.

Yelon JA, Harrigan N, Evans JT. Bicycle trauma: a five-year experience. *Am Surgeon* 1995;61:202–205.

Author: Robert Baker

Warts

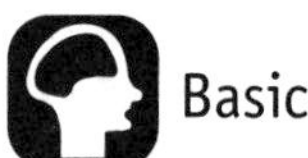

Basics

DEFINITION

A common human papillomavirus (HPV) infection that causes a variety of lesions on the skin and mucous membranes

INCIDENCE/PREVALENCE

- Cutaneous HPV infections. Three types commonly occur: common warts (verruca vulgaris), 70% of cutaneous warts; plantar warts (verruca plantaris), 25% to 30%; and flat warts (verruca plana), 3% to 4%. Warts are uncommon after middle age.
- Mucosal HPV infections. Most common are genital warts (condyloma acuminatum), whose incidence is increasing.

TRANSMISSION AND RISK FACTORS

Cutaneous HPV Infections

- Transmission: direct or indirect contact; minor superficial abrasions of the skin promote infection
- Risk factors: immunocompromised

Mucosal HPV Infections

- Transmission: direct sexual contact; contact with contaminated objects; autoinoculation; during vaginal delivery
- Risk factors: unprotected sexual relations; multiple sex partners

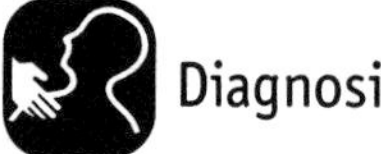

Diagnosis

DIFFERENTIAL DIAGNOSIS

- Verruca vulgaris: corn, guttate psoriasis, molluscum contagiosum, seborrheic keratosis
- Verruca plantaris: callus, corn
- Verruca plana: lichen planus, molluscum contagiosum, seborrheic keratosis
- Condylomata acuminata: lichen planus, pearly penile papules, skin tags, squamous cell carcinoma, syphilis

HISTORY

- Symptoms? Cutaneous and anogenital warts are usually asymptomatic, but plantar warts can cause discomfort during activities.
- Duration of lesion? Without treatment the wart can remain for months to years.
- Diagnosis is usually made by characteristic appearance of lesions.

PHYSICAL EXAM

- Verruca vulgaris (common warts)
  —Skin-colored papule, hyperkeratotic with horny surface
  —Normal skin markings are disrupted.
  —Pathognomonic for warts are red-black dots seen on the surface
  —Can be one or multiple lesions
  —Distribution: fingers, hands (most common), knees, may occur anywhere
- Verruca plantaris (plantar warts)
  —Skin-colored papule with coarse, keratotic surface; has characteristic red-black dots
  —Normal skin markings are disrupted
  —Painful especially over areas of pressure
  —Distribution: plantar surface of foot
- Verruca plana (flat warts)
  —Skin-colored or lightly pigmented; well-defined, smooth, flat or slightly elevated papules
  —Variety of shapes: round, oval, linear
  —Numbers range from a few to hundreds
  —Distribution: face, backs of hands, extremities, especially shins
- Condylomata acuminata (anogenital warts)
  —Skin-colored, slightly pigmented, or pink
  —Range from soft, tiny isolated papules, filiform and often pedunculated sessile papules, to cauliflower resembling masses
  —Distribution: usually on glans penis, prepuce, shaft, labia, vagina, or perianal area; may extend to urethra, bladder, or rectum
  —Subclinical lesions on the genital skin can be visualized as white patches by applying 5% acetic acid to the suspected area
  —Confirmed by biopsy if diagnosis unclear by exam

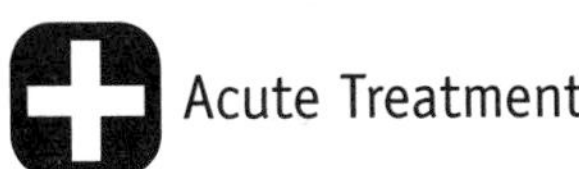

CUTANEOUS LESIONS

- Salicylic acid preparations (10%–40%)
- Cryosurgery (liquid nitrogen): apply to wart and surrounding normal tissue (1 mm) for approximately 10 to 15 seconds; repeat every 4 weeks (may be painful)
- Alternative therapies: electrosurgery; CO_2 laser surgery, or pulsed dye laser (PDL); may be effective for persistent warts

MUCOSAL LESIONS

- Cryosurgery as described above; repeat weekly
- Podophyllin contraindicated during pregnancy
- Trichloroacetic acid 80% to 90%
- Alternative therapies: electrocautery, imiquimod 5%, intralesional interferon, CO_2 laser, PDL

COURSE/PROGNOSIS/ASSOCIATED CONDITIONS

- Cutaneous HPV infection: warts may regress spontaneously; immunocompromised individuals may be refractory to all treatment.
- Condylomata recurs commonly despite therapy.
- Condylomata is associated with cervical dysplasia and cervical squamous cell carcinoma, invasive carcinoma of genitalia, and anal squamous cell carcinoma.

PARTICIPATION/PREVENTION

- Cutaneous lesions: no restrictions for participation; coverage recommended
- Mucosal lesions: condoms recommended but not completely effective
- Anogenital warts: the importance of Pap smears should be stressed; screen for other sexually transmitted diseases

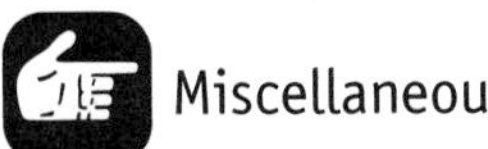

ICD-9 CODE

078.1 Viral warts
078.10 Viral warts, unspecified (verruca: NOS, vulgaris, condyloma NOS)
078.11 Condyloma acuminatum
078.19 Verruca (plana, plantaris)

PROCEDURE CODES

54056 Condylomata cryosurgery
17000 Common or plantar warts (one lesion)
17003 Common or plantar warts (2–14 lesions)
17004 Common or plantar warts (15 or more lesions)
17110 Flat warts (up to 14 lesions)
17111 Flat warts (15 or more lesions)

BIBLIOGRAPHY

Champion RH, Burton JL, Burns DA, et al. *Rook/Wilkinson/Ebling textbook of dermatology*, 6th ed. Oxford, UK: Blackwell Science, 1998.

Fitzpatrick TB, Johnson RA, et al. *Color atlas and synopsis of clinical dermatology*. New York: McGraw-Hill, 1997.

Freedberg IM, Eisen A, et al. *Fitzpatrick's dermatology in general medicine*, 5th ed. New York: McGraw-Hill, 1999.

Goldsmith LA, Lazarus GS, Tharp MD. *Adult and pediatric dermatology: a color guide to diagnosis and treatment*. Philadelphia: FA Davis, 1997.

Monk BJ, Burger RA. Advances in therapy for genital condyloma in women. *Patient Care* 1998;32:53–61.

Authors: Kathleen Weber and Gregory Skaggs

Wolff-Parkinson-White (WPW) Syndrome

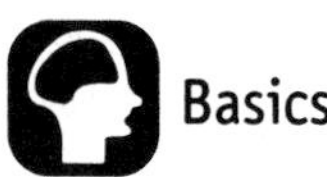

Basics

SIGNS AND SYMPTOMS

- Asymptomatic
- Palpitations
- Dyspnea
- Dizziness
- Nausea
- Abnormal heart rate
  —Rapid and regular (SVT)
  —Irregular (atrial fibrillation)
- Signs of instability
  —Chest pain
  —Hypotension
  —Change in mental status
  —Rales

MECHANISM/DESCRIPTION

- Syndrome caused by ventricular preexcitation via a bundle of Kent
- Type A or orthodromic is the most common (70%)
  —Impulse travels down the A-V node and then up the retrograde pathway
  —A circuit is created that potentiates reentrant tachycardia
- Type B or antidromic
  —Less common than Type A
  —The circuit operates in the opposite direction

ETIOLOGY

N/A

CAUTIONS

- Supplemental oxygen
- Monitor
- Synchronized cardioversion if signs of instability

CONTROVERSIES

- Pre-hospital use of adenosine
  —Stable patients do not require emergent conversion
  —Unstable patients should undergo cardioversion not receive adenosine

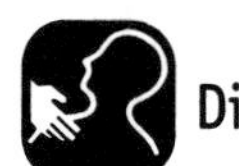

Diagnosis

ESSENTIAL WORKUP

- WPW should be considered as the underlying etiology in all cases of tachydysrhythmias
- The diagnosis should be based on the characteristic EKG findings once the patient has converted to a sinus rhythm
- Electrophysiology studies to assess for radioablation or surgery should be performed as an outpatient

LABORATORY

N/A

IMAGING/SPECIAL TESTS

- EKG
  —Short PR <0.12 seconds
  —Prolonged QRS >0.10 seconds
  —Delta wave
    —Small slurred upstroke at the beginning of the QRS

DIFFERENTIAL DIAGNOSIS

- AV nodal reentry SVT
- Ventricular tachycardia

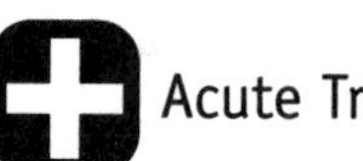

Acute Treatment

INITIAL STABILIZATION

- Unstable patients
  —Synchronized cardioversion starting with 50 J/min
  —Increase incrementally until sinus rhythm is restored

ED TREATMENT

- Stable patients with narrow complex, regular tachycardia
  —Vagal maneuvers such as a Valsalva
  —Right carotid artery massage for no more than 10 seconds

—Auscultate the artery first for a bruit which would contraindicate this procedure
—Fluid replacement and Trendelenburg if the patient has mild hypotension
—Pharmacologic conversion if carotid massage fails
—Adenosine

- Stable patients with irregular wide complex tachycardia
  —Procainamide is the drug of choice
  —Never use calcium channel blockers, β-blockers, or digoxin
  —These medications block the AV node and lead to conduction occurring exclusively down the faster accessory pathway resulting in fatal ventricular dysrhythmias

MEDICATIONS

- Adenosine: 6 mg rapid IV push; if ineffective repeat with 12 mg; peds: 0.1 mg/kg rapid IV push
- Procainamide: 6–13 mg/kg IV at 0.2–0.5 mg/kg/min until arrhythmia controlled, up to a total dose of 1000 mg, then 2–6 mg/min

HOSPITAL ADMISSION CRITERIA

- Patients with signs of instability require admission to a monitored bed
- Failure of outpatient therapy for continuous pharmacological control or ablation

HOSPITAL DISCHARGE CRITERIA

- The majority of patients will be stable and can be discharged once converted to sinus rhythm
- Follow up should be arranged with a cardiologist

Miscellaneous

ICD-9 CODE

426.7

CORE CONTENT CODE

2.4.1.3

BIBLIOGRAPHY

Shah CP. Clinical approach to wide QRS complex tachycardias. *Emerg Med Clin North Am* 1998;16:331–360.

Xie B, Thakur RK, Shah C, et al. Emergency management of cardiac arrhythmias. Clinical differentiation of narrow QRS complex tachycardias. *Emerg Clin North Am* 1998;16: 295–330.

Zipes DP. Specific arrhythmias: Diagnosis and treatment. In: Braunwald E, ed. *Heart disease: A textbook of cardiovascular medicine*. 5th ed. Philadelphia: WB Saunders, 1997:667–675.

Author: Richard Wolfe

SECTION IV

APPENDIX

Office Rehabilitation

Annette Q. Jones and
Kirk D. Jones

Illustrator:
Mariah Steinwinter

The home exercise programs included within this text have been designed to allow the practitioner a means to enable a patient to begin a basic exercise program. The programs consist of a brief introduction of the condition, common causes, signs and symptoms, treatment, and a stretching and strengthening exercise routine with progression. The programs are intended for those patients whose conditions could be managed in this way. For moderate to severe cases, as well as chronic conditions, a referral to a physical therapist is warranted.

Hamstring Strain

WHAT ARE HAMSTRING STRAINS?

A hamstring strain is an injury to the muscles located in the back of the thigh. The injury can consist of a slight tearing of the muscle fibers (first degree) or a moderate tearing (second degree), or be serious enough to cause a complete tear of the muscle (third degree).

COMMON CAUSES

Many factors can cause this type of injury: lack of flexibility, lack of appropriate warm-up and stretching, jumping, fatigue, running mechanics (overstriding, missed step, quick moves), imbalances between the quadriceps and hamstring muscle groups, and/or inadequate rehabilitation following previous injury to this muscle group, causing repetitive trauma.

SIGNS AND SYMPTOMS

Pain and tenderness are felt most commonly in the mid-belly of the muscle. Minor tears involve a smaller area; larger tears would be more widespread. Bruising and swelling at the site of the injury, as well as down the leg even days afterward, can occur. Stiffness with inability to fully extend the knee is associated with the injury. There is weakness of the leg, and walking may be difficult.

TREATMENT

Initially, rest, ice, compression, and elevation above the heart (RICE) treatment is applied for approximately 2 to 3 days following the injury. Icing is performed for 15 to 20 minutes, two to three times during the day. For moderate to severe strains, your physician may prescribe physical therapy for modalities (ultrasound, soft-tissue massage, electrical stimulation), evaluation of weakened/tight muscles, gait analysis, and exercise progression. Crutches should be used if walking is painful. Once walking can be performed without a limp, crutches should be discontinued. Stretching and strengthening exercises, used to promote range of motion and strength, are initiated progressively within 3 to 4 days following injury. Elastic thigh wraps or sleeves can be used for extra support and warmth to the muscles upon returning to sport participation.

STRETCHING

Guidelines for performance and progression of stretching exercises are as follows and/or as prescribed by your physician:

- Keep the stretch to a comfortable level. (Don't force the stretch or cause excessive pain.)
- Do not hold your breath while stretching.
- Hold each stretch for approximately 30 seconds.
- Repeat each stretch three to six times.

STRENGTHENING

Guidelines for performance and progression of strengthening exercises are as follows and/or as prescribed by your physician:

- Do not hold your breath while you lift.
- Stay below the level of pain.
- Do two to three sets of 10 to 15 repetitions two to four times a week. Once you can complete three sets of 15 repetitions easily, increase the weight, reduce the repetitions to 10, and build back up to 15.

HOME EXERCISE PROGRAM

This program is designed to allow you to start with basic exercises. If you should have any questions or difficulties, refer back to your physician.

STRETCHING EXERCISES

Guidelines: Stretch three to six times, holding 30 seconds.
A variety of hamstring stretches are given. Not all have to be performed.

Seated Hamstring Stretch

While seated on the floor or table, extend the injured leg straightforward and bend the opposite leg at the knee into a figure "4" position. Bend forward from the hip over the extended leg with head up. Keep the back and the knee of the injured leg straight.

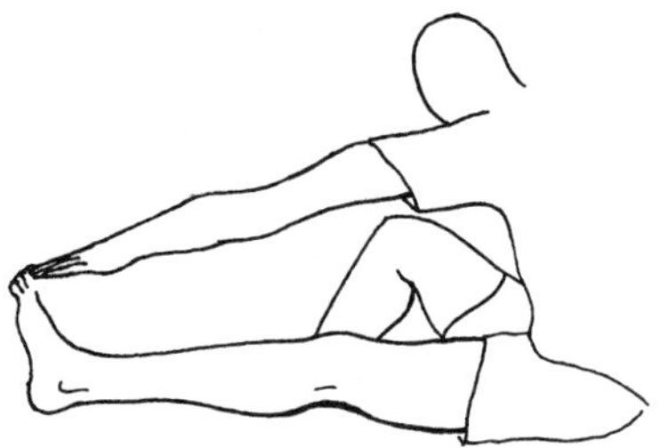

Hamstring Doorway Stretch

Lying on the ground, raise the heel of the injured leg onto the door frame or wall and extend the opposite leg through the doorway. Keep the back and the knee of the injured leg straight. Move closer to the wall to help increase the stretch. Hands can be used to help keep the knee from bending. Keep the upper body and neck relaxed.

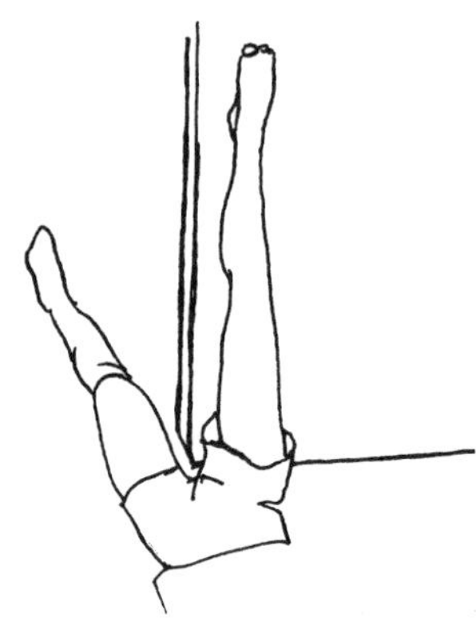

Standing Hamstring Stretch

Place the heel of the injured leg on a bench or stool. Lean forward from the hip over the extended leg. Keep the back and knee of the injured leg straight.

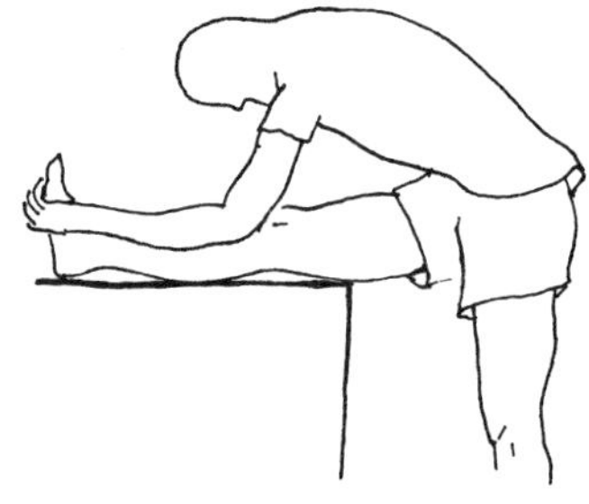

Achilles Stretch

Stand, leaning onto a wall in a lunge position with the injured leg placed further back than the opposite leg. Lunge forward onto the opposite leg while keeping the knee of the injured leg straight and the heel on the ground. Stretch is felt in the calf.

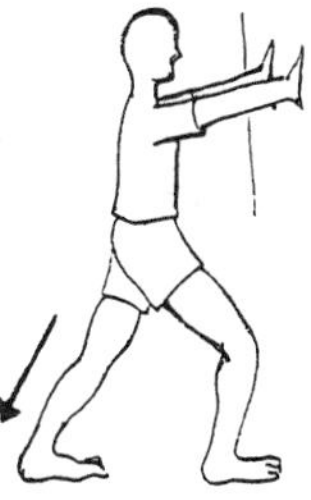

STRENGTHENING EXERCISES

Guidelines: Start with three sets of 10 repetitions, if able (fewer, if unable); progress to three sets of 15 repetitions. Once this is accomplished easily, reduce the repetitions to three sets of 10 and increase the weight intensity.

Standing Hamstring Curls

Support yourself with a chair or counter in front of you. Bend the injured leg at the knee while keeping the thigh pointed straight down. You can begin with no weight and then progress to ankle weights.

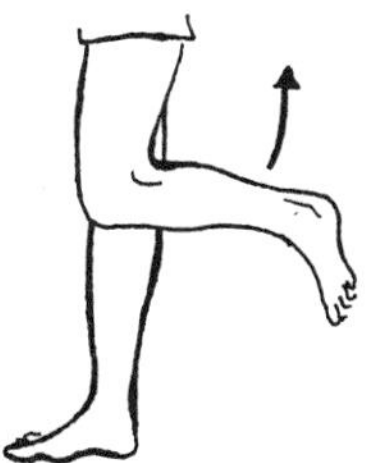

Prone Hamstring Curls

Lying on your stomach, bend the knee of the injured leg toward your buttocks. You can begin with no weight and then progress to ankle weights.

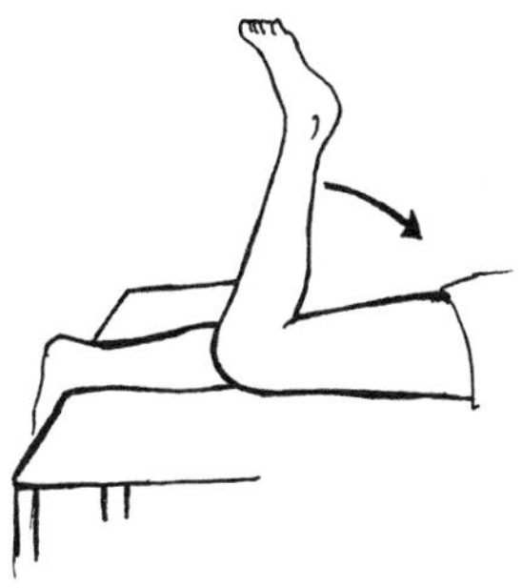

Bilateral Heel Raises

Stand with your feet shoulder-width apart. Raise the heels off the ground onto the balls of the feet. Fingertips can be placed on a counter for light balance.

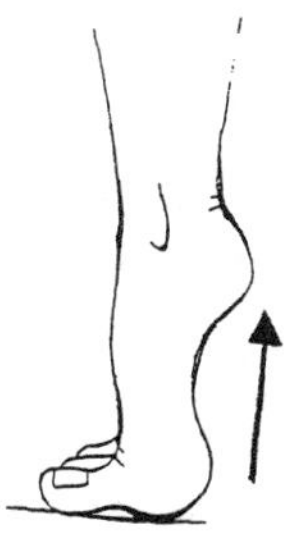

Single Heel Raise

Same as for bilateral heel raises, but using the injured leg only

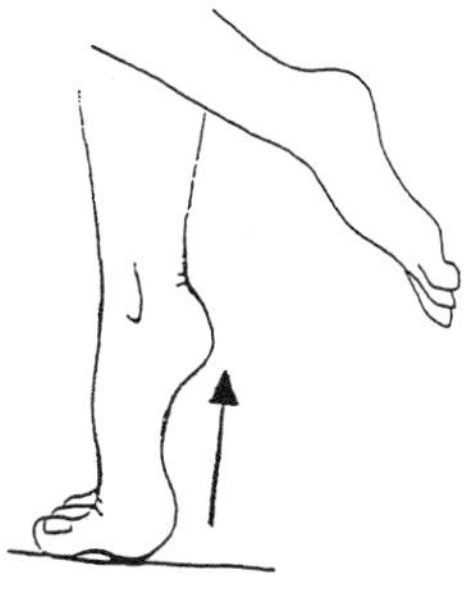

Bicycling

Begin cycling at an easy pace, with progression of speed, resistance, and time.

Jogging, Running, Sprinting (Straight Lines)

Start easy jogging in straight lines first. Progress speed and distances gradually.

Jogging, Running, Sprinting (Figure 8s and Zig-Zag Patterns)

Jog slowly, making a pattern of large figure 8s, and progress to smaller and smaller patterns with increasing speed. Jog in zig-zag patterns with large cuts first and then progress to sharper cuts with increasing speed.

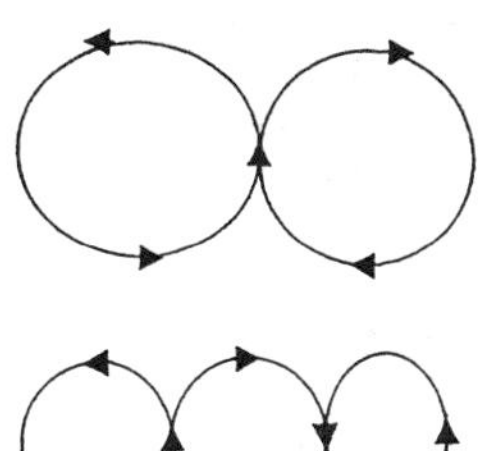

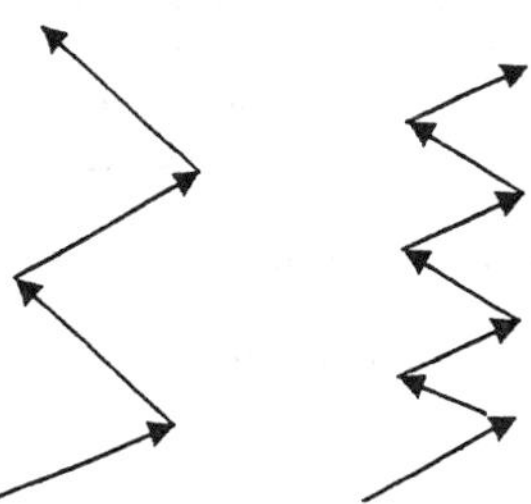

Hopping/Jumping (Front, Back, Side to Side)

Begin by hopping with both feet up and down and progress to front, back, and side-to-side movements. Further progression is achieved by hopping in these same patterns with the affected leg only. Advance to jumping with these same criteria.

Patella Femoral Pain Syndrome

WHAT IS PATELLA FEMORAL PAIN SYNDROME?

Patella femoral pain syndrome is pain localized to the kneecap (patella). The patella is encased within the quadriceps tendon, which is attached to the tibia (shin bone) by way of the patellar tendon. The patella slides back and forth in between grooves located at the end of the femur (thigh bone). Normally, there is a relatively small angle created by the line of the quadriceps muscle pull from the hip, the center of the kneecap, and the insertion of the tendon into the shin bone. With repeated motion in this area, the undersurface of the kneecap can become irritated and inflamed and, eventually, can wear out (chondromalacia), especially if a malalignment is present. The important factor with this condition is to determine the cause.

COMMON CAUSES

Many causes have been attributed to this condition:

- Pronation of the feet (a rolling inward of the feet, with a flattening of the arch), which causes the knees to bend inward (knock-knee)
- Anatomic variance such as wide hips, knock-knees, and/or a lateral placement of the insertion of the patellar tendon onto the shin bone, which increases the angle of muscle pull and then draws the patella toward the outside of the knee
- Anatomic variance in the size and shape of the patella and/or femoral grooves
- Weakness or fatigue of the quadriceps and hamstrings
- Poor mechanics
- Decreased flexibility
- Overuse in activities such as running, jumping, cycling, and walking
- Tightness in the lateral knee structures

SIGNS AND SYMPTOMS

There is pain about the patella, with possible swelling, depending on how much the knee is used. Grinding may be felt or heard with knee movements. Pain occurs with walking, running, and prolonged sitting. Eccentric contractions, such as squatting and walking down stairs or hills, are usually aggravating factors.

TREATMENT

Initially helpful is rest and ice two to three times per day for 15 to 20 minutes. Icing is beneficial as long as the inflammatory condition continues. Ice can be applied after activity and/or rehabilitation to help decrease pain and muscle spasm. Antiinflammatory drugs are sometimes prescribed. Stretching and strengthening exercises, used to promote range of motion and strength, are initiated when pain is decreased. The use of orthotics (a shoe insert, used to help improve malalignments) may be necessary. Physical therapy can be prescribed by your physician to help with evaluation of weakened and/or tight muscles, gait analysis, application of modalities in moderate to severe cases (ultrasound and electrical stimulation), and overall progression of exercises. Knee bracing or patellar taping can be beneficial when attempting to strengthen the knee. If the condition has progressed to severe chondromalacia, surgery may be necessary. Surgical anatomic correction is sometimes performed as well.

STRETCHING

Guidelines for performance or progression of stretching exercises are as follows and/or as prescribed by your physician:

- Keep the stretch to a comfortable level. (Don't force the stretch or cause excessive pain.)
- Do not hold your breath while stretching.
- Hold each stretch for approximately 30 seconds.
- Repeat each stretch three to six times.

STRENGTHENING

Guidelines for performance or progression of strengthening exercises are as follows and/or as prescribed by your physician:

- Do not hold your breath while you lift.
- Stay below the level of pain.
- Do two to three sets of 10 to 15 repetitions two to four times a week. Once you can complete three sets of 15 repetitions easily, increase the weight, reduce the repetitions to 10, and build back up to 15.

HOME EXERCISE PROGRAM

This program is designed to allow you to start with basic exercises. If you should have any questions or difficulties, refer back to your physician.

STRETCHING EXERCISES

Guidelines: Stretch three to six times, holding 30 seconds.

Seated Hamstring Stretch

While seated on the floor or table, extend the injured leg straight forward and bend the opposite leg at the knee into a figure "4" position. Bend forward from the hip over the extended leg, with your head up. Keep the back and the knee of the injured leg straight.

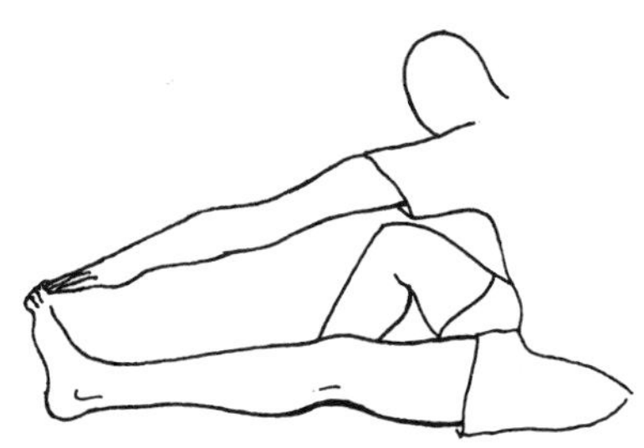

Iliotibial Band Stretch

Stand with the involved leg crossed in back of the opposite leg. Slowly lean toward the "good" leg by bending at the waist. You can lean into a wall or balance by lightly touching a chair. Stretch should be felt at the side of the hip and down the involved leg.

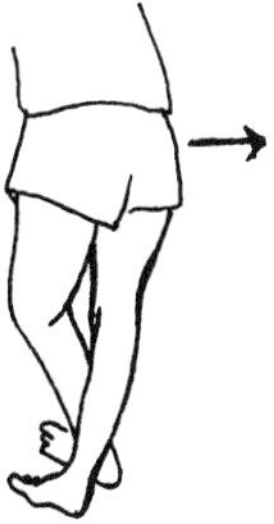

Quadriceps Stretch

Stand in back of a chair for assistance with balance. Hold the top of the foot of the involved leg with the hand of the same side. Slowly bend the knee backward toward the buttocks.

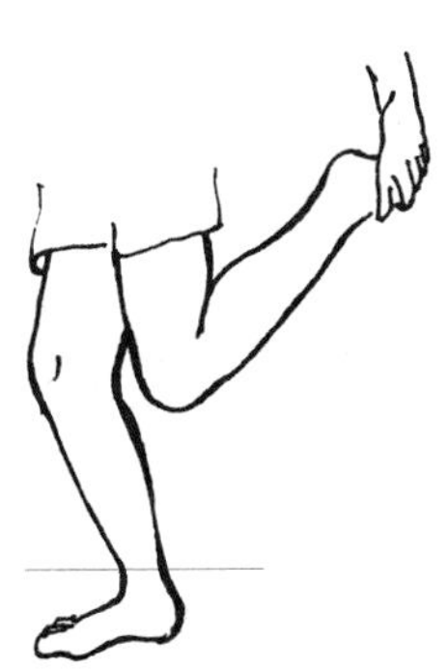

Achilles Stretch

Stand, leaning onto a wall in a lunge position with injured leg placed further back then opposite leg. Lunge forward by bending the good leg while keeping the knee of the injured leg straight and the heel on the ground. Stretch is felt in the calf.

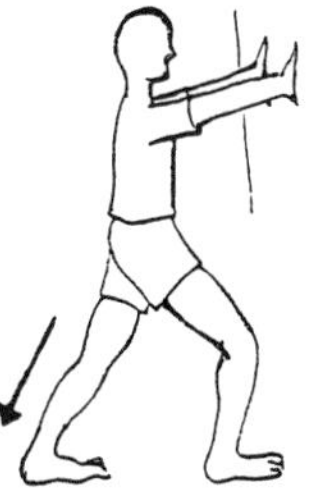

STRENGTHENING EXERCISES

Guidelines: Start with three sets of 10 repetitions if able (less if unable); progress to three sets of 15. Once this is accomplished easily, reduce repetitions to three sets of 10 and increase the weight intensity.

Quadriceps Set (Quad Set)

Place a small, rolled-up towel under the involved knee. Slowly tighten the top thigh muscle while pushing the back of the knee into the towel. The kneecap can be seen to move upward. Stay within pain-free range as you attempt to progress to a full contraction with a fully extended leg. Hold the contraction 6 to 8 seconds and repeat 10 times.

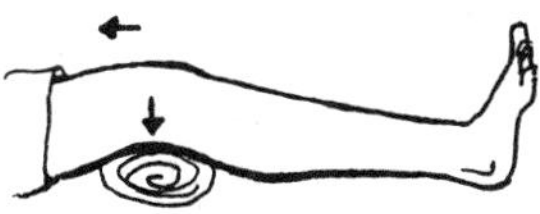

Towel Squeeze

Long sit on a table, with legs extended and a towel roll placed above the knees and between the thighs. Squeeze the towel roll by bringing your thighs together and digging your heels into the table. The feet are in a V position. Hold the contraction for 6 to 8 seconds and repeat 10 times.

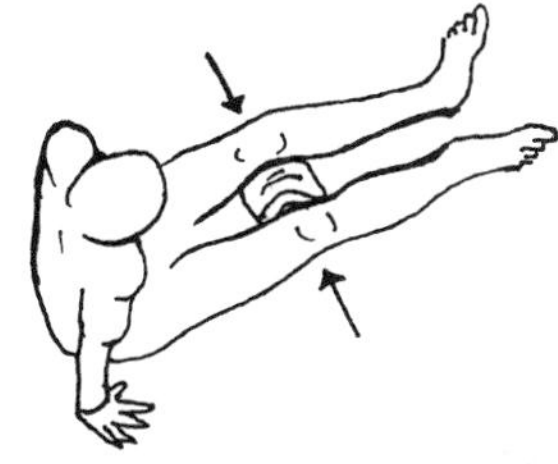

Straight-Leg Raises

Straight-leg raises can be performed once you can maintain a quad set with little to no discomfort.

- Hip Flexion: Lying on your back, bend the uninvolved knee so that the foot is on the table. Perform a quad set with the injured leg, and then lift the leg up to the level of the opposite knee.

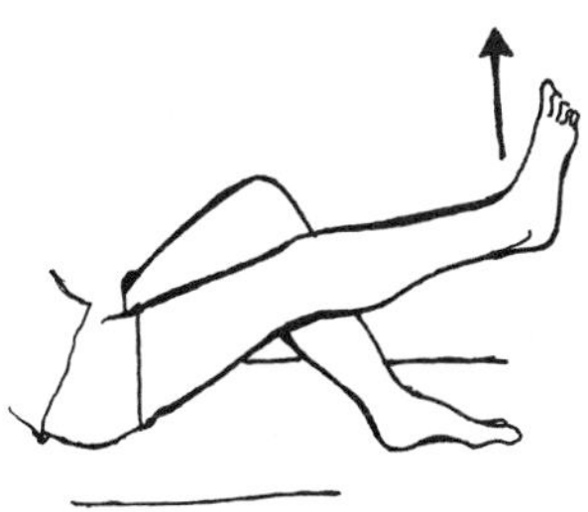

- Hip Abduction: Lying on the uninvolved side, perform a quad set and then raise the leg to a 30-degree angle. You can bend the bottom knee for balance (not shown in illustration).

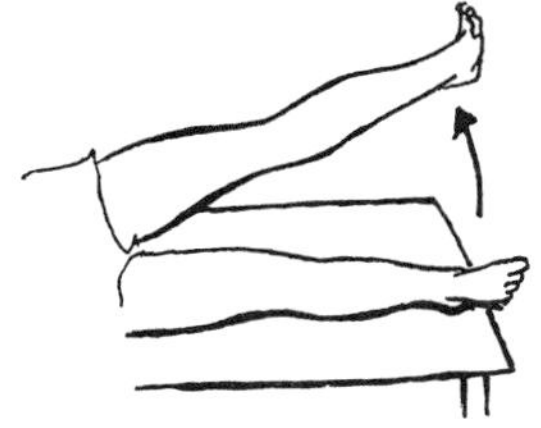

Patella Femoral Pain Syndrome

- Hip Adduction: Lying on the involved side, take the opposite leg, bend the knee, and place the foot on the table in front of you. With the involved leg straight, perform a quad set and lift the leg 4 to 6 inches.

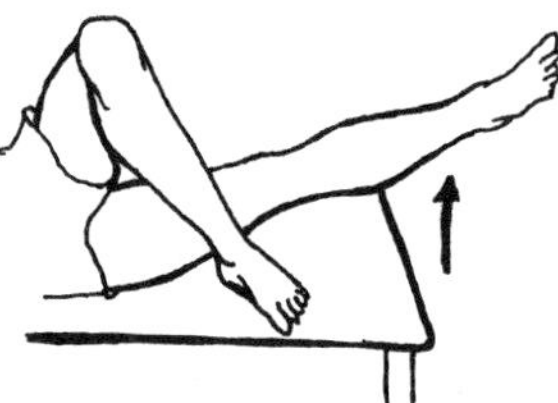

- Hip Extension: Lying flat on your stomach, with both legs straight, perform a quad set with the involved leg and lift the leg 4 to 6 inches. The back should not arch or rotate with this exercise. A small, rolled-up towel could be used under the involved thigh to help prevent compression of the kneecap on the table.

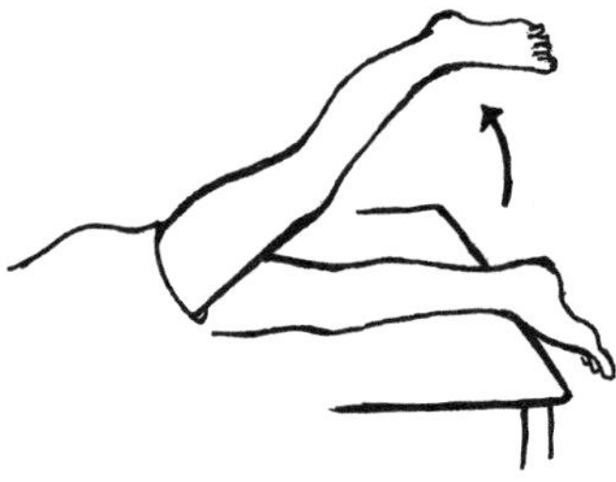

Short-Arc Knee Extension

Long sit on a table. Place a rolled-up towel under the involved leg, allowing the knee to flex to 15 degrees (small bend). Slowly straighten the knee toward full knee extension. Progress to a larger towel roll by increasing the angle of knee bend.

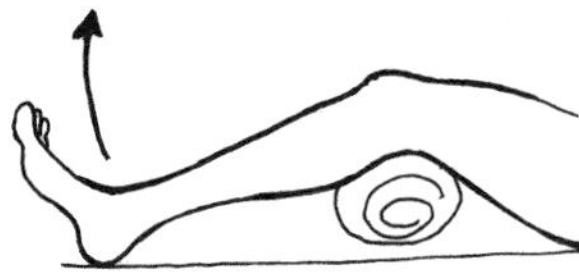

Knee Extension

Seated on the edge of a table, extend the knee through its range. Add ankle weights for progression.

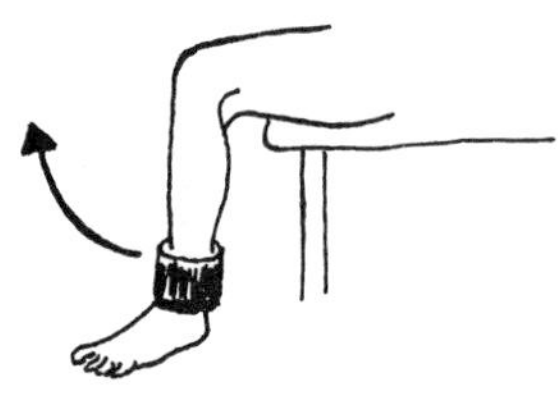

Prone Hamstring Curls

Lying on your stomach, bend the knee of the injured leg toward your buttocks. You can begin with no weight and then progress to ankle weights.

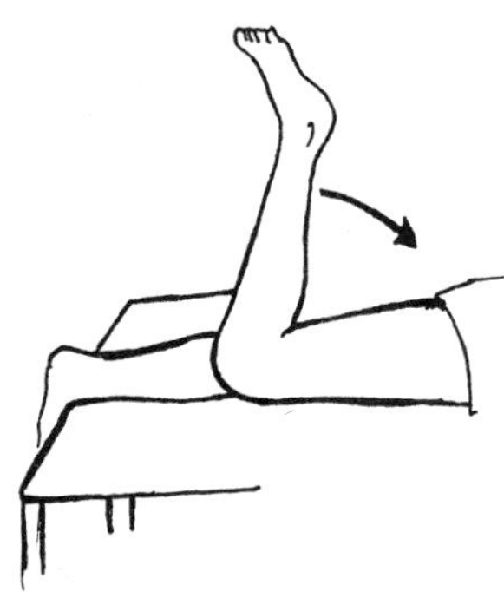

Step Ups

Begin with a 2-inch step. Step up with the involved leg, followed by the good leg. Step down with the good leg, followed by the injured leg. Progress to larger steps, such as 4 inches and then 6 inches. Progression is made only as symptoms allow. No pain should be felt when performing this exercise. Perform one set of 10 repetitions (or fewer, if unable). Progress to three sets of 10, followed by an increase in the height of the step, whereby repetitions are again decreased to one set.

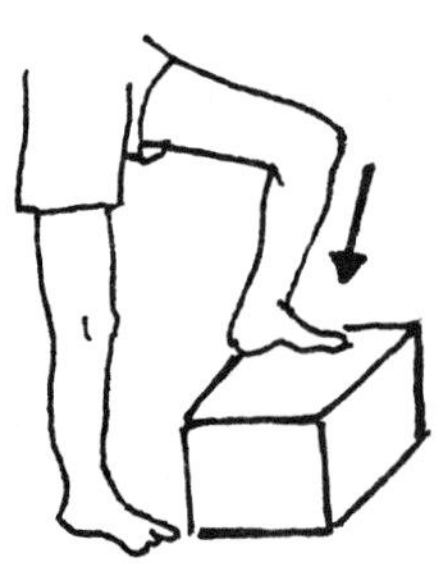

Lateral Step Up

This is a progression of the forward step up. Place the involved leg laterally on a 2-inch step and the uninjured leg on the floor beside it. Raise the toes of the uninjured leg so that the heel of this leg is its only contact with the floor. Raise your body to the level of the step by extending the involved leg. Slowly lower your body by bending the knee of the involved leg so that the heel of the good leg contacts the floor once again. Do not allow the hip to drop to reach the floor. Progress to larger steps, such as 4 inches then 6 inches. No pain should be allowed with this exercise. Perform one set of 10 repetitions (or fewer, if unable). Progress to three sets of 10, followed by an increase in the height of the step, whereby repetitions are again decreased to one set.

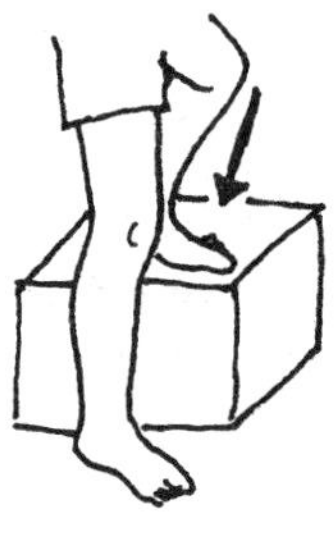

Wall Slides

Stand with your back against a wall and your feet a shoulder-width apart. Slowly squat by sliding down the wall. Progress the squat from one-fourth to one-half as symptoms allow. Placing a ball between thighs and squeezing as you squat can enhance this exercise. Perform one set of 10 repetitions, progressing to three sets of 10 to 15 repetitions. Further strength progression can be achieved by holding progressive weights in your hands.

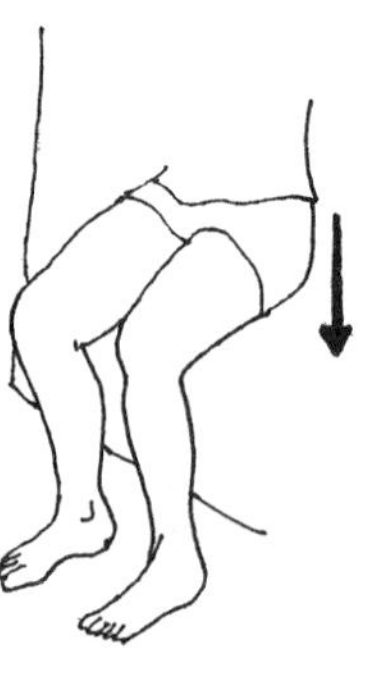

Leg Press

Leg press machines can be utilized, limiting the amount of knee motion to pain-free ranges and then progressing to the full range.

Lunges

Start with a step forward with the involved leg and slowly bend at the knee to a minimal degree, then return to a standing position. Progress this exercise by increasing the degree of knee bend and by utilizing progressive hand weights or bars. Perform one set of 10 repetitions, progressing to three sets of 10 to 15.

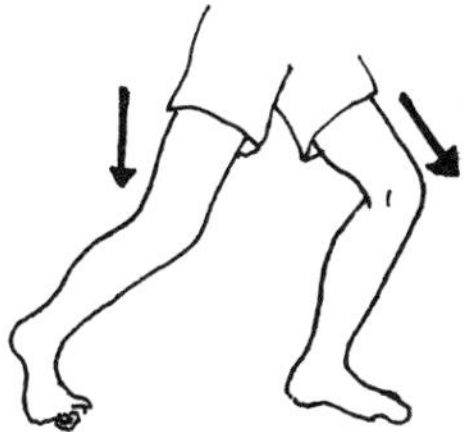

Bilateral Heel Raises

Stand with your feet a shoulder-width apart. Raise your heels off the ground and roll your weight onto the balls of your feet. Fingertips can be placed on a counter for light balance. To continue to improve strength, progress to standing heel raises on weight machines.

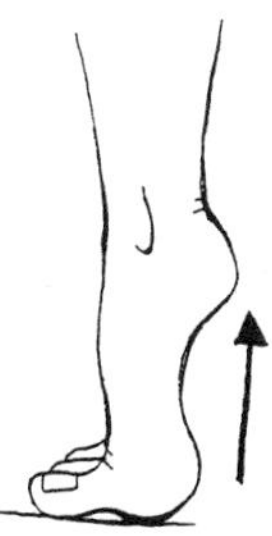

Single-Heel Raise

Same as for bilateral heel raises, but using the injured leg only

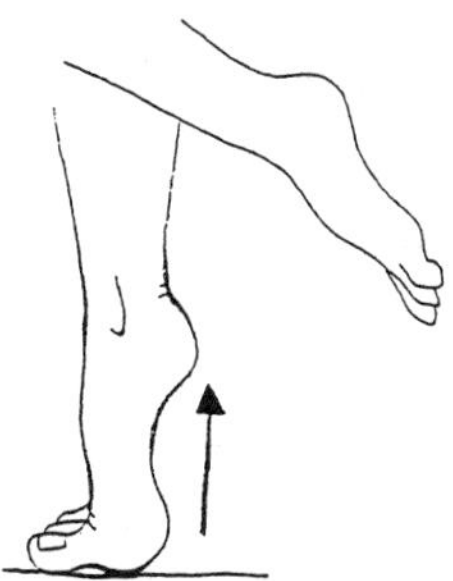

Bicycling

Begin cycling at an easy pace, with progression of speed, resistance, and time.

Jogging, Running, Sprinting (Straight Lines)

Start easy jogging in straight lines first. Progress speed and distances gradually.

Jogging, Running, Sprinting (Figure 8s and Zig-Zag Patterns)

Jog slowly, making a pattern of large figure 8s, and progress to smaller and smaller patterns with increasing speed. Jog in zig-zag patterns with large cuts first and then progress to sharper cuts with increasing speed.

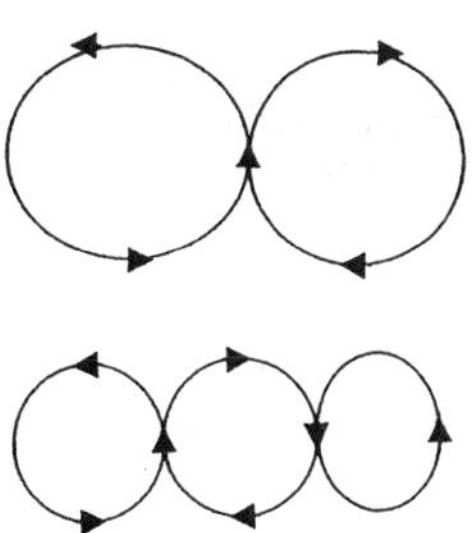

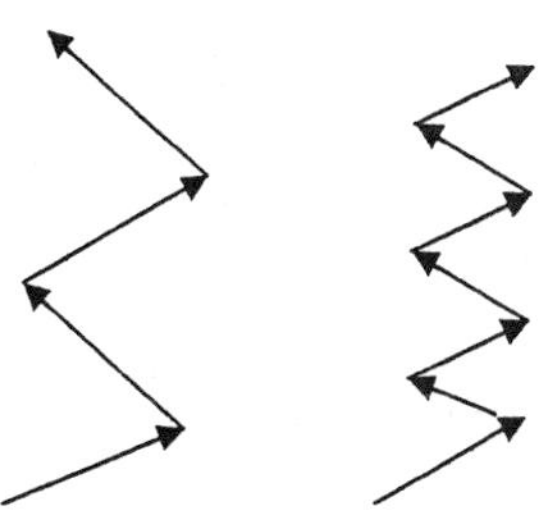

Hopping/Jumping (Front, Back, Side to Side)

Begin by hopping with both feet up and down and progress to front, back, and side-to-side movements. Further progression is achieved by hopping in these same patterns with the affected leg only. Advance to jumping with these same criteria.

Ankle Sprains

WHAT IS AN ANKLE SPRAIN?

An ankle sprain is a tear of the ligaments that help to support the ankle joint. The injury can be minimal, involving microscopic tears, or can completely rupture the supporting structures. The most common type of ankle sprain is termed *inversion* and involves the ligaments on the outside of the joint.

COMMON CAUSES

An ankle sprain occurs when the foot is taken beyond its normal range of motion. This can happen when the foot lands on an uneven surface and the pressure of a person's body weight is forced onto the outside of the foot. An inversion sprain involves the foot turning inward. The foot also can turn outwardly and injure the inside of the ankle, causing an *eversion* type of sprain.

SIGNS AND SYMPTOMS

Pain, swelling, and/or bruising along either the inside or the outside of the ankle joint

TREATMENT

Initially, rest, ice, compression, and elevation above the heart (RICE) treatment is used for approximately 2 to 3 days following the injury. Icing is performed for 15 to 20 minutes two to three times during the day. Antiinflammatory medications may be used to help decrease pain and swelling. Early weight bearing to pain tolerance should be conducted and can be assisted by the use of crutches. When walking can be performed without a limp, use of crutches should be discontinued. Stretching and strengthening exercises, used to promote range of motion and strength, are then initiated. Physical therapy may be prescribed by your physician to help with application of modalities (whirlpool, ultrasound, electrical stimulation, soft-tissue massage), gait analysis, evaluation of ankle range of motion, along with assessment of weak muscles and overall exercise progression in moderate to severe cases. Ankle taping or braces could be used to help with prevention of further episodes but should not be used as a substitute for exercises.

STRETCHING

Guidelines for performance and progression of stretching exercises are as follows and/or as prescribed by your physician:

- Keep the stretch to a comfortable level. (Don't force the stretch or cause excessive pain.)
- Do not hold your breath while stretching.
- Hold each stretch for approximately 30 seconds.
- Repeat each stretch three to six times.

STRENGTHENING

Guidelines for performance and progression of strengthening exercises are as follows and/or as prescribed by your physician:

- Do not hold your breath while you lift.
- Stay below the level of pain.
- Do two to three sets of 10 to 15 repetitions two to four times a week. Once you can easily complete three sets of 15 repetitions, increase the weight, reduce the repetitions to 10, and build back up to 15.

HOME EXERCISE PROGRAM

This program is designed to allow you to start with basic exercises. If you should have any questions or difficulties, refer back to your physician.

STRETCHING EXERCISES

Guidelines: Stretch three to six times, holding 30 seconds.

Ankle Pumps (To Reduce Swelling)

Elevate your foot higher than heart level. Move the ankle up and down 30 times. Rest a minute and then repeat four to five times. Ice the ankle at the same time.

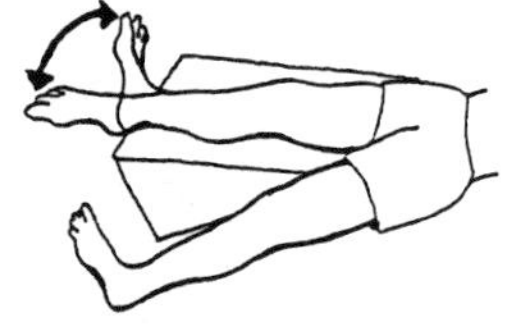

Towel Stretch (Achilles)

Assume a seated position, with legs extended. Place a towel around your foot and hold the ends with both hands. Pull back on the towel, bringing your foot toward you.

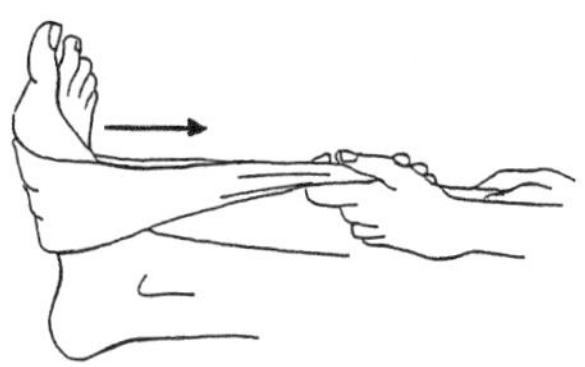

Achilles Stretch

Stand, leaning onto a wall, with the involved foot placed further back than the other foot. Lunge forward onto your uninjured foot while keeping the knee straight and the heel of involved leg on the ground. Stretch is felt in calf.

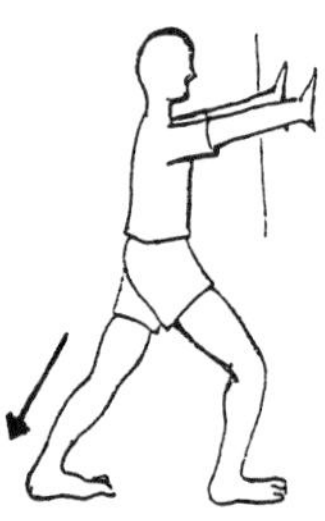

Bent-Knee Stretch

Same as for the Achilles stretch, but the involved leg is bent at the knee. Stretch is felt in the calf.

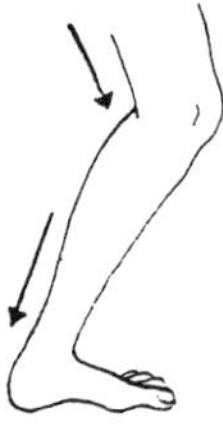

Squats

With your feet shoulder-width apart and your heels remaining on ground, bend your knees until stretch is felt in the calf and ankles.

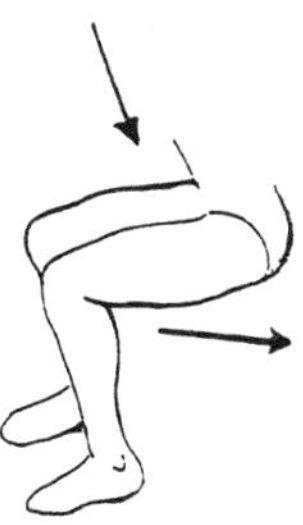

STRENGTHENING EXERCISES—BEGINNING PHASE

Guidelines: Start with three sets of 10 repetitions, if able (fewer, if unable); progress to three sets of 15. When this is accomplished easily, reduce the repetitions to three sets of 10 and increase the weight.

Towel Crunches

Assume a seated position. Place a towel on the floor (not on a carpet). Place the involved foot on top of the towel and curl your toes, gathering the towel underneath and toward you. Repeat 10 times, advance to three sets of 10 to 15 repetitions, and then add weight to the towel. Begin again with fewer repetitions, advancing to three sets of 10 to 15 repetitions.

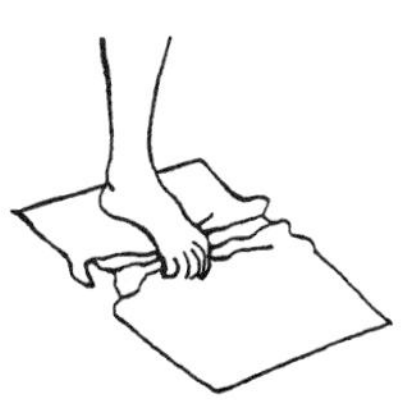

Isometric Inversion/Eversion

Assume a seated position. Place the inside of your foot against an immovable object (e.g., a table leg) and push against it. Then repeat the same exercise with the outside of your foot against the object. Hold the contraction for 6 to 8 seconds and repeat 10 times.

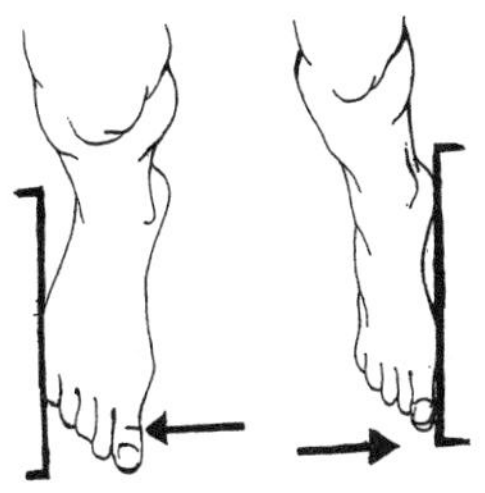

Marble Pick-Up

Assume a seated position. Place several marbles on the floor and attempt to pick them up by curling your toes around them. Once a marble is lifted, turn the foot and place the marble back down on the floor a foot or so away. Repeat for total of 30 repetitions.

Weight Shifts

Stand with your feet a shoulder-width apart. Your hands are placed on a counter or table to help support the weight of your body. Lean your body weight over to the affected ankle and shift your weight back and forth between the two legs. Progress until full weight is placed on the affected ankle. Hold for 10 to 30 seconds; repeat three to six times.

STRENGTHENING EXERCISES—MIDDLE PHASE

Single-Leg Balance (Eyes Open/Closed)

Assume a standing position, with feet a shoulder-width apart. Stand on the affected ankle, as tolerated, working up to 30 seconds with your eyes open. Progress to balancing for 30 seconds with your eyes closed. Repeat three to five times.

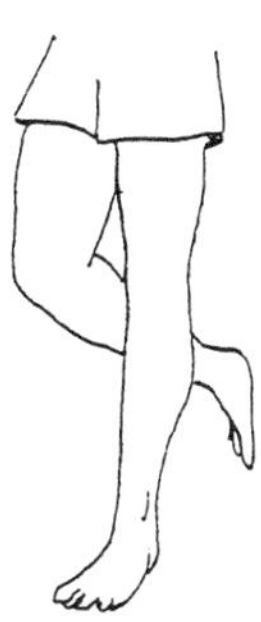

Ankle Sprains

Thera-Band Exercises

With the use of a Thera-Band, wrap one end of the band onto an immovable object and the other end around the mid-foot. Avoid hip movement.

- Ankle movement is toward you.

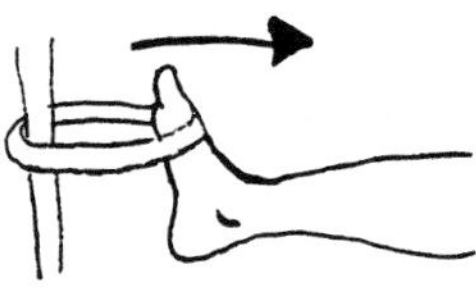

- Ankle movement is toward the little toe side.

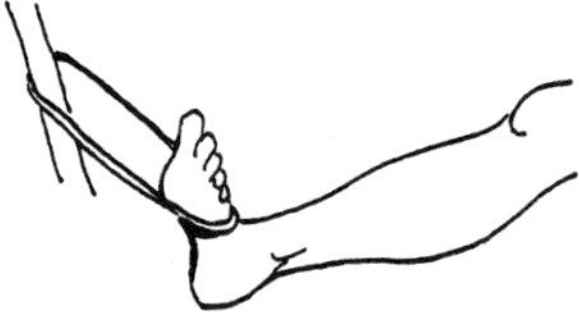

- Ankle movement is toward the big toe side.

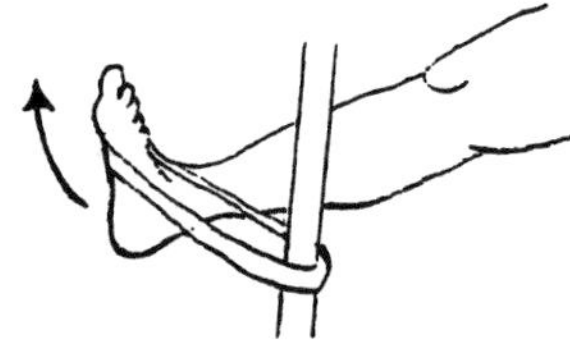

Start with one set of 10 repetitions, progressing to three sets of 10 to 15 repetitions. When you can achieve this easily, advance the color of the Thera-Band and begin again with three sets of 10 to 15 repetitions.

Bilateral Heel Raises

Stand with your feet a shoulder-width apart. Raise your heels off the ground onto the balls of your feet. Fingertips can be placed on a counter for light balance. You can progress to weight machines, performing same action with increasing weight intensity.

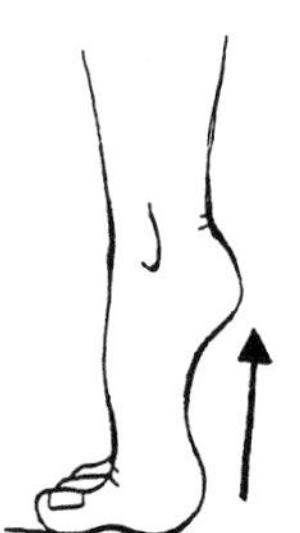

STRENGTHENING EXERCISES—FINAL PHASE

Heel Raise (Single Leg)

Raise the heel of the affected ankle up and down. Fingertips can be placed on a counter for light balance. You can progress to weight machines, performing the same actions with added weight intensity.

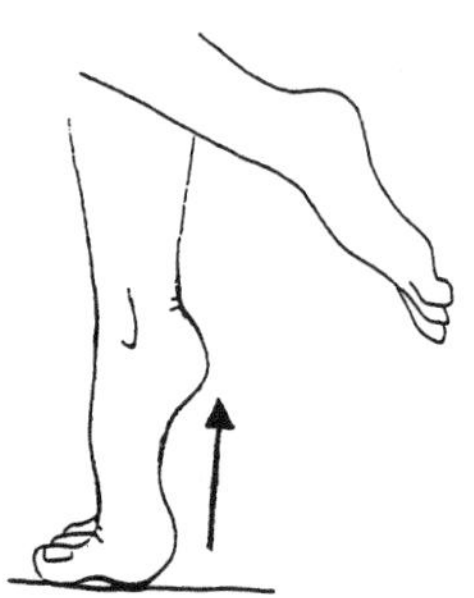

Hopping (Front, Back, Side to Side)

Begin by hopping with both feet up and down and progress to front, back, and side-to-side movements. Further progression is achieved by hopping in these same patterns with the affected ankle only.

Jogging, Running, Sprinting (Straight Lines)

Start easy jogging in straight lines first. Progress speed and distances gradually.

Jogging, Running, Sprinting (Figure 8s and Zig-Zag Patterns)

Jog slowly, making a pattern of large figure 8s, and progress to smaller and smaller patterns with increasing speed. Jog in zig-zag patterns with large cuts first and then progress to sharper cuts with increasing speed.

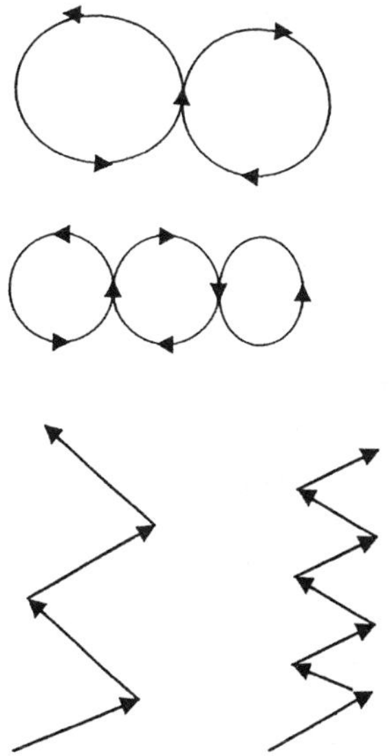

Shin Splints (Medial Tibial Stress Syndrome)

WHAT ARE SHIN SPLINTS?

The term *shin splints* has been a "wastebasket" term used to describe pain about the lower leg. More recently, it has been used to identify pain occurring about the front or medial side of the lower leg. The term *medial tibial stress syndrome,* or *MTSS,* is now being used frequently. The condition itself may be an inflammation of either muscle or bone involving the tibia or shinbone. The involved muscles include the posterior tibialis, flexor hallucis longus, and flexor digitorum longus. Your physician must differentiate this condition from stress fractures or compartment syndromes.

COMMON CAUSES

- Overuse, especially at the start of sport seasons, from excessive running or jumping
- Pronated feet (an inward turning of the foot, which causes stretching of the involved muscles)
- Fallen arches
- Types of training surfaces (softer ground may allow for increased foot pronation)
- Shoes with broken-down medial borders
- Running on slanted surfaces along roads
- Weakness in the involved muscle groups

SIGNS AND SYMPTOMS

Pain can be felt when touching the area just behind the shinbone from above the medial ankle bone and extending upward by more than half way. Pain can be produced with walking and/or running.

TREATMENT

Initially, rest and ice two to three times per day for 15 to 20 minutes is helpful. Icing is beneficial as long as the inflammatory condition continues. Ice can be applied after activity and/or rehabilitation to help decrease pain and muscle spasm. Antiinflammatory medications are used to help decrease pain and swelling. Crutches may need to be used if walking causes pain. Training can continue in the pool or by cycling as long as no pain is felt. Orthotics (a shoe inset used to help correct foot malalignments) may be prescribed if pronation cannot be corrected with strengthening. Supportive taping of the lower leg is of benefit. Physical therapy may be prescribed by your physician to help with application of modalities (ultrasound and/or electrical stimulation), gait analysis, evaluation of weak or tight muscles, and overall exercise progression in moderate to severe cases.

STRETCHING

Guidelines for performance or progression of stretching exercises are as follows and/or as prescribed by your physician:

- Keep the stretch to a comfortable level. (Don't force the stretch or cause excessive pain.)
- Do not hold your breath while stretching.
- Hold each stretch for approximately 30 seconds.
- Repeat each stretch three to six times.

STRENGHTENING

Guidelines for performance or progression of strengthening exercises are as follows and/or as prescribed by your physician:

- Do not hold your breath while you lift.
- Stay below the level of pain.
- Do two to three sets of 10 to 15 repetitions two to four times a week. When you can complete three sets of 15 repetitions easily, increase the weight, reduce the repetitions to 10, and build back up to 15.

HOME EXERCISE PROGRAM

This program is designed to allow you to start with basic exercises. If you should have any questions or difficulties, refer back to your physician.

STRETCHING EXERCISES

Guidelines: Stretch three to six times, holding for 30 seconds.

Achilles Stretch

Stand, leaning onto a wall, with involved foot placed further back than the other foot. Lunge forward onto the uninjured foot while keeping the knee straight and the heel of the involved leg on the ground. Stretch is felt in calf.

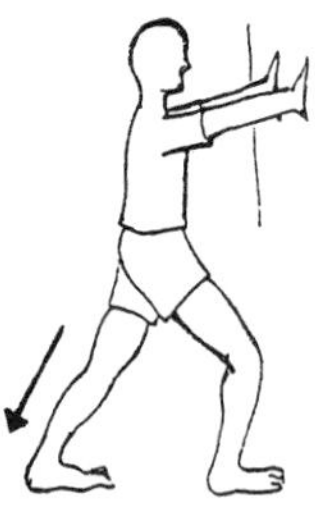

Bent-Knee Stretch

Same as for the Achilles stretch, but the involved leg is bent at the knee. Stretch is felt in the calf.

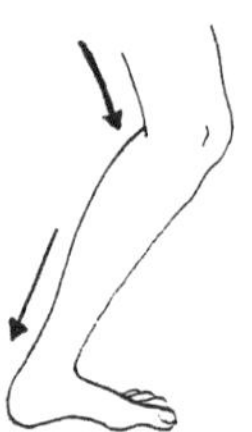

Pointed-Toe Stretch

While seated, with the involved leg bent into a figure 4 position, grasp the top of the foot and stretch the foot downward into a pointed position. Stretch is felt in the top of the foot.

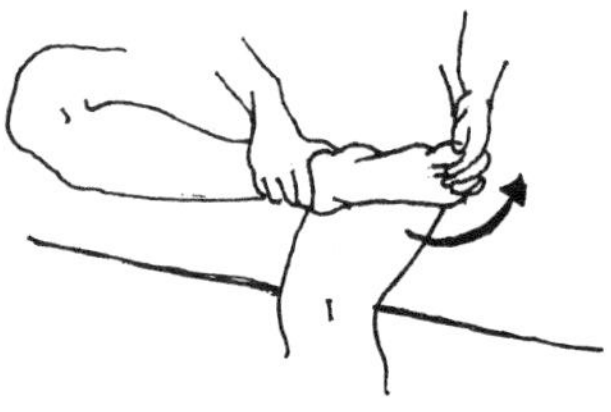

STRENGTHENING EXERCISES

Guidelines: Start with three sets of 10, if able (fewer, if unable); progress to three sets of 15 repetitions. When this is accomplished easily, reduce the repetitions to three sets of 10 and increase the weight.

Towel Crunches

Assume a seated position. Place a towel on the floor (not on a carpet). Place your foot on top of the towel and curl your toes, gathering the towel underneath and toward you.

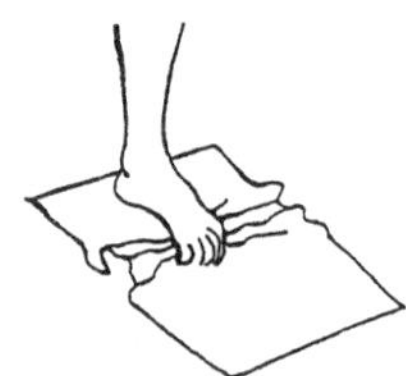

Marble Pick-Up

Assume a seated position. Place several marbles on the floor and attempt to pick up them up by curling your toes around them. Once a marble is lifted, turn your foot and place back down on the floor a foot or so away. Repeat for a total of 30 repetitions.

Heel Walking

Walk on your heels, starting with short distances, such as 10 to 15 feet, progressing to 50 feet.

Thera-Band Exercises

With the use of Thera-Band, wrap one end of the band onto an immovable object and the other end around your mid-foot. Avoid hip movement.

- Ankle movement is toward you.

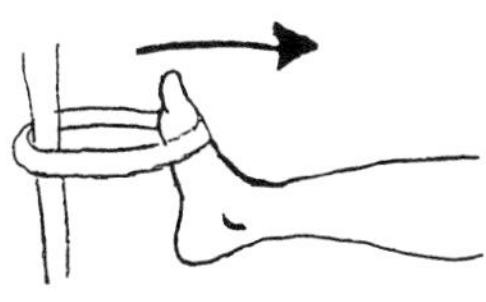

- Ankle movement is toward the little toe side.

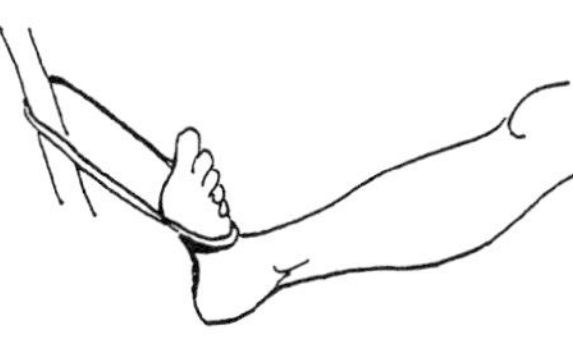

- Ankle movement is toward the big toe side.

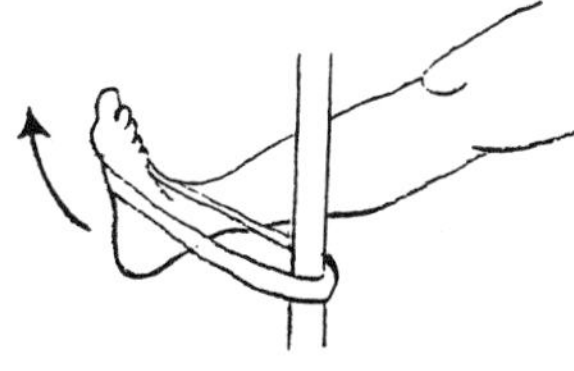

Start with one set of 10 repetitions, progressing to three sets of 10 to 15 repetitions. Once you can achieve this, advance the color of the Thera-Band and begin again toward three sets of 10 to 15 repetitions.

Bilateral Heel Raises

Stand with your feet shoulder-width apart. Raise your heels off the ground and roll your weight onto the balls of your feet. Fingertips can be placed on a counter for light balance. You can progress to weight machines, performing same action, with increasing weight intensity.

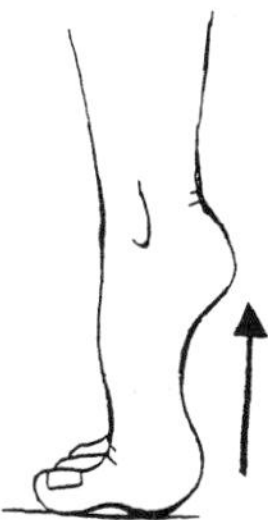

Heel Raise (Single Leg)

Raise the heel of the affected ankle up and down. Fingertips can be placed on a counter for light balance. You can progress to weight machines, performing the same actions for added weight intensity.

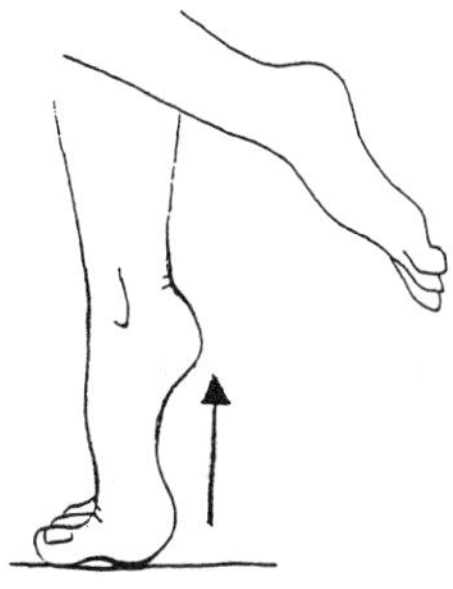

Hopping (Front, Back, Side to Side)

Begin by hopping with both feet up and down and progress to front, back, and side-to-side movements. Further progression is achieved by hopping in same patterns with the affected ankle only.

Jogging, Running, Sprinting (Straight Lines)

Start easy jogging in straight lines first. Progress speed and distances gradually.

Jogging, Running, Sprinting (Figure 8s and Zig-Zag Patterns)

Jog slowly, making a pattern of large figure 8s, and progress to smaller and smaller patterns with increasing speed. Jog in zig-zag patterns with large cuts first and then progress to sharper cuts with increasing speed.

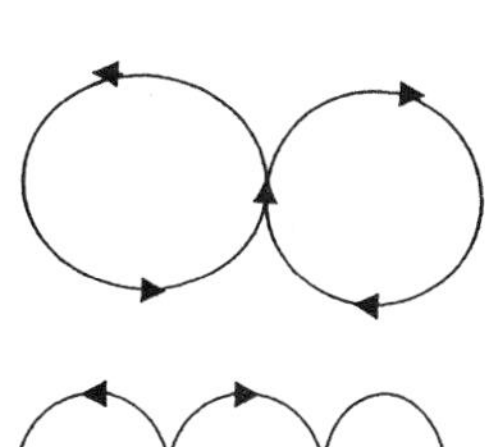

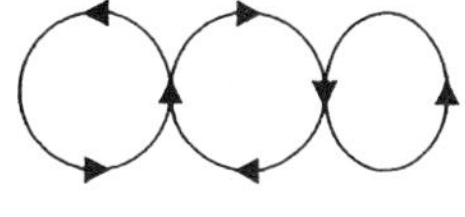

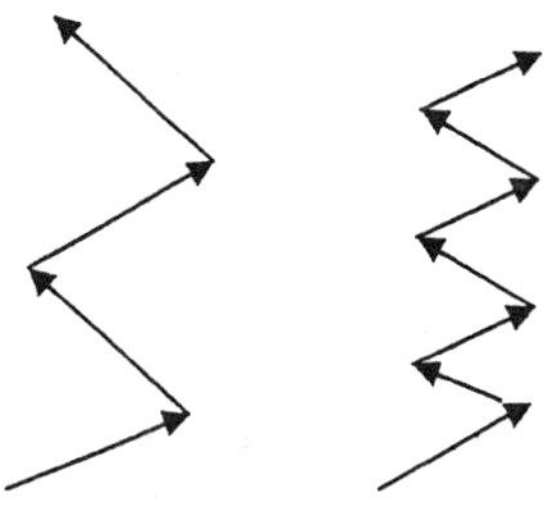

Plantar Fasciitis (Heel Spur Syndrome)

WHAT IS PLANTAR FASCIITIS?

The plantar fascia is a broad band of connective tissue that runs from the calcaneus (heel bone) to the heads of the metatarsal bones in the foot. Its purpose is to provide arch support. This tissue can become inflamed, causing pain to this area.

COMMON CAUSES

- Tight Achilles tendon
- Overuse, especially at the start of sport seasons, from excessive running or jumping
- Pronated feet (an inward turning of the foot, which causes stretching of the involved muscles
- Fallen arches
- Types of training surfaces (softer ground may allow for increased foot pronation)
- Shoes with broken-down medial borders
- Weakness in the involved muscle groups

SIGNS AND SYMPTOMS

Pain is primarily located along the front part of the heel where the connective tissue becomes narrow. Touching this area may produce pain, and it could extend along the tissue into the arch. Upon awakening, the first steps may be very painful to perform due to the stretch being placed on the tissue. Extending the toes upward also causes pain in this area.

TREATMENT

Initially, rest, medication, and ice two to three times per day for 15 to 20 minutes are helpful. Icing is beneficial as long as the inflammatory condition continues. Ice massage to this area is very beneficial. It can be applied after activity and/or rehabilitation to help decrease pain. Antiinflammatory medications are used to help decrease pain and swelling. Sometimes, cortisone injections are administered. Stretching and strengthening exercises, used to promote range of motion and strength, are initiated when pain is decreased. Taping the arch is helpful. Proper footwear is a necessity, and the use of orthotics (a shoe insert used to correct foot malalignments) may be necessary. Physical therapy may be prescribed by your physician to help with evaluation of weakened and/or tight muscles, gait analysis, application of modalities in moderate to severe cases (ultrasound, soft-tissue massage, and electrical stimulation), and overall progression of exercises.

STRETCHING

Guidelines for performance or progression of stretching exercises are as follows and/or as prescribed by your physician:

- Keep the stretch to a comfortable level. (Don't force the stretch or cause excessive pain.)
- Do not hold your breath while stretching.
- Hold each stretch for approximately 30 seconds.
- Repeat each stretch three to six times.

STRENGTHENING

Guidelines for performance or progression of strengthening exercises are as follows and/or as prescribed by your physician:

- Do not hold your breath while you lift.
- Stay below the level of pain.
- Do two to three sets of 10 to 15 repetitions two to four times a week. Once you can complete three sets of 15 repetitions easily, increase the weight, reduce the repetitions to 10, and build back up to 15.

HOME EXERCISE PROGRAM

This program is designed to allow you to start with basic exercises. If you should have any difficulties, refer back to your physician.

STRETCHING EXERCISES

Guidelines: Stretch three to six to times, holding for 30 seconds.

Achilles Stretch

Stand, leaning onto a wall with the involved foot placed further back than the other foot. Lunge forward onto the good foot while keeping the knee straight and the heel of the involved leg on the ground. Stretch is felt in the calf.

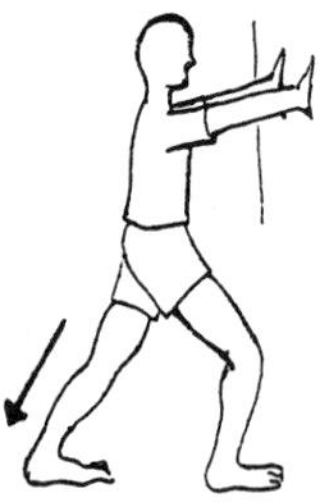

Bent-Knee Stretch

Same as for Achilles stretch, but the involved leg is bent at the knee. Stretch is felt in the calf.

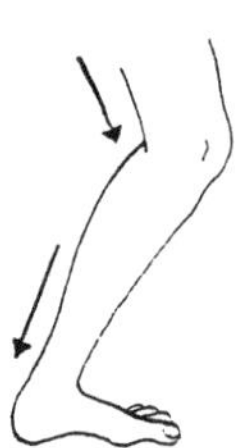

Pointed-Toe Stretch

While seated, with the involved leg bent into a figure 4 position, grasp the top of the foot and stretch the foot downward into a pointed position. Stretch is felt in the top of the foot
.

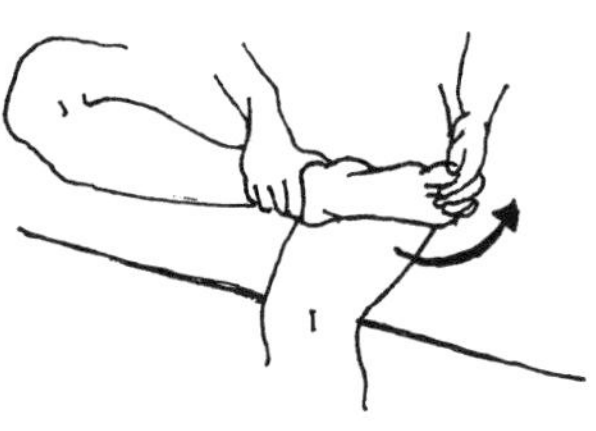

STRENGTHENING EXERCISES

Guidelines: Start with three sets of 10 repetitions, if able (fewer, if unable); progress to three sets of 15. Once this is accomplished easily, reduce the repetitions to three sets of 10 and increase the weight intensity.

Towel Crunches

Assume a seated position. Place a towel on the floor (not on a carpet). Place your foot on top of the towel and curl your toes, gathering the towel underneath and toward you.

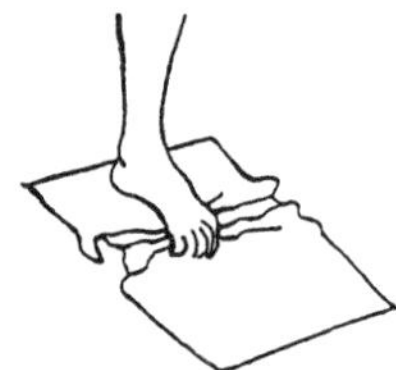

Marble Pick-Up

Assume a seated position. Place several marbles on the floor and attempt to pick them up by curling your toes around them. Once a marble is lifted, turn your foot and place the marble back down on the floor a foot or so away. Repeat for total of 30 repetitions.

Thera-Band Exercises

With the use of Thera-Band, wrap one end of the band onto an immovable object and the other end around your mid-foot. Avoid hip movement.

- Ankle movement is toward you.

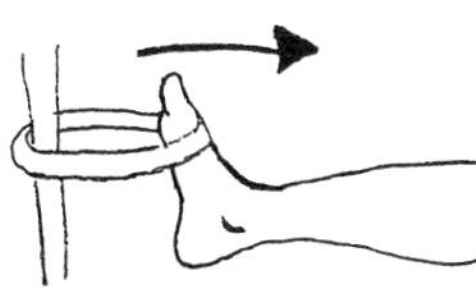

- Ankle movement is toward the little toe side.

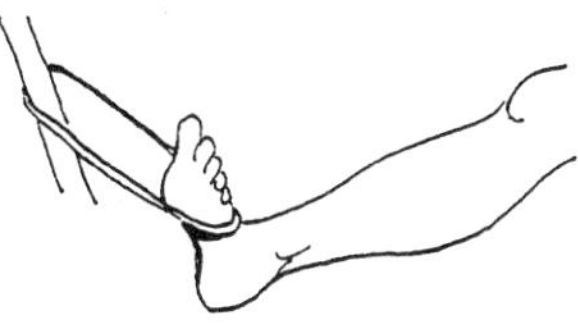

- Ankle movement is toward the big toe side.

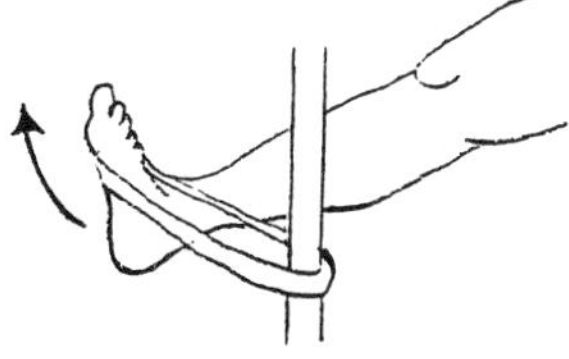

Start with one set of 10 repetitions, progressing to three sets of 10 to 15. Once you can achieve this, advance the color of the Thera-Band and begin again toward three sets of 10 to 15 repetitions.

Bilateral Heel Raises

Stand with your feet shoulder-width apart. Raise your heels off the ground and roll your weight onto the balls of your feet. Fingertips can be placed on a counter for light balance. You can progress to weight machines, performing same action with increasing weight intensity.

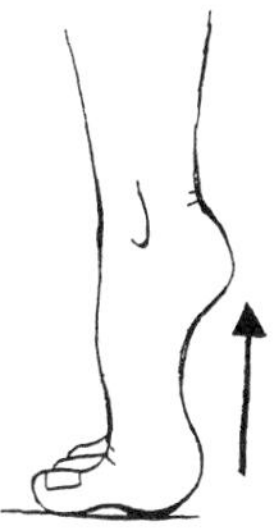

Heel Raise (Single Leg)

Raise the heel of the affected ankle up and down. Fingertips can be placed on a counter for light balance. You can progress to weight machines, performing same actions for added weight intensity.

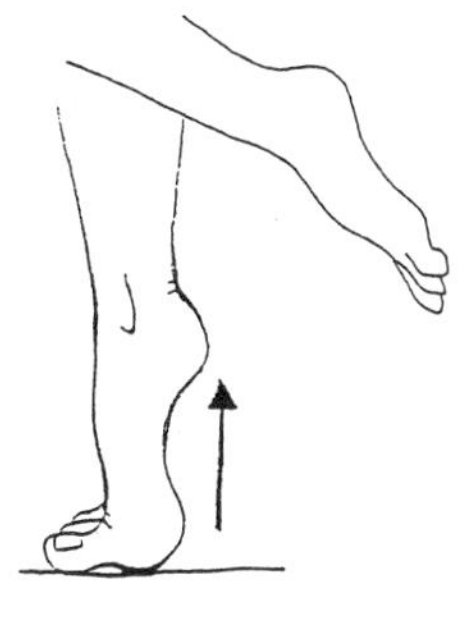

Hopping (Front, Back, Side to Side)

Begin by hopping with both feet up and down and progress to front, back, and side-to-side movements. Further progression is achieved by hopping in same patterns with the affected ankle only.

Jogging, Running, Sprinting (Straight Lines)

Start easy jogging in straight lines first. Progress speed and distances gradually.

Jogging, Running, Sprinting (Figure 8s and Zig-Zag Patterns)

Jog slowly, making a pattern of large figure 8s, and then progress to smaller and smaller patterns with increasing speed. Jog in zig-zag patterns with large cuts first and then progress to sharper cuts with increasing speed.

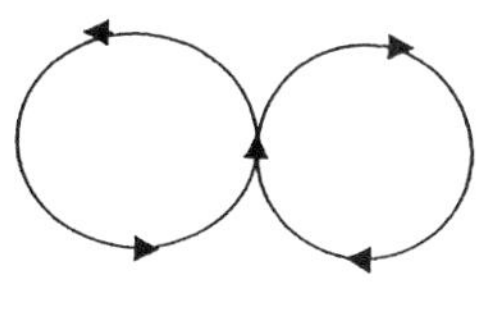

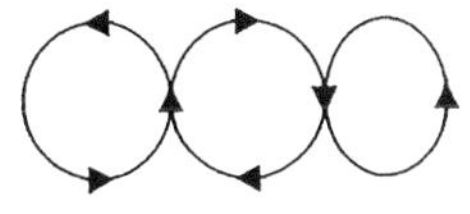

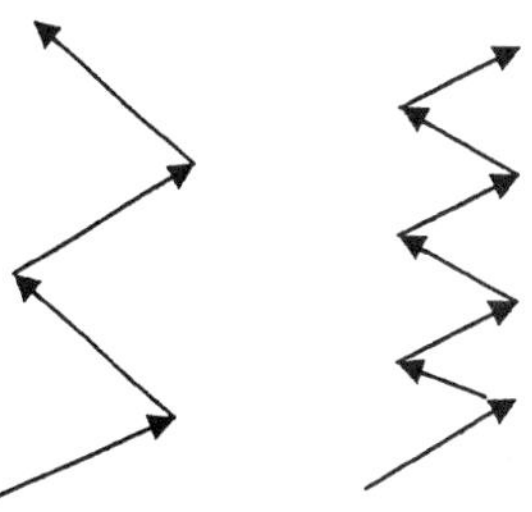

Rotator Cuff Tendinitis

WHAT IS ROTATOR CUFF TENDINITIS?

The rotator cuff is comprised of a group of four flat tendons that surround the front, top, and back of the shoulder. The purpose of these muscles is to rotate the shoulder inward or outward. During elevation of the shoulder, these muscles help to keep the major shoulder bone, the *humerus*, in the socket. Directly above the superior rotator cuff muscle is a sac called a *bursa*, which contains a fluid substance, used to decrease friction between this muscle and the end of the collarbone. Rotator cuff tendinitis is an inflammation of the tendons, which occurs most commonly to the superior tendon, called the *supraspinatus*. An inflammation of the bursa (bursitis) can occur as well.

COMMON CAUSES

The following are common causes of tendinitis:

- Poor posture, usually consisting of rounded shoulders
- Weakness or fatigue of the rotator cuff muscles
- Improper mechanics (throwing, swimming, serving)
- Lack of flexibility
- Overuse (excessive overhead activities)

SIGNS AND SYMPTOMS

Pain or aching about the front and side of the shoulder. The pain can extend down the outside of the shoulder midway to the elbow. Pain usually increases as one elevates the shoulder into overhead positions.

TREATMENT

Initially, rest, medication, and ice two to three times per day for 15 to 20 minutes are helpful. Icing is beneficial as long as the inflammatory condition continues. It can be applied after activity and/or rehabilitation to help decrease pain and muscle spasm. Antiinflammatory medications are used to help decrease pain and swelling. Sometimes, cortisone injections are administered. Stretching and strengthening exercises, used to promote range of motion and strength, are then initiated when pain is decreased. For moderate to severe cases, your physician may prescribe physical therapy for modalities (ultrasound, iontophoresis, soft-tissue massage, electrical stimulation), evaluation of weak/tight muscles, posture analysis, and exercise progression.

STRETCHING

Guidelines for performance or progression of stretching exercises are as follows and/or as prescribed by your physician:

- Keep the stretch to a comfortable level. (Don't force the stretch or cause excessive pain.)
- Do not hold your breath while stretching.
- Hold each stretch for approximately 30 seconds.
- Repeat each stretch three to six times.

STRENGTHENING

Guidelines for performance or progression of strengthening exercises are as follows and/or as prescribed by your physician:

- Do not hold your breath while you lift.
- Stay below the level of pain.
- Do two to three sets of 10 to 15 repetitions two to four times a week. Once you can complete three sets of 15 repetitions easily, increase the weight, reduce the repetitions to 10, and build back up to 15.

HOME EXERCISE PROGRAM

This program is designed to allow you to start with basic exercises. If you should have any questions or difficulties, refer back to your physician.

STRETCHING EXERCISES

Guidelines: Stretch three to six times, holding for 30 seconds.

Posterior Capsule Stretch

Pull the involved arm across your chest, positioning your hand under the opposite shoulder.

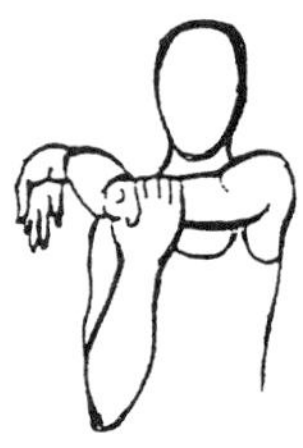

Towel Stretch (Internal Rotation)

This is performed with a towel. Place the uninvolved hand behind your head and the involved hand behind your back while grasping a towel with both hands. Gently pull the towel up toward the ceiling.

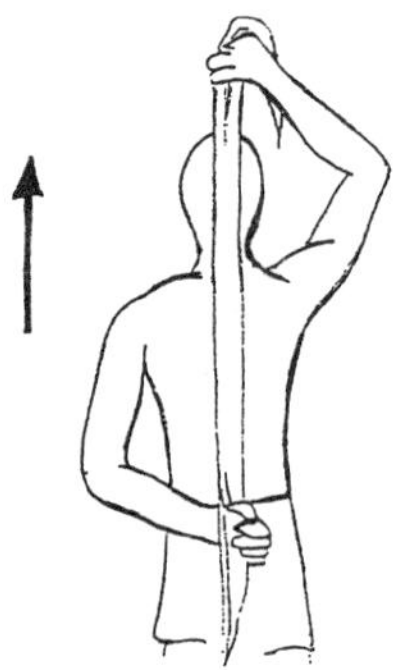

Towel Stretch (External Rotation)

This is performed with a towel. Place the involved hand behind your head and the uninvolved hand behind your back while grasping a towel with both hands. Gently pull the towel down toward the floor.

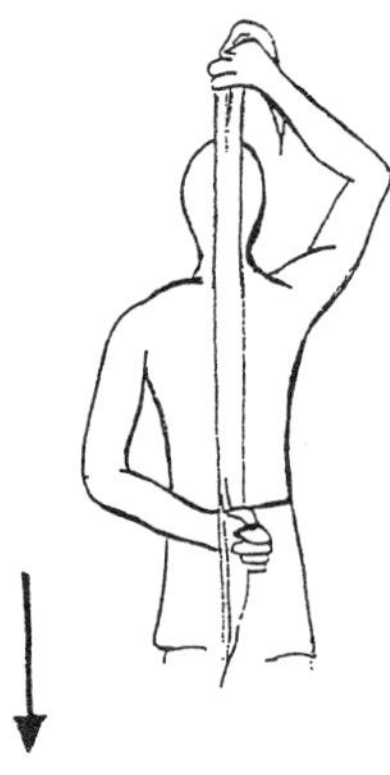

Flexion Stretch

While on your back, clasp your hands together, straighten your elbows, and raise your arms up and over your head.

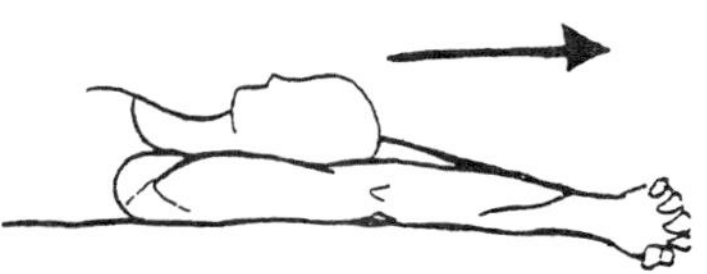

Extension Stretch

When standing, clasp your hands behind your back and gently raise your arms up toward the ceiling.

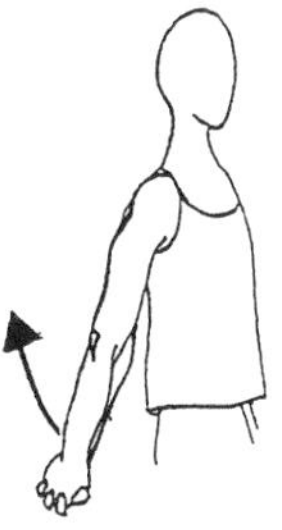

Pectoralis Stretch

Standing in a corner or in a doorway, raise your elbows to shoulder level while supporting your forearms on the door frame or wall. Place one leg in front of the other and gently lunge forward by bending the forward knee. Keep your back straight during the stretch.

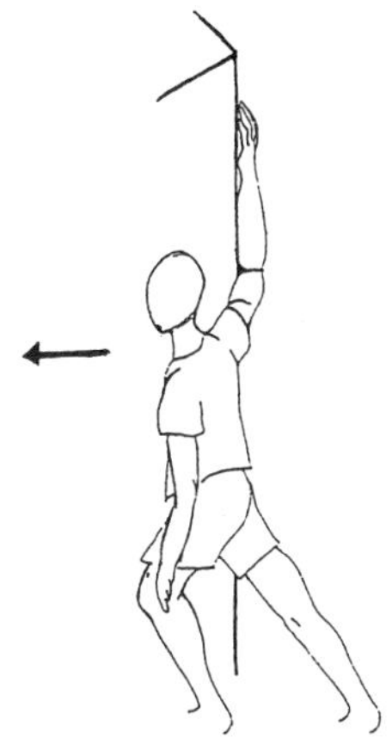

STRENGTHENING EXERCISES

Guidelines: Start with three sets of 10 repetitions, if able (fewer, if unable); progress to three sets of 15 repetitions. Once this is accomplished easily, reduce the repetitions to three sets of 10 and increase the weight intensity.

External Rotation

Lie on the uninvolved side, with involved elbow flexed and held against the side of the body. Bring your hand up toward the ceiling. Add hand weights to progress the exercise.

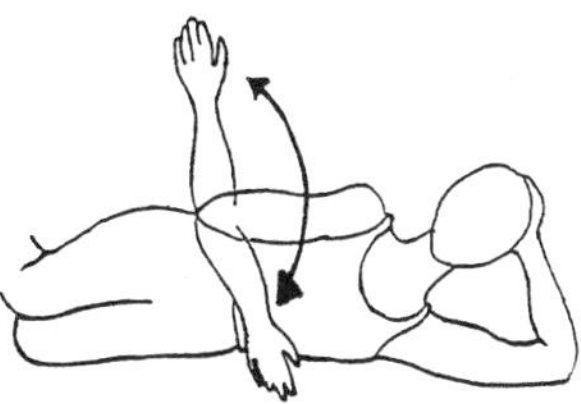

Internal Rotation

While lying on your back, hold the involved elbow flexed to 90 degrees and against the side of your body. Bring your hand toward your stomach. Add hand weights to progress the exercise.

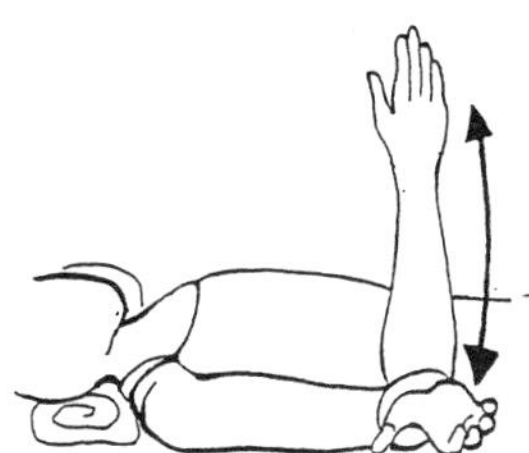

Empty Can

While standing, with your arm extended and the thumb pointed down toward the floor, bring your arm up to 90 degrees or below the pain level. The arm is positioned at an angle of 30 degrees from the side of the body. Progress up to a 5-pound limit with this exercise.

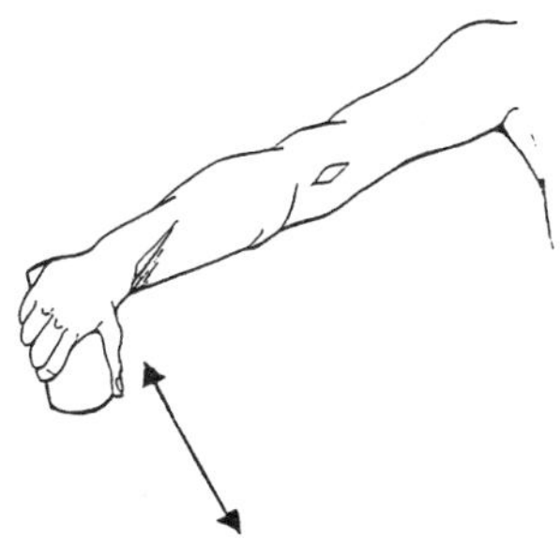

Shoulder Flexion

While standing, raise the involved hand, with the elbow straight toward the ceiling, to shoulder level. Your thumb should be pointed toward the ceiling.

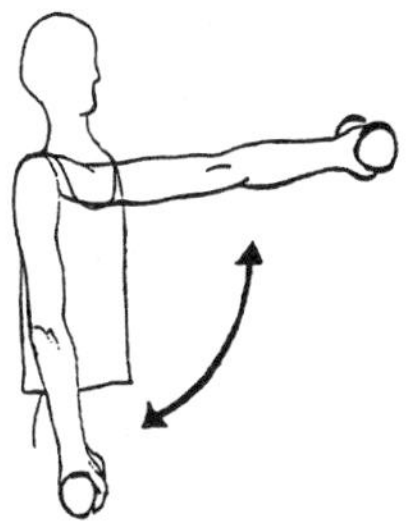

Shoulder Abduction

While standing, raise the involved hand, with the elbow straight out away from the body, to shoulder level.

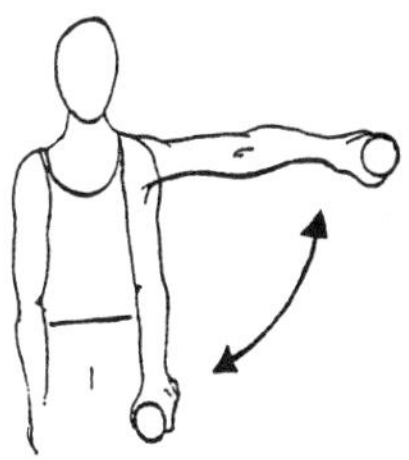

Single Row

Lean forward, bending from the trunk, and support your body with the uninvolved hand on a surface (desk, table). Pull the arm up by bending the elbow toward the ceiling until motion is stopped.

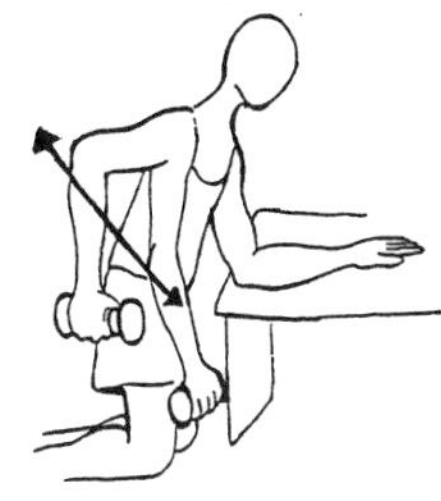

Epicondylitis

WHAT IS EPICONDYLITIS?

Epicondylitis is an inflammatory condition involving the tendons and muscles where they originate along the inside and outside of the elbow. *Tennis elbow* is a term commonly referred to when the condition occurs on the outside or lateral aspect of the elbow. Lateral epicondylitis occurs more frequently than medial epicondylitis.

COMMON CAUSES

Activities that involve forceful and/or continuous wrist motions or a large amount of stabilization applied by the wrist, such as playing racquet sports, swimming, swinging a golf club, throwing, playing tennis, using a computer keyboard, playing piano.

SIGNS AND SYMPTOMS

- Pain and tenderness along either the inside or the outside of the elbow, extending into the same side of the forearm.
- Difficulty gripping without pain; decreased wrist strength
- Tightness/stiffness when stretching elbow and wrist

TREATMENT

Initially, rest, medication, and ice two to three times per day for 15 to 20 minutes are helpful. Icing is beneficial as long as the inflammatory condition continues. Ice can be applied after activity and/or rehabilitation to help decrease pain and muscle spasm. Antiinflammatory medications are used to help decrease pain and swelling. Sometimes, cortisone injections are administered. Stretching and strengthening exercises, used to promote range of motion and strength, are initiated when pain is decreased. A brace worn just below the elbow joint also can be helpful. For moderate to severe cases, your physician may prescribe physical therapy for modalities (ultrasound, iontophoresis, soft-tissue massage, electrical stimulation), evaluation of weak or tight muscles, posture analysis, and exercise progression.

STRETCHING

Guidelines for performance or progression of stretching exercises are as follows and/or as prescribed by your physician:

- Keep the stretch to a comfortable level. (Don't force the stretch or cause excessive pain.)
- Do not hold your breath while stretching.
- Hold each stretch for approximately 30 seconds.
- Repeat each stretch three to six 6 times.

STRENGTHENING

Guidelines for performance or progression of strengthening exercises are as follows and/or as prescribed by your physician:

- Do not hold your breath while you lift.
- Stay below the level of pain.
- Do two to three sets of 10 to 15 repetitions two to four times a week. Once you can complete three sets of 15 repetitions easily, increase the weight, reduce the repetitions to 10, and build back up to 15.

HOME EXERCISE PROGRAM

This program is designed to allow you to start with basic exercises. If you should have any questions or difficulties, refer back to your physician.

STRETCHING EXERCISES

Guidelines: Stretch three to six times, holding for 30 seconds.

Wrist Flexion Stretch

Bend the involved wrist down gently by grasping it with the other hand until a pulling sensation is felt. Keep your elbow straight.

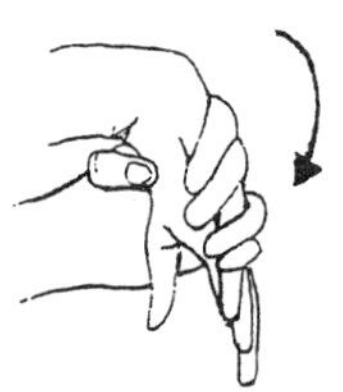

Wrist Flexion Stretch (Advanced)

Same as for the wrist flexion stretch, but with the addition of wrist movement toward the side of the little finger.

Wrist Extension Stretch

Bend the involved wrist up gently by grasping it with the opposite hand until a pulling sensation is felt. Keep your elbow straight.

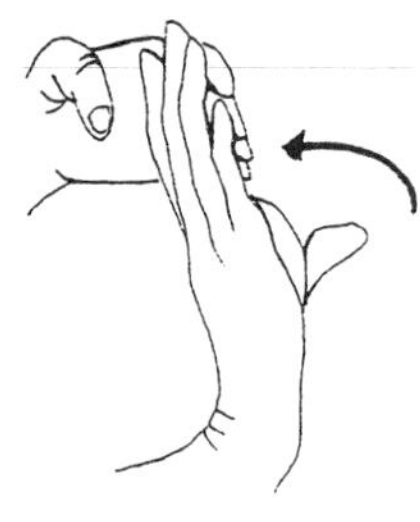

STRENGTHENING EXERCISES

Guidelines: Start with three sets of 10 repetitions, if able (fewer, if unable); progress to three sets of 15 repetitions. Once this is accomplished easily, reduce the repetitions to three sets of 10 and increase the weight intensity.

Wrist Extension Curls

With your forearm supported by your leg or a table and your palm facing downward, lift and lower the weight.

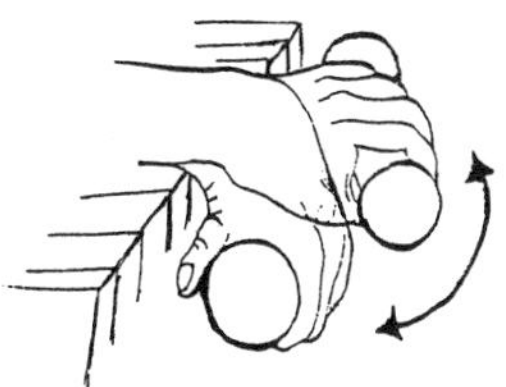

Wrist Flexion Curls

With your forearm supported by your leg or a table and your palm facing upward, lift and lower the weight.

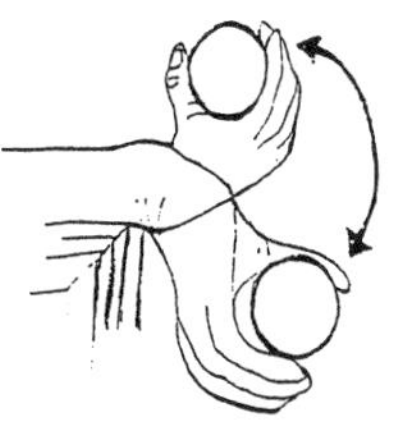

Forearm Pronation/Supination

With your forearm supported by your leg or a table, turn your palm up and then down while holding onto a weight.

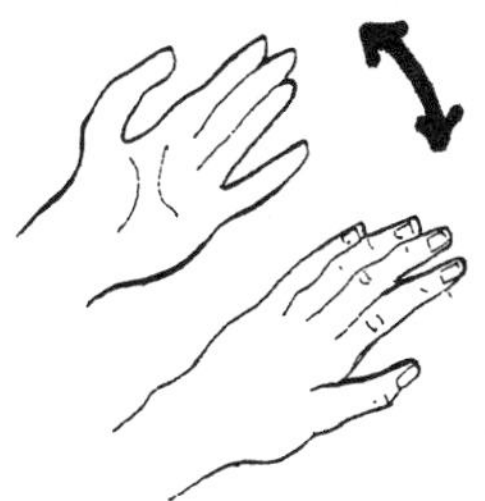

Gripping

To start, gently grip a rubber ball, a towel, or putty and then advance to items with more resistance. Perform 10 to 30 repetitions, increasing in intensity once you are able to perform 30 repetitions.

Finger Extension

Wrap a rubber band around the outside of all your fingers and thumb, gently extend the hand by opening the fingers, and then close the fingers. Perform 10 to 30 repetitions.

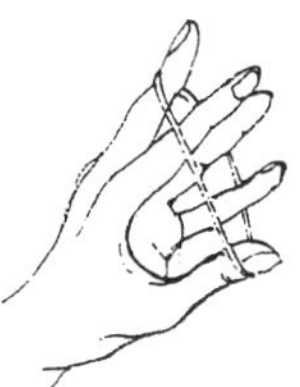

APPENDIX

Algorithms

Greg Nakamoto and Michael Mikus

A NOTE REGARDING THE USE OF THE ALGORITHMS

These algorithms are not intended to be inclusive of all the possible diagnoses that one should consider when evaluating the sports medicine patient. Nor are the particular steps which they follow necessarily the most appropriate manner in which to evaluate a given patient. They are meant to list for the provider some of the more common diagnoses seen in the primary care setting, as well as to prompt the provider to consider some possibly less common diagnoses that have more serious consequences if overlooked. It is not the intent of the algorithms to walk the provider through a work up for a patient and produce a specific diagnosis. The algorithms are meant to help those who are otherwise less familiar with the problems seen in primary-care sports medicine by quickly narrowing the rather large list of possible diagnoses for a given complaint, and by providing a starting point from which to then conduct a more focused evaluation.

The algorithms are organized by body part, and further discriminate as to whether the symptoms are acute or chronic. To help narrow the differential diagnosis based on the localization of symptoms, the diagnoses are listed with references to accompanying figures. For instance, when using the acute shoulder pain algorithm, the "1A" in

-1A: Squared-off shoulder with anterior fullness; arm held in external rotation and partial abduction: *Anterior gleno-humeral dislocation****

refers to the accompanying area labeled 1A in Shoulder Figure 1. Some of the more salient signs and symptoms that may be found are also listed, followed by the diagnosis that they suggest. Also, three asterisks (***) indicate those particular diagnoses that have chapters in this book dedicated to their evaluation. Lastly, for a few of the algorithms, some of the more common radiographic views are shown with accompanying line diagrams to help orient the user to the underlying bony anatomy.

Neck

Acute

? Traumatic, with significant pain

- **Abnormal x-ray - consider:**
  - -1A: *C1-C2 fracture (odontoid, Hangman's, or Jefferson fracture)*
  - -1B: *Lower C-spine vertebral body fracture (teardrop or burst fx)*
  - -1A/B: *Spinous or transverse process fracture*
  - -1A/B: *Vertebral subluxation/dislocation*
- **No obvious fracture or dislocaction on x-ray - consider:**
  - -1A/B: *Herniated nucleus pulposis****
  - -1A/B: *Spinal cord injury*
  - -2A: *Soft tissue injury (carotid dissection, laryngeal injury, etc.)*

? Traumatic, with moderate pain, abnormal neurologic exam, normal x-ray

- **1A/B: Marked deficits:** -*Spinal cord injury*
- **1A/B: Bilateral upper extremity, or upper and lower extremity paresthesias/weakness:** -*Transient quadriplegia/Cervical cord neurapraxia*
- **1D, 2B: Mild unilateral upper extremity paresthesias or weakness:** -*Brachial plexus injury****

? Traumatic, with mild pain, normal neurologic exam

- **1A/B: Laxity on cervical x-rays:** -*Cervical sprain*
- **Cervical x-rays negative for fracture and instability:**
  - -1A/B/C, 2C: *Cervical strain****
  - -1C/D: *Trapezius or levator scapulae strain*

? Atraumatic

- **Consider: Subarachnoid hemmorhage, meningitis, osteomyelitis/discitis**

Chronic

? Neurologic signs/symptoms or radiating pain/paresthesias

- **1B: Disc space narrowing on x-ray:** -Cervical disc disease (with/without *herniated nucleus pulposis****)
- **1A: Neck pain/fatigue and paresthesias, often worse with neck flexion:** -*Atlantoaxial instability****
- **1B: Neck pain/fatigue and paresthesias, positive Spurling's test:** -*Foraminal stenosis with nerve root impingement*
- **1B: Osteoporosis history or risk factors:** -*Compression fracture*
- **1B: Neck pain/fatigue and paresthesias, often worse with neck extension:** -*Cervical stenosis*
- **1A/B: Co-existing constitutional symptoms:** -*Tumor*

? Upper extremity circulatory symptoms

- **Symptoms elicited by elevation of hands overhead, other provocative maneuvers:** -*Thoracic outlet syndrome****
- **Pain, atrophy, and vasomotor hyper-reactivity after previous injury:**-*Reflex sympathetic dystrophy****

? Neither neurological or circulatory symptoms

- **Cervical muscular spasm:**
  - -1A/B/C, 2C: *Cervical strain****
  - -1A/B/C, 2C: *Cervical muscular fatigue*
- **1B: Fused vertebrae on x-ray**: -Klippel-Feil syndrome
- **Consider osteoarthritis, rheumatoid arthritis, SLE, infection, or other medical process**
- **Consider shoulder as source of symptoms**
- **Consider one of the above diagnoses but without neurologic/circulatory signs**

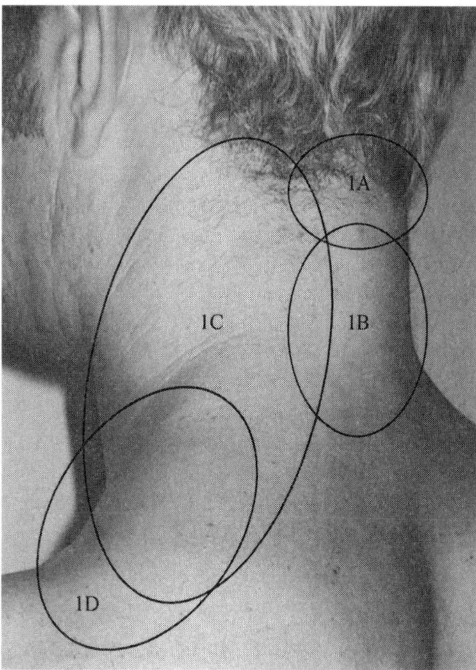

Figure 1

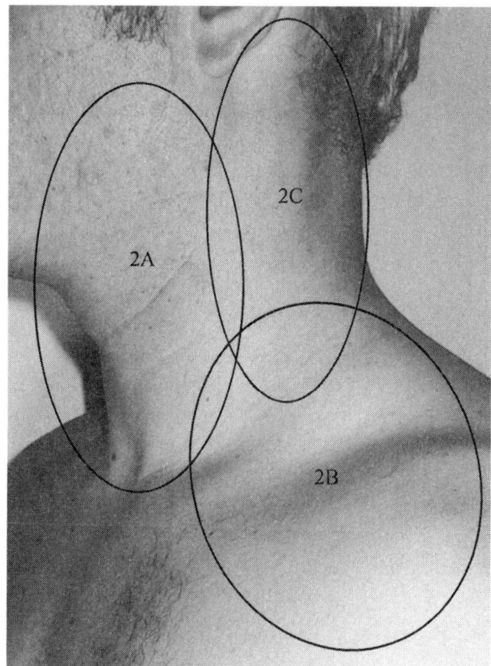

Figure 2

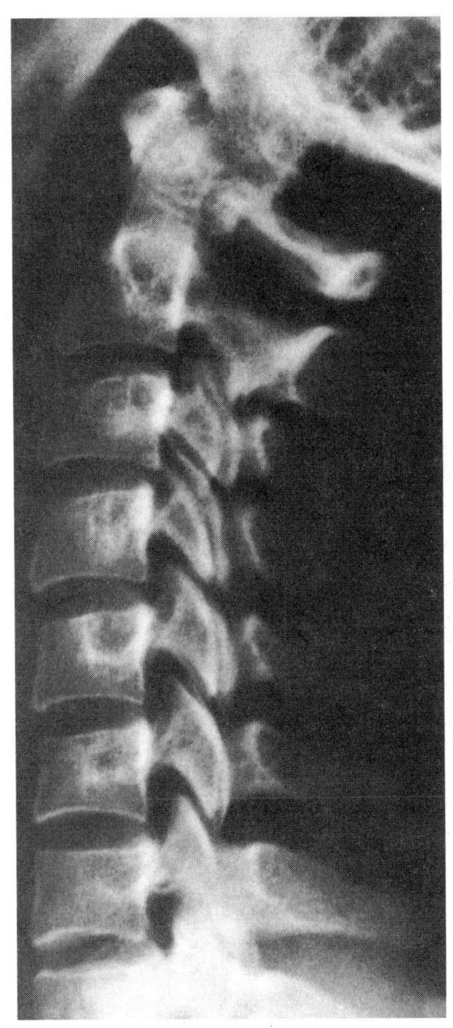

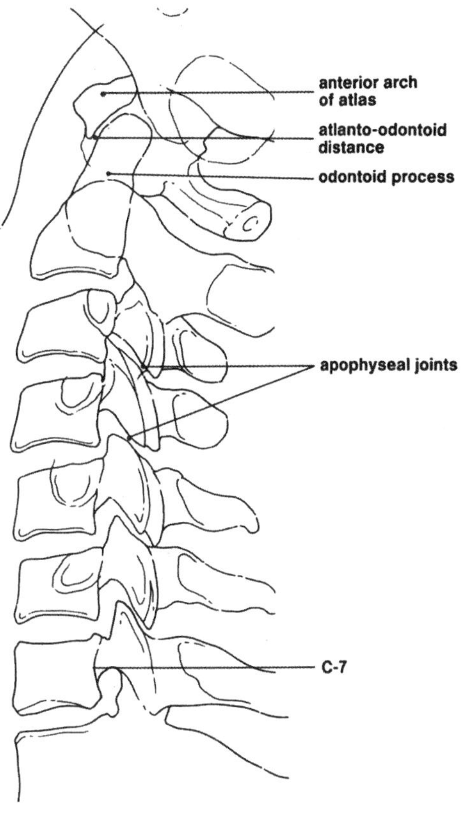

Radiograph 1: Lateral view of the cervical spine

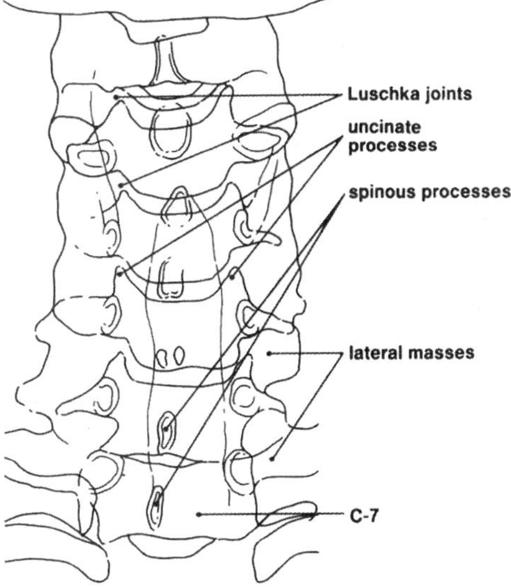

Radiograph 2: AP view of the cervical spine

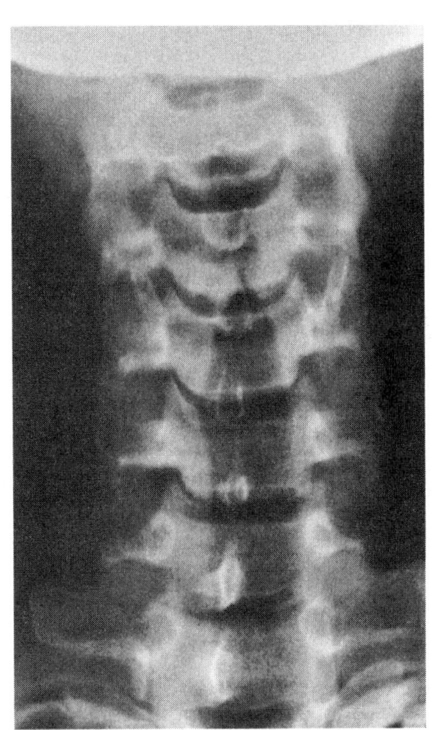

Acute

Trauma with obvious deformity or bony derangement on X-ray

- **Anterior pain:**
  -1A: Squared-off shoulder with anterior fullness; arm held in external rotation and partial abduction: *Anterior glenohumeral dislocation****
  -1B, 2B: Acromioclavicular joint pain and deformity; clavicle displaced superiorly on x-ray: *Acromioclavicular dislocation****
  -1C: Tenting of skin overlying clavicle; most often in middle third: *Clavicle fracture****
- **Lateral pain:**
  -1A, 2A: Humerus fracture evident on x-ray: *Humeral head/neck fracture*
- **Posterior pain:**
  -2A: Arm held in internal rotation and adduction; unable to externally rotate or abduct: *Posterior glenohumeral dislocation****
  -2C: Scapular fracture evident on x-ray: *Scapular fracture*

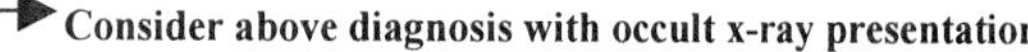

No fracture on X-ray +/- deformity

- **Anterior pain:**
  -1D: Palpable "lump" in mid-upper arm anteriorly: *Biceps tendon rupture****
- **Lateral pain:**
  -1A: Painful arc, positive drop-arm test: *Rotator cuff tear****
- **Generalized pain:**
  -1E: Burning/stinging pain radiating down one arm: *Brachial plexus injury****
- **Consider above diagnosis with occult x-ray presentation**
- **Consider acute exacerbation of CHRONIC injury or medical diagnosis: rheumatoid arthritis, osteoarthritis, SLE, etc...**

Atruamatic

- **Consider: Septic arthritis, or process extrinsic to shoulder joint (MI, zoster, pain referred from visceral source)...**

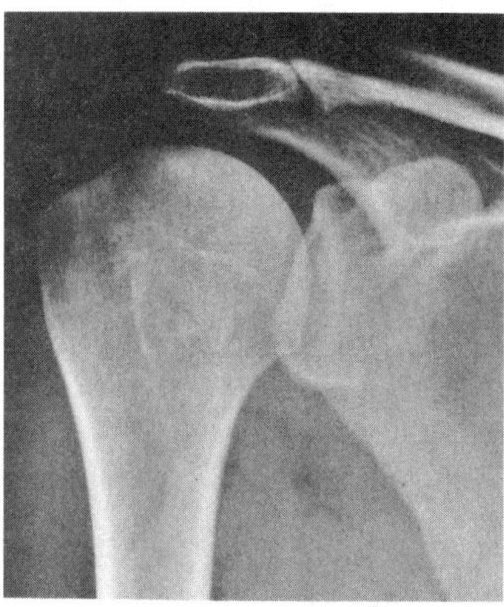

Radiograph 1: AP view of the right shoulder

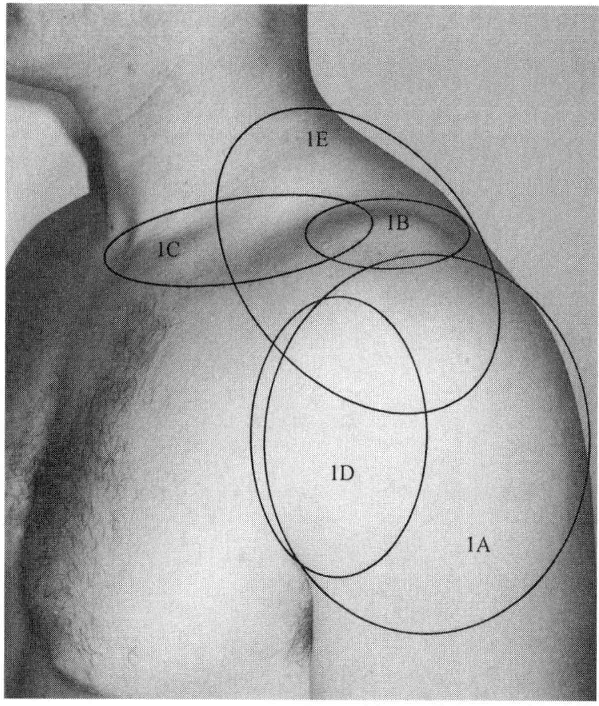

Figure 1

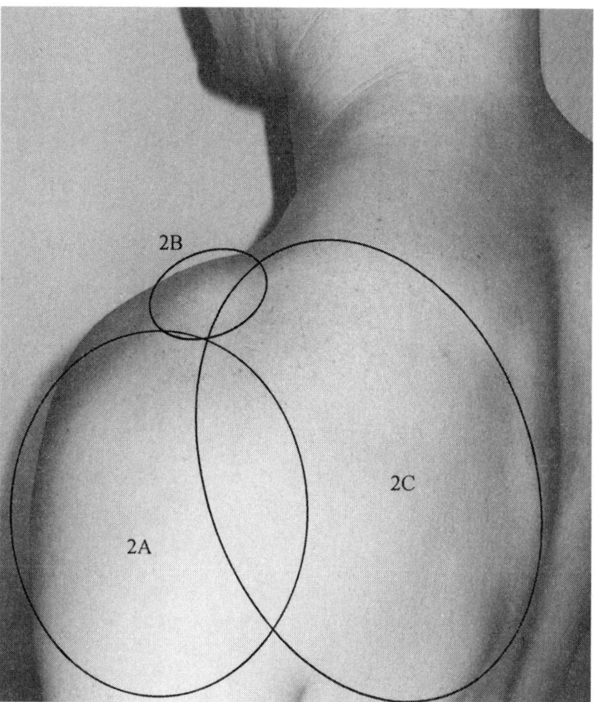

Figure 2

Chronic

History of recent or distant injury, but with chronic symptoms

1A: Positive impingement signs:
*-Impingement, subacromial bursitis,& rotator cuff tendinitis****

1D: Positive Speed's and/or Yergason's signs:
-Biceps tendinitis

1B, 2B: Acromioclavicular joint tenderness:
-Acromioclavicular clavicular arthritis

Decreased range of motion out of proportion to pain:
-Adhesive capsulitis
-Loose body

Signs or symptoms of instability:
*-Anterior instability****
*-Multidirectional instability****

1A: Overhead athlete with painful clicking, possibly with history of instability:
*-Glenoid labral tears/SLAP lesions****

1B/C, 2B: Prior blow to the point of the shoulder; osteolytic changes at acromioclavicular joint:
-Distal clavicular osteolysis

1A, 2A: Humeral head changes on x-ray, often with a history of prior trauma or steroids:
-AVN of the humeral head

Review diagnoses on ACUTE algorithm for possible missed diagnosis

Repetitive stress, usually without history of trauma

1A: Positive impingement signs:
*-Impingement, subacromial bursitis,& rotator cuff tendinitis****

1D: Positive Speed's and/or Yergason's signs:
-Biceps tendinitis

Decreased range of motion out of proportion to pain:
-Loose body

Repetitive stress, usually without history of trauma, continued

Signs or symptoms of instability:
*-Anterior instability****
*-Multidirectional instability****

1A: Overhead athlete with painful clicking, possibly with history of instability:
*-Glenoid labral tears/SLAP lesions****

2A: Overhead athlete with posterolateral pain, atrophy of supra/infraspinatus:
*-Suprascapular nerve palsy****

1B/C, 2B: Prior blow to the point of the shoulder; osteolytic changes at acromioclavicular joint:
-Distal clavicular osteolysis

Insidious onset of pain, swelling, or deformity without trauma or repetitive stress

1A: Positive impingement signs:
*-Impingement, subacromial bursitis,& rotator cuff tendinitis****

1B, 2B: Acromioclavicular joint tenderness:
-Acromioclavicular clavicular arthritis

Signs or symptoms of instability:
*-Anterior instability****
*-Multidirectional instability****

1A, 2A: Humeral head changes on x-ray, often with a history of prior trauma or steroids:
-AVN of the humeral head

Circulatory/vasomotor symptoms:
*-Thoracic outlet syndrome****
*-Reflex sympathetic dystrophy****

Consider osteoarthritis, rheumatoid arthritis, SLE, infection, or other medical process

Associated neck pain or positive Spurling's sign

Consider cervical origin of symptoms

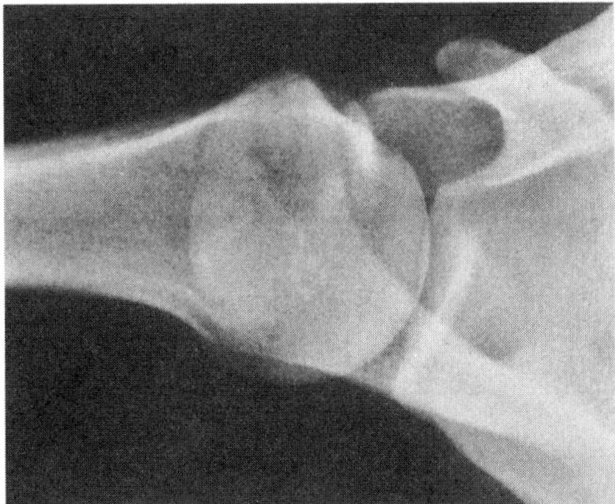

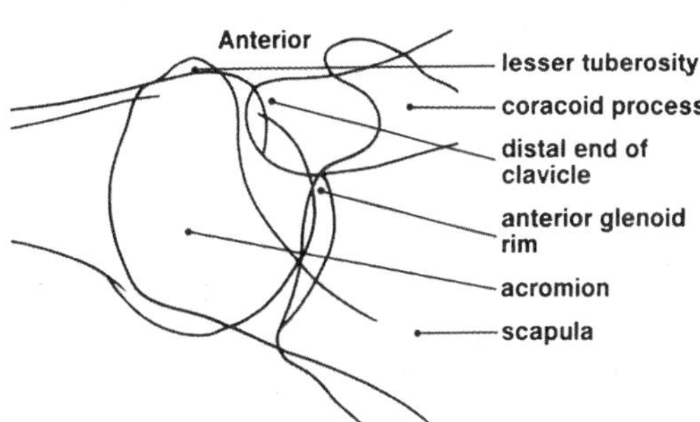

Radiograph 2: Axillary view of the right shoulder

Lower Back

Acute

X-rays not always necessary for acute onset back pain. Consider for significant trauma, neuromotor deficits, history of cancer or drug abuse, age <20 or >55, persistent or systemic symptoms.

? Trauma with obvious deformity or bony derangement on X-ray

- **X-ray reveals possible fracture**:
  - *-Compression fracture****
  - *-Spinous & transverse process fracture****
  - *-Sacral fracture****
  - *-Coccyx fracture****

? Acute pain with radiation +/- neurologic symptoms

- **Low back pain radiating down buttocks/leg**; +/- parasthesias and/or weakness; worse with prolonged sitting or standing and relieved in supine position:
  - *-Possible Herniated nucleus pulposis****
- **Pain localized to lower back with tenderness and muscle spasm**; usually developing a few hours after inciting event:
  - *-Lower back pain & Lumbar strains****

Consider acute exacerbation of CHRONIC injury or medical diagnosis such as:
-neoplasm (wt loss, pain while supine)
-ankylosing spondylitis (AM stiffness in young men)
-infection (fever, history of drug abuse, TB)
-abdominal aortic aneurysm (pulsatile mass)
-degenerative disk disease (↓ disk space; osteophytes on X-ray)

Chronic

History of remote injury, delayed presentation, or persistent pain; generally with symptoms radiating down leg

- ***-Review diagnoses on ACUTE algorithm for possible missed diagnosis***
- **Low back pain radiating down buttocks/leg**; worse with prolonged sitting or standing and relieved in supine position:
  - *-Sciatica****
  - *-Herniated nucleus pulposis****
- **Low back pain, less often radiating down buttocks/leg**; worse with lumbar extension and relieved by flexion (bending forward):
  - *-Spinal stenosis****

Localized low back pain, generally without radiation or neurologic symptoms

- **Young athlete; pain worse with extension and lateral side bending:**
  - *-Spondylolysis and spondylolisthesis****
- **Middle-aged athlete; central or unilateral pain, worse with hyperextension:**
  - *-Facet syndrome****
- **Significant lateral curvature of spine with forward bending; or thoracic kyphosis**:
  - *-Scoliosis and kyphosis****
- **Pain localized to lower back with tenderness and muscle spasm**; usually with tight hamstrings, weak abdominal muscles, and increased lumbar lordosis:
  - *-Lower back pain & Lumbar strains****
- **Sacroiliac joint pain/stiffness**, usually seen in men in their 20s; worse in the morning; elevated ESR; ⊕ HLA B-27, family history:
  - *-Ankylosing spondylitis****

→ (to: Consider acute exacerbation of CHRONIC injury or medical diagnosis)

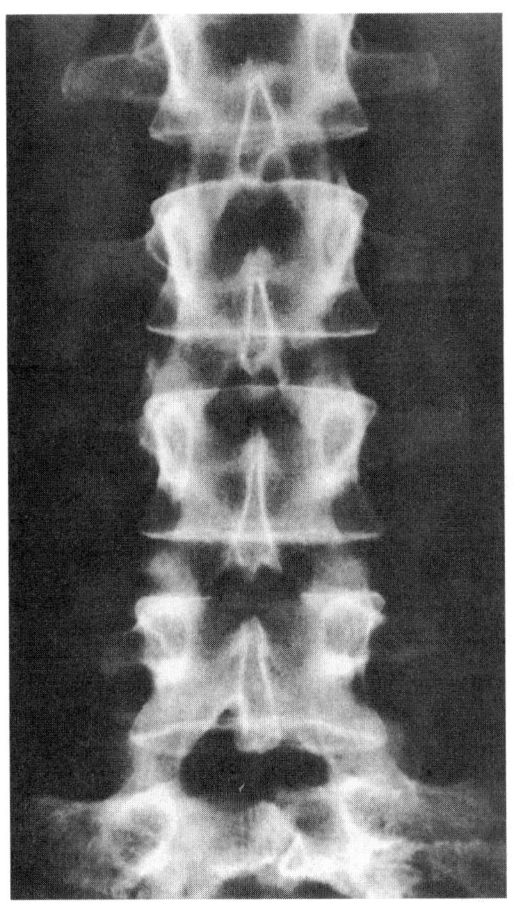

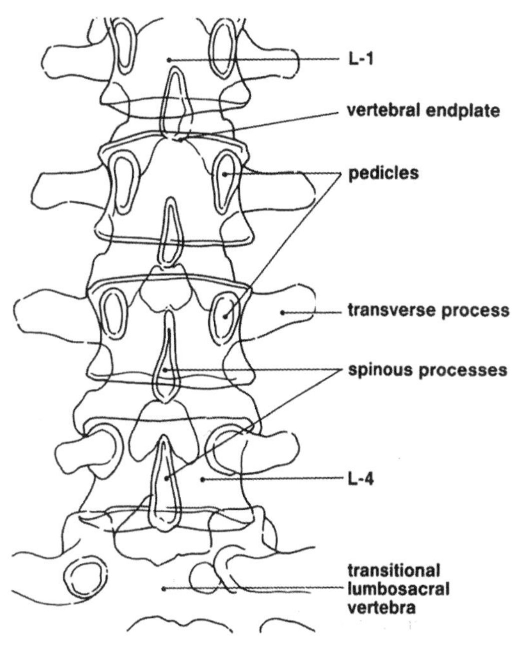

Radiograph 1: AP view of the lumbar spine

Acute Elbow

? Trauma with obvious deformity (obtain X-rays)

- **Dislocation**:
  *-Elbow dislocation****
- **Fracture**:
  *-Coronoid fracture****
  *-Olecranon fracture****
  *-Radial head fracture****
  -Humerus fracture

? X-ray: No fracture, ⊕ effusion

- **1E:Tenderness at radial head**, pain with supination & pronation of forearm:
  *-Occult radial head fx ****

? X-ray: normal, ⊕ tenderness & deformity

- **1A: Localized fluctuance, erythema**, tenderness:
  *-Olecranon bursitis ****
- **2A: Tenderness, loss of biceps strength (flexion, supination)**, biceps tendon not palpable; deformity of upper arm; ecchymosis:
  *-Biceps tendon rupture ****
- **1B: Tenderness loss of triceps strength**, triceps tendon not palpable; defect palpable, ecchymosis:
  *-Triceps tendon rupture ****
- **Consider acute exacerbation of CHRONIC injury or medical diagnosis such as septic arthritis, osteoarthritis or cellulitis**

Forearm Injuries

? Tenderness/pain as pictured

- **1F: Dorsal-radial forearm pain**, +/- swelling and crepitus with "squeaky" sensation 4 to 8 cm proximal to wrist:
  *-Intersection syndrome ****
- **2E: Volar forearm ache radiating to fingers**; median nerve symptoms, ⊕ Tinel's test at area of compression of median nerve, but negative Phalen's test at wrist:
  *-Pronator syndrome ****
- **2F: Volar forearm ache radiating to fingers**; median nerve MOTOR symptoms only (i.e. weakness in thumb and inability to make "OK" sign, but no numbness/parasthesias):
  *-Anterior interosseous nerve syndrome ****

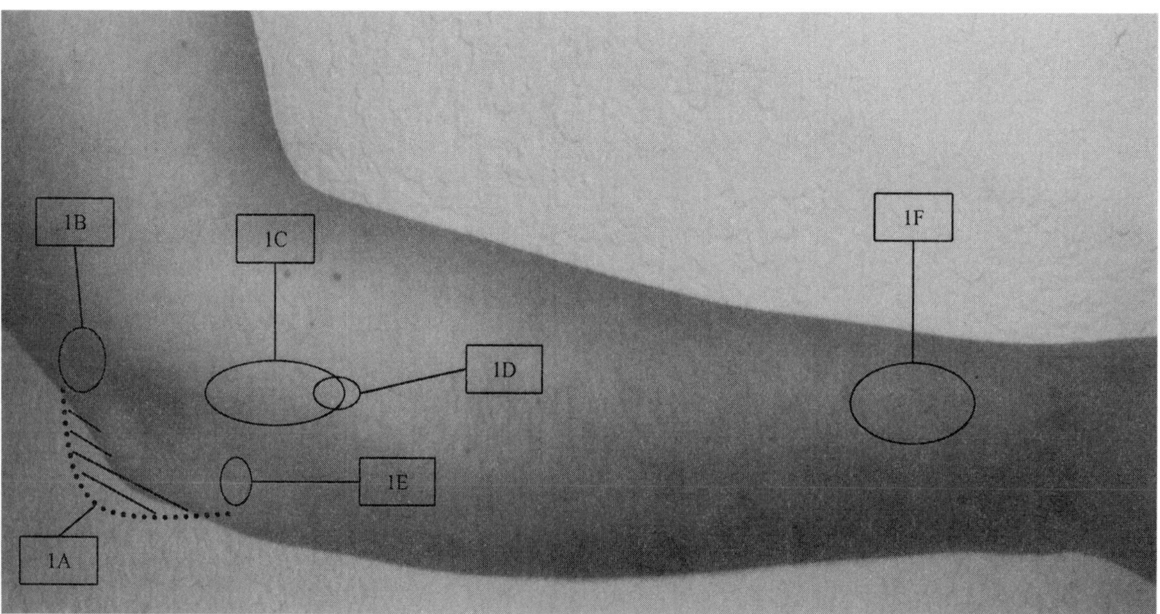

Figure 1

Radiograph 1: AP view of the right elbow

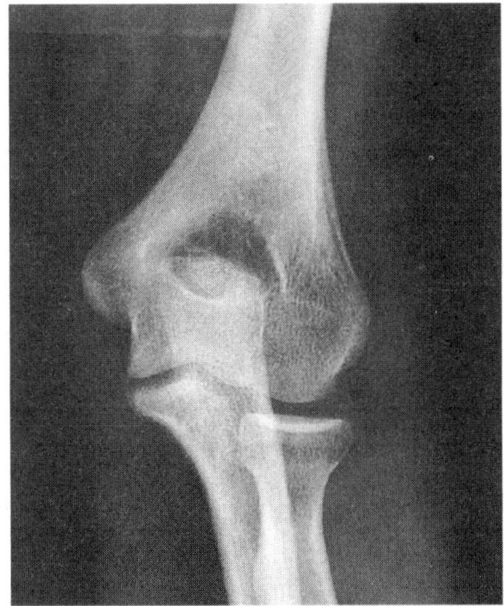

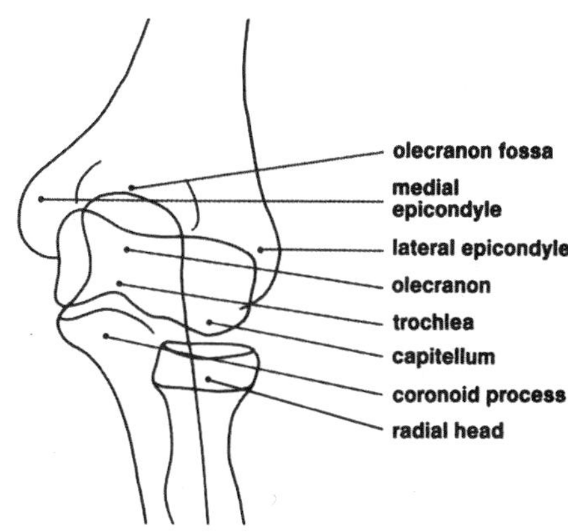

Radiograph 2: Lateral view of the elbow

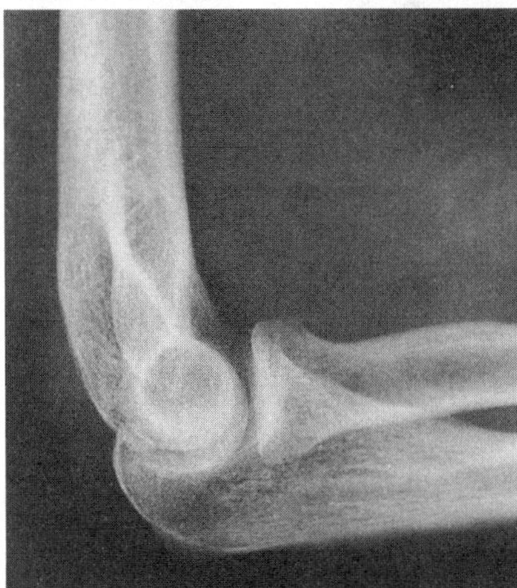

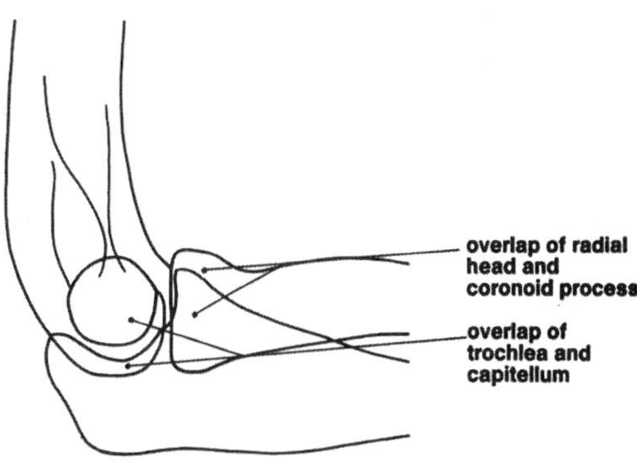

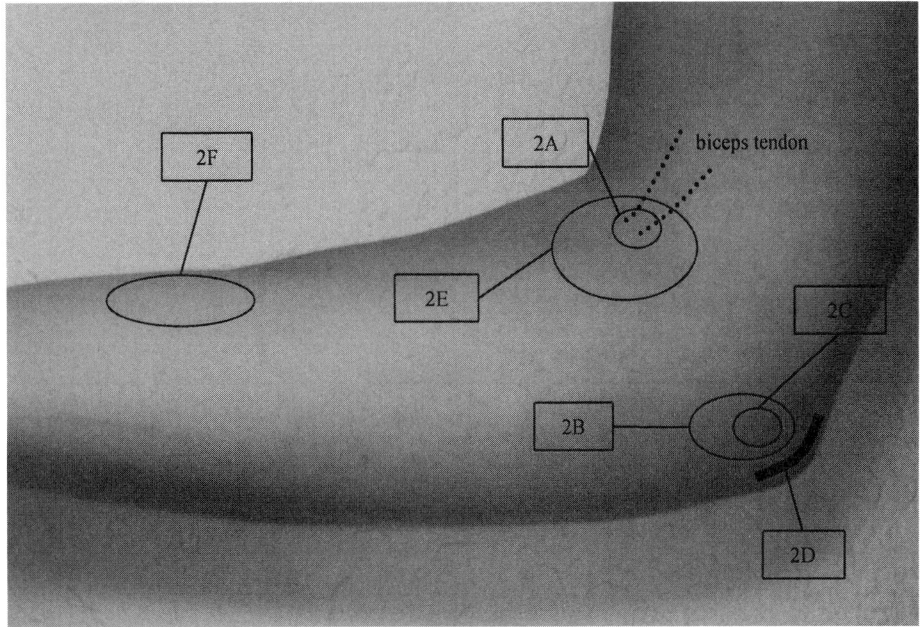

Figure 2

Chronic Elbow

? History of repetitive stress, tenderness as labeled in photos

- **2B: Medial epicondyle and wrist flexor origin tenderness;** worse with resisted wrist FLEXION:
  *-Medial epicondylitis****
- **1C: Lateral epicondyle and wrist extensor origin tenderness;** worse with resisted wrist EXTENSION:
  *-Lateral epicondylitis ****
- **1D: Tenderness ~1-2cm DISTAL to lateral epicondyle**; ⊕Tinel's sign +/- pain with resisted wrist or finger extension, neurologic symptoms:
  *-Posterior interosseous nerve syndrome (rare)****
- **1B: Olecranon tip tenderness**; pain with elbow extension:
  *-Triceps tendinitis ****
- **2A: Biceps tendon tenderness**; pain with elbow flexion:
  -Biceps tendinitis

? Pain +/- laxity with valgus stress, usually seen in throwers/pitchers

- **2C: Medial elbow pain with throwing**; laxity noted in more advanced cases:
  *-Ulnar collateral ligament injury****
  ***In youths**, consider:*
  *-Little League Elbow ****
  *-Panner's disease ****
- **1B: Posterior elbow pain with throwing**; usually in the setting of laxity:
  -Olecranon impingement

? Pain with tenderness and neuropathic symptoms as labeled

- **1D: Tenderness ~1-2cm DISTAL to lateral condyle**; ⊕Tinel's sign +/- pain with resisted wrist or finger extension, neurologic symptoms:
  *-Posterior interosseous nerve syndrome (rare)****
- **2D: Medial elbow pain +/- parasthesias**; ⊕Tinel's sign:
  *-Ulnar nerve palsy (cubital tunnel syndrome) ****

? Locking, catching, foreign body sensation

- **X-rays reveal loose body in joint**:
  -old injury
  *-Panner's disease****

? Chronic warmth, pain with ROM

- **X-rays reveal degenerated joint:**
  Consider rheumatic disease, osteoarthritis or other medical condition.

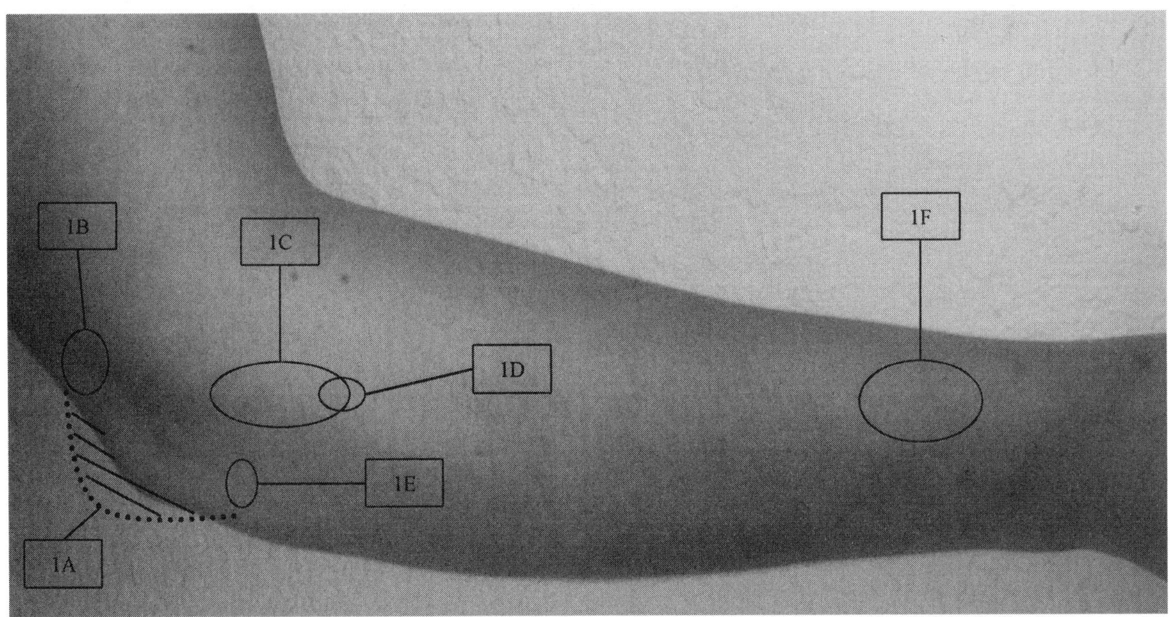

Figure 1

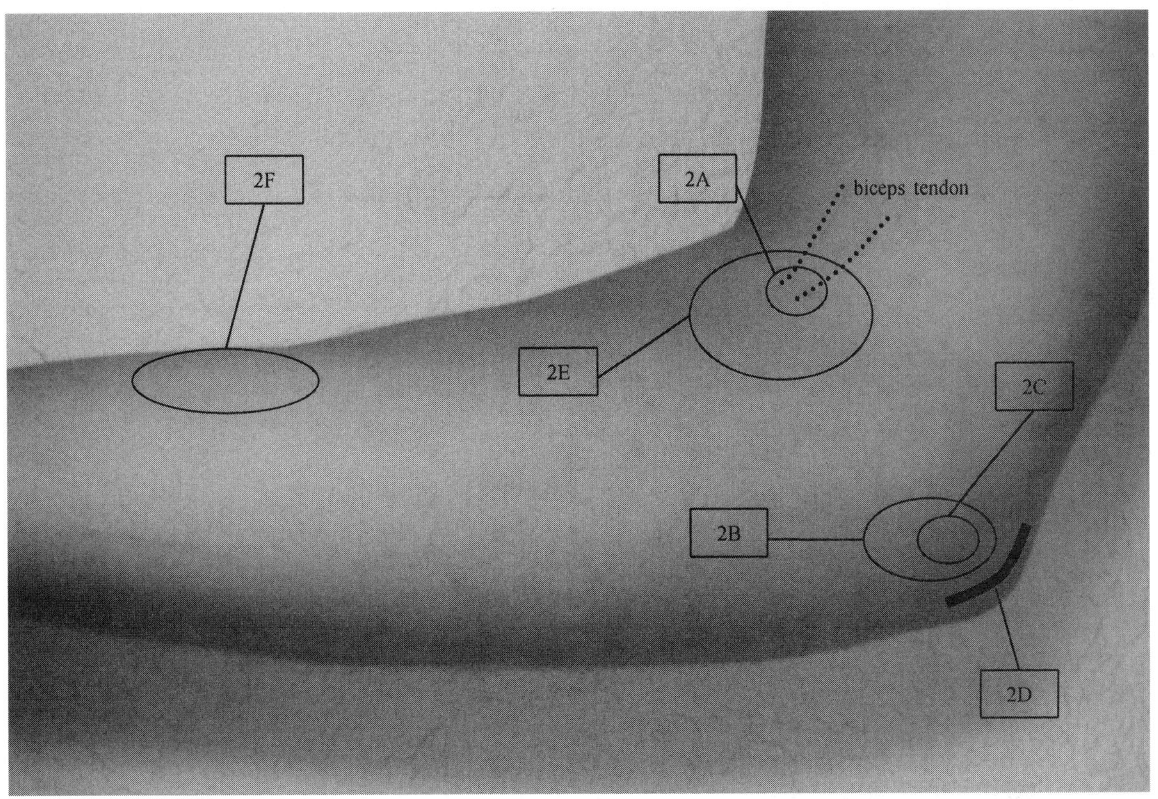

Figure 2

Wrist

Acute

Trauma with obvious deformity or bony derangement on X-ray

- **X-ray reveals possible fracture**:
  - *-Distal radius****
  - *-Scaphoid****
  - *-Lunate****
  - *-Hamate****
  - *-Other carpal bones****
- **1A: Dorsal-radial wrist pain**; gap between scaphoid/lunate on AP X-ray:
  *-Scapho-lunate dissociation****
- **1B: Dorsal-middle wrist pain**; lunate out of place on lateral X-ray
  *-Lunate dissociation****

No fracture on X-ray +/- deformity

- **1A: Anatomic snuffbox** is point of maximal tenderness; pain with axial loading of thumb:
  *-Possible Scaphoid fracture****
- **2C: Ulnar sided pain** with compression across ulnar side of wrist; pain with load and twist of junction between ulna and wrist:
  *-Triangular fibrocartilage complex injury****
- **2D: Ulnar sided pain**, "snapping" on lateral wrist:
  -Extensor carpi ulnaris subluxation
- **Consider acute exacerbation of CHRONIC injury or medical diagnosis such as rheumatoid arthritis, osteoarthritis, SLE or cellulitis**

Chronic

History of acute injury, delayed presentation, or persistent pain

- ***Review diagnoses on ACUTE algorithm for possible missed diagnosis***
- **1A: Dorsal-radial wrist pain**; degeneration of scaphoid on X-ray:
  *-Scaphoid avascular necrosis (see fracture)****
- **1B: Dorsal-middle wrist pain**; degeneration of lunate on X-ray
  *-Kienboch's Disease/AVN of lunate****

Repetitive stress, usually without history of trauma

- **1C: Lateral-radial pain**, tenderness over tendon which forms volar border of snuffbox (APL&EPB), ⊕ Finkelstein's test:
  *-DeQuervain's tenosynovitis****
- **1D or 2E: Volar pain**, ulnar or radial, worse with wrist flexion:
  *-Flexor tendinitis****
- **1E: Proximal dorsal-radial pain**, +/- swelling and crepitus with "squeaky" sensation:
  *-Intersection syndrome****
- **1F: Dorsal-radial pain**, numbness +/- tenderness over dorsum of thumb and hand, ⊕ Tinel's, negative Finkelstein's test:
  -Superficial radial nerve/Wartenberg's disease
- **2A: Volar-middle pain radiating to fingers**; neurologic symptoms; ⊕ Phalen's, Tinel's tests:
  *-Carpal tunnel syndrome****
- **2B: Volar-ulnar pain**, neurologic symptoms in ulnar digits:
  -Ulnar tunnel syndrome

Chronic pain, swelling of joints

- **1B: Dorsal-radial/middle pain**, often with palpable mass:
  -Dorsal ganglion cyst
- **Consider osteoarthritis, rheumatoid arthritis, SLE, cellulitis, or other medical process**

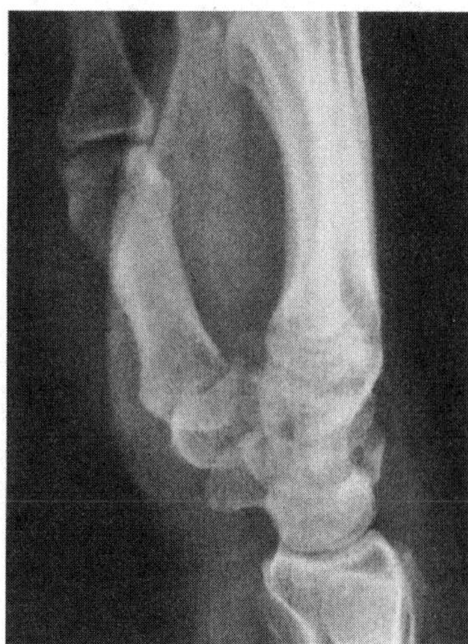

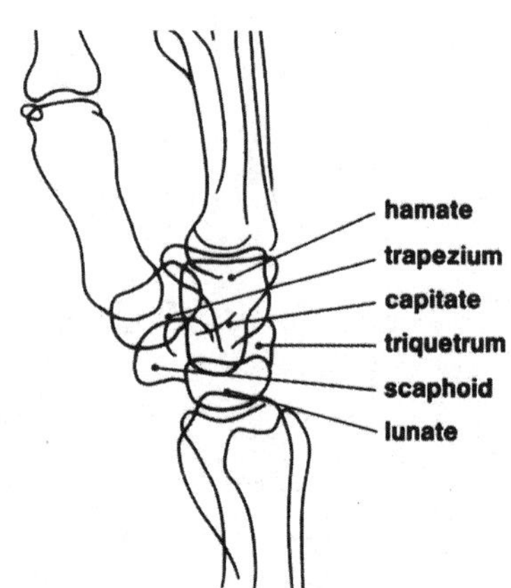

Radiograph 1: Lateral view of the right wrist

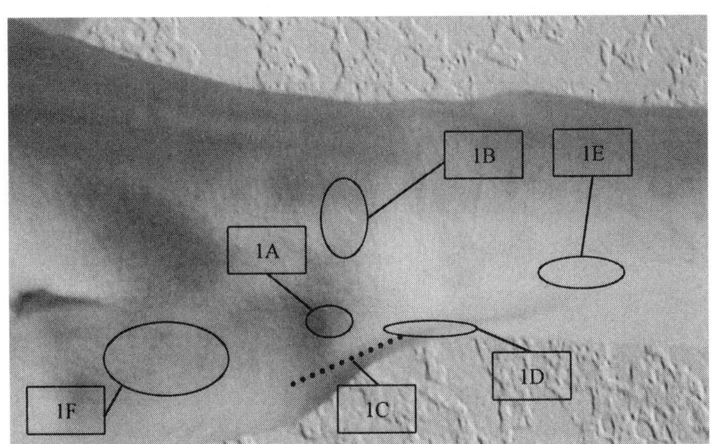

Figure 1

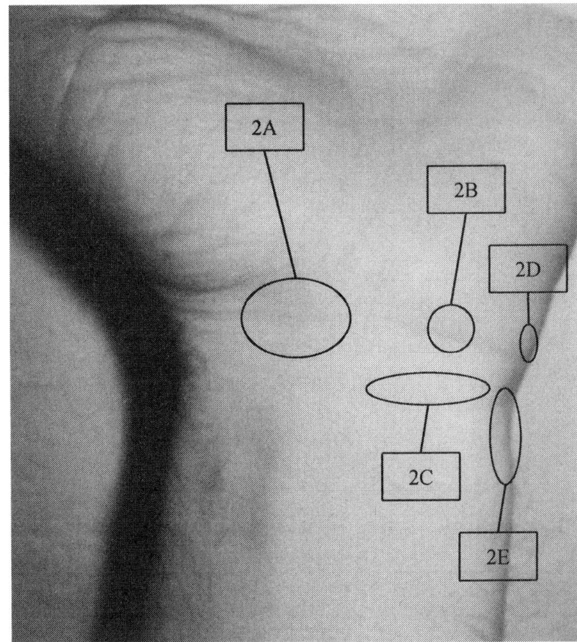

Figure 2

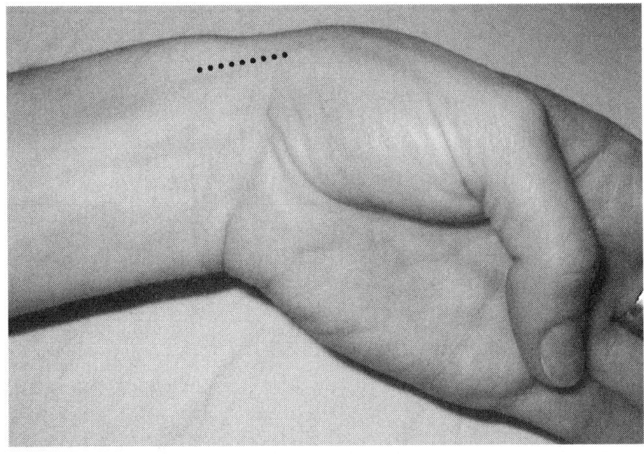

Figure 3: Finkelstein's test - pain and tenderness along abductor pollicis longus (APL) and extensor pollicis brevis (EPB).

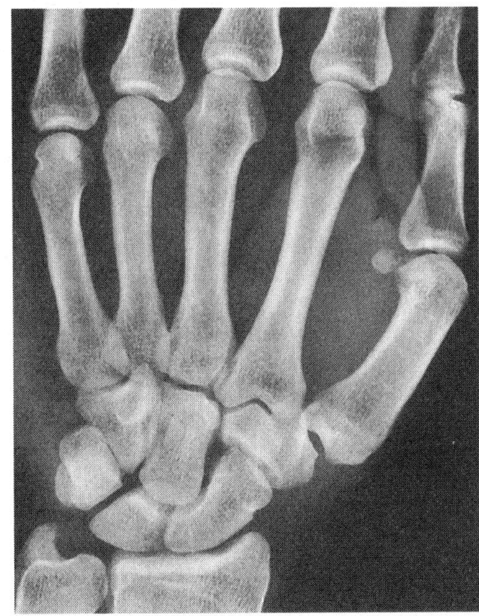

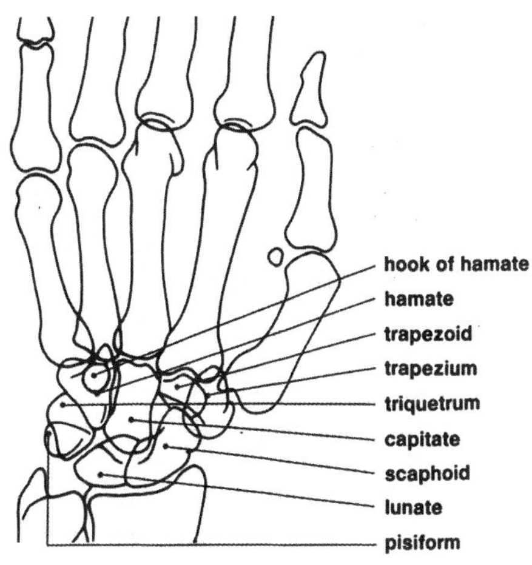

Radiograph 2: PA view of the left wrist

Finger

Acute

? Trauma with obvious deformity and bony derangement on X-ray

- **Dislocation**:
  *-DIP, PIP dislocation ****
  *-MCP dislocation****
- **Fracture**:
  *-Distal phalanx****
  *-Proximal phalanx****
  *-Metacarpal base/shaft****
  *-Middle phalanx****
  *-Metacarpal neck****
- **1A, 2: Inability to *extend* at DIP**, +/- avulsion fracture of dorsum of proximal distal phalanx:
  *-Extensor avulsion/mallet finger****
- **1C: Inability to *flex* at DIP** while holding PIP stable (not due to pain); commonly tender where avulsed tendon stump lies (anywhere from palm to PIP); +/- avulsion of palmar aspect of proximal distal phalanx :
  *-Flexor avulsion/jersey finger****
- **1B: Swollen, tender PIP**; weak extension (not due to pain), tenderness over dorsum of PIP, +/- avulsion of dorsum of proximal middle phalanx :
  *-Central slip avulsion and pseudo-boutonnière deformities (boutonnière deformity usually not visible early)****

? No fracture on X-ray +/- deformity

- ***Extensor avulsion, Flexor avulsion,* and *Central slip avulsions*** as described above commonly occur without fractures.
- **Instability/deformity with active/passive ROM:**
  *DIP, PIP dislocation***, MCP dislocation****
- **Pain, swelling with intact tendons +/- laxity at joints:**
  *-Interphalangeal collateral ligament sprain****
  *-MCP collateral ligament sprain****

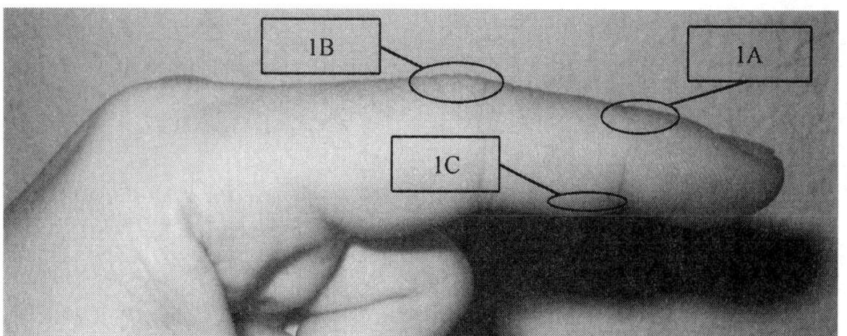

Figure 1

Chronic

? History of acute injury, delayed presentation with deformity +/- pain

- **1A, 2: Inability to *extend* at DIP** :
  *-Extensor avulsion (mallet finger) ****
- **1C: Inability to *flex* at DIP** while holding PIP stable:
  *-Flexor avulsion (jersey finger) ****
- **Boutonnière deformity**: PIP fixed in flexion and DIP in extension:
  *-Central slip avulsion****
- **Swan-neck deformity**: PIP fixed in hyperextension and DIP in flexion:
  -Volar plate injury or
  *-Mallet finger with laxity****

? Locking, catching of fingers

- **PP Fingers locked in flexion contracture** at palmar crease, often with thickened fibrotic cord:
  *-Dupuytren's contracture****
- **Fingers catch with flexion** but not locked:
  -Trigger finger

? Chronic pain, swelling of joints

- **Consider osteoarthritis, rheumatoid arthritis, SLE, infection, other medical process.**

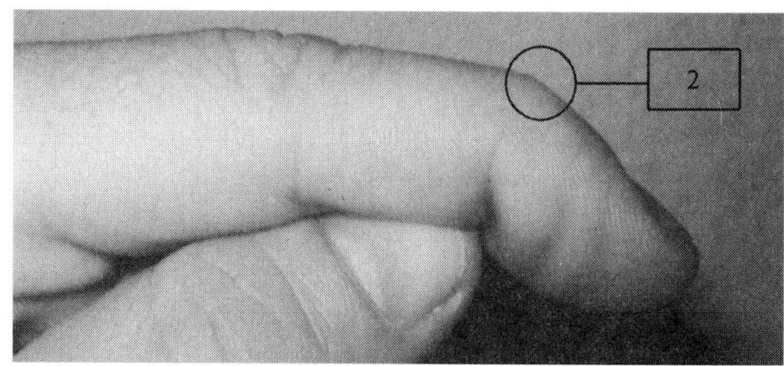

Figure 2: Mallet finger: inability to extend at DIP joint

Acute

? **Trauma with obvious deformity and bony derangement on X-ray**

- **Dislocation**:
  *-DIP, PIP dislocation****
  *-MCP dislocation****
- **Fracture**:
  *-Thumb fracture****
- **Fig 1: Avulsion of ulnar side of proximal phalanx**, tenderness over UCL (ulnar aspect of MCP)
  *-Ulnar collateral ligament injury****

? **No fracture on X-ray +/- deformity**

- **Fig 1: Point of maximal tenderness over ulnar aspect of MCP**; +/- laxity with stress as pictured:
  *-Ulnar collateral ligament sprain****
- **Pain, swelling with intact tendons +/- laxity at IP joint**:
  *-IP Collateral ligament injury****

Chronic

? **History of acute injury, delayed presentation with deformity +/- pain**

- **Fig 1: Impaired grip with laxity of UCL**
  *-Ulnar collateral ligament sprain****

? **Repetitive stress, usually without history of trauma**

- **PP Volar-radial pain**, numbness +/- tenderness over dorsum of thumb and hand, ⊕ Tinel's, negative Finkelstein's test :
  -Superficial radial nerve/Wartenberg's disease ***

? **Chronic pain, swelling of joints**

- **Consider osteoarthritis, rheumatoid arthritis, SLE, infection, other medical process.**

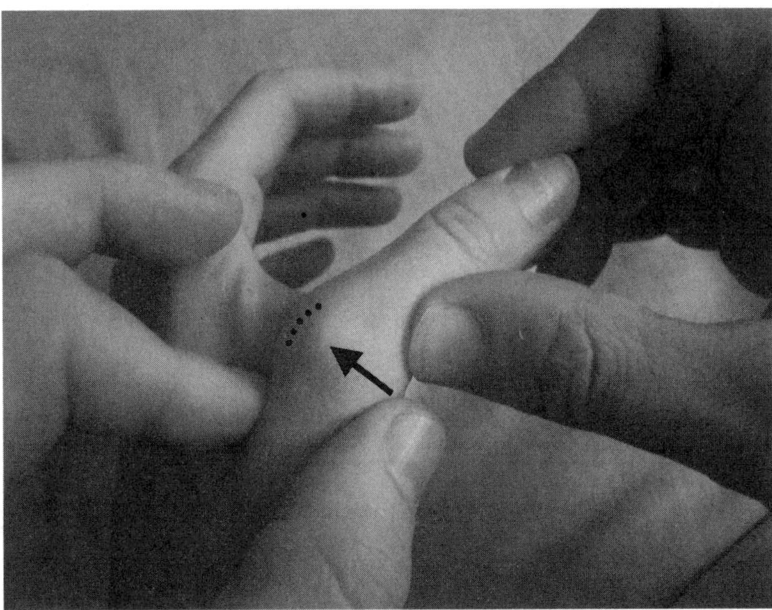

Figure 1: UCL Injury: Apply gentle stress on radial side of MCP in both flexion and extension.

Acute

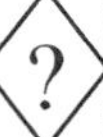

Trauma with obvious deformity or bony derangement on X-ray

Anterior/groin pain:
-High engergy trauma with limb shortening, internal rotation, and adduction: *Hip dislocation (posterior)****, *Hip/pelvis fracture*
-1D: Tenderness at origin of sartoris (ASIS) or rectus femoris (AIIS), usually in adolescent: *Avulsion of ASIS, AIIS****

Posterior/buttock pain:
-2A: Tenderness at origin of hamstring, usually in adolescent: *Ischial tuberosity avulsion****
-2F: Posterolateral or deep pain after direct blow to abdomen or iliac crest; worse with contraction of abdominal muscles or lateral bending: *Iliac crest avulsion****

No fracture on X-ray +/- deformity

Anterior/groin pain:
-1A: Pain with adductor palpation, passive stretch, and resisted contraction: *Adductor strain****
-1B: "Pulling" sensation in anterior thigh while sprinting: *Rectus femoris strain*
-Trauma to anterior thigh with pain, swelling, and decreased range of motion: *Quadriceps contusion****

Lateral pain:
-2B: Pain, soft tissue swelling, ecchymosis after direct blow to iliac crest: *Hip pointer****

Posterior pain:
-2C: "Pop/pull" felt in posterior thigh while sprinting: *Hamstring strain*
-2D: Sharp buttock pain in sprinter: *Gluteus maximus strain*

Consider acute exacerbation of CHRONIC injury or medical diagnosis: rheumatoid arthritis, osteoarthritis, SLE, infection, etc…

Figure 1

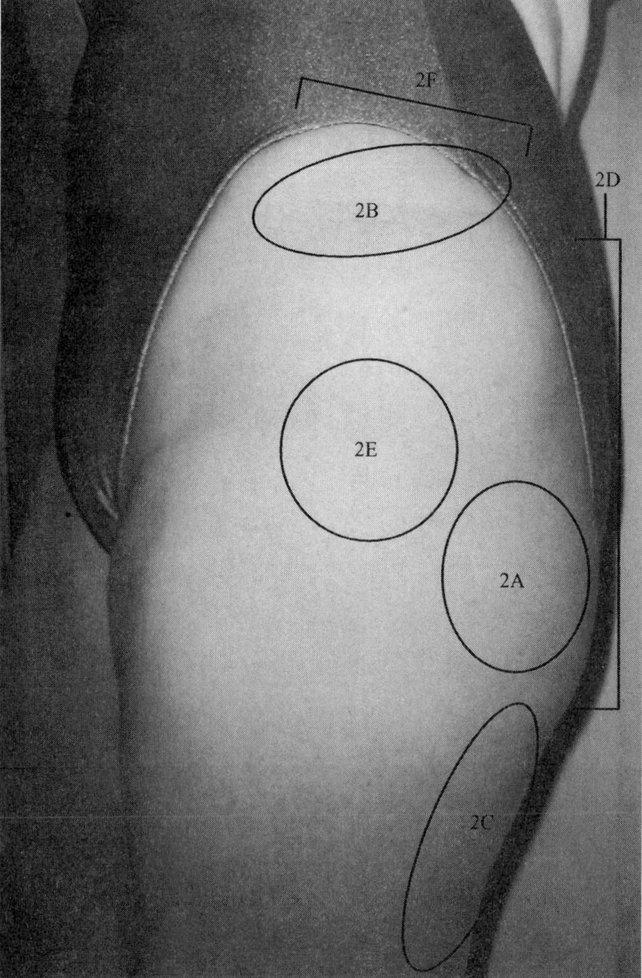

Figure 2

Chronic

History of recent or distant injury, but with chronic symptoms

Anterior/groin pain:
-1A: Pain with muscle palpation, passive stretch, and resisted contraction: *Adductor strain****
-1C: Pain with ipsilateral single-leg stance, Trendelenburg gait; often with a history of prior trauma or steroids: *AVN of the femoral head*
-1C: Deep pain with mechanical symptoms: *Acetabular labral tear*

Posterior/buttock pain:
-Cramping/aching buttock pain worse with sitting: *Piriformis syndrome****

Generalized pain (can localize anywhere depending on prior history):
-Prior contusion with hematoma 2-4 weeks earlier: *Myositis ossificans*

Review diagnoses on ACUTE algorithm for possible missed diagnosis

Repetitive stress, usually without history of trauma

Anterior/groin pain:
-1C: Pain with ipsilateral single-leg stance, Trendelenburg gait: *Femoral neck stress fracture*
-1C: Pain with twisting or cutting in a 20-30 year old: *Osteitis pubis****
-1C: Inferior pubic rim tenderness in athlete with recent change in activity: *Pubic rami stress fracture*
-1C: Groin pain and "snapping" with hip flexion: *Iliopsoas bursitis/tendinitis*
-1C: Pain with sprinting, kicking; work-up otherwise unremarkable: *Sports hernia****

Lateral pain:
-2E: Pain with lying on affected side: *Trochanteric bursitis*
-2E: Tight iliotibial band, "snapping" hip: *Tensor fascia lata syndrome*

Posterior pain:
-Cramping/aching buttock pain worse with sitting: *Piriformis syndrome****
-Tenderness over posterior superior iliac spine, with radiation into buttock or posterolateral thigh: *Sacroiliac joint dysfunction*

Insidious onset of pain, swelling, or deformity without trauma or repetitive stress

Anterior symptoms:
-1C: Pain with ipsilateral single-leg stance, Trendelenburg gait; often with a history of prior trauma or steroids: *AVN of the femoral head*
-Pain/paresthesias radiating down anterior thigh: *Meralgia paresthetica*

Posterior symptoms:
-Cramping/aching buttock pain worse with sitting: *Piriformis syndrome****
-Tenderness over posterior superior iliac spine, with radiation into buttock or posterolateral thigh: *Sacroiliac joint dysfunction*

Consider osteoarthritis, rheumatoid arthritis, SLE, infection, or other medical process

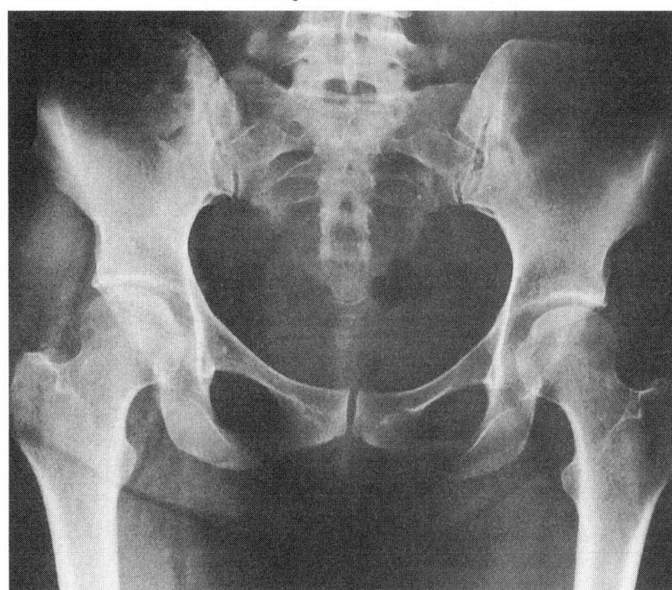

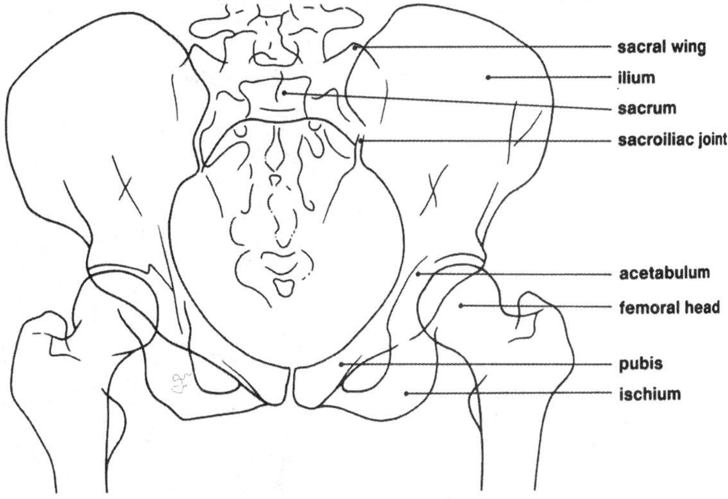

Radiograph 1: AP view of the pelvis

Pediatric Hip

Acute

? Trauma with obvious deformity or bony derangement on X-ray

Anterior/groin pain:
-1C: Groin pain after incidental trauma during adolescent growth spurt, especially in a heavier patient; associated with a limp: *Slipped capital femoral epiphysis*
-1D: Tenderness at origin of sartoris (ASIS) in adolescent: *Avulsion of ASIS****
-1D: Tenderness at origin of rectus femoris (AIIS), in adolescent: *Avulsion of AIIS****

Posterior/buttock pain:
-2A: Tenderness at origin of hamstring, usually in adolescent: *Ischial tuberosity avulsion****
-2F: Posterolateral or deep pain after direct blow to abdomen or iliac crest; worse with contraction of abdominal muscles or lateral bending: *Iliac crest avulsion****

Consider other diagnoses as listed for adult hip pain

? No fracture on X-ray +/- deformity

Anterior/groin pain:
-Trauma to anterior thigh with pain, swelling, and decreased range of motion: *Quadriceps contusion****

Lateral pain:
-2B: Pain, soft tissue swelling, ecchymosis after direct blow to iliac crest: *Hip pointer****

Consider other diagnoses as listed for adult hip pain

Consider acute exacerbation of CHRONIC injury or medical diagnosis: inflammatory arthritis, congenital anomaly, infection, etc...

Chronic

History of recent or distant injury, but with chronic symptoms

Anterior/groin pain:
-1C: Groin pain after incidental trauma during adolescent growth spurt, especially in a heavier patient; associated with a limp: *Slipped capital femoral epiphysis*

Review diagnoses on ACUTE algorithm for possible missed diagnosis

Repetitive stress, usually without history of trauma

Consider other diagnoses as listed for adult hip pain

Insidious onset of pain, swelling, or deformity without trauma or repetitive stress

Anterior pain:
-1C: Groin pain after incidental trauma during adolescent growth spurt, especially in a heavier patient; associated with a limp: *Slipped capital femoral epiphysis*
-1C: Prepubertal patient (2-11y/o) with a limp and decreased internal rotation of the hip: *Avascular necrosis of proximal femoral epiphysis (Legg-Calve-Perthes Disease)****
-Limping child with asymmetric hip abduction test: *Developmental dysplasia of the hip*
-Night pain, worse with activity: *Osteoid osteoma*

Consider other diagnoses as listed for adult hip pain

Consider juvenille arthritis, rheumatoid arthritis, SLE, infection, or other medical process

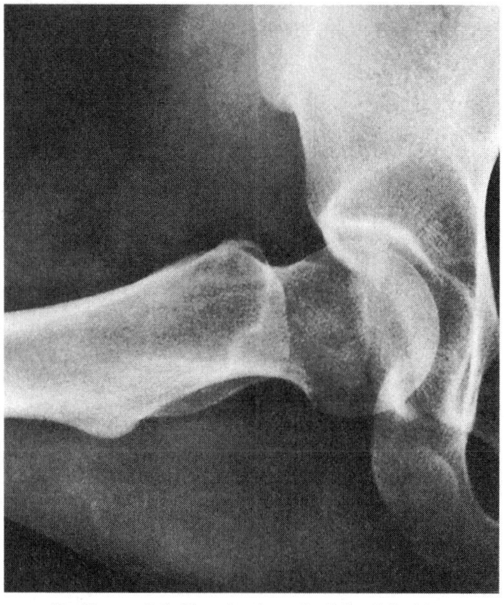

Radiograph 1: Frog leg lateral of the right hip

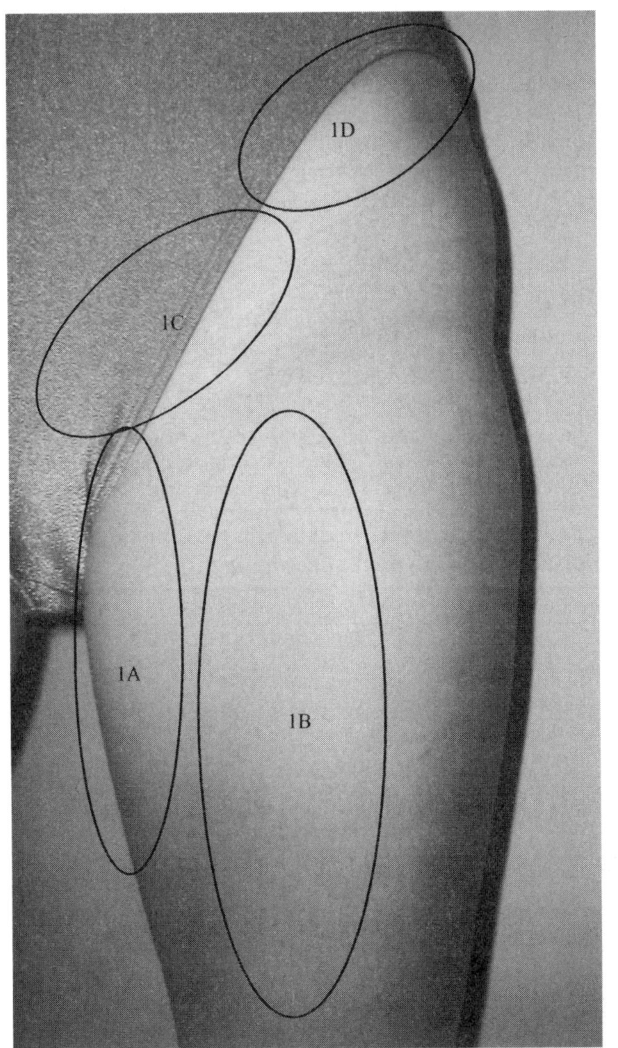

Figure 1

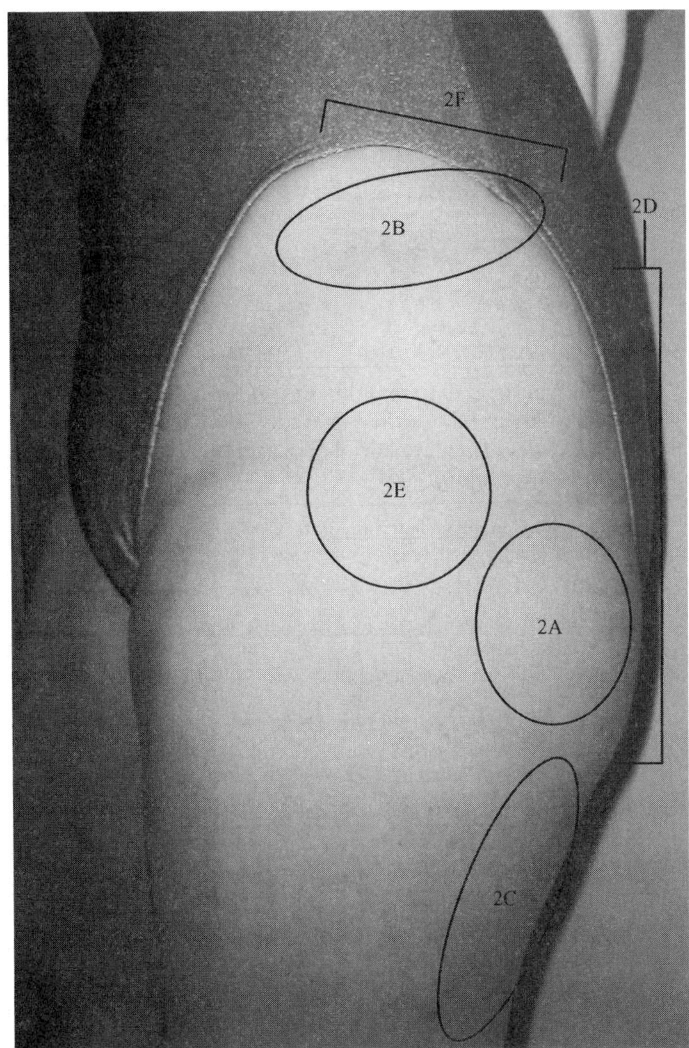

Figure 2

Acute

? Trauma with obvious deformity (obtain X-rays)

- **Dislocation**: Usually reduced in the field, but may have residual pain along medial patella:
  *-Knee dislocation ****
  *-Patellar dislocation****
- **Fracture**:
  *-Avulsion fracture****
  *-Patella fracture****
  *-Femur fracture****
  -Tibia fracture

? No fracture, ⊕ hemarthrosis—if aspirated (controversial)—otherwise may be effusion. (May be difficult to adequately examine for several days after injury.)

- **⊕Lachman, pivot shift, instability**; usually pop felt or heard at time of injury with swelling over a few hours:
  *-Anterior cruciate ligament tear ****
- **1D: ⊕McMurray's test, joint line tenderness**, pain with squatting, twisting:
  *-Meniscal tear (hemarthrosis with peripheral tear)****
- **1K: Tenderness along medial patella**, ⊕ patellar apprehension/instability:
  *-Patellar dislocation (already reduced) ****
- **No specific pattern of tenderness**,
  -Possible osteochondral injury

? No hemarthrosis, +/- effusion (aspiration necessary to distinguish hemarthrosis from effusion but not always recommended)

- **1J: Medial tenderness +/- instability with VALGUS stress**:
  *-Medial collateral ligament injury ****
- **1C: Lateral tenderness +/- instability with VARUS stress**:
  *-Lateral collateral ligament injury ****
  *-Posterolateral capsule injury *** (if laxity with leg in full extension)*
- **⊕ Sag sign, posterior drawer test**:
  *-Posterior cruciate ligament injury ****
- **Consider diagnoses usually associated with hemarthrosis but with concomitant capsular disruption (blood is unable to accumulate in joint if capsule is disrupted)**

? Locking or inability to extend knee fully beyond disability due to pain and swelling

- **1D: Mechanical lock, ⊕McMurray's test, joint line tenderness**: Semi-urgent if unable to fully extend due to locking.
  *-Meniscal tear****
- **1E or 1M: Quad weakness, palpable defect,** ecchymosis:
  *-Patellar/quadriceps tendon rupture ****
- **Consider exacerbation of CHRONIC injury or medical diagnosis such as septic arthritis, osteoarthritis, gout or cellulitis.**
- **Consider HIP injury with pain referred to knee.**

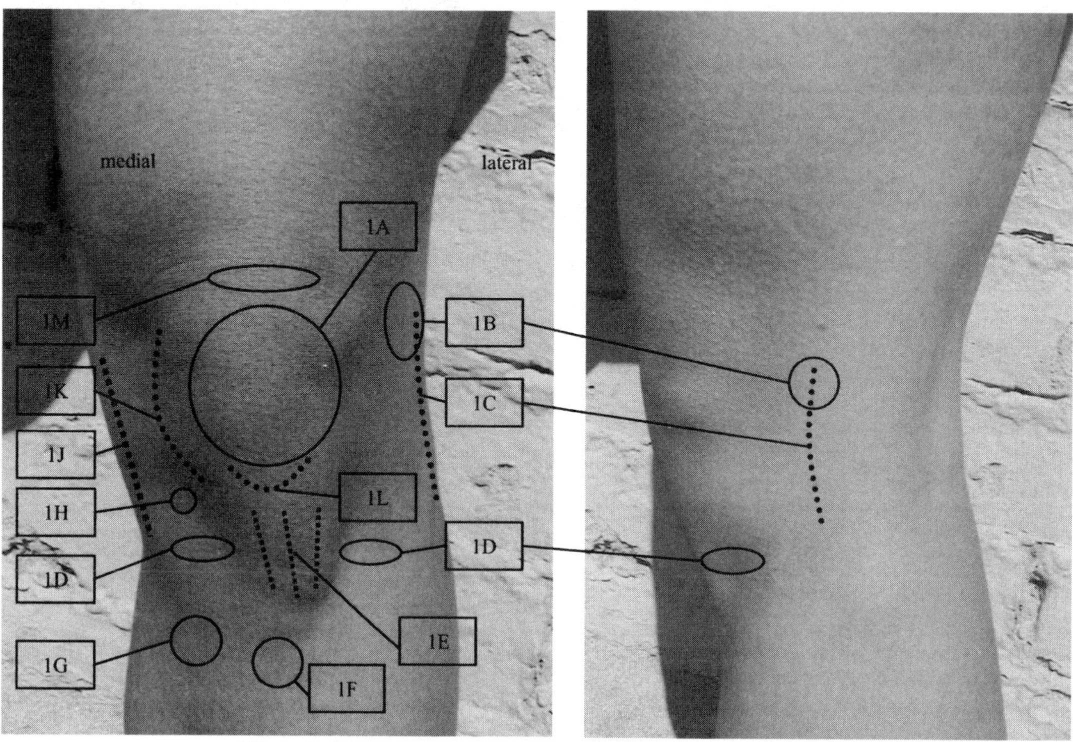

Figure 1   Figure 2

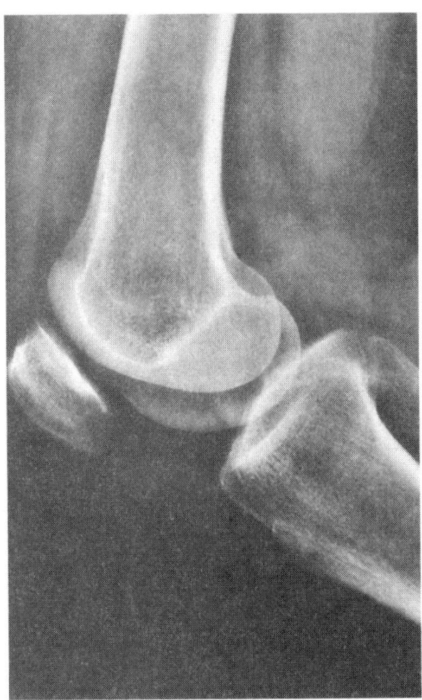

Radiograph 1: Lateral view of the knee

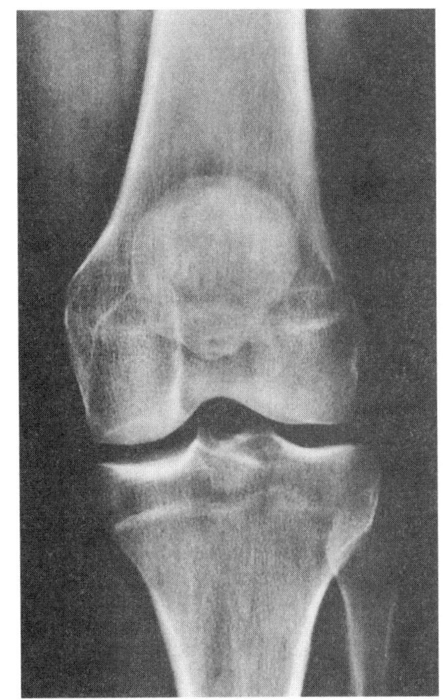

Radiograph 2: AP view of the left knee

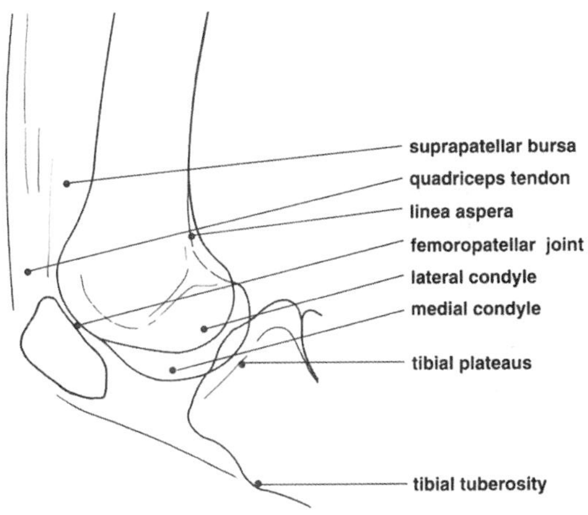

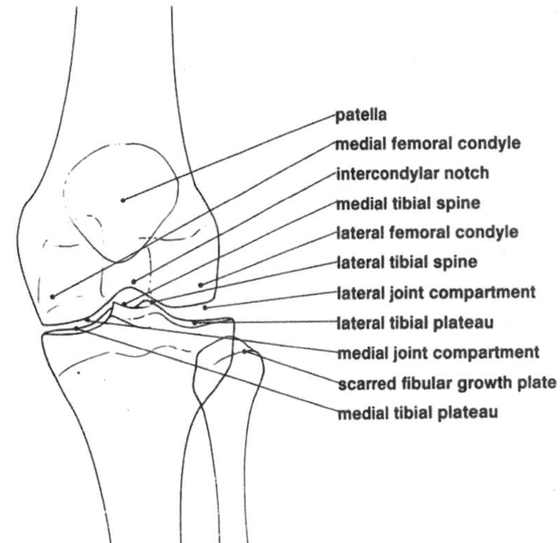

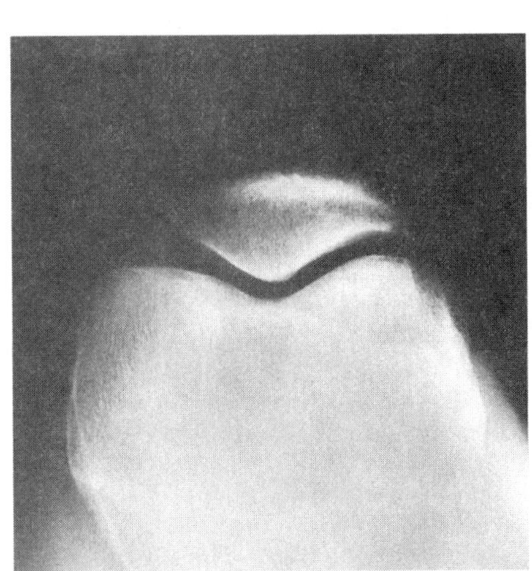

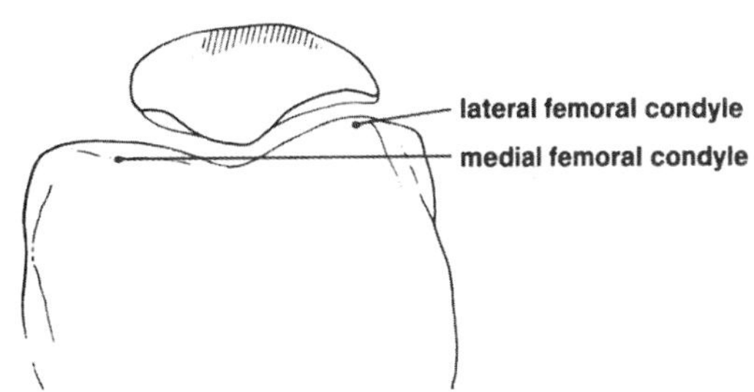

Radiograph 3: Axial (sunrise) view of the patella

Chronic

Remote history of acute injury, but chronic symptoms

- **⊕Lachman, pivot shift, instability**: *-Anterior cruciate ligament tear* ***
- **1D: ⊕McMurray's test, joint line tenderness**, pain with squatting, twisting: *-Meniscal tear* ***
- **⊕ Sag sign, posterior drawer test**: *-Posterior cruciate ligament injury* ***
- **1K: ⊕ patellar apprehension & instability**, +/-tenderness along medial patella: *-Patellar instability* ***
- **Loss of joint space on x-ray**: *-Osteoarthritis*

Localized tenderness as pictured

- **1B: Tenderness along iliotibial band, ⊕ Ober's test**, iliotibial band tightness: *-Iliotibial band syndrome****
- **1E: Tenderness over patellar tendon**: *-Patellar/quadriceps tendinitis****
- **1H: Tenderness & click along medial knee**: *-Redundant plica* ***
- **1G: Tenderness at superior medial tibia**: *-Pes anserine bursitis* ***
- **1A: Patellar tenderness after minor trauma or repetitive athletic activities; bipartite patella on x-ray**: *-Bipartite patella*

Localized swelling (not effusion)

- **Swelling +/-tenderness in popliteal fossa/posterior knee**: *-Baker's cyst* ***
- **PP Swelling +/-tenderness around patella**: *-Bursitis (pre, retropatellar)****

Anterior knee pain—not easily localized

- **1A: ⊕Patellar grind, quad inhibition tests**, pain with going up/down stairs, ↑ Q angle, pes planus: *-Patellofemoral pain syndrome* ***
- **1A: ⊕Non-specific knee pain**; defect on x-ray: *-Osteochondritis dissecans* ***

Locking, catching, foreign body sensation

- Consider loose body or meniscal tear.
- X-rays show DJD: *Consider osteoarthritis.*
- Consider exacerbation of CHRONIC injury or medical diagnosis: septic arthritis, osteoarthritis, gout

Knee work-up otherwise unremarkable

- **Consider hip injury with referred pain to knee or medical problem such as septic arthritis, osteoarthritis, gout, cellulitis, or other medical condition.**

Youth

Tenderness/pain as pictured

- **1F:Tenderness +/-swelling at tibial tubercle**: *-Osgood-Schlatter disease* ***
- **1L: Tenderness +/-swelling at inferior pole of patella**: *-Sindig-Larsen-Johannsen disease (apophysitis of patella)*
- **1D: Lateral joint line tenderness +/- mechanical symptoms**: *-Discoid lateral mensicus*
- **Consider hip injury with pain referred to knee.**

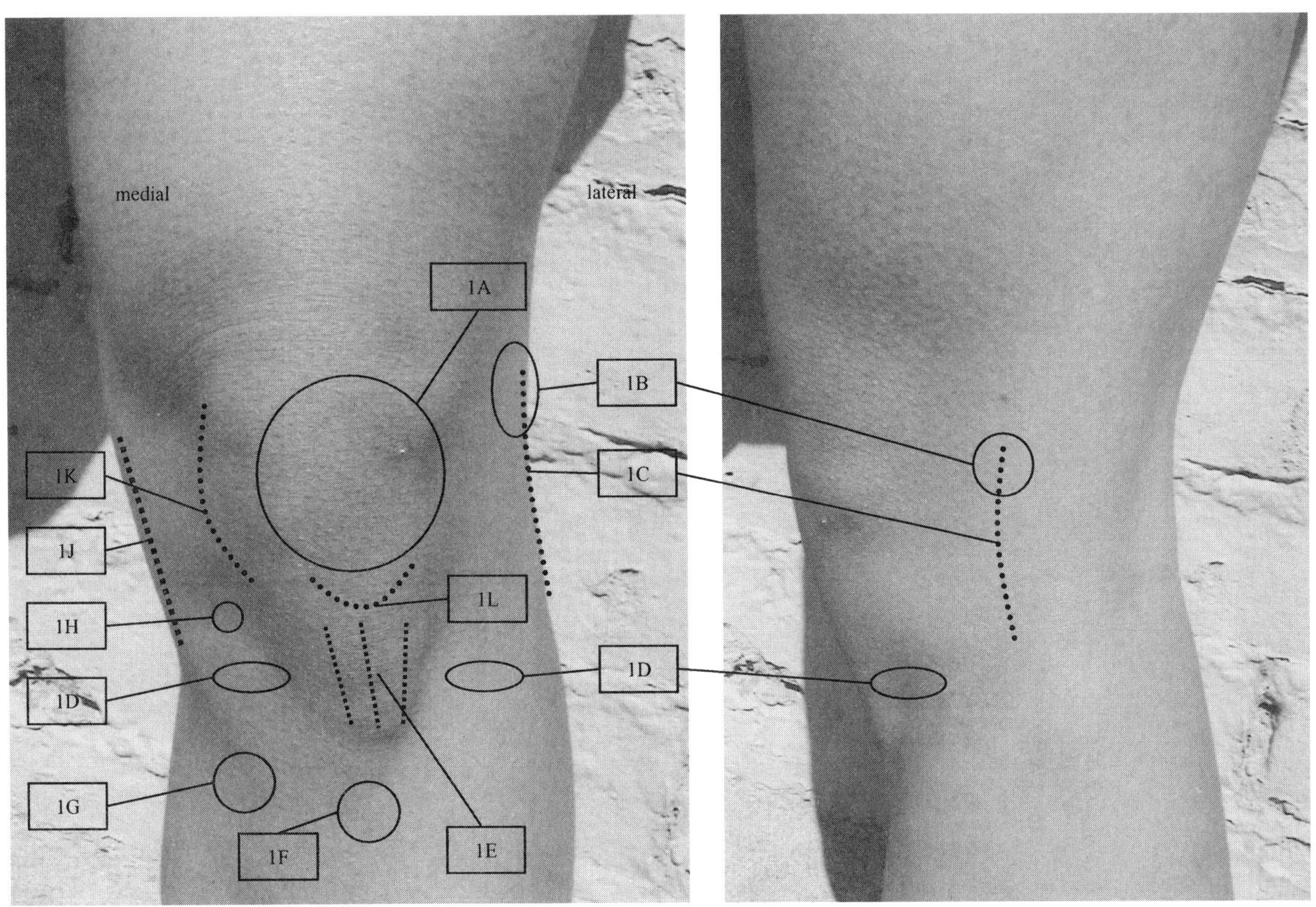

Figure 1

Figure 2

Acute

? Trauma with obvious deformity or bony derangement on X-ray

- **X-ray reveals possible fracture**:
  - *-Tibial fracture* ***
  - *-Fibular fracture* ***

? Negative X-ray

- **Tenderness along lateral border of shin**; history of recent overuse:
  -Acute muscle soreness
- **Progressive unrelenting pain out of proportion to injury**; later developing into symptoms of neurologic and vascular compromise:
  *-Compartment syndrome, anterior *** (surgical emergency)*
- **Calf tenderness +/- palpable defect**; weakness of foot plantarflexion:
  -Gastrocnemius tear
- **Consider acute exacerbation of chronic process**:
  -Review chronic algorithm

Chronic

? Chronic pain (obtain X-rays +/- bone scan or other imaging)

- **Posteromedial tibial pain** over middle and distal thirds; begins with activity and persists progressively longer; X-rays may show periosteal reaction; bone scan shows diffuse uptake:
  *-Medial tibial stress syndrome****
- **Localized tibial pain**; begins with activity and persists progressively longer; usually point tenderness; X-rays may be normal early or show periosteal reaction or stress fracture; bone scan shows localized uptake:
  *-Tibial stress fracture****
- **Exertional shin pain**; predictably begins at certain level of activity; resolves with rest within minutes; X-rays normal; bone scan normal; elevated compartment pressures with exercise:
  *-Compartment syndrome, anterior (chronic exertional type)****
- **Normal X-ray, bone scan, compartment pressures:**
  -Consider rare causes such as lumbosacral radiculopathy, artery/nerve entrapment, fascial defect, or venous thrombosis.

(See ankle algorithm for distal tibia/fibula injuries)

Heel and Ankle

Acute

Trauma with obvious deformity or bony derangement on X-ray

Generalized/diffuse pain (pain can include any or all parts of the heel and ankle):
-1A, 2A, 4A: Generalized heel pain, swelling, ecchymosis: *Calcaneus fracture* ***
-1B, 2B, 3A: Pain at ankle, proximal foot: *Talus fracture****

Posterior pain:
-2C: H/O forced plantar flexion: *Os trigonum fracture*
-2C: Multiple ankle injuries with significant posterior component of pain: consider concurrent *Volkmann's fracture (Posterolateral tibia-fibula ligament avulsion)****
-2C: Fractures of both medial and lateral malleoli with significant posterior component of pain: consider concurrent *Posterior malleolus fracture (trimalleolar fracture)*

Lateral pain:
-2G: Twisting injury, malleolar pain: *Lateral malleolus fracture****

Medial pain:
-1G: Twisting injury, malleolar pain: *Medial malleolus fracture****

Anterior pain:
-3J: Positive squeeze or external rotation tests; increased tib-fib clear space on x-ray, abnormal stress views: *Syndesmosial injury of the lower leg****
-3J: Avulsion of distal tibial epiphysis in 12-15 year old athlete: *Tilleaux fracture: anterior tibia-fibula ligament avulsion****

No fracture on X-ray +/- deformity

Posterior pain:
-1C: Palpable defect in Achilles tendon: *Achilles tendon/gastrocnemius rupture****
-2F: Posterolateral pain/swelling, h/o inversion mechanism: Posterior talo-fibular ligament sprain (see *Lateral ankle sprain****)
-2F: Posterolateral pain/swelling, h/o dorsiflexion-eversion mechanism: *Peroneal tendon dislocation/subluxation*
-1H: Posteromedial pain, weak toe off: *Flexor hallicus longus tear*

Lateral pain:
-2B: Inversion injury, positive drawer test: *Lateral ankle sprain****
-2F: Posterolateral pain/swelling, h/o dorsiflexion-eversion mechanism: *Peroneal tendon dislocation/subluxation*

Medial pain:
-1B: Pronation-external rotation mechanism: Deltoid ligament sprain (*see Medial ankle sprain*)
-1H: Inversion weakness, weak toe rise: *Posterior tibialis tendon rupture*

Anterior pain:
-1I, 3K: Forced plantarflexion mechanism, foot drop: *Tibialis anterior tendon rupture*

Plantar pain:
-1A, 2A, 4A: Ecchymosis at heel: *Heel bruise/heel fat pad syndrome****

Consider occult x-ray presentation of diagnosis usually associated with abnormal x-ray

Consider acute exacerbation of CHRONIC injury or medical diagnosis: rheumatoid arthritis, osteoarthritis, SLE, infection, etc...

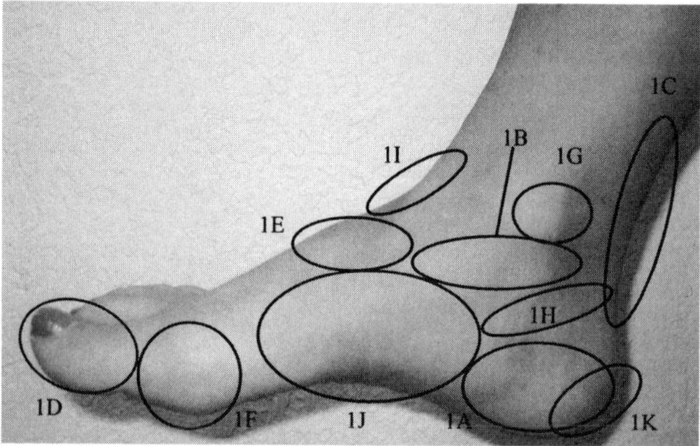

Figure 1

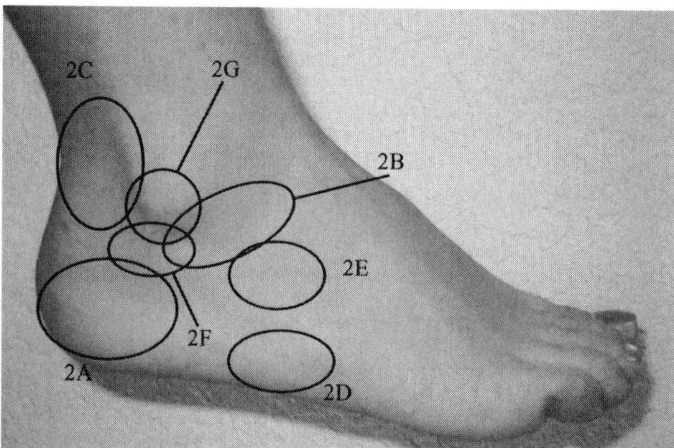

Figure 2

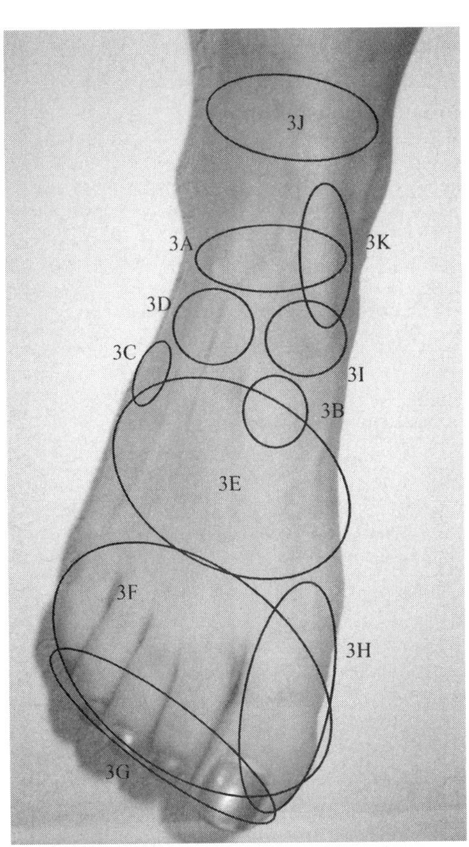

Figure 3

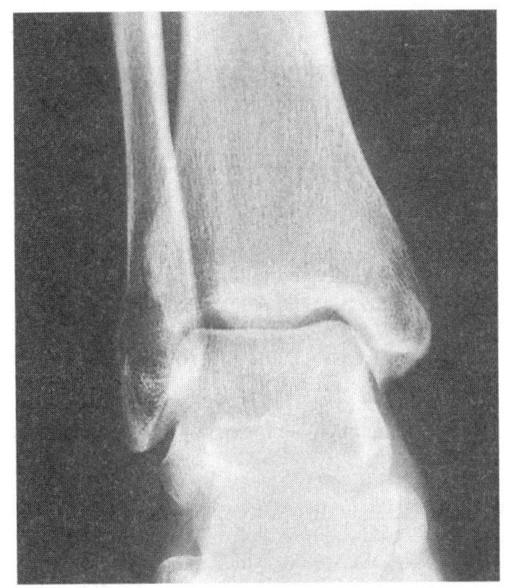

Radiograph 1: AP view of the right ankle

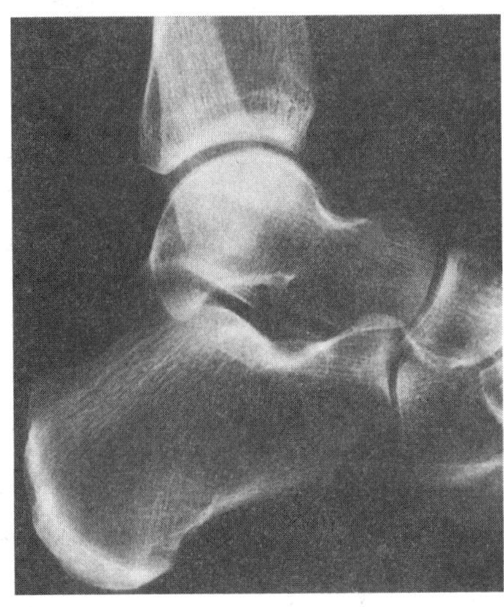

Radiograph 2: Lateral view of the ankle

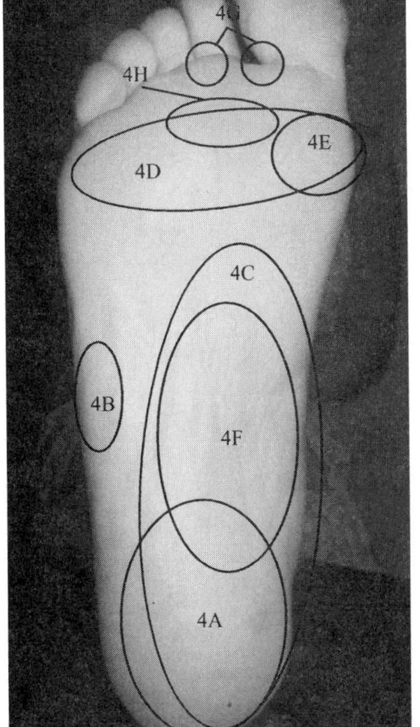

Figure 4

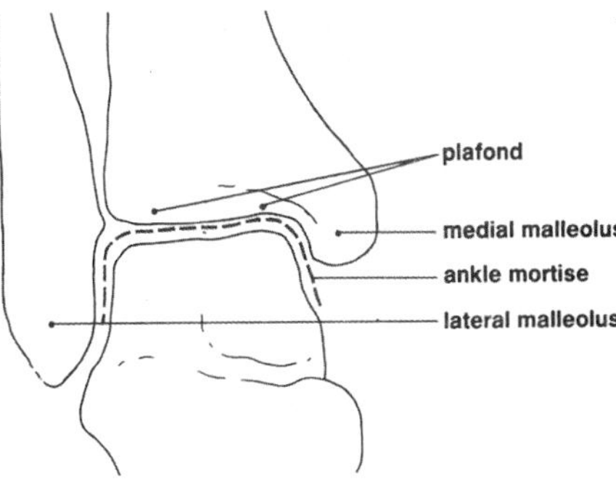

Radiograph 3: Mortise view of the right ankle

Chronic

History of recent or distant injury, but with chronic symptoms

Generalized pain (can localize anywhere or be diffuse):
-1B, 2B, 3A: Unresolved "routine" ankle sprain: OCD of the talar dome (see *Talus fracture****)

Lateral pain:
-2B: Unresolved "routine" ankle sprain: *Chronic ankle instability*
-2F: Posterolateral pain, distant dorsiflexion injury: *Peroneal tendonitis*

Medial pain:
-1B: Unresolved "routine" ankle sprain: *Chronic ankle instability*
-1H: Painful/weak inversion and toe rise: *Posterior tibial tendinitis*

Anterior pain:
-3J: Painful, limited passive dorsiflexion; anterior osteophytes on x-ray: *Anterior bony impingement*
-1I, 3K: Shoelace irritation over anterior ankle: *Tibialis anterior tendonitis*

Plantar pain:
-4C: Plantar hind-to-midfoot paresthesias and pain: *Tarsal tunnel syndrome****

Repetitive stress, usually without history of trauma

Posterior pain:
-1C: Pain 2-6 cm proximal to Achilles insertion into calcaneus: *Achilles tendinitis* ***
-1C: Tenderness posterior to talus but anterior to Achilles tendon: *Retrocalcaneal bursitis*
-1A, 2A, 4A: Recent change in activity, pain with medial-lateral squeeze of calcaneus: *Calcaneal stress fracture*
-2C: Posterolateral pain with forced plantarflexion; os trigonum on x-ray: *Os trigonum tarsi*
-1K: In 7-12 y/o age group: *Calcaneal apophysitis (Sever's disease)*

Medial pain:
-1H: Painful/weak inversion and toe rise: *Posterior tibial tendinitis*

Anterior pain:
-1I, 3K: Shoelace irritation over anterior ankle: *Tibialis anterior tendonitis*

Plantar pain:
-4F: Plantar heel pain, radiating into arch: *Plantar fasciitis****
-4C: Plantar hind-to-midfoot paresthesias and pain: *Tarsal tunnel syndrome****

Insidious onset of pain, swelling, or deformity without trauma or repetitive stress

Posterior symptoms:
-1C: Prominence over posterior calcaneus: *Haglund's deformity****

Lateral symptoms:
-2F: Sinus tarsi pain/swelling in patient with pes planus: *Sinus tarsi syndrome*

Medial symptoms:
-1J: Pes planus, medial loss of arch: *Posterior tibialis tendon rupture, chronic*

Anterior symptoms:
-1I, 3K: Shoelace irritation over anterior ankle: *Tibialis anterior tendonitis*

Plantar symptoms:
-4F: Plantar heel pain, radiating into arch: *Plantar fasciitis****
-4C: Plantar hind-to-midfoot paresthesias and pain: *Tarsal tunnel syndrome****

Consider osteoarthritis, rheumatoid arthritis, SLE, infection, or other medical process

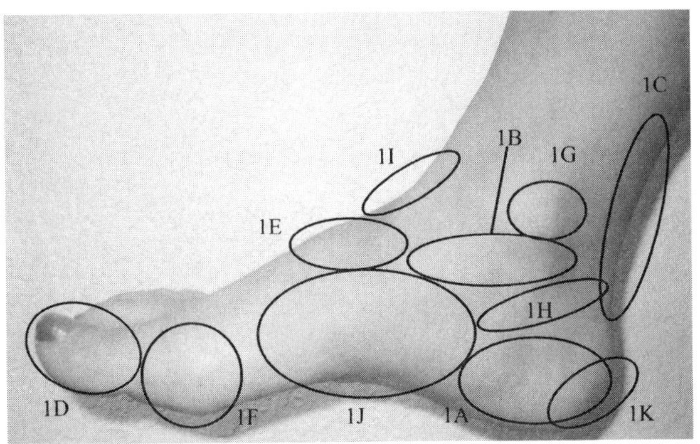

Figure 1

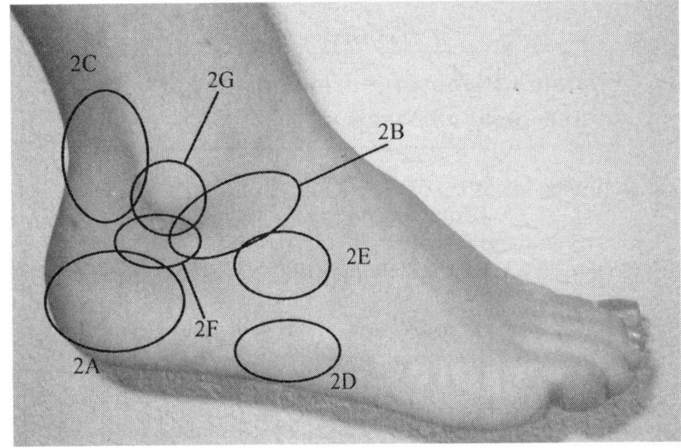

Figure 2

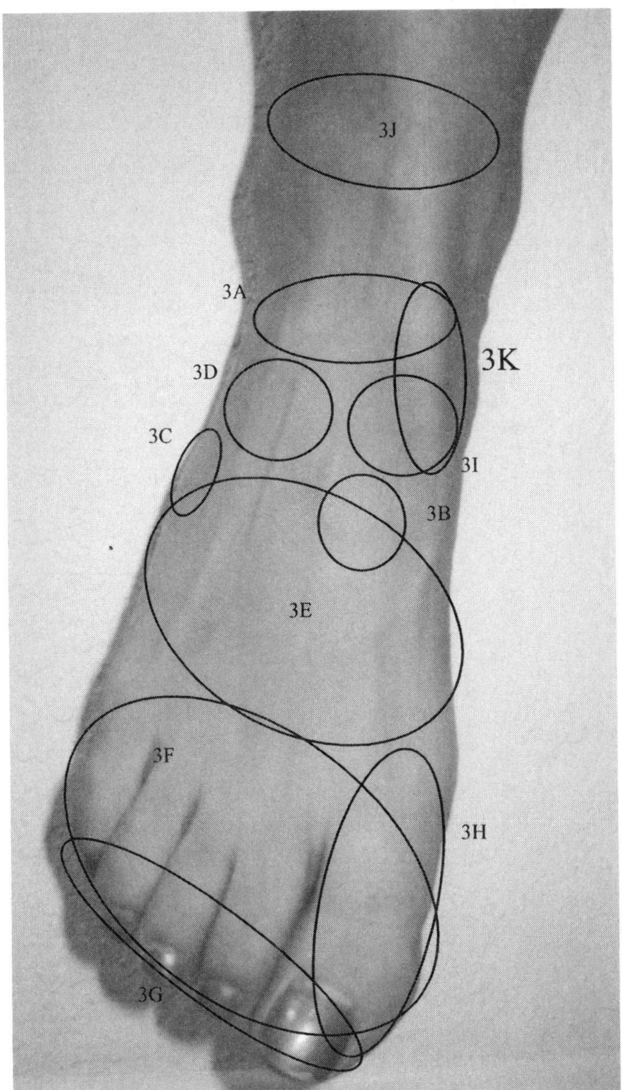

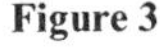
Figure 3

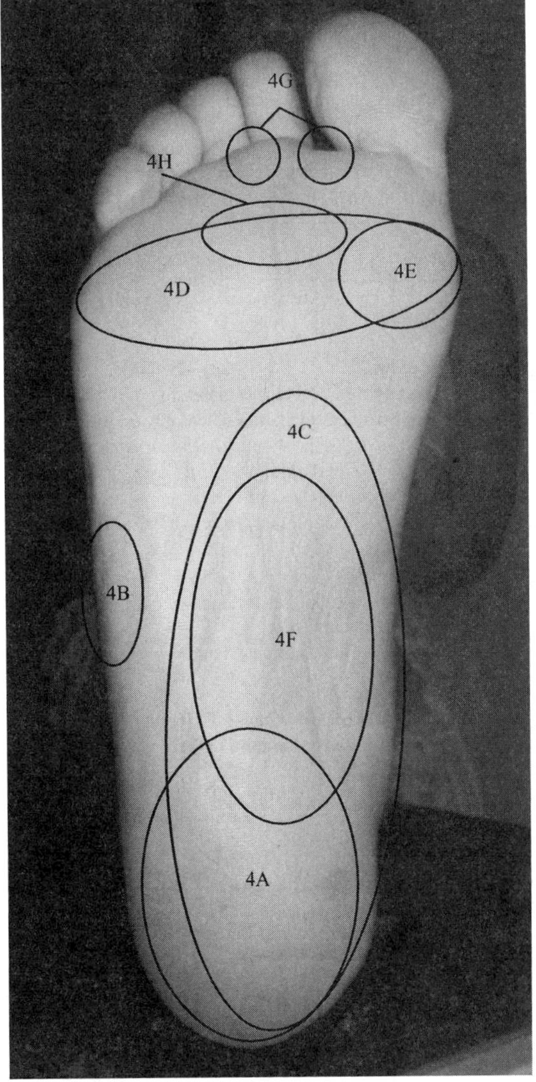

Figure 4

Acute

Trauma with obvious deformity or bony derangement on X-ray

Hindfoot pain:
- -1A, 2A, 4A: Generalized heel pain, swelling, ecchymosis: *Calcaneus fracture* ***
- -1B, 2B, 3A: Pain at ankle, proximal foot: *Talus fracture****
- -2C: Posterolateral ankle pain, worse with plantarflexion of foot: *Os trigonum fracture*

Midfoot pain:
- -3B: Worse with side-to-side compression of midfoot; subtle abnormalities sometimes noted only on weight bearing x-rays or special views: *Lisfranc fracture* ***
- -2D, 3C, 4B: Pain at base of 5th metatarsal, worse with weightbearing: *Fifth metatarsal fracture****
- -2E, 3D: Lateral pain after significant trauma: *Cuboid subluxation and fracture****

Forefoot pain:
- -3E: Pain over metatarsal shafts: *Metatarsal fracture*
- -3F: Pain over phalanxes: *Phalangeal fracture or dislocation*

?

No fracture on X-ray +/- deformity

Hindfoot pain:
- -1A, 2A, 4A: Ecchymosis at heel: *Heel bruise/heel fat pad syndrome****

Midfoot pain:
- -3B: Worse with side-to-side compression of midfoot; subtle abnormalities sometimes noted only on weight bearing x-rays or special views: *Lisfranc fracture* ***
- -3B: History of hyperflexion with soft tissue pain and swelling: *Midfoot ligament sprain*
- -3B: History of direct blow with ecchymosis: *Midfoot contusion*

Forefoot pain:
- -3F: Hyperflexion or lateral deviation of digits: *Phalangeal ligament sprain*
- -3G: Blue/black discoloration of nail: *Subungal hematoma****

Consider acute exacerbation of CHRONIC injury or medical diagnosis: rheumatoid arthritis, osteoarthritis, SLE, infection, etc...

Note: see also "Heel and Ankle Pain" algorithm for additional hindfoot diagnoses

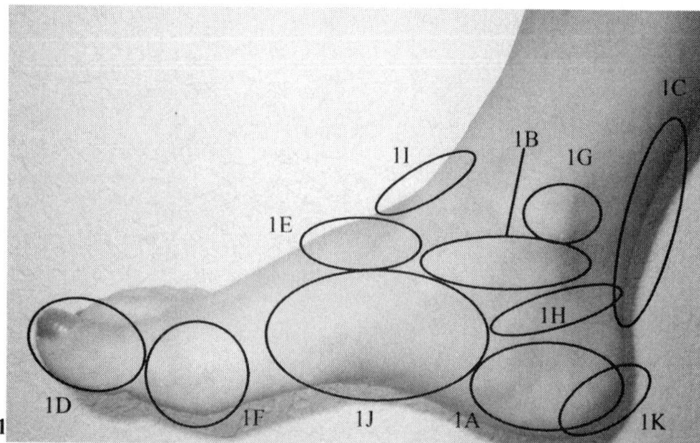

Figure 1

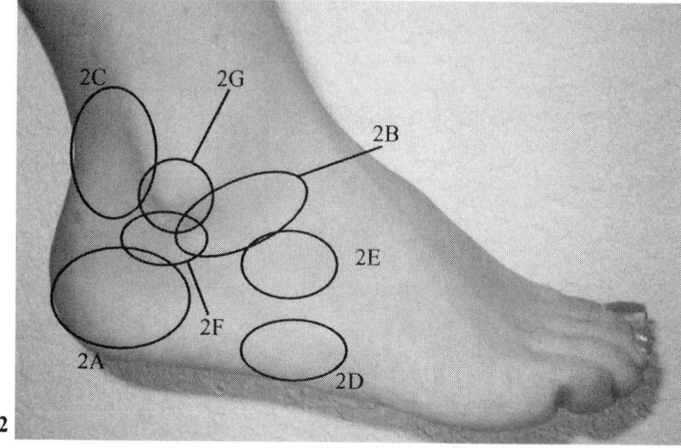

Figure 2

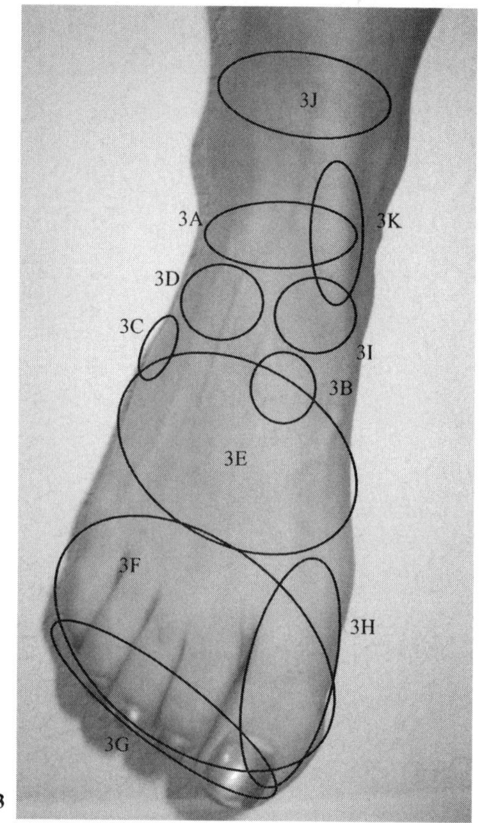

Figure 3

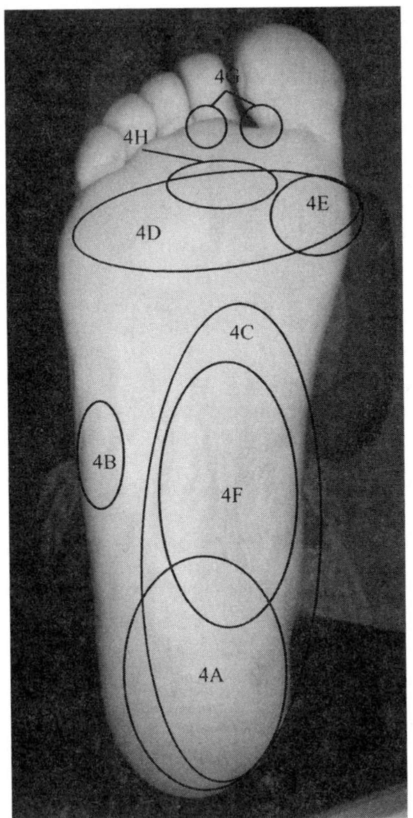

Figure 4

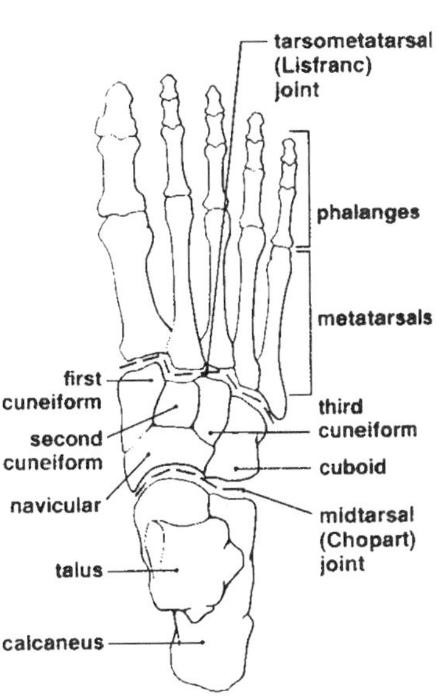

Diagram 1: Bones of the right foot as viewed from above

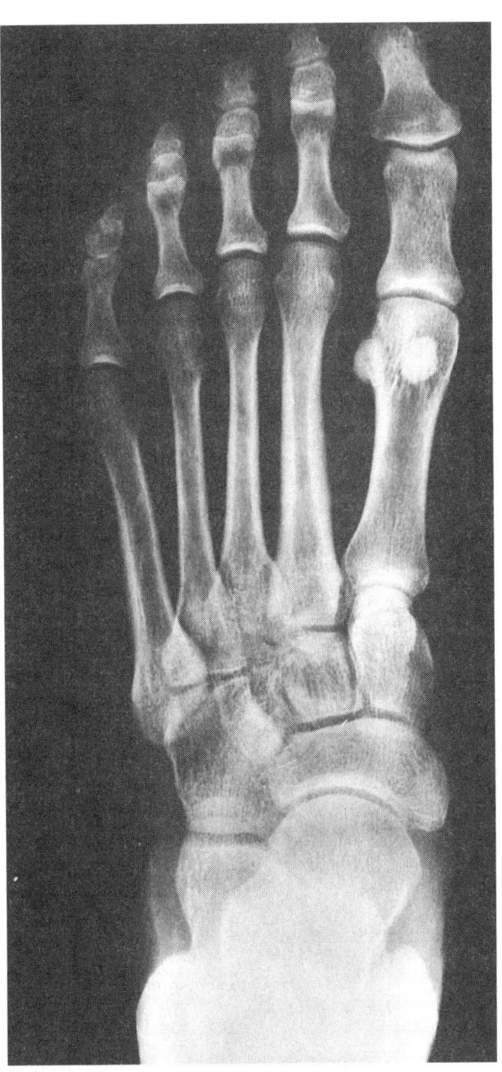

Radiograph 1: AP view of the left foot

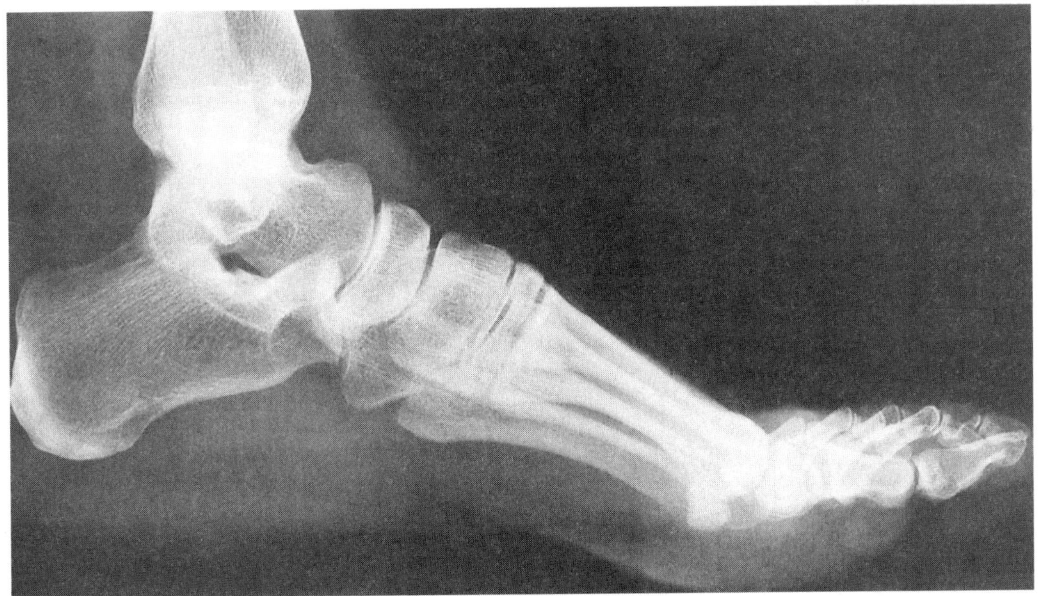

Radiograph 2: Lateral view of the foot

Foot

Chronic

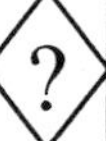

History of recent or distant injury, but with chronic symptoms

Hindfoot pain:
-1C: Pain 2-6cm proximal to Achilles insertion into calcaneus: *Achilles tendinitis* ***

Midfoot pain:
-3B: History of hyperflexion with soft tissue pain and swelling: *Midfoot ligament sprain*

Forefoot pain:
-4D: Pain at plantar metatarsal heads: *Anterior metatarsalgia****
-4E: Pain at 1st MTP during toe-off stage of gait: *Sesamoid dysfunction****
-1D, 3H: Great toe pain, worse with extreme plantar- and dorsiflexion: *Turf toe****

Plantar pain:
-4C: Plantar hind-to-midfoot paresthesias and pain: *Tarsal tunnel syndrome****

Review diagnoses on ACUTE algorithm for possible missed diagnosis

Repetitive stress, usually without history of trauma

Hindfoot pain:
-1C: Pain 2-6 cm proximal to Achilles insertion into calcaneus: *Achilles tendinitis* ***
-4F: Plantar heel pain, radiating into arch: *Plantar fasciitis****

Midfoot pain:
-1E, 3I: Vague dorsal midfoot pain: *Navicular stress fracture****
-1B/E, 3A/D/I:Chronic midfoot/hindfoot pain, worse after activity: *Tarsal coalition*

Forefoot pain:
-4D: Pain at plantar metatarsal heads: *Anterior metatarsalgia****
-3E: Tenderness at base, head, or midshaft of metatarsal: *Metatarsal stress fracture****

Plantar pain:
-4C: Plantar hind-to-midfoot paresthesias and pain: *Tarsal tunnel syndrome****

Insidious onset of pain, swelling, or deformity without trauma or repetitive stress

Hindfoot symptoms:
-1C: Prominence over posterior calcaneus: *Haglund's deformity****
-4F: Plantar heel pain, radiating into arch: *Plantar fasciitis****

Midfoot symptoms:
-1E, 3I: Five to 10 year old with a limp, poorly developed navicular ossification center on x-ray: *Kohler's disease: (aseptic necrosis of tarsal navicular)****

Forefoot symptoms:
-1F: Bony prominence at medial 1st MTP: *Hallux valgus****
-4G: Plantar or interdigital pain or fullness: *Intermetatarsal (Morton's) neuroma****
-4H: Flattening of metatarsal head on x-ray: *Freiberg's disease****
-3G: Painful bony outgrowth of distal phalanx: *Subungal exostosis****
-3F: Flexion/extension contractures of one or more toes: *Hamer/claw/mallet toe****
-3G: Inflammation at medial or lateral nail groove: *Onychocryptosis****
-3G: Nail thickening, yellow-brown discoloration: *Onychomycosis****

Plantar pain:
-4C: Plantar hind-to-midfoot paresthesias and pain: *Tarsal tunnel syndrome****

Consider osteoarthritis, rheumatoid arthritis, SLE, infection, or other medical process

Note: see also "Heel and Ankle Pain" algorithm for additional hindfoot diagnoses

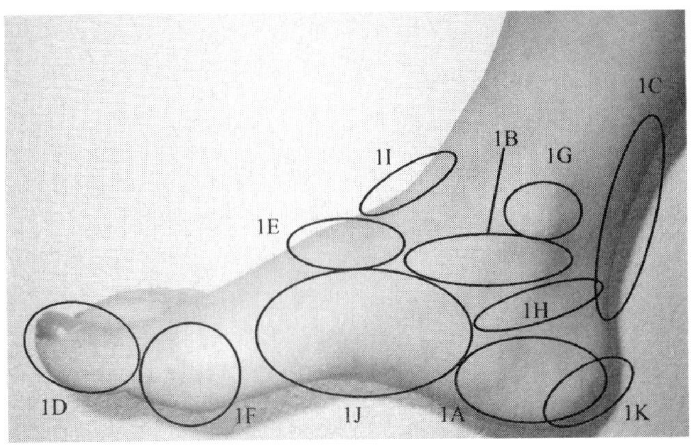

Figure 1

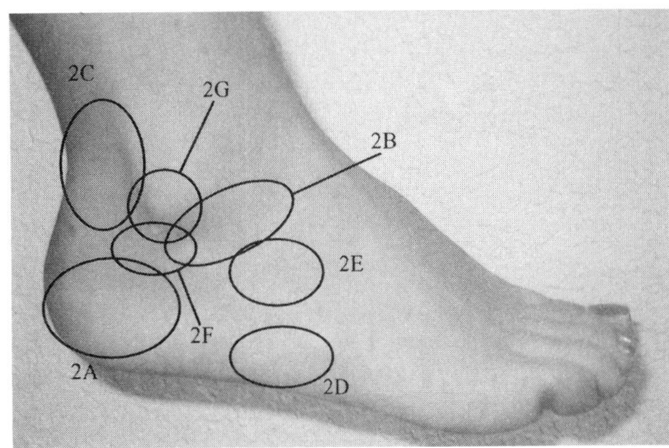

Figure 2

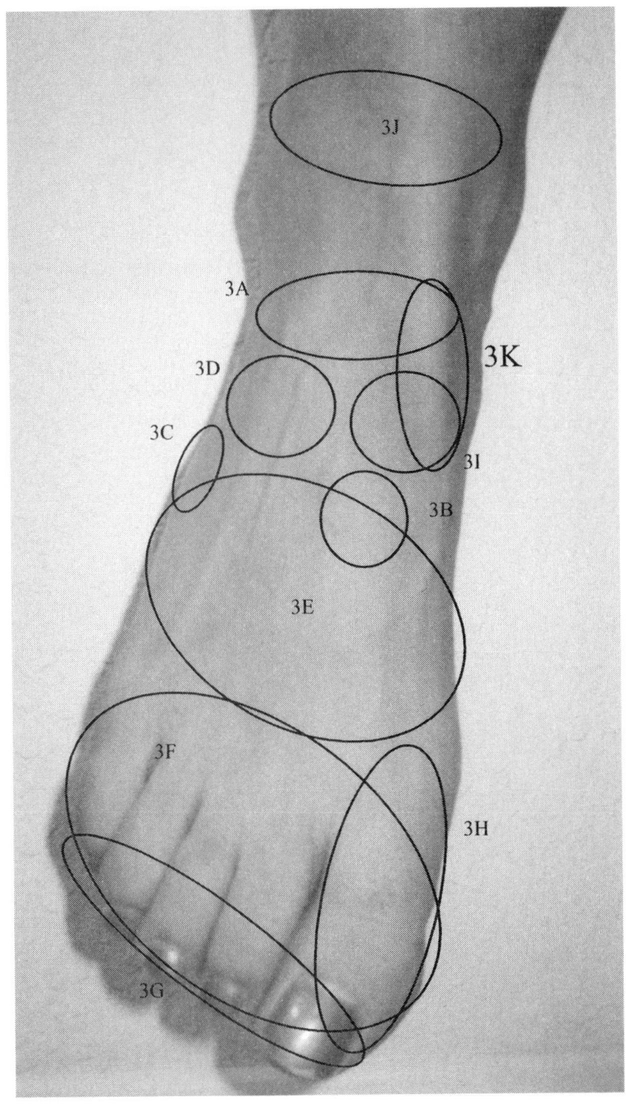

Figure 3

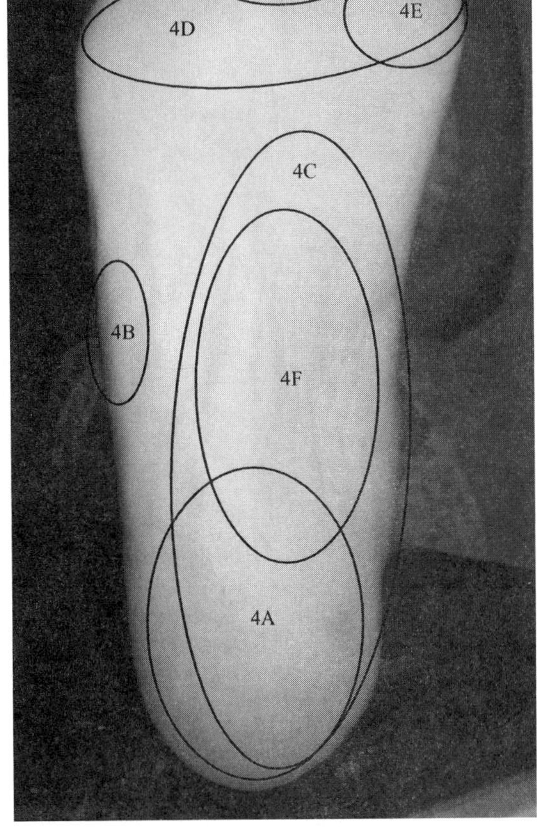

Figure 4

Index

Page numbers in boldface indicate major discussion; page numbers in italics denote figures; those followed by "t" denote tables.

Index

Index

Index